AO CMF

Michael Ehrenfeld | Neal D Futran | Paul N Manson | Joachim Prein

Advanced Craniomaxillofacial Surgery
Tumor, Corrective Bone Surgery and Trauma

Advanced Craniomaxillofacial Surgery—Tumor, Corrective Bone Surgery and Trauma

AO
CMF

Michael Ehrenfeld | Neal D Futran | Paul N Manson | Joachim Prein

Advanced Craniomaxillofacial Surgery
Tumor, Corrective Bone Surgery and Trauma

Includes over 1,300 figures

Library of Congress Cataloging-in-Publication Data is available from the publisher.

Hazards

Great care has been taken to maintain the accuracy of the information contained in this publication. However, the publisher, and/or the distributor, and/or the editors, and/or the authors cannot be held responsible for errors or any consequences arising from the use of the information contained in this publication. Contributions published under the name of individual authors are statements and opinions solely of said authors and not of the publisher, and/or the distributor, and/or the AO Group.

The products, procedures, and therapies described in this work are hazardous and are therefore only to be applied by certified and trained medical professionals in environments specially designed for such procedures. No suggested test or procedure should be carried out unless, in the user's professional judgment, its risk is justified. Whoever applies products, procedures, and therapies shown or described in this work will do this at their own risk. Because of rapid advances in the medical sciences, AO recommends that independent verification of diagnosis, therapies, drugs, dosages, and operation methods should be made before any action is taken.

Although all advertising material which may be inserted into the work is expected to conform to ethical (medical) standards, inclusion in this publication does not constitute a guarantee or endorsement by the publisher regarding quality or value of such product or of the claims made of it by its manufacturer.

Legal restrictions

Distribution by Georg Thieme Verlag, Rüdigerstrasse 14, 70469 Stuttgart, Germany, and Thieme New York, 333 Seventh Avenue, New York, NY 10001, USA

ISBN: 9783132428393
e-ISBN: 9783132428409

1 2 3 4 5 6

Introduction

Seven years after the publication of the manual on *Principles of Internal Fixation of the Craniomaxillofacial Skeleton—Trauma and Orthognathic Surgery*, the second volume entitled *Advanced Craniomaxillofacial Surgery—Tumor, Corrective Bone Surgery and Trauma* is now available. It is a project of AOCMF, a clinical division of the AO Foundation. According to the interdisciplinary nature of AOCMF, this advanced manual includes chapters and contributions from oral and maxillofacial surgeons, plastic surgeons, otolaryngologist oculoplastic surgeons, head and neck surgeons, and researchers.

Medical knowledge is growing rapidly, and the way it is disseminated is changing from printed media toward digital presentations including video channels. On the other hand, principles of operative medicine and surgical standards remain relatively stable and do not change that fast. Therefore, the editors of this book believe that it still makes sense to produce a book that captures current aspects of advanced craniomaxillofacial bone surgery.

This advanced manual is divided into six sections. The first section presents an overview of bone grafts/flaps, bone replacement materials and techniques. Sections two and three cover various aspects of ablative and reconstructive surgery of the mandible, midface, and craniofacial junction. Section four deals with corrections of complex deformities and conditions of the craniofacial skeleton; section five with imaging and planning technologies; and the last section with principles and techniques for facial allotransplantation.

More than 1,300 figures are included to focus on practical surgical details. The combination of text and illustrations is meant to support practical training during surgical specialization, and in addition will allow the experienced surgeon to look up and refresh surgical knowledge.

This advanced manual comprises chapters from many individual surgeons, and great efforts have been made to create a consistent textbook without much overlap. We sincerely hope that the readers will find this book valuable, and we are happy to receive comments and feedback.

Michael Ehrenfeld, MD, DDS

Preface

Seven years after publication of the first volume of the manual on *Principles of Internal Fixation of the Craniomaxillofacial Skeleton—Trauma and Orthognathic Surgery*, in 2012, Professors Ehrenfeld, Prein, and Manson are joined by Professor Futran to produce volume 2 of the manual on advanced techniques in craniofacial surgery, titled *Advanced Craniomaxillofacial Surgery—Tumor, Corrective Bone Surgery and Trauma*. Renowned international experts have contributed to provide one of the most comprehensive works on sophisticated surgical analysis and treatment of complex conditions of the face, head and neck from a multidisciplinary perspective previously not possible except in a worldwide and comprehensive craniomaxillofacial faculty such as that within the interdisciplinary AO Foundation. The past 40 years have witnessed an explosion of progress in the knowledge and treatment of diseases of the head and neck and the craniofacial skeleton, with new methods of surgery, fixation, grafting and especially planning analysis and implants. These advances create new and innovative treatment concepts especially in surgery. Rigid internal fixation techniques, craniofacial exposures as well as modern planning algorithms are today applied to trauma, tumor surgery, orthognathic and craniofacial surgery for the benefit and improvement of all reconstructive and esthetic skeletal procedures in the head and neck region.

This advanced manual and companion to the *Principles of Internal Fixation of the Craniomaxillofacial Skeleton* adds to the information of the first volume sophisticated techniques in skeletal and soft-tissue analysis for the disciplines of craniofacial surgery, trauma, tumors, orthognathic, facial and esthetic skeletal surgery. This volume 2 complements the basic principles in volume 1. It covers information required to manage the challenging problems beyond the basic information and procedures presented in volume 1 and permits the acquisition of comprehensive treatment planning techniques and improvements required to achieve good results in more challenging specialty procedures throughout the entire region.

The expertise of several disciplines offers a comprehensive and unique interdisciplinary perspective necessary to create the "team" approach fundamental to achieving the progress required and expected in sophisticated medical centers: Oral and Maxillofacial Surgery, Plastic and Reconstructive Surgery, Otolaryngology and Facial Plastic and Reconstructive Surgery, Ophthalmology and Oculoplastic Surgery, Neurosurgery, and Head and Neck Surgery. The focused expertise of each discipline is assembled and combined to produce an all-inclusive volume which delivers excellent insight into the developments of the past 40 years in all techniques of facial bone surgery. Indeed, the advent of microvascular surgery, skeletal analysis, computed surgical planning, sophisticated personalized implant creation, comprehensive radiographic analysis, and thorough planning such as model surgery, patient-specific implants, detailed preoperative computerized planning and analysis have brought new principles, techniques, and possibilities that allow the individual surgical practitioner to achieve sophisticated goals more efficiently with reduced surgical time, frustration, and revolutionary outcomes.

Importantly, these new techniques of radiographic analysis and computerized planning permit a wide range of less common and highly sophisticated operations to be undertaken by all practitioners. The same techniques of analysis, when used postoperatively, generate data from results which directly translate into improvements and recommendations for new and better treatments, permitting a cycle of constant improvement which continues to generate new and better operations. The vast volume of this new material may at first seem overwhelming to the individual practitioner, but these chapters segment the knowledge into compartments which seem scalable and possible for the individual practitioner to incorporate into his or her own treatment algorithms.

It has been an enormous task to collect and to coordinate this talented group of international experts and specialty communities into this volume. The production of uniform detailed and comprehensive artwork itself is far beyond the limited quality of the usual contributions available in standard multiauthor textbooks, and the quality and numerous illustrations allow a knowledge and mastery of the principles discussed so that individual practitioners can predictably improve their knowledge and skill in any of the areas covered. The references indicate further enhancements in knowledge and practice through additional study.

Today, the wide range of surgical possibilities, implant materials, and techniques of planning and analysis allow our patients better outcomes through easier and more straightforward surgery for the practitioners who despite the added expense of the implants, analysis and techniques can even offer their patients less costly operations made possible by reduced operative time, reduced possibility of complications, reduced secondary or revisional surgery, and the improved outcomes that fully justify the results achieved.

It has been our privilege to benefit from the associations with multiple generations of surgeons worldwide in multiple disciplines through the unique structure of the AO Foundation. All specialties have been united to produce the comprehensive interdisciplinary knowledge available in these volumes. We believe we have learned as much by editing and organizing this advanced volume as anyone having this textbook.

We the editors thank the AO Foundation and its sponsors for providing the educational network that has made the interdisciplinary exchange of this knowledge advancing progress possible.

Good luck and good learning as you appreciate the special treat offered by this international multidisciplinary effort of the AOCMF.

Michael Ehrenfeld, MD, DDS, Prof
Neal D Futran, MD, DMD, Prof
Paul N Manson, MD, Prof
Joachim Prein, MD, DDS, Prof

Acknowledgment

The editors express their appreciation to the authors for contributing chapters to this book and sharing their knowledge and experience with the reader. We are convinced that this effort will contribute significantly to the education of craniomaxillofacial surgeons. We are also grateful to the authors for understanding that the editors needed to update the original manuscripts in order to exclude overlap and ensure consistency throughout the book.

Special thanks go to Almuth Nussbaumer who has been of invaluable help to the editors in the coordination of this book project.

The AO Education Institute team has provided significant resources and expertise without which this book would not have been possible. We thank Vidula H Bhoyroo for the overall planning and management of this project, as well as Urs Rüetschi, Robin Greene, Carl Lau, and Jecca Reichmuth for their dedicated support.

Many thanks to all illustrators, especially the main illustrator Marcel Erismann. And our appreciation to Roman Kellenberger who did a tremendous job in typesetting the book.

We convey our appreciation and deep gratitude to Prof Hans F Zeilhofer and Prof Christoph Kunz for their logistical support to Prof Prein in the production of this project by generously providing the infrastructure within their unit.

We are also grateful to the former and current Executive Directors of AOCMF, Tobias Hüttl and Erich Roethlisberger for their unwavering support of this very important project.

Finally, we thank our families for their patience, help, and support during the production of this book.

Contributors

Editors

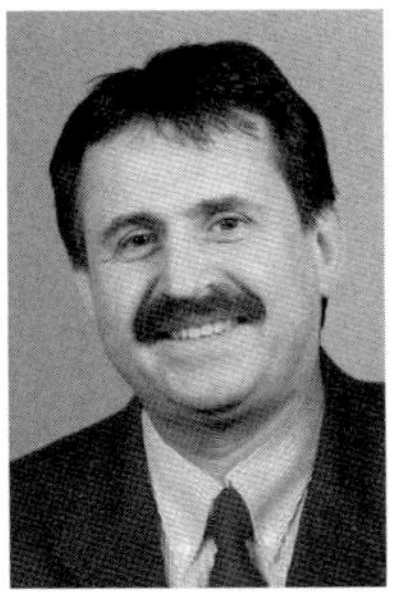

Michael Ehrenfeld, MD, DDS, Prof
Professor and Chair Department for Oral and Maxillofacial Surgery
Ludwig-Maximilians-University
Lindwurmstrasse 2a
80337 Munich
Germany

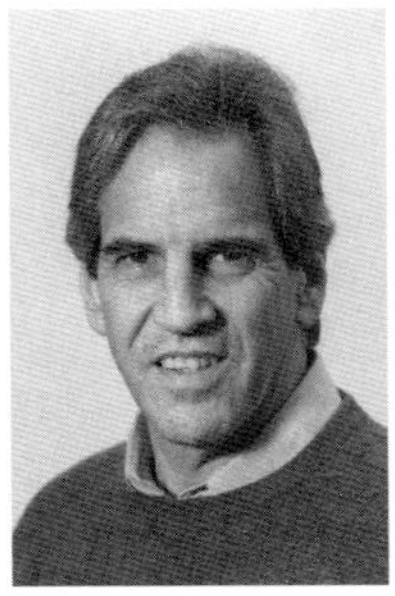

Neal D Futran, MD, DMD, Prof
Professor and Chair of Otolaryngology-HNS
Director of Head and Neck Surgery
University of Washington
1959 NE Pacific Street
Box 356515
Seattle, WA 98195
USA

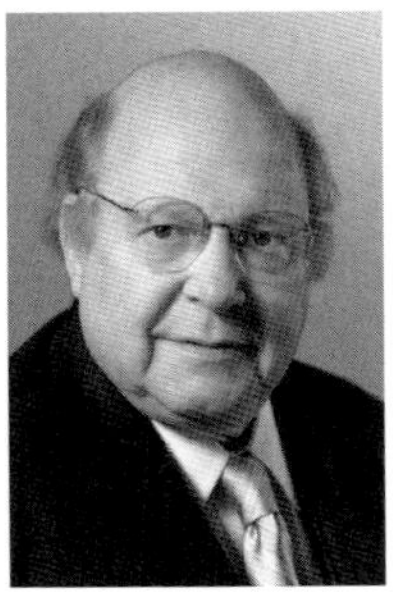

Paul N Manson, MD, Prof
Johns Hopkins
Plastic, Reconstructive and Maxillofacial Surgery
8152 R McElderry Wing
601 North Caroline Street
Baltimore, MD 21287-0981
USA

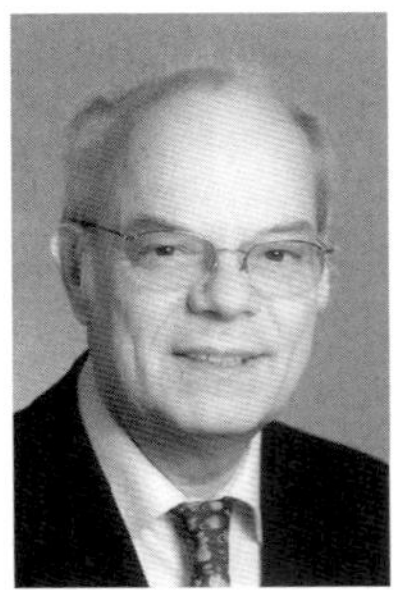

Joachim Prein, MD, DDS, Prof
University Hospital
Reconstructive Surgery
Spitalstrasse 21
4031 Basel
Switzerland

Authors

Gregorio Sánchez Aniceto, MD, PhD
Hospital Doce de Octubre
Maxillofacial Surgery Service
Ctra. Andalucía Km. 5.4
28041 Madrid
Spain

Suad Aljohani, DMD
Department of Oral and Maxillofacial Surgery
Ludwig Maximilian Universität
Lindwurmstrasse 2a
80337 Munich
Germany

Faisal Al-Mufarrej, MD
Seattle Children's Hospital
Division of Craniofacial & Plastic Surgery
4800 Sand Point Way NE
Seattle, WA 98105
USA

Jörg Beinemann, MD
University-Hospital Basel
Clinic of Oral-, Cranio- and Maxillo-Facial Surgery
Spitalstrasse 21
4031 Basel
Switzerland

R Bryan Bell, MD, DDS, FACS
Oral and Maxillofacial Surgery
Oregon Health & Science University/
Providence Cancer Center
1849 NW Kearney Suite #300
Portland, OR 97209
USA

Gido Bittermann, MD
Universitätsklinikum Freiburg
Department für Zahn-, Mund- und Kieferheilkunde
Klinik für Mund-, Kiefer- und Gesichtschirurgie
Hugstetter Strasse 55
9106 Freiburg
Germany

Remy H Blanchaert, Jr, MD, DDS
1919 N Webb Road
Wichita, KS 67206-3405
USA

Marc Bohner, MSc, EOFL, PhD
Robert Mathys Foundation
Skeletal Substitutes roup
Bischmattstrasse 12, POB 203
2544 Bettlach
Switzerland

Rolf Bublitz, Dr, Ltd Oberarzt
Klinikum Stuttgart, Katharinenhospital
Klinik für MKG-Chirurgie Zentrum f. Implantologie
Kriegsbergstrasse 60
70174 Stuttgart
Germany

Daniel Buchbinder, DMD, MD, Prof
Continuum Health Partners
Institute for Head and Neck and Craniofacial
Diseases
10 Union Square East, Suite 5B
New York, NY 10003
USA

Peter Bucher, CDT
CFC Hirslanden
Hirslanden Medical Center
Rain 34
5000 Aarau
Switzerland

Carl-Peter Cornelius, MD, DDS, Prof
Ludwig Maximilians-Universität, Klinikum Innenstadt
Klinik und Poliklinik für Mund-, Kiefer-,
Gesichtschirurgie
Lindwurmstrasse 2a
80337 Munich
Germany

Marcin Czerwinski, MD, FRCS
Scott & White Memorial Hospital
Section Cleft-Craniofacial Surgery
2401 S 31st Street
Temple, TX 76508
USA

Stéphanie Dakpé, MD
Department of Maxillofacial Surgery
University Hospital
Avenue Laennec
CHU Amiens-Picardie
80000 Amiens
France

Bernard Devauchelle, MD, Prof, Dr, FRCS(Eng)
Chirurgie Maxillofaciale
Hôpital Nord
Place Victor Pauchet
80054 Amiens cedex 1
France

Edward Ellis III, DDS, MS, Prof
University of Texas Health Science Center
at San Antonio
Department Oral Maxillofacial Surgery
7703 Floyd Curl Drive, MC-7908
San Antonio, TX 78229-3900
USA

Gregory RD Evans, MD, FACS, Prof
University of California, Irvine
Aesthetic and Plastic Surgery Institute
200 S Manchester Suite 650
Orange, CA 92868
USA

Jamie Gateno, MD, DDS
Chairman Oral and Maxillofacial Surgery Department
Houston Methodist Hospital
6560 Fannin
Suite 1280
Houston, TX 77030
USA

Nils-Claudius Gellrich, MD, DDS, Prof
Medical University Hannover
Department of Oral and Maxillofacial Surgery
Carl-Neuberg-Strasse 1
30625 Hannover
Germany

Michael P Grant, MD, PhD, FACS
Division Head, Oculoplastic Surgery Director
Ocular and Orbital Trauma Center
Wilmer Ophthalmological Institute
The Johns Hopkins Hospital
600 North Wolfe Street
Maumenee 505
Baltimore, MD 21287
USA

Raquel Guijarro-Martínez, MD, DMD
Maxillofacial Institute
Quirón-Teknon Hospital
Vilana St 12, D-185
08022 Barcelona
Spain

Patrick J Gullane, CM, MB, FRCS, FACS, Prof
University of Toronto
Department of Otolaryngology/
Head and Neck Surgery
Room 8N-877
200 Elizabeth Street
Toronto, ON M5G 2C4
Canada

Ralf Gutwald, MD, Prof
University Hospital Freiburg
Department of Oral and Maxillofacial Surgery
Hugstetter Strasse 55
79106 Freiburg
Germany

Christine Hagenmaier, DMD
Herkomerplatz 2
81679 Munich
Germany

Jeffrey Haller, MD
Rocky Mountain Eye Center
700 W Kent Ave Ste 1
Missoula, MT 59801
USA

Beat Hammer, MD, DMD, Prof
Hirslanden Medical Center
Cranio-Faciales-Centrum
Rain 34
5000 Aarau
Switzerland

Henning Hanken, MD
Wilhelm-Bock-Weg 5
22297 Hamburg
Germany

Max Heiland, MD, DMD, PhD
Klinik für Mund-, Kiefer- und Gesichtschirurgie CVK
Charité - Campus Virchow-Klinikum
Augustenburger Platz 1
13353 Berlin
Germany

Alexander Hemprich, MD, DMD, Prof
Universität Leipzig
Klinik und Poliklinik für Mund-, Kiefer- und Plastische Gesichtschirurgie
Liebigstrasse 10-14
04103 Leipzig
Germany

Thomas Hierl, MD, DDS, PhD
Department of Oral and Maxillofacial Surgery/
Plastic Facial Surgery
Helios Vogtland-Klinikum Plauen
Roentgenstrasse 2
08529 Plauen
Germany

Jürgen Hoffmann, MD, DMD, Prof
Department of Oral and Maxillofacial Surgery
National Cancer Center
University Hospital Heidelberg
Im Neuenheimer Feld 400
69120 Heidelberg
Germany

Dominik Horn, MD, DMD
Ärztlicher Mitarbeiter
Klinik und Poliklinik für Mund-, Kiefer- und Gesichtschirurgie
Universitätsklinikum Heidelberg
Im Neuenheimer Feld 400
69120 Heidelberg
Germany

Richard A Hopper, MD, Prof
University of Washington
Seattle Children's Hospital
Craniofacial Center Division of Pediatric Plastic Surgery
4800 Sand Point Way NE
Seattle, WA 98105
USA

Keith A Hurvitz, MD
Long Beach Medical Center
2880 Atlantic Avenue
Suite 290
Long Beach, CA 90806
USA

Keith Jones, MD, BDS, FRCS
The Old Rectory
Main Street
Tatenhill, Staffs DE13 9SD
UK

Leonard B Kaban, DMD, MD, FACS, Prof
Harvard School of Dental Medicine
Massachusetts General Hospital
Department of Oral and Maxillofacial Surgery
55 Fruit Street
Warren 1201
Boston, MA 02114
USA

Robert M Kellman, MD, FACS, Prof
SUNY Upstate Medical University
Department of Otolaryngology &
Communication Sciences
750 East Adams Street
Syracuse, NY 13210-2339
USA

Douglas W Klotch, MD, FACS
Tampa General Hospital
Department of Craniomaxillofacial Surgery
3450 East Fletcher Avenue
Suite 260
Tampa, FL 33613
USA

Christoph Kunz, MD, DMD, Prof
Head Oral and Craniomaxillofacial Surgery
Department of Surgery
University Hospital
Spitalstrasse 21
4031 Basel
Switzerland

Risto Kontio, MD, DDS, PhD
Helsinki University Hospital
Department of Oral and Maxillofacial Surgery
Kasarminkau 11-13, POB 263
00029 HUS Helsinki
Finland

Chen Lee, MD, FRCSC, FACS
Aesthetica MD
Clinique de Chirurgie Plastique & Esthétique
4055 Ste-Catherine Ouest
Suite 100
Westmount, Quebec H3Z 3J8
Canada

Nicholas R Mahoney, MD
Assistant Professor of Ophthalmology
Johns Hopkins University
Wilmer Eye Institute
600 N Wolfe Street
Maumenee 505
Baltimore, MD 21287
USA

Gerson Mast, Dr med, Dr med dent, PhD
Klinikum der Universität München Innenstadt
Klinik für Mund-, Kiefer-, Gesichtschirurgie
Lindwurmstrasse 21
80337 Munich
Germany

Alexander Metz, MD
Kliniken Essen Mitte, Evang. Huyssens-Stiftung/
Knappschaft GmbH
OMF Surgery, Plastic Surgery
Henricistrasse 92
45136 Essen
Germany

Marc C Metzger, MD, DDS, Prof
University Hospital Freiburg
Oral and Maxillofacial Surgery
Hugstetter Strasse 55
79106 Freiburg
Germany

Christopher Mohr, Prof, Dr med, Dr med dent
Kliniken Essen-Mitte Evangelische Huyssens-
Stiftung/Knappschaft
Klinik für Mund-, Kiefer-, Gesichtschirurgie
Henricistrasse 92
45136 Essen
Germany

Reid V Mueller, MD, Prof
Oregon Health Sciences University
Division of Plastic and Reconstruction Surgery
3303 SW Bond Ave, CH5P
Portland, OR 97239-4501
USA

Peter C Neligan, MB, FRCSC(I), FRCS, FACS, Prof
University of Washington
Department of Surgery, Division of Plastic Surgery
1959 NE Pacific Street
Box 356410
Seattle, WA 98195-6410
USA

Christine B Novak, PhD, Prof
Hand Program
Division of Plastic and Reconstructive Surgery
399 Bathurst Street, EW2-422
Toronto, ON M5T 2S8
Canada

Sven Otto, PD, Dr med, Dr med dent
Department of Oral and Maxillofacial Surgery
Ludwig Maximilian Universität
Lindwurmstrasse 2a
80337 Munich
Germany

Nicholas J Panetta, MD
Department of Plastic Surgery
University of Pittsburgh Medical Center
3550 Terrace Street
6B Scaife Hall
Pittsburgh, PA 15261
USA

Maria E Papadakis, MD, DMD, PhD
Harvard School of Dental Medicine
Massachusetts General Hospital
Department of Oral and Maxillofacial Surgery
55 Fruit Street Warren 1201
Boston, MA 02114
USA

Roman P Pförtner, MD
Kliniken Essen Mitte, Evang Huyssens-
Stiftung/Knappschaft
OMF Surgery, Plastic Surgery
Henricistrasse 92
45136 Essen
Germany

Jeffrey C Posnick, DMD, MD
Posnick Center
Facial Plastic Surgery
5530 Wisconsin Avenue, Suite 1250
Chevy Chase, MD 20815
USA

Florian A Probst, MD, DMD, PhD
Facharzt für Mund-, Kiefer- und Gesichtschirurgie
Klinikum der Universität München
Klinik und Poliklinik für Mund-, Kiefer- und
Gesichtschirurgie
Lindwurmstrasse 2a
80337 Munich
Germany

Berton Rahn†, MD, DMD
Professor of Maxillofacial Surgery
Vice-Director AO Research Institute
Clavadelerstrasse 8
7270 Davos
Switzerland
† Deceased

Majeed Rana, PD, Dr med, Dr med dent
Facharzt für Mund-, Kiefer- und Gesichtschirurgie
Plastische und Ästhetische Operationen
Fachzahnarzt für Oralchirurgie
Klinik für Mund-, Kiefer- und Plastische Gesichtschirurgie
Zentrum für operative Medizin II (ZOM II)
Heinrich-Heine-Universität Düsseldorf
Moorenstrasse 5
40225 Düsseldorf
Germany

Ignacio Ismael García Recuero, MD
Oral & Maxillofacial Surgery Department
Craniofacial Surgery Unit
HU 12 deOctubre, HU Quirón
Madrid
Spain

Geoff Richards, Dr Sci, MSc
AO Research Institute
Clavadelerstrasse 8
7270 Davos
Switzerland

Michel Richter, Prof, Dr med, Dr med dent
Former Chairman of Oral and
Maxillofacial Surgery Clinic
Hôpitaux Universitaires de Genève
Rue Gabrielle-Perret-Gentil 4
1205 Genève
Switzerland

Dennis Rohner, Prof, Dr med, Dr med dent
Hirslanden Medical Center
Craniofacial Center
Rain 34
5000 Aarau
Switzerland

Martin Rücker, Prof, Dr med, Dr med dent
Zentrum für Zahnmedizin
Privatpraxis für Mund-, Kiefer- und Gesichtschirurgie
Pestalozzistrasse 10
8032 Zurich
Switzerland

Larry A Sargent, MD
Sargent Plastic Surgery of Utah
620 East Medical Drive
No. 310
Bountiful, UT 84010
USA

Sebastian Sauerbier, PD, Dr med, Dr med dent
Mund-, Kiefer- und Gesichtschirurgie
Pacelliallee 4
36043 Fulda
Germany

Rainer Schmelzeisen, MD, DDS, Prof, FRCS
(London)
University Hospital Freiburg
Department Oral Maxillofacial Surgery
Hugstetter Strasse 55
79106 Freiburg im Breisgau
Germany

Maximillian Schöllchen, Dr med
Arzt in der Fortbildung zum Facharzt für
Mund-, Kiefer- und Gesichtschirurgie
Klinik und Poliklinik für Mund-, Kiefer und
Gesichtschirurgie
Universitätsklinikum Hamburg-Eppendorf
Martinistrasse 52
20246 Hamburg
Germany

Ralf Schumacher, Dipl Ing
Leiter Medical Additive Manufacturing
Hochschule für Life Sciences - FHNW
Gründenstrasse 40
4132 Muttenz
Switzerland

Alexander Schramm, Prof, Dr med, Dr med dent
Military Hospital Ulm, Academic Hospital,
University of Ulm
Oral and Maxillofacial Surgery
Oberer Eselsberg 40
89081 Ulm
Germany

Warren Schubert, MD, FACS, Associate Prof
Regions Hospital
Department of Plastic and Hand Surgery
Mail Stop 11503 B
640 Jackson Street
St Paul, MN 44101
USA

Navin K Singh, MD
Washingtonian Plastic Surgery
5454 Wisconsin Ave, Ste 1710
Chevy Chase, MD 20815
USA

Martin Stoddart, MD, PhD
AO Research Institute
Clavadelerstrasse 8
7270 Davos
Switzerland

E Bradley Strong, MD, Prof
University of California, Davis
Department of Otolaryngology-Head and Neck
Surgery
2521 Stockton Blvd, Suite 7200
Sacramento, CA 95817
USA

Adrian Sugar, Dr. h.c., FRCS
Morriston Hospital
Maxillofacial Unit
West Glamorgan
Swansea, SA6 NL, Wales
UK

James Q Swift, DDS, Associate Prof
University of Minnesota School of Dentistry
Division of Oral and Maxillofacial Surgery
515 Delaware Street SE
7-174 Moos Tower
Minneapolis, MN 55455-0329
USA

Jesse A Taylor, MD, Assistant Prof
The University of Pennsylvania
Children's Hospital of Philadelphia
Plastic, Reconstructive and Craniofacial Surgery,
Co-Director, CHOP Cleft Team
3400 Spruce St
10 Penn Tower
Philadelphia, PA 19104
USA

John F Teichgraeber, MD, Prof
Division of Pediatric Plastic Surgery
Department of Pediatric Surgery
University of Texas
Houston Health Science Center
6410 Fannin Street
Suite 950
Houston, TX 77030
USA

Sylvie Testelin, PhD, MD
Department of Maxillofacial Surgery
University Hospital
Avenue Laennec
Chu Amiens Picardie
80000 Amiens
France

Florian M Thieringer, MD, DDS, MHBA
Oral and Cranio-Maxillo-Facial Surgery
University Hospital Basel
Spitalstrasse 21
4031 Basel
Switzerland

Maria J Troulis, MD
Chief Oral and Maxillofacial Surgery
Massachusetts General Hospital
Walter C. Guralnick Professor and Chair
Oral and Maxillofacial Surgery
Harvard School of Dental Medicine
Warren 1201
55 Fruit Street
Boston, MA 02114
USA

Dieter Weingart, Prof, Dr med, Dr med dent
Klinikum Stuttgart, Katharinenhospital
Aerztlicher Direktor Klinik für Mund-, Kiefer- und Gesichtschirurgie
Plastisch-ästhetische Operationen
Zentrum für Implantologie Leiter Kopfzentrum
Kriegsbergstrasse 60
70174 Stuttgart
Germany

Frank Wilde, MD, DMD
Military Hospital Ulm
Academic Hospital Ulm University
Oberer Eselsberg 40
89081 Ulm
Germany

Hans-Florian Zeilhofer, Prof, Dr med, Dr med dent
University Hospital Basel
Clinic and Policlinic for Maxillofacial Surgery
Spitalstrasse 21
4031 Basel
Switzerland

James J Xia, MD, PhD, MS, Prof
Professor of Oral and Maxillofacial Surgery Director of Surgical Planning Laboratory
Houston Methodist Hospital
6560 Fannin Street
Suite 1280
Houston, TX 77030
USA

Table of Contents

1.1 Types and harvest of bone grafts and bone flaps

Michael Ehrenfeld, Christine Hagenmaier, Remy H Blanchaert Jr

1 Introduction

In craniomaxillofacial (CMF) surgery bone grafts and bone flaps are used to replace missing bone. Bone deficits or defects may result from congenital malformations and developmental disorders, or originate from tumor surgery, trauma, medication-related bone diseases, irradiation or infections. Bone grafts may also be indicated in esthetic surgery.

Today fresh autogenous bone is still the gold standard among all available bone replacement materials [Axhausen, 1962; Schweiberer, 1970; Tessier et al, 2005]. However, nonresorbable alloplastic materials (eg, porous polyethylene, silastic, ceramic materials) are preferred for contour augmentation procedures because they do not undergo the unpredictable initial remodeling and resorption seen with nonvascularized autogenous bone grafts. Bone graft harvest itself may be associated with complications and undesired adverse effects [Tessier et al, 2005].

Fresh autogenous bone in principle can be harvested as nonvascularized bone grafts, pedicled bone grafts, and microvascular bone flaps [Bardenheuer, 1892; Sykoff, 1900; Krause, 1907; Axhausen, 1908; Lexer, 1908; Rydygier, 1908; Lindemann, 1916; Matti, 1932; Converse, 1945; Conley, 1972; Boyne, 1973; Taylor et al, 1975; O'Brien, 1977; Taylor et al, 1979; Quillen, 1979; Ariyan, 1980; Swartz et al, 1986]. Pedicled bone grafts today are rarely used in CMF reconstructive surgery; thus they are not further discussed in this chapter. Nonvascularized autogenous bone can be harvested as cancellous bone and marrow, cortical bone, corticocancellous bone, and so-called bone dust, which is small particles of cortical bone.

In the preoperative planning phase, the surgeon must assess the patient carefully to determine the needed type of bone based on the characteristics of the defect, the quality and quantity of the surrounding soft tissues, and the specific clinical indication for surgery. Potential donor sites must then be considered and a surgical plan developed that balances the risk-benefit ratio of each of the suitable donor sites and graft/flap types. This chapter reviews the most commonly used bone graft and bone flap donor sites used in CMF reconstruction. The intent is to provide the surgeon with a review of the potential donor sites and an outline of the techniques used for bone graft/flap harvest and donor site management.

2 Nonvascularized bone grafts

Nonvascularized bone grafts are typically harvested from certain preferred donor sites. In the recipient site the bone must be revitalized mainly via tissue ingrowth. Therefore, the recipient site must be of good biological quality, especially well perfused, and allow for complete 360° coverage of the bone graft(s) to avoid exposure, contamination, and healing disturbances [Axhausen, 1962; Schweiberer, 1970; Axhausen, 1951; Axhausen, 1952; Chalmers, 1959; Williams, 1962; Heiple et al,1963; Ray, et al, 1963; Burwell, 1965]. Revitalization of a nonvascularized bone graft goes along with a process of resorption, remodeling, and maturation, which is typically associated with a loss of bone volume. The amount of resorption depends on many factors, such as the dimensions and the density of the grafted material (it takes longer to revitalize large and more dense bone grafts, and therefore they show a greater percentage of bone loss), the type of the bone (cortical, cancellous, corticocancellous, bone dust), tissue qualities at the recipient site (vascularization), biomechanical properties (functional loading), and fixation of the bone graft to surrounding bone [Lexer, 1908; Lentrodt et al, 1976; Eitel et al, 1980; Schweiberer et al, 1981; Lentrodt et al, 1987]. The amount of bone loss after nonvascularized bone transplantation is unpredictable.

Indications for nonvascularized bone grafts

Nonvascularized bone grafts are indicated for filling bone defects, for example, after extirpation of large cysts (see chapter 2.3). Another widespread indication is for ridge augmentation procedures in preprosthetic surgery and dental implantology (see chapter 4.4). Small mandibular or maxillary continuity defects can be treated with nonvascularized bone grafts; other indications include osteotomy gaps in orthognathic surgery, defect zones in fractures, and facial clefts (see chapters 4.6 and 4.7) [Steinhäuser, 1968]. Nonvascularized bone grafts have been used for augmentation procedures in esthetic surgery (malar augmentation, chin augmentation), but because of the potential loss of bone volume nonresorbable grafting materials like ceramic implants or porous polyethylene should be considered instead [Reuther, 1979; Bell, 1992].

2.1 Cancellous bone and marrow

Cancellous bone and marrow is commonly used in CMF reconstruction of small defect areas. It may be harvested from either the ilium or tibia using a trocar, when only small amounts of bone graft are needed, or via open techniques. Grafts obtained by trocar may be suitable for small defects, such as in a fracture nonunion or for sinus floor elevation procedures. Harvest of the bone graft is generally simple; however, proper selection of the most appropriate donor site and careful execution of the harvest are required to minimize donor site morbidity and potential complications. Recipient site preparation for cancellous grafting is perhaps more critical. Development of a well-vascularized, appropriately sized pocket of soft tissue is critical to containment of the graft and a prerequisite for revascularization. Avoidance of oral exposure and therefore bacterial contamination is also vital. Grafted sites, which require extensive soft-tissue dissection and creation of potential dead space, should be drained with a closed suction technique to avoid hematoma and seroma formation. Perioperative antibiotics are administered in the standard fashion. Compressed cancellous bone and marrow can be handled nicely and can be shaped and molded to achieve anatomically adequate filling of appropriate defects.

This chapter outlines the most commonly used donor sites for maxillofacial bone graft reconstruction, which are the ilium and tibia. General characteristics of each site are described. A description of open harvesting techniques for the anterior and posterior ilium and the tibia are provided in the subsequent sections of this chapter.

2.1.1 Ilium

The ilium is a common donor site for autogenous cancellous bone used in CMF reconstruction. Bone can be harvested from either the anterior or posterior ilium. The anterior site is most often used because of its ease of access in comparison with the posterior ilium that requires the patient to be placed in a prone position. However, when large amounts of cancellous bone (> 35 cc compressed) are required, the posterior ilium is a more suitable donor site and a viable alternative to bilateral anterior harvests. The character of the bone is different from these two locations, which is, however, more important for the harvest of corticocancellous grafts. Major CMF reconstruction procedures typically require open techniques for harvest of appropriate and adequate amounts of bone. The posterior ilium provides a thin monocortical element and cancellous material, which often contains visible fat in adult patients. The anterior ilium may be harvested as either cancellous bone and marrow, or as a monocortical or bicortical graft. It has a much thicker cortical component and a less fatty appearing cancellous bone and marrow component.

2.1.1.1 Ilium—anterior technique (medial harvest)

The patient is positioned supine. In some cases, a folded sheet under the ipsilateral hip may make medial visualization easier. The ilium should be outlined on the skin with a surgical marker from the anterior superior iliac spine (ASIS) to the iliac tubercle. The site should be widely prepared and draped. The length of the incision depends on the volume of the harvest required. In general, a 2–6 cm incision is made parallel to the iliac crest either over or slightly lateral to the crest (**Fig 1.1-1**).

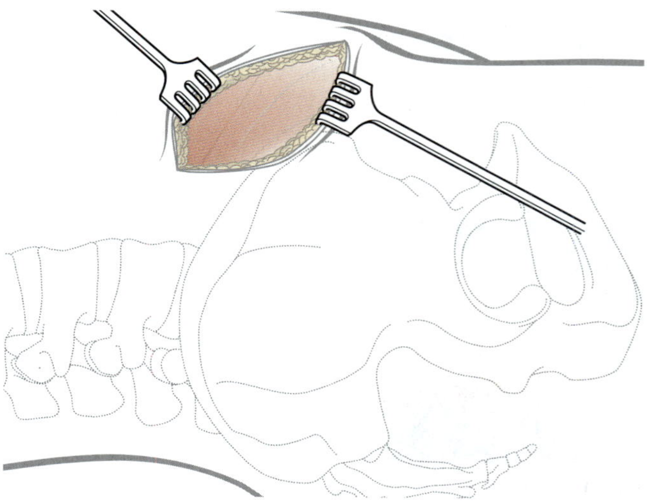

Fig 1.1-1 Approach to the anterior ilium.

The incision should be no closer than 1 cm to the ASIS to minimize injury to the lateral cutaneous femoral nerve. Incision is made through the skin and subcutaneous tissue, then through Scarpa fascia. Dissection is continued to the aponeurosis overlying the iliac crest (**Fig 1.1-2**).

Being careful to incise the aponeurosis minimizes bleeding and facilitates reapproximation. Careful subperiosteal dissection allows excellent exposure. Avoid overzealous soft-tissue retraction, as this is the likely cause of injury to the lateral femoral cutaneous nerve. For the harvest of cancellous material only, the crest may be split with chisels and the cancellous material removed with gouges and/or curettes (**Fig 1.1-3**).

In pediatric patients the iliac crest is still covered with cartilage. The cartilage can be easily separated from the bone with a scalpel and reflected medially pedicled on the adjacent soft tissues to allow access to the bone. The collected cancellous bone can be placed in a 30 cc syringe and compressed to better delineate the volume harvested (**Fig 1.1-4**).

The syringe can then be placed in a lap sponge moistened with chilled saline solution and set aside. This simplifies the collection of the bone, reveals the actual volume obtained, and facilitates the delivery of the bone to the recipient site. However, it must be noted that cancellous bone and marrow should never be placed in saline solution or similar or washed out with saline solution to avoid loss of cells and proteins.

Placement of a resorbable hemostatic agent in the harvest site often controls hemorrhage such that there is no need for a closed suction drain. The wound is then closed in layers.

2.1.1.2 Ilium—posterior technique

The patient is positioned prone. Extreme care in positioning with placement of appropriate lateral chest support and careful rotation of the arms is important to avoid elevated ventilation pressures and nerve injury. The bed is flexed, and reverse Trendelenburg applied to keep the upper body parallel to the floor (**Fig 1.1-5**).

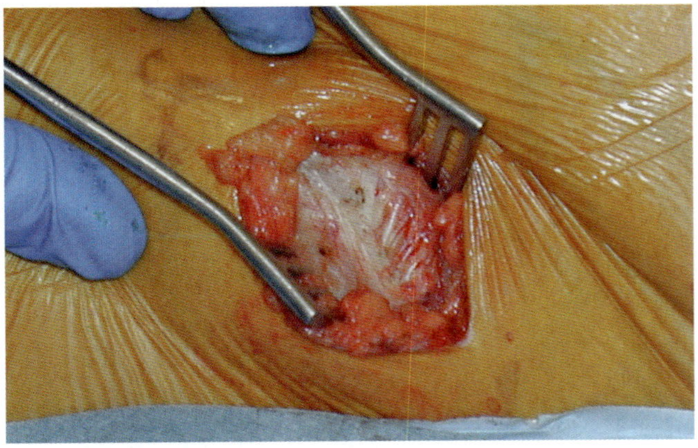

Fig 1.1-2 After incision of the skin and subcutaneous tissue, the fascia is exposed.

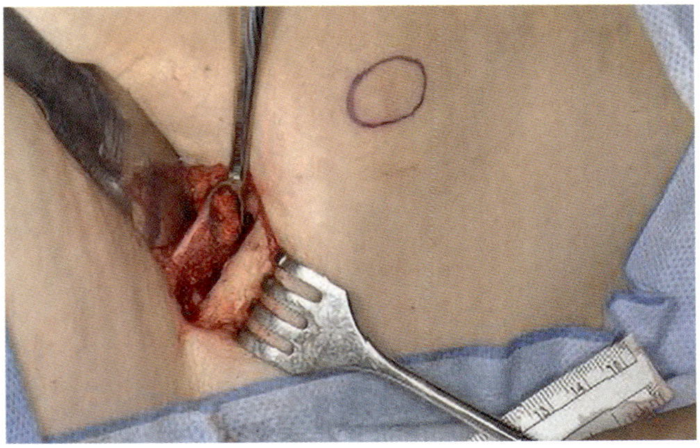

Fig 1.1-3 Harvesting of cancellous bone and marrow with a curette.

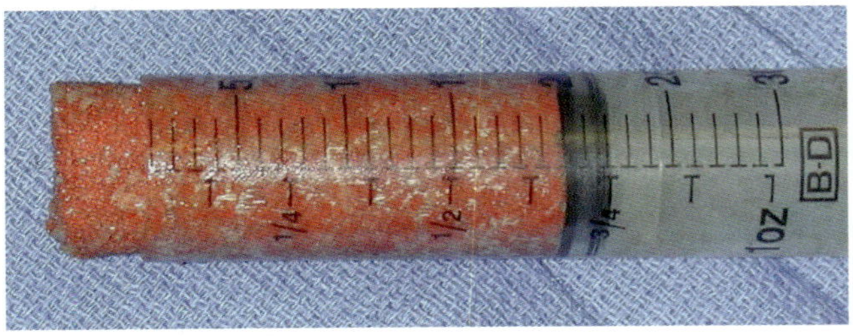

Fig 1.1-4 The cancellous bone graft material has been placed in a 30 cc syringe and compacted.

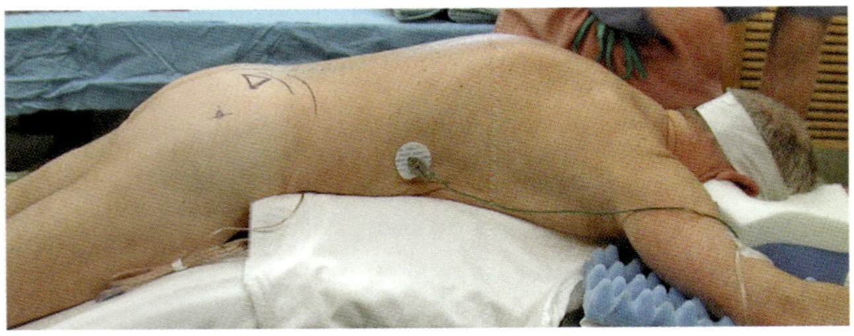

Fig 1.1-5 Proper positioning for harvest of bone from the posterior ilium is critical. Note the lateral padding.

The surgical anatomical landmarks are then outlined with a marker to include the iliac crest, sacrum, and the insertion of the gluteus maximus muscle (**Fig 1.1-6**). Next, the operative field is scrubbed and then prepared and draped excluding the anal region from the field.

A curvilinear incision inferior to and parallel to the posterior iliac crest is then created. The incision should be placed 1–2 cm lateral to the sacroiliac joint to avoid the cluneal nerve. The dissection is deepened through fascia to the insertion of the gluteus maximus muscle. The periosteum is then incised and elevated exposing a triangular protuberance at the site of the muscle insertion. It is recommended that the location of the sciatic notch be determined by manual palpation to assure that no retractor is placed in its vicinity. A retractor is then placed to facilitate harvest. The lateral iliac cortex is removed with a saw and/or chisel and the underlying cancellous material collected with gouges and/or curettes (**Fig 1.1-7**).

Avoid violation of the medial cortex and the sacroiliac joint. If pure cancellous bone and marrow are needed, the cortical bone may be replaced and fixed with miniplates. Often times, the application of a resorbable hemostatic agent obviates the need for a closed suction drain. The wound is closed in layers using resorbable sutures.

2.1.2 Tibia

The proximal tibial metaphysis has reemerged in recent years as an alternative site for the harvest of cancellous bone. After description of the harvest procedure and its applications in CMF surgery, the tibia has become an accepted and frequent alternative to the anterior ilium for defects requiring only small amounts of bone. The major reported advantage is decreased morbidity. Reports of tibial bone harvest with local anesthesia and deep sedation demonstrate the simplicity of the procedure and the utility of the technique in CMF surgery. Cancellous harvests of 15–25 mL uncompressed bone have been reported. This volume is perfectly suited for dentoalveolar reconstructions in preparation for implant placement (sinus augmentation, etc) and management of fracture nonunion where only cancellous material is needed [Herford et al, 2003].

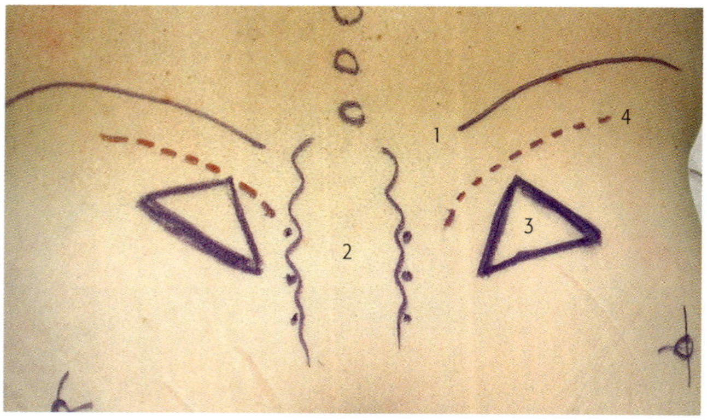

Fig 1.1-6 Upper borders, iliac crest, sacrum, and tubercle where musculus gluteus maximus inserts. Incision line (4).
1 = upper border
2 = sacrum
3 = tubercle
4 = incision line

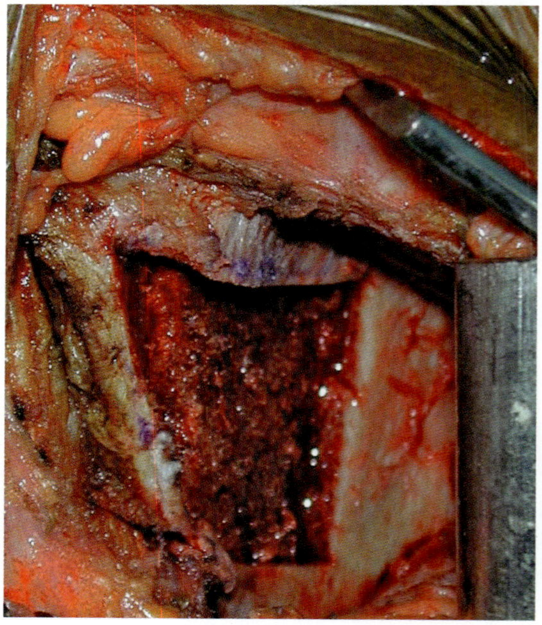

Fig 1.1-7 After removal of a portion of the lateral cortex, excellent access to the cancellous bone and marrow is provided.

2.1.2.1 Harvest technique

Approaches lateral or medial to the patellar tendon are possible. The anatomy of the proximal lower leg should be outlined with a surgical marker to include the insertion of the patellar tendon and the tibial plateau (**Fig 1.1-8**).

The incision length depends on the harvest technique. A small stab is required if a trocar is used. Otherwise the incision is carried down to the periosteum which is incised and reflected. A bone window is then created with a sagittal saw or piezotome and removed (**Fig 1.1-9**).

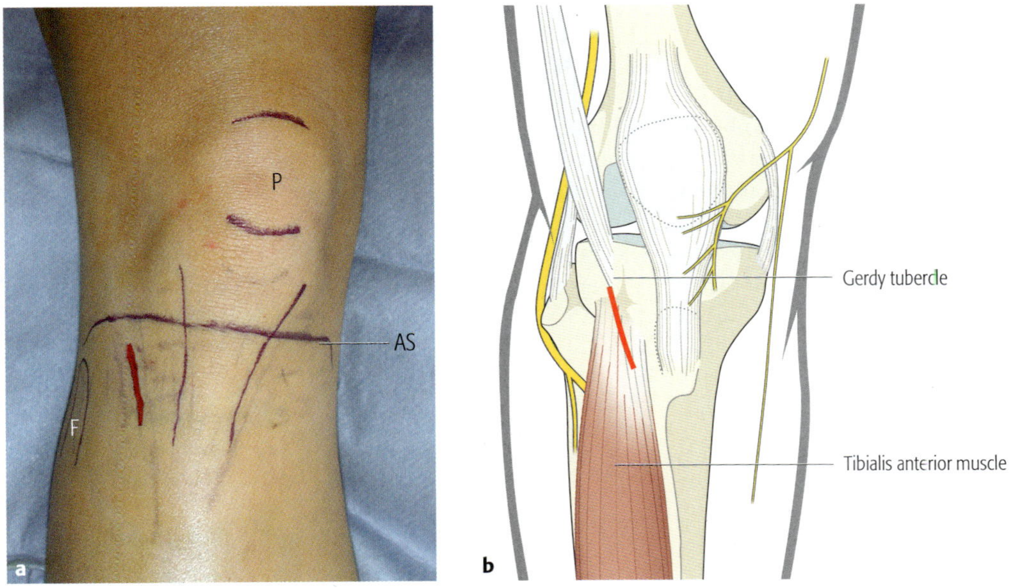

Fig 1.1-8a–b Planning for a lateral bone harvest from the tibial head. The incision line (red) is obliquely orientated to the joint plane and is placed just above and over Gerdy tubercle. P indicates patella; AS, articulation surface, plane of the femoral tibial joint; and F, fibular head.

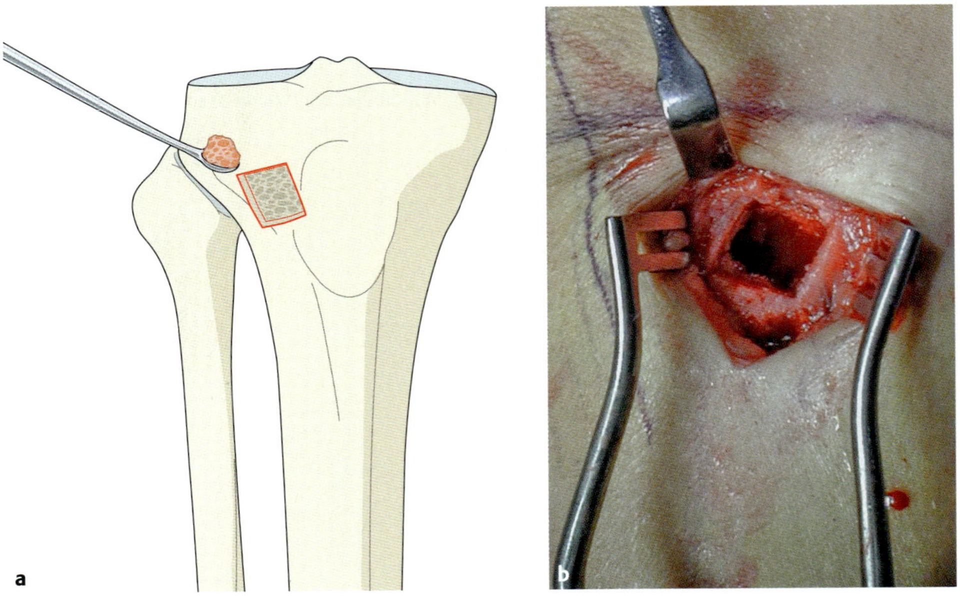

Fig 1.1-9a–b After osteotomy of the tibial cortex, cancellous bone and marrow can be harvested.

The cancellous bone is harvested with a curette, placed in a small container, and set aside. Operative site hemostasis is facilitated by the placement of a topical hemostatic agent. The wound is then closed in layers. After application of a wound dressing, the leg is covered in a soft roll and a gently compressive elastic bandage is applied. Ambulation is allowed immediately with a rapid return to normal exercise activities in a few weeks.

2.2 Cortical bone

Cortical bone grafts are used in CMF reconstruction for structural support and onlay augmentation. Examples of use of these grafts for structural support include maxillary lengthening with loss of bone contact and for restoration of the pillars of the facial skeleton in high-energy CMF trauma. In orthognathic surgery, cortical bone grafts are often available from the distal portion of the proximal segments after sagittal ramus osteotomies. These bone grafts can be used to augment the maxilla and to bridge gaps after maxillary advancements or maxillary lengthening procedures in bimaxillary cases. Cortical outer table bone grafts from the cranial vault or hip are alternatives, among others. Cortical bone grafts may be used for onlay augmentation in dentoalveolar reconstruction, for instance, after atrophy or traumatic bone loss, to allow placement of osseointegrated implants.

Cortical bone grafts require rigid fixation for optimal results. Whenever possible, a lag screw technique should be used for stabilization of the grafts after appropriate contouring. Miniplate/microplate fixation is an alternative. Failure to fixate the graft can result in migration, movement, infection, and rapid resorption.

2.2.1 Mandible

The harvest of cortical bone from the mandible is used for the purpose of onlay bone grafting in preparation for dental implant placement. The procedure is commonly performed with the patient under local anesthesia or local anesthesia and sedation. Patient acceptance of an oral donor site is high in comparison to a distant donor site.

Cortical bone from the mandible is typically harvested from either the ramus or symphysis (**Fig 1.1-10**).

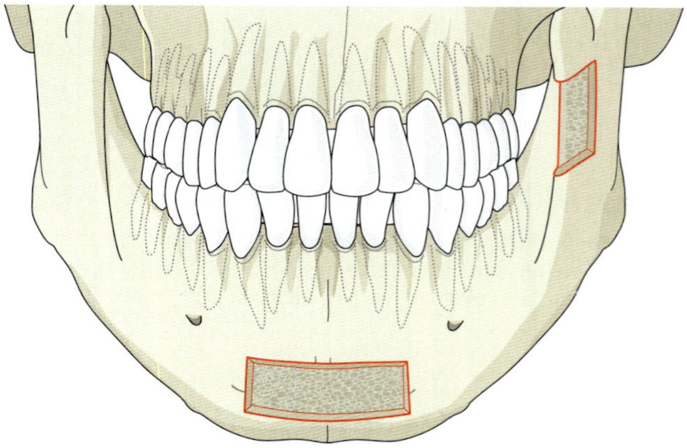

Fig 1.1-10 Potential mandibular bone harvest sites.

2.2.1.1 Ramus

The ramus of the mandible is exposed through a standard posterior vestibular access identical to that used for orthognathic surgery. The mucosa is incised along the external oblique line and the soft tissues are reflected by subperiosteal dissection. Thus, a wide exposure is obtained. A small drill bit, a specially designed right-angle rotating saw or a piezotome is used to outline the graft harvest along the lateral portion of the ramus. A small curved chisel allows elevation of the graft. The graft is then immediately placed at the recipient site and rigidly stabilized or placed in a saline moistened sponge and placed aside. The site is thoroughly irrigated and closed in a single layer. A gentle compressive dressing can be placed on the face to assist in closure of the dead space created by the dissection.

2.2.1.2 Symphysis

The symphysis of the mandible is exposed through a standard vestibular access incision. It is important to maintain a suitable cuff of the unattached tissue by placing the incision labial to the junction of the attached and unattached mucosa. The mentalis muscles must be elevated, and the dissection completed widely to obtain adequate exposure. It is often best to dissect circumferentially around the mental nerve and release the periosteum at the mental foramina to avoid traction injury to the mental nerves. The bone harvest is then outlined with either a small fissure bur, a piezotome, or a specially designed rotating saw. Care must be taken to stay a few millimeters below the apices of the teeth. A curved osteotome is required to elevate the bone graft. For wound closure suturing in two layers, ie, muscle and mucosa, is required. Proper support of the mentalis muscles is necessary to achieve an esthetic outcome. If the mentalis muscle is not resuspended, chin ptosis will likely occur. Additional support of the mentalis muscle and closure of the dead space can be provided with tape or compressive dressing support of the chin. It appears that postoperative pain and local wound complications are more common when the symphysis is used to obtain cortical bone from the mandible.

2.2.2 Maxilla

From the maxilla small amounts of mostly cortical bone can be taken from the nasal aperture (**Fig 1.1-11**) or from the tuber maxillae. The maxilla is approached via transoral incisions in the upper vestibular mucosa.

Other than swelling and pain for a few days, there is no significant donor site morbidity. The bone volume is sufficient for small defects, such as localized ridge augmentations in dental implantology.

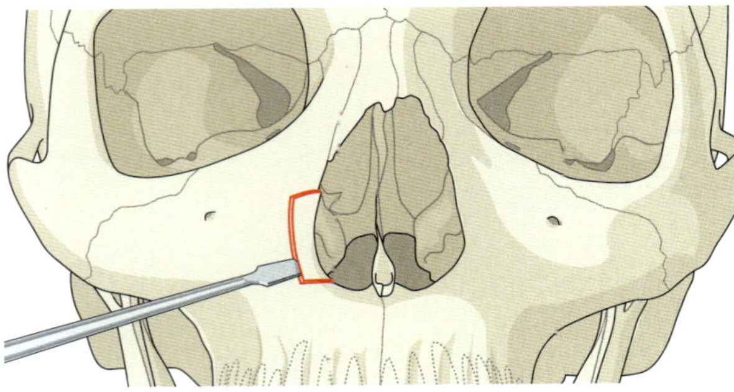

Fig 1.1-11 Bone harvest from the nasal aperture.

2.2.3 Cranial bone

In adult patients the harvest of split thickness calvarium is typically accomplished by removal of the outer cortex; however, the inner cortex may also be separated from a previously elevated full thickness calvarial bone flap as it is commonly performed in craniofacial surgery. The description here will focus on the former technique (**Fig 1.1-12**). The well-developed diploe allows for easy harvest of the outer table. Donor site morbidity is low with proper technique [Jackson et al, 1986]. Younger children typically do not have a layered skull with outer table, diploe, and inner table. Here, harvest of outer table bone grafts is not possible; however, full thickness cortical bone grafts may be taken and split in two layers. One layer is usually replanted to maintain skull continuity for brain protection.

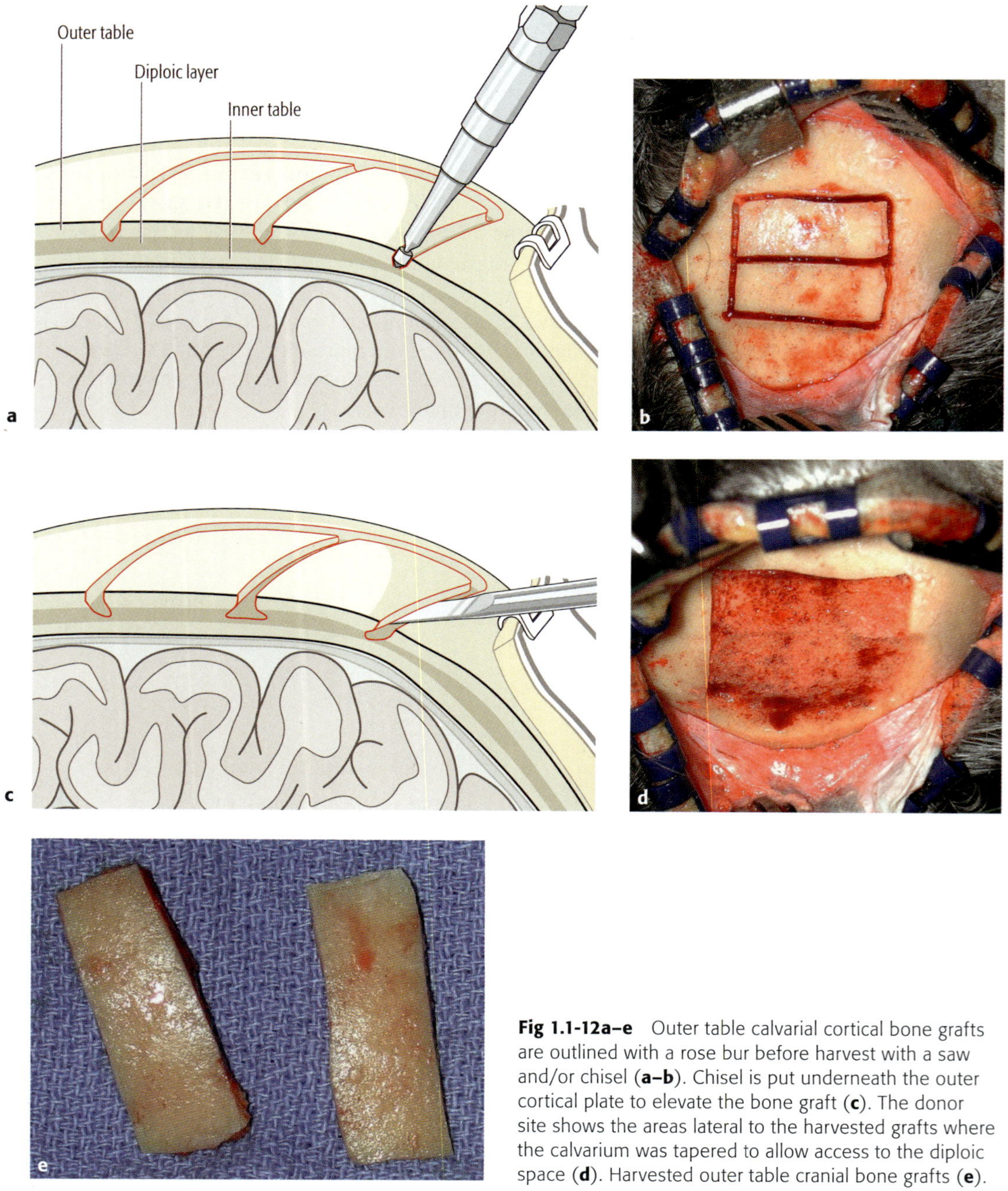

Fig 1.1-12a–e Outer table calvarial cortical bone grafts are outlined with a rose bur before harvest with a saw and/or chisel (**a–b**). Chisel is put underneath the outer cortical plate to elevate the bone graft (**c**). The donor site shows the areas lateral to the harvested grafts where the calvarium was tapered to allow access to the diploic space (**d**). Harvested outer table cranial bone grafts (**e**).

Access to the parietal bone is accomplished through either a curvilinear incision directly over the parietal area or by a coronal incision. Dissection widely beneath the galea allows wide exposure with gentle retraction. The planned bone harvest is outlined with a rose burr taking care to completely osteotomize the outer cortex without perforation of the inner cortex.

A saw or chisel is then used in the diploic space to complete the osteotomy. Angled saw blades may further facilitate the bone graft harvest. The cortical bone can be brittle; therefore, it is best to gently elevate the entire bone graft taking care to free the graft evenly. Excessive force on any portion of the graft will result in fracture or create cracks that will fracture while the graft is being stabilized or recontoured. The harvested bone graft should be wrapped in a saline moistened sponge and placed aside or immediately placed into the recipient site and stabilized rigidly. The donor site is closed over a closed suction drain after copious irrigation.

2.2.4 Ilium

The ilium is a rarely used donor site for the harvest of cortical bone only. Clinical conditions (ie, closed head injury), or operator experience may necessitate the use of this site in some instances. Cortical bone harvest from the ilium requires the identical exposure described in section 2.1.1. The most important modification of the technique is the utilization of a saw or piezotome for creation of the osteotomies. The cortex can then be easily removed with a straight or slightly curved chisel. The inner cortex is preferred to avoid deformity. The technique is similar to the one shown in **Figs 1.1-1–1.1-13**, but only the cortical bone is harvested. The cancellous bone exposed following removal of the cortical bone will tend to bleed. This technique, therefore, requires extreme attention to hemostasis before donor site closure, a suction drain may be indicated [Hall et al, 1981].

2.3 Corticocancellous bone grafts

2.3.1 Ilium

The exposure for harvest of corticocancellous bone from the ilium is outlined completely in section 2.1.1. In the anterior approach, corticocancellous blocks of bone may be harvested from the inner or outer aspect (**Fig 1.1-13**).

Bone blocks may be harvested with one or both cortices. The harvest can be performed including parts of the iliac crest or underneath the crest (**Fig 1.1-14**).

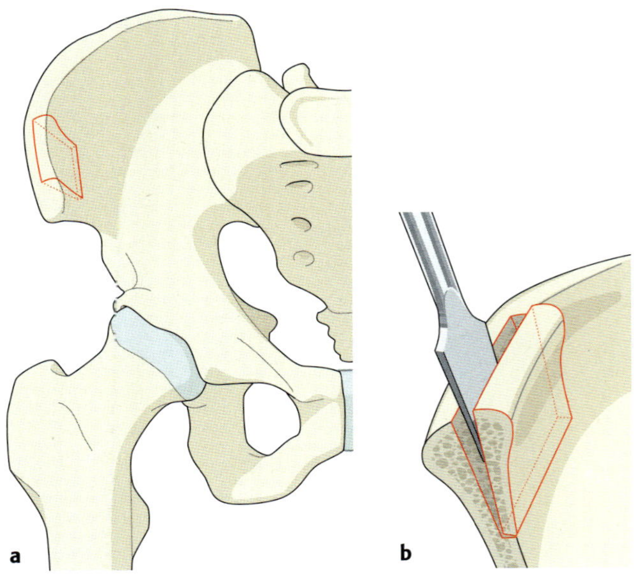

Fig 1.1-13a–b After outlining the desired style and height of a cortico-cancellous graft from the inner aspect of the ilium, the block is elevated with a chisel.

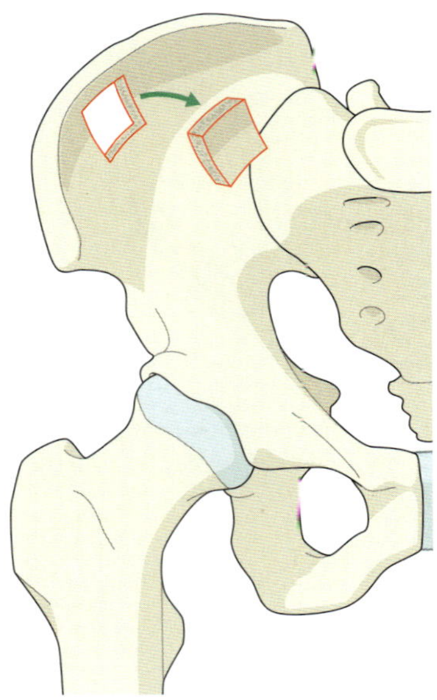

Fig 1.1-14 By taking bicortico-cancellous bone from underneath the iliac crest, the outer contour of the iliac crest is preserved.

To routinely assure harvest of a complete corticocancellous block, it is recommended that saws be used. The saw provides a tactile sense of when the opposite cortex is encountered. It is important that the vertical and inferior bone cuts be made with diverging walls to allow easy and gentle elevation of the graft from the donor site. If the inferior cut is made first, hemorrhage will not complicate visualization of the field while the vertical and then superior horizontal cuts are made. The entire corticocancellous block may be transferred directly to the recipient site and stabilized with plate(s) and screws (**Fig 1.1-15**).

For segmental mandible reconstruction, a reconstruction plate placed along the lateral surface of the mandible provides stability. Additional cancellous bone and marrow may be placed at the intersection of the graft and native bone as well as into osteotomy gaps to improve contact and assure osseous union.

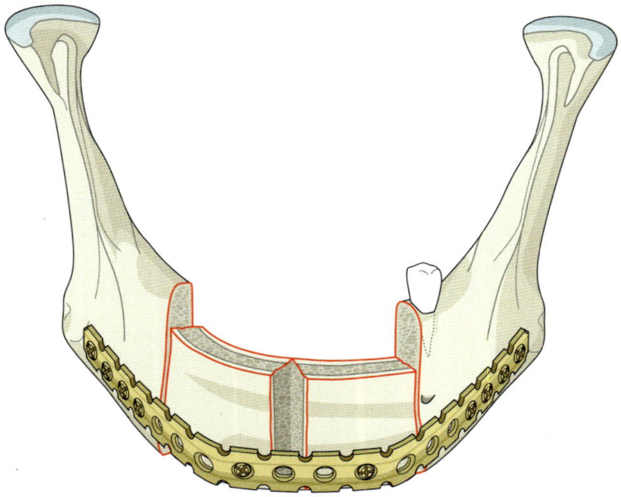

Fig 1.1-15 Stabilization of the bone graft in the chin area with a reconstruction plate. Cancellous bone and marrow may later be used to fill the osteotomy gap.

2.3.2 Rib

The ribs provide a significant donor site for the elective reconstruction of the orbit, calvarium, mandibular condyle, and ramus. For condylar head reconstruction, a costochondral graft, which is a variation of a rib graft, is indicated. In this setting a composite graft with a 5 mm cartilage cap is harvested. The perichondrium must be maintained on the junction of the bone graft and cartilage to provide stability to the cartilage cap/rib construct.

Some avoid the rib donor site in the setting of trauma because of concerns regarding postoperative splinting and less effective ventilation or atelectasis. Harvest of the 4th–6th rib is common. The shape of the ribs in this region is most suitable. Whenever possible, the opposite side rib should be used for mandible reconstruction to take full advantage of the natural curvature of the rib.

Harvest of the rib is completed with the patient in supine position. A small folded towel underneath the donor site is of assistance in gaining adequate exposure. Elective incision in the inframammary crease provides excellent exposure and an acceptable scar (**Fig 1.1-16a**).

Dissection requires incision and reflection of the fascia of the intercostal muscles. The rib is exposed in a subperiosteal plane laterally which facilitates rapid dissection (**Fig 1.1-16b**). For harvest of composite grafts, the medial harvest must be accomplished superficial to the periosteum/perichondrium at the costocartilage junction. This transition requires a precise and delicate approach. The cartilage is then incised with a blade and the deep dissection along the costocartilage junction completed. The rib is then gently retracted laterally and a piezotome or a saw is used to cut the rib at the lateral extent of the required harvest. Rib cutters tend to fracture the rib at the site of the osteotomy and should therefore not be used.

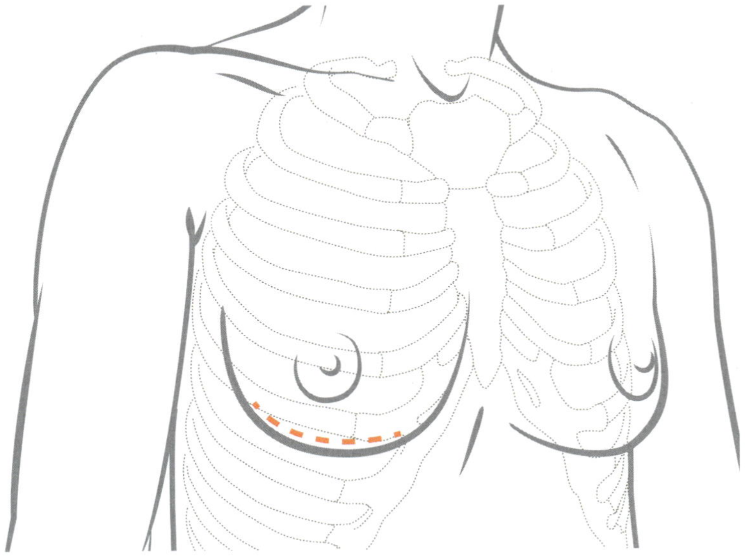

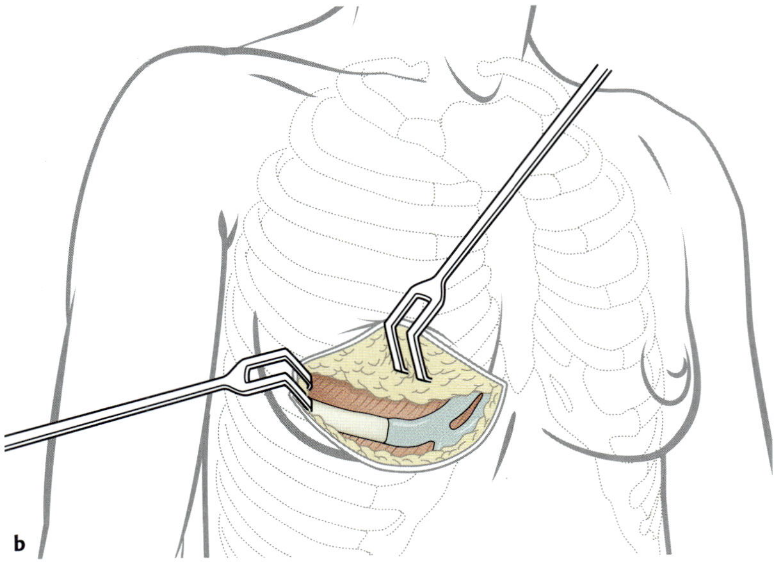

Fig 1.1-16a–b

a Outline of a planned incision in the inframammary crease for harvest of a composite costochondral graft.

b Exposure of the rib at the bone/cartilage junction.

Rigid stabilization of the graft with lag screws should typically be completed after appropriate contouring. It is important to use a bone plate segment as a washer at each screw placement site to prevent splitting of the rib graft. Likewise, the screw sites selected should be staggered to prevent splitting the rib (**Fig 1.1-17**).

2.4 Bone dust

Small quantities of small particle nonvascularized bone, also called bone dust, can be harvested through bone scraping and bone dust collection from the surface areas of cortical bone. Bone dust can be used for defect filling of minor bone defects, periimplant augmentation, or filling of osteotomy gaps and burr holes.

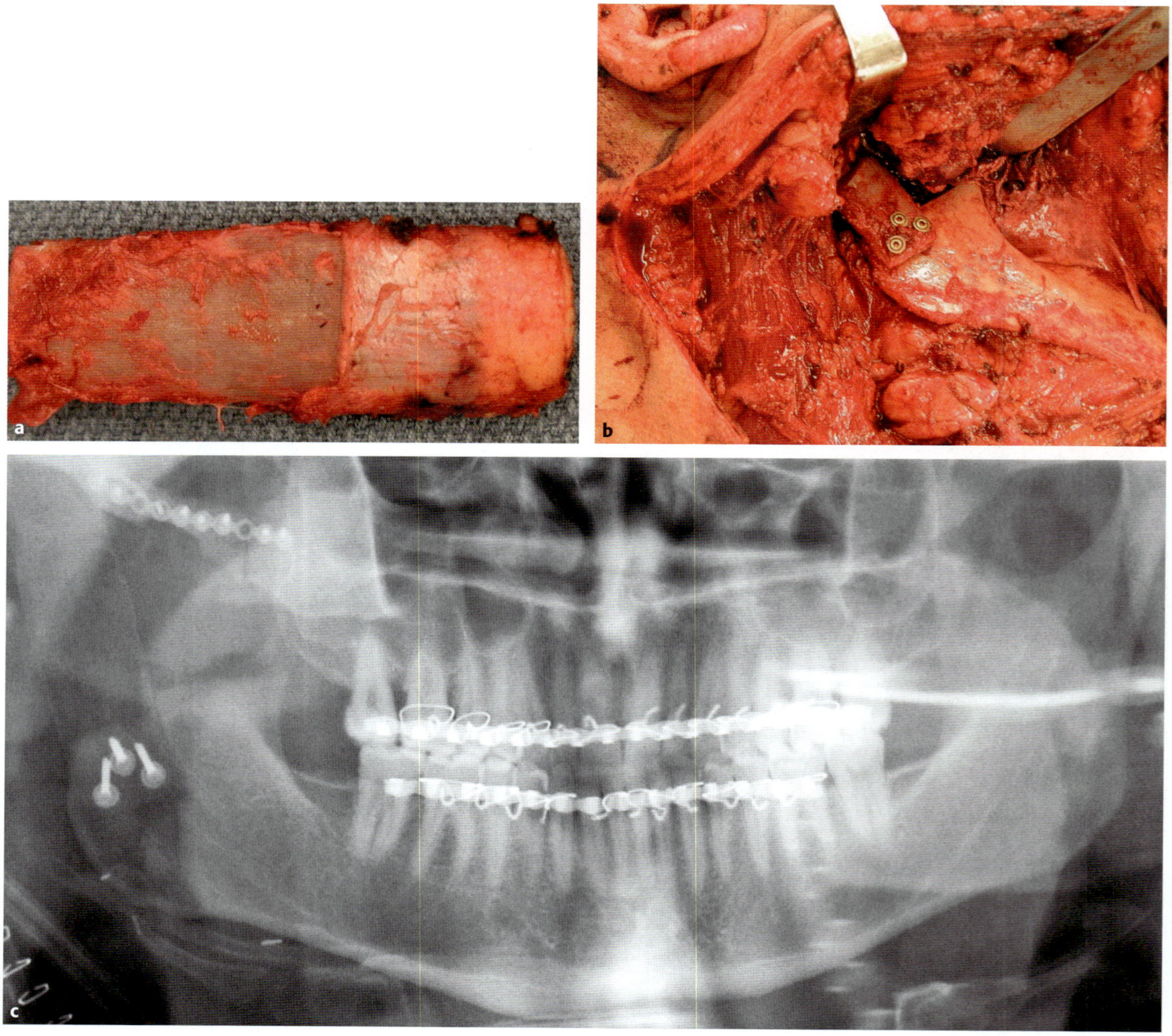

Fig 1.1-17a–c

a Costochondral graft. Note the intact perichondrium/periosteum at the junction.

b The costochondral graft has been inserted. Segments of a bone plate have been used as washers to help distribute the forces of the lag screw over the weak bone.

c Placement and fixation of the graft and hardware can be seen in this postoperative image.

Bone scraping has been introduced with the advent of piezoelectric surgery. Special bone scrapers are available for piezotomes. They look like small chisels and are used to scrape off bone particles from cortical bone areas, such as the chin region, the mandibular body and angle, the zygomatic alveolar crest, or the cranial vault. The scraped off small cortical bone particles are collected in a bone collector, which is integrated into the suction device (**Fig 1.1-18**) [Benninger et al, 2012; Alt et al, 2003; Zaffe et al, 2007; Kainulainen et al, 2006; Graziani et al, 2007; Jackson et al, 1988].

Bone dust collection with a bone collector may also be used in conjunction with almost any bone cutting technology, such as a rose or Lindemann burr.

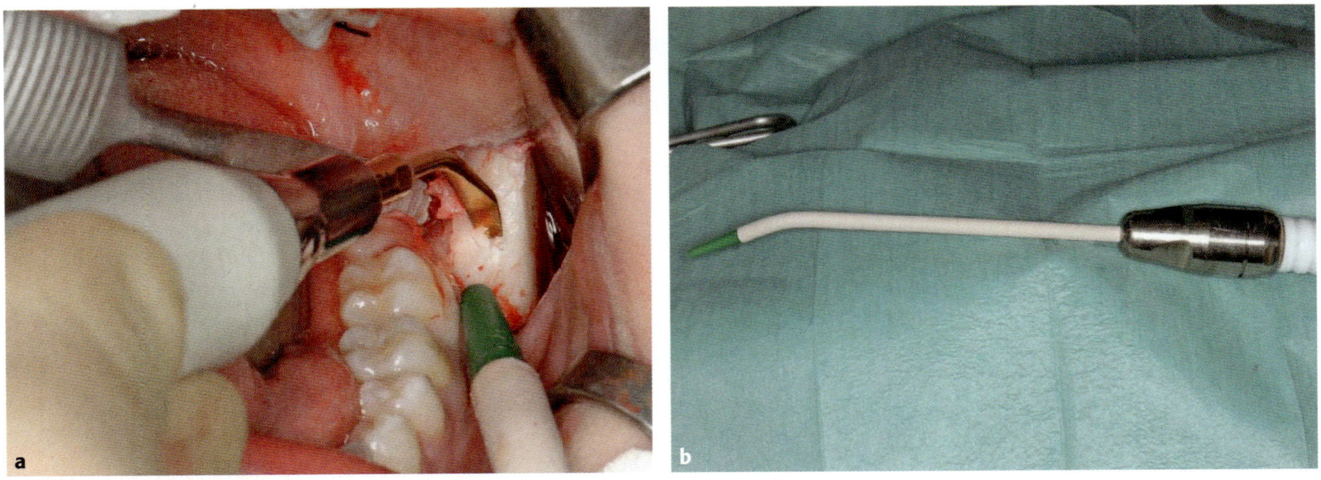

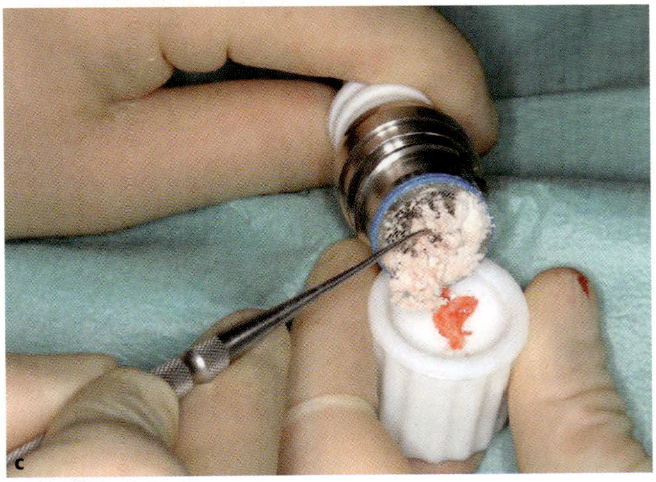

Fig 1.1-18a–c
- **a** Bone dust collected with a piezotome and bone scraper from the oblique ridge of the mandible.
- **b** Bone collector (metal piece) connected to suction device.
- **c** Bone collector opened, bone dust removed.

3 Microvascular bone flaps

3.1 Ilium

The microvascular iliac bone flap is based on the deep circumflex iliac artery (DCIA) and accompanying veins. The DCIA leaves the external iliac artery on its medial aspect normally 1–3 cm cranially to the inguinal ligament. Venous drainage is usually by two accompanying veins, which mostly form a common trunk 1–2 cm before the external iliac vein is reached. The two veins have complex connective branches and sometimes rather resemble a vascular network than two distinct vessels. The DCIA and accompanying veins run superior to the inguinal ligament and reach the inner aspect of the ilium underneath the fascia of the iliac muscle 1–3 cm from the inner cortex of the anterior ileum. An ascending branch of the DCIA supplies the internal oblique muscle allowing simultaneous transfer on one vascular pedicle (**Fig 1.1-19**). This tissue is most commonly used for replacement of missing mucosa or skin because of the thickness and immobility of the skin portion of the flap that is available. A skin island can also be harvested together with a microvascular iliac bone flap. The vascular supply to the skin is via musculocutaneous perforator vessels (**Fig 1.1-20**).

One significant advantage of the iliac free flap is that the surgeon can harvest bone of whatever height is necessary. This results in the ability to tailor the height of the reconstruction, which facilitates dental implant-based maxillofacial rehabilitation [Urken et al, 1991].

The patient is positioned supine, the donor area should be lifted by underlying sheets or a cushion (**Fig 1.1-21**). The operative field is prepared widely and draped. The area exposed should extend medially to the linea semilunaris, superiorly to the level of the lower ribs, laterally as far as possible (at least past the iliac tubercle), and inferior about 4 cm below the groin. If a skin paddle is desired, it must be created from directly over the iliac crest. Landmarks for dissection are the reliably palpable femoral vessels, the ASIS, and the iliac crest (**Fig 1.1-22**). Identification and preservation of the musculocutaneous perforators that supply the skin may be difficult intraoperatively. The perforators can be identified by Doppler ultrasound and marked on the skin before surgery. Many surgeons prefer to use the internal oblique muscle instead of a skin island for intraoral soft-tissue reconstruction.

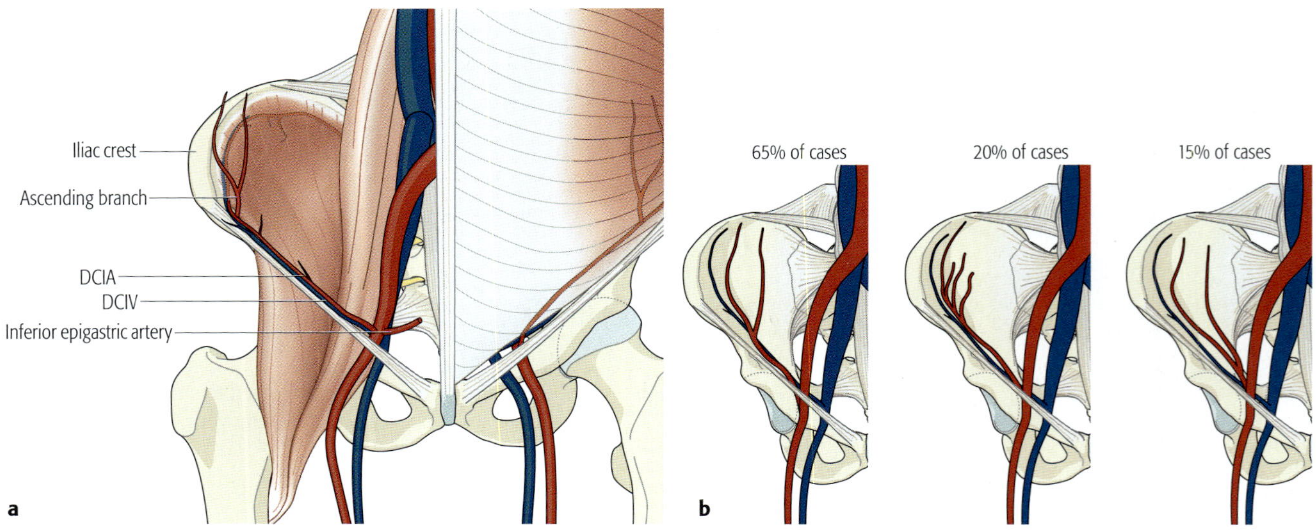

Fig 1.1-19a–b

a The vascular supply of the flap depends on the deep circumflex iliac artery (DCIA) and vein(s) (DCIV). The vessels originate from the external iliac vessels and run laterally and upward underneath and parallel to the inguinal ligament. They reach the ilium underneath the anterior superior iliac spine and continue in a groove between the transverse abdominis and iliacus muscle. An ascending branch runs upward underneath the internal oblique muscle.

b An ascending branch from the DCIA is running superiorly underneath the obliquus abdominis muscle. Three main anatomical variations of the ascending branch have been described, which need to be respected during flap harvest. In 65% of cases, the ascending branch originates from the DCIA within 1 cm medial to the ASIS. In 20% of cases there is no single dominant ascending branch. The internal oblique is supplied by a series of small branches of the DCIA. In 15% of cases, the ascending branch originates in a more medial and proximal location.

The flap can be harvested in two different sequences. After identification of the deep circumflex iliac vessels, the dissection can be performed by identification and dissection of the vascular pedicle, followed by separation of the soft-tissue flap components before finally the osteotomy is made to mobilize the bony portion (center to periphery). It is also possible to harvest the soft-tissue flap components (skin, internal oblique muscle) first, then follow the vascular pedicle down to its origin at the external iliac vessels, and then perform the osteotomy (periphery to center).

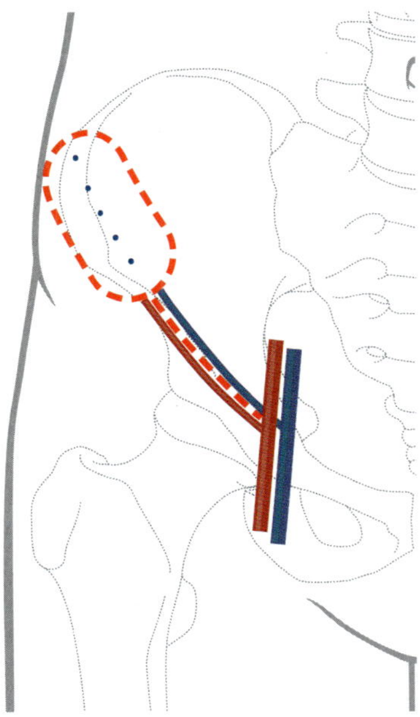

Fig 1.1-20 The skin island of an osteomusculo-cutaneous flap is nourished via perforating vessels, which are located medial to the iliac crest. They should be located centrally within the skin portion.

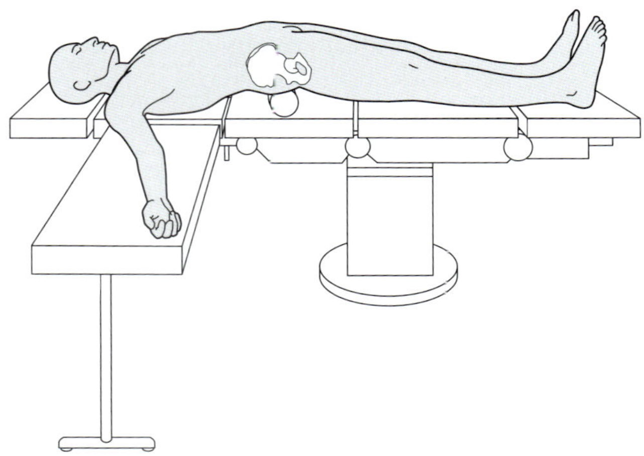

Fig 1.1-21 Patient position for iliac bone flap harvest.

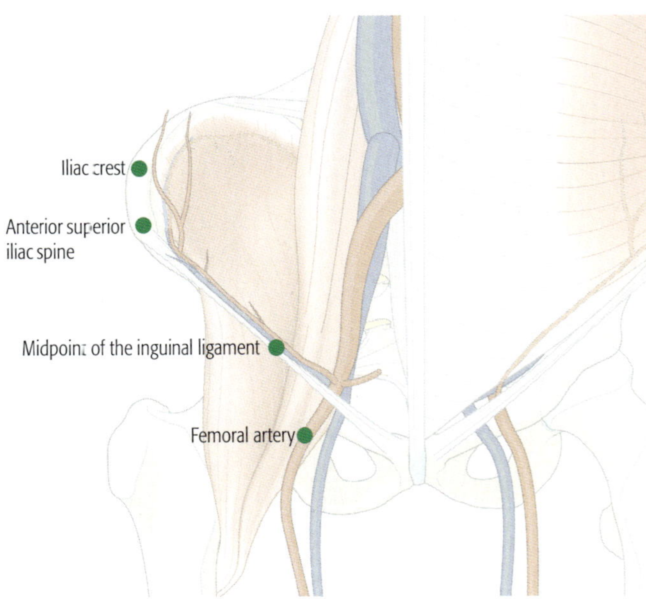

Fig 1.1-22 Landmarks for dissection are the femoral artery, which can be reliably palpated, the anterior superior iliac spine (ASIS) and the iliac crest.

For a center to periphery approach, the vascular pedicle is identified through a skin incision, which follows the course of the inguinal ligament on a line between pubic tubercle and ASIS (**Fig 1.1-23**).

The femoral artery can be palpated and is exposed. Below the inguinal ligament the superficial circumflex artery usually leaves the femoral artery on its lateral aspect and is useful for intraoperative orientation. 2–3 cm above the superficial artery the DCIA will leave the external iliac artery in a lateral and upward direction. Medially, the inferior epigastric artery exits the external iliac artery and is another landmark for dissection. The deep circumflex iliac venous drainage system usually consists of two concomitant veins, which are also exposed. After identification of the vascular pedicle the aponeurosis of the abdominal wall musculature will be divided layer by layer within or above the inguinal ligament. The vascular pedicle is freed until immediately below the ASIS (**Fig 1.1-24**). In this area the lateral cutaneous femoral nerve needs to be identified to preserve it during further dissection.

To harvest an osteomusculo-cutaneous flap, the desired and previously marked skin portion is now incised down to the fascia of the external oblique muscle. The muscles are transsected 3–4 cm away from their bone attachment to preserve a muscle cuff containing the perforators (**Fig 1.1-25**).

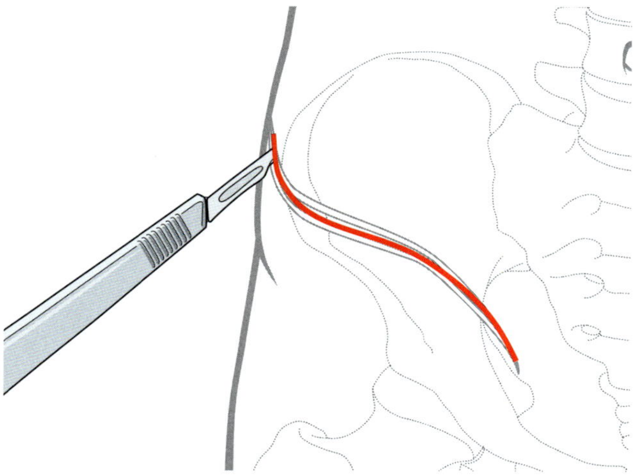

Fig 1.1-23 Skin incision for harvest of an osteomuscular flap with or without additional internal oblique muscle.

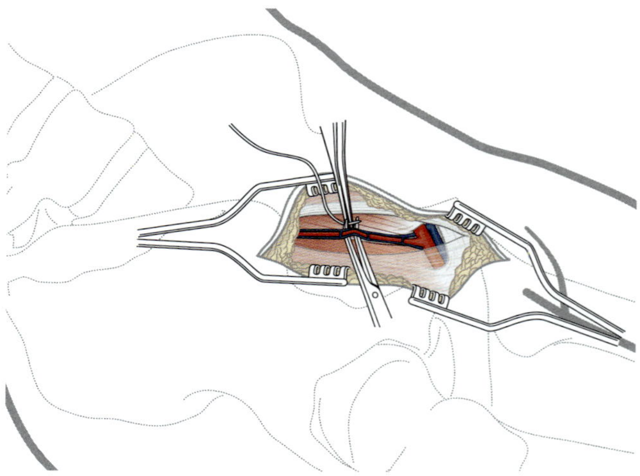

Fig 1.1-24 The deep circumflex iliac vessels are dissected after identification of the external iliac vessels and division of the fascias of the abdominal wall.

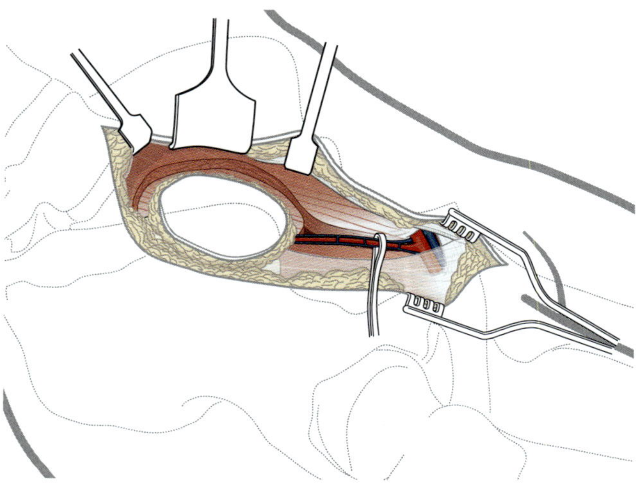

Fig 1.1-25 Transection of the abdominal wall muscles 3–4 cm away from their attachment to the iliac bone to preserve the perforators to the skin.

The vascular pedicle itself is located close to the junction between transverse abdominal muscle and iliac muscle. The fascia of the iliacus muscle is incised approximately 2 cm away from the inner ilium surface to protect the vascular pedicle. A strip of iliacus muscle is included into the flap. After division of the fascia and superficial muscle fibers the caudally located portion of the iliacus muscle is freed from the bone with a periosteal elevator (**Fig 1.1-26**).

Finally, the lateral surface of the anterior ilium is exposed by stripping the relevant part of the gluteus medius muscle in a subperiosteal manner (**Fig 1.1-27**).

If an osteomuscular iliac bone flap with an additional internal oblique muscle component is desired, a curved incision is created 2–3 cm medial to the iliac crest and superior to the groin crease. The incision is carried through the skin, subcutaneous tissue, and the external oblique muscle fascia. The external oblique fascia is thin. After incision, it is retracted and the internal oblique muscle is widely exposed (**Fig 1.1-28**).

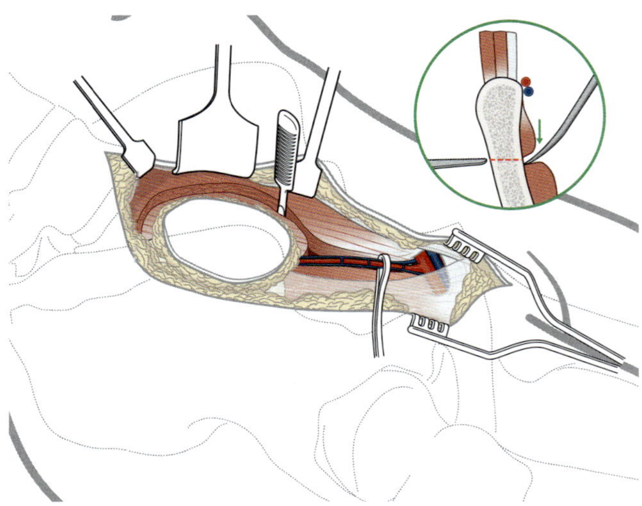

Fig 1.1-26 After transection the iliacus muscle is stripped caudally to expose the medial surface of the iliac bone.

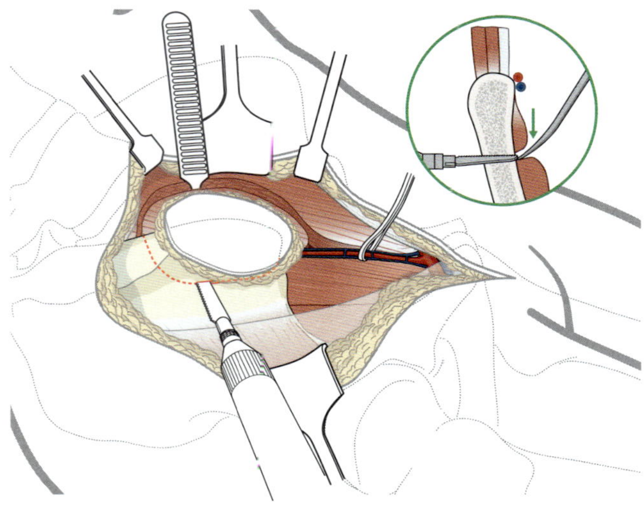

Fig 1.1-27 Before bone flap harvest, muscles attached to the lateral side of the ileum are stripped from the bone surface subperiosteally to expose the lateral aspect of the ilium.

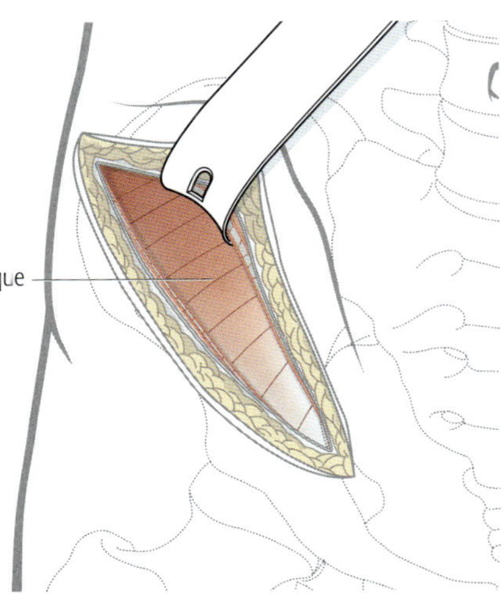

Fig 1.1-28 The thin external oblique fascia is incised and retracted to expose the internal oblique muscle.

The internal oblique muscle is incised in the desired size and reflected laterally. The ascending branch of the DCIA running on the undersurface of the muscle is identified (**Fig 1.1-29**). A retrograde dissection is now performed along the ascending branch to the main vascular pedicle until the deep circumflex iliac vessels are reached (**Fig 1.1-30**).

The vessel dissection is now completed until the whole pedicle is isolated. Care must be taken to avoid injury to the lateral femoral cutaneous nerve. Alternatively, the ascending branch can arise directly from the external iliac artery In this case two arteries need to be dissected and two arterials anastomoses performed. After isolation of the vascular pedicle the distal end of the DCIA is ligated (**Fig 1.1-31**).

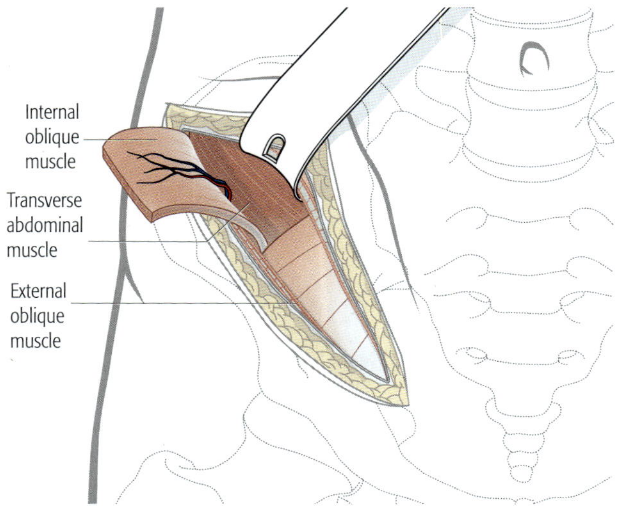

Fig 1.1-29 The internal oblique muscle is incised as needed and raised laterally. The ascending branch of the DCIA, running on the undersurface of the muscle, is identified.

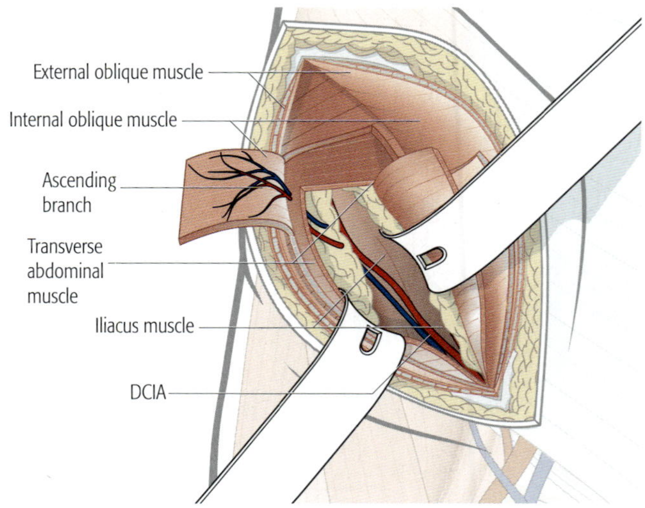

Fig 1.1-30 After isolation of the desired portion of the internal oblique muscle and identification of the ascending branch retrograde dissection is performed along the ascending branch to the deep circumflex iliac vessels.

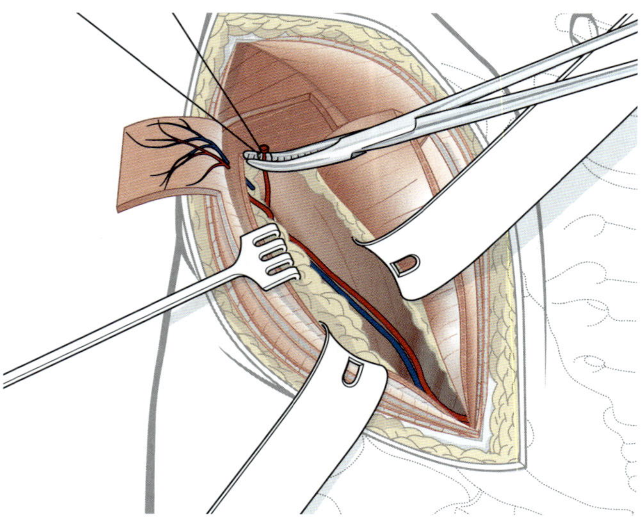

Fig 1.1-31 After dissection of the vascular pedicle is completed, the distal end of the DCIA is ligated.

After dissection and before the flap is isolated, the vascular pedicle is ligated and divided close to the external iliac vessels as soon as the recipient site is prepared for flap inset (**Fig 1.1-32**). If no additional soft-tissue components (eg, skin, internal oblique muscle) are needed, only a small portion of the muscles of the abdominal wall respectively their fasciae (transversalis, external oblique, internal oblique) together with a strip of iliacus muscle are included into the flap to protect the vascular pedicle. In doing so an osteomuscular iliac bone flap is created (**Fig 1.1-33a**). If the flap is harvested with a skin island from the groin it is called an osteo-musculo-cutaneous iliac bone flap (**Fig 1.1-33b**).

Depending on amount and shape of the bone needed and according to the preoperative planning, the ASIS can either be preserved or included into the flap. If it is possible to preserve the ASIS, this should be done and a minimum of 2–3 cm bone adjacent to the spine should be maintained to minimize the risk of anterior iliac spine fractures. If it is feasible to maintain the ASIS and the bone is therefore harvested more posteriorly it has the positive side-effect that the vascular pedicle will be longer. If the ASIS needs to be included into the flap, the sartorius and tensor fascia latae muscles need to be detached from the bone. After that the lateral surface of the ilium is exposed subperiosteally and the osteotomy is performed from the lateral side. Care must be taken to preserve the vascular pedicle on the medial side during the bone cutting process.

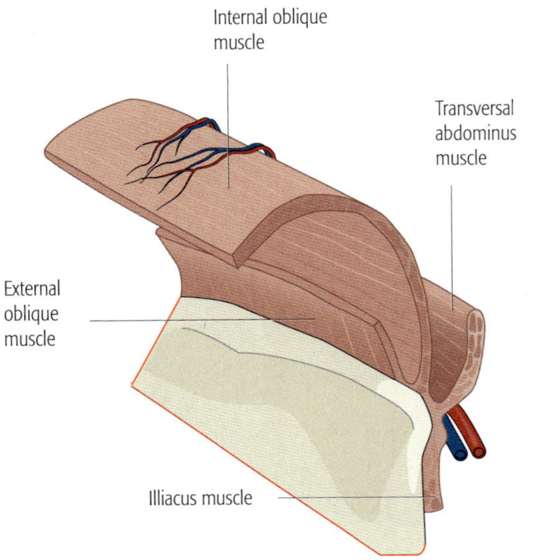

Fig 1.1-32 Isolated iliac bone flap with additional internal oblique muscle.

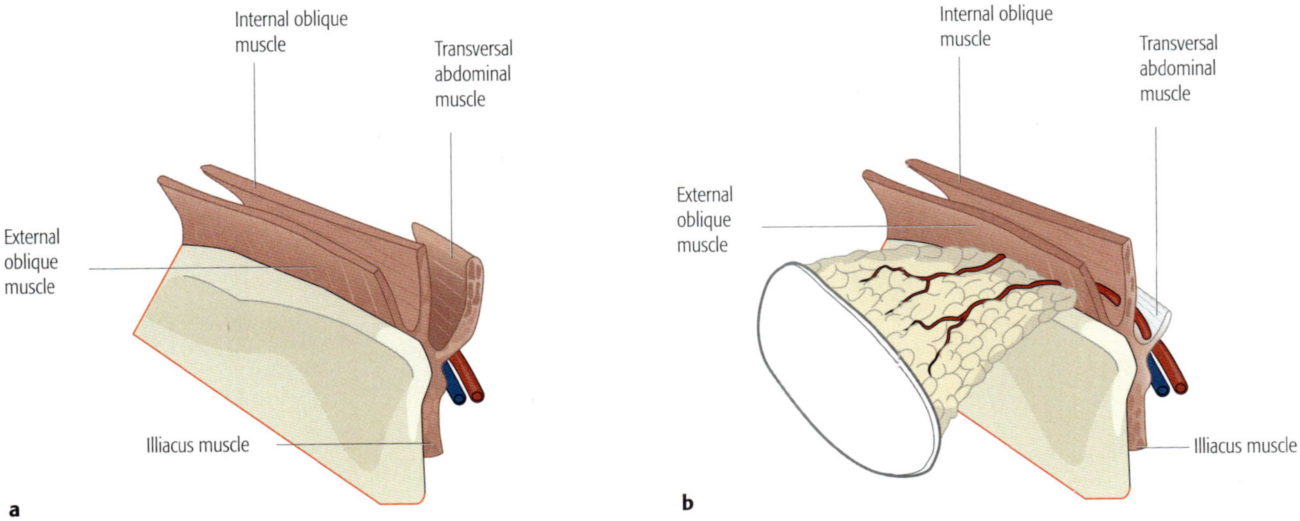

Fig 1.1-33a–b

- **a** Iliac bone flap without additional soft-tissue components (internal oblique muscle and/or skin). A thin strip of muscles needs to be included to protect the vascular pedicle.
- **b** Iliac bone flap with a skin island.

After complete isolation of the flap it should immediately be transferred to the recipient side to avoid longer periods of nonperfusion. The flap may be irrigated with saline solution but is not routinely rinsed with anticoagulants.

Flap contouring may require osteotomies, which can be done as opening or closing osteotomies. As a rule, opening osteotomies will add to bone length, closing osteotomies will reduce length of the bony portion. Inset of a bone flap is typically carried out after opening osteotomies. The osteotomies are always performed through the lateral cortex of the ilium and in a monocortical fashion in order not to harm the vascular pedicle and the soft-tissue components, which are located close to the medial surface of the ilium, respectively the iliac crest. The medial bone is greenstick fractured with finger pressure to allow adaptation of the bone flap (**Fig 1.1-34**).

Bone flap stabilization with osteosynthesis plates and screws is also always performed on the lateral side of the ilium (see chapter 2.6) (**Fig 1.1-35**). Flap contouring may be performed while the flap is still connected to the external iliac vessels and perfused.

Meticulous management of the donor site is crucial to avoid complications. To avoid profuse bleeding from the cancellous portion of the remaining ilium, the donor site is sealed with bone wax, fibrin glue, or other local hemostatic agents. The donor site must be reconstructed to avoid hernia formation. The closure of the abdominal wall must be precisely completed in layers. Hernia formation is reduced if support of the closure is provided with polypropylene mesh or similar. The muscles should be reinserted to the bone using sutures through drill holes in the remaining iliac bone (**Fig 1.1-36**). The muscles and fascia of the abdominal wall should be closed over a suction drain and the skin approximated.

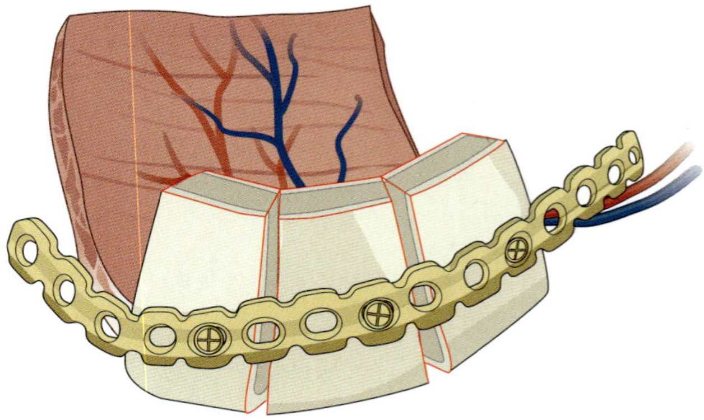

Fig 1.1-35 The flap is fixed to a reconstruction plate with monocortical screws, bicortical screw placement may damage the vascular pedicle especially during the drilling process. The vascular pedicle lies on the medial side of the ilium, respectively the neomandible.

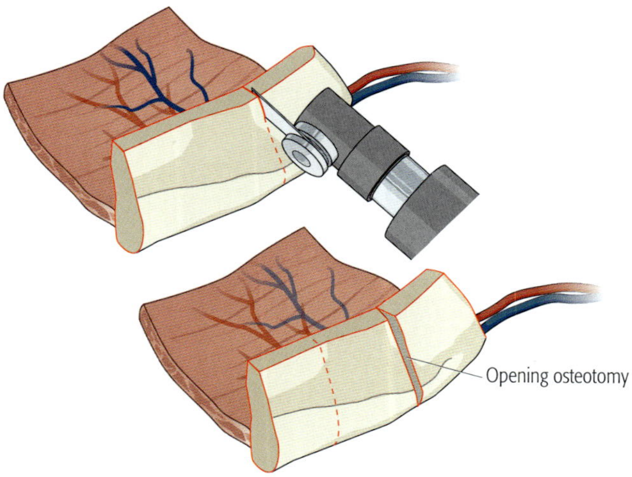

Fig 1.1-34 For flap contouring, monocortical osteotomies are performed on the lateral aspect of the ilium (flap). The medial cortex is then greenstick fractured to avoid damage to the vascular pedicle.

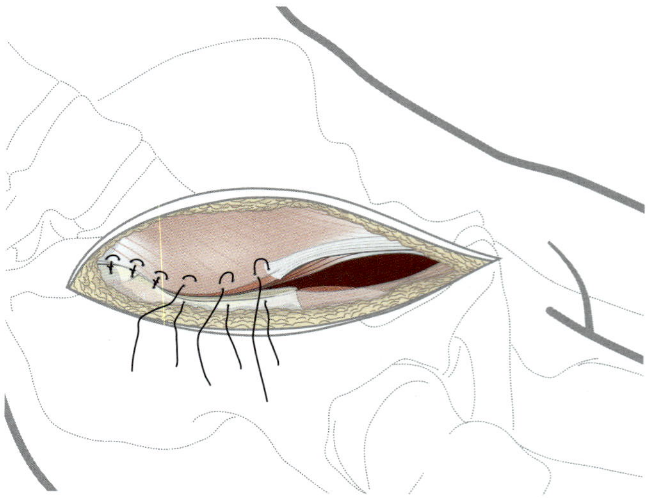

Fig 1.1-36 For better stability of the abdominal wall during wound closure, the muscles of the abdominal wall may be anchored directly to the bone using multiple drill holes.

3.2 Fibula

The microvascular free fibula flap has earned a reputation as a reliable and straightforward means of achieving successful reconstruction of bone defects in the maxillofacial region [Hidalgo et al, 1995]. The flap has been used extensively in mandible reconstruction. Most commonly the flap is used for reconstruction after ablative defects (tumor surgery) or avulsive defects (gunshot wounds). The flap has also been proven to be suitable for maxillary reconstruction (after infrastructure maxillectomy).

Recognized advantages of the flap include large diameter flap vessels, abundant length of available bone, reliable skin paddle, and distant donor site with little donor site morbidity. The most cited criticism of the fibula flap is that the height of the bone is too small for mandible reconstruction. The height of the fibula, in fact, closely approximates that of an edentulous mandible. However, it must be noted that numerous large case series exist, where successful mandibular rehabilitation has been accomplished.

The fibula is the smaller tubular bone of the lower leg. Most important is its role in forming the lateral component of the upper jump joint. Above that it carries only approximately 6% of the load on the lower leg. It has thick cortical layers and not much cancellous bone. In a cross-section, the fibula shows three edges which define the lateral, medial, and posterior facies (see chapter 2.6). The fibula contains an intraosseous artery, but the blood supply to the fibula flap is via the attached muscles and the periosteum. Except for the fibular head and the lateral malleolus, the whole fibula is covered with muscles. From the medial facies of the fibula the margo interosseus arises, to which the interosseous membrane is attached. The lower leg usually contains three vessel nerve bundles, but variations such as a 2-vessel situation are possible. The anterior and the posterior intermuscular septae are running from the superficial fascia of the lower leg to the fibula. Together with the interosseous membrane and the lamina profunda of the fascia cruris, they form well-defined anatomical compartments, which contain the three vascular bundles (**Fig 1.1-37**).

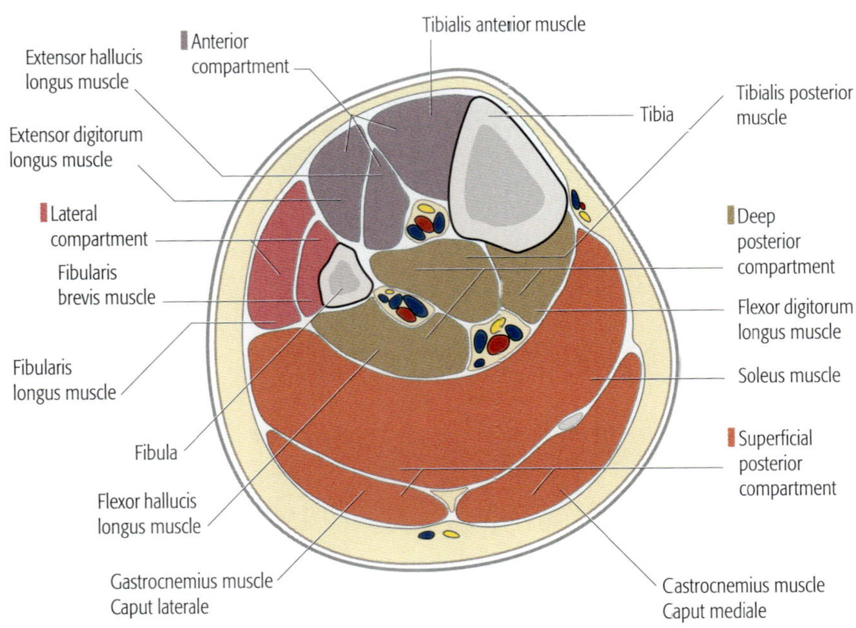

Fig 1.1-37 Cross-section from the middle portion of the lower leg, view from below. Compartments, fascias and neurovascular bundles.

The flexor hallucis longus muscle plays a key role in fibula flap harvest. The muscle parts close to the vascular pedicle need to be incorporated into the flap to protect the vascular bundle and to guarantee periosteal blood supply to the bone. For additional volume, extended flexor hallucis longus muscle components and additional segments of the adjacent soleus muscle can be included into the flap. For a fibula bone flap with skin component (osteomusculocutaneous flap), a skin island over the lateral aspect of the fibula with perforating septocutaneous vessels can be included. The perforators are typically located within the posterior intermuscular septum but may also run through the adjacent musculature (**Fig 1.1-38**).

The flap is based on the peroneal vessels. Preoperative assessment of the donor site is extremely important. Clinical assessment should be corroborated with imaging studies whenever the status of the vasculature is uncertain. If clinical examination reveals any sign of peripheral vascular disease, a magnetic resonance angiogram, CT angiogram or standard angiography should be performed. Congenital abnormalities may also contraindicate the use of the flap, particularly a peroneal dominant circulation (**Fig 1.1-39**).

For flap harvest, the patient is positioned supine and the entire lower extremity is prepared and draped. The recipient site should first be evaluated and appropriate recipient vessels dissected. The presence of good blood flow within those vessels should be demonstrated before commencing flap elevation. This is especially important in the setting of secondary reconstruction, prior neck surgery, and reconstructions for osteoradionecrosis. In some circumstances, such as tumor resection and neck dissection, the harvest can take place simultaneously.

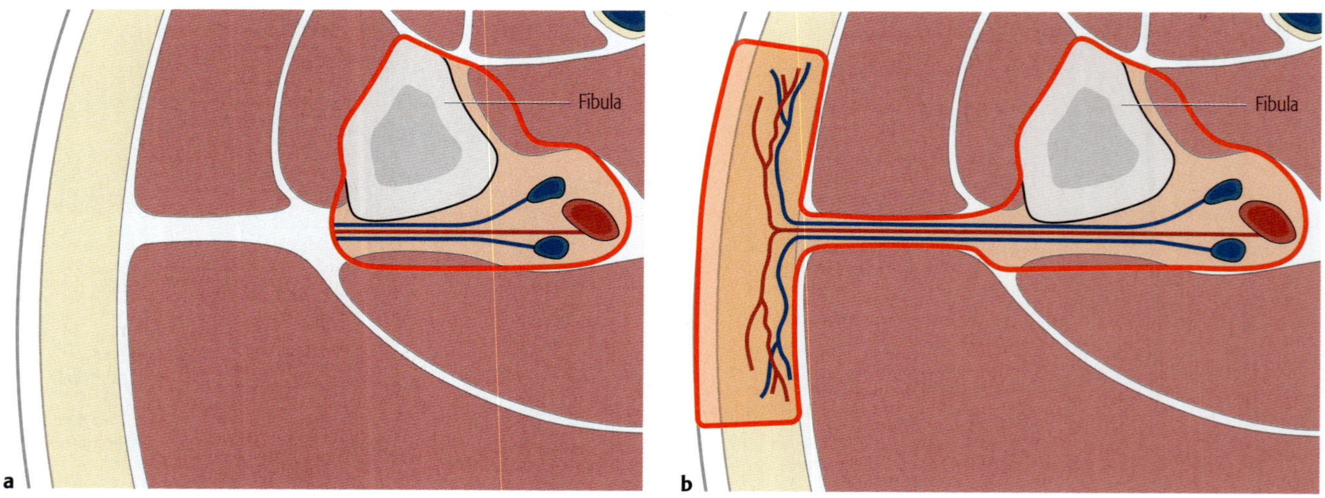

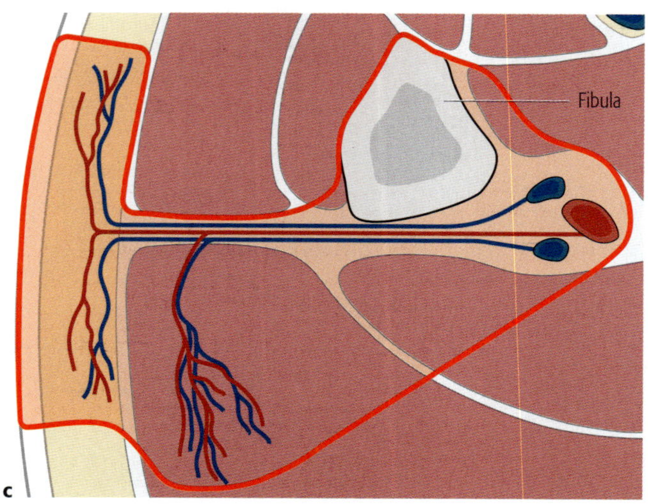

Fig 1.1-38a–c Variations of fibula flap design.
- **a** Fibula bone flap with small muscle components of flexor hallucis longus muscle and tibialis posterior muscle.
- **b** Osteoseptocutaneous fibula flap (with small components).
- **c** Osteomusculocutaneous fibula flap with extended components of flexor hallucis longus and soleus muscles.

The flap can most easily be harvested after application of a sterile tourniquet above the knee (**Fig 1.1-40**). However, some surgeons prefer to harvest the flap without tourniquet to be able to see the bleeding. If the recipient site is not ready for flap inset at the time of flap harvest the flap should stay connected to the peroneal vessels until the recipient side is fully prepared. The flap can then be allowed to perfused before transfer to the recipient site. Some clinicians elect to perform osteotomies and plating of the fibula flap while it remains pedicled to minimize ischemia time (see chapter 2.7). Flap contouring today is often done using CAD/CAM cutting guides (see chapter 5.3.12).

If a skin paddle is needed, it is oriented over the lateral intramuscular septum (**Fig 1.1-41**). Most perforating vessels to the skin are located at the junction of the middle and lower third of the fibula. These vessels may be identified with the use of Doppler ultrasound.

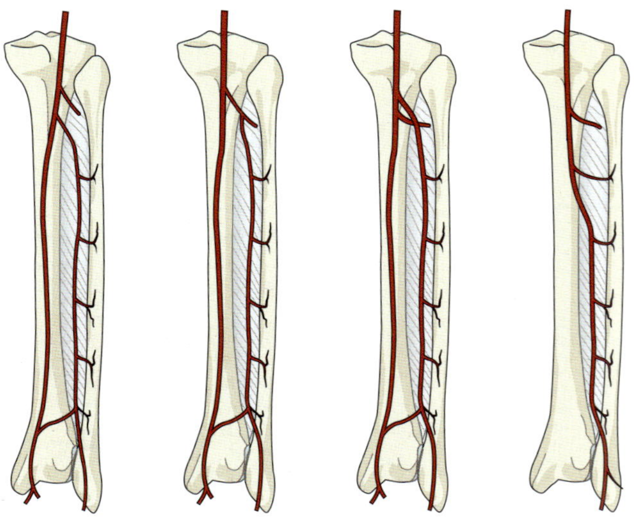

Fig 1.1-39 Variations of the peroneal artery. The use of a fibula free flap is contraindicated in patients with inadequate anterior or posterior tibial vessels to avoid compromise of the blood supply to the foot (approximately 8% of the patients).

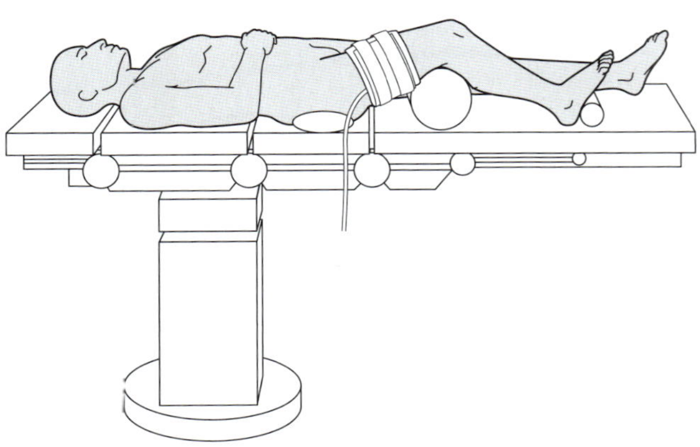

Fig 1.1-40 For flap harvest the patient is placed in a supine position with the knee of the donor leg flexed. If a tourniquet is used, it is placed at the middle of the thigh and inflated (up to 90 minutes) to twice the systolic pressure.

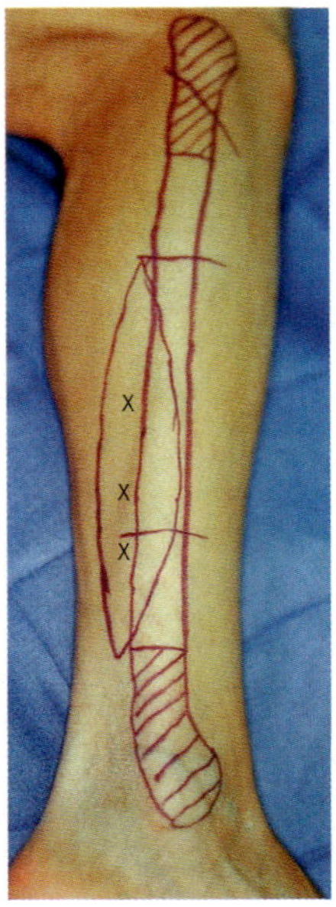

Fig 1.1-41 The fibula free flap donor site and planned harvest of skin flap are outlined in this image. Perforators have been identified by Doppler ultrasound and are marked on the skin.

During fibula flap harvest the proximal and distal 6–7 cm of the fibula needs to be preserved to ensure stability of the lower leg, especially of the superior jump joint.

For flap harvest an incision is performed along the lateral aspect of the fibula in a straight or slightly curved manner. The incision should start at least 2 cm inferior to the fibular head to avoid damage to the common peroneal nerve. If a skin island is going to be included, it should have been previously marked and the perforators should have been identified by Doppler ultrasound. The anterior border of the skin island is included into the incision line (**Fig 1.1-42**).

The skin is incised including the superficial fascia of the lateral compartment. The dissection is continued until the posterior intermuscular septum is reached. Within the septum the perforators are identified (**Fig 1.1-43**).

The peroneal muscles are elevated from the periosteum of the fibula and retracted anteriorly to expose the fibular bone. Care should be taken to preserve the periosteum over the bone, especially in the area of the perforators (**Fig 1.1-44**). Sharp dissection is then carried to the interosseous membrane leaving a thin layer of the extensor hallucis longus muscle attached to the fibula (**Fig 1.1-45**).

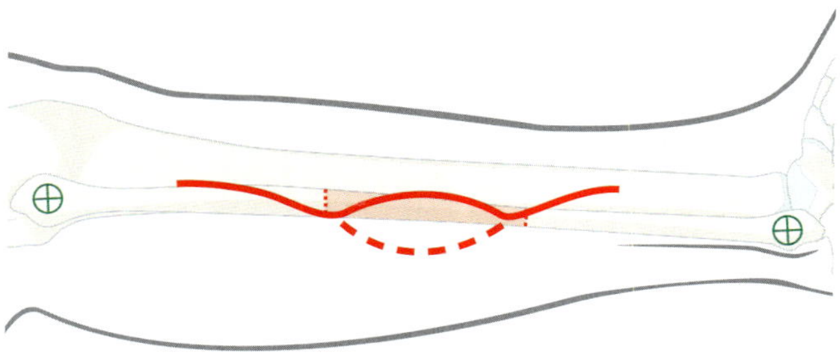

Fig 1.1-42 The shape of the incision may be curved or a straight line. At the distal end, the desired skin flap is incorporated into the incision. The incision starts 2 cm inferior to the fibular head to avoid damage to the common peroneal nerve.

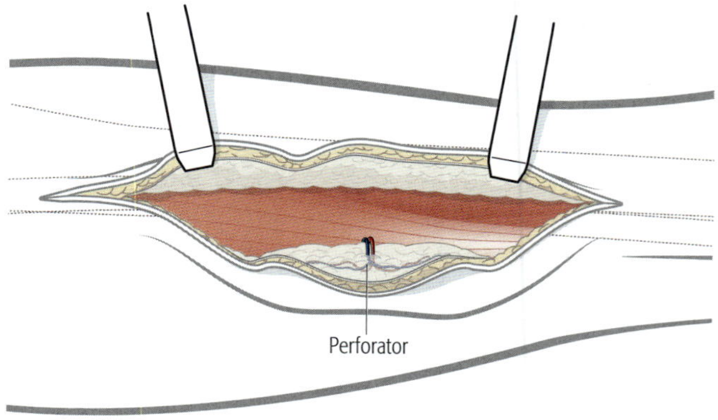

Fig 1.1-43 The skin is incised including the fascia of the lateral compartment. The muscles are exposed and the dissection continued posteriorly to identify the perforators to the skin island.

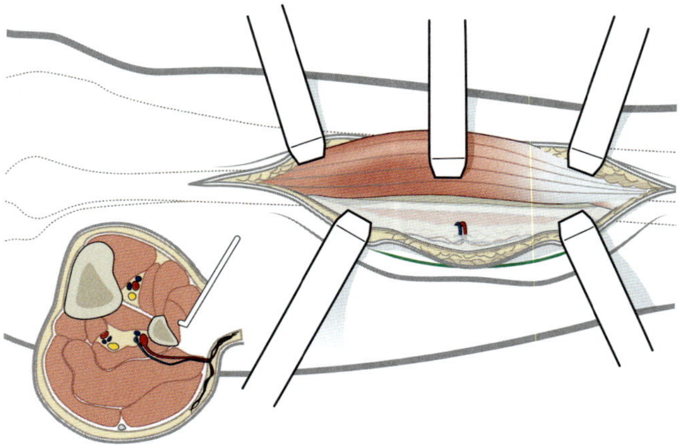

Fig 1.1-44 The peroneal muscles are separated from the periosteum of the fibula and retracted anteriorly to expose the fibular bone. Take care to preserve the periosteum over the bone, especially in the area of the perforator(s).

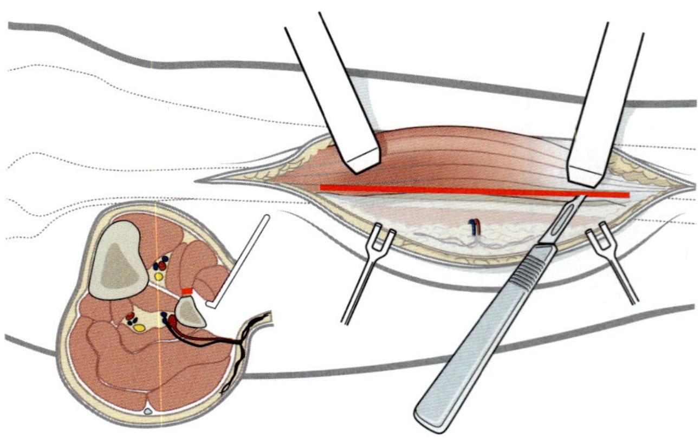

Fig 1.1-45 Sharp dissection is then carried to the interosseous membrane leaving a thin layer of the extensor hallucis longus muscle attached to the fibula.

To be able to mobilize the bone and for better access the desired bone segment is now osteotomized. To expose the bone a subperiosteal dissection is performed 360° around the fibula only at the planned osteotomy sites (**Fig 1.1-46**). During the osteotomies the vascular pedicle needs to be protected, for example with periosteal elevators to avoid damage. The osteotomies are performed with oscillating or reciprocating saws (**Fig 1.1-47**).

The interosseous membrane is now cut, and the posterior tibialis muscle divided to expose the vascular pedicle (**Fig 1.1-48 and Fig 1.1-49**).

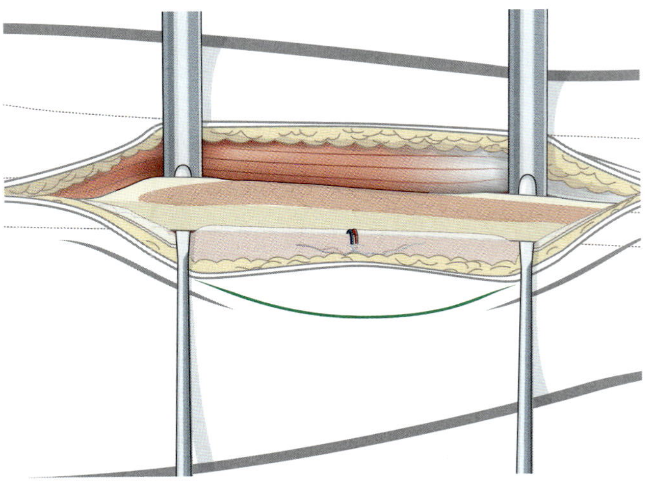

Fig 1.1-46 In preparation for the necessary osteotomies, a subperiosteal dissection is performed 360° around the fibula only at the osteotomy sites.

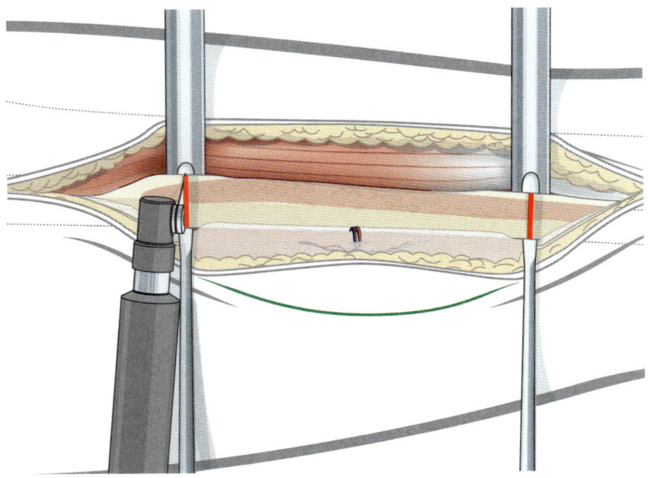

Fig 1.1-47 The osteotomies are performed with a saw. During the bone-cutting process the peroneal vessels are protected with periosteal elevators.

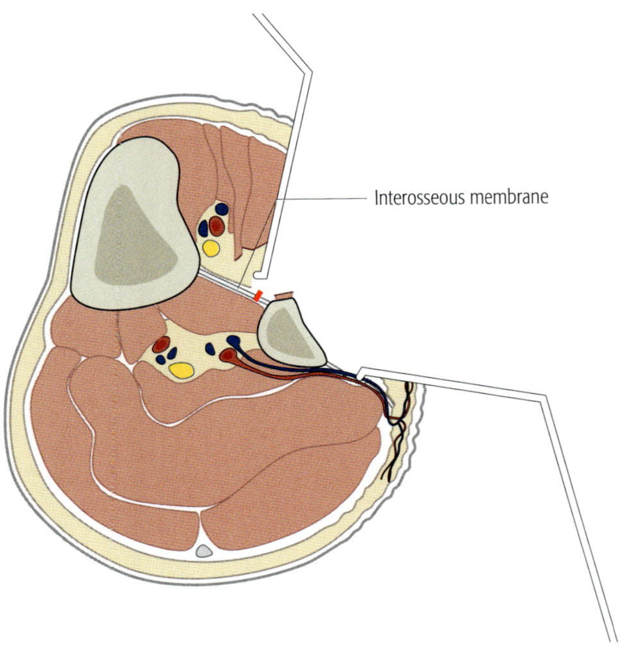

Fig 1.1-48 The interosseous membrane is cut leaving a few millimeters of the membrane attached to the fibula.

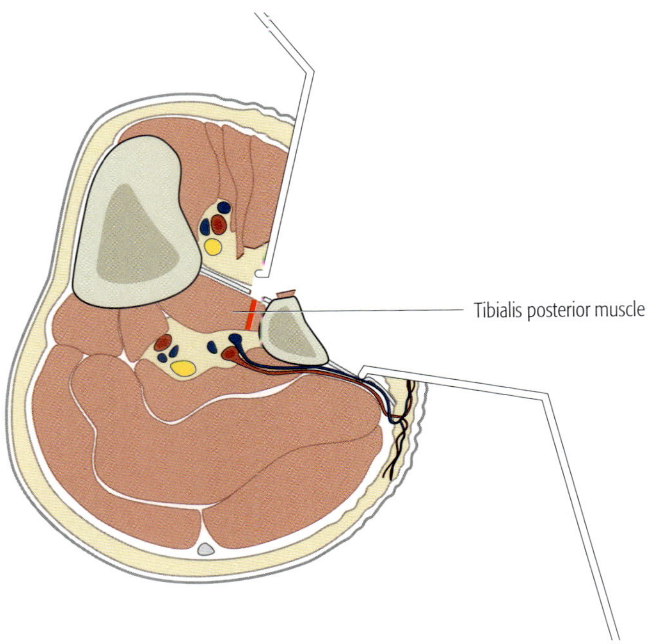

Fig 1.1-49 Dissection is continued into the posterior compartment. The tibialis posterior muscle is divided to expose the pedicle, and a cuff of muscle tissue is left attached to the bone.

The osteotomized bone segment is now mobile and is retracted laterally to have access to the vascular bundle. The distal branches of the pedicle are now identified and ligated (**Fig 1.1-50**).

When harvesting an osteoseptocutaneous flap, the posterolateral skin incision is now made down to the fascia and a subfascial elevation of the skin from the soleus muscle is made. Care must be taken to protect the perforators from the peroneal artery during this step. For perforator protection a thin strip of soleus muscle may be included into the flap. (**Fig 1.1-51**). The fibula segment is rotated laterally and the flexor hallucis is transected from inferior to superior leaving a thin muscle cuff to protect the vascular pedicle (**Fig 1.1-52**).

If the skin flap is not needed, the skin perforators can be sacrificed.

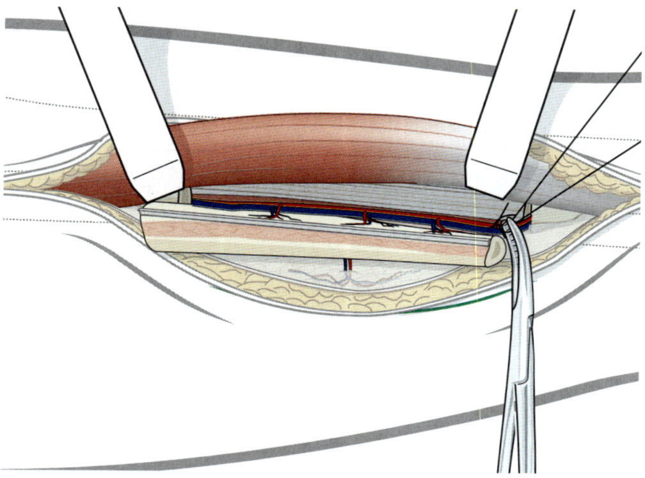

Fig 1.1-50 The osteotomized bone segment is retracted and rotated laterally to expose the peroneal vessels. The distal branches of the pedicle are now identified and ligated.

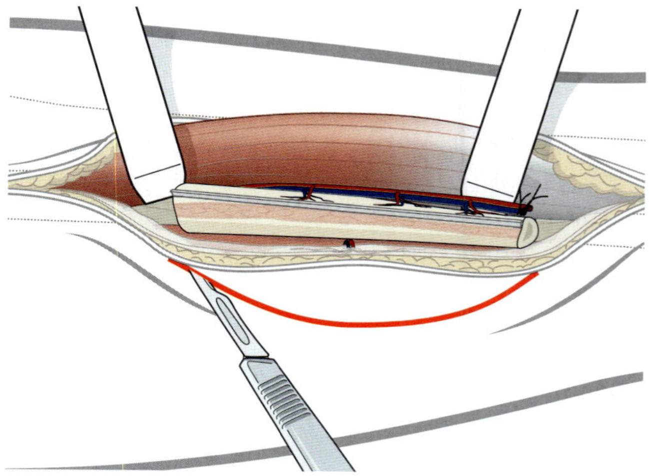

Fig 1.1-51 To harvest an osteoseptocutaneous flap, the posterolateral skin incision is now made down to the fascia and a subfascial elevation of the skin from the soleus muscle is made. Be careful to protect the perforators from the peroneal artery during this step.

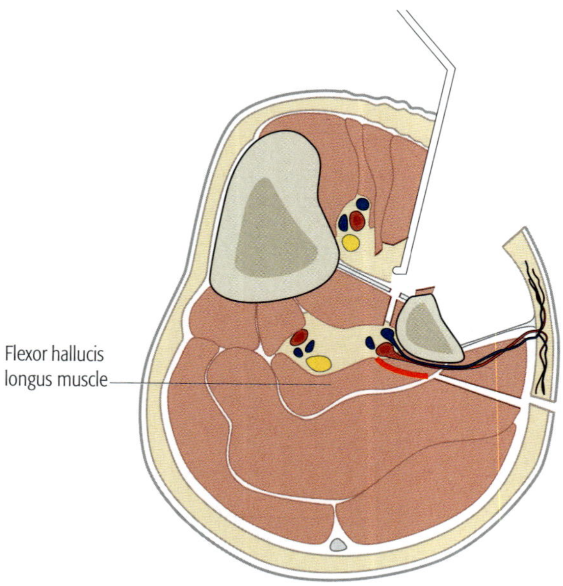

Fig 1.1-52 While retracting the bone segment, the flexor hallucis longus muscle is transected from inferior to superior leaving a thin muscle cuff to protect the vascular pedicle.

The flap is now mobile and for maximum pedicle length the vascular pedicle is dissected in a proximal direction until the bifurcation of the posterior tibialis and the peroneal vessels is reached (**Fig 1.1-53**). If bone flap contouring through osteotomies is required some surgeons prefer to do this while the flap is still connected and perfused, while others prefer to perform necessary osteotomies on a side table shortly before the recipient site is ready for flap inset. Ligation of the vascular pedicle is the last step of flap harvest (**Fig 1.1-54**) (see chapter 2.7).

After harvest of an osteomuscular fibula flap the donor site can usually be closed primarily. However, it is vital to avoid tension after donor site closure, especially after skin portions have been included into the flap in order to not create a compartment syndrome. If tension is present, a split thickness or thin full thickness skin graft should be used (**Fig 1.1-55**).

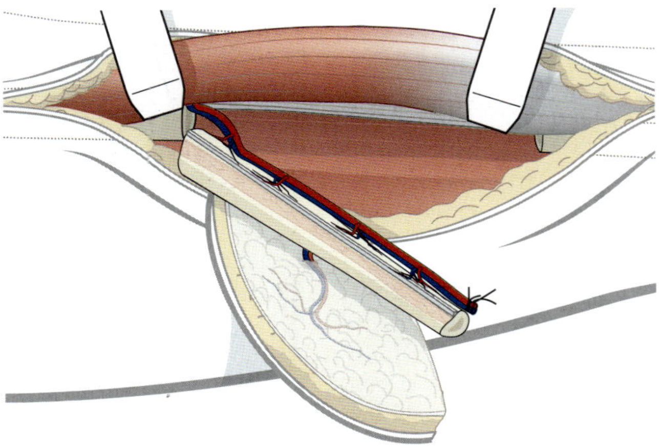

Fig 1.1-53 The proximal pedicle is dissected up to the bifurcation area of the posterior tibialis and the peroneal vessels.

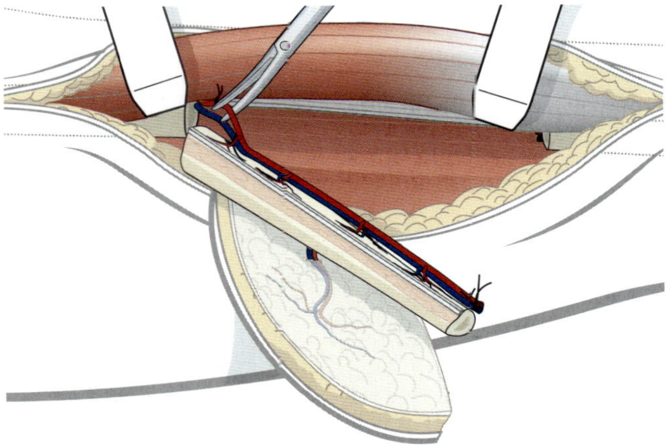

Fig 1.1-54 After identification of the bifurcation, the peroneal vessels are ligated and the pedicle is transected.

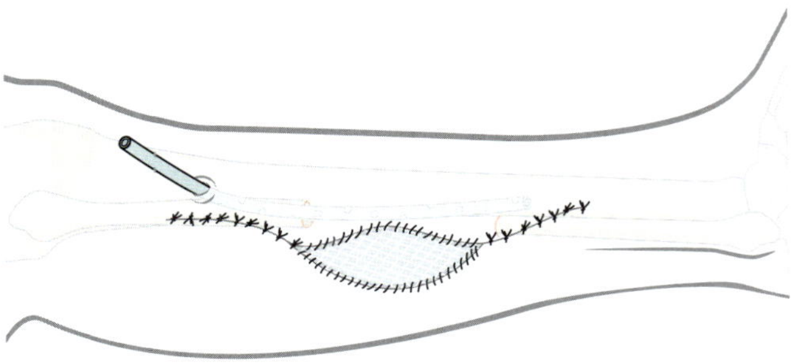

Fig 1.1-55 Wound closure needs to be performed without tension to avoid compartment syndrome. In case of the slightest tension a split thickness or thin full thickness skin graft should be used. A drain is inserted.

Inset of the flap requires assessment of the necessary pedicle length and contouring of the skin paddle. The vessels should be oriented along the medial aspect of the flap. Osteotomies are created after minimal periosteal reflection and are followed by excision of bone wedges with a saw. Refinement of these osteotomies is often necessary and is completed with a burr. The flap can be adapted free hand, with the use of a template or directly to a bone plate. The latter technique offers significant advantage in that the shape of flap has already been determined and the surgeon must simply match it (**Fig 1.1-56 and Fig 1.1-57**).

Bone contouring can also be done with cutting guides produced with CAD/CAM technology (see chapter 5.3.12). The bone flap is first stabilized with monocortical screws in the flap and bicortical screws in the neighboring mandible, after that the soft-tissue inset is performed. Microvascular anastomosis is then completed and the flap evaluated for appropriate perfusion.

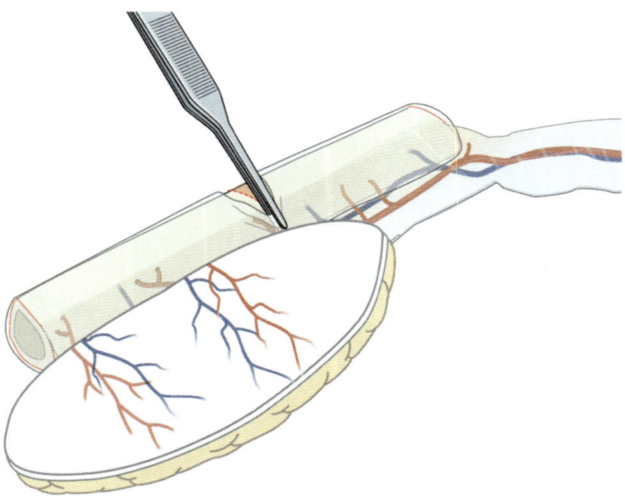

Fig 1.1-56 If osteotomies need to be performed be careful not to injure the vascular pedicle. Typically, closing osteotomies are performed. This means that a wedge of bone is taken out, after that the remaining fibular segments are realigned at an angle defined through the wedge. For the planned osteotomies the periosteum should be freed from the bone resected during the closing ostectomy and retracted carefully during the bone cuts. Stripping of excess periosteum for the closing ostectomy will put vascular supply to the segment at risk.

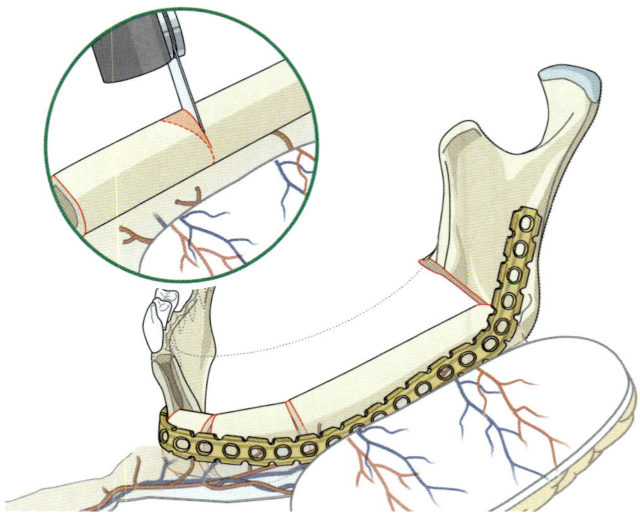

Fig 1.1-57 The bone is adapted to the overlaying plate as much as possible to avoid large bone-plate gaps. The individual fibula segments should not be less than 2.5 cm in length.

3.3 Scapula

The scapula is a triangular-shaped bone with a thin center portion, whereas the lateral border of the scapula has a corticocancellous structure. Scapula bone flaps are shorter compared to iliac and especially fibula flaps, although with interindividual variations. The scapula bone flap is less commonly used in maxillofacial bone reconstruction because it requires intraoperative repositioning of the patient. It offers, however, a significant advantage over the other free bone flaps as it can be harvested with several separately mobile skin paddles [Sullivan et al, 1989]. Usually the lateral border of the scapula provides enough bone even for segmental mandible reconstruction. The lateral border has a slightly helical shape (**Fig 1.1-58**).

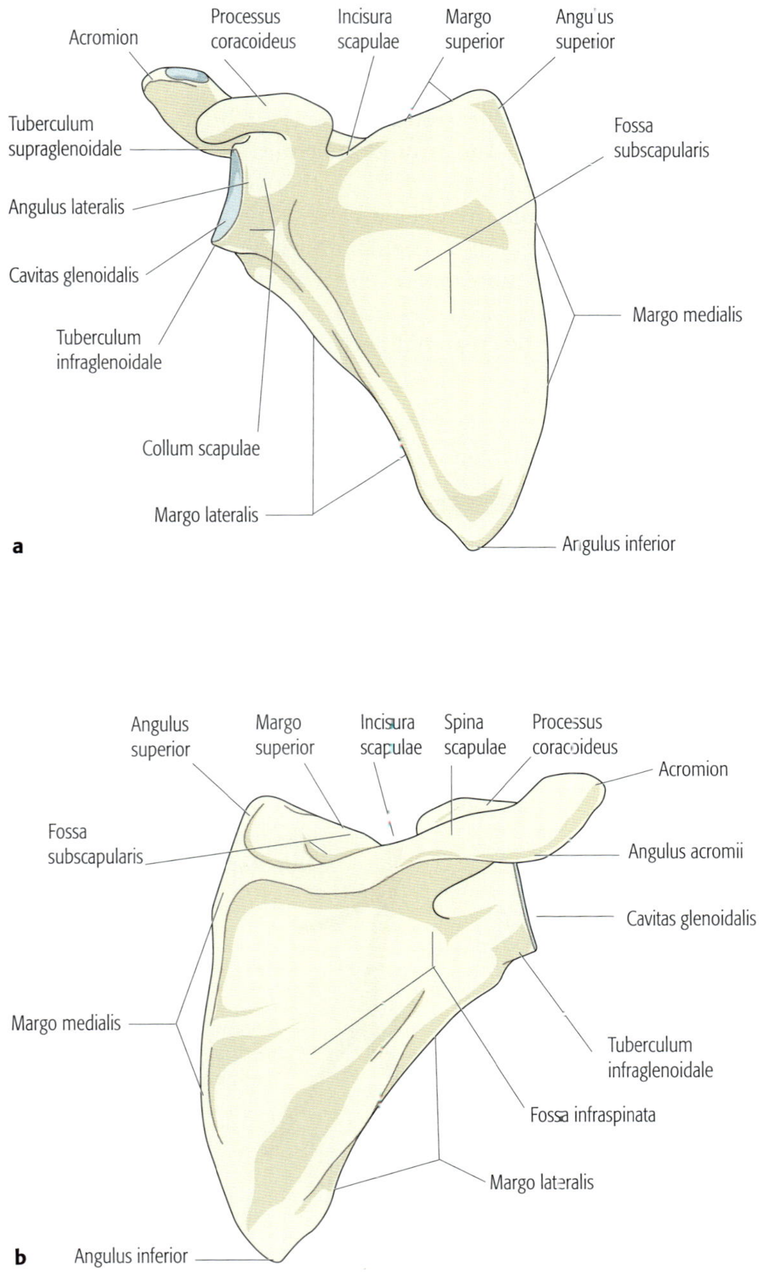

Fig 1.1-58a–b Anatomy of the scapula.

The individual size can be assessed through preoperative computed tomographic imaging. Pedicled on the circumflex scapular artery and frequently two accompanying veins, bone flaps with a thickness of approximately 1.5 cm, a width of approximately 3 cm, and a length of 10–14 cm can be harvested. The bone quality is, however, variable and may not always be relied on to support dental implant-based rehabilitation. The flap is often used in reconstruction of large maxillectomy defects and through and through defects involving the mandible. Blood supply to the scapula bone flap is through the circumflex scapular vessels, which mostly originate from the subscapular vessel system (**Fig 1.1-59**).

As a variation the circumflex scapular vessels can originate from the axillary artery. The arteries are typically accompanied by veins. It is important to know that veins of the scapular drainage system may have valves. The vascular axis containing the circumflex scapular artery can be elongated in dissecting the subscapular vessels up to the axilla. Through this technique a long vascular pedicle of approximately 12–14 cm can be created if necessary. On the subscapular vascular axis, the scapular bone flap can be combined with a scapular or parascapular fasciocutaneous or a musculocutaneous flap from the latissimus dorsi muscle. Various flap combinations are possible. Most frequently a parascapular, scapular, and/or latissimus dorsi soft-tissue flap is combined with a bone flap from the lateral border of the scapula, a serratus anterior flap may also be included. From the tip of the scapula a vascularized bone flap pedicled on the angular branch from the thoracodorsal vessels can be isolated. This angular bone flap can be used alone or in combination with a bone segment from the superior portion of the lateral border. In the latter case this allows for a more independent insert of the two separate bone segments (**Fig 1.1-60**).

The scapula has multiple muscle attachments on both sides. The blood supply to the bone is via attached muscles and the periosteum. Therefore, a muscle cuff along the lateral border of the scapula needs to be preserved during bone flap harvest (**Fig 1.1-61**).

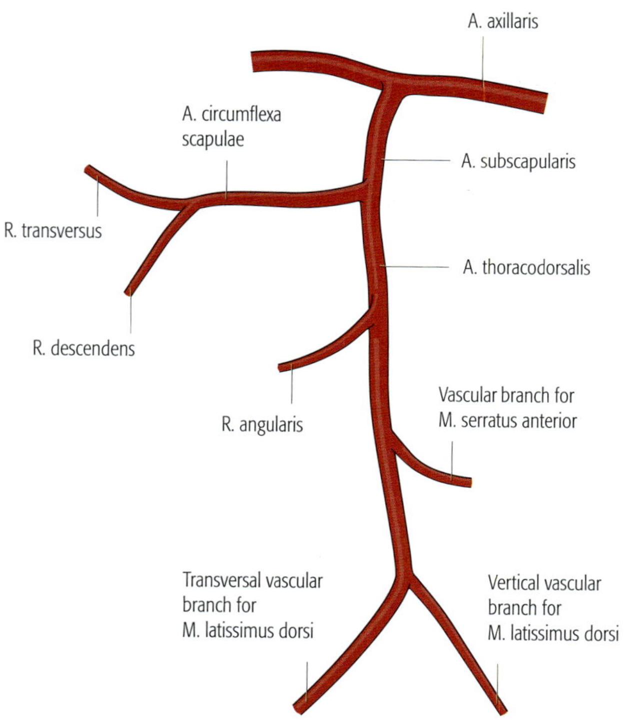

Fig 1.1-59 Subscapular arterial system.

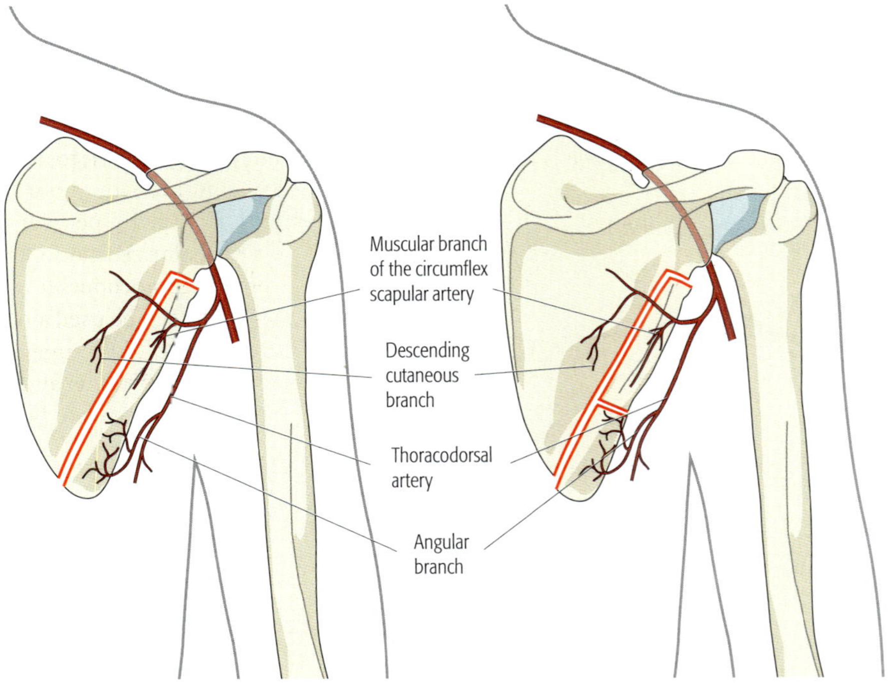

Fig 1.1-60 From the lateral border of the scapula two bone flaps with independent vascular supply can be harvested. The superior part of the lateral border is supplied via the circumflex scapular artery, while the tip region is supplied via the angular branch coming from the thoracodorsal artery.

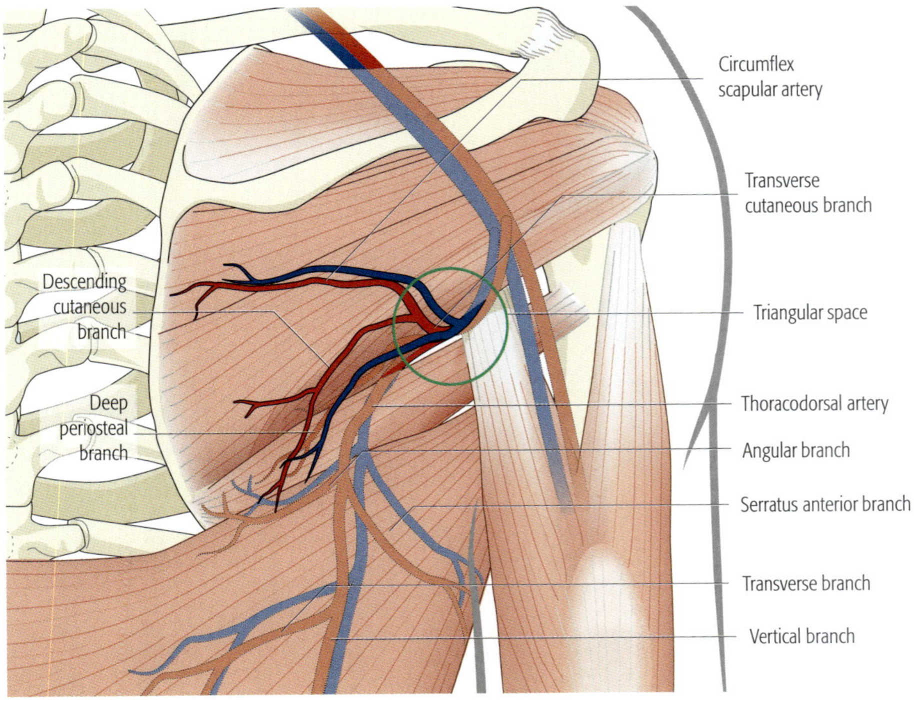

Fig 1.1-61 View from posterior with muscles attached to the scapula. The circumflex scapular artery goes through the triangular space. Finally, it will bifurcate into two cutaneous branches (scapular and parascapular artery).

The scapular flap is harvested with the patient in lateral position. The cutaneous branches of the circumflex scapular artery run horizontally about midway between the scapular spine and tip and vertically parallel to the lateral border of the scapula. These cutaneous branches can be located at the triangular intersection (triangular space) of the teres major, teres minor and the long head of the triceps brachii muscles. Dissection landmarks are the acromion, the lateral border of the scapula, and the tip. The triangular space is located and marked through palpation (**Fig 1.1-62**).

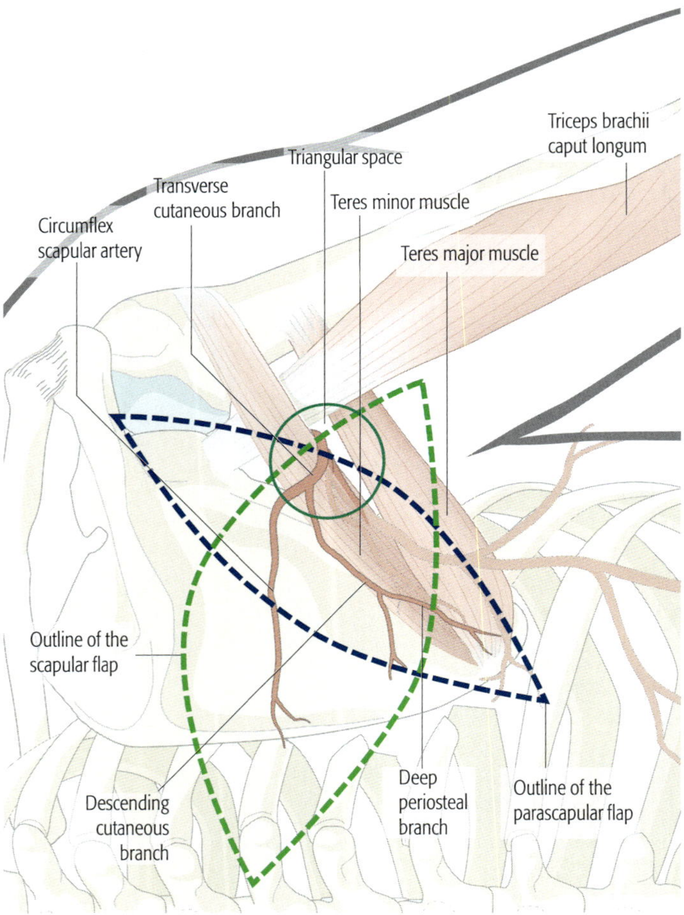

Fig 1.1-62 A scapular flap is raised with the patient positioned on his or her side. Landmarks for dissection are the scapular tip, the acromion, the lateral border of the scapula and the usually palpable triangular space.

For harvest of a combined scapular (fascio)cutaneous and a scapula bone flap, the scapular flap is raised over a vascular axis that runs parallel to the scapular spine approximately in the middle between scapular tip and scapular spine. If the bone is going to be harvested together with a parascapular flap, it is important to know that the parascapular vessel axis lies parallel to the lateral margin of the scapula, and the vessels to the skin run in a subcutaneous plane. The flap is marked on the skin and the skin incisions and subfascial dissection are completed first.

For harvest of a scapular bone flap the dissection starts laterally and continues in a medial direction toward the triangular space and the vascular axis (**Fig 1.1-63**). The inferior and/or medial aspect flaps should be elevated toward the triangular space to allow visualization of the branches before completing the superior skin incision (**Fig 1.1-64**).

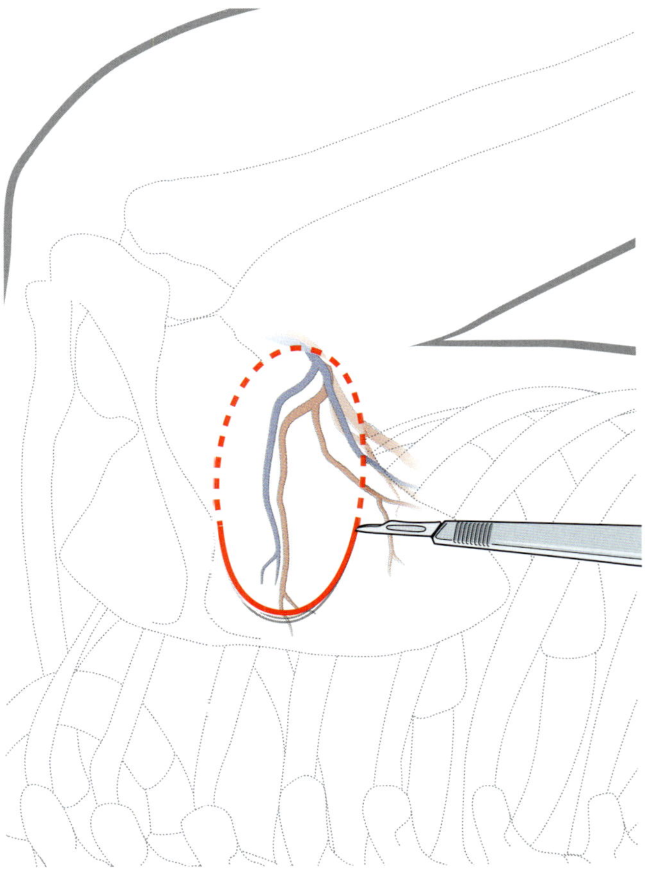

Fig 1.1-63 Starting medially, the skin is incised down to the deep fascia of the skin and a subfascial elevation from the infraspinatus muscle is performed.

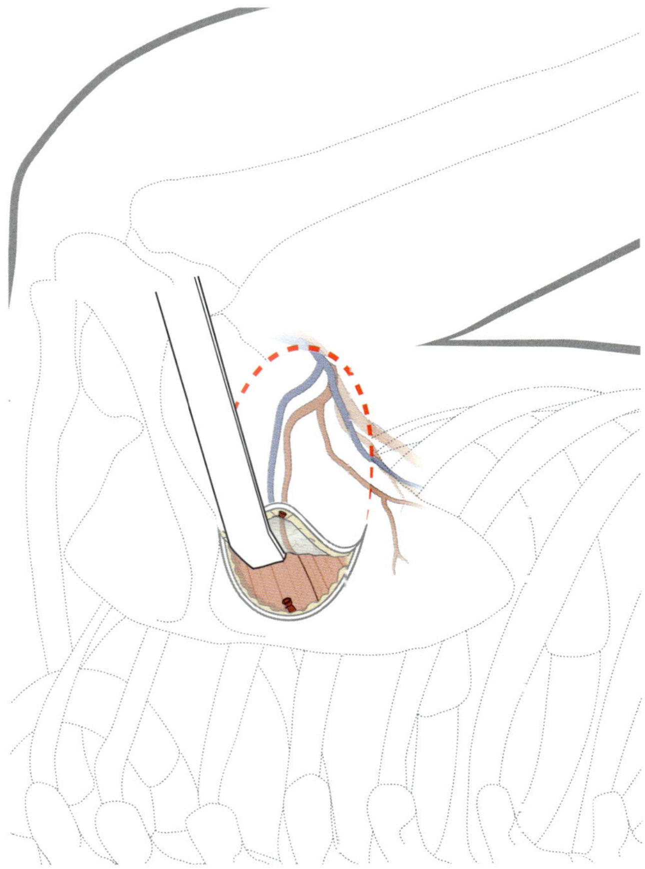

Fig 1.1-64 As the flap is raised, the pedicle on the undersurface of the cutaneous layer can be identified.

For bone flap harvest, the skin incision is extended vertically and inferiorly to provide a better overview over the operation field and to allow for dissection of the vascular pedicle of the scapular soft-tissue flap into the triangular space until its origin from the circumflex scapular artery is identified. Vessel dissection continues until the bifurcation of the subscapular artery and the circumflex scapular artery has been identified (**Fig 1.1-65**).

The skin incision is completed, and the flap is mobilized from the underlying muscles.

The blood is supplied to the lateral scapula by many small periosteal branches of the circumflex scapular artery. To preserve these branches, a small cuff of teres major and minor muscle is maintained with the scapula. The latissimus dorsi muscle is then identified and retracted allowing excellent visualization of the thoracodorsal, circumflex scapular and angular vessels. The thoracodorsal artery is then ligated (unless the latissimus muscle is also being transferred).

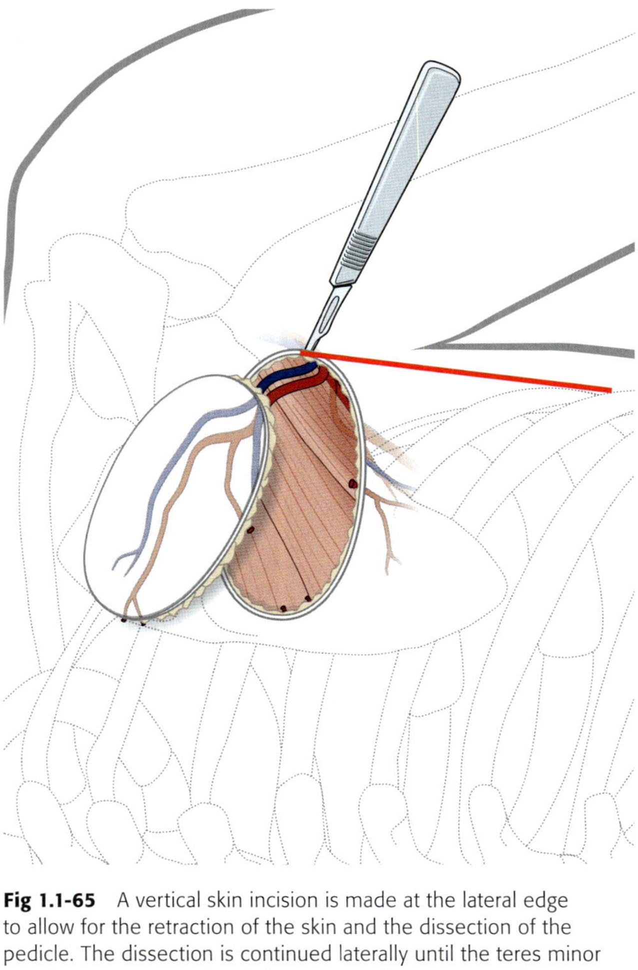

Fig 1.1-65 A vertical skin incision is made at the lateral edge to allow for the retraction of the skin and the dissection of the pedicle. The dissection is continued laterally until the teres minor muscle is encountered and the origin of the pedicle can be found in the triangular space. Meticulous dissection is performed to expose the circumflex scapular artery up to the bifurcation (maximum limit) of the subscapular artery.

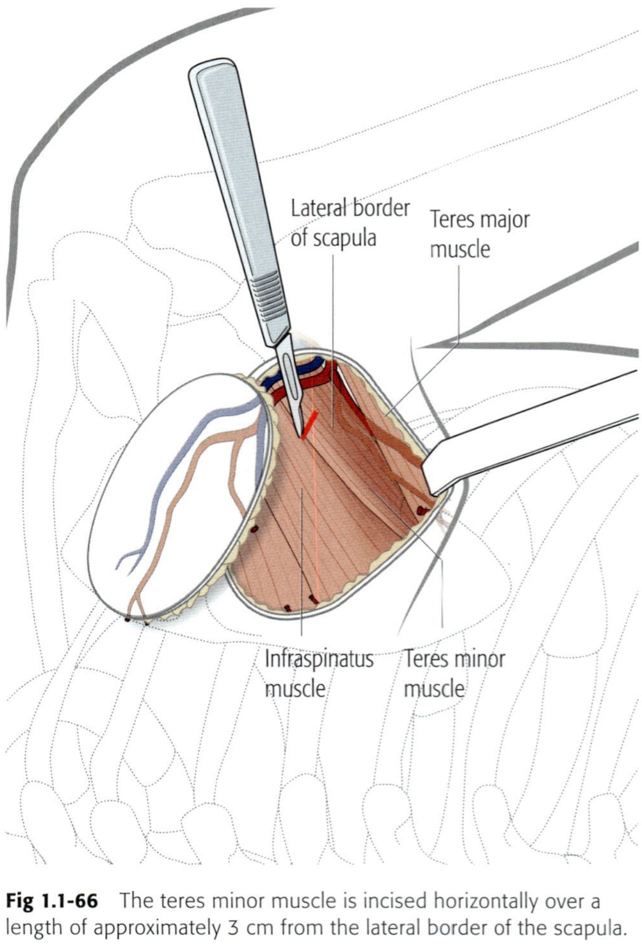

Fig 1.1-66 The teres minor muscle is incised horizontally over a length of approximately 3 cm from the lateral border of the scapula.

The teres minor muscle is incised first horizontally in a length of approximately 3 cm medially from the lateral border of the scapula (**Fig 1.1-66**). Then the teres minor and major muscles are incised and divided parallel to the lateral border of the scapula (**Fig 1.1-67**). A small cuff of the teres minor and major muscles is left attached to the scapular bone to protect the blood supply of the bone flap. The medial parts of teres major and minor muscles are retracted, and an osteotomy is performed as planned with a saw (**Fig 1.1-68**).

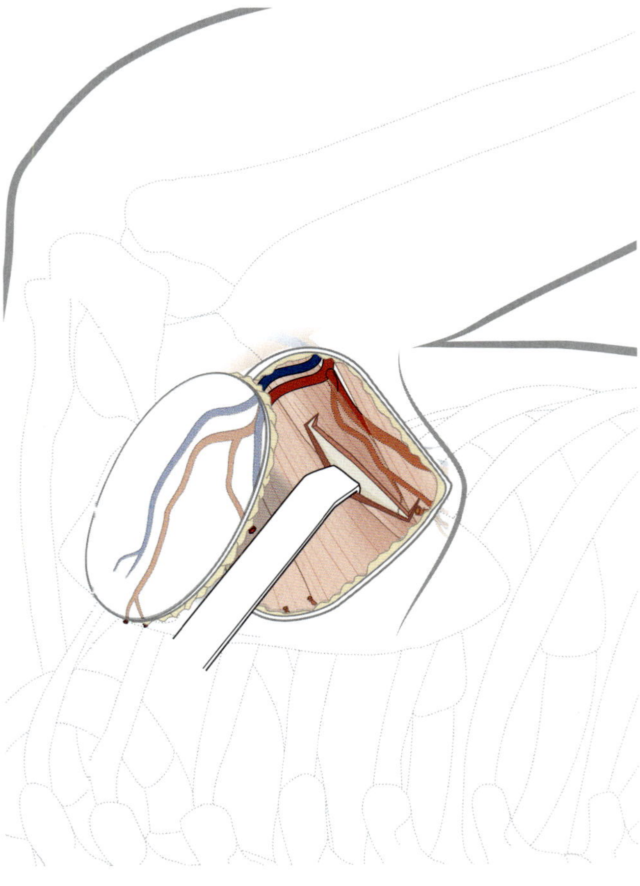

Fig 1.1-67 The teres major and teres minor muscles are then transected parallel to the lateral border of the scapula. After that the medial parts of the muscles are retracted and the bone is exposed.

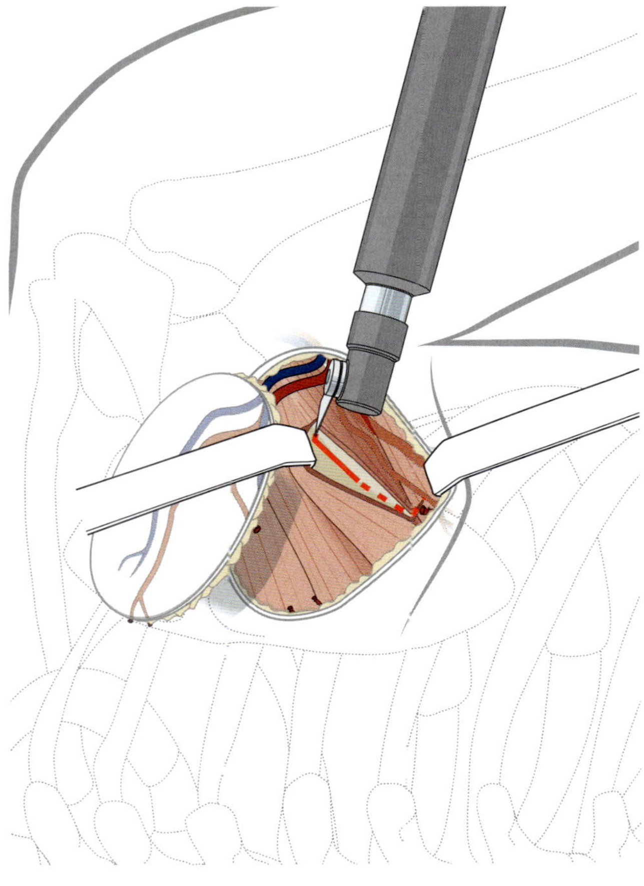

Fig 1.1-68 Osteotomies performed as planned with a saw.

The scapular osteotomies are completed after transecting the infraspinatus muscle maintaining a 2 cm cuff along the lateral edge of the scapula.

The upper osteotomy line remains just below the insertion of the long head of the triceps brachii corresponding to a point approximately 2 cm caudal to the lower edge of the glenoid fossa. The medial osteotomy is performed approximately 2 cm medial to the lateral border of the scapula. For reconstruction of the palate a wider strip of bone can be harvested. The tip of the scapula can be harvested separately if the angular vessels are preserved. Following completion of the osteotomies, the bone is rotated and a 2 cm cuff of the subscapularis muscle is maintained on the deep surface of the scapula completing the flap elevation (**Fig 1.1-69**). The flap pedicle is then dissected proximally to achieve the desired length before vessel ligation. The bone or combined bone and soft-tissue flap is now completely isolated on its vascular pedicle (**Fig 1.1-70**). The harvest is then completed, the flap set aside, and the donor site closed.

The teres major muscle should be directly sutured to the scapula through drill holes placed for that purpose. The overlying skin is then mobilized and approximated in layers over a closed suction drain. The teres major muscle is responsible for internal rotation, extension and adduction of the arm. The morbidity of the flap harvest is not insignificant. Even when repaired well, significant limitation of mobility may remain.

The patient is then repositioned, and the bone flap inserted and stabilized with monocortical screws before inset of the skin and microvascular anastomosis. It is important to work quickly to avoid prolonged ischemia of the flap.

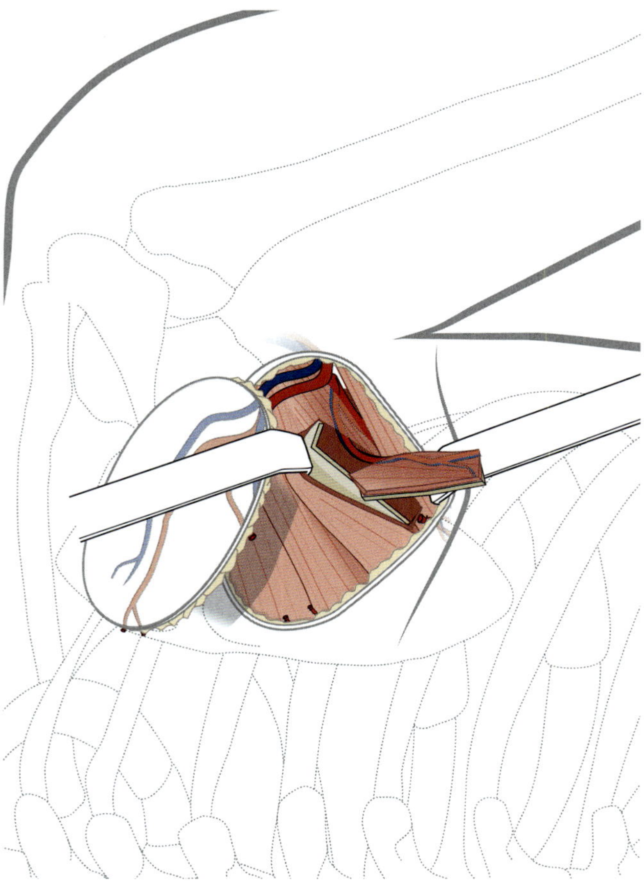

Fig 1.1-69 The bone is retracted laterally and freed from the subscapularis muscle inserting into the anterior surface of the scapula. A muscle cuff is left attached to the bone.

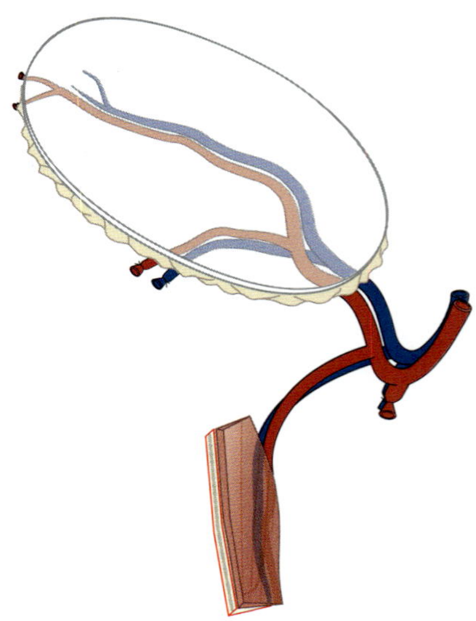

Fig 1.1-70 The flap is now completely mobilized and the pedicle is transected.

Pedicled on the thoracodorsal vessels, more flap combinations can be harvested including components of the latissimus dorsi muscle and/or a separate tip flap from the scapula. In addition, a parascapular flap can be included. If no vessel variation is present all the flaps can be raised based on the subscapular vessel system (**Fig 1.1-71**). Those complex flaps are also called chimeric flaps.

3.4 Radial forearm osteoseptocutaneous free flap

Although the radial forearm free flap is most commonly harvested as a fasciocutaneous flap, perforators to the radius allow it to be developed as an osteoseptocutaneous radial forearm free flap. The radial forearm osteoseptocutaneous free flap (RFOFF) has waxed and waned in popularity. This flap has high survival rates and is technically not difficult to harvest. The main limitations compared with other bone flaps are the thinness of the bone stock and the potential donor site morbidity. The latter issue has been overcome by prophylactically plating the radial bone donor site [Schnayder et al, 2011]. The soft-tissue attributes are superior for oral cavity defects and the main indications in using this flap are for lateral mandibular defects that require a large soft-tissue component, and anterior palatomaxillary defects [Villaret et al, 2003].

The donor arm is assessed with an Allen's test to determine the integrity of the palmar arch and ability to harvest the radial artery and venous system (**Fig 1.1-72**). In a right-handed person the left arm should be chosen for flap harvest, provided that the vessel situation allows for this.

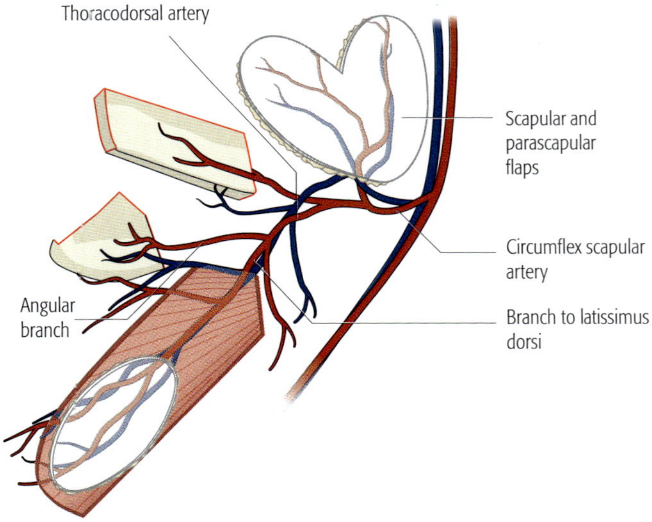

Fig 1.1-71 Chimeric flap with multiple tissue components pedicled on the subscapular vessels. It includes a (fascio)cutaneous scapular and parascapular flap, two independent scapular bone flaps and a latissimus dorsi flap.

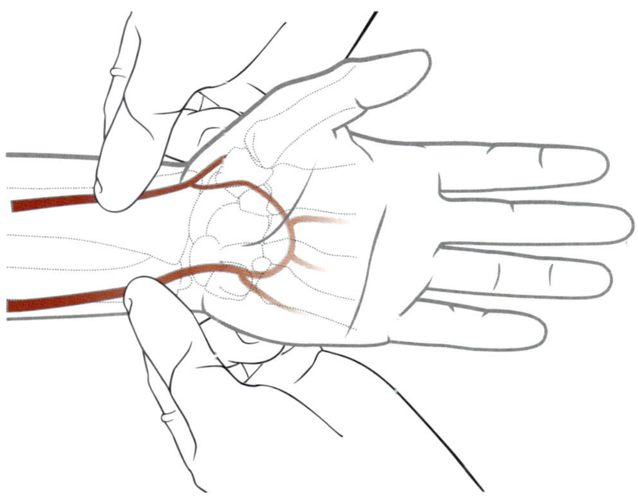

Fig 1.1-72 An Allen test is performed to ensure the integrity of the palmar circulation before the harvest of the radial forearm flap. The Allen test is a clinical test to assess perfusion of the hands. At the beginning the radial and the ulnar artery are located by palpation proximal and close to the wrist. Both arteries are digitally compressed to completely block arterial blood supply to the respective hand. With both arteries compressed, the patient is asked to clench and unclench the hand several times. After that the hand is then held open, the palm should be blanched. The ulnar artery is released, and the time taken for the palm and especially the thumb and thenar eminence to refill is recorded. If the capillary refill time is less than 6 seconds, the test is considered positive. The test is then completed with the radial artery tested in a similar fashion. If the hand does not refill through the ulnar artery alone with the radial artery blocked, a radial forearm flap should not be taken in order not to compromise perfusion of the hand. Alternatively, the radial artery can be reconstructed with a vein graft after flap harvest.

The flap is raised with the patient in a supine position and the arm abducted. The arm may be exsanguinated with a wrap and then the tourniquet is inflated to 250 mm Hg (**Fig 1.1-73**). However, some surgeons prefer flap harvest under perfusion.

The soft-tissue component is marked and the flap outline is drawn on the volar aspect of the forearm. The soft-tissue component of the flap can be harvested in a size up to 8 x 16 cm. The flap should be centered between the cephalic vein (if this vein is to be used) and the radial artery. If the cephalic vein is not reliable or if radial concomitant veins are selected, the flap will be centered over the radial artery. The palmar border of the flap should be placed over the flexor carpi radialis (**Fig 1.1-74**).

Flap harvest starts with distal part of the incision, the radial artery and the deep concomitant veins are identified, and the distal part of the skin flap is reflected. In a subfascial manner the skin paddle is then outlined and raised, including the deep fascia, to the level of the brachioradialis muscle on the radial and flexor carpi radialis tendon/muscle on the ulnar side of the lateral intermuscular septum. This septum contains the perforating vessels to the skin. On the radial side the cephalic vein and the superficial branch of the radial nerve are identified. The cephalic vein may be included into the flap for venous drainage.

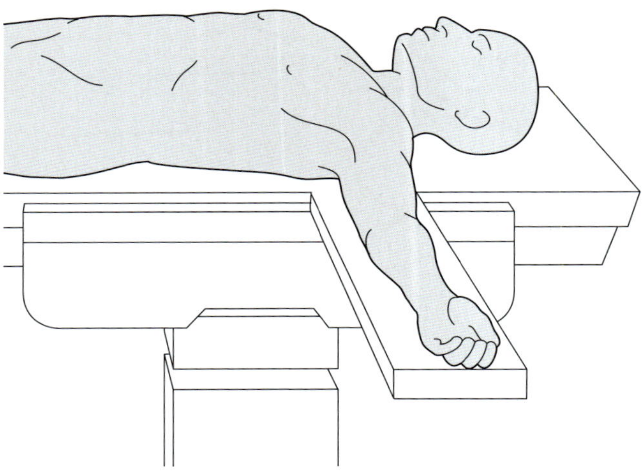

Fig 1.1-73 For flap harvest the patient's arm is abducted and positioned on a side table. A tourniquet is placed on the upper arm and inflated to a pressure of 1.5x patient's systolic pressure (usually 250 mm Hg). The tourniquet should not be applied for more than 60 minutes.

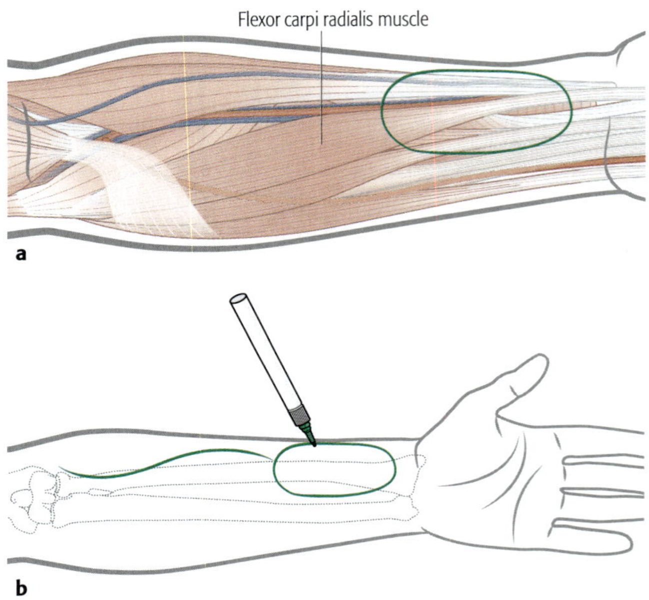

Fig 1.1-74a–b The flap outline is marked on the skin together with a proximal lazy S extension of the incision toward the antebrachial fossa.

The radial artery and the venae comitantes are ligated distally, and the pedicle and the fascia are raised approximately 1–2 cm (**Fig 1.1-75**).

On the ulnar side the flexor pollicis longus muscle and, depending on the length of the bone segment, parts of the flexor digitorum superficialis muscle are exposed and divided with, for example, a Bovie electrocautery until the necessary length of radial bone is exposed (**Fig 1.1-76 and Fig 1.1-77**).

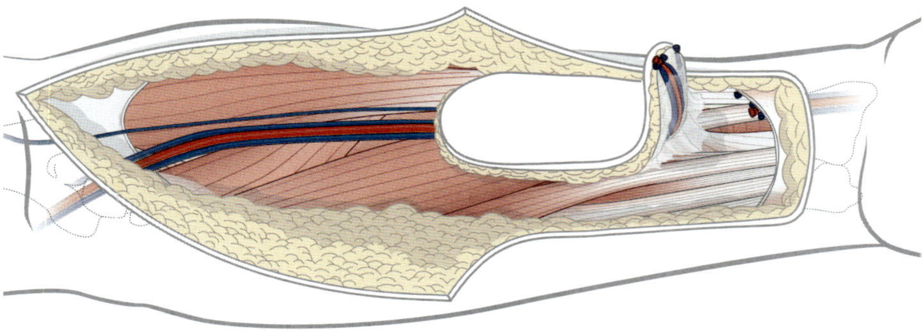

Fig 1.1-75 The proximal part of the incision is made, and the skin flap is reflected. Careful dissection medial to the cephalic vein and radial to the vascular pedicle preserves the superficial branch of the radial nerve intact. The radial artery and the venae comitantes are ligated distally and the pedicle and the fascia are raised approximately 1–2 cm.

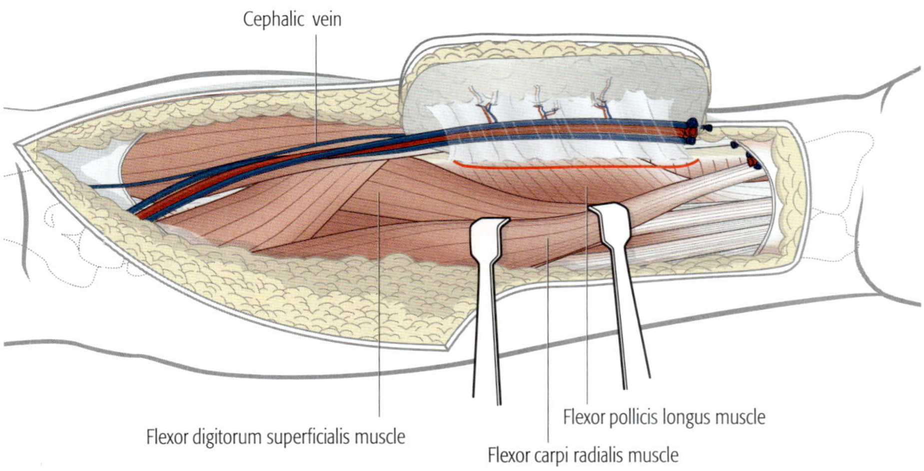

Fig 1.1-76 On the ulnar aspect the flexor carpi radialis muscle is identified and medial to it the flexor digitorum longus and the flexor pollicis longus muscle are exposed.

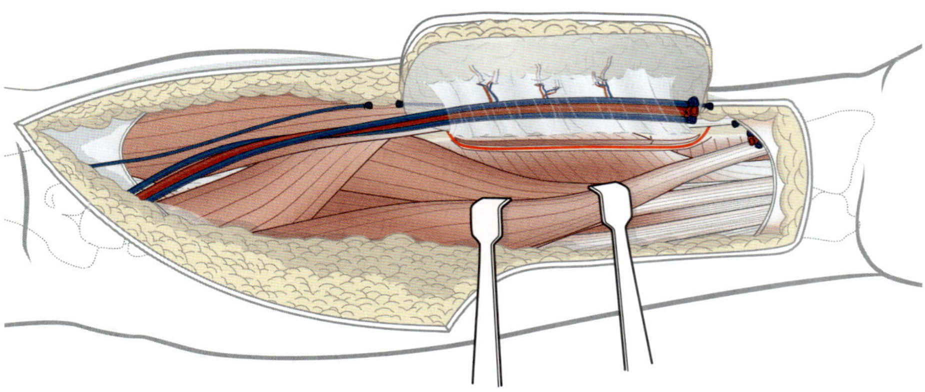

Fig 1.1-77 After determination of the desired length of the bone segment the flexor digitorum longus and the flexor pollicis longus muscle are incised leaving a muscle cuff attached to the radius. The cephalic vein is ligated, and venous drainage will now be through the deep comitant veins.

The bone available lies in between the insertion of the pronator teres and the insertion of the tendon of the brachioradialis muscle. Lateral retraction of the brachioradialis tendon exposes the radial surface of the bone and the area of the radius to be osteotomized is marked. A sagittal saw is used to remove a maximum of 40% of the cross-section of the radial bone with beveled cuts at the proximal and distal end (**Fig 1.1-78 and Fig 1.1-79**).

The deep vascular pedicle and the cephalic vein are skeletonized up to the antecubital fossa and the flap is harvested (**Fig 1.1-80**).

A 10- to 14-hole radial forearm plate 3.5 is adapted across the radial bone defect, with screws placed only through areas with two cortices (**Fig 1.1-81**).

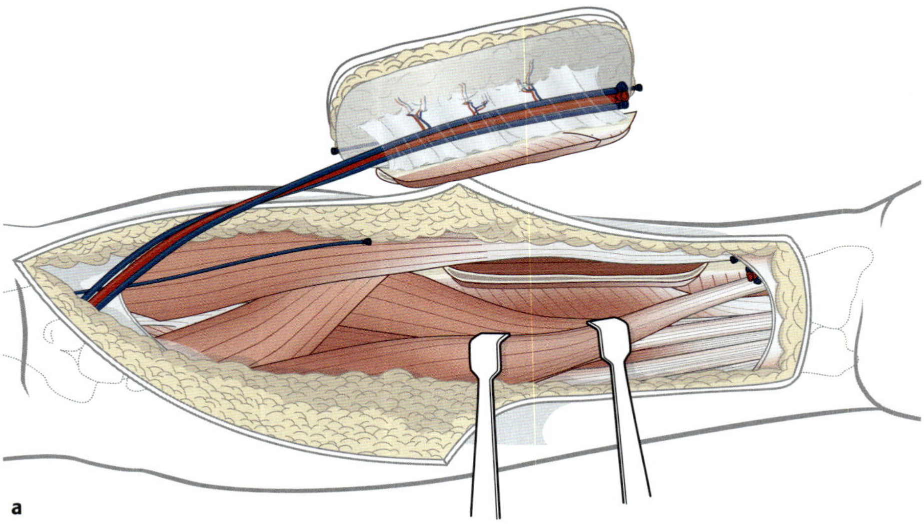

a

Fig 1.1-78 After exposure of the radius from the radial side, the osteotomy is performed with a saw. The osteotomy should be performed keel shaped to avoid sharp angles within the remaining bone, which may be predilection sites for forearm fractures.

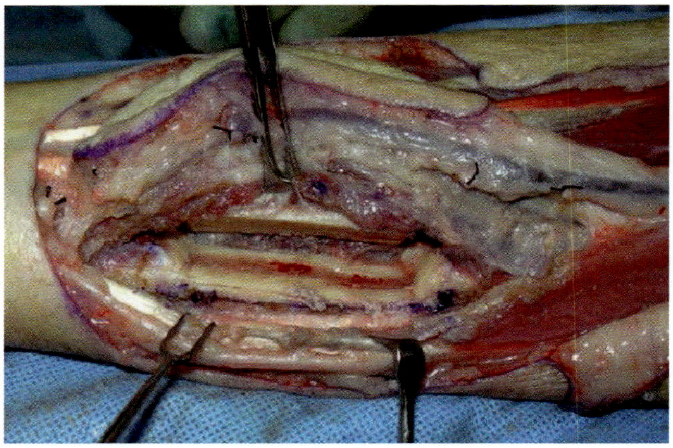

Fig 1.1-79 Lateral retraction of the brachioradialis tendon exposes the radial surface of the bone. A segment of radius has been osteotomized and is part of the flap.

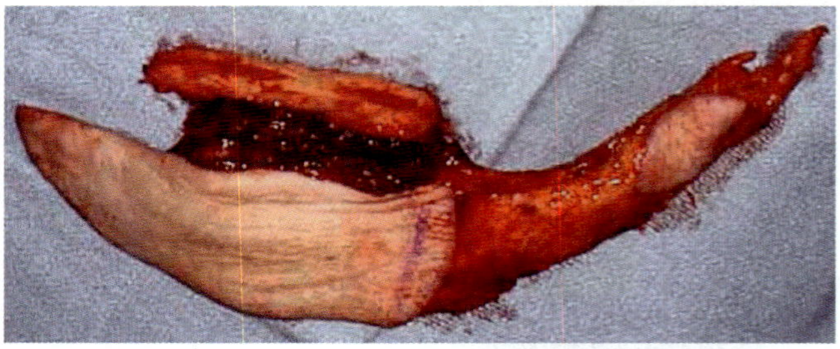

Fig 1.1-80 Harvested radial forearm osteocutaneous free flap.

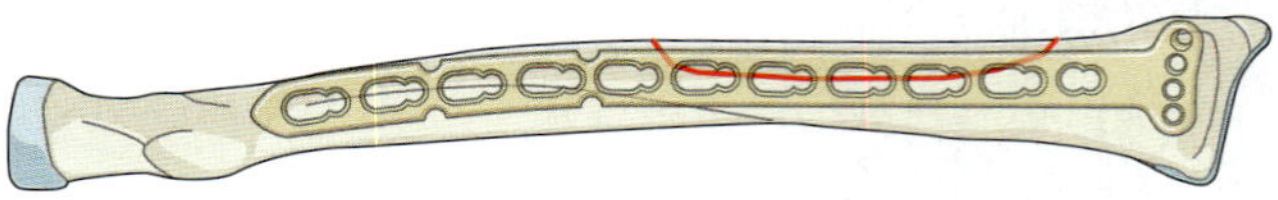

Fig 1.1-81 A radial forearm plate is adapted across the radial bone defect so that at least two to three holes are on either side of the radial bone defect.

At least two, preferably three bicortical screws are placed on either side of the bone defect. The adjacent muscles are approximated over the plate and a skin graft and splint are applied in the same manner as a soft tissue but only radial forearm free flap. The postoperative care is identical as well.

Due to the fragile blood supply to the harvested radial bone, a maximum of one osteotomy should be made when insetting it into the bone defect, with at least two screws to fix each segment to the plate (**Fig 1.1-82**).

Efforts should be made to osteotomize the edges of the bone to maximize bone-to-bone contact and allow for optimal healing. The soft tissues of the flap are draped over the plate and bone and sutured into the defect. Fortunately, pedicle length is not an issue for this flap and the anastomoses can be created to any suitable neck vessels.

If a soft-tissue radial forearm flap was harvested together with the bone, closure is typically done using a split thickness or thin full thickness skin graft (**Fig 1.1-83**).

4 Summary

The utilization of bone grafts and/or bone flaps in craniomaxillofacial reconstruction is common. The selection of the most appropriate donor site and type of bone graft/bone flap for each clinical challenge is important. The craniomaxillofacial surgeon must therefore be familiar with as many available donor sites, grafts, and flaps as possible to select the most suitable donor site and graft/flap.

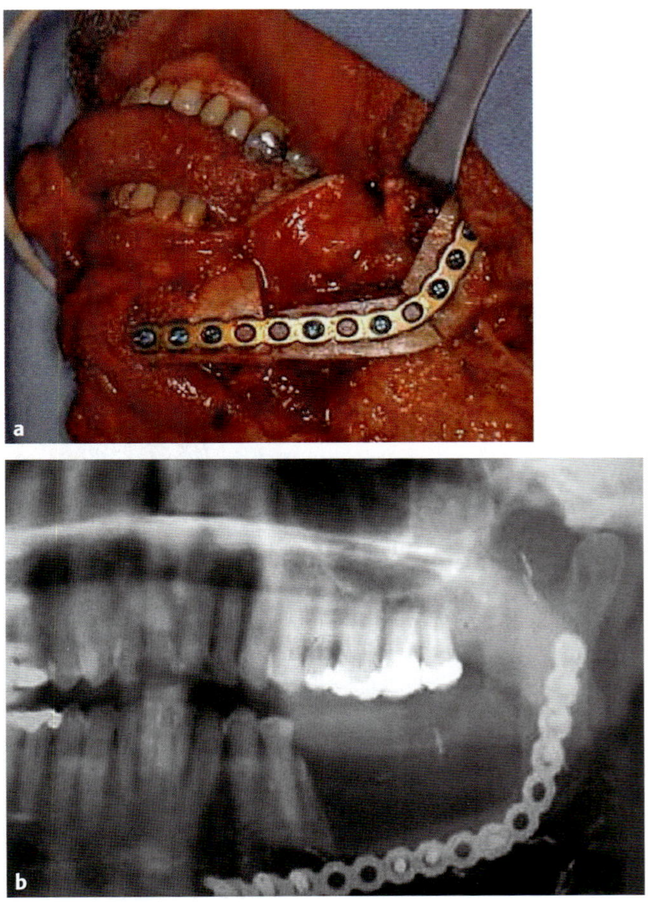

Fig 1.1-82a–b
a Radial bone with one osteotomy fixed to a reconstruction plate.
b Postoperative panoramic radiograph of the reconstructed mandible.

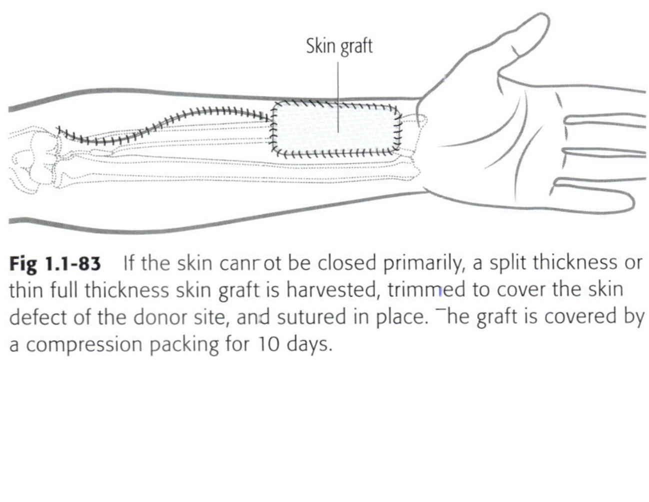

Fig 1.1-83 If the skin cannot be closed primarily, a split thickness or thin full thickness skin graft is harvested, trimmed to cover the skin defect of the donor site, and sutured in place. The graft is covered by a compression packing for 10 days.

5 References and suggested reading

Alt V, Meeder PJ, Seligson D, et al. The proximal tibia metaphysis: a reliable donor site for bone grafting? *Clin Orthop Rel Res.* 2003 Sep;(414):315–321.

Ariyan S. The viability of rib grafts transplanted with the periosteal blood supply. *Plast Reconstr Surg.* 1980 Feb;65(2):140–151.

Axhausen G. Histologische Untersuchungen über Knochentransplantationen am Menschen. *Dtsch Z Chi.* 1908;91:388–428. German.

Axhausen W. Die Quellen der Knochenneubildung nach freier Transplantation. *Langenbecks Arch Klin Chir.* 1951;279:439– 443. German.

Axhausen W. Die Knochenregeneration—ein zweiphasiges Geschehen. *Zentralbl Chir.* 1952;77(11):435–442. German.

Axhausen W. Die Bedeutung der Individual- und Artspezifitaet der Gewebe fuer die freie Knochenueberpflanzung. *Hefte Unfallheilkunde.* 1962;72.1. German.

Bardenheuer B. Ueber Unter- und Oberkieferresektion. *Verh Dtsch Ges Chir.* 1892;21:123–130. German.

Bell RB, Weimer KA, Dierks EJ, et al. Computer planning and intraoperative navigation for palatomaxillary and mandibular reconstruction with fibular free flaps. *J Oral Maxillofac Surg.* 2011;69(3):724–732.

Bell WH. *Modern Practice in Orthognathic and Reconstructive Surgery.* Philadelphia: WB Saunders; 1992.

Benninger B, Ross A, Delamarter T. Approaches to proximal tibial bone harvest techniques. *J Oral Maxillofac Res.* 2012 Jul 1;3(2):e2.

Bergeron L, Tang M, Morris SF. The anatomical basis of the deep circumflex iliac artery perforator flap with iliac crest. *Plast Reconstr Surg.* 2007 Jul;120(1):252–258.

Boyne P. Methods of osseous reconstruction of the mandible following surgical resection. *J Biomed Mat.* 1973;4:195.

Burwell RG. Osteogenesis in cancellous bone grafts: considered in terms of cellular changes, basic mechanisms and the perspective of growth control and its possible aberrations. *Clin Orthop.* 1965;40:35–47.

Chalmers J. Transplantation immunity in bone homografting. *J Bone Joint Surg.* 1959;41B:160–179.

Conley J. Use of composite flaps containing bone for major repairs in the head and neck. *Plast Reconstr Surg.* 1972 May;49(5):522–526.

Converse JM. Early and late treatment of gunshot wounds of the jaw in French battle casualties in North Africa and Italy. *J Oral Surg.* 1945;3:112–137.

Eitel F, Schweiberer K, Saur K, et al. Theoretische Grundlagen der Knochentransplantation: Osteogenese und Revaskularisation als Leistung des Wirtslagers. In: Hierholzer G, Zilch H, eds. *Transplantatlager und Implantatlager bei verschiedenen Operationsverfahren.* Berlin: Springer; 1980. German.

Esser E, Mrosk T. Langzeitergebnisse nach Unterkieferrekonstruktionen mit avaskulaerem Spongiosatransfer und Titangitter. In: Schwenzer N, ed. *Fortschritte Kiefer- Gesichts Chir.* Stuttgart: Thieme; 1994;39:90–92. German.

Essig H, Rana M, Kokemueller H, et al. Pre-operative planning for mandibular reconstruction—a full digital planning workflow resulting in a patient specific reconstruction. *Head Neck Oncol.* 2011 Oct 3;3:45.

Feenstra L, Uges DR. The bone collector: a new device. *Arch Otolaryngol.* 1978 Jan;104(1):57.

Frodel JL Jr, Marentette LJ, Quatela VC, et al. Calvarial bone graft harvest: techniques, considerations, and morbidity. *Arch Otolaryngol Head Neck Surg.* 1993 Jan;119(1):17–23.

Freudlsperger C, Bodem JP, Engel E, et al. Mandibular reconstruction with a prefabricated free vascularized fibula and implant-supported prosthesis based on fully three-dimensional virtual planning. *J Craniofac Surg.* 2014 May;25(3):980–982.

Frohberg U, Mazock JB. [A review of morbidity associated with bone harvest from the proximal tibial metaphysis.] *Mund Kiefer Gesichtschir.* 2005;9:63–65. German.

Grätz KW, Sailer HF, Haers PE, et al. Mandibular reconstruction with full thickness calvarial bone and temporal muscle flap. *Br J Oral Maxillofac Surg.* 1996 Oct;34(5):379–385.

Graziani F, Cei S, Ivanovski S, et al. A systematic review of the effectiveness of bone collectors. *Int J Oral Maxillofac Implants.* 2007 Sep–Oct;22(5):729–735.

Geideman W, Early JS, Brodsky J. Clinical results of harvesting autogenous cancellous graft from the ipsilateral proximal tibia for use in foot and ankle surgery. *Foot Ankle Int.* 2004;25:451–455.

Hall MB, Smith RG. The medial approach for obtaining iliac bone. *J Oral Surg.* 1981 Jun;39(6):462–465.

Hammer B, Prein J. Differentialindikation mikrochirurgischer Knochentransplantate fur die Rekonstruktion des Unterkiefers. In: Bootz F, Ehrenfeld M, eds. *Aktuelle Ergebnisse des mikrovaskulaeren Gewebetransfers im Kopf-Hals-Bereich.* Stuttgart: Thieme; 1995:149. German.

Heiple KG, Chase SW, Herndon CH. A comparative study of the healing process following different types of bone transplantation. *J Bone Joint Surg.* 1963 Dec;45:1593–1616.

Herford AS, King BJ, Audia F, et al. Medial approach for tibial bone graft: anatomic study and clinical technique. *J Oral Maxillofac Surg.* 2003 Mar;61(3):358–363.

Hidalgo DA, Rekow A. A review of 60 consecutive fibula free flap mandible reconstructions. *Plast Reconstr Surg.* 1995 Sep;96(3):585–596.

Hoelzle F, Riediger D, Ehrenfeld M. Mikrochirurgische Transplantate. In: Hausamen JE, Machtens E, Reuther J, et al, eds. *Mund-, Kiefer- und Gesichtschirurgie.* Heidelberg: Springer; 2012:645–707.

Hoppenreijs TJM, Nijdam ES, Freihofer HPM. The chin as a donor site in early secondary osteoplasty: a retrospective clinical and radiological evaluation. *J Craniomaxillofac Surg.* 1992;20:119–124.

Jack U. *Vergleichende Untersuchung zahnaerztlicher Implantatsysteme auf ihre Eignung zur Implantation in Rippentransplantate.* Thesis. Germany: University of Tuebingen; 1994. German.

Jackson AT, Helden G, Marx R. Skull bone grafts in maxillofacial and craniofacial surgery. *J Oral Maxillofac Surg.* 1986 Dec;44(12):949–955.

Jackson IT, Sullivan C, Shiele UU. A simple bone dust collector. *Plast Reconstr Surg.* 1988 Jun;81(6):967–969.

Kainulainen VT, Kainulainen TJ, Oikarinen KS, et al. Performance of six bone collectors designed for dental implant surgery. *Clin Oral Implants Res.* 2006 Jun;17(3):282–287.

Kim HS, Kim BC, Kim HJ, et al. Anatomical basis of the deep circumflex iliac artery flap. *J Craniofac Surg.* 2013 Mar;24(2):605–609.

Klapp R. Ueber chirurgische Behandlung der Kieferschussbrueche. *Z Arztl Fortbild.* 1916;13:225–232. German.

Krause F. Unterkiefer-Plastik. *Zentralbl Chir.* 1907;34:1045–1046. German.

Leiggener C, Messo E, Thor A, et al. A selective laser sintering guide for transferring a virtual plan to real time surgery in composite mandibular reconstruction with free fibula osseous flaps. *Int J Oral Maxillofac Surg*. 2009 Feb;3882):187–192.

Lentrodt J, Fritzemeier CU, Bethmann I. Erfahrungen bei der osteoplastischen Unterkieferrekonstruktion mit autologen freien Knochentransplantaten. In: Kastenbauer E, Wilmes E, Mees K, eds. *Das Transplantat in der Plastischen Chirurgie*. Rotenburg: Sasse; 1987:59–61. German.

Lentrodt J, Holtje WJ. Tierexperimentelle Untersuchungen zur Revaskularisation autologer Knochentransplantate. In: Schuchardt K, Scheunemann H, eds. *Fortschritte Kiefer- und Gesichts-Chir*. Stuttgart: Thieme; 1976;20:17–21. German.

Levine JP, Bae JS, Soares M, et al. Jaw in a day: total maxillofacial reconstruction using digital technology. *Plast Reconstr Surg*. 2013;131:1386–1391.

Lexer E. Die Verwendung der freien Knochenplastik nebst Versuchen ueber Gelenkversteifung und Gelenk-transplantation. *Arch Klin Chi*. 1908;86:939. German.

Lindemann A. Ueber die Beseitigung der traumatischen Defekte der Gesichtsknochen. In: Bruhn C, ed. *Die gegenwartigen Behandlungswege der Kieferschussverletzungen*. Hefte IV-VI. Wiesbaden: Bergmann; 1916. German.

Matti H. Ueber freie Transplantation von Knochenspongiosa. *Langenbecks Arch Clin Chir*. 1932;168:236. German.

Maves MD, Matt BH. Calvarial bone grafting of facial defects. *Otolaryngol Head Neck Surg*. 1986 Nov;95(4):464–470.

Michel C, Reuther J, Meier J, et al. Die Differentialindikation mikrochirurgischer und freier autogener Knochentransplantate zur Rekonstruktion des Unterkiefers. In: Schwenzer N, ed. *Fortschritte Kiefer- Gesichts Chir*. Stuttgart: Thieme; 1994;39:96–100. German.

Modabber A, Ayoub N, Mohlhenrich SC, et al. The accuracy of computer-assisted primary mandibular reconstruction with vascularized bone flaps: iliac crest bone flap versus osteomyocutaneous fibula flap. *Medical Devices*. 2014;7:211–217.

O'Brien BMcC. *Microvascular Reconstructive Surgery*. Edinburgh: Churchill Livingstone; 1977.

O'Keeffe RM Jr, Riemer BL, Butterfield SL. Harvesting of autogenous cancellous bone graft from the proximal tibial metaphysis. A review of 230 cases. *J Orthop Trauma*. 1991;5(4):469–474.

Payr E. Ueber osteoplastischen Ersatz nach Kieferresektion (Kieferdefekten) durch Rippenstuecke mittels gestielter Brustwand-lappen oder freier Transplantation. *Zentralbl Chir*. 1908;35:1065–1070. German.

Quillen CG. Latissimus dorsi myocutaneous flaps in head and neck reconstruction. *Plast Reconstr Surg*. 1979 May;63(5):664–670.

Ray RD, Sabet TY. Bone grafts: cellular survival versus induction. *J Bone Joint Surg*. 1963;45A:337.

Rehrmann A. Das freie Knochentransplantat zum Unterkieferersatz unter besonderer Beruecksichtigung der Kinnrekonstruktion. In: Schuchardt K, Schilli W, eds. *Fortschritte Kiefer- Gesichts Chir*. Stuttgart: Thieme; 1978:23:39.

Reuther JF. *Druckplattenosteosynthese und freie Knochentransplantation zur Unterkieferrekonstruktion*. Berlin: Quintessenz; 1979. German.

Riediger D, Ehrenfeld M. Der vaskularisierte Knochenspan, experimentelle Grundlagen und klinische Anwendung. In: Kastenbauer E, Wilmes E, Mees K, eds. *Das Transplantat in der Plastischen Chirurgie*. Rotenburg: Sasse; 1987:4–9.

Riediger D, Schmelzle R. Modifizierte Anwendung des myokutanen Latissimus dorsi-Lappens zur Defektdeckung im Mund-Kiefer-Gesichtsbereich. *Dtsch Z Mund Kiefer Gesichts Chir*. 1986;10:364–374. German.

Roser SM, Ramachandra S, Blair H, et al. The accuracy of virtual surgical planning in free fibula mandibular reconstruction: comparison of planned and final results. *J Oral Maxillofac Surg*. 2010;68:2824–2832.

Rozen WM, Ting JW, Baillieu C, et al. Stereolithographic modeling of the deep circumflex iliac artery and its vascular branching: a further advance in computed tomography-guided flap planning. *Plast Reconstr Surg*. 2012 Aug;130(2):380e–382e.

Rydygier LRV. Zum osteoplastischen Ersatz nach Unterkieferresektion. *Zentralbl Chir*. 1908;35:1321–1322. German.

Sailer HF, Pajarola GF. Plastische Korrekturen an Weichteilen und Knochen. In: *Orale Chirurgie*. Stuttgart: Thieme; 1996:308–309. German.

Schliephake H. Entnahmetechniken autologer Knochentransplantate. *Implantologie*. 1994;4:317–327. German.

Schweiberer L, Brenneisen R, Dambe LT, et al. Derzeitiger Stand der auto-, hetero- und homoplastischen Knochentransplantation. In: Cotta H, Martini AK, eds. *Implantate und Transplantate in der Plastischen und Weider her stel- lungschirurgie*. Berlin: Springer; 1981:115–127. German.

Schweiberer L. Experimentelle Untersuchungen von Knochentransplantaten mit unveraenderter und denaturierter Knochengrundsubstanz. Hefte Unfallheilk 103. Berlin: Springer; 1970. German.

Shnayder Y, Tsue T, Toby EB, et al. Safe osteocutaneous radial forearm flap harvest with prophylactic internal fixation. *Craniomaxillofac Trauma Reconstr*. 2011 Sep;4(3):129–136.

Soutar DS. The radial forearm flap in intraoral reconstruction. In: Riediger D, Ehrenfeld M, eds. *Microsurgical Tissue Transplantation*. Chicago: Quintessence; 1989:31–38.

Steinhäuser EW. Unterkieferrekonstruktion durch intraorale Knochentransplantate–deren Einheilung und Beeinflussung durch Funktion—eine tierexperimentelle Studie. *Schweiz Monatsschr Zahnheilk*. 1968;78:213. German.

Strauch B, Yu HL. *Atlas of Microvascular Surgery*. New York: Thieme; 1993.

Sullivan MJ, Baker SR, Crompton R, et al. Free scapular osteocutaneous flap for mandibular reconstruction. *Arch Otolaryngol Head Neck Surg*. 1989 Nov;115(11):1334–1340.

Swartz WM, Banis JC, Newton ED, et al. The osteocutaneous scapular flap for mandibular and maxillary reconstruction. *Plast Reconstr Surg*. 1986 Apr;77:530– 545.

Sykoff V. Zur Frage der Knochenplastik am Unterkiefer. *Zentralbl Chir*. 1900;27:81. German.

Taylor GI, Miller GD, Ham FJ. The free vascularized bone graft. A clinical extension of microvascular techniques. *Plast Reconstr Surg*. 1975;55:553–554.

Taylor GI, Townsend P, Corlett R. Superiority of the deep circumflex iliac vessels as the supply for free groin flaps. *Plast Reconstr Surg*. 1979 Dec;64(6):745–759.

Tessier P. Autogenous bone grafts from the calvarium for facial and cranial application. *Clin Plast Surg*. 1982 Oct;9(4):531–538.

Tessier P, Kawamoto H, Matthews D, et al. Autogenous bone grafts and bone substitutes—tools and techniques: I. A 20,000-case experience in maxillofacial and craniofacial surgery. *Plast Reconstr Surg*. 2005 Oct;116(5 Suppl):6S–24S; discussion 92S–94S.

Tessier P, Kawamoto H, Matthews D et al. Taking long rib rafts for facial reconstruction—tools and techniques: III. A 2900-case experience in maxillofacial and craniofacial surgery. *Plast Reconstr Surg*. 2005 Oct;116(5 Suppl):38S–46S; discussion 92S–94S.

Tessier P, Kawamoto H, Posnick J, et al. Taking calvarial grafts, either split in situ or splitting of the parietal bone flap ex vivo—tools and techniques: V. A 9650-case experience in craniofacial and maxillofacial surgery. *Plast Reconstr Surg.* 2005 Oct;116(5 Suppl) :54S–71S; discussion 92S–94S.

Ting JW, Rozen WM, Grinsell D, et al. The in vivo anatomy of the deep circumflex iliac artery perforators: defining the role for the DCIA perforator flap. *Microsurgery.* 2009;29:326–329.

Urken ML, Weinberg H, Vickery C, et al. The internal oblique-iliac crest free flap in composite defects of the oral cavity involving bone, skin, and mucosa. *Laryngoscope.* 1991 Mar;101(3):257–270.

Villaret DB, Futran NA. The indications and outcomes in the use of the osteocutaneous radial forearm free flap. *Head Neck.* 2003 Jun; 25(6):475–481.

Wilde F, Cornelius CP, Schramm A. Computer-assisted mandibular reconstruction using a patient-specific reconstruction plate fabricated with computer-aided design and manufacturing techniques. *Craniomaxillofac Trauma Reconstr.* 2014 Jun;7(2):158–166.

Williams R. Comparison of living autogeneous and homogeneous grafts of cancellous bone heterotopically placed in rabbits. *Anat Rec.* 1962;143:93–105.

Zaffe D, D'Avenia F. A novel bone scraper for intraoral harvesting: a device for filling small bone defects. *Clin Oral Implants Res.* 2007 Aug;18(4):525–533.

Michael Ehrenfeld, Christine Hagenmaier, Remy H Blanchaert Jr

1.2 Bone lengthening by distraction

Leonard B Kaban, Maria E Papadaki, Maria J Troulis

1 Introduction

Distraction osteogenesis (DO) is a method of bone lengthening in which the body is induced to create new bone, thereby avoiding the need for a bone graft. An osteotomy or a corticotomy is made and a device is rigidly fixed to the bone across the cut. A callus is allowed to develop and then the device is activated to gradually produce tension in the overlying soft tissue and to separate the bone segments. New bone is generated in response to the tension that is applied across the bone gap. Distraction osteogenesis has been described as "in vivo tissue engineering". Some surgeons use the term "distraction histogenesis" alluding to the fact that not only bone but also soft tissues are generated, whereas others refer to it as "callus distraction" pointing out that callus is a tissue that is primarily manipulated.

In 1905, Codivilla was the first to describe limb lengthening by DO. Illizarov [1988, 1989] reintroduced and popularized the technique in the 1950s by reporting its use in large numbers of patients and by publishing the results of his experimental studies in large animals. Ilizarov is considered to be the father of DO. Snyder et al [1973] were the first to use DO to expand the mandible in a canine model. Subsequently, McCarthy et al [1992] used DO for mandibular lengthening in four syndromic patients and Perrott et al [1993] reported mandibular widening by DO.

Distraction osteogenesis is now a commonly used technique for skeletal expansion of the lower jaw including symmetric and asymmetric mandibular lengthening in the vertical, sagittal and transverse planes, and correction of mandibular continuity defects (transport DO). Expansion of the midface by DO has also been frequently reported at the Le Fort I and III levels. Distraction osteogenesis has become one of the standard treatment methods to correct syndromic and nonsyndromic congenital deformities (eg, craniofacial [hemifacial] microsomia, Treacher Collins syndrome, Nager syndrome, midface hypoplasia secondary to cleft lip/palate, and syndromic craniosynostosis) and acquired midface and mandibular deficiencies that require advancement of more than 10 mm.

2 Distraction protocol

Long-bone and craniomaxillofacial distraction protocols currently in use are based on the pioneering clinical and experimental work of Ilizarov. The latency period is defined as the time from the corticotomy or osteotomy to the start of activation of the distraction device. A latency period of 7–21 days has been reported in long-bone DO, and 4–10 days has been the standard for craniomaxillofacial DO. The rationale for a latency period is to permit soft-callus formation and upregulation of angiogenesis and bone metabolism to facilitate osteogenesis. However, the anatomy of the craniomaxillofacial region, especially its rich blood supply, is significantly different from that of long bones. Hypothetically, that would permit a distraction protocol with zero latency in order to shorten the duration of treatment. Experiments in our laboratory demonstrated that mandibular and maxillary DO could be successfully accomplished with no latency period in 6-month-old minipigs.

Distraction period is defined as the duration of active skeletal lengthening, ie, traction forces being applied by the device. Rate refers to the total lengthening in millimeters per day and the number of times per day (rhythm) the distractor is activated. The typical rate in both long bones and the maxillofacial skeleton is 1 mm/day divided into two activations (rhythm = 2). Based on Ilizarov's reports [1988, 1989] that a 1 mm/day rate produces superior bone formation compared with 2 mm/day and 4 mm/day, this rate has become the standard for distraction in the craniomaxillofacial and axial skeletons.

Rhythm may vary from one to four activations per day or the distraction device may be activated continuously. The latter requires a device that activates independently without the patient performing the task. The hypothesis that continuous DO may decrease the treatment period is accepted by many investigators. Magill et al [2009], Goldwaser et al [2012] and Peacock et al [2013] have reported on the successful use of a new automated continuous distraction device in minipigs. Continuous bone distraction is not yet available for clinical application.

Finally, the fixation or consolidation period as part of a distraction protocol extends from the end of active distraction to the removal of the device when adequate bone fills the gap. This is usually twice the number of millimeters of distraction in days. Empirically, fixation is usually maintained for approximately 6–12 weeks.

3 Biology of distraction osteogenesis

There is considerable active research to improve our understanding of the biology and mechanism of bone formation as a result of distraction. Numerous authors hypothesize that osteogenesis occurs via intramembranous bone formation. However, others counter that the mechanism is endochondral, or perhaps a combination of endochondral and intramembranous formation. Finally, it may be that neither intramembranous nor endochondral bone formation occurs but rather a distinct and unique process. Li et al [1999] have used histology, immunohistochemistry, and nonradioactive in situ mRNA (in a rabbit model) to document the presence of an overlapping cartilage-bone phenotype in cells of the transitional areas in the DO gap. In this study [Li et al, 1999] chondrocytes appeared to be directly transformed into cells that form bone matrix. The cellular events that regulate tissue generation during DO are still not clear. An understanding of the biology of the facial DO wound might allow surgeons to manipulate it to increase the quality and quantity of bone formation while decreasing the treatment period.

To date, the molecular mechanisms that govern bone formation during DO are poorly understood. In recent studies, growth factor expression in small animal models of DO has been documented. It was reported that transforming growth factor beta (TGF-β) mRNA was elevated during latency, distraction and fixation periods in the rat mandible and bone morphogenic protein-4 (BMP-4) mRNA was slightly elevated during latency but increased further with DO in the rat femur. Yates et al [2002] using a porcine model found that TGF-β and BMP-4 were at the highest levels during the earliest periods (ie, latency and active distraction) and continued to decrease throughout the treatment period, reaching the lowest concentrations during fixation. BMP-4 was also found at highest levels at the middle and the end of the active distraction period in a minipig model by mid-DO and end-DO [Hansen et al, 2012].

Biomechanical properties and stability of the distraction wound are related to the quality and quantity of bone formed. They are affected by intrinsic biomechanical parameters (eg, geometric shape, cross-sectional area, density of the distracted bone segments, the length of the distraction regenerate, and the tension developing within the soft-tissue envelope), extrinsic biomechanical factors (eg, number, length and diameter of pins or screws, the rigidity and material properties of the distraction device), and the device orientation and vector.

Additionally, biological factors determine the biomechanical properties of the regenerate bone. They include the technique used for the osteotomy, the latency period, the rate and rhythm of distraction, and the duration of the fixation period. Kaban et al [2003] studied the biomechanical stiffness of an experimental mandibular distraction wound and correlated it with radiographic and ultrasound data. Twenty-four Yucatan minipigs underwent unilateral mandibular distraction. The protocol used was 0-day latency, rates of 1, 2, and 4 mm/day (12 mm distraction gap) and 24-day fixation period. Radiographic and ultrasound bone fill scores were obtained at 0, 8, 16, and 24 days of the neutral fixation. At the time of sacrifice, biomechanical stiffness was estimated using an Instron machine to produce a downward force of 2 mm/min at the premolar occlusal surface. Force (kilo-Newton) and displacement (millimeter) were recorded at a rate of 10,000 points/second. The results of this study [Kaban et al, 2003] indicated that stiffness of the DO wound increased with duration of neutral fixation regardless of the rate of distraction. The stiffness values of the wounds at all time points were greater in the group of animals distracted at 1 mm/day versus those distracted at 2 and 4 mm/day. In addition, greater bone fill by plain radiographs and ultrasonography was correlated with increased biomechanical strength. However, at the end of 24 days neutral fixation, even in the most clinically stable group, stiffness across the distraction wound was only 25.5% of control. This raises questions regarding the management of patients at the time of removal of distraction devices.

The relationship between histomorphometric bone fill and clinical stability of a mandibular distraction wound in an animal model (20 minipigs) was investigated by Glowacki et al [2004]. Variables in the distraction protocol included 0-day or 4-day latency, 1 mm, 2 mm, or 4 mm daily distraction rates; gap size of 7 mm or 12 mm and evaluation after neutral fixation for various lengths of time. Histological examination showed equivalent bone fill with or without 4 days latency. It also showed that osteogenesis was nearly complete with 1 mm/day when assessed at the end of a standard neutral fixation period (twice the duration of distraction at 1 mm/day). However, mandibles that had been distracted for 3 days at 4 mm/day showed moderate osteogenesis and clinical stability with increasing time of neutral fixation.

Zimmermann et al [2004] documented the progression of bone formation with mandibular distraction in the same animal model, at various distraction rates and fixation times, using 3-D computed tomography (CT) and plain x-ray. In this study they demonstrated that the mean percentage of bone volume in the distraction wound that was calculated on the CT scans increased with fixation time from 16.7% at 0 days, to 64% at 24 days of fixation. The radiographic bone fill scores were 0.17 at 0 days and 2.0 at 24 days of fixation (0 = no bone fill; 1 = bone fill > 0 < 50%; 2 = bone fill > 50 < 100%; 3 = complete bone fill). They also demonstrated that bone fill scores were higher with a distraction rate of 1 mm/day compared with rates 2 and 4 mm/day. The maximum bone volume in the gap at the end of the fixation period (24 days) was found to be only 64% (1 mm/day) and remained below control values (81.3%). However, clinical stability and radiographic bone fill scores were high. In all these studies, the best biomechanical properties for the newly formed bone were achieved with a distraction rate of 1 mm/day. Latency period had no effect on the quantity of bone formation or stiffness of the new bone. Stiffness of the regenerate increased with duration of fixation.

Skeletal advancement by DO is potentially more stable than traditional techniques because concurrent soft-tissue expansion may improve long-term skeletal stability. Castano et al [2001] documented that increased muscle length in a minipig distraction model was due to increase in masseter muscle size by myocyte proliferation (hypertrophy). The animal model for the study comprised 16 Yucatan minipigs who underwent an osteotomy at the junction of the body and ramus unilaterally and fixation of the device perpendicular to the osteotomy. Distraction was carried out according to the following protocols: group 1 (12 animals): 0 or 4 latency and 1, 2, or 4 mm/day (n = 2 animals in each group) for an elongation of 12 mm and 24 days fixation and group 2 (4 animals): 0- or 4-day latency and 1 mm distraction per day (n = 2 animals in each group) for 7 days and 14 days of fixation. At the end of the fixation period, tissues were harvested from masseter muscle overlying the osteotomy and the nonoperated side. Proliferation of myocytes was estimated using immunohistochemical localization with antibodies against proliferating cell nuclear antigen (PCNA). Numerous PCNA-positive myocytes were observed in the muscle samples on the distracted side (16.8% of myocyte nuclei were PCNA positive, with higher results in the group with 12 mm elongation) compared to the contralateral control side (2.3%). Similarly, Lawler et al [2012] examined the anterior digastric muscle with hematoxylin and eosin staining and immunohistochemical staining for PCNA (total cell proliferation), paired Box-7 gene protein (Pax7; satellite cells) and myogenic differentiation 1 protein (MyoD; differentiating myoblasts) in 19 Yucatan minipigs that underwent unilateral mandibular DO. Proliferating cells, satellite cells, and differentiating myoblasts were significantly increased at the middle and the end of the active distraction period indicating that digastric muscle response to DO consist of proliferation and hypertrophy. Hypertrophy of the soft-tissue envelope has clinical significance in long-term stability for patients undergoing distraction procedures.

Biology of DO in the maxilla at the Le Fort I level was studied by Papadaki et al [2012]. The anatomy of the midface is significantly different from both the mandible and the long bones in that it lacks a distinct marrow cavity and source of precursor cells for bone formation. The maxilla represents a nonmobile bone with only small muscle attachments and transmits occlusal forces in a unique pattern through the buttresses. Nine Yucatan minipigs in the mixed dentition stage underwent modified Le Fort I osteotomy through a vestibular incision under general anesthesia. An intraoral distraction device was fixed across the osteotomy bilaterally. The distraction protocol was 0-day latency, 1 mm/day rate for 12 days, and 24 days of fixation. Maxillary specimens (n = 9) were harvested and divided in half at end-DO (n = 6 sides), mid-fixation (n = 6), and end-fixation (n = 6). The zone of advancement was examined with hematoxylin and eosin staining, collagen II, CD 34, PCNA, and tartrate-resistant acid phosphatase staining at the above-mentioned time points. The percentage surface area (PSA) of the advancement zone occupied by fibrous tissue, vessels, proliferating cells, osteoid, and bone was determined under microscope. At end-DO, in the advancement zone, PSA of proliferating cells was 33.16%; fibrous tissue, 52%; vessels, 4.35%; and new bone 5.45%. At end-fixation, PSA of proliferating cells decreased to 10.53%, fibrous tissue to 2.3%, vessels to 1.5%, and PSA of new bone increased to 44.9%. No cartilage was found in the advancement zone in the maxilla at any time point.

A similar study in the minipig mandible by Lawler et al [2012] using the same distraction protocol and the same methodology, as the above study, showed fibrous tissue decrease from the middle of the active DO period (53.12 ± 8.59 PSA) to end-fixation (25.00 ± 0.83 PSA). Cartilage was present in end-DO (1.72 ± 2.71 PSA) and mid-fixation (5.82 ± 6.64 PSA) in the mandible. In the mandible, bone increased from the middle of the active DO period (25.18 ± 0.99 PSA) to end-fixation (64.89 ± 0.79 PSA).

Understanding the biology of the craniomaxillofacial DO wound is not only of scientific and academic interest but is also a prerequisite for the improvement of the technique and its clinical outcomes. Once the cellular and tissue processes are understood, it may be possible to refine the method and develop shorter distraction protocols.

3.1 Clinical application

Craniomaxillofacial skeletal deformities may require correction by skeletal expansion. In the past, this was achieved by osteotomies, acute bone repositioning, and autogenous bone transplantation. Complications, such as infection, skeletal relapse, bone graft loss or nonunion, asymmetry, and less than satisfactory esthetic and functional results were reported in some of these cases. In contrast, DO offers unique clinical benefits that include the possibility of significant bone advancement, simultaneous soft-tissue histogenesis and decreased risk of damaging structures like nerves, temporomandibular joint, and tooth buds. Furthermore, DO is less invasive, requires shorter operating time, and eliminates donor site morbidity.

Distraction osteogenesis is classified into monofocal, bifocal, and trifocal distraction. Monofocal distraction is defined as a distraction wound with one site of new bone formation. This is the model for lengthening of hypoplastic bone, eg, mandible. One area of bone formation and one area of bone fusion exist in bifocal DO. In bifocal DO, an osseous segment, "the transport disc" is cut from one end of a mandibular defect and is moved to fuse with the other side of the bone. Trifocal DO is also used for bone reconstruction and consists of two transport discs, one on each side of the defect. The two discs are transported toward each other to fuse together.

Monofocal DO is also subdivided into unidirectional, bidirectional, and multidirectional by the dimensions or directions in which bone lengthening is required (vertically, horizontally, or sagittally). Multidirectional distraction is required for most corrections. Curvilinear distraction is a 3-D reconstruction and may be accomplished by: (1) external complex devices, (2) reorientation of the distal bony segment and reattachment of the device, or (3) a novel, curvilinear semiburied, fixed-trajectory device. With this device all 3-D movements can be resolved into a simple movement about a unique axis. Seldin et al [1999] evaluated such a distractor in two minipigs. They combined translation and rotational movement and achieved 12 mm elongation and 11° angulation of the distal segment.

Kaban et al [2009] reported early results in a series of 13 patients who underwent bilateral curvilinear distraction for mandibular advancement, ramus lengthening, and counterclockwise rotation. The subjects' diagnoses were posttraumatic micrognathia (n = 1), Treacher Collins syndrome (n = 3), Nager syndrome (n = 3), craniofacial microsomia (n = 2), syndromic micrognathia (n = 3), and nonsyndromic micrognathia (n = 1). The mandible was successfully expanded in multiple dimensions with the partially buried curvilinear device. In three patients the regenerate had to be "molded" and the jaw fixed in the desired position. In the other 10 patients correct jaw position was achieved at the end of the distraction.

3.2 Devices

Currently, two classes of distraction devices are available. External distractors are attached to the bone through percutaneous pins. These devices can achieve unidirectional, bidirectional, and multidirectional distraction. Disadvantages include the complexity of the devices with their multiple joints, pin-track scars, and the discomfort to the patient (**Fig 1.2-1**).

Semi-buried devices place the distraction mechanism beneath the skin or mucosa. They generally incorporate an activating arm that protrudes through the skin (percutaneous) or the mucosa (transmucosal) so that the surgeon or the patient can activate the buried distraction mechanism (**Fig 1.2-2**).

A 3-D distraction can be accomplished by curvilinear, semi-buried devices (**Fig 1.2-3**).

In the future, totally buried, remotely activated devices capable of 3-D movements will probably be used in most cases.

4 Preoperative planning

Accurate preoperative planning is vital for the successful outcome of a distraction procedure to correct a skeletal deformity. When planning is inadequate, it is possible to create a secondary deformity worse than the original defect. Precise determination of the location and orientation of the osteotomy, position of the device in relation to the osteotomy,

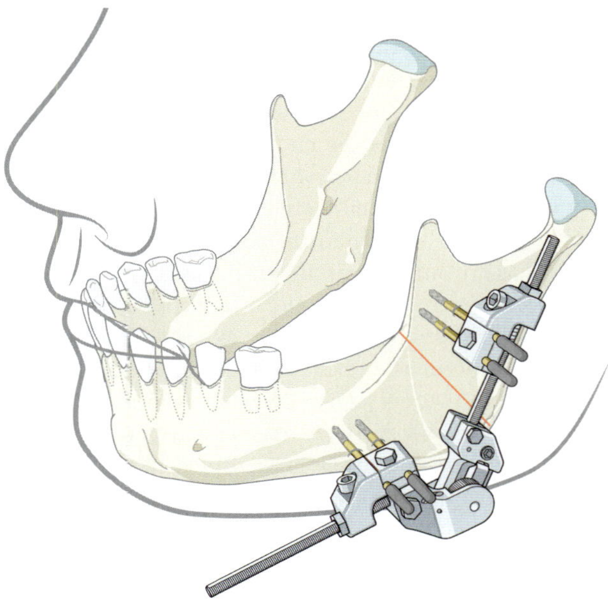

Fig 1.2-1 A multidirectional external mandible distractor. This device is attached to the bone using percutaneous pins.

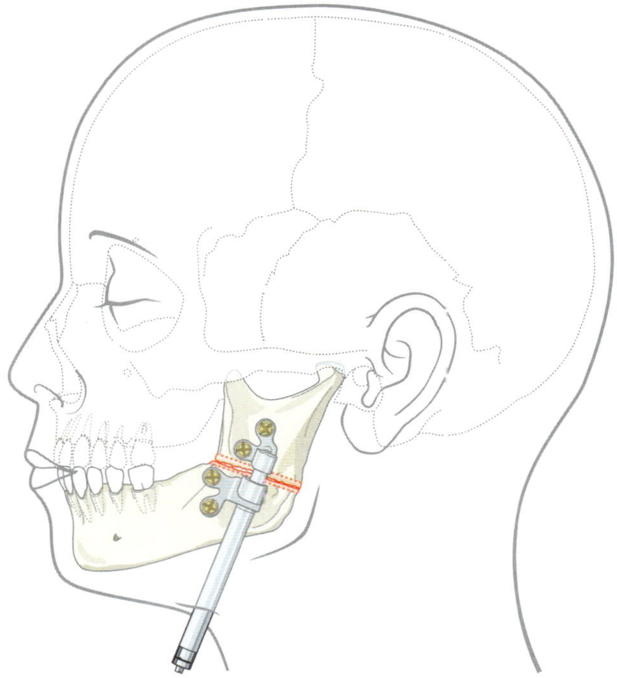

Fig 1.2-2 A unidirectional, semi-buried device.

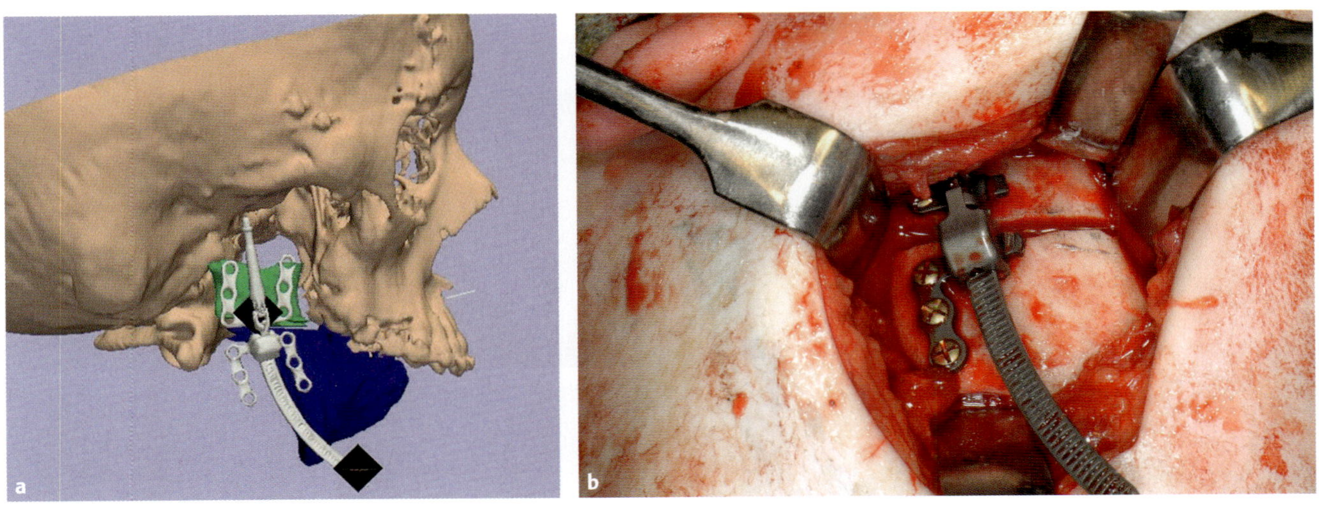

Fig 1.2-3a–b

a A curvilinear device fit on the 3-D image of the patient's skull. Based on the fit, the surgeon chooses the footplate to use and the one to cut off and discard.

b Intraoperative photo showing the device placed on the right side of the mandible (two footplates have been removed) across the osteotomy.

and the proper overall distraction vector are all critical to achieve the desired result.

Diagnostic workup includes clinical examination, analysis of photographs (frontal, frontal smile, right and left lateral, and submental views), radiographs (lateral and anteroposterior cephalograms, orthopantomogram, 3-D CT images), and anatomically articulated dental casts. Cooperation with an orthodontist is mandatory. Furthermore, with semi-buried devices, preoperative planning is particularly critical because mid-treatment course corrections are not possible. A 3-D software-driven treatment planning system for accurate determination of skeletal movements has been developed. A 3-D CT scan is obtained and planning software for the craniofacial skeleton is used to plan the procedure (**Fig 1.2-4** and **Fig 1.2-5**). A 3-D visualization of the facial skeleton, selection of landmarks, measurement of angles and distances, simulation of osteotomies, repositioning of bones, prediction of movements (even of the proximal mandibular segment), detection of collisions, and superimposition of scans can be accomplished with this technique. Furthermore, the vector required to correct the deformity is determined and the perception for required devices rendered.

5 Assessment of DO process

Common methods of assessment of the clinical DO process consist of serial physical examinations, plain x-rays, ultrasound, and CT. Panoramic radiograph and lateral cephalogram are obtained immediately preoperatively, immediately postoperatively, at the end of distraction phase, and at the end of the fixation period. Ultrasound is an inexpensive, noninvasive, and efficient method of imaging that provides detailed assessment of bone formation across a defect. It has proved to be useful for the evaluation of long-bone DO healing and additionally it lacks the disadvantage of exposing the patient to radiation. We confirmed the validity of ultrasound as a reliable technique to measure the osteotomy/corticotomy gap, to detect new bone formation, and to assess the bone maturity. It is repeated every 2 weeks during the fixation period and guides the clinician in deciding when to remove the distraction device (**Figs 1.2-6–1.2-11**).

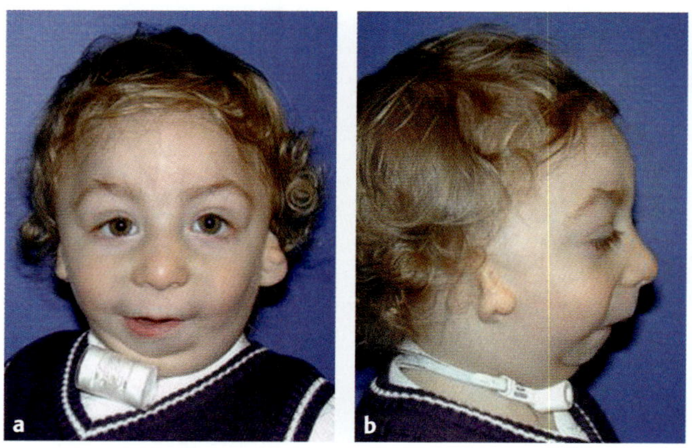

Fig 1.2-4a–b
a Frontal view.
b Lateral view of a tracheostomy-dependent child with bilateral craniofacial microsomia. He had obstructive apnea because of severe mandibular retrognathia.

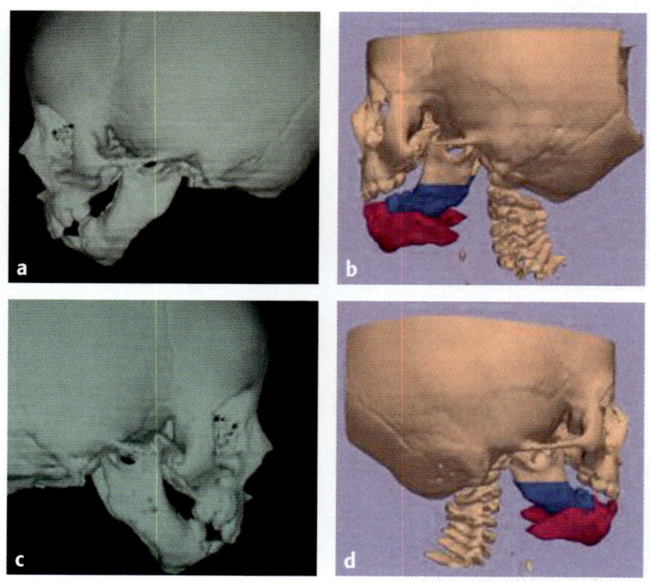

Fig 1.2-5a–d Preoperative lateral 3-D computed tomographic images (left, top, and bottom) and planned skeletal movements (right, top, and bottom) seen in red and determined using a commercially available 3-D treatment planning system. The system helps to define the radius of curvature of the device.

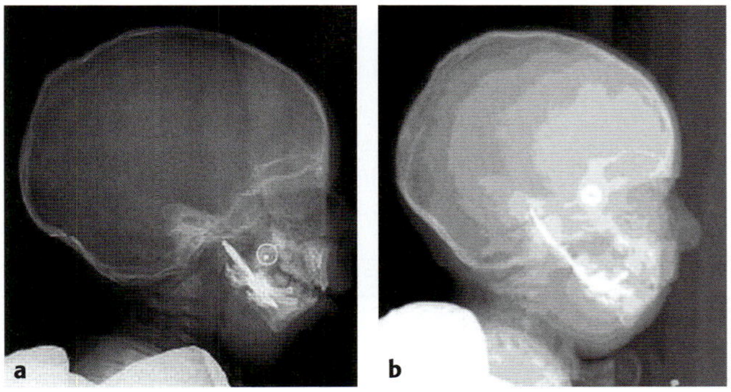

Fig 1.2-6a–b Lateral cephalograms taken immediately postoperatively.

a After device placement.

b At end-distraction. The device used is a custom-made, curvilinear semi-buried distractor capable of 3-D movements.

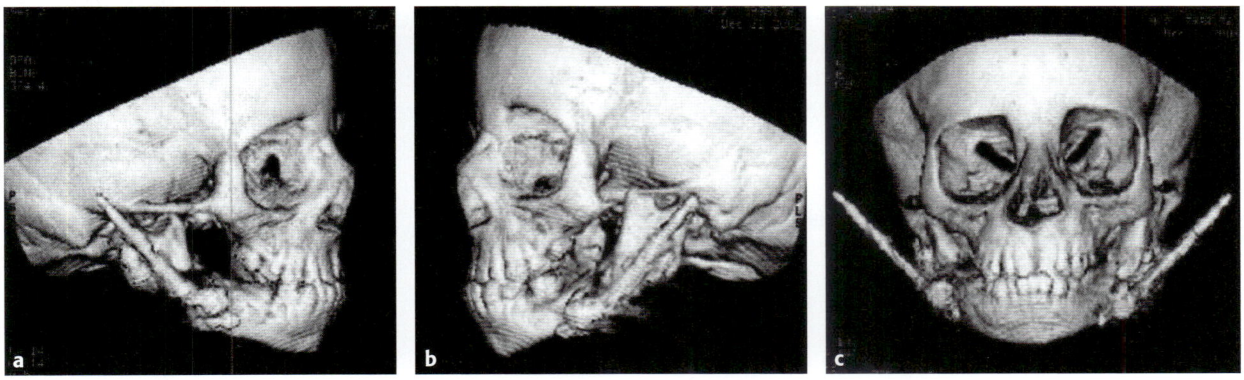

Fig 1.2-7a–c Lateral and AP postoperative 3-D computed tomographic images demonstrate the elongation.

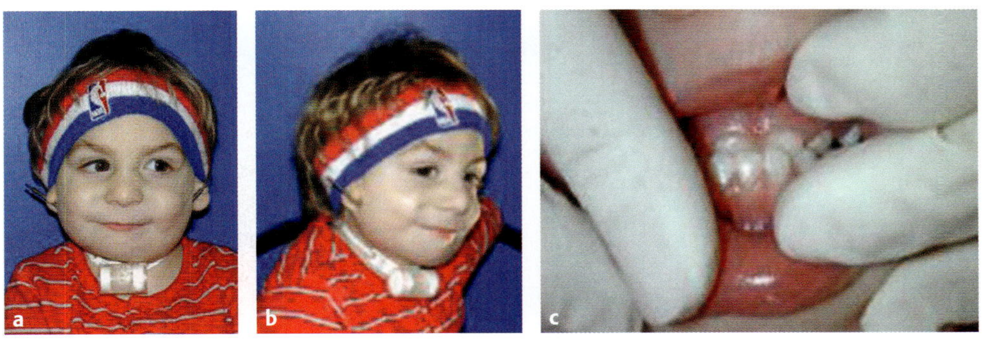

Fig 1.2-8a–c Frontal and intraoral views at end-distraction (during fixation).

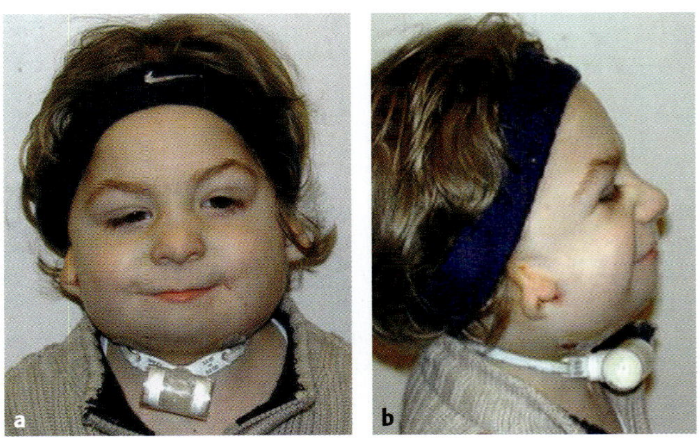

Fig 1.2-9a–b Frontal and lateral views of the child after device removal.

6 Complications

Complications of DO may occur as a result of inaccurate treatment planning, incorrect placement of the osteotomy/corticotomy or the distraction device, mistakes during the active distraction phase, and problems with fixation. Technical problems with the devices, such as deformation, have also been reported. The surgeon must select patients who are willing to comply and capable of activating the device on a daily basis. The noncompliant or unprepared patient may turn the device in the wrong direction, fail to keep the wounds clean, activate the device too frequently or not frequently enough, and fail to comply with dietary, hygiene, and physical activity instructions. Thus, loosening or dismantling of the device, premature union of the segments, malocclusion, wound dehiscence, and infection may result.

Considerations that the surgeon should keep in mind during the operation to avoid complications are to make a complete osteotomy or corticotomy to activate the device to ensure bony separation, to execute the planned osteotomy in the desired location, place the distractor with the proper orientation relative to the osteotomy, and fix it properly.

7 Limitations of DO

Limitations of DO arise from the cumbersome nature and complexity of distraction devices, cutaneous incisions and pin-track scars, lengthy treatment protocols, and lack of accurate 3-D control of the distraction vector. Better devices and better understanding of the biological events that regulate osteogenesis will improve DO in the future for patients.

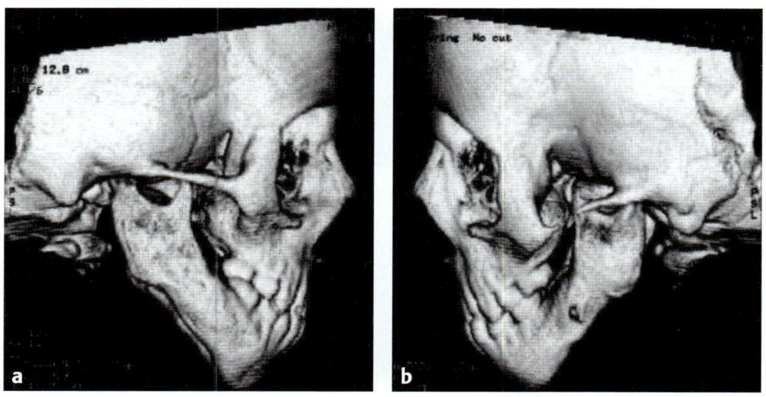

Fig 1.2-10a–b Postoperative lateral 3-D computed tomographic images show the mandibular expansion and bone formation. At this point the child was scheduled to have his tracheostomy removed.

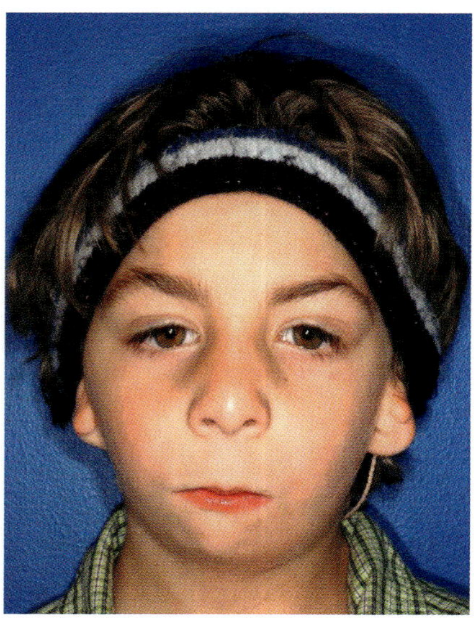

Fig 1.2-11 Four years postoperatively the child without tracheostomy and doing well (with permission from *Journal of Oral and Maxillofacial Surgery*).

8 References and suggested reading

Ayoub AF, Richardson W, Barbenel JC. Mandibular elongation by automatic distraction osteogenesis: the first application in humans. *Br J Oral Maxillofac Surg*. 2005 Aug;43(4):324–328.

Block MS, Brister GD. Use of distraction osteogenesis for maxillary advancement: preliminary results. *J Oral Maxillofac Surg*. 1994 Mar;52(3):282–286; discussion 287–288.

Castano FJ, Troulis MJ, Glowacki J, et al. Proliferation of masseter myocytes after distraction osteogenesis of the porcine mandible. *J Oral Maxillofac Surg*. 2001 Mar;59(3):302–307.

Codivilla A. On the means of lengthening, in the lower limbs, the muscles and tissues which are shortened through deformity. *Am J Orth Surg*. 1905;2:353–357.

Constantino PD, Friedman CD. Distraction osteogenesis. Applications for mandibular regrowth. *Otolaryngol Clin North Am*. 1991 Dec;24(6):1433–1443.

Glowacki J, Shusterman EM, Troulis M, et al. Distraction osteogenesis of the porcine mandible: histomorphometric evaluation of bone. *Plast Reconstr Surg*. 2004 Feb;113(2):566–573.

Goldwaser BR, Magill J, Papadaki ME, et al. Continuous mandibular distraction osteogenesis: novel device and preliminary results in minipigs. *J Oral Maxillofac Surg*. 2013 Apr;71(4):e168–177.

Goldwaser BR, Papadaki ME, Kaban LB, et al. Automated continuous mandibular distraction osteogenesis: review of the literature. *J Oral Maxillofac Surg*. 2012;70(2):407–416.

Hansen GM, Lawler ME, Williams WB, et al. BMP4 localization and PCNA expression during distraction osteogenesis of the porcine mandible. *Int J Oral Maxillofac Surg*. 2012 Jul;41(7):867–873.

Ilizarov GA. The principles of the Ilizarov method. *Bull Hosp Jt Dis Orthop Inst*. 1988;48(1):1–11.

Ilizarov GA. The tension-stress effect on the genesis and growth of tissues: Part I. The influence of stability of fixation and soft-tissue preservation. *Clin Orthop Relat Res*. 1989 Jan;(238):249–281.

Kaban LB, Seldin EB, Kikinis R, et al. Clinical application of curvilinear distraction osteogenesis for correction of mandibular deformities. *J Oral Maxillofac Surg*. 2009 May;67(5):996–1008.

Kaban LB, Thurmüller P, Troulis MJ, et al. Correlation of biomechanical stiffness with plain radiographic and ultrasound data in an experimental mandibular distraction wound. *Int J Oral Maxillofac Surg*. 2003 Jun;32(3):296–304.

Kessler P, Wiltfang J, Neukam FW. A new distraction device to compare continuous and discontinuous bone distraction in mini-pigs: a preliminary report. *J Craniomaxillofac Surg*. 2000 Feb;28(1):5–11.

Lawler ME, Hansen GM, Williams WB, et al. Serial histologic and immunohistochemical changes in anterior digastric myocytes in response to distraction osteogenesis. *J Oral Maxillofac Surg*. 2012 Jan;70(1):168–178.

Lawler ME, Tayebaty FT, Williams WB, et al. Histomorphometric analysis of the porcine mandibular distraction wound. *J Oral Maxillofac Surg*. 2010 Jul;68(7):1543–1554.

Li G, Simpson AH, Triffitt JT. The role of chondrocytes in intramembranous and endochondral ossification during distraction osteogenesis in the rabbit. *Calcif Tissue Int*. 1999 Apr;64(4):310–317.

Losken HW, Mooney MP, Zoldos J, et al. Coronal suture response to distraction osteogenesis in rabbits with delayed-onset craniosynostosis. *J Craniofac Surg*. 1999 Jan;10(1):27–37.

Magill JC, Byl MF, Goldwaser B, et al. Automating skeletal expansion: an implant for distraction osteogenesis of the mandible. *J Med Device*. 2009 Mar;3(1):14502.

McCarthy JG, Schreiber J, Karp N, et al. Lengthening of the human mandible by gradual distraction. *Plast Reconstr Surg*. 1992 Jan;89(1):1–8; discussion 9–10.

McCarthy JG, Stelnicki EJ, Mehrara BJ, et al. Distraction osteogenesis of the craniofacial skeleton. *Plast Reconstr Surg*. 2001 Jun;107(7):1812–1827.

Mofid MM, Manson PN, Robertson BC, et al. Craniofacial distraction osteogenesis: a review of 3278 cases. *Plast Reconstr Surg*. 2001 Oct;108(5):1103–1114; discussion 1115–1157.

Papadaki ME, Kaban LB, Troulis MJ. Minipig model of maxillary distraction osteogenesis: immunohistochemical and histomorphometric analysis of the sequence of osteogenesis. *J Oral Maxillofac Surg*. 2012 Nov;70(11):2629–2640.

Papadaki ME, Troulis MJ, Glowacki J, et al. A minipig model of maxillary distraction osteogenesis. *J Oral Maxillofac Surg*. 2010 Nov;68(11):2783–2791.

Peacock ZS, Tricomi BJ, Murphy BA, et al. Automated continuous distraction osteogenesis may allow faster distraction rates: a preliminary study. *J Oral Maxillofac Surg*. 2013 Jun;71(6):1073–1084.

Perrott DH, Berger R, Vargervik K, et al. Use of a skeletal distraction device to widen the mandible: a case report. *J Oral Maxillofac Surg*. 1993 Apr;51(4):435–439.

Perrott DH, Rahn B, Wahl D, et al. Development of a mechanical testing system for a mandibular distraction wound. *Int J Oral Maxillofac Surg*. 2003 Oct;32(5):523–527.

Ploder O, Mayr W, Schnetz G, et al. Mandibular lengthening with an implanted motor-driven device: preliminary study in sheep. *Br J Oral Maxillofac Surg*. 1999 Aug;37(4):273–276.

Rachmiel A, Potparic Z, Jackson IT, et al. Midface advancement by gradual distraction. *Br J Plast Surg*. 1993 Apr;46(3):201–207.

Schmelzeisen R, Neumann G, von der Fecht R. Distraction osteogenesis in the mandible with a motor-driven plate: a preliminary animal study. *Br J Oral Maxillofac Surg*. 1996 Oct;34(5):375–378.

Seldin EB, Troulis MJ, Kaban LB. Evaluation of a semiburied, fixed-trajectory, curvilinear, distraction device in an animal model. *J Oral Maxillofac Surg*. 1999 Dec;57(12):1442–1446.

Snyder CC, Levine GA, Swanson HM, et al. Mandibular lengthening by gradual distraction: preliminary report. *Plast Reconstr Surg*. 1973 May;51(5):506–508.

Thurmüller P, Troulis M, O'Neill MJ, et al. Use of ultrasound to assess healing of a mandibular distraction wound. *J Oral Maxillofac Surg*. 2002 Sep;60(9):1038–1044.

Troulis MJ, Everett P, Seldin EB, et al. Development of a three-dimensional treatment planning system based on computed tomographic data. *Int J Oral Maxillofac Surg*. 2002 Aug;31(4):349–357.

Troulis MJ, Glowacki J, Perrott DH, et al. Effects of latency and rate on bone formation in a porcine mandibular distraction model. *J Oral Maxillofac Surg*. 2000 May;58(5):507–513; discussion 514.

Troulis M, Kaban L. Complications of mandibular distraction osteogenesis. *Oral Maxillofacial Surg Clin N Am*. 2003 May;15(2):251–264.

Wiltfang J, Kessler P, Merten HA, et al. Continuous and intermittent bone distraction using a microhydraulic cylinder: an experimental study in minipigs. *Br J Oral Maxillofac Surg*. 2001 Feb;39(1):2–7.

Yates KE, Troulis MJ, Kaban LB, et al. IGF-I, TGF-beta, and BMP-4 are expressed during distraction osteogenesis of the pig mandible. *Int J Oral Maxillofac Surg*. 2002 Apr;31(2):173–178.

Zimmermann CE, Harris G, Thurmüller P, et al. Assessment of bone formation in a porcine mandibular distraction wound by computed tomography. *Int J Oral Maxillofac Surg*. 2004 Sep;33(6):569–574.

1.3 Ceramic bone substitute materials

Marc Bohner, Berton Rahn†

1 Introduction

In 1892, Dreesman performed the first implantation of a synthetic ceramic (plaster of Paris = calcium sulphate hemihydrate) as bone substitute. In 1920, Albee and Morrison investigated the use of a calcium phosphate (CaP) paste to accelerate bone fracture healing. Since then, the field of ceramic bone substitutes and available products has expanded dramatically. Despite this development, it is still not clear for many users what they are implanting and in which ways implanted materials differ. This chapter describes the physical, chemical, and biological differences of CaPs, the main class of ceramic bone graft substitute materials. Particular attention is paid to the new developments in the field, ie, the so-called "calcium phosphate cements" (CPCs) and calcium phosphate "putties" (or "pastes").

Sections 2, 3, and 4 of this chapter cover the chemical and physical aspects of CaPs, apatites, and CPCs, respectively. The fifth section summarizes the in vivo properties of CaPs. The sixth section briefly discusses new trends in the field.

2 Calcium phosphates

CaPs, as suggested by their name, consist of calcium (Ca^{2+}) and (ortho)phosphate (PO_4^{3-}) ions. For example, one of the most common bone graft substitutes is β-tricalcium phosphate (β-TCP) with the chemical formula: β-$Ca_3(PO_4)_2$. Calcium phosphates may contain bound water, such as in dicalcium phosphate dihydrate (DCPD): $CaHPO_4 \cdot 2H_2O$. In the latter case, the water molecules are an inherent part of the crystal structure. Phosphate ions can be either unprotonated (PO_4^{3-}), or protonated with one or two protons (HPO_4^{2-}, $H_2PO_4^-$, respectively). As such, there are not only two or three CaP compounds but more than ten (**Table 1.3-1**) [Bohner, 2000].

Since protonation modifies the acidity of the phosphate ion, some of these compounds are acidic, eg, monocalcium phosphate monohydrate (MCPM; $Ca(H_2PO_4)_2 \cdot H_2O$), whereas other compounds are basic, eg, tetracalcium phosphate (TetCP; $Ca_4(PO_4)_2O$). Generally, the higher the Ca/P molar ratio, the more basic the compound is. All these chemical differences lead to CaPs with diverse solubilities (**Fig 1.3-1**), some CaPs being soluble over a broad pH range (eg, MCPM) whereas other compounds are poorly soluble at neutral pH but highly soluble in acidic conditions (eg, β-TCP) [Vereecke et al, 1990]. These differences explain variations in biological response, as is found in detail in the chapter.

The large range of chemical properties also affects the physical properties. Some CaPs are only stable at high temperature (> 600–1400°C), such as β-tricalcium phosphate (β-TCP; β-$Ca_3(PO_4)_2$), α-tricalcium phosphate (α-TCP; α$Ca_3(PO_4)_2$), or TetCP [Bohner, 2000]. These compounds are typically used in the composition of CPCs. Other compounds, such as dicalcium phosphate (DCP; $CaHPO_4$), DCPD, octacalcium phosphate (OCP; $Ca_8H_2(PO_4)_6 \cdot 5H_2O$) and hydroxyapatite (HA; $Ca_5(PO_4)_3OH$) precipitate (= crystallize) at room temperature, and hence can be found in the human body [Elliott, 1994].

3 Apatites

Although apatites belong to the CaP family, and some are found in the body, their variety and importance in the field of mineralization require elaboration. The most famous apatite is hydroxyapatite (HA) because it is the main component of bone. Bone consists of a mineral that has practically the same crystallographic structure as HA, but a different composition. Bone mineral typically contains "impurities", such as Na, K, Mg, Sr, carbonates, sulfates, F, or Cl [Elliott, 1994]. These impurities can be easily incorporated into the HA structure by replacing calcium, hydroxyde, or phosphate ions. As a result, apatites represent a family of materials (to which HA belongs) that have been the subject of numerous publications and books. Note, in the text "HA" will be used for "apatite".

Name	Abbreviation	Formula	Ca/P	Mineral name	End product (EP)/ raw material (RM) for the following commercial products
Monocalcium phosphate	MCP	$Ca(H_2PO_4)_2$	0.50	-	-
Monocalciumphosphate monohydrate	MCPM	$Ca(H_2PO_4)_2{\cdot}H_2O$	0.50	-	RM: Chronos Inject, Eurobone, Jectos, Norian CRS, Vitalos
Dicalcium phosphate	DCP	$CaHPO_4$	1.00	Monetite	RM: Calcibon, Rebone
Dicalcium phosphate dihydrate	DCPD	$CaHPO_4{\cdot}2H_2O$	1.00	Brushite	EP: Chronos Inject, Eurobone, Jectos, Vitalos
Octacalcium phosphate	OCP	$Ca_8H_2(PO_4)_6{\cdot}5H_2O$	1.33	-	-
α-Tricalcium phosphate	α-TCP	$\alpha\text{-}Ca_3(PO_4)_2$	1.50	-	EP: Biobase RM: Biobon, Biopex, Calcibon, Callos, Cementek, Graftys, Hydroset, Kyphos, Mimix, Norian CRS
β-Tricalcium phosphate	β-TCP	$\beta\text{-}Ca_3(PO_4)_2$	1.50	-	EP: Calciresorb, Cerasorb, Ceros, Chronos, Conduit TCP, Vitoss RM: Chronos Inject, Eurobone, Jectos, Vitalos
Calcium-deficient hydroxyapatite* ("tricalcium phosphate")	CDHA	$Ca_{10-x}(HPO_4)_x(PO_4)_{6-x}(OH)_{2-x}$	1.50-1.67	-	EP: Biobon, Bonesource, Calcibon, Cementek, Hydroset, Mimix, Norian CRS
Biphasic calcium phosphate	BCP	Mixture of β-TCP and HA	1.50-1.67	-	EP: BCP, BoneCeramic, BoneSave, Ceraform, mBCP, OsSatura, Triosite
Hydroxyapatite	HA	$Ca_5(PO_4)_3OH$	1.67	Hydroxyapatite	EP (high T): Actifuse, Cerapatite, Endobon EP (low T): BioOss, Pro Osteon 200 and 500
Oxyapatite†	OXA	$Ca_{10}(PO_4)_6O$	1.67	-	-
Tetracalcium phosphate	TetCP	$Ca_4(PO_4)_2O$	2.00		RM: Bonesource, Cementek, Rebone

Table 1.3-1 List of CaPs with their name, abbreviation, chemical formula, Ca to phosphate molar ratio, mineral name and finally a nonexhaustive list of commercial products based on these CaP compounds.

* Generally, the Ca/P molar ratio is 1.50. Importantly, the end product of CPC reactions is chemically and physically close to CDHA. CDHA can be considered as a typical LT-HA.
† This phase is reactive in the presence of water, so it is difficult to produce pure oxyapatite.

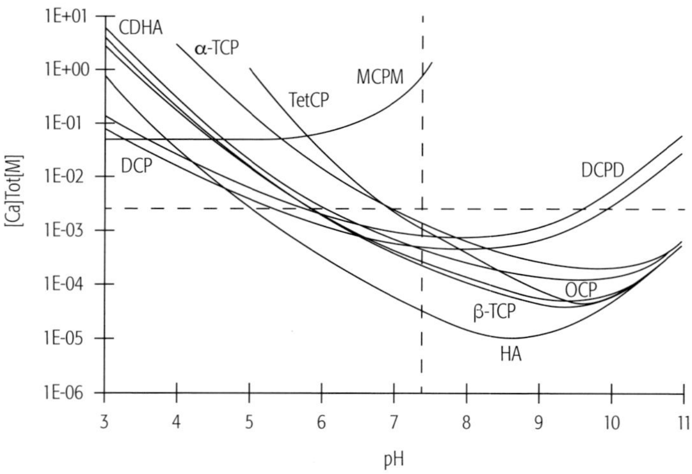

Fig 1.3-1 Solubility of calcium phosphates in pure water at 25°C. The solubility is expressed as the calcium concentration present in the aqueous medium after equilibration. At physiological pH (vertical line), the solubility decreases in the order of: MCPM > α-TCP > TetCP > DCPD > DCP > OCP > CDHA > β-TCP > HA.

Another important point concerning HA is that it can be synthetized at low and high temperature. Low temperature HA (LT-HA) is obtained by precipitation in an aqueous solution at or close to room temperature, and has deviations from the stoichiometry of pure HA. Typically, LT-HA contains impurities (eg, Mg, Sr, or Fe ions, silicates, carbonates) present in the raw materials used for their synthesis, and may also contain deficiencies, for example in calcium. Calcium-deficient hydroxyapatite or tricalcium phosphate (CDHA or TCP; $Ca_9(HPO_4)(PO_4)_5OH$; **Table 1.3-1**) may be readily produced by hydrolysing α-TCP in water [Monma et al, 1976];

$$3\ \alpha\text{-}Ca_3(PO_4)_2 + H_2O \rightarrow Ca_9(HPO_4)(PO_4)_5OH \quad (1)$$

LT-HA is characterized by a small crystalline dimension, typically below 100 nm. Since the solubility of nanoparticles increases when their size decreases, LT-HA is markedly more soluble than high-temperature apatites. This effect is increased by the presence of impurities and deficiencies in the apatite structure. The solubility of LT-HA is probably close to that of β-TCP. However, there is a lack of reliable solubility data.

Commercially, all "apatite" CPCs (see hereafter) are LT-HA. Typical commercial products include Biobon, Bonesource, Calcibon, Cementek, Hydroset, Mimix, or Norian CRS. Pastes (or "putties") may also consist of such particles, eg, "Ostim" (**Table 1.3-1**).

High temperature apatites (HT-HA) are obtained by heating stoichiometric LT-HA at high temperature, typically above 700–800°C. At such temperatures, atomic diffusion is large enough to produce a macroscopic change of crystal size and form: crystals become rounder and much bigger, hence decreasing their surface energy (**Fig 1.3-2**).

The high atomic diffusion taking place at high temperature can also be exploited to produce HT-HA by reactive sintering of, eg, DCP and calcium carbonate according to the following reaction:

$$3CaHPO_4 + 2CaCO_3 \rightarrow Ca_5(PO_4)_3OH + H_2O + 2\ CO_2 \quad (2)$$

Since HT-HA crystals/particles are much larger than LT-HA particles, their solubility is greatly reduced, leading to a much lower resorption rate if implanted in vivo (see hereafter).

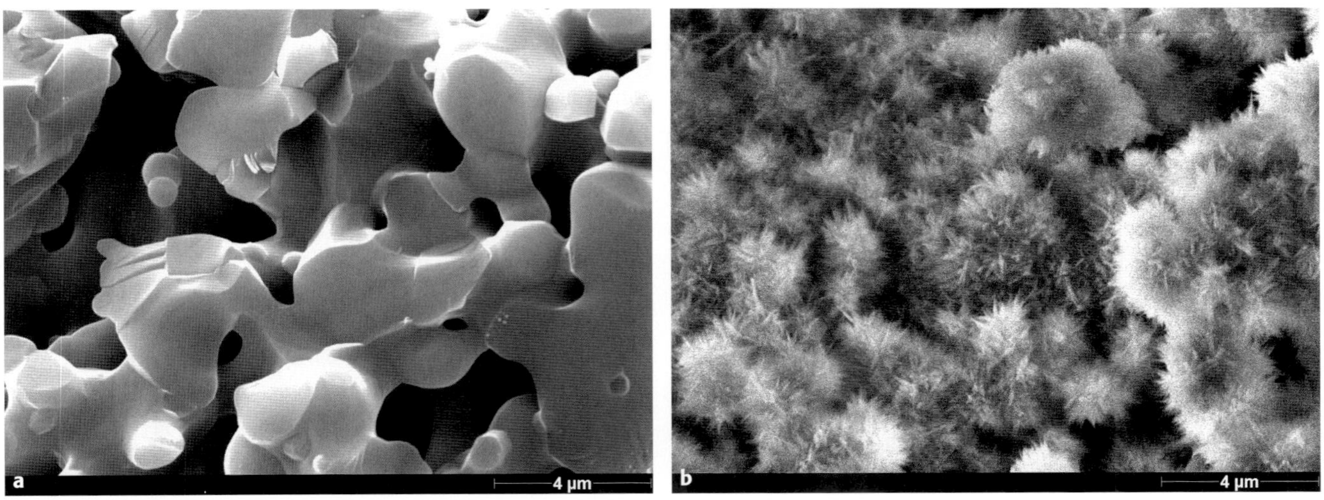

Fig 1.3-2a–b Microstructure of a sintered compound (eg, β-tricalcium phosphate; left) and of a LT-HA (right). In the present example, the left structure (**a**) is obtained by sintering the right structure (**b**) for 5 minutes at 1250°C (cooling and heating rate: 1°C/min). The scale bar has a length of 4 µm.

4 Calcium phosphate cements

Calcium phosphate cements were first proposed by LeGeros et al [1982], but really discovered and patented by Brown and Chow [1983]. As indicated by their name, CPCs harden with time. The starting point of the setting reaction is the mixture of an aqueous solution with one or several CaP powder(s). This can be schematically written:

CaP powders + Water -> CaP solid (3)

Contrary to polymer cements, such as polymethylmethacrylate (PMMA), CPCs do not harden via polymerization, ie, by the growth and entanglement of polymer chains. The CPCs harden via a dissolution-precipitation reaction that can be divided into four phases: (1) initiation of the dissolution of the cement components; (2) dissolution of the cement components in the mixing liquid; (3) nucleation of small crystals in the mixing liquid; and (4) growth of the latter crystals until all starting components are consumed. Mechanical stability is provided by the entanglement of crystals (**Fig 1.3-2b**). Generally, the paste becomes solid beyond 10% reaction grade at an early stage of the CPC reaction. Even though some early hardening may occur within a few minutes, the overall setting/hardening reaction can easily last 24 hours, therefore early loading is prohibited. Due to their ceramic nature, CPCs are brittle. As a result, their mechanical properties are much stronger in compression than in traction. Specifically, CPC's compressive strength is typically five to ten times larger than their tensile strength.

There are two main types of CPCs depending on the end product of the reaction:

DCPD cements or apatite cements. The DCPD cements are more resorbable than HA cements due to the larger solubility of DCPD compared with HA. There are only few commercial cements belonging to the first category (eg, Chronos Inject, Eurobone, Jectos, Vitalos) (**Table 1.3-1**). Most commercial CPC belong to the second class of cements (Biobon, Bonesource, Calcibon, Cementek, Hydroset, Mimix, Norian CRS etc).

Most CPCs are exothermic, sometimes even more than PMMA cements. However, heat release is slow (over several days), resulting in an absence or only a minor temperature increase during setting, therefore all CPCs can be considered to harden isothermally.

4.1 In vivo behavior of calcium phosphates

The planned function of an implant determines which material and design characteristics are required to produce adequate results. Many defective bone structures can be treated satisfactorily by temporary substitutes that will be replaced gradually by site-specific bony tissue. In this case the implant material has to maintain its characteristics as long as function demands but preferably it has to disappear after regional tissue has taken over function. The clinical indication must respect the fact that mechanical loading characteristics of the bone substitute ceramics have reasonable strength in compression but are weak in tension and shear. The use of ceramic material must avoid such regions, or be used with additional protection provided by metal implants (plates, cages, meshes and so on) to avoid acute or fatigue failure.

Many parameters affect the resorption rates of CaPs, such as CaP solubility, crystal size, or geometry, and despite in vivo studies much is still unknown; however, what is known will be conveyed.

The main factor affecting the in vivo behavior of CaPs is their solubility. Solubility differences span several orders of magnitude [Vereecke et al, 1990]. For example, HT-HA is roughly ten times less soluble than LT-HA, CDHA, and β-TCP, which are roughly ten times less soluble than DCPD. Such solubility differences lead to different in vivo behaviors. High-temperature HA can be considered to be inert whereas LT-HA, CDHA, and β-TCP are readily resorbed (roughly 1–10 µm/week) [Bashoor-Zadeh et al, 2011]. In general, one may roughly assume that the resorption rate is a function of the solubility at pH 7.4 [Driessens et al, 1987]:

HT-HA $<$ LT-HA $\approx$ CDHA $\approx$ β-TCP $<$ OCP $\approx$ DCP $<$ DCPD $<$ α-TCP $<$ TetCP $<$ MCPM

In practice, the situation is different because rather soluble CaPs, such as DCPD and α-TCP, may not only dissolve but also react in vivo to form a low-temperature apatite. This type of behavior has also been reported for OCP, DCPD (**Fig 1.3-3**) [Bohner et al, 2003; Constantz et al, 1998], and α-TCP (reaction (3) [Merten et al, 2001].

The conversion reaction of DCPD into CDHA can be written:

$$9CaHPO_4 \cdot 2H_2O \rightarrow Ca_9(HPO_4)(PO_4)_5OH + 3H_3PO_4 + 17H_2O \quad (4)$$

Once conversion has occurred, CaP resorption rate is strongly reduced. Similarly α-TCP (eg, BioBase) which is one order of magnitude more soluble than β-TCP (eg, Cerasorb, Ceros, Chronos) has been reported to resorb at a similar rate as β-TCP [Merten et al, 2001]. In this context, Gbureck et al [2007] demonstrated that DCPD did not resorb faster in vivo than DCP as predicted from the solubility data but slower. Similarly α-TCP (eg, BioBase) which is one order of magnitude..."

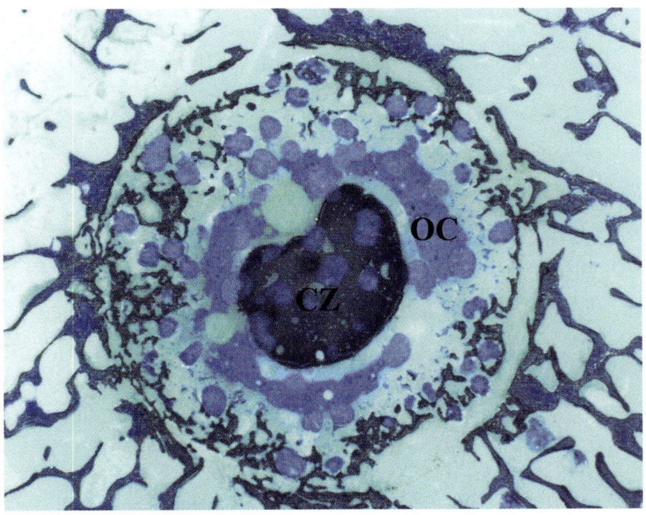

Fig 1.3-3 Dicalcium phosphate dihydrate to calcium-deficient hydroxyapatite conversion in the center of chronOS Inject cement after 3 months implantation in a sheep model (courtesy D Apelt, MD, University of Zurich, Zurich, Switzerland). The converted zone (CZ) is the darker zone present in the cement center. The nonconverted zone (original cement [OC]) is surrounding the converted zone. The edges of the 8 mm cylindrical drill hole are visible.

Less soluble or poorly soluble CaPs, such as HT-HA, LT-HA, and β-TCP, are insoluble in standard physiological conditions (serum or blood, pH 7.4). Indeed, body fluids contain such large Ca and phosphate ion concentration that they are saturated toward HA and β-TCP. While these materials are known as "bioinsoluble," these bioinsoluble CaPs can be resorbed in vivo because certain cells, such as macrophages or osteoclasts, can reduce the local pH down to values close to pH 3 [Silver et al, 1988] and hence increase CaP solubility. At low pH values, HA, and β-TCP are not bioinsoluble anymore (**Fig 1.3-1**).

As a rule, soluble (= biosoluble) CaPs, such as DCPD and α-TCP, are generally converted in vivo to a bioinsoluble CaP, and bioinsoluble CaPs are resorbed by cells. The extent of cellular resorption is a direct function of the material solubility. Whereas β-TCP (eg, Cerasorb, Ceros, chronOS) and LT-HA (eg, Biobon, Bonesource, Calcibon, Cementek, Hydroset, Mimix, or Norian CRS) are resorbed at a rate of roughly 1–10 μm per week [Bashoor-Zadeh et al, 2011], HT-HA can be considered to be "inert" and to remain in place long after the lifespan of the patient [Linhart et al, 2004].

The differences between a biosoluble and a bioinsoluble CaP have been linked to the materials, OCP [Driessens et al, 1987; Eidelman et al, 1987] and DCP [Bohner et al, 2009]. CaP phases that are more soluble than OCP/DCP will spontaneously dissolve and convert in vivo, whereas CaP phases that are less soluble than OCP/DCP will be resorbed by cells. Interestingly, OCP [Suzuki et al, 2006] and DCPD [Bohner et al, 2003; Constantz et al, 1998] have been reported to convert to CDHA in vivo, contrary to DCP [Gbureck et al, 2007]. As these three compounds have solubilities that are close to each other, OCP, DCPD, and DCP are close to the limit between biosoluble and bioinsoluble CaPs. Therefore, and based on the present results, DCP-based bone replacement materials appear to provide the fastest transition between a bone defect and mature new bone.

Among all commercial products, there are a few biphasic materials, ie, material consisting of a mixture of two or more CaPs. In biphasic materials the component with the higher solubility, usually the matrix, starts to degrade first. The matrix gradually disappears and the slower degrading filler component continues its function resulting in a creeping substitution of the implant (**Fig 1.3-4** and **Fig 1.3-5**, [Gisep et al, 2003]), which finally results in an adequate bony structure. This concept is used in CPCs, eg, chronOS Inject where the matrix (DCPD) resorbs much faster than the filler (β-TCP granules), as do "biphasic calcium phosphates" (eg, BCP, MBCP, Triosite, Bone Save) which consist of a mixture of β-TCP and HA.

■ Bone ingrowth
■ Ceramic cement

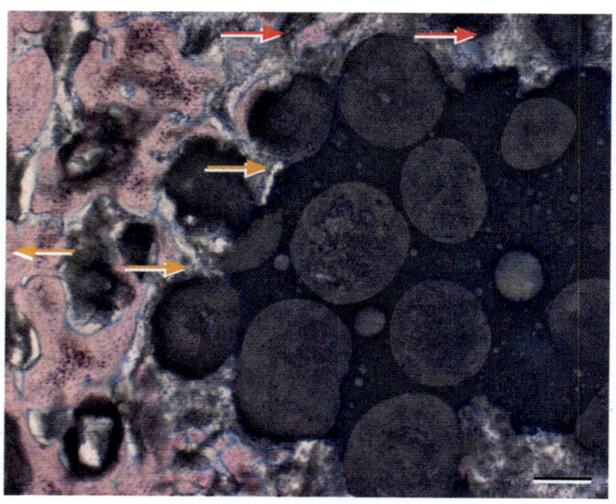

Fig 1.3-4 Creeping substitution of biphasic ceramic cement. Differences in solubility of the two phases result in different degradation speeds. This allows bone to grow into the space previously taken by the more rapidly degrading matrix while slower degrading filler granules maintain shape and function (courtesy Armando Gisep, PhD, AO Research Institute Davos).

■ Connective tissue
■ Bone
■ Ceramic cement

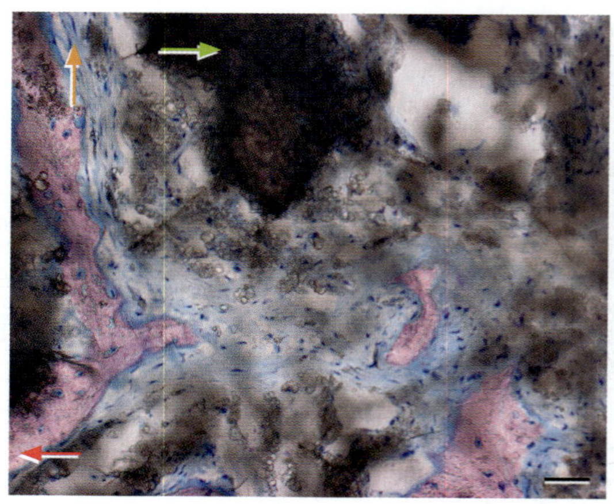

Fig 1.3-5 Replacement of ceramic matrix by local tissue. In a biphasic ceramic cement the matrix disappears and is replaced by connective tissue that is gradually differentiating into bone (courtesy Armando Gisep, PhD, AO Research Institute Davos).

In addition to solubility, there are many factors that have been reported to modify the resorption rate of a material. Some are patient related (eg, implant location, social habits), and some are material related. One important material-related aspect is the material geometry. Because CaP resorption is surface mediated, a more porous and open structure is resorbed faster than more compact structures [Bashoor-Zadeh et al, 2011]. As CPCs are compact, resorption of their volume is much lower than that of macroporous blocks or granules, which lead to slow resorption times [Frankenburg et al, 1998]. Continuous loading of CPCs in vivo may result in fatigue cracks [Gisep et al, 2004], permitting ingrowth of soft tissue and of bone (**Fig 1.3-6**) [Gisep et al, 2003].

Regarding biocompatibility, an "affinity" between bone and material or at least an inertness (eg, high-temperature HA) is required. The CPCs harden isothermally and rapidly attain a physiological pH value after setting, and no relevant tissue response occurs from the setting process. In the early phase following implantation the appearance of inflammatory cells, like granulocytes, and in the later phase lymphocytes are a normal finding, which is attributed to the surgical trauma. These cells occur in relatively low numbers, and achieve a steady state within a few weeks and normal host tissue will be found at the interface. In the case of an infection with continuing inflammation, the pH may drop, which may lead to a more rapid resorption of ceramic implants. During resorption, soluble as well as particulate resorption products result. The soluble compounds, ie, calcium and phosphate ions, have been shown to modify the functions of osteoblasts and osteoclasts [Wu et al, 2003; Meleti et al, 2000; Kanatani et al, 1991; Zaidi et al, 1989; Habibovic et al, 2011]. The particles produced are engulfed by macrophages and foreign body giant cells, and the cytotoxic effect that particles in a micrometer range may have is unknown. Some suggest that release of microparticles make CaP ceramics osteoinductive [Le Nihouannen et al, 2005].

In general, CaP ceramics have an excellent biocompatibility [Kurashina et al, 1997] and final resorption products (calcium and phosphate ions) are not harmful. The presence of capillaries and fibroblasts/fibrocytes in close vicinity to ceramic crystallites (**Fig 1.3-7**), the absence of inflammatory cells, and the incorporation of crystallites into newly formed bone (**Fig 1.3-8**) support its characterization as inert.

- Tissue ingrowth into cracks
- Ceramic cement
- Cracks

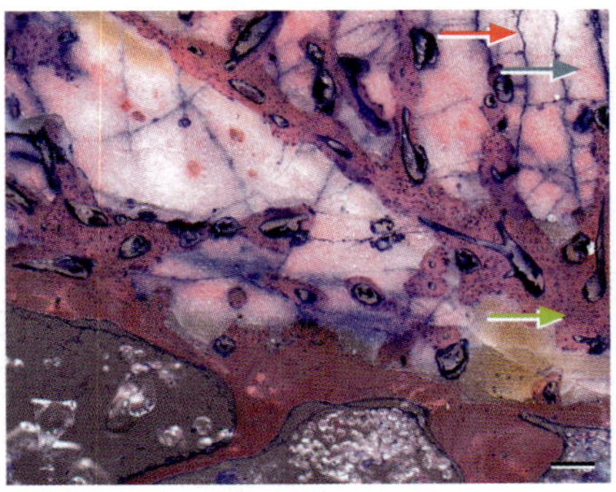

Fig 1.3-6 Gradual replacement of slowly resorbing ceramic cement. Cracks of mechanical origin permit bone ingrowth into the otherwise compact apatite cement (Courtesy Armando Gisep, PhD, AO Research Institute Davos).

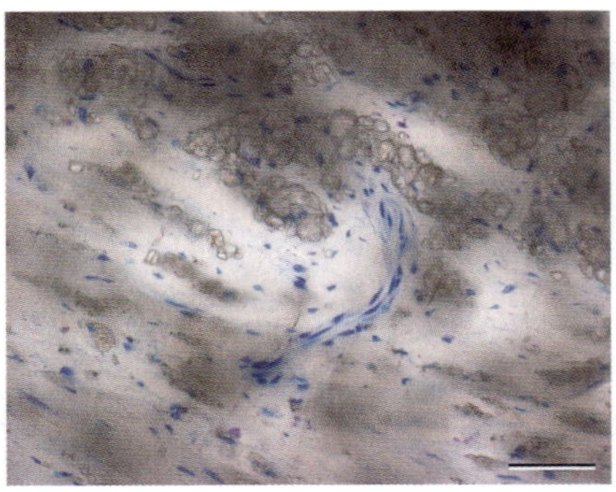

Fig 1.3-7 Crystallites of resorbing ceramic cement in soft tissues. The presence of capillaries and fibroblasts/fibrocytes in close vicinity to the ceramic crystallites, and the absence of inflammatory cells give evidence of an excellent biocompatibility of the resorption products (courtesy Armando Gisep, PhD, AO Research Institute Davos).

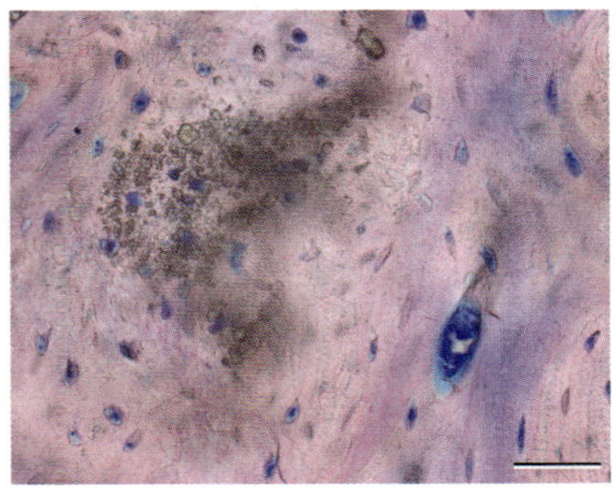

Fig 1.3-8 Crystallites incorporated into bone. Newly formed bone has grown around the remnants of the resorbed ceramic cement, making them a part of a ceramic-bone composite (courtesy Armando Gisep, PhD, AO Research Institute, Davos, Switzerland).

5 New trends

While most CaP ceramic bone substitutes are sold as granules or beads, in the range of 0.5–5 mm in diameter, recently new formulations such as CPCs (see section 4) and putties (= nonhardening pastes) have been introduced [Bohner, 2010]. These new formulations offer better handling but are more expensive compared with granules. Also, most CPCs and some putties possess a slow resorption rate. Despite the fact that putties do not harden, putties seem to be more successful commercially than CPCs, possibly due to their handling characteristics, lower cost, and resorption properties.

A third trend beside the development of CPCs and putties in the field of ceramic bone graft substitutes is the appearance of so-called ion-substituted CaPs. Since it is easy to replace calcium or phosphate ions present in the crystallographic structure of CaP ceramics by foreign ions, the use of CaP ceramics as delivery system for biologically active ions has been tried [Habibovic et al, 2011; Bohner, 2009]. A long list of ions, such as Si or Sr ions, have been proposed and used. Currently, there is no scientific evidence demonstrating that the link between the release of these ions correlates with an improved biological response [Bohner, 2009].

Several companies have claimed that their product is osteoinductive, ie, that it induces bone formation in an ectopic site (eg, in a muscle or subcutaneously). Some companies have even claimed equivalence between their material and a BMP-2 loaded product [Yuan et al, 2010]. While evidence has shown that such osteoinductive CaPs are more effective in orthotopic locations [Yuan et al, 2010] compared with less osteoinductive materials; all materials can be osteoinductive and ectopic bone formation has also been observed in polymers and metal [Barradas et al, 2011], as a function of implantation time. The postulated mechanisms proposed to explain ectopic bone formation [Barradas et al, 2011] do not explain the currently published data (explanations include the release of Ca and phosphate ions or the activation of macrophages via the release of microparticles (diameter $< 5\ \mu m$) [Le Nihouannen et al, 2005].

In conclusion, ceramics, and among them CaPs, are the most potent synthetic bone graft substitute materials. Over the last 40 years, numerous commercial formulations have been launched and used. However, further improvements are desirable, such as ceramic handling characteristics (eg, ready-to-use injectable pastes and cements) and especially in the in vivo response (eg, osteoinductivity).

6 References and suggested reading

Albee FH. Studies in bone growth: triple calcium phosphate as a stimulus to osteogenesis. *Ann Surg.* 1920 Jan;71(1):32–39.

Bashoor-Zadeh M, Baroud G, Bohner M. Simulation of the in vivo resorption rate of β-tricalcium phosphate bone graft substitutes implanted in a sheep model. *Biomaterials.* 2011 Sep;32(27):6362–6373.

Barradas AM, Yuan H, van Blitterswijk CA, et al. Osteoinductive biomaterials: current knowledge of properties, experimental models and biological mechanisms. *Eur Cell Mater.* 2011 May 15;21:407–429.

Bohner M, Theiss F, Apelt D, et al. Compositional changes of a dicalcium phosphate dihydrate cement after implantation in sheep. *Biomaterials.* 2003 Sep;24(20):3463–3474.

Bohner M. Calcium orthophosphates in medicine: from ceramics to calcium phosphate cements. *Injury.* 2000 Dec;31Suppl(4):D37–47.

Bohner M, Luginbühl R, Reber C, et al. A physical approach to modify the hydraulic reactivity of alpha-tricalcium phosphate powder. *Acta Biomater.* 2009 Nov;5(9):3524–3535.

Bohner M, Brunner TJ, Stark WJ. Controlling the reactivity of calcium phosphatecements. *J Mater Chem.* 2008;18(46):5669–5675.

Bohner M, Gbureck U, Barralet JE. Technological issues for the development of more efficient calcium phosphate bone cements: a critical assessment. *Biomaterials.* 2005 Nov;26(33):6423–6429.

Bohner M, Lemaître J. Can bioactivity be tested in vitro with SBF solution? *Biomaterials.* 2009 Apr;30(12):2175–2179.

Bohner M. Design of ceramic-based cements and putties for bone graft substitution. *Eur Cell Mater.* 2010 Jul 1;20:1–12.

Bohner M. Silicon-substituted calcium phosphates—a critical view. *Biomaterials.* 2009 Nov;30(32):6403–6406.

Brown WE, Chow LC. A new calcium phosphate setting cement. *J Dent Res.* 1983;62:672.

Constantz BR, Barr BM, Ison IC, et al. Histological, chemical, and crystallographic analysis of four calcium phosphate cements in different rabbit osseous sites. *J Biomed Mater Res.* 1998;43(4):451–461.

Dreesman H. [Ueber Knochenplombierung.] *Beitr Klin Chir.* 1892;9:804–810. German.

Driessens FCM, Verbeeck RMH. Relation between physicochemical solubility and biodegradability of calcium phosphates. In: Implant materials in biofunction. Proceedings of the Seventh European Conference on Biomaterials: September 8–11, 1987; Amsterdam, The Netherlands.

Elliott JC, ed. Structure and chemistry of the apatites and other calcium orthophosphates. In: *Studies in Inorganic Chemistry.* Amsterdam: Elsevier; 1994:1–389.

Eidelman N, Chow LC, Brown WE. Calcium phosphate saturation levels in ultrafiltered serum. *Calcif Tissue Int.* 1987 Feb;40(2):71–78.

Frankenburg EP, Goldstein SA, Bauer TW, et al. Biomechanical and histological evaluation of a calcium phosphate cement. *J Bone Joint Surg Am.* 1998 Aug;80(8):1112–1124.

Gbureck U, Hölzel T, Klammert U, et al. Resorbable dicalcium phosphate bone substitutes prepared by 3D powder printing. *Adv Funct Mater.* 2007 Dec;17(18):3940–3945.

Gisep A, Wieling R, Bohner M, et al. Resorption patterns of calcium-phosphate cements in bone. *J Biomed Mater Res.* 2003 Sep 1;66(3):532–540.

Gisep A, Kugler S, Wahl D, et al. Mechanical characterisation of a bone defect model filled with ceramic cements. *J Mater Sci Mater Med.* 2004 Oct;15(10):1065–1071.

Habibovic P, Barralet JE. Bioinorganics and biomaterials: bone repair. *Acta Biomater.* 2011 Aug;7(8):3013–3026.

Kanatani M, Sugimoto T, Fukase M, et al. Effect of elevated extracellular calcium on the proliferation of osteoblastic MC3T3-E1 cells: its direct and indirect effects via monocytes. *Biochem Biophys Res Commun.* 1991 Dec;181(3):1425–1430.

Kurashina K, Kurita H, Kotani A, et al. In vivo study of a calcium phosphate cement consisting of alpha-tricalcium phosphate/dicalcium phosphate dibasic/tetracalcium phosphate monoxide. *Biomaterials.* 1997 Jan;18(2):147–151.

LeGeros RZ, Chohayeb A, Shulman A. Apatitic calcium phosphates: possible dental restorative materials. *J Dent Res.* 1982 Mar;61(Suppl:1);343.

Le Nihouannen D, Daculsi G, Saffarzadeh A, et al. Ectopic bone formation by microporous calcium phosphate ceramic particles in sheep muscles. *Bone.* 2005 Jun;36(6):1086–1093.

Linhart W, Briem D, Amling M, et al. [Mechanical failure of porous hydroxyapatite ceramics 7.5 years after implantation in the proximal tibial]. *Unfallchirurg.* 2004 Feb;107(2):154–157. German.

Merten HA, Wiltfang J, Grohmann U, et al. Intraindividual comparative animal study of alpha- and beta-tricalcium phosphate degradation in conjunction with simultaneous insertion of dental implants. *J Craniofac Surg.* 2001 Jan;12(1):59–68.

Meleti Z, Shapiro IM, Adams CS. Inorganic phosphate induces apoptosis of osteoblast-like cells in culture. *Bone.* 2000 Sep;27(3):359–366.

Monma H, Kanazawa T. The hydration of α-tricalcium phosphate. *Yogyo-Kyokai-Shi.* 1976;84(4):209–213.

Monma H, Kanazawa T. Hydration of α-tricalcium phosphate. *J Ceram Soc Jpn.* 2000;108:575–580.

Suzuki O, Kamakura S, Katagiri T, et al. Bone formation enhanced by implanted octacalcium phosphate involving conversion into Ca-deficient hydroxyapatite. *Biomaterials.* 2006 May;27(13):2671–2681.

Silver IA, Murrills RJ, Etherington DJ. Microelectrode studies on the acid microenvironment beneath adherent macrophages and osteoclasts. *Exp Cells Res.* 1988 Apr;175(2):266–276.

Vereecke G, Lemaître J. Calculations of the solubility diagrams in the system Ca(OH)2-H3PO4-KOH-HNO3-CO2-H2O. *J Crystal Growth.* 1990;104(4):820–832.

Wu X, Itoh N, Taniguchi T, et al. Requirement of calcium and phosphate ions in expression of sodium-dependent vitamin C transporter 2 and osteopontin in MC3T3-E1 osteoblastic cells. *Biochim Biophys Acta.* 2003 Jun;1641(1):65–70.

Yuan H, Fernandes H, Habibovic P, et al. Osteoinductive ceramics as a synthetic alternative to autologous bone grafting. *Proc Natl Acad Sci USA.* 2010 Aug 3;107(31):13614–13619.

Zaidi M, Datta HK, Patchell A, et al. 'Calcium-activated' intracellular calcium elevation: a novel mechanism of osteoclast regulation. *Biochem Biophys Res Commun.* 1989 Sep;163(3):1461–1465.

1.4 Growth factors for craniomaxillofacial applications

Martin Stoddart, Geoff Richards

1 Introduction

The natural process of bone repair and regeneration is macroscopically divided into three phases: (1) the inflammatory phase, (2) the repair phase; (3) the remodeling phase (**Fig 1.4-1**). Each of these phases is recognized with microscopic evaluation of histological sections. All phases depend upon a carefully coordinated sequence of events controlled by growth factors and the cells they attract. Failure of early recruitment and differentiation of cells into the defect leads to a delay in healing, or in the worst case, a nonunion. Nonunions are commonly associated with infection, poor reduction, or poor mechanical stability, such as incorrect use of implants generate too much motion and increased interfragmentary strain. Healing is also impaired by biological disease processes, such as diabetes and the nicotine from smoking. The critical initial event is the development of a functional vascular supply that provides nutritional exchange and an access route by which mesenchymal stromal cells and the hematopoietic stem cells, required for healing, gain access to the defect.

Bone healing can be direct or indirect and this depends greatly on the mechanical environment to which the cells are exposed [Rahn, 1987].

Indirect bone healing occurs when the initial hematoma is replaced within the first week by fibrous granulation tissue and subsequently a fibrocartilaginous template. Mesenchymal stem cells proliferate and migrate through callus, differentiating into fibroblasts and chondrocytes producing an extracellular matrix. After the fracture ends are linked by soft callus at 2–3 weeks, the template is invaded by blood vessels, calcifies, and the hard callus stage begins and lasts until the fragment ends are firmly united by new bone at 3–4 months. This occurs through a process of endochondral ossification, converting the callus to woven bone. It begins from fragment ends and progresses to the center, forming a bony callus sponge (ie, woven immature bone). The remodeling period begins when there is no further interfragmentary motion. The woven bone is slowly replaced by lamellar bone through surface erosion and osteonal remodeling, which may take a few months to years depending upon the bone and patient. The surfaces of resorption spaces are covered with lamellar bone, thereby forming new bone trabeculae. Further bone deposition combined with local resorption leads to a reshaping of those trabeculae and lasts until the bone has returned to its original morphology. Healing in trabecular bone occurs without the formation of significant external callus. After the inflammatory stage, bone formation is dominated by intramembranous ossification, which is attributed

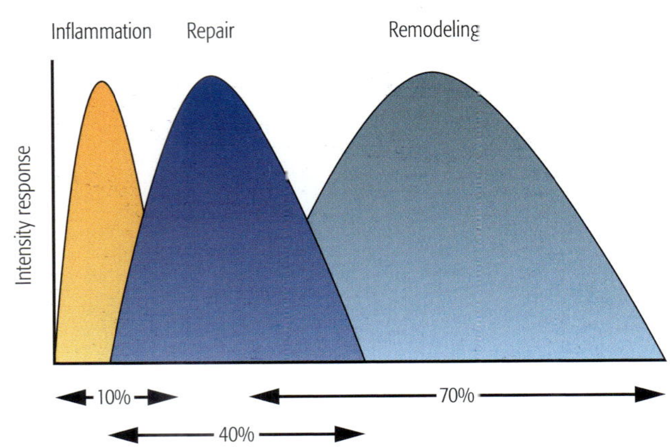

Fig 1.4-1 The three main phases in bone healing after fracture. The approximate duration of the response is set against the activity of that particular phase. The time taken for each phase varies for pediatric and geriatric patients, and is different for various craniomaxillocial bones. The mechanical environment will also modify the duration of each phase. Additionally, each of these phases is stringently controlled by the balance of growth factor concentrations within the cellular microenvironment, and as such can be modified by the application of growth factors or inhibition of their signaling pathways.

to tremendous angiogenic potential. It has been proposed that the delayed healing seen in patients with diabetes is a result of increased sensitivity to tumor necrosis factor-α leading to increased FOX01 transcription factor mediated apoptosis. This would negatively affect the production and remodeling of the cartilaginous template.

Direct bone healing occurs in a mechanically rigid defect where there is anatomical alignment of the fracture ends. Initially, it occurs through resorption (temporary phase of reduced density) followed by the slow deposition of laminar bone through intramembranous ossification. The "cutter head" is responsible for intracortical remodeling. A group of osteoclasts resorb a canal into the compact bone; they are located in scalloped concavities at the head of the cutter cones at the bone surface and release H+ ions that maintain a low pH of 3.5 that dissolves the bone mineral. They also secrete proteolytic enzymes to remove the organic phase of the bone matrix. This process is followed by a group of osteoblasts that are again arranged in a conical shape that enter this canal to slowly refill it with lamellar bone. The intracortical remodeling cannot take place without previous resorption of the bone. The cutter cones cross the fracture zone from each direction and establish new osteons behind. For more details on direct/indirect bone healing refer to *Bone in Clinical Orthopedics* [Rahn, 2002]. Differences in the healing process are in part due to the growth factor environment to which the cells are exposed. The cells themselves play a role in conditioning the microenvironment and this can be a direct result of the mechanical forces applied to the cells. Mechanical forces modify the cellular response leading to a sequential cascade of events and ultimately bone healing.

The repair of large craniomaxillofacial (CMF) bone defects presents unique challenges. As bone regeneration is most commonly associated with mechanical strength, it is often strength and mechanical stability that are primary outcome measurements used to assess the quality of bone repair. However, during the repair of CMF defects, form is as critical as function to maintain the appearance and psychological health of the patient.

Current approaches for the replacement of large CMF bone defects rely heavily on bone transplantation techniques, either autograft or allograft. Both tissue sources have potential drawbacks due to the limited availability of bone tissue. In the case of autogenous tissue, there is the added problem of morbidity, including pain and potential for infection at the harvest site. For allograft tissue, there are additional ethical considerations along with the risks of immunological rejection, disease transmission, and lesser potential for survival as efficient replacement.

To improve the outcomes, tissue-engineering approaches are gaining interest. A number of approaches are currently available and each relies to varying extents on osteoconduction and osteoinduction. Osteoconductive scaffolds allow for the differentiation of invading progenitor cells into osteoblasts. Osteoinduction involves direct stimulation of invading osteoprogenitor cells to differentiate into osteoblasts, so that new bone formation begins. The most widely studied type of osteoinductive molecules are bone morphogenetic proteins (BMPs). In summary, their properties have led to the development of a new field of orthobiologics which is developing novel biological approaches to bone repair and regeneration.

The most simple tissue-engineering approach is the use of bone substitutes as a bulking/filling agent to provide a rapid off-the-shelf solution for a large CMF bone defect to be used in combination with implants for mechanical support. Osteoconductive fillers like β-tricalcium phosphate have been used widely with some degree of success, yet more effective methods are still sought. This has led to a greater investigation into how grafts can be combined with biological factors to enable a more rapid repair of a bony defect or more rapid integration of an implanted material with the host bone. One option is the addition of autogenous cells, commonly stem cells, either freshly isolated or monolayer expanded. This increases complexity and the issues regarding good manufacturing practices lead to a large increase in associated costs. A cell-based therapy is also considered to be more of a patient-specific medicine approach, and for some extreme cases it may be the ideal solution. However, an attractive alternative is the off-the-shelf option, which can be routinely used as is currently the case with acellular bone substitutes.

2 Growth factors: an overview

One biological approach which allows for an off-the-shelf solution is the use of growth factors, with the goal of improving the endogenous response. Bone induction is a sequential multistep cascade whose key steps are chemotaxis, mitosis, and differentiation. Growth factors can be used to enhance each of these steps and some factors affect multiple steps. The remainder of this chapter covers the various growth factors under consideration and their biological mode of action. Only a few growth factors are approved for clinical use including BMP-2, BMP-7, and plate-derived growth factor (PDGF).

A number of growth factors have been investigated preclinically for their ability to modify cellular responses within the musculoskeletal system. **Table 1.4-1** gives a summary of those most commonly investigated factors and their roles. Often, the same factor is postulated to be beneficial for bone as well as cartilage. This dual utility for both tissues suggests that the actual cellular response to a particular growth factor depends on the local milieu of signals from other cells as well as matrix adhesions, and is a balance of the numerous factors present in a particular tissue. As bone often develops through a process of endochondral ossification, it is also likely that any factor which leads to the formation of a cartilaginous template will also be effective in repairing bone defects by this mechanism.

2.1 Platelet-rich plasma

An easily accessible source of growth factors for biological stimulation has been platelet-rich plasma (PRP). Numerous growth factors are available in autogenous form in PRP with few problems associated with the harvest of the blood used to prepare the PRP. Devices are now available which are able to produce PRP relatively quickly within the operating room, and the application of PRP has become widespread and used for multiple indications. The growth factors known to be present within PRP include PDGF, transforming growth factor-β (TGF-β), fibroblast growth factor, insulin-like growth factor 1 and 2, vascular endothelial growth factor, epidermal growth factor, and connective tissue growth factor. While all these factors are invariably present, their absolute amounts vary greatly. Donor variation and the exact preparation method used lead to the differences. The variation in the final product has also made the determination of efficacy and indications difficult. Although the use of PRP has become common, its effectiveness is still debated and its exact effects are still unclear. The differences seen are likely to be due to a difference in preparation, final platelet count, indication, and surgical technique. These confounding factors are further complicated by the various platelet-rich preparations being investigated. In addition to PRP, there are autogenous growth factor concentrates that also contain the buffy coat and PRGF that can be used in liquid or gel form. The exact activation mechanism, degree of concentration, and site of implantation will each have an effect on the result. This level of variability has made the determination of mechanism and effectiveness impossible.

While it is generally accepted that platelet-rich preparations may have beneficial effects for soft-tissue injuries, such as tendon, its effects on bone regeneration are not as clear. It has been suggested that too high a concentration of platelets (more than a 2.5x concentrate) may actually be inhibitory for osteoblast proliferation and function in vitro [Graziani et al, 2006]. While several clinical studies have demonstrated a clinical benefit of PRP, other studies have shown no effect or an inhibitory effect. It has been shown that in lumbar intertransverse fusion, the addition of autogenous growth factor to the autogenous bone graft led to a reduced fusion rate [Weiner et al, 2003].

Growth factor	Function
Transforming growth factor-β	Recruits progenitor cells. Differentiation into chondroblast and osteoblast lineages. Inhibits later stages of osteoblast development.
Bone morphogenetic proteins	Differentiation into chondroblast and osteoblast lineages.
Vascular endothelial growth factor	Recruitment and differentiation of endothelial cells. Promotes angiogenesis and vasculogenesis. Stabilization of blood vessels.
Fibroblast growth factor	Mitogen. Important in early granulation tissue formation. Enhanced angiogenesis.
Platelet-derived growth factor	Mitogen. Recruitment of progenitor cells. Promotes angiogenesis.

Table 1.4-1 Summary of the main functions of growth factors known to modulate bone regeneration.

There have also been suggestions of adverse effects based on supraphysiological doses of growth factors found within the preparations. Although completely autogenous, reported adverse effects include pain (normally associated with the injection site when being used to treat inflammatory soft-tissue injuries), infection, worsening of symptoms, blood clots, nerve injury, skin discoloration, calcification, scarring, and allergic reaction.

2.2 Transmission of growth factor signal

Due to numerous different growth factors and their isoforms, detailing the specific pathways used by each individual growth factor is beyond the scope of this chapter; however, a general mode of action is summarized in **Table 1.4-1** and there are similarities in their mode of action. Often one growth factor is able to bind multiple transmembrane receptors, each of which leads to a different response. Alternatively, multiple factors may compete for the same receptor, again leading to a modulation of the response. In many cases, binding of the growth factor leads to receptor dimerization, whereby the receptors are held in physical proximity and form a complex which is required for activation. The activation of a receptor commonly leads to receptor phosphorylation and subsequent phosphorylation of downstream proteins to increase their activity. The receptors may form homodimers or heterodimers, and the response generated will be dependent on the type of interaction formed. The activation of receptors initiates a signal cascade to amplify the signal and to provide multiple steps at which the signal can be modified or potentially blocked. Ultimately, intracellular proteins which interact with gene promoter sequences will be activated to change gene transcription activity, and hence the phenotype of the cell.

Further complexity is added as the response of each factor is modulated by the local milieu and the other factors that are present. Thus, application of a particular growth factor may lead to one response when applied in isolation but a different response may be seen if it is applied in combination therapy or if other factors are present in the environment at the time of application. These clinically relevant issues imply caution in the use of growth factors, especially where cofactors are required to produce the desired response. Each pathway produces part of the activation signals required; if any of the pathways are not activated due to lack of ligand or are attenuated, the response is not observed. Local conditions, such as the presence of inflammatory factors, may have large consequences on the effect of the growth factor applied, and yet these areas have been largely unexplored.

2.3 Species differences

The effects of various growth factors vary with the species used for the preclinical studies. It has been demonstrated that rhBMP2 has an osteoinductive effect and leads to an increase in alkaline phosphatase expression on bone marrow-derived stem cells of rodent origin. rhBMP-2 does not have the same effect on human cells, which do not respond in the same manner [Osyczka et al, 2004]. Human cells are more responsive to rhBMP-6 [Friedman et al, 2006]. This raises the question: how does rhBMP-2 function in the clinical setting? The answer is not clear. rhBMP-2 is known to have an angiogenic effect, and this may be partly responsible for the increased bone formation. Critical issues arise when translating preclinical studies into the clinical setting: do they behave in a similar manner on human and animal cells? How is the dosage controlled relative to size, ie, if 1 mg is required for a 1 mm defect in rats, how much is required for a 3 cm defect in humans? The efficacy of any growth factor is likely to be dependent on the species used. Consider these possible differences when translating the use of these factors into human clinical applications. Other BMP proteins, such as rhBMP-6, may obtain a similar bone-forming response at lower doses, an issue relevant in clinical practice.

3 Transforming growth factor-β superfamily

The transforming growth factor beta (TGF-β) superfamily is a large family of structurally related cell regulatory proteins that have been extensively investigated for their ability to modulate the development of cartilage and bone. The TGF-β superfamily consists of the TGF-β subfamily, the decapentaplegic-Vg-related subfamily (including the bone morphogenetic proteins and the growth differentiation factors), and the activin/inhibin subfamily, a group encompassing various divergent members, such as Nodal and Lefty. Ligands of the TGF- β superfamily form dimers that bind to heterodimeric receptor complexes consisting of type I and type II receptor subunits containing serine/threonine kinase domains.

3.1 Transforming growth factor-βs

The TGF-βs bind to higher affinity type II receptors, leading to recruitment of the lower affinity type I receptor. This physical interaction of the two receptor types is crucial in generating a downstream signaling response and determining which outcome is observed. Following ligand binding, the type II receptor phosphorylates and activates the type I receptor, initiating a SMAD-dependent signaling cascade

(SMADs are the human homologues of the Drosophila Mothers against decapentaplegic genes that control developmental patterning) that induces or represses transcriptional activity. Various TGF-βs and their receptors activate different SMAD pathways. The TGF-β is known to exist in three different isoforms in humans TGF-β1, 2, and 3, and each is synthesized as a latent precursor molecule containing a propeptide that requires cleavage for activation. The differences in functions between these isoforms are not clear but interesting insights can be seen in expression patterns found in cranial sutures. The TGF-β1, β2, and β3 all use the same cell surface receptors yet have differing effects on suture patency and cell proliferation. It has been proposed that TGF-β2 induces suture closure through phosphorylation of extracellular-signal-regulated kinases 1 and 2 (Erk1/2-intracellular molecules that are responsible for transmitting extracellular signals into an intracellular response by way of protein kinase intracellular signaling). The TGF-β3 has been shown to downregulate expression of TGFBR1 that would reduce its availability for all TGF-βs, in particular TGF-β2 that would lead to reduced suture fusion. The balance between stabilizing suture signals TGF-β1, TGF-β3, and TGF-β2, which promotes the recruitment of osteoblasts and osteogenesis at the bone fronts, is essential for normal suture morphogenesis.

However, TGF-β3 has been shown to have potent bone-forming capabilities in osteoconductive scaffolds in ectopic and orthotopic sites in nonhuman primates by way of endochondral ossification, a result not seen in rodents [Ripamonti, 2006]. These differences again highlight the role of species and site-specific responses caused by the local microenvironments in the final result obtained. The TGF-β3 has also shown promise in periodontal tissue regeneration in nonhuman primates [Teare et al, 2008].

3.2 Bone morphogenetic proteins

Bone morphogenetic proteins were initially identified by the pioneering work of Marshall Urist in the mid-1960s when he discovered demineralized bone contained a protein that was osteoinductive. While BMPs were initially discovered due to their ability to induce the formation of bone and cartilage, they are known to modulate many developmental processes. There are currently 20 known BMPs, most of which are members of the TGF-β superfamily (BMP-1 is a metalloproteinase) and were originally isolated from demineralized bone matrix.

Despite their well-established propensity to induce robust bone formation, only two, BMP-2 and BMP-7/ OP-1, are clinically available. Members of the BMP family bind to high-affinity type I receptors and then recruit low-affinity type II kinase receptors. The kinase domains of type II receptors are constitutively active, and upon ligand binding they phosphorylate Gly-Ser domains in the type I receptors. This process leads to the activation of type I receptors and a transmission of the signal to intracellular signaling molecules. The specificity of the intracellular signals is mostly determined by type I receptors. The BMPs bind to three distinct type II receptors: BMP type II receptor (BMPR-II), activin type II receptor (ActR-II) and activin type IIB receptors (ActR-IIB). There are also three type I BMP receptors: activin receptor-like kinase 2 (ALK-2), BMP receptor 1A (BMPR1A/ ALK-3), and BMP receptor 1B (BMPR1B/ ALK-6) which phosphorylate SMAD 1/5/8 (see below). Activation of BMP signaling leads to transcription of a number of osteoblast-specific genes leading to osteogenic differentiation.

The BMP types I and II receptors are also present on human endothelial cells. The BMP-2 induces endothelial cell proliferation and tube formation but not migration. This suggests that BMP-2 is able to enhance angiogenesis, playing a role in enhanced osteogenic response observed.

The BMPs are known to be modulated by numerous factors including noggin, Nell 1 and Sclerostin (also known as SOST). Each of these factors is interesting for its ability to modify or enhance the osteogenic response. Sclerostin in particular is known to modulate signaling and be antagonistic to bone formation. This has led to the development of antisclerostin antibodies which are currently being investigated for their effect on inhibiting osteoporosis.

3.3 SMAD signaling

The SMADs are the human homologues of the drosophila Mothers against decapentaplegic genes that are involved in developmental patterning. Upon binding of a member of the TGF-β superfamily, SMAD signaling is activated. There are three classes of SMAD: the receptor-regulated SMADs (R-SMAD), the common-mediator SMAD (co-SMAD), and the antagonistic or inhibitory SMADs (I-SMAD). The balance of signals between the TGF-β family ligands and subsequent downstream SMAD signals tightly regulates osteochondral differentiation and maintenance. Of the eight known SMAD proteins, SMAD1, SMAD5, and SMAD8 are R-SMADs activated by type I BMP receptors, whereas SMAD2 and SMAD3 are activated by activin and TGF-β type I receptors. SMAD4 is a co-SMAD shared by both BMP and TGF-β/activin signaling pathways. SMAD6 acts as a negative regulator of TGF-β signaling both in the cytoplasm and in the nucleus. SMAD7 is a TGF-β type 1 receptor antagonist which blocks both BMP and TGF-β signaling. It forms a complex with the type I receptors, preventing access of downstream signaling SMADS (**Fig 1.4-2**; **Table 1.4-2**).

The balance between SMAD 1/5/8 and SMAD 2/3 activation plays a major role in the endochondral ossification process. While the activation of both pathways is believed to be a requirement for the initiation of chondrogenesis, inhibition of SMAD 1/5/8 phosphorylation (hence, inhibition of BMP signaling through ALK-2,-3,-6) has been shown to prevent termination differentiation and hypertrophy [Hellingman et al, 2011], leading to reduced deposition of calcified tissue and delayed bone healing.

4 Clinically available growth factors

Of many growth factors investigated within the laboratory setting, few have been developed to a standard where they are approved for clinical use. The US Food and Drug Administration (FDA) has approved the use of two recombinant BMPs, rhBMP-2, and rhBMP-7 (rhBMPs-recombinant proteins are produced from cloned DNA sequences, allowing for ease of production and purification) for well-defined medical conditions in limited patient populations. Both are approved for limited clinical applications but have grown

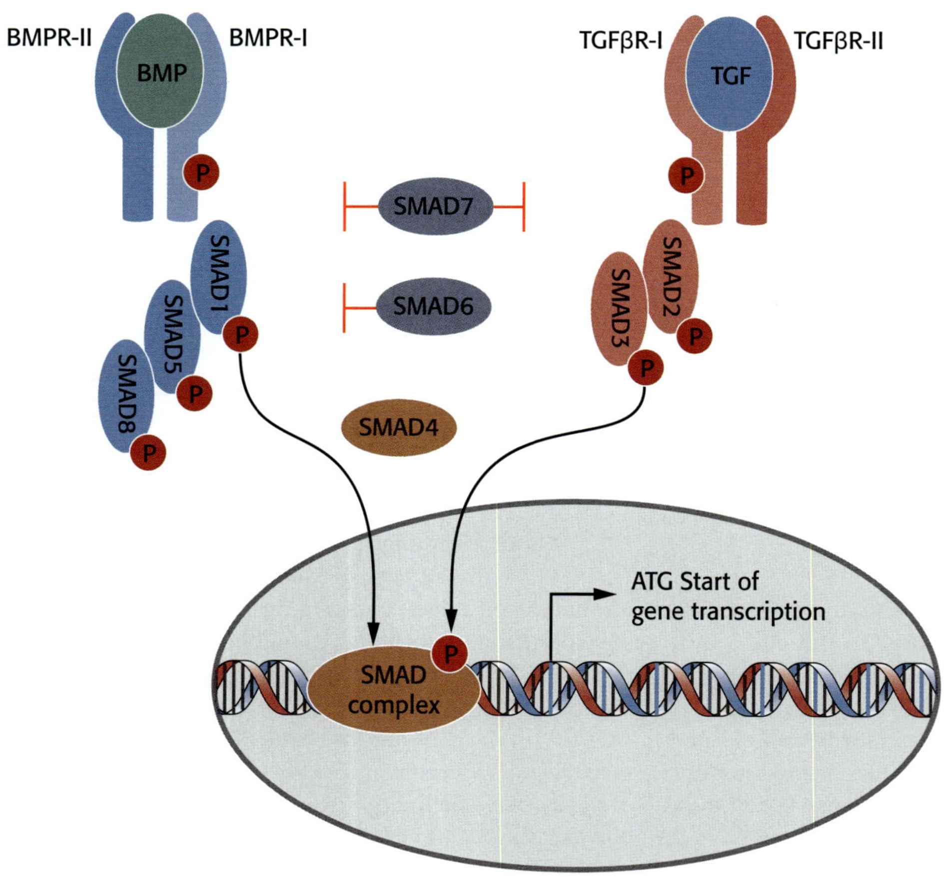

Fig 1.4-2 Transforming growth factor-β (TGF-β) superfamily signals are transmitted via activation receptors I and II complexes upon ligand binding. The bone morphogenetic protein (BMP) signals are mediated through SMAD 1, 5, 8 while TGF-β are mediated through SMAD 2, 3. Both SMAD complexes combine with SAMD4 co-SMAD and translocate to the nucleus where gene transcription is activated. The signals can be prevented by activation of SMAD6 (BMP signals only) or SMAD7 (both BMP and TGF-β signals). Proteins are activated by phosphorylation (P).

in "off-label" use, especially in the case of rhBMP-2. rhBMP-2 is available, impregnated into a bovine collagen I scaffold, while rhBMP-7 is used in the form of a putty for posterolateral fusion of the lumbar spine.

4.1 Recombinant BMP-2

Recombinant BMP-2 has received premarket FDA approval for fusion of the lumbar spine in skeletally mature patients with degenerative disc disease at one level from L2-S1. It also has FDA approval for the healing of acute, open tibial shaft fractures stabilized with an intramedullary nail and treated within 14 days of the initial injury. rhBMP-2 is also approved for certain oral and maxillofacial uses. Recombinant BMP-2 is indicated as an alternative to autogenous bone graft for sinus augmentations and for localized alveolar ridge augmentations for defects associated with extraction sockets. The efficacy of rhBMP-2 in CMF applications is still to be determined.

4.2 Recombinant BMP-7

Recombinant BMP-7 (rhBMP-7, referred to as OP-1 and contained in OP-1 Implant and OP-1 Putty) has received humanitarian device exemption approval as an alternative to autograft in difficult-to-manage long-bone nonunions where use of autograft is not feasible and alternative treatments have failed. It is also approved as an alternative to autograft in compromised patients requiring revision posterolateral (intertransverse) lumbar spinal fusion for patients where autogenous bone and bone marrow harvest are not feasible or are not expected to promote fusion. Examples of compromising factors include osteoporosis, smoking, and diabetes. While not approved for CMF applications, rhBMP-7 is considered investigational when used as an alternative or adjuvant to bone grafting procedures during CMF surgeries.

Both rhBMPs are contraindicated for all uses in patients who are skeletally immature (younger than 18 years) or pregnant, and in those with a known hypersensitivity to the specific rhBMP, bovine type 1 collagen or to other components of the formulations.

Recombinant human platelet-derived growth factor-BB (rhPDGF-BB) has been approved for periodontal-related defects, such as intrabony periodontal defects, furcation periodontal defects, and gingival recession associated with periodontal defects. It is sold as a completely synthetic grafting system for bone and periodontal regeneration composed of rhPDGF-BB and a synthetic calcium phosphate matrix.

A major issue in the use of these factors is the control of their effects to guide healing while eliminating unwanted adverse effects. The use of these factors has not been without complications, in particular those associated with rhBMP-2. This factor has been shown to lead to multiple complications and in some cases the reported complication rate has been as high as 40%.

4.3 Adverse effects

The clinical use of growth factors has not been without controversy. Experience has, with the use of these factors, revealed adverse effects that were not apparent at the time of approval. rhBMP-2 in particular has produced a number of complications, some of which are life-threatening: nerve damage, swelling, ectopic bone formation, retrograde ejaculation, and cancer. A warning was issued by the FDA on July 1, 2008 (FDA Public Health Notification: Life-threatening Complications Associated with Recombinant Human Bone Morphogenetic Protein in Cervical Spine Fusion [FDA, 2008]) and some practitioners question their continued use.

TGF-β superfamily ligand	Type I receptor	Type II receptor	R-SMADs
Activin A	ACVR1B (ALK4)	ACVR2A	SMAD2, SMAD3
BMPs	ACVR1 (ALK2) BMPR1A (ALK3), BMPR1B (ALK6)	BMPR2	SMAD1 SMAD5, SMAD8
GDF-5	BMPR1B (ALK6)	BMPR2	SMAD1 SMAD5, SMAD8
TGF-βs	TGFβRI (ALK5)	TGFβRII	SMAD2, SMAD3

Table 1.4-2 Details of the receptors and SMAD molecules used by the various TGF-β superfamily involved in bone repair.*

*Each factor uses SMAD4 as a coSMAD. SMADs are the human homologues of the drosophila Mothers against decapentaplegic genes that control developmental patterning; TGF-β indicates transforming growth factor-β; ACVR, activin A receptor; ALK, activin receptor-like kinase; BMP, bone morphogenetic protein; and GDF, growth differentiation factor.

In 2011 a controversial review detailed a number of problems associated with rhBMP-2 use [Carragee et al, 2011]. It was claimed that surgical technique played a role in the discrepancies but the general belief is that the supraphysiological dose is the cause of the complications. It is clear that the application of rhBMPs for bone regeneration still needs further research to identify its mode of action and the cause of the adverse effects. The most prevalent adverse effect is ectopic bone formation in the tissues surrounding the defect. It has been proposed that rhBMP-2 has the potential to induce endothelial cells to become osteoblasts via a mesenchymal intermediate [Medici et al, 2012]; however, the frequency of occurrence and the exact mechanisms are not known.

In fibrodysplasia ossificans progressiva there is a tendency for muscle to ossify and become bone. This is known to be caused by a constitutively active mutation within the gene for activin receptor type 1 (also known as activin-like kinase 2) which is a BMP type-1 receptor. This may also be the underlying mechanism by which ectopic bone formation occurs during the application of rhBMP-2 in clinical situations.

5 New horizons: other factors of interest

5.1 Delivery mechanism

Potentially, the most critical aspect in the use of growth factors is how and when they are applied. Growth factors function in combination with other factors, eg, the concentration in relation to the other factors within the cellular microenvironment modifies the response obtained. Therefore, the delivery system used directly effects the required response. Different delivery systems can lead to different durations and doses of exposure (**Fig 1.4-3**). In many cases, the half-life of growth factors in vivo is measured in minutes. For example, in vivo studies have shown that rhBMP-2 has a half-life of 7–16 minutes when injected systemically, and up to 8 days locally when implanted on a collagen sponge. This may account for supraphysiological concentrations of factors in the clinical environment. Applying a physiologically relevant dose in a certain way means it will only be available for a short period at the critical level.

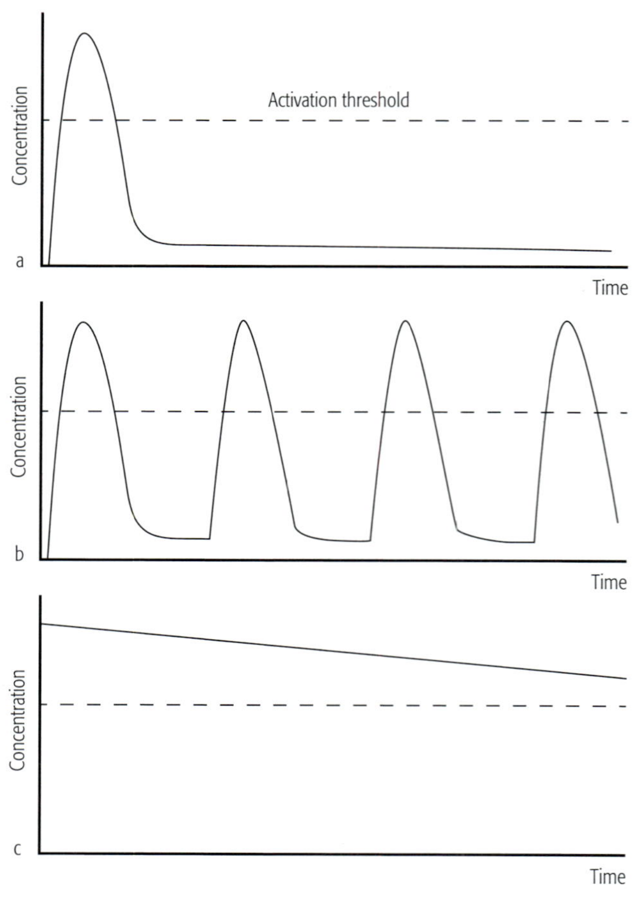

Fig 1.4-3a–c Release characteristics showing concentration over time in relation to the threshold required to obtain a response.
- **a** Classic burst release where all the growth factor is rapidly released and cleared.
- **b** Repeated administration of the same factor applied in **a**. Multiple peaks of availability are seen, which rapidly drop below threshold levels.
- **c** A sustained release system that enables levels to be maintained above threshold levels. In each of the three cases, the peak concentration achieved is similar, yet the response obtained is varied.

The cellular response obtained requires that the activation threshold is reached and then maintained for a sufficient duration to induce the required change. In the absence of a suitable slow-release carrier system, a "burst" release followed by a subactivation concentration is observed. In cases where multiple doses are applied, this results in temporal peaks of extremely high concentration followed by longer periods where no additional factor is present. In the case where a threshold is required for activation, this may lead to short periods of activation followed by longer periods of inactivity. In some cases, this variation may even lead to a different result than that seen when the factor is constantly above the threshold level. This can be seen in the action of parathyroid hormone which exhibits differential effects depending on intermittent versus continuous elevation in serum. Intermittent parathyroid hormone increases bone formation and bone mass and is being investigated as a therapy for osteoporosis, whereas constant parathyroid hormone is associated with bone loss [Lombardi et al, 2011]. An optimum response is obtained when a carrier is able to provide a sustained release of a low dose over long periods. For this reason, lots of work is focusing on the development of release systems able to offer some level of control. For example, 1 mg recombinant protein applied directly is relatively rapidly dispersed, whereas 1 mg recombinant protein in a slow-release hydrogel leads to the tissue being exposed to lower local doses over a longer period. The simplest release systems are those that control the degradation rate, while complex systems are investigating cell-mediated release of factors to release factors only when cells are present to receive the signal.

5.2 Genetically modified proteins

Clinically, growth factors used within the clinic may be improved by genetically modifying a factor to enhance its properties. For example, it may be possible to increase the half-life of the protein, or reduce binding to its inhibitor ligands. These reduce the dose required and potentially reduce adverse effects. They could also be combined with, or incorporated into, novel scaffold systems that allow for a greater control of the release of the factor.

5.3 Vascular endothelial growth factor

The powerful stimulation of angiogenesis by vascular endothelial growth factor has attracted much attention in the field of enhancement of bone repair. While it is able to induce the formation of new vessels, there have been problems associated with dosing and the development of a physiological vascular network. When given in too high a dose, the vessels formed have a tendency to be unstable.

5.4 NEL-like molecule-1

NEL-like molecule-1 is an osteogenic inducer which functions downstream of Runx2 and has been shown to reduce the transcription of early osteogenic regulators while inducing intermediate and late markers of differentiation. Nell-1 has been shown to induce osteogenic differentiation in vitro and increased bone formation in mouse calvarial defects [Aghaloo et al, 2006]. In low dose it enhances the bone-forming potential of low-dose rhBMP-2 in rat calvarial defects compared with low- or high-dose rhBMP-2 alone [Aghaloo et al, 2010]. This may offer a mechanism by which lower doses of rhBMP-2 can be used to provide a more physiological response with fewer adverse effects, but as rhBMP-2 has been shown to behave differently on rat and human cells, this needs to be confirmed with human cells. NEL-like molecule-1 has also been shown to inhibit adipogenesis [James et al, 2011] and in combination with CD146 human perivascular stem cells from adipose tissue has shown promise in forming new bone.

5.5 Blocking strategies

Rather than stimulate pathways using recombinant growth factors, a number of groups are now looking for factors which may be targets for strategies that involve inhibition. Denosumab is a monoclonal antibody against receptor activator of nuclear factor κB-ligand (a key molecule in osteoclastogenesis) that targets biological pathways as a therapy for osteoporosis. This treatment appears to have a similar mechanism of action as bisphosphonates but potentially has greater patient compliance as it is administered by way of subcutaneous injection twice a year. However a condition similar to bisphosphonate-related osteonecrosis of the jaw in denosumab-treated patients has been reported.

5.6 Mechanobiology

The interfragmentary strain applied to a fracture gap is known to play a major role in the final healing outcome. It has been demonstrated that the type of load applied to progenitor cells can modify their cytokine expression profile, including among other things, an upregulation of TGF-β expression. A greater understanding of this process, and mechanisms by which the strain applied to a defect may be accurately controlled, may offer therapies that lead to an enhanced natural healing by way of rehabilitation protocols alone. This would have the potential to greatly reduce costs while at the same time lead to a safer, more natural healing environment.

5.7 Gene therapy

As stated previously, one of the most challenging aspects of the delivery of growth factors is the ability to reliably release a constant low dose over a longer period. In this problem, gene therapy may offer solutions. Viral vectors for gene therapy are broadly divided into integrating and nonintegrating vectors. The integrating vectors, such as retrovirus and lentivirus, are more commonly investigated for chronic diseases such as rheumatoid arthritis where a more sustained release is required over years. As they integrate their DNA into the nucleus of the host cell, there are also some serious safety aspects that are yet to be overcome. For the repair of a traumatic bone defect, shorter-term expression is desirable and adenovirus or adeno-associated virus (AAV) may be more appropriate. Both adenovirus and AAV are nonintegrating viruses, meaning the foreign viral nucleic acids are lost over time, a process more rapid during cell division. Adenovirus infections are most commonly associated with respiratory diseases, whereas there are currently no known diseases caused by AAV, and for this reason AAV has come into particular focus over the last few years. Both viruses have the advantage that they can infect dividing and nondividing cells. To be used for gene therapy applications, viral capsid genes are removed rendering the virus replication deficient. As the technology has matured, further viral genes have been removed. The removal of viral genes has the added advantage of producing space within the viral genome into which foreign genes, such as those encoding for growth factors, can be incorporated. While adenovirus can lead to an inflammatory immune response depending on how many viral genes remain in the vector, AAV has a much reduced immune response making it promising for use in clinical applications. In July 2012, the European Medicines Agency recommended the approval of an AAV gene therapy treatment for the first time. The treatment, Glybera (alipogene tiparvovec), is intended for lipoprotein lipase deficiency in patients with severe or multiple pancreatitis attacks.

The great advantage that gene therapy offers is the ability to produce a sustained low dose over weeks to months. Protocols are being developed to allow for 3-D transduction that would allow for the use of vectors intraoperatively. Thus the levels obtained are more physiological and this will reduce the adverse effects seen when using supraphysiological doses of the recombinant protein. While there is still much work to be done to confirm the safety of viral vectors, the recent successes obtained with this technology suggests it may be on the cusp of becoming more mainstream. Alternatively, there is the option of nonviral vectors, which while more inefficient, are currently considered to be much safer. Tissue-engineering scaffolds which have the vector and gene of interest incorporated into the scaffold itself are being developed as an "off-the-shelf" approach. These systems are devised to allow the release of the vector only when the cells are present to provide a more controlled release that is more effective.

6 The future of growth factors

Growth factors offer undoubted promise for improving fracture repair, regeneration of large bone defects and improving integration of implants with the surrounding live bone. However, for them to become clinically relevant, a more reproducible control of factor release needs to be developed. While growth factors can be used to increase bone formation, it is still unclear in which form they should be applied. Whether it be direct, in a slow-release system or in the form of gene therapy will be dependent on which can overcome the adverse effects most effectively. It is also intriguing to speculate that regulating the strains being applied to the developing tissue might be a mechanism by which the granulation tissue and invading progenitors might be directed to produce their own growth factors.

7 References and suggested reading

Aghaloo T, Cowan CM, Chou YF, et al. Nell-1-induced bone regeneration in calvarial defects. *Am J Pathol*. 2006 Sep;169(3):903–915.

Aghaloo T, Cowan CM, Zhang X, et al. The effect of NELL1 and bone morphogenetic protein-2 on calvarial bone regeneration. *J Oral Maxillofac Surg*. 2010 Feb;68(2):300–308.

Carragee EJ, Hurwitz EL, Weiner BK. A critical review of recombinant human bone morphogenetic protein-2 trials in spinal surgery: emerging safety concerns and lessons learned. *Spine J*. 2011 Jun;11(6):471–491.

Friedman MS, Long MW, Hankenson KD. Osteogenic differentiation of human mesenchymal stem cells is regulated by bone morphogenetic protein-6. *J Cell Biochem*. 2006 Jun;98(3):538–554.

Graziani F, Ivanovski S, Cei S, et al. The in vitro effect of different PRP concentrations on osteoblasts and fibroblasts. *Clin Oral Implants Res*. 2006 Apr;17(2):212–219.

Hellingman CA, Davidson EN, Koevoet W, et al. Smad signaling determines chondrogenic differentiation of bone-marrow-derived mesenchymal stem cells: inhibition of Smad1/5/8P prevents terminal differentiation and calcification. *Tissue Eng*. 2011;Part A 17:1157–1167.

James AW, Pan A, Chiang M, et al. A new function of Nell-1 protein in repressing adipogenic differentiation. *Biochem Biophys Res Commun*. 2011 Jul 22;411(1):126–131.

Lombardi G, Di Somma C, Rubino M, et al. The roles of parathyroid hormone in bone remodeling: prospects for novel therapeutics. *J Endocrinol Invest*. 2011 Jul;34(7 Suppl):18–22.

Medici D, Olsen BR. The role of endothelial-mesenchymal transition in heterotopic ossification. *J Bone Miner Res*. 2012 Aug;27(8):1619–1622.

Osyczka AM, Diefenderfer DL, Bhargave G, et al. Different effects of BMP-2 on marrow stromal cells from human and rat bone. *Cells Tissues Organs*. 2004;176(1-3):109–119.

Rahn BA. Direct and indirect bone healing after operative fracture treatment. *Otolaryngol Clin North Am*. 1987 Aug;20(3):425–440.

Rahn BA. Bone healing: histologic and physiologic concepts. In: Summer-Smith G, ed. *Bone in Clinical Orthopedics*. 2nd ed. Stuttgart: Georg Thieme; 2002; 287–326.

Ripamonti U. Soluble osteogenic molecular signals and the induction of bone formation. *Biomaterials*. 2006 Feb;27(6):807–822.

Teare JA, Ramoshebi LN, Ripamonti U. Periodontal tissue regeneration by recombinant human transforming growth factor-beta 3 in Papio ursinus. *J Periodontal Res*. 2008 Feb;43(1):1–8.

US Food and Drug Administration Web site. Available at: http://www.fda.gov/MedicalDevices/Safety/AlertsandNotices/PublicHealthNotifications/ucm062000.htm). Accessed July 1, 2008.

Weiner BK, Walker M. Efficacy of autologous growth factors in lumbar intertransverse fusions. *Spine (Phila Pa 1976)*. 2003 Sep 1;28(17):1968–1970.

2.1 Access osteotomies in the mandible in tumor surgery and osteosynthesis

Keith Jones

1 Introduction

The provision of optimal surgical access is a fundamental requirement in head and neck surgery. Mandibular access osteotomies facilitate the management of many head and neck tumors and various types of mandibulotomies are described. The procedure should have minimal morbidity and a minimal effect on appearance and function, including speech and swallowing. The choice of a mandibular access procedure is dictated by the clinical and imaging findings, and the degree of access required to successfully ablate the tumor.

2 Indications and contraindications for mandibulotomy

Mandibular access procedure are used:

- In the treatment of tumors of the oral cavity, oral tongue and tongue base, oropharynx and hypopharynx.
- With modification, the technique can be used to gain access to tumors of the parapharyngeal space and infratemporal fossa.
- As a route to gain access to an anterior approach to the cervical spine.
- In conjunction with marginal mandibulectomies if indicated.

With the advent of transoral laser resection (TOLR) for oropharyngeal tumors, and the current vogue to treat oropharyngeal squamous cell carcinoma with chemoradiotherapy, the requirement for mandibulotomy has diminished.

- Where there is involvement of the more distal mandibular bone by tumor, a segmental resection is recommended.
- Previously irradiated patients and patients who have received high-dose antiresorptive medication (bisphosphonates, RANK-ligands) are seen as a relative contraindication.

3 Preoperative imaging

As part of the preoperative evaluation, in addition to the full imaging workup for the head and neck tumor, the following is required:

- A full preoperative dental evaluation, including dental x-rays where necessary. It is important to identify and if necessary eliminate any dental pathology and identify any teeth that have a poor prognosis which could potentially complicate the access procedure.
- Panoramic digital radiographs of the mandible orthopantomography to rule out the existence of synchronous pathology of the mandible and to identify root shape and position.
- High-resolution computed tomography (CT), cone beam CT, or magnetic resonance imaging scan of the mandible to rule out any involvement of the mandible by tumor, especially if the tumor lies in direct proximity to the mandible.

4 Anatomical considerations

4.1 Lip splitting/associated incisions

A mandibular osteotomy may be used alone or in conjunction with a complete or partial lip-splitting technique. A partial lip-splitting technique can still provide adequate surgical access. In this technique, the soft tissues around the chin point are divided through but the division stops at the base of the labiomental fold, thus preserving the orbicularis function and maintaining oral continence. The lip-splitting incisions in common use are illustrated in **Fig 2.1-1**.

Mandibulotomy can also be successfully performed without a lip- or chin-splitting procedure, however access is then more limited.

To provide optimal exposure of the tumor site, the mandibular access procedure will invariably be combined with either a unilateral or bilateral lingual soft-tissue release procedure (**Fig 2.1-2**).

Vascular control

Most mandibular access procedures will be associated with a neck dissection procedure or a direct transcervical approach. This provides access for complete vascular control of the major vessels in the neck.

Mental and inferior alveolar nerves

The osteotomy and subsequent osteosynthesis must not injure the mental or inferior alveolar nerves. The mental foramen is most frequently located in line with the longitudinal access of the second premolar root. The next most common position is between the roots of the first and second premolar but the location can vary from canine to first molar position.

Muscle attachments

The muscle attachments that need to be considered when planning a mandibular access procedure include the following:

- The paired anterior bellies of the digastric muscles arise from a depression on the lower lingual border of the mandible, near the midline.
- The paired mylohyoid muscles form the muscular diaphragm of the floor of mouth, which are attached along the complete length of the mylohyoid line of the mandible with the posterior fibers being inserted into the body of the hyoid bone.
- The genioglossus and geniohyoid muscles are attached to the genial tubercles on the lingual aspect of the mandible in the midline and are located in the lower half of the basal bone in the dentate mandible. The medial pterygoid muscle is attached as a strong tendinous sheet into the medial and posteromedial mandibular ramus below the level of the lingula.
- The bone in the symphyseal and parasymphyseal region of the mandible is vascular and receives its blood supply via the attached musculature; terminal branches of the lingual artery may penetrate the bone directly.

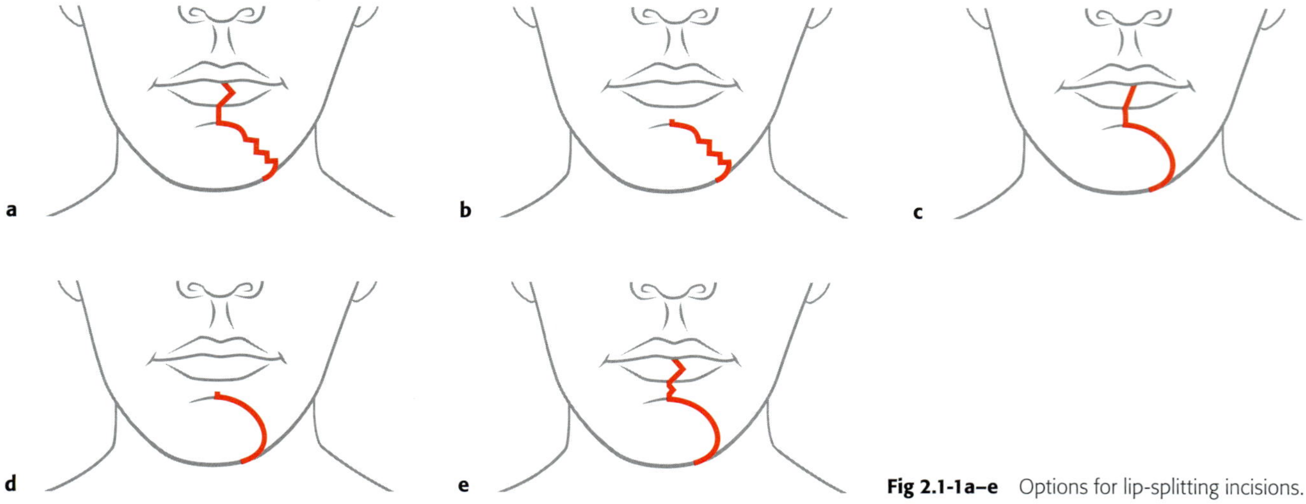

Fig 2.1-1a–e Options for lip-splitting incisions.

4.2 Surgical approach

Following completion of a neck dissection procedure, or following cervical flap elevation as an access procedure, the lower border of the mandible in the submental area is isolated and exposed. A mandibulotomy procedure alone without any form of lip splitting can provide a significant improvement in access without incurring the additional morbidity of the soft-tissue division of the lip and its associated functional and esthetic effects. However, even though lip splitting provides direct access to the osteotomy site, the surgical approach to the mandibulotomy is essentially the same. The soft-tissue attachments of the chin point are all stripped by subperiosteal dissection, exposing approximately 3–4 cm of the mandible at the approximate site of the mandibulotomy. The mental nerve site is clearly identified and protected.

Intraorally, the labial and lingual sulcus at the site of the osteotomy is infiltrated with local anesthesia. Using a scalpel a gingival crevicular incision is made on both lingual and buccal aspects of the mandible. The attached mucosa is elevated using a Freer elevator so that a subperiosteal communication can be produced from the oral cavity to the chin. After soft-tissue dissection, the mandibulotomy is performed (see next section). Before wound closure, the mucosa in the labial sulcus is divided and a releasing incision is made into the labial sulcus at least 1 cm away from the mandibulotomy site so as to avoid closure of the wound directly over the osteotomy cut.

Depending on the location of the tumor, choices exist regarding the extent of the lingual release. In the dentate mandible, a gingival crevicular incision is preferred and this incision extends from the area of the osteotomy to the retromolar region (**Fig 2.1-2**).

In the edentulous mandible, the incision is taken along the crest of the ridge. The use of a crevicular and crestal incision is preferred over a sulcular incision for two main reasons:

- Ease of closure
- Reduces the risk of leakage and fistulation by locating the incision away from the buccal and lingual sulcus

The mobile segments of the mandible are then separated and the mylohyoid muscle is divided along its complete length adjacent to the mandible. When dealing with posterior tongue, oropharyngeal, or parapharyngeal tumors access can be improved by a release incision that extends posteriorly into the anterior pillar and if necessary into the soft palate (**Fig 2.1-3**).

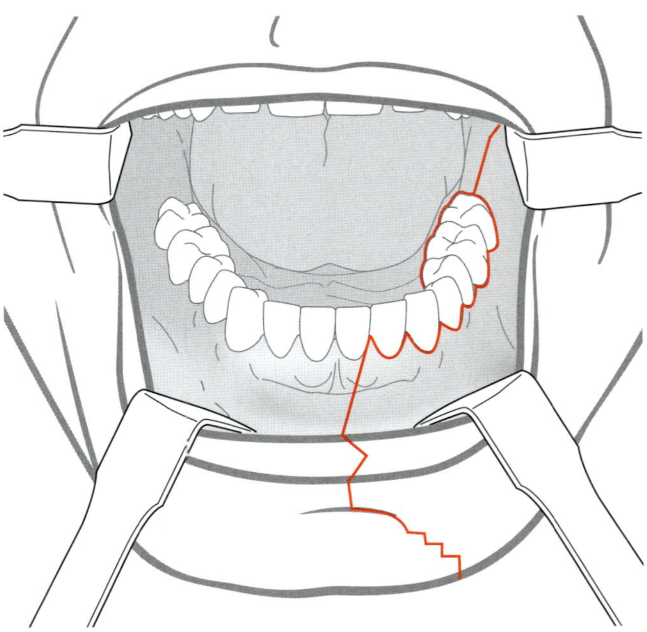

Fig 2.1-2 Buccal and lingual release incisions with lip split.

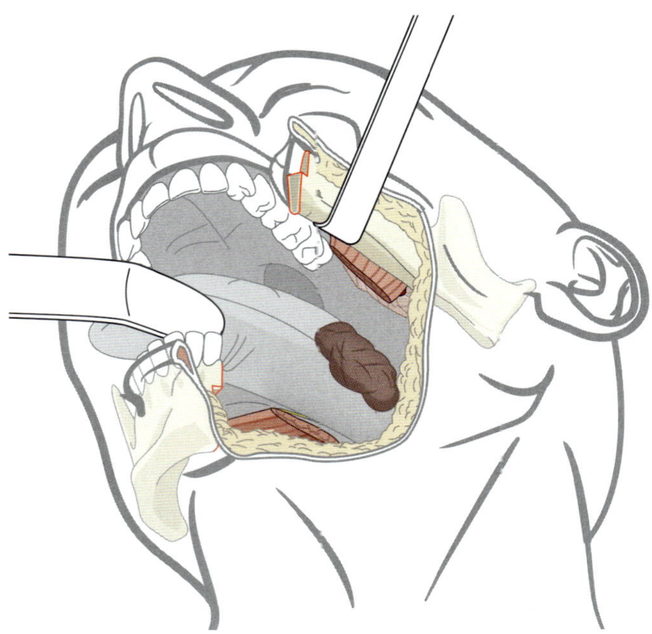

Fig 2.1-3 Lip and mandibular split in the chin area. Lateral rotation of the mandible exposing the floor of the mouth and the tongue.

Lateral rotation of the mandible exposes the lingual nerve coursing medially and dependent on the individual tumor and the access required, resection or division of the lingual nerve may be necessary. Increased access by further rotation of the mandible can be provided by stripping the attachment of the medial pterygoid from the medial surface of the mandible.

5 Types of access osteotomies and osteosynthesis

5.1 Osteosynthesis in mandibular access osteotomies

In this type of access surgery the planned bone cuts are usually marked on the bone and the plates adapted and prelocalized onto the bone with screws before the osteotomy is undertaken. The plate and screws are then removed and can then be carefully stored in the sterile field until the tumor ablation procedure is completed.

Depending on the biomechanical and biological situation, the choice of hardware can range from load-sharing miniplates to rigid load-bearing plates. In certain situations the lag screw technique can also be used. The weaker and more compromised the bone is, the stronger the fixation should be.

5.2 Midline and paramedian mandibulotomies

These osteotomies provide good exposure with acceptable morbidity. A vertical osteotomy cut is marked onto the bone below and in between the roots of the teeth. The osteotomy cut is initially scored using a fine saw blade in a reciprocating saw or a piezotome. At this stage, the titanium plates, which will be used for the final fixation, are prelocalized onto the mandible and temporarily screwed into place. The plates are removed and safely stored. The mandibulotomy cut is then completed using the fine saw blade with a fine spatula osteotome utilized to complete the cut between the dental roots. The lingual periosteum is elevated and protected during this process. The mental nerve is preserved but separation of the genial muscles invariably occurs. During wound closure, muscle repair should be performed to avoid a drooping chin. The site, however, is favorable as it is likely to lie in the periphery of planned radiotherapy (**Fig 2.1-4** and **Fig 2.1-5**).

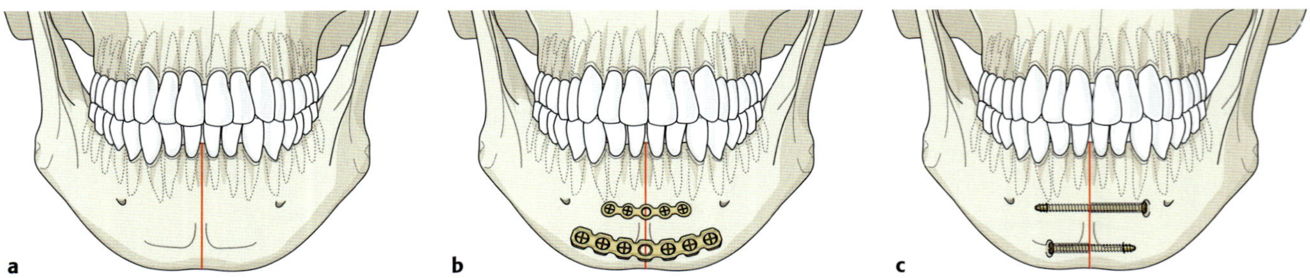

Fig 2.1-4a–c
a Midline osteotomy.
b Fixation of midline osteotomy with plates.
c Fixation of midline osteotomy with lag screws.

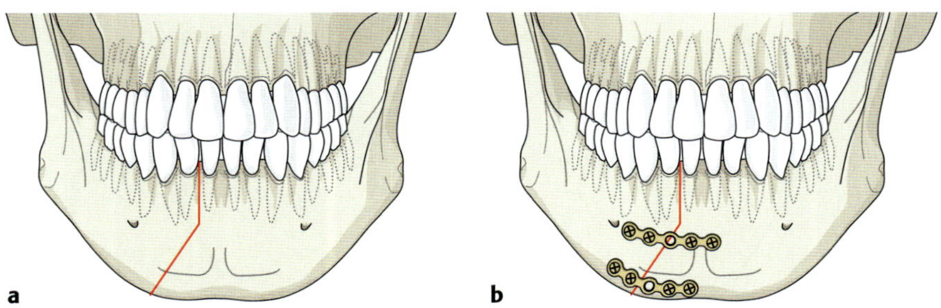

Fig 2.1-5a–b
a Paramedian osteotomy on the right.
b Fixation of paramedian osteotomy with miniplates.

5.3 Symphyseal or parasymphyseal stepped mandibulotomy

In a stepped osteotomy the upper cut is taken down and below root level and is then completed as a stepped osteotomy to the lower border of the mandible anterior to the mental nerve. The lower limb of the step can be taken anteriorly if a lip split is being used or posteriorly if a non-lip-splitting technique is used. The stepped osteotomy can be fixated with plates as described. The fixation tends to be more stable as the stepped cut limits horizontal and vertical movements of the bone. And there is broader surface of contact between the edges of the bone. With this technique, the attachments of the genial and digastric muscles are preserved, as is the inferior alveolar nerve (**Fig 2.1-6**).

Lateral mandibulotomy

This approach involves an osteotomy through the body or angle of the mandible. This procedure is rarely indicated as it involves transsection or extended neurolysis of the inferior alveolar nerve without much added benefit.

Chin point osteotomy

This technique is used in conjunction with the lingual release technique and can be used for tongue base and pharyngeal tumors. The complete chin point of the mandible is osteotomized by a horizontal subapical bone cut linked to the lower border of the mandible by bilateral divergent bony cuts which pass anterior to the mental foramen. The horizontal cut passes above the level of the genial tubercles and the chin point is pedicled on the anterior bellies of the digastric and geniohyoid and genioglossus muscles. Miniplate and lag screw fixation can be done in a variable pattern (**Fig 2.1-7**).

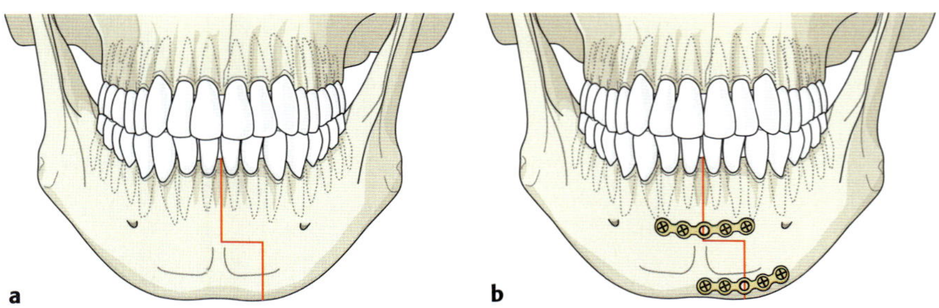

Fig 2.1-6a–b
a Stepped parasymphyseal mandibulotomy.
b Fixation of stepped parasymphyseal mandibulotomy with miniplates.

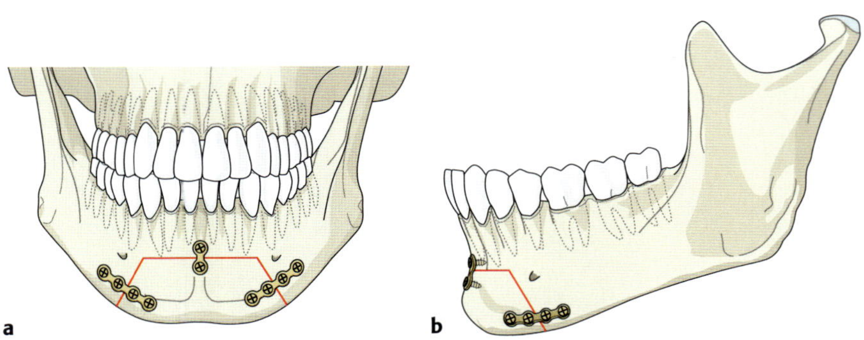

Fig 2.1-7a–b
a Fixation of chin point osteotomy with miniplates from anterior.
b Fixation of chin point osteotomy with miniplates from lateral.

6 Complications and pitfalls

Published complication rates in different series vary between 10.5% and 47.6% with approximately 50% of those patients experiencing minor complications and 50% major complications [Dai et al, 2003; Nam et al, 2006].

Complications associated with mandibulotomy are many and varied, and include:

- Fistulation
- Malocclusion
- Mandibular malunion
- Bone exposure/plate exposure
- Postoperative infection
- Osteoradionecrosis
- Lingual nerve and inferior alveolar nerve injury

Paramedian stepped osteotomies and those osteotomies fixed rigidly with monocortical and bicortical screws and plates are associated with fewer complications [Shinghal et al, 2013].

Radiation therapy was a major factor causing complications (range, 11–30%) [Dziegielewski et al, 2009; Sharan et al, 2008]. Anterior mandibulotomy located at the periphery of the radiotherapy portal carries a decreased risk of osteoradionecrosis, therefore close cooperation with the radiation oncologist in the preoperative planning phase is recommended.

Infection is also reported as a common complication. This needs to be actively managed in the perioperative phase using antibiotics.

7 References and suggested reading

Baek CH, Lee SW, Jeong HS. New modification of the mandibulotomy approach without lip splitting. *Head Neck.* 2006 Jul;28(7):580–586.

Biedlingmaier JF, Ord R. Modified double mandibular osteotomy for tumours of the parapharyngeal space. *J Oral Maxillofac Surg.* 1994 Apr;52(4):348–352.

Boyle JO, Reid V. Complications of surgery of the oral cavity. In: Eisele DW, Smith, RV, eds. *Complications in Head and Neck Surgery.* 2nd ed. Philadelphia: Elsevier; 2009:257–266.

Brown JS, Lowe D, Kalavrezos N, et al. Patterns of invasion and routes of tumor entry into the mandible by oral squamous cell carcinoma. *Head Neck.* 2002 Apr;24(4):370–383.

Chatni SS, Sharan R, Patel D, et al. Transmandibular approach for excision of maxillary sinus tumours extending to pterygopalatine and infratemporal fossae. *Oral Oncol.* 2009 Aug;45(8):720–726.

Collin J, McLennan A. Oblique paramedian mandibulotomy with fixation by lag screws. *Br J Oral Maxillofac Surg.* 2009 Oct;47(7):560–561.

Dai TS, Hao SP, Chang KP, et al. Complications of mandibulotomy: midline versus paramidline. *Otolaryngol Head Neck Surg.* 2003 Jan;128(1):137–141.

Devine JC, Rogers SN, McNally D, et al. A comparison of aesthetic, functional and patient subjective outcomes following lip split mandibulotomy and mandibular lingual releasing access procedures. *Int J Oral Maxillofac Surg.* 2001 Jun;30(3):199–204.

Dziegielewski PT, Mlynarek AM, Dimitry J, et al. The mandibulotomy; friend or foe? Safety outcomes and a literature review. *Laryngoscope.* 2009 Dec;119(12):2369–2375.

Engroff SL, Blanchaert RH, von Fraunhofer JA. Mandibulotomy fixation: a laboratory analysis. *J Oral Maxillofac Surg.* 2003 Nov;61(11):1297–1301.

Gallet P, Gangloff P, Mastronicola R, et al. Combined transoral and suprahyoid approach for oropharyngeal cancers: an alternative to mandibulotomy. *Rev Laryngol Otol Rhinol (Bord).* 2011;132(2):95–102.

Judson BL, Adam SI, Lowlicht R, et al. Transcervical double mandibular osteotomy approach to the infratemporal fossa. *World Neuro Surg.* 2012 Dec;78(6):715.

Kolokythas A, Eisele DW, El-Sayed I, et al. Mandibular osteotomies for access to select parapharyngeal space neoplasms. *Head Neck.* 2009 Jan;31(1):102–110.

Lazaridis N, Antoniades K. Condylotomy or vertical subsigmoid osteotomy with a mandibulotomy anterior to the mental foramen for improved access to parapharyngeal space tumours. *J Oral Maxillofac Surg.* 2008 Mar;66(3):597–606.

Mehanna P, Devine J, McMahon J. Lip split and mandibulotomy modifications. *Br J Oral Maxillofac Surg.* 2010 June;48(4):314–315.

Merrick GD, Morrison RW, Gallagher JR, et al. Pedicled genial osteotomy modification of the mandibular release access operation for access to the back of the tongue. *Br J Oral Maxillofac Surg.* 2007 Sept;45(6):490–492.

Moore EJ, Olsen KD. Complications of surgery of the parapharyngeal space. In: Eisele DW, Smith RV, eds. *Complications in Head and Neck Surgery.* 2nd ed. Philadelphia: Elsevier; 2009:241–250.

Na HY, Choi EJ, Choi EC, et al. Modified mandibulotomy technique to reduce posteroperative complications: 5 year results. *Yonsei Med J.* 2013 Sept 1;54(5):1248–1252.

Nabil S, Samman N. Risk factors for osteoradionecrosis after head and neck radiation: a systematic review. *Oral Surg Oral Med Oral Path Oral Radiol.* 2012 Jan;113(1):54–69.

Nam W, Kim HJ, Choi EC, et al. Contributing factors to mandibulotomy complications: a retrospective study. *Oral Surg Oral Med Oral Path Oral Radiol Endod.* 2006 Mar;101(3):65–70.

Sharan R1, Iyer S, Chatni SS, et al. Increased plate and osteosynthesis related complications associated with postoperative concurrent chemoradiotherapy in oral cancer. *Head Neck.* 2008 Nov;30(11):1422–1430.

Shinghal T, Bissada E, Chan HB, et al. Medial mandibulotomies: is there sufficient space in the midline to allow a mandibulotomy without compromising the dentition? *J Otolaryngol Head Neck Surg.* 2013 May 2;42:32.

Smith GI, Brennan P, Ilankovan V. Vertical ramus osteotomy combined with parasymphyseal mandibulotomy for improved access to the parapharyngeal space. *Head Neck.* 2003;25:1000–1003.

2.2 Mandible resections without loss of continuity (rim resections)

Sebastian Sauerbier, Ralf Gutwald, Rainer Schmelzeisen

1 Introduction

Malignant tumors may be located in proximity, adjacent to, or involve the mandible. Until the latter part of the 20th century, segmental resection was considered state of the art when a tumor was close to the mandible or when an actual infiltration of the bone occurred. Loss of continuity of the mandible frequently results in esthetic and functional impairment and/or reduction in quality of life for the patient. If rim resection is performed when oncologically sound, no significant statistical difference in survival and recurrence rates are observed between this approach and mandibular continuity resections. Quality of life is also better for patients with rim resections than for those who undergo segmental resections. Therefore, whenever possible, a marginal rim mandibulectomy should be performed.

A rim resection is indicated if the carcinoma is only clinically adjacent or superficially infiltrating the mandible and if no signs of deep bone infiltration are visible in fine-cut computed tomographic (CT) scans or scintigraphy.

2 Imaging

2.1 Conventional x-rays

Typically tumors are detected by clinical examination. Panoramic x-ray can give a general picture of whether the mandible is invaded by tumor. Early states of tumor infiltration into the mandible are not easily detected by conventional x-ray because at least 30% demineralization has to occur to permit detection by conventional x-rays. There is 82% accuracy in diagnosing bony invasion with panoramic x-rays. The rate of false-negative (2–46%) exceeds the rate of false-positive (0–16%) findings [Brown et al, 1994]. Periodontal diseases, apical and marginal inflammations, and overlay of the spinal column complicate the interpretation. Conventional x-rays should be taken in the second plane for the mandible in a posteroanterior view as described by Clementschitsch [1955].

2.2 3-D imaging

When a malignant lesion is suspected or confirmed by biopsy, an axial and coronal CT scan of the midface and mandible is taken routinely. The images can be reconstructed in multiplanar or in 3-D format. The multi-detector row computed tomography (MDCT) with slices as thin as 0.5 mm have improved sensitivity and specificity. Artifacts from dental restorations can cause false-positive findings; their rate is lower than that of false-negative findings. Tsue et al [1994] believe a CT scan is accurate in exclusion of bone infiltration.

Cone beam CT (CBCT) may also be used to detect bone destruction adjacent to tumor spread. It is not likely to be disturbed by metal artefacts compared to CT, but does not allow differentiation of tumor tissues from other soft tissues.

The neck, thorax, and abdomen are also examined by CT scan to screen for metastasis. When the soft-tissue relation of the tumor to the bone cannot be verified by a conventional contrast-enhanced CT scan, magnetic resonance imaging (MRI) may be used. The high-signal intensity of fatty tissue in T1 images makes MRI ideal to judge bone marrow infiltration. In a study of 22 patients treated with mandibular resection, Chung et al [1994] found a high sensitivity with no false-negative MRI results for tumor invasion. Magnetic resonance imaging has been shown to be prone to false-positive results (range, 73–77%) because lesions from tooth extractions, infectious odontogenic diseases, and osteoradionecrosis cannot be differentiated from tumor invasion. For Bolzoni et al [2004] and Vidiri et al [2010] MRI scans are helpful to differentiate between tumor and fibrosis in irradiated patients. In an MRI case-series of 15 patients, Bolzoni et al [2004] found sensitivity, specificity, and an accuracy of 93% each. The negative predictive value was 96% and the positive predictive value was 87.5%. An MRI study virtually excludes cortical or bone marrow invasion. In contrast to the previous data, Vidiri et al [2010] compared MRI to MDCT in a more recent study in 36 patients and found no statistical difference in sensitivity, specificity, and accuracy (MRI: 93%, 82%, and 86%; MDCT: 79%, 82%, and 81%), respectively. The negative predictive value was 73% for MRI and 86% for MDCT. The positive predictive value was 76% for MRI and 95% for MDCT. The MRI results depend on the researchers and their technique. An MRI also determines tumor volume more accurately.

2.3 Bone scintigraphy and single-photon emission CT

Bone scintigraphy and single-photon emission CT (SPECT) have been used to help screening for metastasis and bone infiltration but the results are disappointing. Isotope imaging is not specific for bone invasion. There is a higher rate of false positive (26–35%) than of false-negative results (0–7%). This means that a negative scanning result makes an extensive bony infiltration unlikely [Brown, 2003; Brown et al, 1994; Shaha, 1991; Zupi et al, 1996] but cannot guarantee for a mandible free of tumor.

3 Anatomical considerations and planning

The decision for a mandibular resection with or without loss of continuity depends on the infiltration mode of the carcinoma which can be estimated by the described imaging methods.

In dentate patients, carcinomas may reach the mandibular bone at the point of contact of the fixed gingiva and Sharpey fibers. The histological image of bone invasion consists of osteoclasts in front of the actual tumor frontier. Direct contact between tumor cells and bone does not exist until later stages of the disease. There are two types of tumor invasion into the mandible. In the first form, "the irregular invasive diffuse infiltration" breaks through the cortical bone and often quickly infiltrates the canal of the inferior alveolar nerve followed by wide horizontal spreading into the mandible's marrow space. Large tumor masses invading the mandibular body can disseminate perineurally. Perineural spread demands a continuity resection when either the inferior alveolar nerve or the mandibular foramen is reached.

The second form of bony invasion was described by Müller et al [1990] as "erosive and expansive." It shows a compact broad tumor front which erodes the bone from its area of contact. This form is considered less aggressive than irregular invasion. The thorough study by Brown and Browne [1995] supports the presumption that the erosive infiltration pattern occurs at the lesion's periphery and later during progression transforms into the irregular invasive one.

Alveolar and retromolar tumors arising from the alveolar crest more often enter the bone via periodontal spaces, while tumors of the floor of the mouth and the tongue enter into the bone directly at the point of contact. In some cases the foramina of the mandible are entry points for squamous cell carcinomas. Invasion into the radiated mandible varies from case to case and is generally characterized by multiple foci. This makes it difficult to predict the mode of infiltration and justifies an extensive continuity resection.

Histological examinations of oral cavity tumors involving the mandible reveal an infiltration rate ranging from 22–48%. Barttelbort et al [1987] found histological bone infiltration in 3 of 21 patients who underwent rim mandibulectomy. Ord et al [1997] described an infiltration rate of 65% in segmental and 7.6% in marginal bony resections of the mandible. The grade of tumor differentiation does not correlate with the invasion rate. The invasive type is found more often with increasing depth of the bony invasion. On average the invasive type infiltrates 12 mm wider than the erosive type. Even though carcinoma invasion of bone occurs in both edentulous and dentate regions of the mandible, extent and depth of bony invasion were greater in dentate regions.

An adequate preoperative assessment of possible bone infiltration helps to decide whether to perform a rim or a segmental mandibulectomy. Using clinical and radiological examination, infiltration can be determined with an accuracy of 82–88%.

Small and shallow carcinomas in proximity to the mandible but without cortical infiltration should be removed with a rim resection. This should include a bone block including the cortex underlying the tumor.

Following the assumption that carcinomas reach the mandible via the attached mucosa, it is important to plan enough bone resection to achieve adequate margins. A caudal rim with height of at least 1 cm should be preserved. Brown et al [2005] introduced a guide to mandibular resection based on the Cawood and Howell classification of the mandible [1991]. It helps to judge whether a rim or segmental resection is necessary (**Table 2.2-1**). Clear margins with at least > 5 mm of normal tissue between the tumor front and the edge of the resection should be achieved because tumor-free margins are essential for survival and local tumor control.

4 Types of rim resections and techniques

Barttelbort et al [1993] postulate three basic requirements for the optimum technique: (1) It must adequately remove the primary tumor as well as those tissues that are also at risk for tumor infiltration. (2) It should be technically simple, biomechanically sound, and have a low complication rate. (3) It should preserve or permit reconstruction of the mandibular arch particularly in anterior lesions to restore normal function and facial appearance.

The access of choice for most of the rim resections is a transoral approach. If needed, it can be combined with an extraoral submandibular approach.

Mandible continuity can be preserved with vertical, horizontal, or oblique rim resection.

The vertical (sagittal) mandibulectomy (**Fig 2.2-1a–b**), including the removal of the lingual plate is technically demanding, and a fracture of the mandible may occur. To prevent a fracture, it is crucial to outline the osteotomy at the mandible's base with a burr, a saw, or a piezosurgery device. In dentate regions the teeth should be extracted before a sagittal resection is carried out.

The horizontal rim resection is indicated for tumors on the alveolar crest (**Fig 2.2-1c–d**). It permits selective removal of all the tissues at risk based on sound pathological evidence. It is easy to perform, has few complications, and permits maximal form and function for the patient. Osteotomies with sharp edges should be avoided because they function as points of stress concentration and increase the risk of a fracture. Smooth curved osteotomies are biomechanically superior. The length of the osteotomy depends on clinical necessity. Technically, the osteotomy can include the anterior part of the ascending ramus and the coronoid process. Brown et al [2005] favor an oblique saw-cut from cranial-vestibular to caudal-lingual (**Fig 2.2-1e–f**).

Cawood and Howell classification	OPG-, MRI-, BS- No invasion/periosteal invasion	OPG-, MRI+ or BS+ early invasion (< 5 mm)	OPG+, MRI+, BS+ late invasion (> 5 mm)
I-II (dentate or immediately postextraction)	Rim	Rim	Rim/segment
III-IV (round or knife edge)	Rim	Rim/segment	Segment
V-VI (flat or depressed ridge)	Rim/segment	Segment	Segment

Table 2.2-1 Guide to mandibular resection for oral squamous cell carcinoma based on the Cawood and Howell classification of the mandible [Brown et al, 2005].*
*OPG indicates orthopantomogram; MRI, magnetic resonance imaging; and BS, bone scintigraphy.

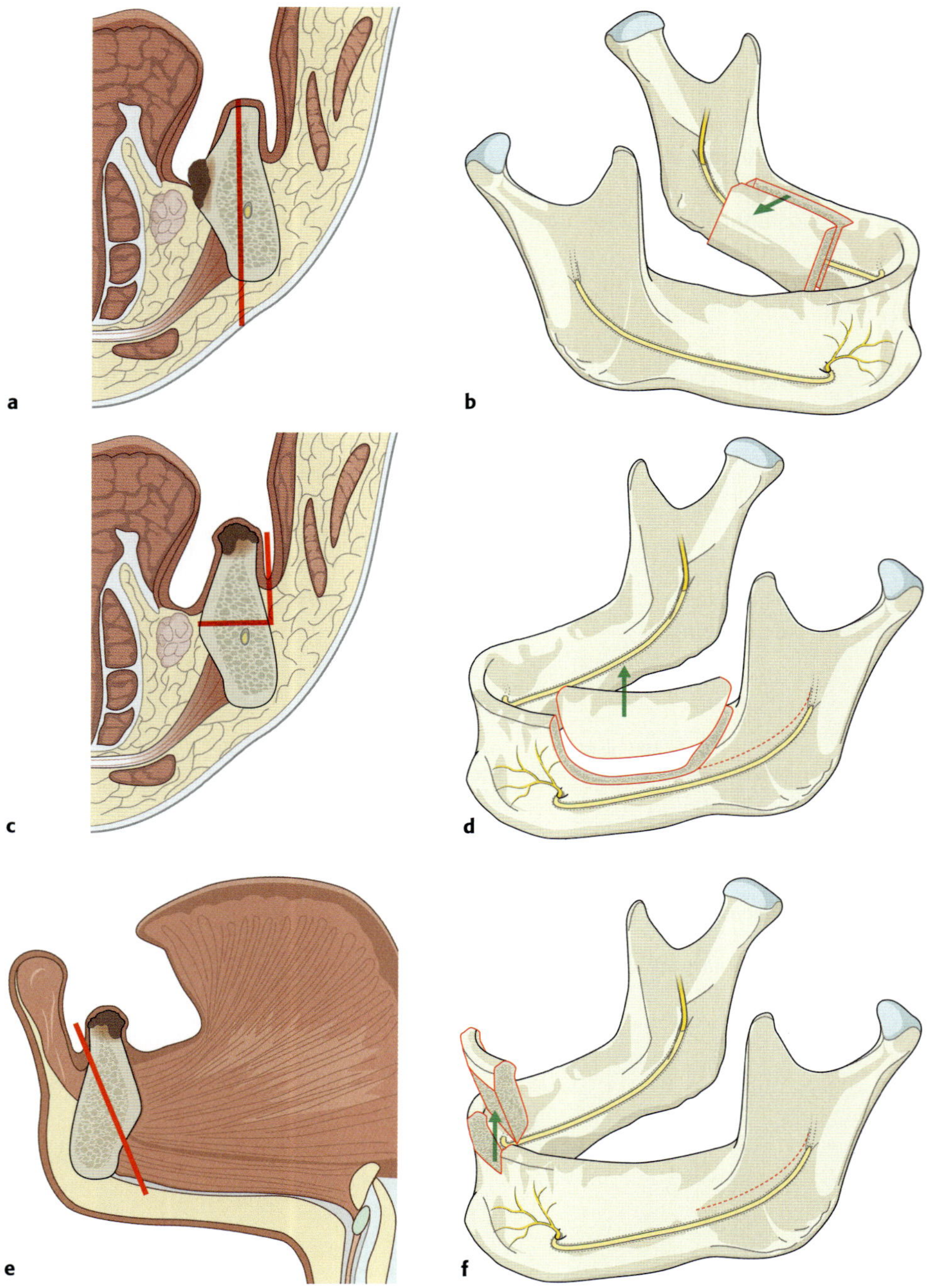

Fig 2.2-1a–f
a–b Vertical (sagittal) rim resection.
c–d Horizontal rim resection.
e–f Oblique rim resection, chin area.

A rim resection procedure is performed with the patient under general anesthesia in nasal intubation. The patient is placed in the supine position. The mouth and neck are properly washed and disinfected. In addition to the usual head and neck instruments, an oscillating saw, a Lindemann drill, round burrs, various osteotomes, a piezosurgery unit, and a headlamp should be available. Preoperative antibiotics are administered. The mouth is inspected and palpated. Mucosal incisions are outlined with a sterile pen and should have 1–1.5 cm distance to the boundary of the tumor. Local anesthetic with vasoconstrictor is injected into the planned soft-tissue incision line. Biopsies for frozen section histopathology are taken from the whole circumference of the soft tissues surrounding the resected specimen. In case of a positive result the area is resected further. This helps to obtain tumor-free soft-tissue margins during surgery. The planned osteotomy can be outlined with a small round burr and carried out with a saw or piezotome. The amount of bone resection depends on the proximity of tumor tissue to the bone (**Fig 2.2-2**). If the resection has to be performed in dentate areas, the teeth including their roots and periodontal spaces should be removed en bloc together with the specimen. The aim of a rim resection procedure is to protect the mental and the inferior alveolar nerve if they do not have to be removed for oncological reasons. Piezosurgery may be helpful to protect soft-tissue structures, such as nerves.

Approximately 1 cm in height should be preserved of the mandible's base. Saw-cuts should be tapered, as right-angled osteotomies should be avoided (**Fig 2.2-3**).

The extension of the resection depends on the location and the size of the tumor. Intraoperative palpation helps to assess this issue. Functions of speech and swallowing are better if some attachment of the tongue to the residual mandible can be preserved or reestablished. If the lingual nerve is involved or within the resection margin of the carcinoma, it should be resected. After completing the resection, the specimen is marked with sutures (**Fig 2.2-4**) and biopsies for frozen section are harvested from the deep margins.

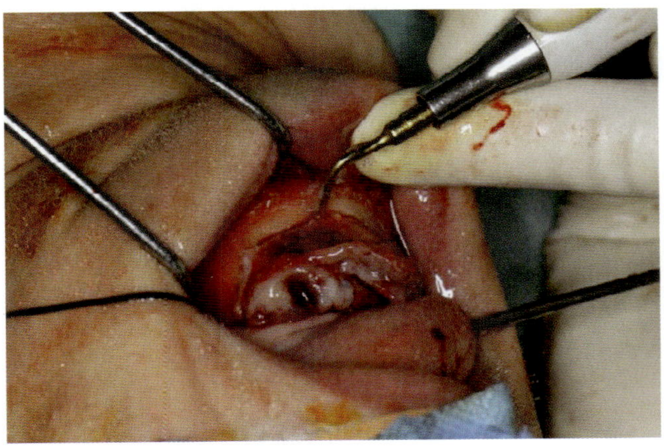

Fig 2.2-2 The osteotomy is performed with a piezotome.

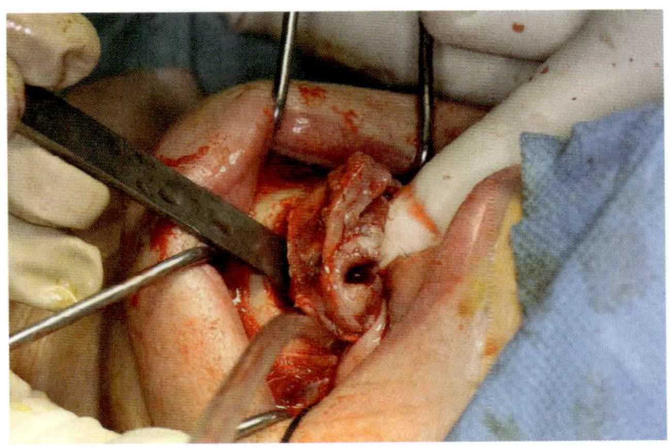

Fig 2.2-3 Osteotomes can help to mobilize the segment. Care must be taken not to fracture the mandible.

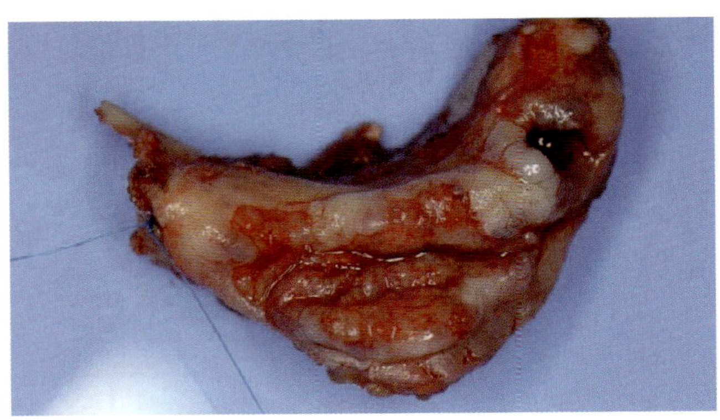

Fig 2.2-4 The specimen after resection.

Finally, hemostasis is obtained. Intraoperative markings of the resection margins with titanium vessel clips allow generating a virtual model of tumor margins from postoperative CT data. If the pathologist localizes problem areas with uncertain margins, the oncologist can plan with this data a focused delivery of radiation to the remaining tissues. Finally, the edges of the remaining bone should be smoothed by a round burr to obtain a boat-shaped defect (**Fig 2.2-5**).

For reconstruction of smaller mucosal defects, a collagen membrane or split skin graft can be used (**Figs 2.2-6–2.2-10**). The preoperative and postoperative panoramic radiographs is shown in **Fig 2.2-11**. Local mucosa flaps work well when tension-free closure can be obtained. Regional or free tissue transfers are typically used to cover larger soft-tissue defects.

If a graft or flap is used, a nasogastric feeding tube is inserted at the end of surgery. Oral diet should not be allowed until postoperative day 7 to 10 to prevent dehiscence and infection.

Further reconstruction aims at improving masticatory function and speech. Bone grafting is performed as a secondary procedure when there is sound histological evidence of tumor control (**Figs 2.2-12–2.2-18**). In selected cases distraction osteogenesis may be considered. Dental implant insertion usually requires vestibuloplasty and mobilization of the tongue. This can be done for instance with split skin grafts.

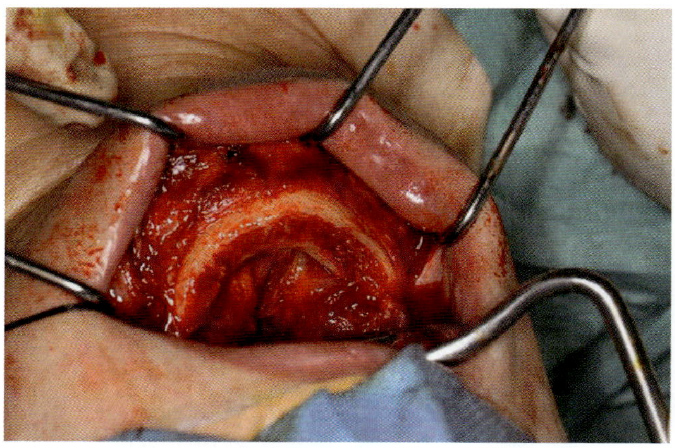

Fig 2.2-5 Defect after resection. The edges are smoothened with a round burr.

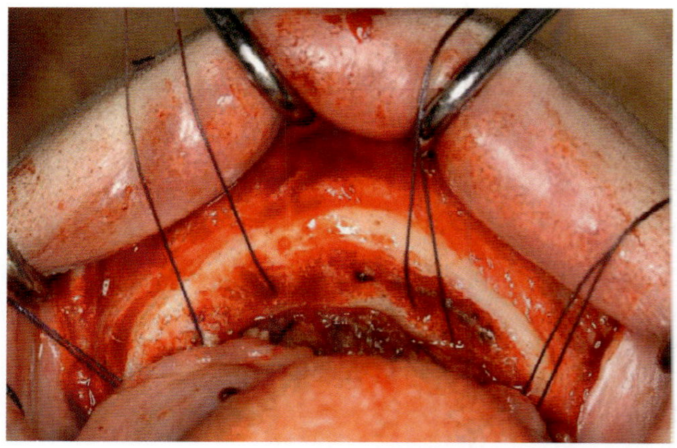

Fig 2.2-6 Suturing the floor of the mouth to the lingual cortex of the mandible. Tension-free closure is crucial to prevent dehiscence. In this case primary closure is not possible. The cortical bone is covered because granulation tissue can only emerge from the medulla but not from the cortex of the mandible.

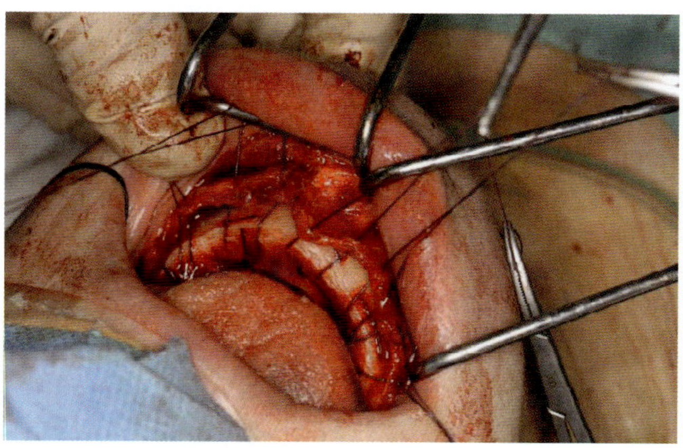

Fig 2.2-7 Fixation of the vestibular mucosa to the cortex of the mandible.

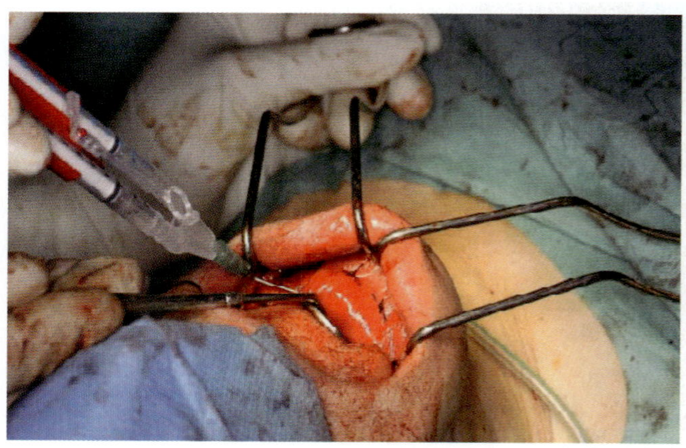

Fig 2.2-8 A split skin graft or in this case a collagen membrane is sutured into the defect. The collagen membrane was underlined with fibrin glue for better stability.

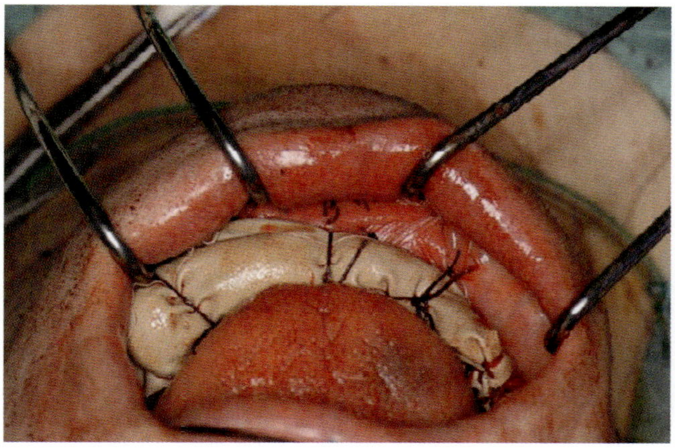

Fig 2.2-9 A finger of a surgical glove is filled with a cotton gauze and fixated with sutures to form the vestibule and the floor of the mouth.

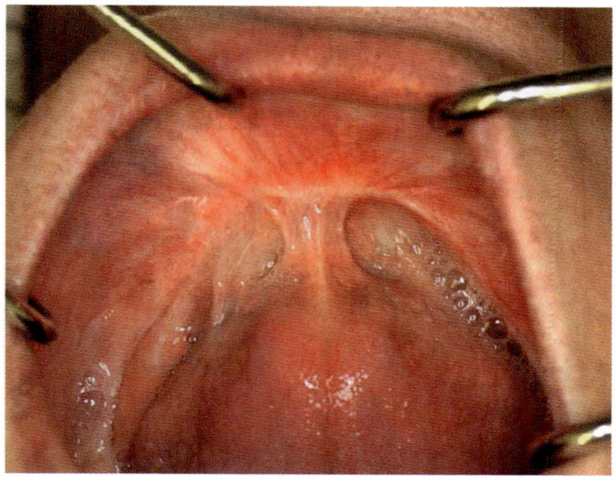

Fig 2.2-10 An 8-month postoperative result.

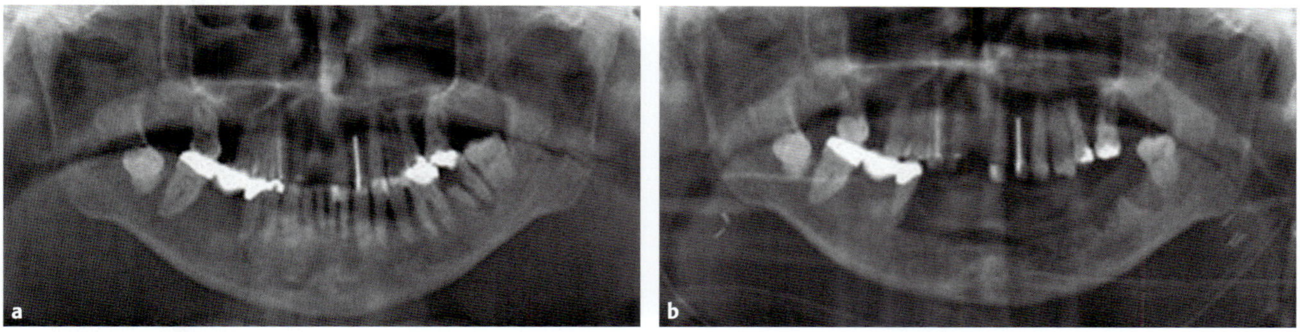

Fig 2.2-11a–b Preoperative and postoperative panoramic radiographs before and after rim resection in the chin area.

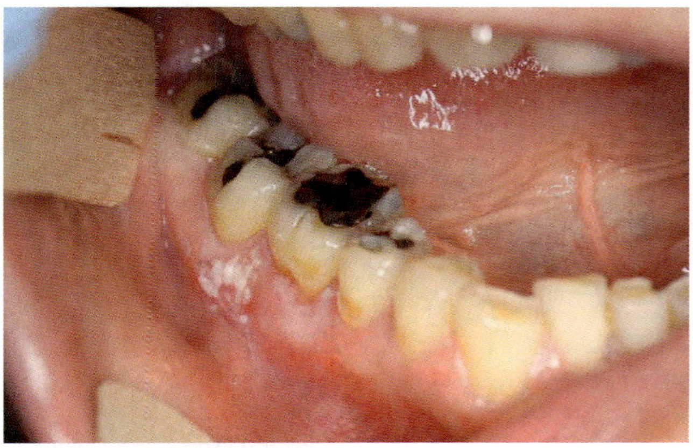

Fig 2.2-12 Intraoral view of tumor erosion in region 46 to 47 by a pathologically confirmed squamous cell carcinoma.

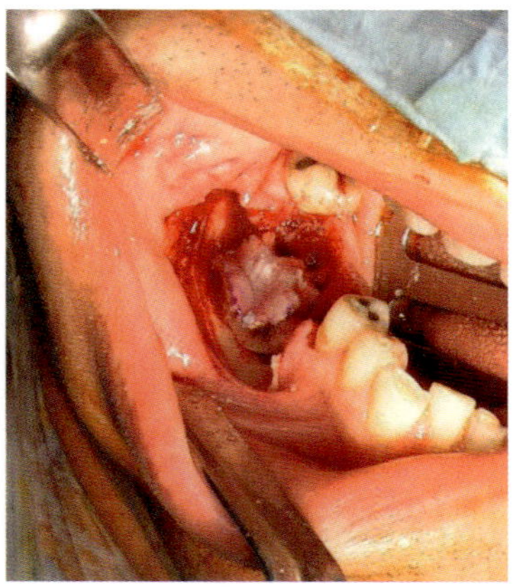

Fig 2.2-13 Intraoperative situation after tumor resection.

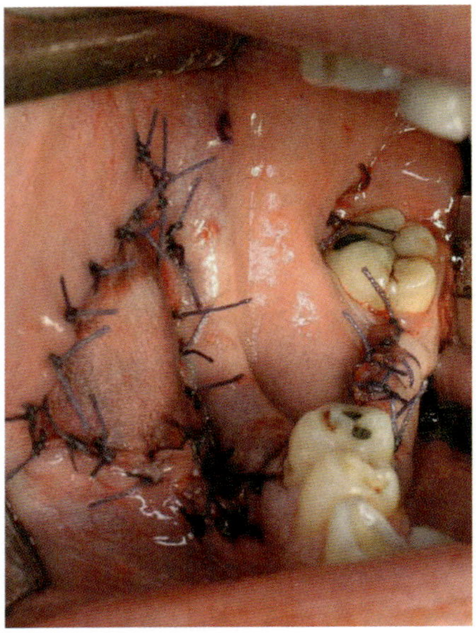

Fig 2.2-14 Closure is achieved with a local pedicled flap. The secondary defect is covered with a collagen membrane.

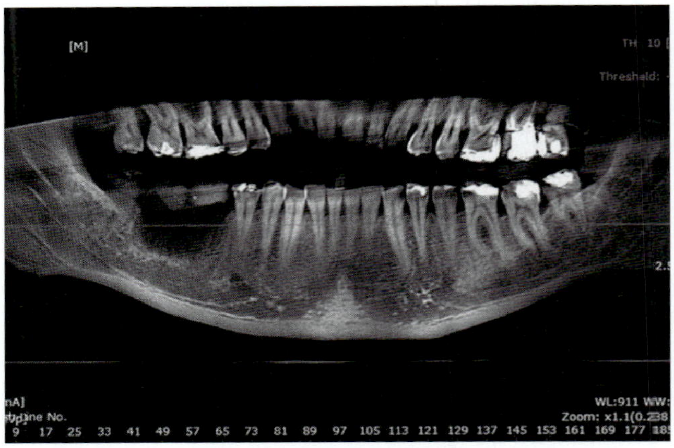

Fig 2.2-15 Panoramic view of the mandible after tumor resection. Note the curved, round edged defect. An interim bridge was inserted after healing to replace the removed teeth 46 and 47.

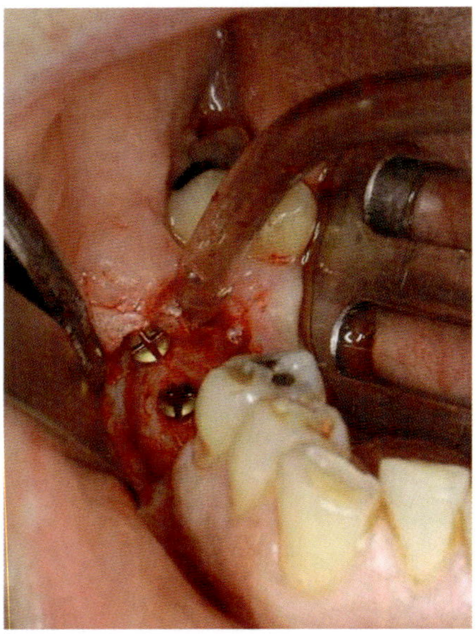

Fig 2.2-16 The alveolar ridge was reconstructed with a free bone graft from the iliac crest. The image shows the integrated bone block after healing at the stage of osteosynthesis hardware removal and dental implant insertion.

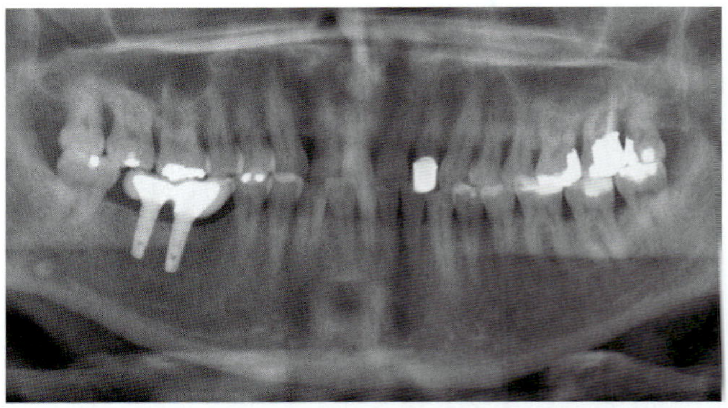

Fig 2.2-17 Panoramic x-ray after osseointegration of dental implants and prosthetic loading.

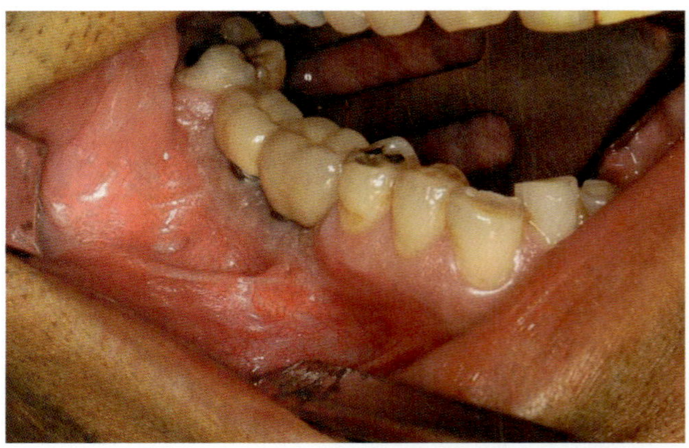

Fig 2.2-18 Final reconstruction after bone transplantation, dental implant insertion and vestibuloplasty with a split-skin graft from the lateral thigh. The prosthetic work was performed in collaboration with the patient's referring dentist. The soft tissue adjacent to the implants shows no sign of inflammation.

5 Protection plate concept

In cases when the remaining mandibular bone stock is less than 1 cm in height after rim resection, a "protection plate" can be used to stabilize the residual bone. Bone grafting may be done when appropriate to strengthen the residual mandible. In treatment of benign lesions, like cysts or giant cell granulomas, extensive cortical thinning and bone loss can occur by curettage or partial resection. If a weak mandibular strut is suspected or if a fracture of the mandible occurs during resective surgery, a load-bearing conventional or locking reconstruction plate may be used (**Figs 2.2-19–2.2-21**). Depending on the case the locking plate has to be applied via an extraoral approach. If the necessity of a reconstruction plate is likely, the plate should be contoured and provisionally attached to the mandible before the actual resection takes place (**Fig 2.2-20**). After positioning the plate, it is secured to the mandible by the plate holding forceps. The holes are drilled and the screw length is measured with a depth gauge, and the screw is inserted. Anatomically preformed reconstruction plates, like the MATRIX mandible preformed reconstruction plates, save application time and prevent plate failure following weakening caused by the plate bending process. Depending on the lesion, the plate is removed before tumor resection. Rim resections of the lower border of the mandible may be indicated to treat tumor invasion from submandibular gland tumors or lymph nodes (**Fig 2.2-22**).

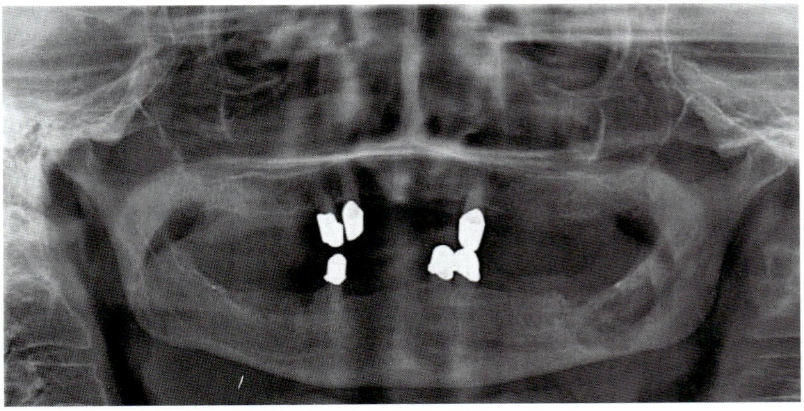

Fig 2.2-19 Panoramic x-ray of a bisphosphonate-induced lesion at the left mandibular angle. After resection, instability is to be suspected.

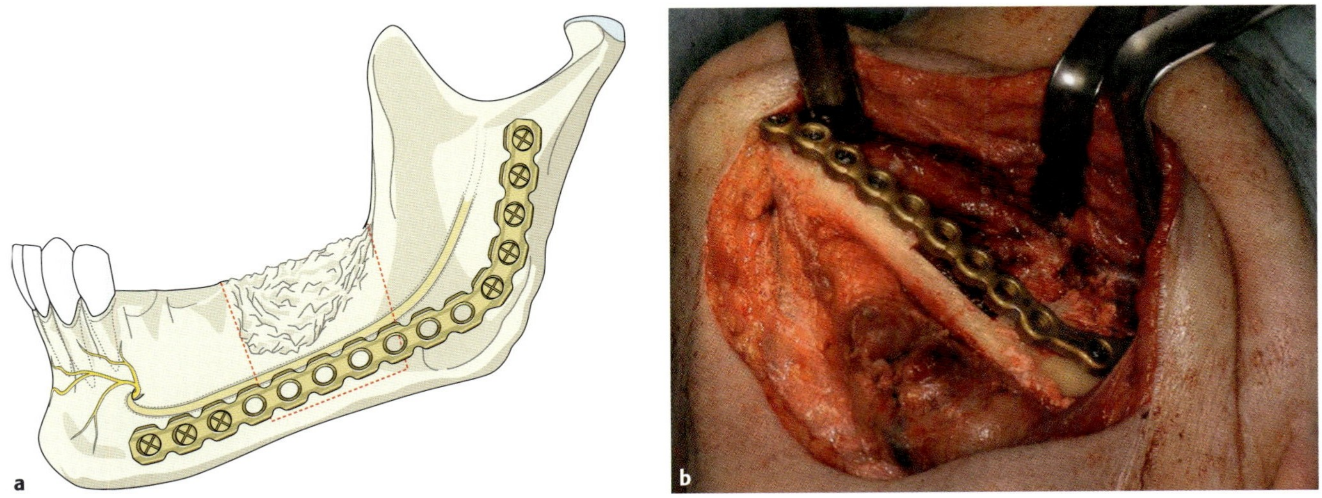

Fig 2.2-20a–b

a A load-bearing reconstruction plate is applied before bone removal.

b Operation site after marginal rim mandibulectomy and protection plate insertion via a submandibular approach.

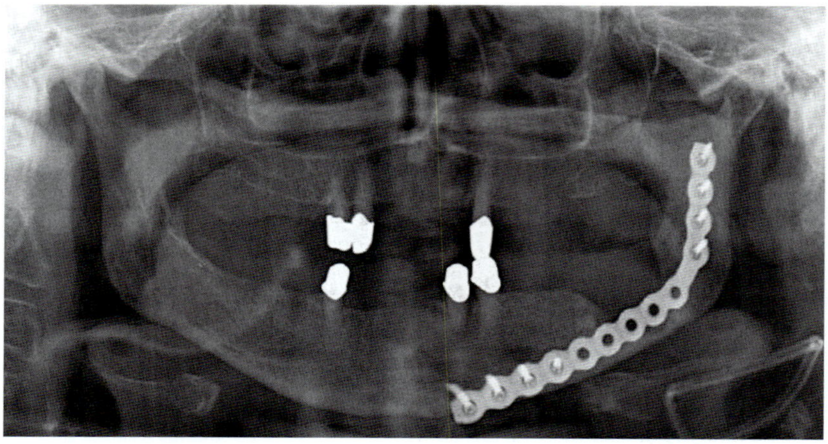

Fig 2.2-21 Panoramic x-ray after tumor resection and protection plate insertion.

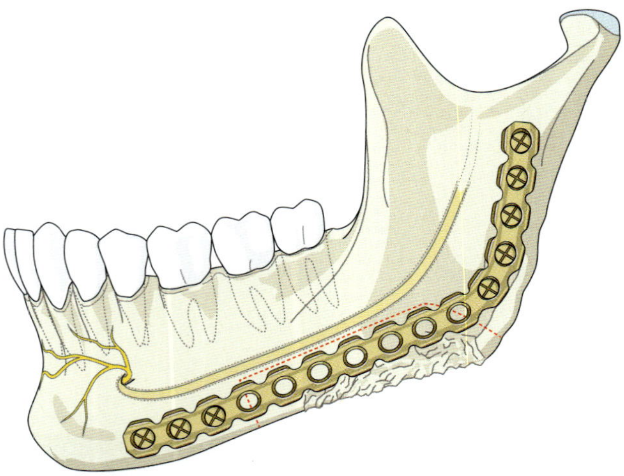

Fig 2.2-22 Lower border rim resection outlined with a protection plate in situ.

6 Complications and pitfalls

Marginal rim resection may be complicated by a fracture, which can occur intraoperatively or postoperatively under functional loads. To prevent this, it is important to smoothen and to round the edges at the anterior and posterior osteotomy sites.

Depending on the tumor location, patients should expect some degree of inferior alveolar nerve hypesthesia/anesthesia due to traction and proximity to the tumor resection. If the continuity of the nerve is intact, this should resolve within 6–12 months.

Unfavorable soft-tissue situations or previous radiation can cause an increase in complication rates. These problems begin with a decreased accuracy of tumor imaging, impaired wound healing, impaired wound vascularity, wound dehiscence, fractures of the residual bone, and a higher rate of reconstructive failures. A tension-free soft-tissue closure is crucial to prevent wound dehiscence, which typically occurs between postoperative day 4 and 10. When reconstruction of the floor of the mouth is performed, it is often a problem to avoid dehiscence followed by infection due to tongue movements. A vascularized tissue flap helps to achieve abundant soft tissues and good coverage in movable areas.

Only superficially located invasive bony lesions should be treated with a rim resection. In the case that the hard tissue histology turns out to have tumor involved bony margins, it is necessary in a second surgery to extend the resection, which necessitates a complete segmental resection.

Extractions of teeth in contact to a carcinoma should not be done before resective surgery because tumor tissue could be translocated into the extraction sockets. Removal of teeth should take place at the actual tumor surgery. So far there is no correlation between histological evidence of bone infiltration and the risk of local recurrence. It is more frequent in the soft tissues than in bone.

It is difficult to compare survival and recurrence rates in the literature because case numbers are often low. Another reason is the pre-selection of patients for rim or continuity resection depending on the tumor size and location. Smaller tumors are often treated with rim resections. Deeply invading tumors require mostly a segmental resection. Wolff et al [2004] did not find a significantly different 5-year survival rate of 135 patients with marginal (70%) vs segmental (57%) resection. Also local relapses, metastases and second primary tumors did not show significant differences. Pathak et al [2009] compared patients with vestibular cancer to patients with a tumor in the floor of the mouth. All 179 patients were treated with marginal rim mandibulectomy. The 5-year survival rate was significantly better for patients with buccal cancer. Patients with cancer of the floor of the mouth had a lower survival rate.

In summary, rim resection of the mandible is a sound technique for appropriately selected patients with oral cavity carcinomas. Careful attention to the geometry and details of the bone resection, preservation of the inferior alveolar nerve, and soft-tissue closure optimize results.

7 References and suggested reading

Abler A, Roser M, Weingart D. [On the indications for and morbidity of segmental resection of the mandible for squamous cell carcinoma in the lower oral cavity]. *Mund Kiefer Gesichtschir.* 2005 May;9(3):137–142. German.

Ahuja RB, Soutar DS, Moule B, et al. Comparative study of technetium-99m bone scans and orthopantomography in determining mandible invasion in intraoral squamous cell carcinoma. *Head Neck.* 1990 May–Jun;12(3):237–243.

Barttelbort SW, Ariyan S. Mandible preservation with oral cavity carcinoma: rim mandibulectomy versus sagittal mandibulectomy. *Am J Surg.* 1993 Oct;166(4):411–415.

Barttelbort SW, Bahn SL, Ariyan SA. Rim mandibulectomy for cancer of the oral cavity. *Am J Surg.* 1987 Oct;154(4):423–428.

Bittermann G, Scheifele C, Prokic V, et al. Description of a method: computer generated virtual model for accurate localisation of tumour margins, standardised resection, and planning of radiation treatment in head & neck cancer surgery. *J Craniomaxillofac Surg.* 2013 Jun;41(4):279–281.

Bolzoni A, Cappiello J, Piazza C, et al. Diagnostic accuracy of magnetic resonance imaging in the assessment of mandibular involvement in oral-oropharyngeal squamous cell carcinoma: a prospective study. *Arch Otolaryngol Head Neck Surg.* 2004 Jul;130(7):837–843.

Brown J. Mechanisms of cancer invasion of the mandible. *Curr Opin Otolaryngol Head Neck Surg.* 2003 Apr;11(2):96–102.

Brown J, Chatterjee R, Lowe D, et al. A new guide to mandibular resection for oral squamous cell carcinoma based on the Cawood and Howell classification of the mandible. *Int J Oral Maxillofac Surg.* 2005 Dec;34(8):834–839.

Brown JS, Browne RM. Factors influencing the patterns of invasion of the mandible by oral squamous cell carcinoma. *Int J Oral Maxillofac Surg.* 1995 Dec;24(6):417–426.

Brown JS, Griffith JF, Phelps PD, et al. A comparison of different imaging modalities and direct inspection after periosteal stripping in predicting the invasion of the mandible by oral squamous cell carcinoma. *Br J Oral Maxillofac Surg.* 1994 Dec;32(6):347–359.

Brown JS, Lowe D, Kalavrezos N, et al. Patterns of invasion and routes of tumor entry into the mandible by oral squamous cell carcinoma. *Head Neck.* 2002 Apr;24(4):370–383.

Carter RL, Tanner NS, Clifford P, et al. Direct bone invasion in squamous carcinomas of the head and neck: pathological and clinical implications. *Clin Otolaryngol Allied Sci.* 1980 Apr;5(2):107–116.

Cawood JI, Howell RA. Reconstructive preprosthetic surgery. I. Anatomical considerations. *Int J Oral Maxillofac Surg.* 1991 Apr;20(2):75–82.

Chung TS, Yousem DM, Seigerman HM, et al. MR of mandibular invasion in patients with oral and oropharyngeal malignant neoplasms. *AJNR Am J Neuroradiol.* 1994 Nov;15(10):1949–1955.

Clementschitsch F. [Roentgenography in disease and injuries of the jaws]. *Dtsch Zahnarztl Z.* 1955 Mar;10(5):380–396. German.

Dubner S, Heller KS. Local control of squamous cell carcinoma following marginal and segmental mandibulectomy. *Head Neck.* 1993 Jan–Feb;15(1):29–32.

Eley KA, Watt-Smith SR, Golding SJ. Magnetic resonance imaging-based tumor volume measurements predict outcome in patients with squamous cell carcinoma of the mandible. *Oral Surg Oral Med Oral Pathol Oral Radiol.* 2013 Feb;115(2):255–262.

Gilbert S, Tzadik A, Leonard G. Mandibular involvement by oral squamous cell carcinoma. *Laryngoscope.* 1986 Jan;96(1):96–101.

Hirsch DL, Dierks EJ. Use of a transbuccal technique for marginal mandibulectomy: a novel approach. *J Oral Maxillofac Surg.* 2007 Sep;65(9):1849–1851.

Klotch DW, Prein J. Mandibular reconstruction using AO plates. *Am J Surg.* 1987 Oct;154(4):384–388.

Kondoh T, Hamada Y, Kamei K, et al. Transport distraction osteogenesis following marginal resection of the mandible. *Int J Oral Maxillofac Surg.* 2002 Dec;31(6):675–676.

Lydiatt DD. Mandibular resection. *Head Neck.* 1995 May–Jun;17(3):247–251.

Mazzarella LA Jr, Friedlander AA. Sagittal ostectomy of the mandible for floor of mouth cancer. *Arch Otolaryngol.* 1981 Apr;107(4):245–248.

McGregor AD, MacDonald DG. Patterns of spread of squamous cell carcinoma to the ramus of the mandible. *Head Neck.* 1993 Sep–Oct;15(5):440–444.

Müller H, Slootweg PJ. Mandibular invasion by oral squamous cell carcinoma. Clinical aspects. *J Craniomaxillofac Surg.* 1990 Feb;18(2):80–84.

O'Brien CJ, Carter RL, Soo KC, et al. Invasion of the mandible by squamous carcinomas of the oral cavity and oropharynx. *Head Neck Surg.* 1986 Mar–Apr;8(4):247–256.

O'Sullivan GJ, Carty FL, Cronin CG. Imaging of bone metastasis: an update. *World J Radio.* 2015, Aug 28;7(8):202–211.

Ord RA, Sarmadi M, Papadimitrou J. A comparison of segmental and marginal bony resection for oral squamous cell carcinoma involving the mandible. *J Oral Maxillofac Surg.* 1997 May;55(5):470–477; discussion 477–478.

Pathak KA, Shah BC. Marginal mandibulectomy: 11 years of institutional experience. *J Oral Maxillofac Surg.* 2009 May;67(5):962–967.

Prein J, Kellman RM. Rigid internal fixation of mandibular fractures—basics of AO technique. *Otolaryngol Clin North Am.* 1987 Aug;20(3):441–456.

Probst FA, Mast G, Ermer M, et al. MatrixMANDIBLE preformed reconstruction plates—a two-year two-institution experience in 71 patients. *J Oral Maxillofac Surg.* 2012 Nov;70(11):e657–666.

Rogers SN, Devine J, Lowe D, et al. Longitudinal health-related quality of life after mandibular resection for oral cancer: a comparison between rim and segment. *Head Neck.* 2004 Jan;26(1):54–62.

Sader R, Noror B, Horch HH, eds. [*Lehrbuch der Ultraschalldiagnostik im Kopf-Hals-Bereich*]. Reinbeck, Germany: Einhorn-Presse Verlag; 2001. German.

Sauerbier S, Gutwald R, Wiedmann-Al-Ahmad M, et al. Clinical application of tissue-engineered transplants. Part I: mucosa. *Clin Oral Implants Res.* 2006 Dec;17(6):625–632.

Schmelzeisen R, Hausamen JE, Neukam FW, et al. Combination of microsurgical tissue reconstruction with osteointegrated dental implants. Presentation of a technique. *Int J Oral Maxillofac Surg.* 1990;19(4):209–211.

Schmelzeisen R, Rahn BA, Brennwald J. Fixation of vascularized bone grafts. *J Craniomaxillofac Surg.* 1993 Apr; 21(3):113–119.

Shaha AR. Preoperative evaluation of the mandible in patients with carcinoma of the floor of mouth. *Head Neck.* 1991 Sep–Oct;13(5):398–402.

Shaha AR. Marginal mandibulectomy for carcinoma of the floor of the mouth. *J Surg Oncol.* 1992 Feb;49(2):116–119.

Slootweg PJ, Müller H. Mandibular invasion by oral squamous cell carcinoma. *J Craniomaxillofac Surg.* 1989 Feb;17(2):69–74.

Söderholm AL, Lindqvist C, Hietanen J, et al. Bone scanning for evaluating mandibular bone extension of oral squamous cell carcinoma. *J Oral Maxillofac Surg*. 1990 Mar;48(3):252–257.

Totsuka Y, Usui Y, Tei K, et al. Results of surgical treatment for squamous carcinoma of the lower alveolus: segmental vs marginal resection. *Head Neck*. 1991 Mar–Apr;13(2):114–120.

Tsue TT, McCulloch TM, Girod DA, et al. Predictors of carcinomatous invasion of the mandible. *Head Neck*. 1994 Mar–Apr;16(2):116–126.

van den Brekel MW, Castelijns JA, Snow GB. The role of modern imaging studies in staging and therapy of head and neck neoplasms. *Semin Oncol*. 1994 Jun;21(3):340–348.

Vidiri A, Guerrisi A, Pellini R, et al. Multi-detector row computed tomography (MDCT) and magnetic resonance imaging (MRI) in the evaluation of the mandibular invasion by squamous cell carcinomas (SCC) of the oral cavity. Correlation with pathological data. *J Exp Clin Cancer Res*. 2010;29:73.

Wolff D, Hassfeld S, Hofele C. Influence of marginal and segmental mandibular resection on the survival rate in patients with squamous cell carcinoma of the inferior parts of the oral cavity. *J Craniomaxillofac Surg*. 2004 Oct;32(5):318–323.

Wolff KD, Hoelzle F. *Raising of Microvascular Flaps*. Berlin Heidelberg: Springer-Verlag; 2011.

Zupi A, Califano L, Maremonti P, et al. Accuracy in the diagnosis of mandibular involvement by oral cancer. *J Craniomaxillofac Surg*. 1996 Oct;24(5):281–284.

2.3 Benign noncontinuity intraosseous lesions

Michel Richter

1 Introduction

Benign noncontinuity intraosseous mandibular and maxillary lesions are likely to be treated by curettage and/or enucleation. They include odontogenic cysts (ie, dentigerous cysts), non-odontogenic cysts (ie, aneurismal cysts, solitary bone cysts), benign osteolytic neoplasms (ie, keratocysts, unicystic ameloblastoma, giant cell granuloma), and some fibroosseous lesions (ie, ossifying fibroma, fibrous dysplasia). These pathologies have the common attribute that they usually can be adequately treated without segmental resection of the mandible or maxilla.

These lesions have a distinct potential to grow to a considerable size producing thinning and sometimes erosion of both the inner or outer mandibular or maxillary cortex. Nerve function is usually intact.

A pathological fracture of the structurally weakened bone may occur either before treatment, at the time of tumor removal, or any time after surgery, especially if the mass extends to the inferior mandibular border.

2 Clinical diagnosis and imaging

The pathologies discussed in this chapter typically grow without symptoms until they are either randomly detected by a routine x-ray or have grown to such a size that contour changes are detectable.

Necessary imaging usually includes an orthopantomogram for smaller lesions (**Fig 2.3-1**). For larger lesions and those in proximity to specific anatomical structures like the inferior alveolar nerves, maxillary sinuses, or condyles, a computed tomography (CT) or cone beam CT is indicated (**Fig 2.3-2**). A magnetic resonance imaging scan may be complementary for vascular lesions.

3 Treatment considerations

3.1 Biopsy

While smaller lesions can be removed in a 1-stage procedure, it is recommended to take biopsies of larger lesions to establish a diagnosis as part of treatment planning. The reason for this is that some lesions like keratocysts or unicystic ameloblastoma require a locally more aggressive treatment.

3.2 Treatment

Removal of the lesion from the bony cavity by enucleation of the cystic membranes and/or curettage is the treatment of choice for most of the lesions with the exception of keratocysts or unicystic ameloblastoma.

A transoral vestibular approach is indicated for lesions arising in the tooth-bearing area and is best accomplished by using an extended broad-based full-thickness mucoperiosteal flap to expose the lateral cortex overlying the lesions. A transcutaneous approach is indicated for mandibular lesions when much of the ramus and the condyle are involved by the pathological process.

Keratocysts or unicystic ameloblastomas, require a thorough curettage complemented by removing a thin layer of bone adjacent to the pathology with a burr. In addition, the modified Carnoy solution may be used to better facilitate removal of those pathologies and avoid recurrences.

There should also be wide access to the mass, which frequently needs a large lateral decortication so that all the pathology can be directly visualized and totally removed.

In most mandibular cases, preservation of the inferior alveolar nerve is possible because the pathological process displaces the neurovascular bundle and the mandibular canal rather than invading the nerve. Nerve function is usually intact before treatment.

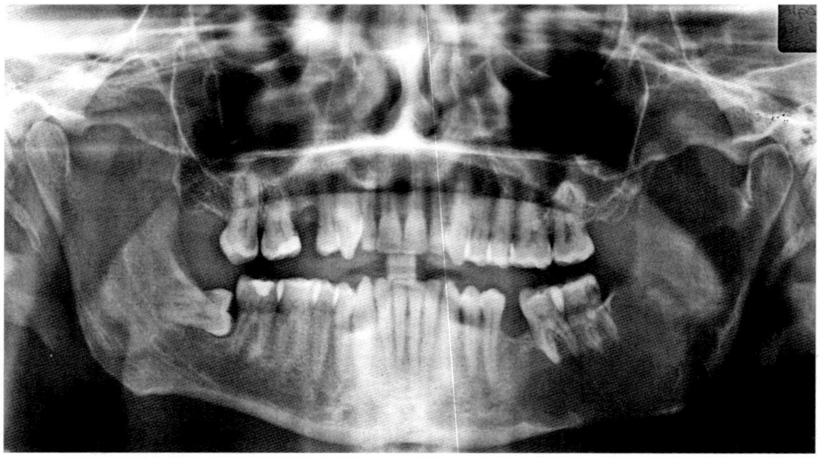

Fig 2.3-1 Orthopantomogram. Large odontogenic keratocyst confirmed by an intraoral biopsy before definitive treatment. The well-defined radiolucent area involves half of the mandibular body and the whole ramus on the left. The anterior margins of the cavity are smooth with a thin cortex left at the posterior border. The lesion is adjacent to the erupted teeth but without resorption of their roots. The canal of the inferior alveolar nerve is displaced to the inferior border.

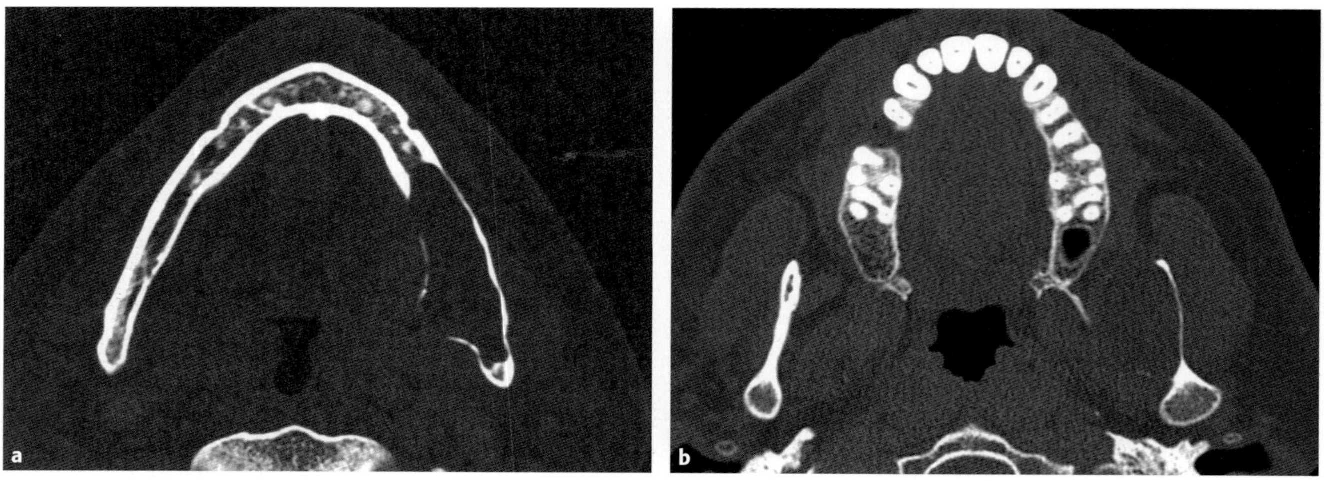

Fig 2.3-2a–b Computed tomographic (CT) scan. Expansion of the lesion has thinned the vestibular cortical plate. The lingual cortex of the posterior mandibular body and the ascending ramus perforated. The head of the condyle is intact. In general, the keratocyst herniates out of bone but does not infiltrate the soft tissues adjacent to the mandible.

3.3 Autogenous or alloplastic bone replacement

Large residual cavities are best grafted primarily with autogenous bone. This remains the gold standard in the treatment of large bone defects. Immediate grafting with autogenous cancellous bone chips will provide bone to improve strength and add bone stock for insertion of dental implants and dental rehabilitation. Autogenous bone provides a good osteoconductive, osteoinductive, and osteogenic substrate able to induce new bone formation at the recipient sites.

The iliac crest and the proximal tibia are possible donor sites, which can be selected according to the expected volume of bone required [Engelstad et al, 2010].

To minimize the amount of graft required to fill large cavities, a mixture of autogenous cancellous bone chips and alloplastic materials like hydroxylapatite (HA) or β-tricalcium phosphate can be used.

3.4 Protection plating

For large mandibular defects, autogenous cancellous bone grafting does not provide immediate stability for the weakened mandible. Although the mandibular bony walls are preserved they are usually thinned, and there is loss of internal resistance and capacity to sustain forces and strains, which act on the mandibular body during mastication.

Postoperative mandibulomaxillary fixation (MMF) may be a preventive measure. Immobilization may be necessary for about 4 weeks to prevent a fracture. On the other hand, MMF has adverse effects, which imply that it is a procedure not as benign as commonly thought [Ellis et al, 1989].

Inserting and fixing a load-bearing reconstruction plate to protect the weakened area of the mandible can avoid a pathological fracture during or after the procedure instead of MMF. The plate must be applied in the same manner as for a comminuted or defect fracture. An angulated or preformed plate can be selected for large lesions. This process is called "protection plating".

The length of the plate depends on the radiographic and clinical extension of the disease, but a minimum of three screws should be used in each segment on either side of the lesion. Adapting the plate to the mandibular contour before the removal of the lesion is preferred. In case an expansive pathology has changed the original contour of the mandible, an initial adaptation of the protection plate is not recommended. In those scenarios the lesion needs to be removed first, then a reconstruction plate is placed secondarily, usually with the patient in MMF. An alternative is manufacturing of an individual patient-specific protection plate following a CAD/CAM planning and manufacturing process (see chapter 5.3.10).

After complete removal of the pathology, larger defects are filled with autogenous bone, a mixture of autogenous bone and alloplastic material, or alloplastic material alone depending on the biomechanical situation and surgeons and patients preferences (**Fig 2.3-3**).

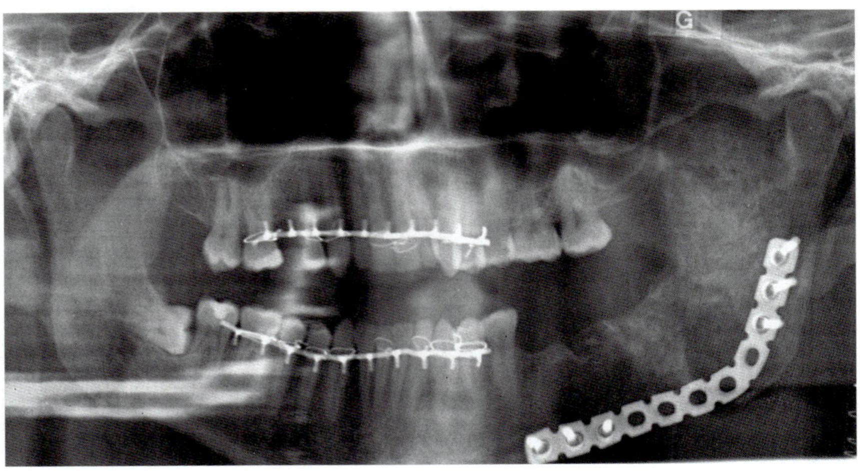

Fig 2.3-3 Orthopantomogram 2 days postoperatively. A reconstruction plate was fixed before removal of a keratocyst with three screws on each side and the cavity was filled with cancellous bone chips taken from the iliac crest. Arch bars were applied for intraoperative mandibulomaxillary fixation.

If a transoral vestibular approach was chosen, suturing of the mucosal flaps must create a tight seal to minimize contamination from the oral flora.

A therapeutic course of antibiotics is preferred after surgery. The patient is instructed to maintain good oral hygiene, which can be supplemented using chlorhexidine solution.

If a transcutaneous approach has been used, a suction drain helps to avoid the formation of a dead space or a hematoma. The closure is done in layers with resorbable and nonresorbable suture material depending on the surgeon's preference. A short course of prophylactic antibiotic therapy (maximum 48 hours) is adequate only if any intraoral contamination by the saliva can be excluded. If not, a 10-day therapeutic course of antibiotics should be considered. Protection plating to reinforce a curetted and grafted mandibular defect is functionally stable, thus a soft diet is not necessary in the postoperative period.

3.5 Plate removal

The reconstruction plate can be left in place permanently in adults but patients may request its removal for personal or cosmetic reasons. If screws interfere with the insertion of dental implants, this could also be a reason for screw or plate removal. In any event, the plate should not be removed for a minimum of 6 months after the original surgery.

3.6 Dental implants

In case of tooth loss in the area of the pathology, placement of dental implants in grafted bone may be considered after a 3-month period of initial bone healing (**Fig 2.3-4**).

4 Complications and pitfalls

If a plate has not been adapted before the removal of the lesion and there is an incidental fracture during the curettage procedure, the patient must be placed in temporary MMF before adaptation and fixation of the reconstruction plate. The procedure is comparable with an osteosynthesis of a fracture in bone of reduced quality.

Early intraoral exposure of cancellous bone chips or alloplastic material because of wound dehiscence should be treated by superficial curettage, revision of the wound, and secondary closure.

Contamination of the graft can lead to infection with swelling and drainage. Management consists of reopening the original wound, taking samples for bacteriology, debridement of the wound, and removal of all sequestra. A therapeutic course of antibiotics is prescribed and if necessary modified according to the results of the bacterial cultures.

The plate should not be removed if it is stable with no loose screws.

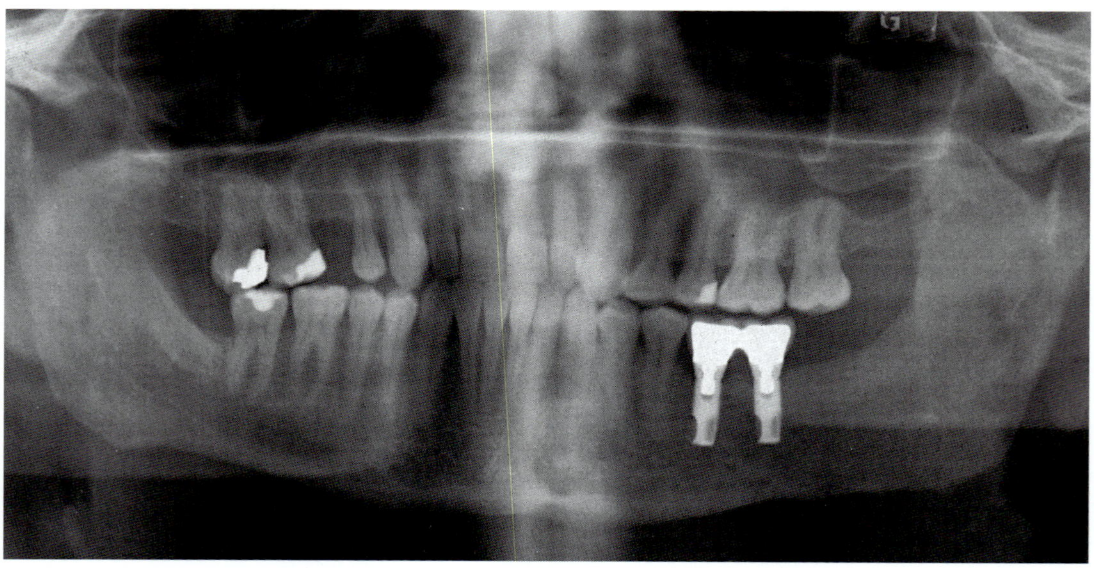

Fig 2.3-4 Orthopantomogram 2 years postoperatively (same case as in **Fig 2.3-3**). The plate was removed on the patient's request. Two dental implants were placed 1 year after the operation, followed by over-denture 6 months later for rehabilitation of the occlusion.

5 References and suggested reading

Adamopoulos O, Papadopoulos T. Nanostructured bioceramics for maxillofacial applications. *J Mater Sci Mater Med*. 2007 Aug;18(8):1587–1597.
Ellis E 3rd, Carlson DS. The effects of mandibular immobilization on the masticatory system: a review. *Clin Plast Surg*. 1989 Jan;16(1):133–146.
Engelstad ME, Morse T. Anterior iliac crest, posterior iliac crest, and proximal tibia donor sites: a comparison of cancellous bone volumes in fresh cadavers. *J Oral Maxillofac Surg*. 2010;68:3015–3021.

2.4 Segmental defects, defect bridging, reconstruction with free nonvascularized bone grafts

Edward Ellis III

1 Introduction—segmental resection of mandibular tumors

If a tumor extends close to the inferior border of the mandible, a discontinuity will be created with resection of the tumor. It will therefore be necessary to bridge the defect with a load-bearing reconstruction bone plate, bone graft or bone flap to maintain the position of the residual mandibular fragments and the mandible [Alpert et al, 2012]. The following points will affect the way that surgery is performed:

When a continuity defect is created, the muscles of mastication attached to the residual mandibular fragments will distract the fragments in different directions unless efforts are made to stabilize the remaining mandible in its normal position at the time of partial resection. Maintaining relationships with the remaining mandible fragments after resection of portions of the mandible is a key principle of mandibular reconstruction. This is important for occlusal and temporomandibular joint positioning. When the residual fragments are left to drift, significant facial distortions can occur from deviation of the residual mandibular fragments. Reconstruction (load-bearing) bone plates inserted at the time of resection are useful for controlling the position of the mandibular fragments [Alpert et al, 2012]. These plates are of sufficient strength to obviate the need for mandibulomaxillary fixation, permitting active use of the mandible in the immediate postoperative period. When the mandibular symphysis has been removed, the tongue can be sutured to the plate, maintaining its forward position to prevent airway obstruction. The bone plate can be left in place when the mandible is secondarily reconstructed with bone grafts, permitting mobility of the mandible during the healing phase of the bone graft. If the condyle requires removal with the surgical specimen and delayed bone reconstruction is chosen, the reconstruction bone plate may need to have a prosthetic condylar process attached until bony reconstruction is performed (see chapter 2.5).

If the resection requires intraoral exposure of the site, delayed bone reconstruction is usually chosen because of the high-infection risk of an immediate nonvascularized bone graft from oral contamination. Alternatively, microvascular bone flaps are an option.

The position of the mandible must be reestablished after the resection procedure to maintain proper occlusion of the remaining teeth. Pre-plating is the best option when possible (see Case 3). If pre-plating is not possible and when adequate teeth are present on each side of the resection defect, arch bars applied to the upper and lower teeth or intermaxillary fixation screws can maintain the occlusion after resection, with the patient in mandibulomaxillary fixation, when the reconstruction bone plate is being adapted. If the patient has inadequate teeth present on one or both sides of the resection defect, pre-plating (if possible) or plates spanning between the maxilla and mandible in areas away from the resection can be applied before resection and reapplied afterward to maintain the proper position of the mandible while the reconstruction bone plate is applied. Alternatively, a fix-bridge temporary plating system can be applied from one side to the other to maintain the position of the fragments until a reconstruction plate is adapted. The fix-bridge is then removed.

If the tumor has not expanded the buccal cortex of the mandible, in situ adaptation of the reconstruction bone plate can be performed before resection (pre-plating), especially if the tumor is benign and the outer cortex intact. This provides perfect positioning of the mandibular fragments so the occlusion should not be affected.

If the tumor has expanded or destroyed the buccal cortex, preadaptation of a bone plate can be performed by making a stereolithographic model of the affected mandible, burring down the involved area, and adapting a reconstruction bone plate to the model. The plate is sterilized and used during surgery, saving time intraoperatively. CAD/CAM technology is another option (see chapter 5.3.12).

2 Principles of defect bridging

When a discontinuity of the mandible is created, a reconstruction bone plate will be required to maintain the position of the residual mandibular fragments and the position of the mandible in space. These plates are strong (load-bearing) and can function for months until bone can be successfully transplanted to obtain osseous reconstruction across the defect. When applying reconstruction bone plates to a mandibular discontinuity, several factors are important:

- A reconstruction bone plate 2.4 or similar is recommended because it has sufficient strength to transfer all forces of mastication across to the opposite side, ie, it is load-bearing [Alpert et al, 2012].
- A minimum of three screws on each side of the defect are necessary for defect bridging. It is always better to have more (**Fig 2.4-1**).
- Reconstruction bone plates using locking screws are preferable because the chance of a screw loosening with resultant inflammation and (potentially) infection is minimized [Herford et al, 1988]. Loss of fixation is less likely than when nonlocking screws are used because attaching screws to the plate increases the rigidity of the fixation across the defect.
- The occlusion of any remaining teeth must be reestablished before attaching a reconstruction bone plate (**Fig 2.4-1** and **Fig 2.4-5**).

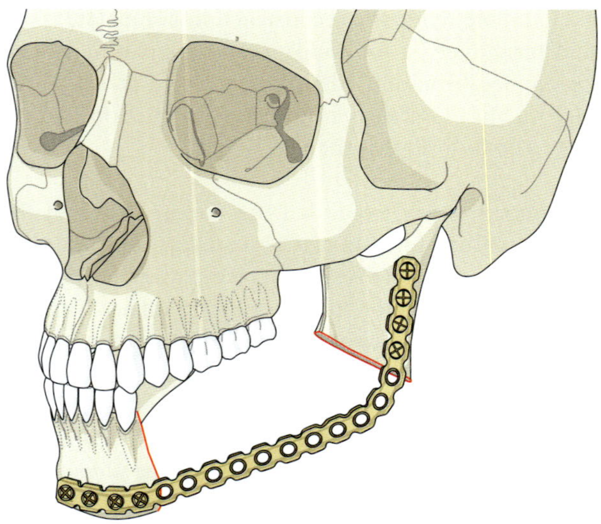

Fig 2.4-1 Bridging of a lateral mandibular defect with a reconstruction plate. Fixation with four screws on each side.

2.1 Examples

For purposes of this chapter, it is assumed that the tumors that are being removed are benign tumors requiring segmental resection because of involvement of both the alveolar process as well as encroachment on the inferior border. It is further assumed that stable internal fixation of the mandible will occur with a reconstruction bone plate primarily and osseous reconstruction will occur secondarily using nonvascularized bone.

Case 1: Segmental resection of an ameloblastoma in the posterior mandibular region where condyle can be maintained and there is expansion of buccal cortex: pre-plating is not possible (**Fig 2.4-2**).

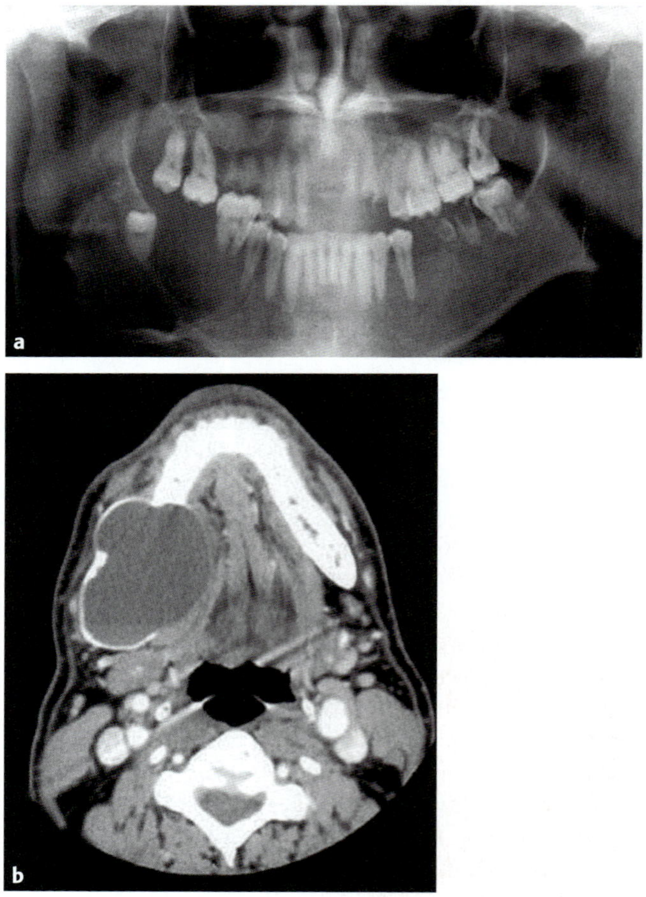

Fig 2.4-2a–b

a Ameloblastoma in the right angle of the mandible.

b A computed tomographic scan of tumor showing the expansion of the lateral cortex.

Expansion of the buccal cortex precludes pre-plating. Segmental resection of an expanding benign tumor in the posterior mandible/ramus region of the mandible is performed in one of three ways. The following steps highlight these procedures:

1. Exposure of the site is performed via a transoral approach. The soft-tissue incisions around the resection will vary depending on tumor involvement and location of previous biopsy site. All mucosa surrounding the biopsy must be excised with the specimen (**Fig 2.4-3**).
2. For dentate patients, arch bars or intermaxillary fixation screws are placed.
3. If there will be ample bone remaining in the mandibular ramus after tumor resection, a condyle-positioning plate spanning between the zygoma and the mandibular ramus can be applied (**Fig 2.4-5**).
4. The resection is performed with burrs, saws, piezoelectric devices, etc (**Fig 2.4-4**).

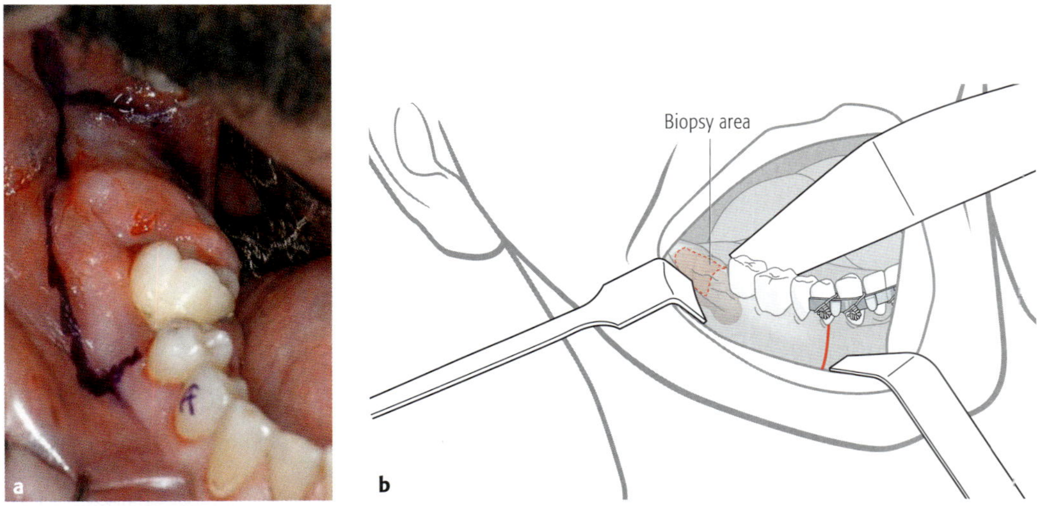

Fig 2.4-3a–b A biopsy specimen was taken in the retromolar area. Mucosa surrounding biopsy site is excised at the same time. An extraoral approach may be used simultaneously to facilitate resection and application of the reconstruction bone plate.

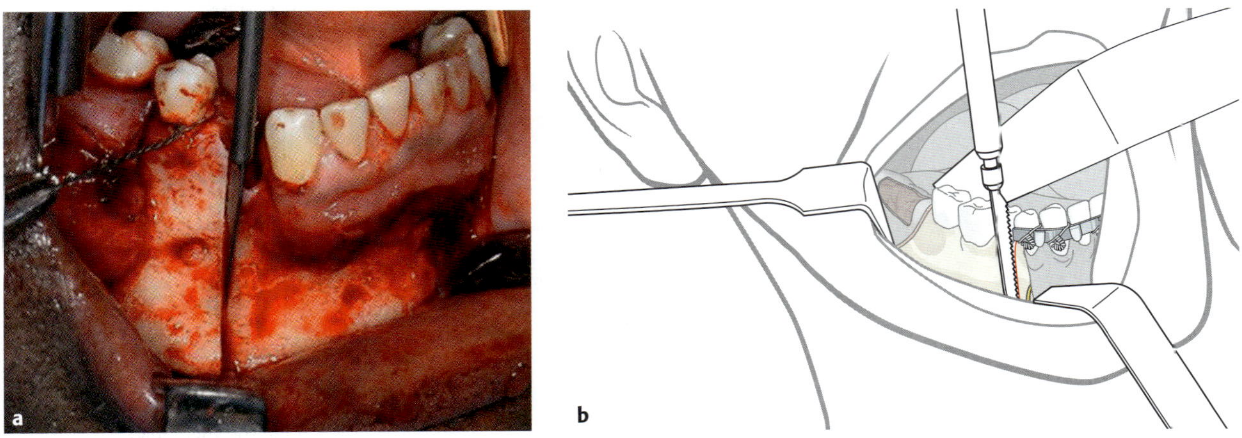

Fig 2.4-4a–b The mandible is cut anterior to the tumor through the alveolus of the second premolar with a reciprocating saw.

5. The occlusion is reestablished by maxillomandibular fixation (MMF). Wire ligatures are used in the clinical case (**Fig 2.4-5**). Some surgeons prefer MMF via arch bars as shown in the drawings.
6. If a condyle positioning plate was adapted, it is now replaced to maintain the preoperative position of the mandibular ramus.
7. A reconstruction bone plate is adapted and secured across the defect. The MMF is released and the occlusion verified (**Fig 2.4-6**).
8. The soft tissues are closed.
9. Alternatively, a stereolithographic model can be made prior to surgery and the expanded buccal cortex shaved down to mirror the opposite side. A reconstruction bone plate can be preadapted on the model, sterilized and used during surgery (**Fig 2.4-7**).

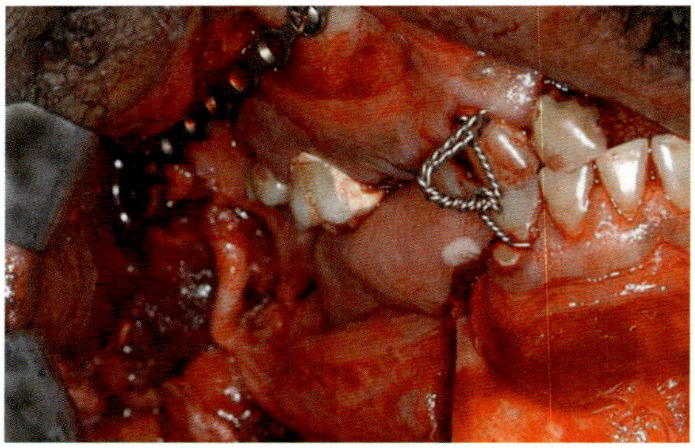

Fig 2.4-5 Tumor resected. Patient in maxillomandibular fixation and a bone plate adapted between zygoma and ramus of the mandible is shown.

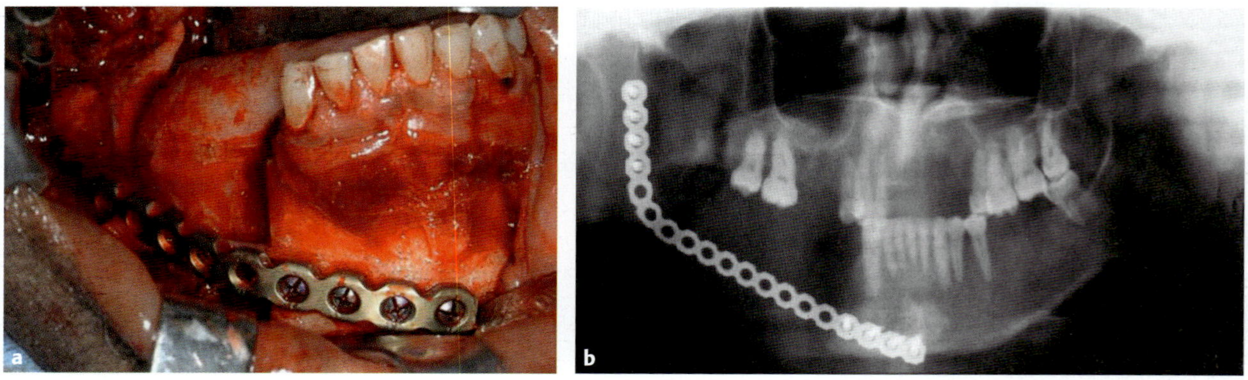

Fig 2.4-6a–b
a Reconstruction plate in place after tumor resection.
b Postoperative view with reconstruction plate bridging the defect.

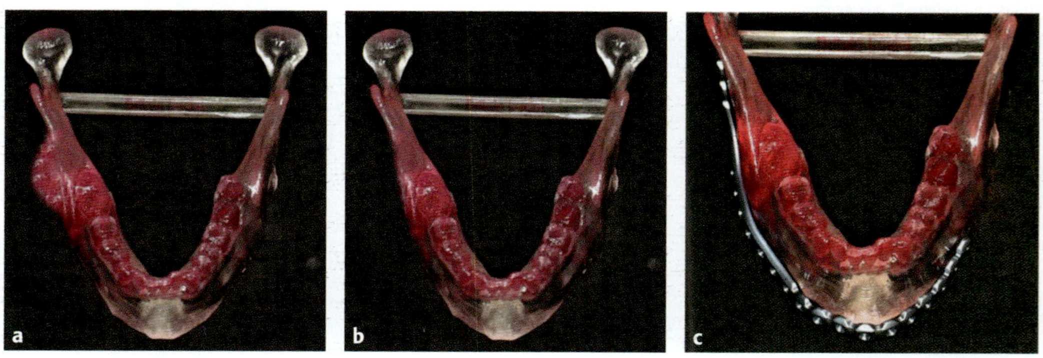

Fig 2.4-7a–c
a STL model of an expanded buccal cortex.
b Buccal expansion of the cortex removed.
c Adaptation of the reconstruction plate after removal of buccal expansion.

Case 2: Segmental resection of an ameloblastoma in the posterior mandible/ramus region of the mandible that necessitates removal of the mandibular condyle requires that a reconstruction bone plate with a prosthetic condyle be available **(Fig 2.4-8)**.

The following steps highlight this procedure:

1. Exposure of the site is performed via a transoral approach. The soft-tissue incisions around the resection will vary depending on tumor involvement. An extraoral approach may be used simultaneously to facilitate resection and application of the reconstruction bone plate.
2. For dentate patients, arch bars or intermaxillary fixation screws are placed. For non-dentate patients, bone plates spanning between the maxilla and mandible are applied before resection and replaced after resection but before adaptation of the reconstruction bone plate. To increase the efficiency during surgery, a stereolithographic model that includes the temporal component of the temporomandibular joint can be made before surgery and the anticipated resection performed so that the reconstruction bone plate/condyle unit can be preadapted.
3. The anterior margin osteotomy is performed with burrs, saws, piezoelectric devices, etc. The dissection includes the entire ramus into the articular capsule. The inferior alveolar vessels require ligation at the mandibular foramen. The specimen is removed with the condyle attached and the articular disc is left in situ.
4. The MMF is reestablished.
5. A reconstruction bone plate that contains a prosthetic condyle is positioned into the glenoid fossa and adapted to the residual mandible. It is attached with a minimum of three screws (**Fig 2.4-9**).
6. The MMF is released and the occlusion verified.
7. The soft tissues are closed. A drain may be needed.

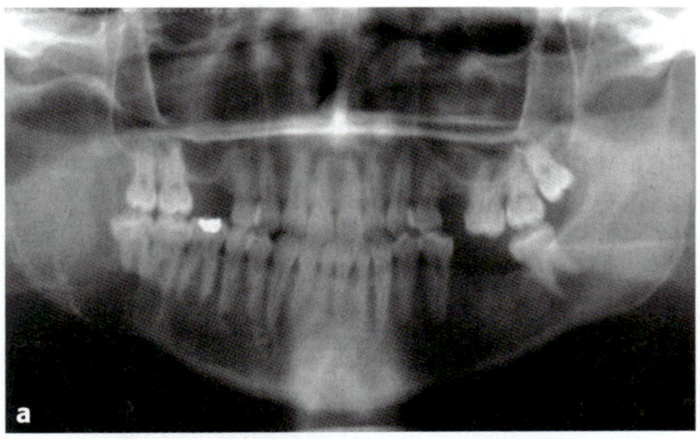

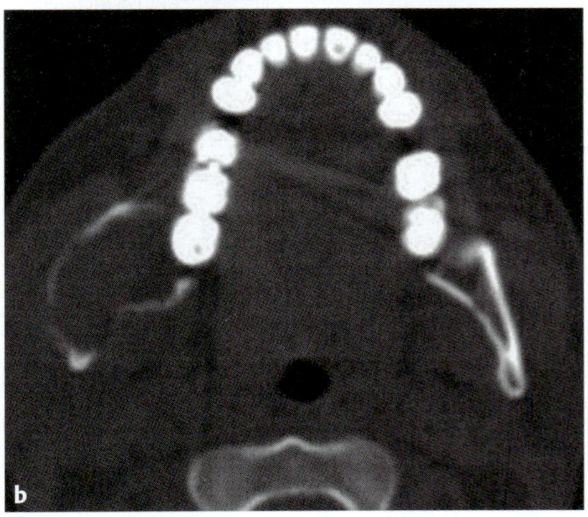

Fig 2.4-8a–b
a Ameloblastoma in the right angle of the mandible.
b The cortex is expanded and the tumor is encroaching on the condylar process.

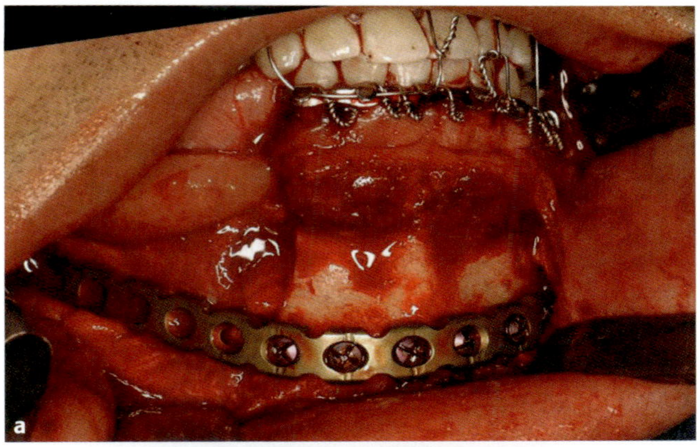

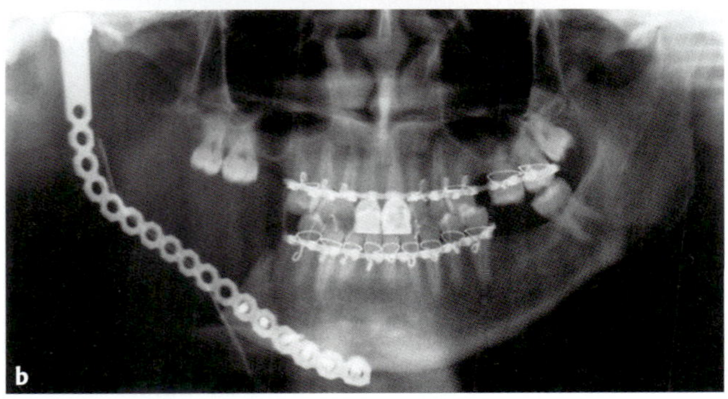

Fig 2.4-9a–b
a The patient is in maxillomandibular fixation (MMF) and the reconstruction plate is in place.
b Postoperative image showing the reconstruction plate with condylar head in place and MMF.

8. Once the mucosa has healed (approximately 8 weeks), bony reconstruction can proceed.
9. Because the mandibular condyle has been removed, a costochondral bone graft with approximately 3–4 mm of cartilage can be used to reconstruct the missing condyle (**Fig 2.4-10**). The occlusion is re-established and secured by MMF, and a transfacial approach to the posterior mandibular body and ramus is used to access the defect. After dissection of the bone plate and the creation of a surgical pocket for the bone graft, the condylar portion of the reconstruction bone plate is removed by cutting through the plate with a burr. The costochondral graft is slotted with a fissure burr to allow it to slide around the vertical portion of the bone plate, taking care to assure firm seating into the mandibular fossa (**Fig 2.4-11**). Bone screws through the rib graft are used to secure the graft to the bone plate. The mandibular ramus and posterior body are then reconstructed by first securing a solid piece of corticocancellous iliac bone to the bone plate, angling the superior portion of the graft toward the lingual side to provide space for reconstruction of the basal bone and alveolus using particulate bone. The particulate bone is packed tightly to provide good bone density and the soft tissues are closed (**Fig 2.4-12** and **Fig 2.4-13**).
10. Because the rib graft has thin bony cortices, MMF is maintained for 6 weeks to allow the bone grafts to solidify.

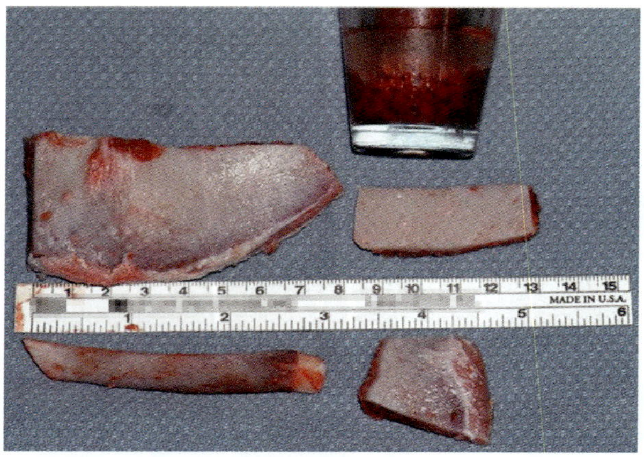

Fig 2.4-10 Bone grafts after harvesting from iliac crest and rib.

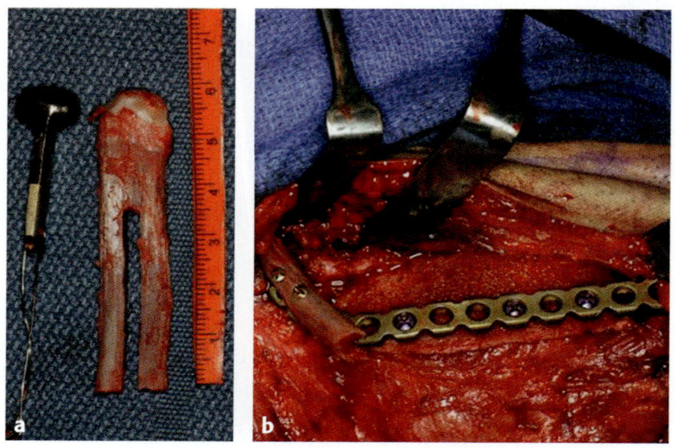

Fig 2.4-11a–b Condylar prosthesis is removed, and the rib graft is slotted to adapt around the posterior portion of the bone plate.

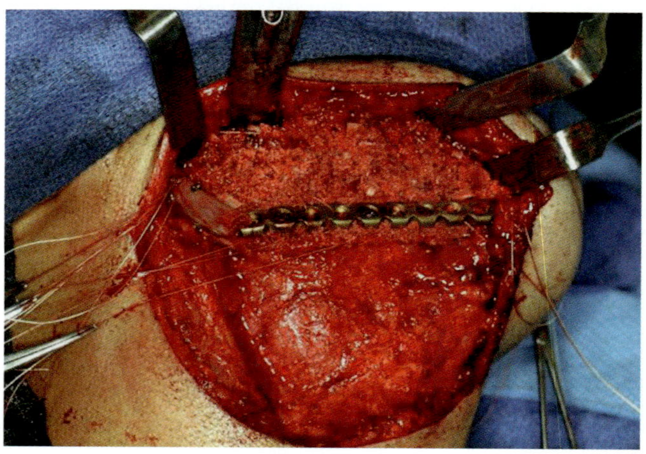

Fig 2.4-12 Corticocancellous bone graft is attached to the reconstruction plate in the area of the mandibular ramus/body. The wound is closed in layers, and a suction drain is installed. X-rays are taken directly after surgery and at an interval of some months to check bone healing and bone graft take.

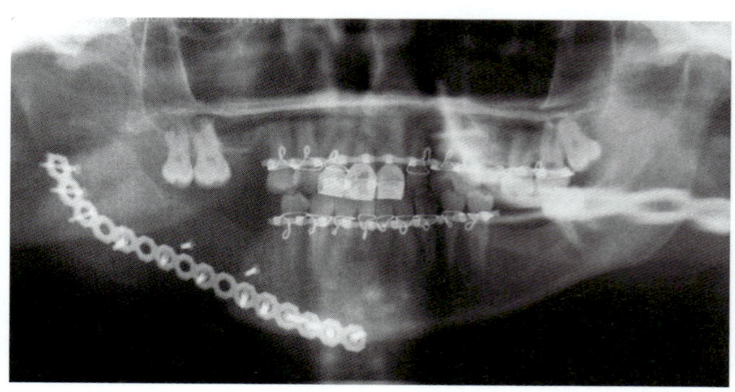

Fig 2.4-13 Orthopantomogram showing the reconstruction 3 months after tumor resection.

Case 3: Segmental resection of a nonexpanding ameloblastoma in the body and symphysis region of the mandible is perhaps the most routine and uncomplicated of all resection procedures (**Fig 2.4-14**).

The following steps highlight this procedure:

1. Exposure of the site is performed via a transoral approach (**Fig 2.4-15**). The soft-tissue incisions in the area of resection will vary depending on tumor involvement. An extraoral approach can be used simultaneously if needed to facilitate resection and application of the reconstruction bone plate.

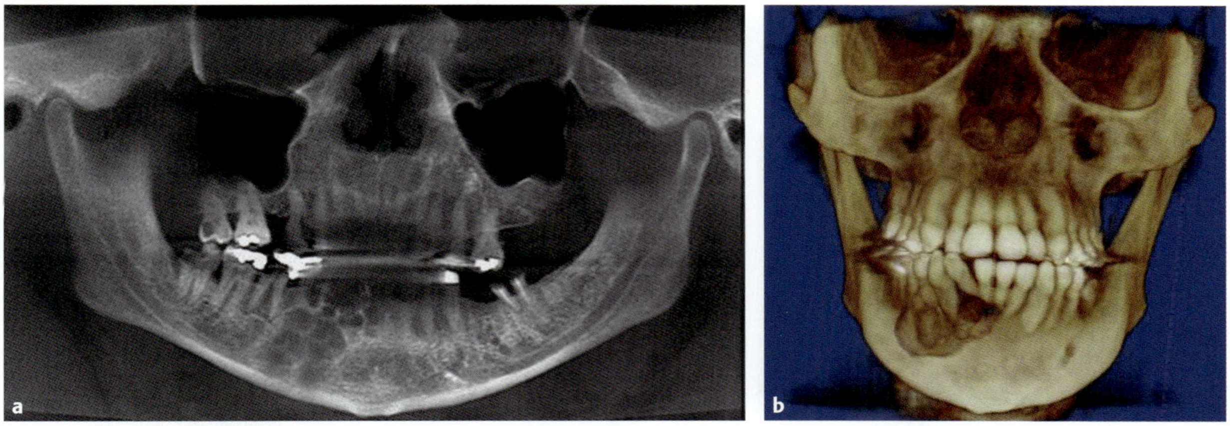

Fig 2.4-14a–b Orthopantomogram of the mandible showing an ameloblastoma in the right mandibular body. There is no expansion of the buccal cortex at the inferior border, where the reconstruction plate will be applied.

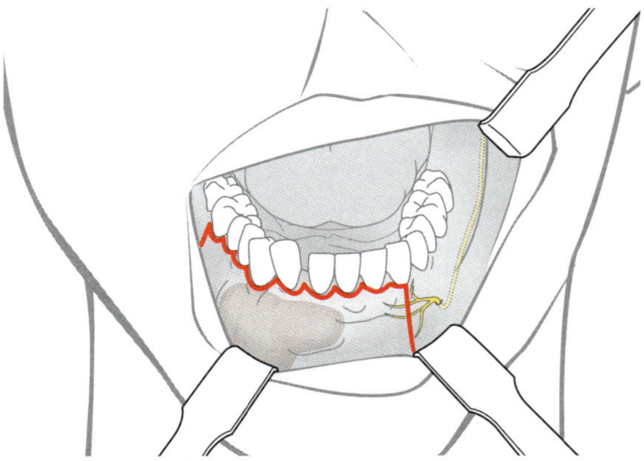

Fig 2.4-15 Transoral incisions for segmental resection of the mandible.

2. The mandible is preplated. The plate can either be removed or left attached during the resection depending on access (**Fig 2.4-16**).
3. The resection is performed with burrs, saws, piezoelectric devices, etc.
4. If the plate was removed, it is now reapplied and the occlusion verified (**Fig 2.4-17** and **Fig 2.4-18**).
5. If the symphysis has been removed, the tongue musculature is sutured to the bone plate to prevent glossoptosis (**Fig 2.4-19**).
6. The soft tissues are closed.

3 Secondary reconstruction of the mandible with nonvascularized autogenous bone

Each bone defect poses a unique set of problems that reconstructive surgical intervention must address. In each of these instances, restoration of normal structure is usually possible, with resultant improvement in function and appearance. When an osseous structure is defective in size, shape, position, or amount, reconstructive surgery can replace the defective structure.

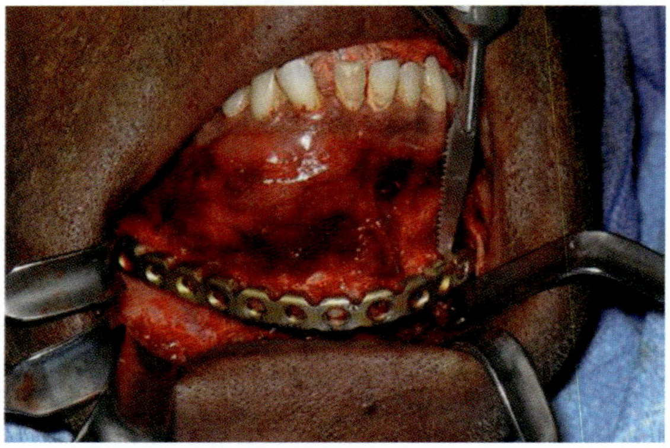

Fig 2.4-16 Intraoral exposure of the inferior lateral mandible in the tumor area. The reconstruction plate is attached with screws on both sides of the resection defect before the resection is performed. Now the anterior osteotomy is performed with a reciprocating saw.

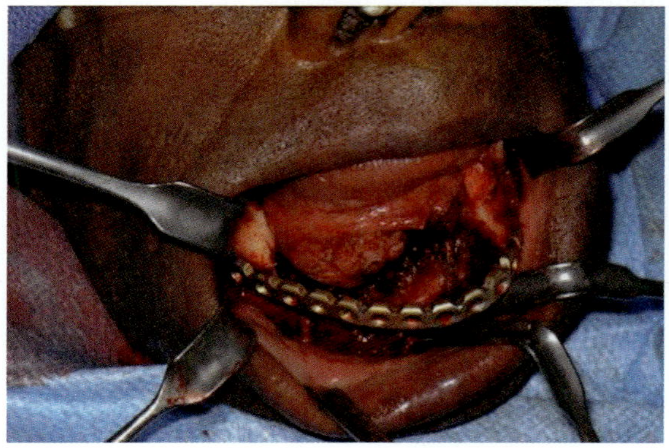

Fig 2.4-17 After resection the defect is shown.

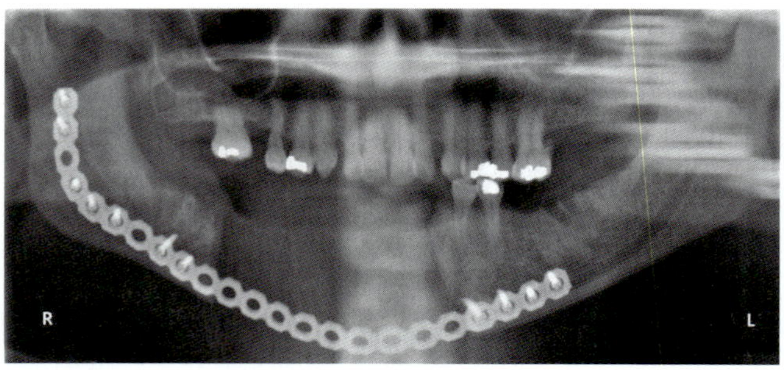

Fig 2.4-18 Orthopantomogram showing the reconstruction plate in place after the tumor resection.

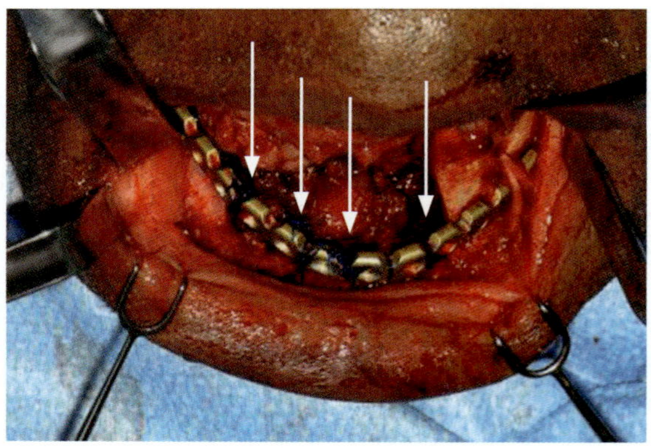

Fig 2.4-19 The tongue musculature is sutured (white arrows) to the bone plate.

Several types of grafts are available to the surgeon. In this chapter, the use of nonvascularized autogenous bone is presented.

3.1 Assessment of osseous defect

Each patient must be thoroughly evaluated because no two patients have the exact same problems. Analysis of the patient's problem must consider the hard-tissue defect, any soft-tissue defects, and any associated problems that will affect treatment.

3.1.1 Hard-tissue defect

Several factors concerning the actual osseous defect must be thoroughly assessed to help formulate a viable treatment plan. Adequate radiographs are necessary to evaluate the full extent of the osseous defect. The site of the defect may be just as important as the size of the defect when dealing with mandibular osseous problems. For example, if the mandibular condyle is missing, treatment is relatively more difficult. A residual portion of the ramus with the condyle still attached makes osseous reconstruction easier because the temporomandibular articulation is difficult to restore.

The mandible has powerful muscles attached to it that usually direct functional movements. When the continuity of the mandible is broken, these muscles no longer work in harmony and may severely displace mandibular fragments into unnatural positions. Therefore, the position of the residual mandibular fragments must be ascertained. For example, if a portion of the mandible around the molars is missing, the muscles of mastication still attached to the mandibular ramus may rotate the ramus anteriorly-superiorly and medially, which may allow penetration into the oral cavity and compound the difficulty of planned treatment. Ideally, maintenance of the position of the residual mandibular fragments will have occurred during the extirpative surgery with a reconstruction bone plate, simplifying bone reconstruction.

3.1.2 Soft-tissue defect

Proper preparation of the soft-tissue bed that is to receive the bone graft is just as important to the success of bone grafting as the bone graft material itself. Cells close to the graft surface are initially nourished by diffusion of nutrients from the surrounding soft tissues. Revascularization of the bone graft through the development of new blood vessels from the soft-tissue bed must then occur. Thus, an essential factor for the success of any bone-grafting procedure is the availability of an adequately vascularized soft-tissue bed. Fortunately, this essential factor is usually obtainable in the lush vascular tissue of the head and neck region. However, occasionally the soft-tissue bed is not as good as it should be, such as after radiotherapy or excessive scarring from trauma or infection. In those cases, vascularized bone flaps must be used. Therefore, a thorough assessment of the quantity and quality of the surrounding soft tissues is necessary before undertaking bone graft procedures. In an environment of poor soft-tissue quality and quantity, macrovascular tissue transfer should be considered.

An intraoral examination helps the clinician determine how much oral mucosa is present and the condition of the tissues. If the patient received cancericidal doses of radiation to the area of the osseous defect, the clinician can assume that the patient's soft tissues have undergone extreme atrophy and scarring and will be nonpliable and fragile. The soft tissues in this instance will provide a poor bed for a bone graft because the environment is hypovascular, hypoxic, and hypocellular [Marx et al, 1986]. Similarly, if the patient's defect was caused by a severe infection, it is likely that an excess of scar tissue formation occurred, which will result in nonpliable, poorly vascularized tissue.

After a thorough evaluation, a decision must be made about the adequacy of the soft tissues. If the quantity of tissue is deficient, soft-tissue flaps from the neck containing muscle and skin can be used to enhance the amount of tissue available to close over the bone graft. Soft-tissue free flaps, such as the radial forearm flap, may be considered. If the soft tissues are deficient in quality, one can improve the quality of the soft tissues present using hyperbaric oxygen (HBO). The HBO method improves tissue oxygenation by the administration of oxygen to the patient under higher-than-normal atmospheric pressures. Tissue oxygenation has been shown to improve to acceptable levels after 30 HBO treatments; however, this is still controversial among clinicians [Herford et al, 1998]. After HBO treatment, bone-grafting procedures can be performed with good success. Another course of HBO treatment is then recommended after the bone-grafting procedure [Marx et al, 1982].

3.2 Source of graft

The bone can be obtained from various donor sites in the body and can be taken in several different forms. Block grafts are solid pieces of both cortical and underlying cancellous bone. The iliac crest is often used as a source of this type of graft. The entire thickness of the ilium can be obtained, or the ilium can be split to obtain a thinner piece of block graft. Ribs also constitute a form of block graft but are used less frequently for mandibular reconstruction because of their size and the morbidity from their harvest. However, taken as a costochondral graft, they are used for replacement of the mandibular condyle when missing. Particulate marrow cancellous bone grafts are obtained by harvesting the medullary bone and the associated endosteum and hematopoietic marrow. Particulate marrow cancellous bone grafts produce the greatest concentration of osteogenic cells, and due to the particulate nature more cells survive transplantation because of the access they have to nutrients in the surrounding graft bed [Gray et al, 1982]. The most common site for the procurement of this type of graft is again the ilium.

3.3 Goals of mandibular reconstruction

Marx and Saunders [1986] have identified several major goals for mandibular reconstruction that one should strive for and achieve before considering any grafting procedure a success.

3.3.1 Restoration of continuity

Because the mandible is a bone with two articulating ends acted on by muscles with opposing forces, restoration of continuity is the highest priority when reconstructing the mandible. Achieving this goal provides the patient with better functional movements and improved facial esthetics by realigning any deviated mandibular segments.

3.3.2 Restoration of alveolar bone height

The functional rehabilitation of the patient rests on the ability to masticate efficiently and comfortably. Prosthetic dental appliances are frequently necessary in patients who have lost a portion of their mandible. To facilitate prosthetic appliance usage, an adequate alveolar process must be provided during the reconstructive surgery.

3.3.3 Restoration of osseous bulk

Any bone-grafting procedure must provide enough osseous tissue to withstand normal function. If too thin an osseous strut is provided, fracture of the grafted area may occur.

3.4 Surgical principles of maxillofacial bone-grafting procedures

Several important principles should be followed during any grafting procedure. They must be strictly adhered to if a successful outcome is desired. The following are a few that pertain to reconstructing mandibular defects:

1. **Control of residual mandibular segments:** If control of the residual mandibular fragments was not performed during the extirpative surgery (eg, by reconstruction bone plate), it will have to be performed at the time of bone grafting. Over time the muscles of mastication become atrophic, fibrotic, and nonpliable, which makes realignment of the fragments extremely difficult. During the reconstructive surgery, it may be necessary to strip several muscles off the mandibular fragments to release the bone from their adverse pull. A coronoidotomy or a coronoidectomy is usually performed to remove the superior pull of the temporalis muscle. Before inserting a bone graft, the clinician must be sure to reach the desired position of the remaining mandibular fragments because what is achieved at surgery is what the patient must live with in the future.
2. **A good soft-tissue bed for the bone graft:** All bone grafts must be covered on all sides by soft tissues to avoid contamination of the bone graft and to provide the vascularity necessary for revascularization of the graft. Areas of dense scar should be excised until healthy tissue is encountered. Incisions should be designed so that when the wound is closed, the incision will not be over the graft, which means that the initial incision may be low in the neck. A multilayered soft-tissue closure is performed to reduce any space that might allow collection of blood or serum and to provide a tight closure.
3. **Immobilization of the graft:** Immobilization of bone is necessary for osseous healing to progress. In dealing with mandibular defects, the graft must be secured to remaining mandibular fragments, and these fragments must be rigidly immobilized to ensure that no movement exists between them. When the defect has healthy teeth on each side, immobilization can be provided using MMF. However, several other methods are possible, such as using a bone plate between the residual bone fragments.

4. **Aseptic environment:** Even when transplanting autogenous osseous tissue, the bone graft is avascular, which means that the graft has no way of fighting any amount of infection. Therefore, a certain percentage of bone grafts become infected and must be removed. Several measures can be taken to improve the success of bone-grafting procedures. The first is to use an extraoral incision where possible. The skin is much easier to cleanse and disinfect than is the oral cavity. Bone grafts inserted through the mouth are exposed to the oral flora during the grafting procedure. Second, one should take care not to perforate into the oral cavity during the dissection. Ideally, dissection to the level of the oral mucosa without perforation is preferred.
5. **Systemic antibiosis:** The prophylactic use of antibiotics may be indicated when transplanting osseous tissue. Prophylaxis may be beneficial in helping reduce the incidence of infection.

4 Complications and pitfalls

There are many complications that can occur when resecting and/or reconstructing the mandible. The usual surgical complications, such as bleeding, infection, and nerve injuries, are inherent in surgery of this type but can be minimized by careful surgery. Recurrence of pathology is always a possibility so the tumor must be totally removed and the patient should be monitored carefully. Malocclusion is usually second to improper technique, such as not properly reestablishing the occlusion or seating the condyle before reconstruction with a plate and/or bone. Dehiscence of the mucosa and exposure of the bone graft is one of the most feared complications and often results in total loss of a block type of nonvascularized bone graft. Particulate bone grafts may survive, in part, after oral exposure if they have been partially revascularized at the time of exposure.

5 References and suggested reading

Alpert B, Kushner GM. Fractures in bone of reduced quality. In: Ehrenfeld M, Manson PN, Prein J, eds. *Principles of Internal Fixation of the Craniomaxillofacial Skeleton: Trauma and Orthognathic Surgery.* Stuttgart: Thieme; 2012:178.

Gray JC, Elves MW. Donor cells' contribution to osteogenesis in experimental cancellous bone grafts. *Clin Orthop Relat Res.* 1982 Mar;(163):261–271.

Herford AS, Ellis E 3rd. Use of a locking reconstruction bone plate/screw system for mandibular surgery. *J Oral Maxillofac Surg.* 1998 Nov;56(11):1261–1265.

Marx RE, Saunders TR. Reconstruction and rehabilitation of cancer patients. In: Fonseca RJ, Davis WH, eds. *Reconstructive Preprosthetic Oral and Maxillofacial Surgery.* Philadelphia: WB Saunders; 1986.

Marx RE, Ames JR. The use of hyperbaric oxygen therapy in bony reconstruction of the irradiated and tissue-deficient patient. *J Oral Maxillofac Surg.* 1982 Jul;40(7):412–420.

2.5 Reconstruction of the condyle

James Q Swift

1 Introduction

To perform normal oral functions an intact, supporting, and mobile mandible is essential. For symmetry, projection, speech, and for masticatory function the articulation should be bilateral.

The articulation of the temporomandibular joint (TMJ) consists of the proximal mandible and the temporal bone of the skull base bilaterally. The proximal mandible is composed of the condylar process of the mandible, sometimes named the condylar "neck" and the condyle itself often called the "head" of the mandibular condyle. Muscles associated with mandibular function, the temporalis, masseter, and medial pterygoid attach to the coronoid process of the mandible (temporalis) and the mandibular ramus, angle, posterior border and inferior border (medial pterygoid, masseter, also termed the pterygomasseteric "sling"). They suspend the proximal mandible and condyle in close approximation to the glenoid fossa of the temporal bone and skull base so as to allow closing of the mouth for mastication, speech, and other oral functions. The lateral pterygoid muscle attaches to the proximal mandible on the medial aspect of the condyle and condylar process or neck. When contracting, the lateral pterygoid provides anterior translation of the condyle to the anterior aspect of the head.

The fibrocartilaginous disc of the TMJ is located between the condyle of the mandible and the glenoid fossa. The disc is attached to the lateral pterygoid muscle on its medial and anterior aspect, posteriorly to the joint capsule and to the glenoid fossa.

The joint space is lined by synovia. There is a superior and an inferior joint space. The two joint spaces are potential spaces and do not communicate.

Opening movement of the mouth with separation of the maxillary and mandibular dentition is accomplished primarily by gravity with some assistance from the suprahyoid musculature in the anterior neck and from the lateral pterygoid. The closing movement of the mouth with approximation of the maxillary and mandibular dentition is accomplished by the contraction of the temporalis, medial pterygoid, and masseter muscles. The overall force of muscle contraction is much greater in the closing movement of the mouth than the opening movement. The normal muscular contraction for mouth closure is a bilateral phenomenon. Closure of the mouth can still be accomplished in the presence of nonfunction or paralysis of some of the muscles of closure.

Presence of anatomically normal mandibular condyles is an important component of TMJ function. Loss of volume or dimension of the condyle of the mandible may result in skeletally induced malocclusion and lateral changes of the teeth resulting in premature dental occlusion on the side of volume loss, and open bite on the side contralateral to the volume loss. Volume loss in skeletally immature patients due to tumor extirpation or trauma (comminution of condyle and/or displacement of proximal mandible) may result in facial asymmetry and will likely adversely affect the development of the contralateral maxilla and mandible. If there is volume loss of the condyles of the mandible bilaterally, the result may be dental contact in the posterior dentition, usually the molars, with no contact in the anterior dentition. If there is increase in volume in the condyle of the mandible associated with enlargement, the result may be an open bite on the side of the lesion with laterognathia away from the enlarged condylar head.

2 Disease processes necessitating reconstruction of the mandibular condyle

There are several pathological processes that result in destruction or alteration of the mandibular condyle resulting in a consideration for reconstruction of the condyle for normal oral function.

2.1 Trauma—immediate and delayed

2.1.1 Immediate

Condylar fractures of the mandible are frequently encountered. There is a wide array of fracture patterns, from "low" or inferior condylar neck fractures, to "high" condylar head fractures with severe comminution. In rare situations, part of the proximal mandible may be avulsed. The condyle of the mandible also may be forced into the middle cranial fossa through the glenoid fossa, with or without fracture of the condylar neck and/or head.

There are many techniques and procedures for reconstruction of the fractured or displaced mandibular condyle, including no reduction with stabilization of occlusion and range of motion of the mandible, to open reduction from different approaches, both transoral and transcutaneous. Fracture reduction and fixation to premorbid anatomy are desired goals of the operations. Reduction and fixation of fractures of the mandibular condyle are reviewed and discussed [Ehrenfeld et al, 2012].

If the condyle is severely comminuted or avulsed, consideration can be given to immediate reconstruction of the condyle with autogenous free grafting, vascularized bone, or the use of an alloplastic material, either temporarily or on a permanent basis.

2.1.2 Delayed

With both surgical treatment and fixation of condylar fractures as well as those treated non-surgically without fixation and/or reduction, there are treatment failures. This may be detected at some point in the postoperative course when occlusion is no longer controlled or influenced by inter-arch dental elastics and the patient complains of open bite or malocclusion compared with premorbid condition, occlusal premature contacts, facial asymmetry, and change in facial appearance.

If a malocclusion occurs after trauma resulting in a mandibular condyle fracture with or without surgical intervention, and the patient desires normal oral function and occlusion, reconstruction of the condyle may be indicated. There are generally two approaches in this situation.

Some surgeons will allow the fracture to heal, empirically 6 months. Rather than retreat the condyle directly, they then treat the malocclusion by using conventional orthognathic surgical techniques, with or without presurgical orthodontics. This is possible in patients free of pain and with an acceptable range of motion. In the case of bilateral mandibular condyle fractures, which has resulted in retrognathia, anterior open bite and displaced condyles (usually medial and anterior displacement), they will prescribe and perform a Le Fort I osteotomy to close the anterior open bite. This concept precludes attempting to approach, reduce, and stabilize the condyle fractures to save the patient from facial scars, grafting, and potential for facial nerve injury associated with the surgical approach. However, the result may be a compromise, as the plane of the occlusion will be changed to the pathologically repositioned traumatized mandible, and the retrognathic appearance will remain or perhaps worsen.

The other approach is to directly operate on the condyle(s). In this case, both the proximal and distal segments will have remodeled, the fracture lines will not be detectable and will not serve as a guide for fragment positioning. There may be a gap between proximal and distal segments once the condyle is repositioned in relation to the glenoid fossa. This may necessitate the need for bone grafting, which increases the complexity of procedure.

2.2 Tumor

As with any region of the body, benign and malignant tumors may present in the TMJ area and/or skull base/temporal bone. Tumors of bone, cartilage, synovium, muscle, salivary gland, blood vessels, nerves, and connective tissue can develop and grow in or around the TMJ.

Benign tumors include osteoma, osteochondroma, chondroma, synovial chondromatosis, pigmented villonodular synovitis, giant cell granuloma, pleomorphic adenoma, and chondromyxoid fibroma.

Malignant tumors in the TMJ area include adenocarcinoma, adenoid cystic carcinoma, osteosarcoma, chondrosarcoma, synovial sarcoma, and adjacent tissue malignant disease including squamous cell carcinoma, basal cell carcinoma, and metastatic disease (eg, thyroid carcinoma, pancreatic carcinoma, mamma, renal carcinoma, and prostate carcinoma).

Benign lesions of the mandibular body, angle, and ramus can expand into the mandibular condyle as they enlarge, including ameloblastoma, keratocystic odontogenic tumor, central giant cell granuloma, and follicular cyst. If surgical treatment planning requires fixed and determined surgical margin beyond the margin of the tumor for best outcomes, the management of the mandibular condyle becomes important regarding the need for disarticulation, or complete resection of the condyle versus maintaining the mandibular condyle in place.

When the temporomandibular articulation can be preserved without undue risk, it must be done. Reconstruction of the proximal mandible with attachment to a residual condylar head is favored to inserting an autogenous graft, free flap, or alloplastic metal condylar head or total joint. If at least 1.5 cm of condylar head can be preserved, it can be fixed to the mandible and/or to a graft. Any condylar head preservation and fixation is preferred over a graft or alloplast contacting the glenoid fossa in hopes of developing a functional articulation.

3 Degenerative disease/arthritis spectrum of disease/autoimmune disease

Resorptive processes, many times associated with antibodies to antinuclear antigens, may result in degeneration and loss of the condylar head and sometimes the neck. If left untreated, or if the disease process is aggressive, resorption of the proximal mandible continues to the sigmoid notch, leaving nothing proximal to the mandibular ramus. This resorptive process can occur with osteoarthritis/degenerative joint disease, although the resorption is usually less severe. Idiopathic condylar resorption may result in unilateral or bilateral resorption of the proximal mandible. This entity generally occurs in women in the second decade of life. These diseases may result in a need for reconstruction of the proximal mandible, condyle, and glenoid fossa.

3.1 Congenital anomalies

Failure of the proximal mandible to develop normally occurs in multiple congenital anomalies. Probably the most frequent and potentially the most severe is hemifacial macrosomia (craniofacial microsomia, Goldenhar syndrome, see chapter 4.5), showing unilateral mandibular hypoplasia of varying degrees, sometimes with an absence of a TMJ articulation. The condylar head is often diminutive, malformed and malpositioned. The glenoid fossa can be absent, and the articulation of the mandible is inferiorly positioned compared with the contralateral normally developed side.

Mandibulofacial dysostosis (Treacher Collins syndrome) may also present with a missing or malformed proximal mandible, with disruption of position and contour of the glenoid fossa.

Pierre Robin sequence usually presents with a hypoplastic mandible and associated airway compromise. In most patients afflicted, the TMJ may be normal in its appearance but the condyle/fossa relationship and anatomy may be hypoplastic.

Syngnathia, congenital TMJ ankylosis, a rare congenital anomaly may require reconstruction of the condyle of the mandible in association with release of the ankylosis.

3.2 Surgically mutilated TMJs

Surgically mutilated TMJs may be created in several ways. Perhaps one of the most frequent surgical situations resulting in the need for reconstruction of the condyle and TMJ may result from multiple surgical operations for temporomandibular disorders. The etiology of temporomandibular disorder was presumed to be mechanical with displacement or dislocation of the TMJ disc especially in an anterior/posterior dimension. Once this displacement occurred, usually the result of some form of trauma, it is presumed that continuous degeneration would occur over time, resulting in osteoarthrosis and degeneration of the condylar head and disc. Some surgeons would provide surgical intervention to reposition displaced discs, mostly related to mechanical disc malposition interfering with mandibular mobility to reduce the pain presumably associated with the displacement of the disc. Progression of the disease, associated in some situations with frequent surgical intervention, may result in severe degeneration of the condyle. This results in volume loss with associated malocclusion and reduced range of motion. It may be difficult to separate the pathology of the disease process itself from the pathology associated with multiple operations.

In addition, during the 1970s and 1980s when treating disc malpositions in the TMJ many surgeons would excise the disc if it was not possible to reposition or repair it. Some surgeons believed that if the disc was removed, there was a need to replace it. Some surgeons used autogenous free grafts, including fascia, dermis, and cartilage. Others used alloplastic materials. Two of the most popular materials were silicone and polytetrafluoroethylene. They were shaped comparably in size and configuration to the natural disc that had been removed and were placed between the condyle of the mandible and the temporal bone. Unfortunately, these materials disintegrated in most patients, resulting in fracture and/or transit to adjacent lymph nodes. In some situations, foreign body giant cell reactions ensued, with formation of osteoclasts which resulted in osteolysis and bone degeneration beyond normal anatomical confines of the TMJ.

This type of process resulted in the need to remove the implanted materials that were involved with the osteolysis. This resulted in the need for reconstruction of the condyles and in necessary situations the glenoid fossa.

3.3 TMJ hypomobility/ankylosis/heterotopic bone formation

Hypomobility of the mandible may cause significant disability. Reduction in the range of motion is detected typically as the afflicted person has problems eating and chewing. Further limits on mobility restrict access and can be a challenge to attain an airway for ventilation.

Ankylosis of the TMJ can be a result of frequent operations, trauma to the condyle, and hemorrhage in the TMJ space. It may be due to the formation of heterotopic bone, a vigorous and aggressive growth of bone outside of normal anatomical confines resulting in fusion of the mandible to the temporal bone.

Ankylosis is also seen after reconstruction of the condyle when using costochondral grafting, a technique that is described later in this chapter. It may also result from ramus lengthening using distraction osteogenesis.

Treatment of ankylosis is described in chapter 4.3.

4 Goals for reconstruction of the mandibular condyle/TMJ

- Maximum interincisal opening of 40 mm or more (vertical measurement between edge of maxillary central incisor and mandibular central incisor without restriction)
- Pain-free motion with opening of the mouth, lateral movements, protrusive movements, and excursive movements
- Maximum intercuspation of teeth
- Normal and/or restored articulation of speech
- Unrestricted voice projection
- Masticatory efficiency for nutrition
- Facial symmetry
- Minimal or absent facial scarring
- Normal facial animation

4.1 Techniques to reconstruct the mandibular condyle

4.1.1 Malocclusion/malfunction after trauma

Condylar displacement may result in a loss of vertical dimension of the condyle, condylar process, and ramus. Malocclusion may be a consequence. If a patient presents with malocclusion he/she is evaluated to determine if premorbid occlusion can be obtained by mandibular movement. If so, many clinicians will decide to treat the fracture with mandibulomaxillary fixation (MMF). This fixation is often provided by arch bars, fixation screws or dental wiring, to which elastics are applied to guide the patient into preinjury occlusion. However, this technique may result in a malunion of the displaced condyle. If the patient can continue to function normally, this is of no consequence in most situations. In the case of bilateral mandibular condylar fractures with displacement of the proximal segments, the likelihood of after-treatment malocclusion, specifically anterior open bite, is higher.

The planning of condylar reconstruction initially requires dental impressions to construct dental models. The position of the mandible for maximum intercuspation of teeth is determined by evaluating and positioning the dental casts.

A computed tomographic (CT) scan is obtained and a stereolithographic model of the skull base inferior to the mandible may be constructed.

In the model the condyle is separated from the condylar neck if it is attached. An assessment must be made to determine if the mandibular condyle can be salvaged. This is determined by the size of the remaining condylar process and the amount of bone remaining to retain an osteosynthesis plate. The condyle is placed in the anticipated premorbid anatomical position. The gap between the proximal and distal mandible is evaluated. A rigid bone plate is contoured to fit from the proximal to distal mandible with at least two fixation screws on each side of the fracture gap. If the gap is wider than 1–2 mm, autogenous cancellous bone graft is used to fill it (**Fig 2.5-1**).

Surgical approaches are determined. Most frequently, a posterior ramus/transparotid incision is used for access. After the dissection and release of the mandibular condyle, the patient is placed in MMF. The condyle is then reduced, sometimes an osteotomy needs to be performed to release it, and fixed with the precontoured bone plate(s). Bone graft is applied if necessary. The MMF is removed and the occlusion is checked.

Postoperatively, training elastics may be used to control occlusion. Physical therapy is necessary to rehabilitate to normal oral function. A regimen of 12 visits to a physical therapist staged over 6 weeks is the normal course.

This technique may be used at any time after it has been determined that closed reduction treatment has failed. The longer the interval between trauma and definitive treatment with reconstruction of the condyle, the higher the likelihood for condylar degeneration, and increased need for bone grafting.

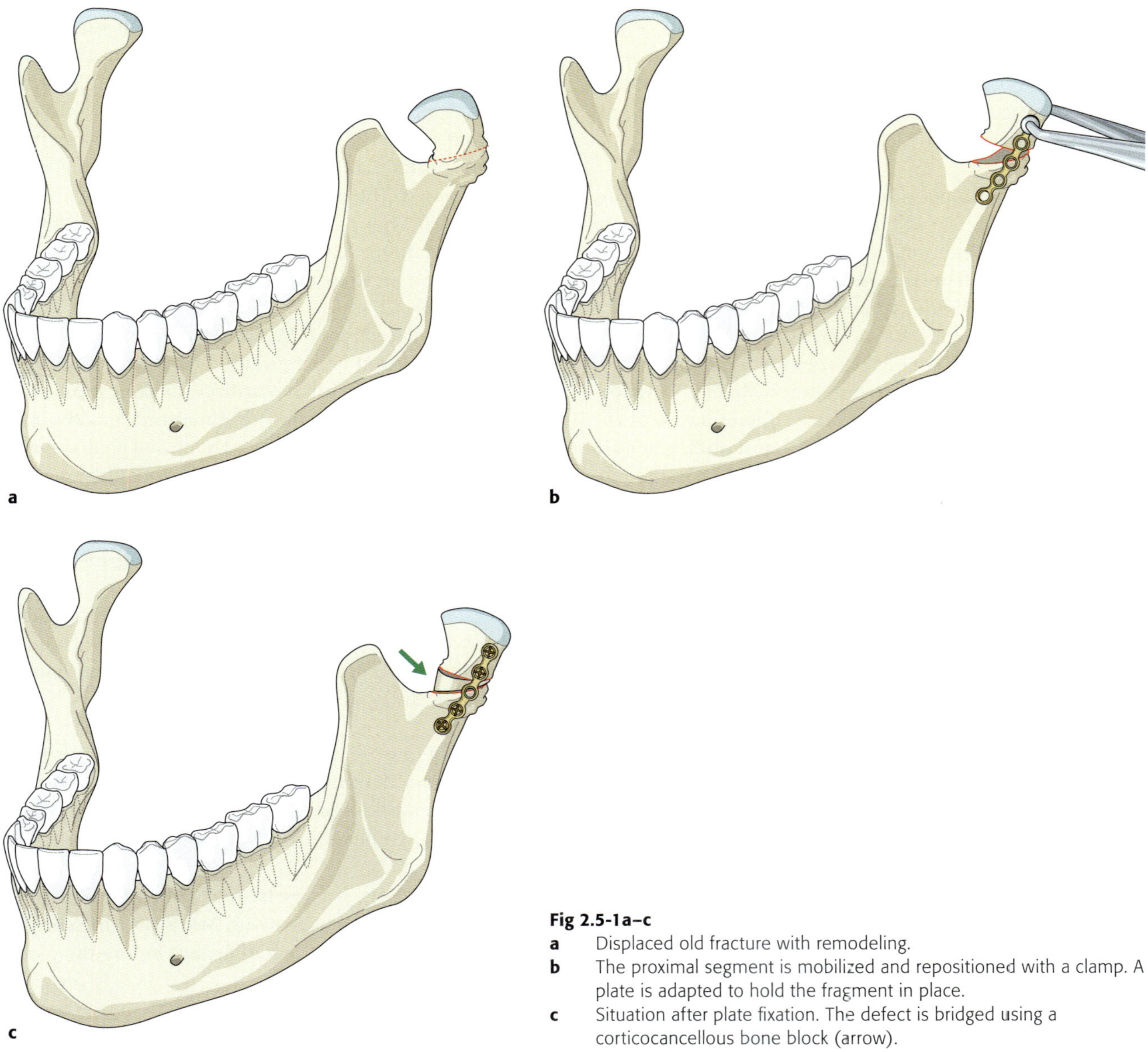

Fig 2.5-1a–c

a Displaced old fracture with remodeling.

b The proximal segment is mobilized and repositioned with a clamp. A plate is adapted to hold the fragment in place.

c Situation after plate fixation. The defect is bridged using a corticocancellous bone block (arrow).

4.1.2 Avulsive/volume loss

If there is a loss of the condyle or proximal mandible from avulsion, degeneration, resorption, resection, previous surgery or other pathology, consideration may be given to reconstruction of the condyle and proximal mandible.

First the clinician must assess the disability and suffering caused by the absence of the condyle and proximal mandible. In certain situations, patients can accommodate to the unilateral loss of the proximal mandible and still be able to occlude dentally with sufficient bite force to masticate a bolus of food with minimal dysfunction. Often there is a significant deviation to the side of the absence of the condyle with maximum opening of the mouth, which for many patients is an acceptable consequence. Bilateral loss of the condylar head and proximal mandible most often results in anterior open bite with posterior dental contact in the molar region with resultant disabilities of speech and insufficient mastication.

If there is intolerable disability with proximal mandible absence, proximal mandibular reconstruction may be offered. The reconstruction may be provided unilaterally or bilaterally.

4.1.3 Costochondral grafting

The use of a costochondral rib graft is an established technique of condyle reconstruction. It allows the utilization of a vertical strut to lengthen the mandibular ramus/condyle complex to the desired height. The procedure has been used for grafting in skeletally immature patients as it is postulated that the rib bone/cartilage graft will grow with the patient in accordance with facial skeletal growth. It is difficult to determine and predict when, how, and to what degree growth will occur.

The technique has been utilized to treat patients with craniofacial microsomia as well as patients with ankylosis of the TMJ, resection of the proximal mandible and reconstruction in primarily adolescent subjects but in skeletally mature patients as well [Kaban et al, 2009].

The planned and predicted reconstruction is determined by CT scans and the use of stereolithographic models. In patients with craniofacial microsomia, there is generally a reduction in length of the condyle and ramus on the affected side. The anticipated dental relationship, which is generally a lateral open bite on the side of lengthening, is planned with the use of dental impressions and dental casts. An interocclusal splint is constructed that will be used during the operation to determine the dimension of vertical augmentation.

A retromandibular or submandibular approach is used. This can be challenging in craniofacial microsomia as the external ear is generally dysmorphic and there is significant absence of normal soft tissues compared with the contralateral normal side of the face. The facial nerve may also be in an unusual position. Dissection to the lateral proximal mandible is obtained. The harvested autogenous costochondral graft is shaped. Approximately 1 cm of cartilage is left attached to the bone. Around the costochondral junction, periosteum and perichondrium are left attached.

The patient is placed into MMF, if indicated, using the dental splint constructed presurgically. The graft is positioned flat against the ramus with the cartilage abutting the glenoid fossa. Note that in the patient with craniofacial macrosomia, there is dysmorphia of the temporal bone and glenoid fossa. In many situations, there is not a depression of the glenoid and the graft is placed in a position that could be assumed to be anatomically normal. The graft is fixed into place with three bicortical screws or with bone plates (**Fig 2.5-2**).

The surgical site is closed routinely. If the proximal mandible has been lengthened considerably, closure will require undermining adjacent tissue to allow the soft-tissue dimensional change at the angle region.

The MMF is removed. If a splint has been used, it is fixed to the maxillary dentition to keep the intraocclusal space until an orthodontic appliance can be used. Elastic traction may be used to guide the newly established occlusion.

In cases of ankylosis, it must be released and the planned occlusion must be established with MMF after the surgical dissection to the proximal mandible, but before the placement of the graft(s).

With ankylosis, a temporalis fascia flap may be used as interpositional material to prevent reankylosis. Other surgeons use abdominal fat or acellular dermis as an interpositional material for the same purpose.

Costochondral grafting has also been used for reconstruction of the condyle in cases of idiopathic condylar resorption. The technique has also been utilized for primary reconstruction of the condyle and proximal mandible in trauma cases with avulsion or comminution of the mandibular condyle.

In cases of mandibular disarticulation for the treatment of tumor or when pathology cannot be resected with proper margins and the condyle is removed, costochondral grafting may be utilized to reconstruct the proximal mandible including the condyle. This technique is sometimes used in combination with bone plates and screws, vascularized free flaps, iliac crest cortical grafts, and other techniques used in the reconstruction of the mandible.

4.1.4 Partial joint replacement with alloplast

Consideration may be given to the utilization of a titanium plate with a metal condyle cast as part of the plate, or with a metal condyle attached with screws. The metal condyle approximates the glenoid fossa and the plate is attached to the distal mandible at a point where adequate fixation screws can be applied to stabilize the plate (**Fig 2.5-3**).

Application of this technique has not been extensively studied. In case studies of condylar replacements, migration of the condyle through the glenoid fossa into the middle cranial fossa has been reported. A glenoid fossa implant may alleviate concerns regarding possible prosthetic condylar migration through the temporal bone into the middle cranial fossa (**Fig 2.5-4**).

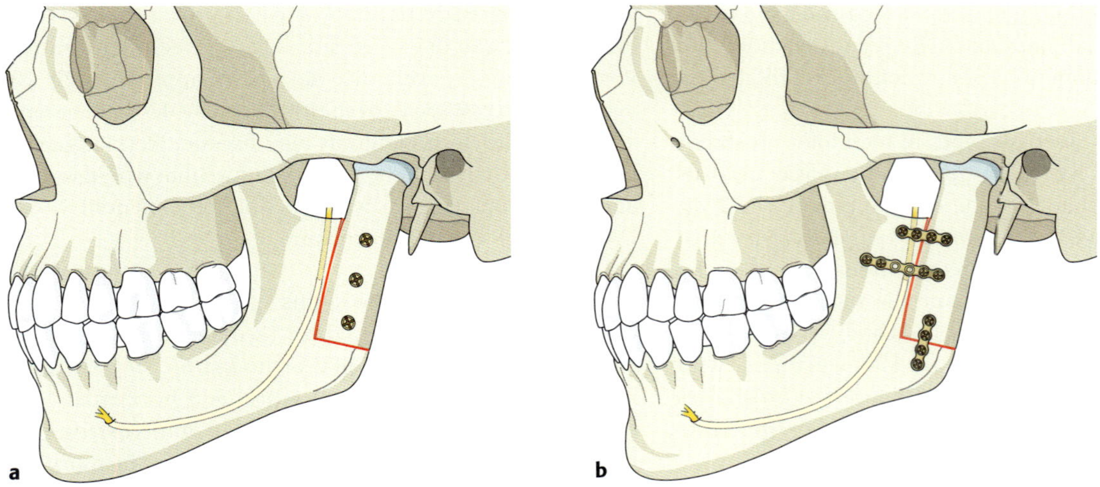

Fig 2.5-2a–b
a Costochondral rib graft fixed with three lag screws.
b Costochondral rib graft fixed with plates and screws.

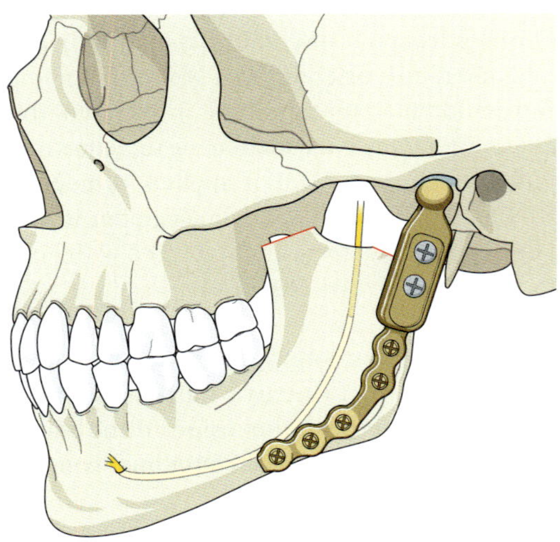

Fig 2.5-3 Reconstruction of the temporomandibular joint with a metal condyle fixed with screws to the ascending ramus. The metal head is placed against the articular disc. The coronoid process has been resected.

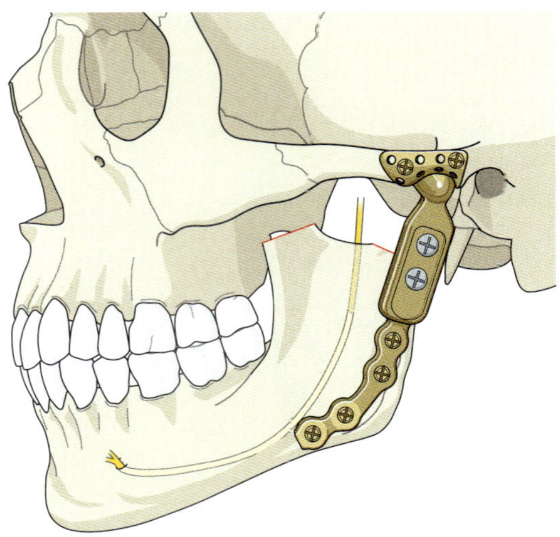

Fig 2.5-4 The glenoid component is fixed to the zygomatic process of the temporal bone.

Because of the lack of studies related to long-term use and longevity, the use of a bone plate with a condyle must be considered temporary or short term. In this context, a plate with a condyle may be used as a "space maintainer" until there is definition of pathology or tissue recovery in staged resection and reconstruction cases.

4.1.5 Total joint replacement with alloplast

Reconstruction of the mandibular condyle can be accomplished with an alloplastic total joint reconstruction (**Fig 2.5-5**).

The term "total" signifies that an alloplastic articulating surface is implanted and fixed to the temporal bone, and a proximal condylar component is implanted and fixed to the ramus of the proximal mandible. Any reconstruction with fewer than two components is not by definition a total joint.

Currently, there are two basic types of total joint prosthesis available. One type is a "stock" prosthesis that comprised various anatomical shapes of the components of the TMJ. These shapes are based on anatomical norms and can be fitted in almost all cases. The glenoid component is fixed to the lateral aspect of the glenoid fossa and the zygomatic process of the temporal bone with screws. The condylar component of the stock prosthesis is attached to the lateral mandible with screws as well. The MMF is applied before the prostheses components are fitted and fixed. After placement, the MMF is removed and the occlusion is tested for reproducibility.

For planning and manufacturing of a custom-made TMJ prosthesis, a high-resolution CT scan is needed. A stereolithographic model is constructed. The appropriate occlusion is established on the model. The surgeon determines what if any bone needs to be resected in the glenoid fossa region and determines if the proximal mandible and/or condylar head needs to be resected or altered. The devices are then constructed with a glenoid fossa component and a condylar component. Both are fixed and stabilized by screws comparable to a stock prosthesis. An advantage of the patient-fitted device is assured adaptation of the device in situ. A disadvantage is that the fabrication process is time-consuming. Also, to obtain an accurate model, if the surgical site to be reconstructed has significant metal (prior metal alloplastic implant) in the area, it must be removed before an accurate CT scan is made [Sanovich et al, 2014].

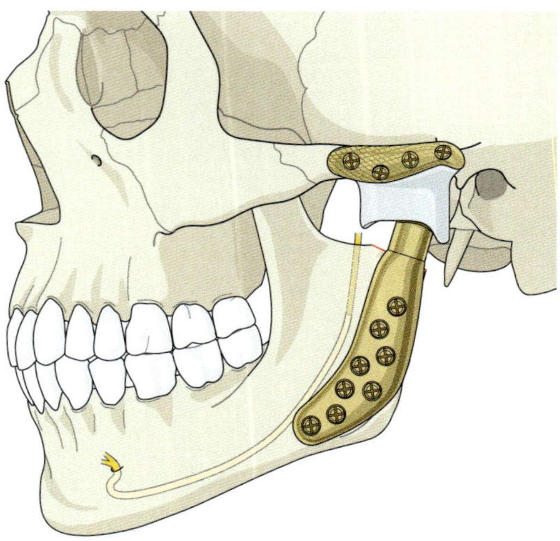

Fig 2.5-5 Total reconstruction of the mandibular joint with an alloplastic joint.

One challenge with the alloplastic TMJ prosthesis is that the longevity of the device in situ has not been determined. Post-placement surveillance has shown approximately 20-year longevity [Mercuri, 2013]. However, the devices are metal and plastic. Both materials may harden, fret, fatigue, or fragment with time to the point of failure that would require another reconstruction with possible replacement versus utilization of some other technique.

4.1.6 Osteotomies of the ramus

Other techniques advocated for reconstruction of the occlusion include conventional orthognathic surgical techniques that can increase the vertical and horizontal component of the mandible. Various types of ramus osteotomies have been utilized. It is important to ascertain the morphology and surface area of the condylar component of the proximal mandible if there is an expectation that it can bear functional load transmitted to the condylar head.

The vertical sliding osteotomy is used frequently. This procedure is performed from a transcutaneous approach. It is like vertical oblique ramus osteotomies used for mandibular setback for mandibular repositioning in orthognathic surgery. A vertical osteotomy is made from the sigmoid notch to the antegonial notch area. MMF is applied intraoperatively. The proximal mandibular condylar segment is then repositioned into the glenoid fossa and stabilized with bone plates or with plates and screws (**Fig 2.5-6**).

Transcutaneous inverted L osteotomy has also been used in craniofacial microsomia cases to increase the posterior facial height and increase the vertical dimension of the ramus (**Fig 2.5-7**). Rigid fixation plates hold the proximal segment in the extended position.

Sagittal split ramus osteotomy (SSRO) can also allow repositioning of the proximal component and condyle of the mandible into the glenoid fossa (**Fig 2.5-8**).

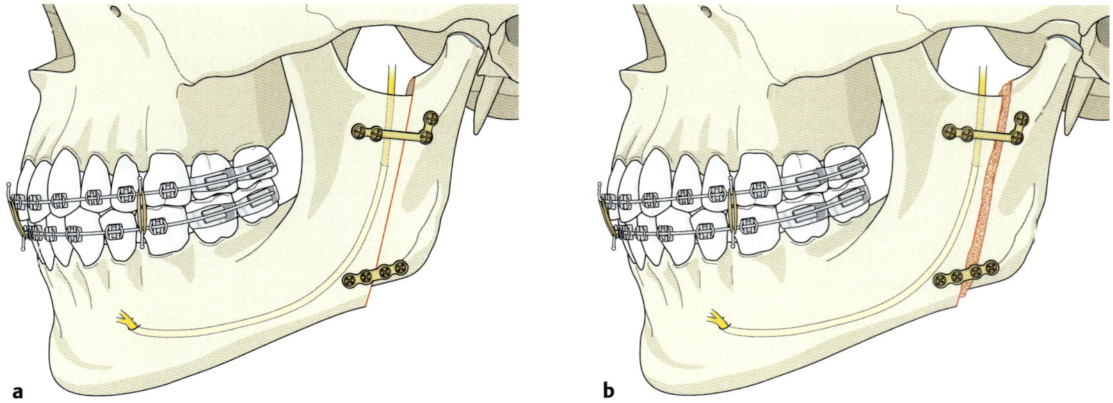

Fig 2.5-6a–b

a Vertical oblique sliding ramus osteotomy with repositioning.

b Additional placement of bone graft to enhance contact and lateral augmentation.

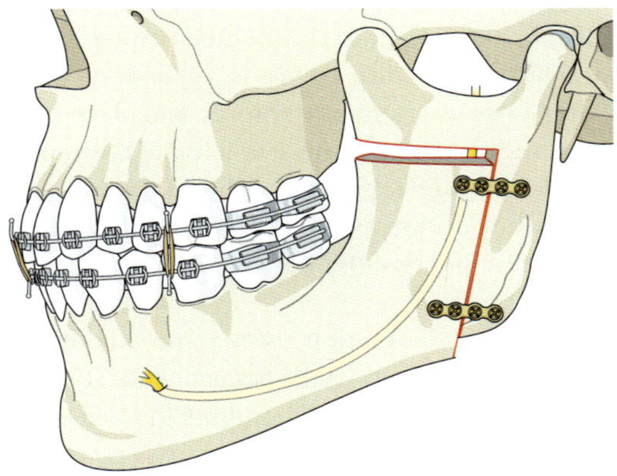

Fig 2.5-7 Inverted L osteotomy to increase the vertical dimension of the ramus.

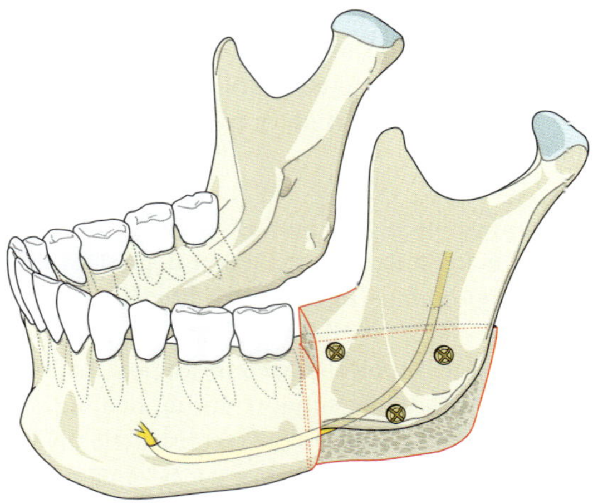

Fig 2.5-8 Sagittal split ramus osteotomy for reposition of the ramus.

There may be a limitation, however, to the degree of lengthening. In general, more vertical length can be gained from the inverted L or vertical oblique osteotomy. Yet the SSRO can be accomplished from an intraoral approach thus avoiding facial scarring.

Whatever vertical ramus lengthening technique is utilized, rigid fixation must be used for stability of outcome. With the inverted L and vertical oblique procedures, bone plates and screws must be used. With the SSRO, position screws or plates and screws can be used.

When using the inverted L or vertical oblique osteotomy, bone grafting to provide lateral facial contours or to provide stability to the vertical lengthening may be utilized. In this case, it is recommended that these procedures be provided transcutaneously to minimize contamination of the bone grafts.

4.1.7 Vascularized tissue grafting/free flap

Autogenous transplantation of vascularized bone with or without adjacent soft tissue has been utilized for large avulsive defect tissue wounds secondary to either trauma or extirpation of tumors.

The fibula is the most used graft because of its versatility to reconstruct most mandibular defects. Other bone flaps may also be utilized if appropriate (**Fig 2.5-9**) (see also chapter 2.6).

A reconstruction plate is typically used to support a microvascular bone flap to provide support during healing. An alloplastic condyle may be added to the reconstruction plate. If no condylar add-on is used, a gap must be maintained between the end of the bone flap and the glenoid fossa. This gap should be filled with a separate layer of tissue, for instance temporal fascia, to prevent ankylosis.

There may be considerable scarring associated with the wound from resection and potential irradiation, as well as the approximation and healing of the flap. This fibrosis may lead to limited range of motion. Physical therapy is extremely important to provide the best opportunity to return to normal oral function.

4.1.8 Distraction osteogenesis

Distraction osteogenesis has been described to elongate the ramus and lengthen the condyle. It has been utilized for condylar reconstruction in patients with craniofacial microsomia. The technique has also been used for patients with Pierre Robin sequence to allow unobstructed airway and may preclude tracheostomy in some patients.

The technique is like previously described ramus osteotomies (inverted L, vertical oblique). Rather than extending the condylar or proximal segment to the glenoid fossa and stabilizing it, an active distraction device is applied after the osteotomy. After a vertical ramus osteotomy and placement of the distractor, the distraction device is activated, expanding the proximal and distal segments. Around the osteotomy, bone generation occurs as the device is activated, in most situations 1 mm per day (**Fig 2.5-10**) (see chapter 4.5).

Another indication for distraction osteogenesis is ramus lengthening in ankylosis cases [Stucki-McCormick, 1997]. This requires osteotomy of the proximal mandible to release the bone ankylosis with subsequent distraction to elongate the ascending ramus.

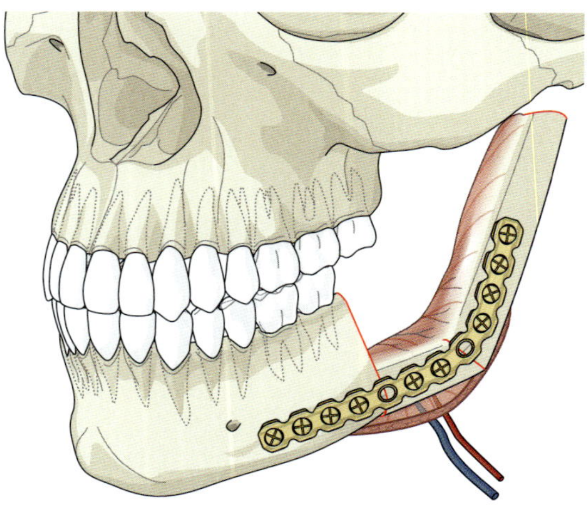

Fig 2.5-9 Reconstruction of ascending ramus with a free fibula flap.

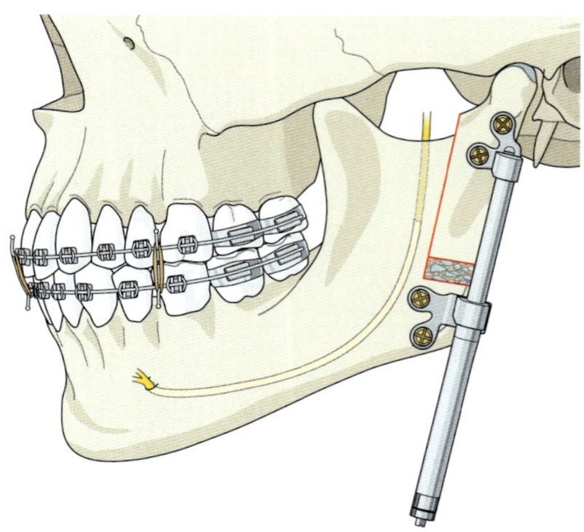

Fig 2.5-10 Osteotomy of the proximal ramus with distraction device for lengthening of the ramus.

4.2 Adjunctive procedures and therapies

Reconstruction of the condyle and proximal mandible requires an assessment of the range of motion of the mandible, as described. Normal or functional range of motion is generally considered to be 40–50 mm between the incisors with lateral excursions of 6 mm or more and protrusion of 6 mm or more as well.

Detachment of the temporalis muscle from the proximal mandible may allow a greater increase in the range of motion. In addition, any restriction in mobility due to coronoid impingement may be remedied by coronoidectomy. If unsure that the coronoid process and temporalis are contributing to restriction of range of motion, surgical sequence would suggest that there be release of the condyle from the glenoid as the initial procedure with intraoperative assessment of range of motion. If still restricted, the contralateral contribution to restricted range of motion must be determined. If based on imaging and clinical examination restriction of range of motion is not due to contralateral disease, then elective coronoidectomy may be performed.

Aggressive physical therapy should be used in all cases of condylar reconstructions as surgical entry into the TMJ space may result in hemorrhage, hematoma, and subsequent fibrosis. A suggested course of therapy is 12 visits administered within a 6-week period. The first few visits are used for pain abatement and passive range of motion exercises. Active range of motion exercises can be used as tolerated. With condylar reconstruction, a range of motion with 35 mm interincisor distance can be accepted as appropriate postsurgical outcome.

5 Conclusion

Reconstruction of the mandibular condyle is necessary in numerous clinical situations. Maintenance or reestablishment of the temporomandibular articulation will allow restoration of oral function including mastication and speech. The ultimate goals are to restore occlusion and preserve or restore facial symmetry both at rest and in function, thereby improving or restoring the quality of life for the patient.

6 References and suggested reading

American Academy of Oral and Maxillofacial Surgeons. Parameters of care: clinical practice guidelines for oral and maxillofacial surgery (AAOMS ParCare 07) temporomandibular joint surgery. *J Oral Maxillofac Surg*. 2007;(4.0).

Ehrenfeld M, Manson PN, Prein J, eds. *Manual Principles of Internal Fixation of the Craniomaxillofacial Skeleton: Trauma and Orthognathic Surgery*. Stuttgart: Thieme; 2012.

Chung CJ, Choi YJ, Kim IS, et al. [Total alloplastic temporomandibular joint reconstruction combined with orthodontic treatment in a patient with idiopathic condylar resorption.] *Orthod Fr*. 2012 Sep;83(3):225–238. In French.

Holmlund A, Lund B, Weiner CK. Response to letter to editor on publication: "mandibular condylectomy with osteoarthrectomy with and without temporalis muscle transfer." *Br J Oral Maxillofac Surg*. 2013 Oct;51(7):671–672.

Hsu JE, Keenan MA. Current review of heterotopic ossification. *Univ Penn Orthop J*. 2010;20:126–130.

Idebottom AJ. How do I manage restricted mouth opening secondary to problems with the temporomandibular joint? *Br J Oral Maxillofac Surg*. 2013;51(6):469–472.

Potter JK, Dierks EJ. Vascularized options for reconstruction of the mandibular condyle. *Semin Plast Surg*. 2008 Aug; 22(3):156–160.

Kaban LB, Bouchard C, Troulis MJ. A protocol for management of temporomandibular joint ankylosis in children. *J Oral Maxillofac Surg*. 2009 Sep;67(9):1966–1978.

Leiggener C, Jaquiery C, Kunz C, et al. Transparotid approach for tumor excision from the infratemporal space in temporomandibular joint reconstruction: a 3-year follow-up. *Oral Surg Oral Med Oral Pathol Oral Radiol Endod*. 2010 Jan;109(1):e1–4.

Mercuri LG. Avoiding and managing temporomandibular joint total joint replacement surgical site infections. *J Oral Maxillofac Surg*. 2012 Oct;70(10):2280–2289.

Mercuri LG. Silicone elastomer implants in surgery of the temporomandibular joint. *Br J Oral Maxillofac Surg*. 2013 Oct;51(7):584–586.

Mercuri LG, Swift JQ. Considerations for the use of alloplastic temporomandibular joint replacement in the growing patient. *J Oral Maxillofac Surg*. 2009 Sep;67(9):1979–1990.

Mercuri LG, Westermark A, Holmlund A, et al. Mandibular condylectomy with osteoarthrectomy with and without transfer of the temporalis muscle. *Br J Oral Maxillofac Surg*. 2013 Oct;51(7):671.

Psutka DJ. Surgical reconstruction of the temporomandibular joint part II: alloplastic materials. *Ontario Dentist*. 2007 Oct;18–24.

Quinn PD. Lorenza prosthesis. *Oral Maxillofac Surg Clin North Am*. 2000;12(1):93–103.

Saeed A, Muhammad AB, Arsalan W, et al. Viability of costochondral graft in temporomandibular joint ankylosis. *Pakistan Oral Dental J*. 2014 Mar;34(1):25–29.

Sanovich R, Mehta U, Abramowicz S, et al. Total alloplastic temporomandibular joint reconstruction using Biomet stock prostheses: the University of Florida experience. *Int J Oral Maxillofac Surg*. 2014 Sep;43(9):1091–1095.

Schiopu D, Girard J, Soenen M, et al. Metal ions levels measurements for early total hip replacement malfunction diagnosis with «plasma-sprayed ceramic» bearings couple. *Orthop Traumatol Surg Res*. 2010 Feb;96(1):75–79.

Shaker AA. The use of costochondral grafts in the management of temporomandibular. *Joint Ankylosis Egypt J Plastic Reconstruct Surg*. 2003 Jan;(27):73–83.

Sidebottom AJ, Gruber E. One-year prospective outcome analysis and complications following total replacement of the temporomandibular joint with the TMJ concepts system. *Br J Oral Maxillofacial Surg*. 2013 Oct;51(7):620–624.

Sidebottom AJ, Speculand B, Hensher R. Foreign body response around total prosthetic metal-on-metal replacements of the temporomandibular joint in the UK. *Br J Oral Maxillofac Surg*. 2008 Jun;46(4):288–292.

Stucki-McCormick SU. Reconstruction of the mandibular condyle using transport distraction osteogenesis. *J Craniofac Surg*. 1997;8(1):48–52; discussion 53.

Westermark A, Heden P, Aagaard E, et al. The use of TMJ concepts prostheses to reconstruct patients with major temporomandibular joint and mandibular defects. *Int J Oral Maxillofac Surg*. 2011 May;40(5):487–496.

2.6 Mandible reconstruction with microvascular free flaps

Michael Ehrenfeld, Keith A Hurvitz, Gregory RD Evans

1 Introduction

Reconstruction of the mandible following ablative surgery continues to be a challenge for craniomaxillofacial (CMF) surgeons. Patient quality of life is a significant factor to consider in the overall treatment plan. The goal of reconstructive efforts is to provide patients with a fully functional result allowing resumption of normal life activities. Vascularized bone transfer has become the standard of care for reconstruction of large mandibular defects [Hidalgo et al, 2002; Mehta et al, 2004]. Its use in mandible reconstruction has proven successful over the past two decades, and results from long-term radiographic studies on transferred vascularized bone flaps have shown minimal loss of bone volume [Hidalgo et al, 2002; Disa et al, 1999]. In addition, functional results following free flap surgery to the mandible have shown resumption of normal diet and retention of intelligible speech postoperatively in most patients [Hidalgo et al, 2002; Jones et al, 2003].

Nonvascularized bone grafts have been used successfully for years for the reconstruction of small bone defects of the mandible. For longer bone defects and those associated with overlying skin or mucosa defects, nonvascularized grafts have a higher potential to fail. Free bone grafts require a well vascularized bed and must be protected from secretions from the oral cavity by a tension free closure and tight mucosal lining. A factor unique to cancer surgery is that a large percentage of patients with tumors require adjuvant radiation therapy. Ionizing radiation can be damaging to surrounding soft tissue and bone, which can result in devascularization of the recipient bed with scarring and fibrosis. If a patient lacks a dependable soft-tissue bed for support of a nonvascularized bone graft, failure is more prone to occur. Foster et al [1999] compared the use of nonvascularized bone grafts versus vascularized bone flaps in mandible reconstruction. They observed a high failure rate for bone grafts when placed in previously irradiated patients. In addition, patients repaired with nonvascularized bone grafts were found to have a lower rate of bony union compared with patients reconstructed with vascularized bone flaps. Nonvascularized bone grafts still have a role in mandible reconstruction but should be limited to smaller defects without significant oral contamination. In all other situations, especially when patients have a history of or a planned radiation therapy, a vascularized free flap is the preferred method of reconstruction.

The four most commonly used donor sites for microvascular reconstruction of the mandible include the fibula, iliac crest, scapula, and radial forearm. This chapter presents clinical aspects of managing mandible defects using these vascularized soft tissue and bone flaps. Flap harvest is described in chapter 1.1.

2 Donor sites

2.1 Fibula

Since Hidalgo first published his series in 1989 on the use of the fibula flap for mandible reconstruction, the fibula has become the workhorse for mandibular reconstruction. Based upon the peroneal artery and its associated veins, the flap provides a long bone segment approximately 25 cm in length. The segmental periosteal blood supply to the bone allows multiple osteotomies to be performed without major risk of bone devascularization [Cordeiro et al, 1999; Hidalgo et al, 1998; Shpitzer et al, 1997, 2000; Takushima et al, 2001; Hidalgo, 1989; Chana et al, 2004]. These qualities make the fibula flap well suited for adapting to the angulation of the chin region and allow it to be used for almost every mandible defect. Height and width of the fibula are relatively small with considerable interindividual variations. The cross section of a fibula resembles the bone stock of a highly atrophic mandible, the bone cross sections vary in different segments of the fibula. Dental implant placement is usually possible, but not always in thin and small fibulae (**Fig 2.6-1**).

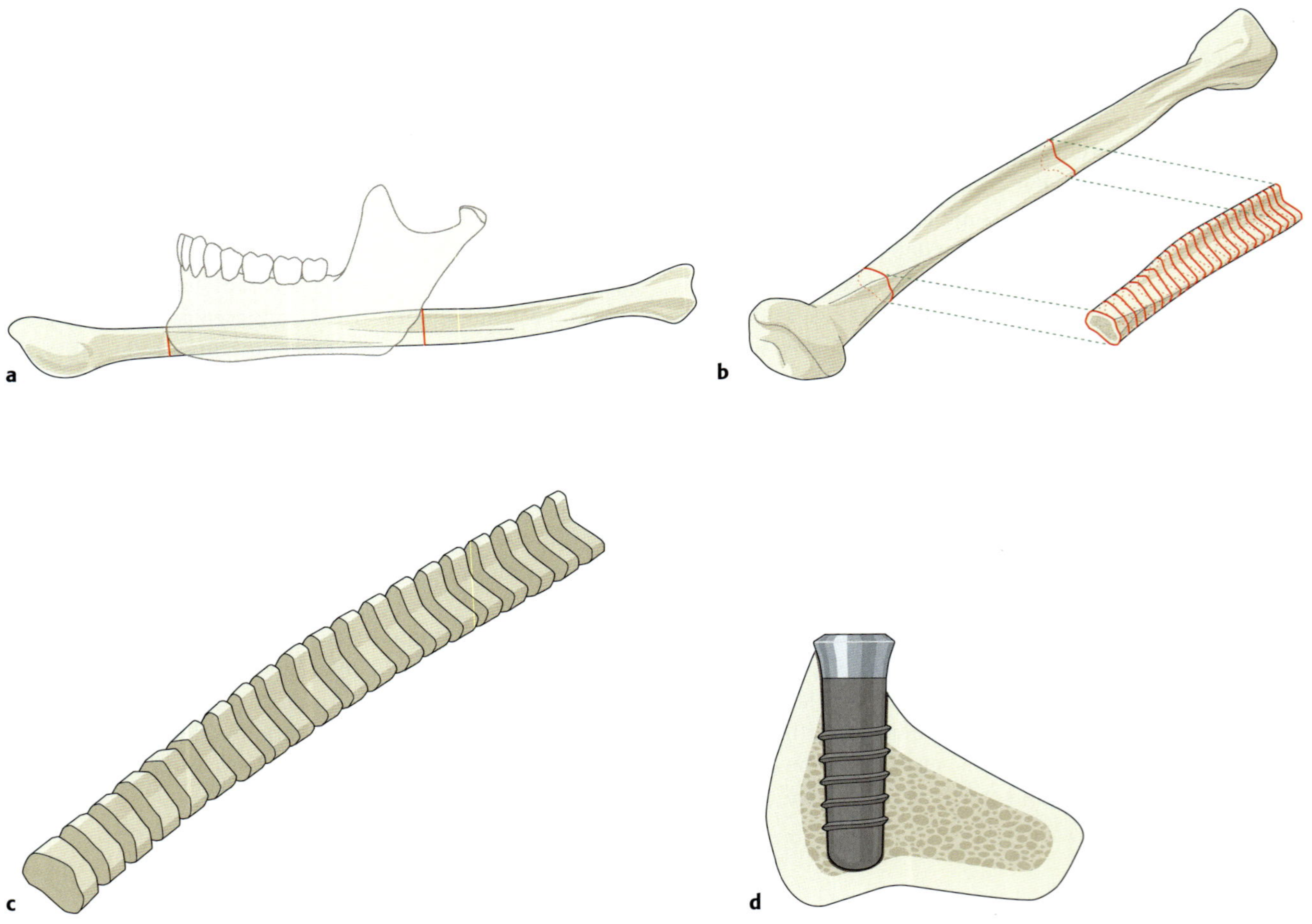

Fig 2.6-1a–d Fibula bone stock.

a Distal half of fibula for mandible reconstruction. Bone stock resembling a highly atrophic mandible.

b Fibular bone that is twisted in a helical fashion.

c Cross sections vary in their individual shape and may not always present with enough bone stock for dental implants.

d Cross section of fibula with dental implant.

The individual amount of bone in a specific patient can be assessed by preoperative computed tomography (CT). To overcome limited bone height and width a fibula flap may also be folded upon itself in a double-barrel or over and under barrel fashion to recreate full mandible height (see chapter 5.3.12). Another option to increase bone stock is primary (at the time of flap transplantation) or secondary distraction osteogenesis [Zhang et al, 2002]. The flap can be harvested with a reliable skin paddle so that internal or external lining can be achieved [Zenn et al, 1997; Jones et al, 2003]. A portion of the soleus muscle is then included in the design to ensure incorporation of the septocutaneous perforators for skin perfusion. When additional bulk is required for filling defects, a portion of the flexor hallucis longus muscle can also be harvested with the flap. The fibula has also been shown to effectively sustain the placement of osteointegrated implants [Foster et al, 1999; Cordeiro et al, 1999; Gabr et al, 2004; Kuzon et al, 1998].

2.2 Iliac crest

The iliac crest free flap has the advantage of providing a large stock of bone. The natural shape of the flap resembles that of a hemimandible and readily accepts dental implants (**Fig 2.6-2**).

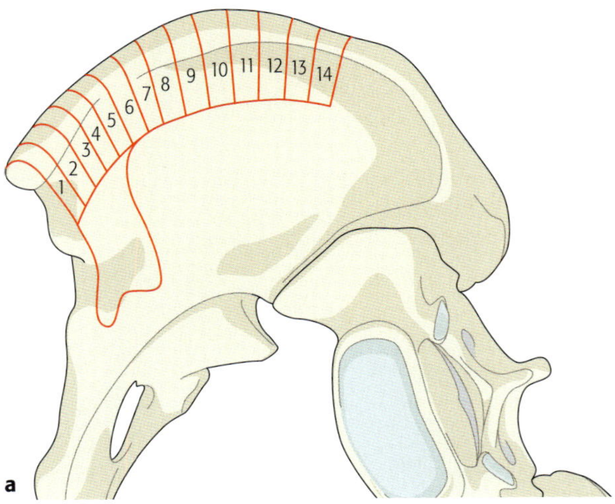

a

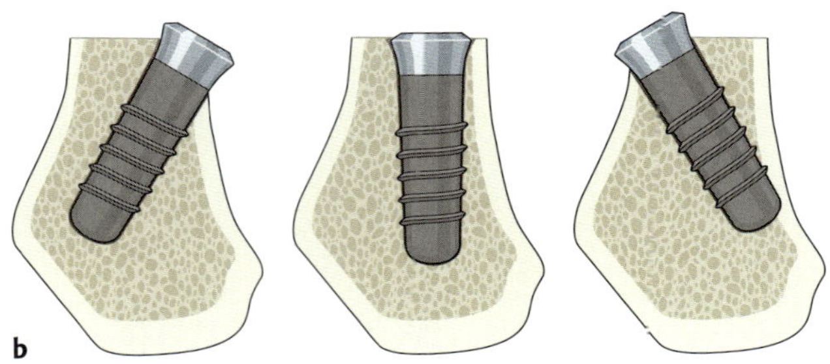

b

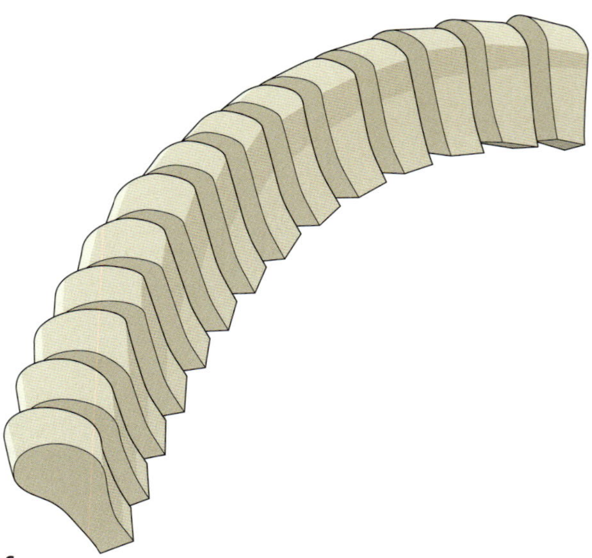

c

Fig 2.6-2a–c Bone stock iliac crest.

- **a** The anterior iliac crest provides enough bone stock to reconstruct a hemimandible, the natural curvature including the anterior superior iliac spine is well suited to reconstruct the angle of the mandible.
- **b** Thin layers of cortical bone line a huge quantity of cancellous bone and marrow. Bone width and height are always enough to receive dental implants.
- **c** Cross sections of the iliac crest.

It is based on the deep circumflex iliac artery and its associated veins. The flap can be raised with or without a skin paddle and the donor site scar can be well hidden within the garment line. It can also incorporate the internal oblique muscle for additional soft-tissue coverage.

This makes it useful for young dentate patients with the wish for implant-retained dental rehabilitation [Hidalgo, 1989; Kildal et al, 2001]. Early on, this flap was used extensively for mandible reconstructions, however since the description of the fibula flap for mandible reconstruction its use has somewhat diminished. Although the bone stock of this flap is some of the best available, particularly when osteointegrated implants are being considered, it still has limited length [Disa et al, 1999; Cordeiro et al, 1999]. Furthermore, the skin paddle is bulky and must be oriented parallel to the bone flap to prevent potential constriction of the perforating vessels, thereby limiting the flexibility of reconstruction, unless the perforators to the skin are dissected separately, which allows for a thinner skin portion which can be inserted with more flexibility. An alternative is the harvest of an additional portion of the internal oblique muscle, which is highly suited for the reconstruction of mucosal lining.

2.3 Scapula

The scapula flap is based on the circumflex scapular artery and its associated veins. Length and volume of the bone stock are limited, maximum length is up to 14–16 cm with wide interindividual variations (**Fig 2.6-3**).

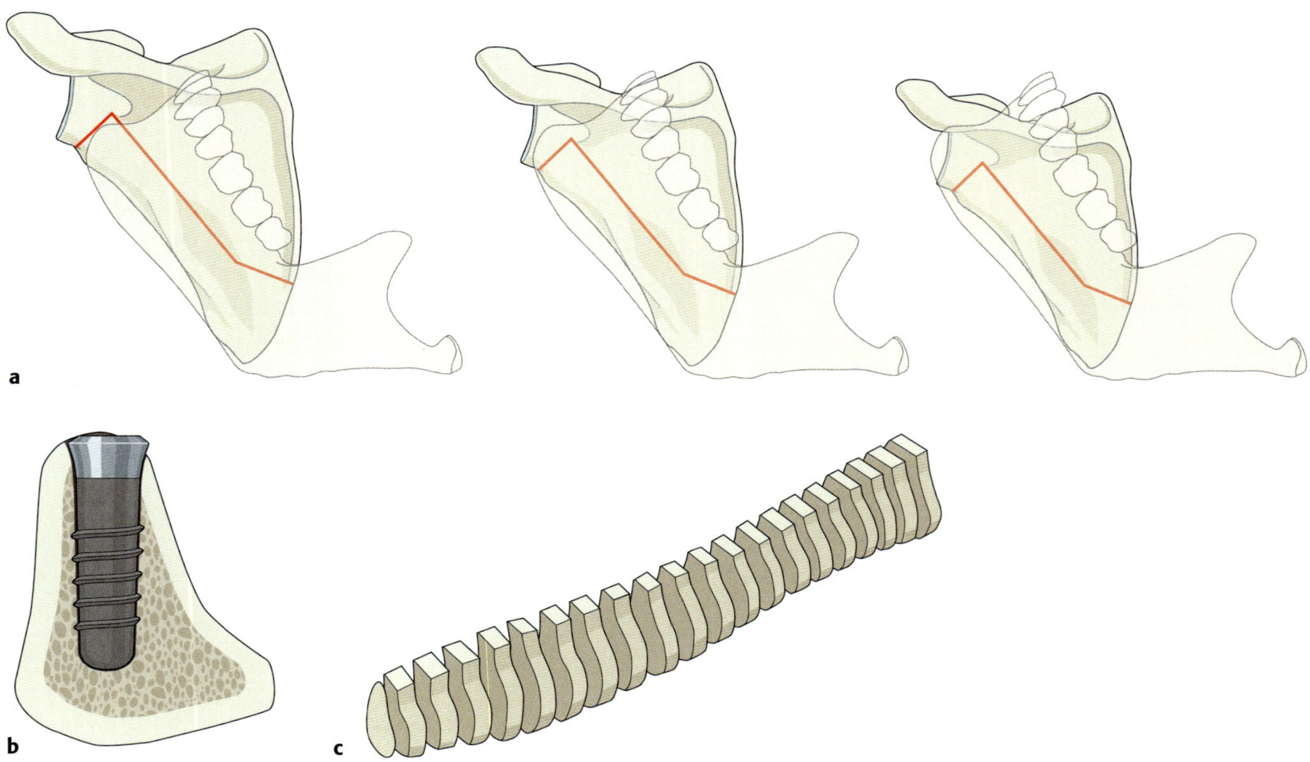

Fig 2.6-3a–c Bone stock lateral scapula.
From the lateral border of the scapula bone segments including the scapular tip can be harvested. Bone stock shows significant interindividual variations depending on the individual build and muscle mass (**a**). The bone often shows a slightly twisted or helical shape. The cortical layers are thicker close to the glenoid fossa, whereas the tip has a thin cortical layer and contains cancellous bone and marrow. The cross sections do not always have enough width and height for dental implant placement (**b**). Cross section of the lateral scapula (**c**).

A segment of bone along with large independent and reliable skin paddles can be harvested on a single pedicle. If dissected proximally up to its origin at the axillary artery and vein, the pedicle is long and the vessels usually have a large caliber. Because of these unique features, the flap is primarily used for situations which require a small bone component and large soft-tissue components, such as through and through defects of the lower face including the mandible (see chapter 1.1). Elevation of the serratus anterior or latissimus dorsi muscles upon the same pedicle can be performed to increase tissue bulk if required [Disa et al, 2000; Urken et al, 2001]. Pedicled on the angular branch originating from the thoracodorsal vessels a bone segment from the scapular tip with independent blood supply can be harvested. Some have argued that the scapular bone does not readily tolerate osteotomies or osteointegrated implants and is not suited for anterior mandibular reconstruction [Disa et al, 2000; Cordeiro et al, 1999]. The major disadvantage of the scapula flap is the need to alter patient position during harvest. The location of the donor site prevents a two-team approach, and therefore adds time to the operation. However, in situations that preclude the use of either the fibula or iliac crest (ie, patients suffering from severe bilateral peripheral vascular disease or preoperative gait difficulties), the scapula flap may be the best option [Urken et al, 1998].

2.4 Radial forearm

The radial forearm flap is based on the radial artery and its associated venae comitantes of the volar forearm. This flap has a long vascular pedicle and can be harvested with a large skin paddle. It is thin and pliable, making it perfect for molding and shaping. The radial forearm flap can also be raised as an osteocutaneous flap by incorporating a monocortical segment of radial bone (see chapter 1.1). Up to 14 cm can be safely harvested from the radius, however the bone is thin and may not tolerate osteointegrated implants or multiple osteotomies [Disa et al, 2000; Cordeiro et al, 1999]. In addition, a potential drawback is the possibility of a delayed fracture in the donor site of the radial bone following harvest [Villaret et al, 2003]. Prevention of a potential fracture is possible by plating the radius donor site [Jones et al, 2003]. Sensation to the flap may be restored by raising the medial or lateral antebrachial cutaneous nerves and performing a primary nerve coaptation to the available sensory head and neck nerves. Most reconstructive CMF surgeons consider a radial forearm bone flap not a good option for functional mandible reconstruction because of limited bone height and length, and consider it a reserve flap for special cases.

3 Classification of mandible defects

Several authors have published mandible defect classifications based on location and extent of segmental mandible defects [Jewer et al, 1989; Urken et al, 1991; Boyd et al, 1993; Schultz et al, 2015]. Defect classification systems are helpful, especially for scientific studies, but unfortunately there is no classification that is universally accepted. Additionally, it is generally accepted that not only bone loss but also additional soft-tissue loss, scarring, respectively mobility and neurological deficits, all have an important impact on the functional result after ablative tumor surgery and subsequent reconstruction. Consequently, Urken et al [1991] published a classification system that addresses not only bone defects but also soft-tissue defects and neurological deficits. The mandible is divided into the regions C (condyle, bilaterally) R (ramus, bilaterally), B (body, bilaterally) and S (symphysis). The symphysis is subdivided in two halves (SH) because the resection of the complete symphysis may have a significant impact on postoperative functional results following the complete detachment of the extrinsic muscles of the tongue and the suprahyoid muscles (**Fig 2.6-4** and **Tables 2.6-1** and **2.6-2**).

Defect	Abbreviation
Mucosa	
Labial	L
Buccal	B
Soft palate	SP
Hemi	SP^H
Total	SP^T
Floor of mouth	FOM
Anterior	FOM^a
Lateral	FOM^L
Pharynx	PH
Lateral	PH^L
Posterior	PH^P
Tongue	
Mobile	
One-quarter	$T^M_{1/4}$
One-half	$T^M_{1/2}$
Three-quarters	$T^M_{3/4}$
Nonfunctional	T^M_{NF}
Tongue base	
One-quarter	$T^B_{1/4}$
One-half	$T^B_{1/2}$
Three-quarters	$T^B_{3/4}$
Nonfunctional	T^B_{NF}
Total glossectomy	TG
Cutaneous defects	C
Cheek	C^C
Neck	C^N
Mentum	C^M
Lips	C^L
Upper (C^{UL})	$C^{UL}_{1/4}$ $C^{UL}_{1/2}$ $C^{UL}_{3/4}$ C^{UL}_T
Lower (C^{LL})	$C^{LL}_{1/4}$ $C^{LL}_{1/2}$ $C^{LL}_{3/4}$ C^{LL}_T

Table 2.6-1 Classification of soft-tissue defects potentially associated with mandible resection.

Neurological
Hypoglossal = N^H
Lingual = N^L
Facial = N^F
Inferior alveolar = N^{IA}
Bilateral defects = N_B

Table 2.6-2 Classification of nerve lesions potentially associated with mandible resection.

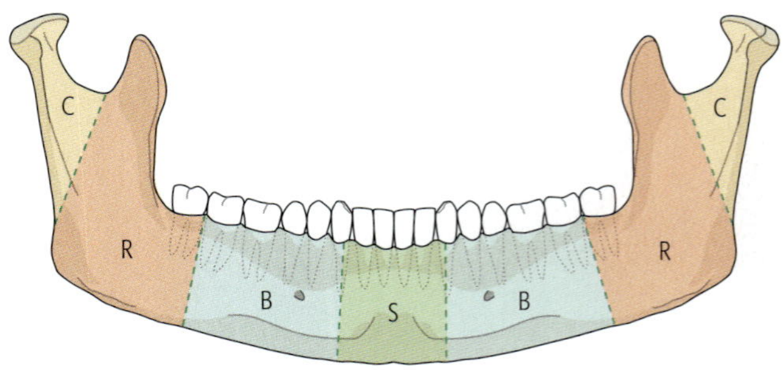

Fig 2.6-4 Mandible defect classification [Urken et al, 1991]. The mandible is divided into the regions C (condyle, bilaterally), R (ramus, bilaterally), B (body, bilaterally), and S (symphysis). The symphysis is subdivided in two halves (SH).

4 Considerations for flap selection

Several clinical aspects need to be taken into consideration to select the bone flap best suited for a specific patient, and the appropriate donor site for flap harvest.

4.1 Type of bone defect

Long mandible defects up to a complete mandible can be reconstructed with a single fibula flap (**Fig 2.6-5**).

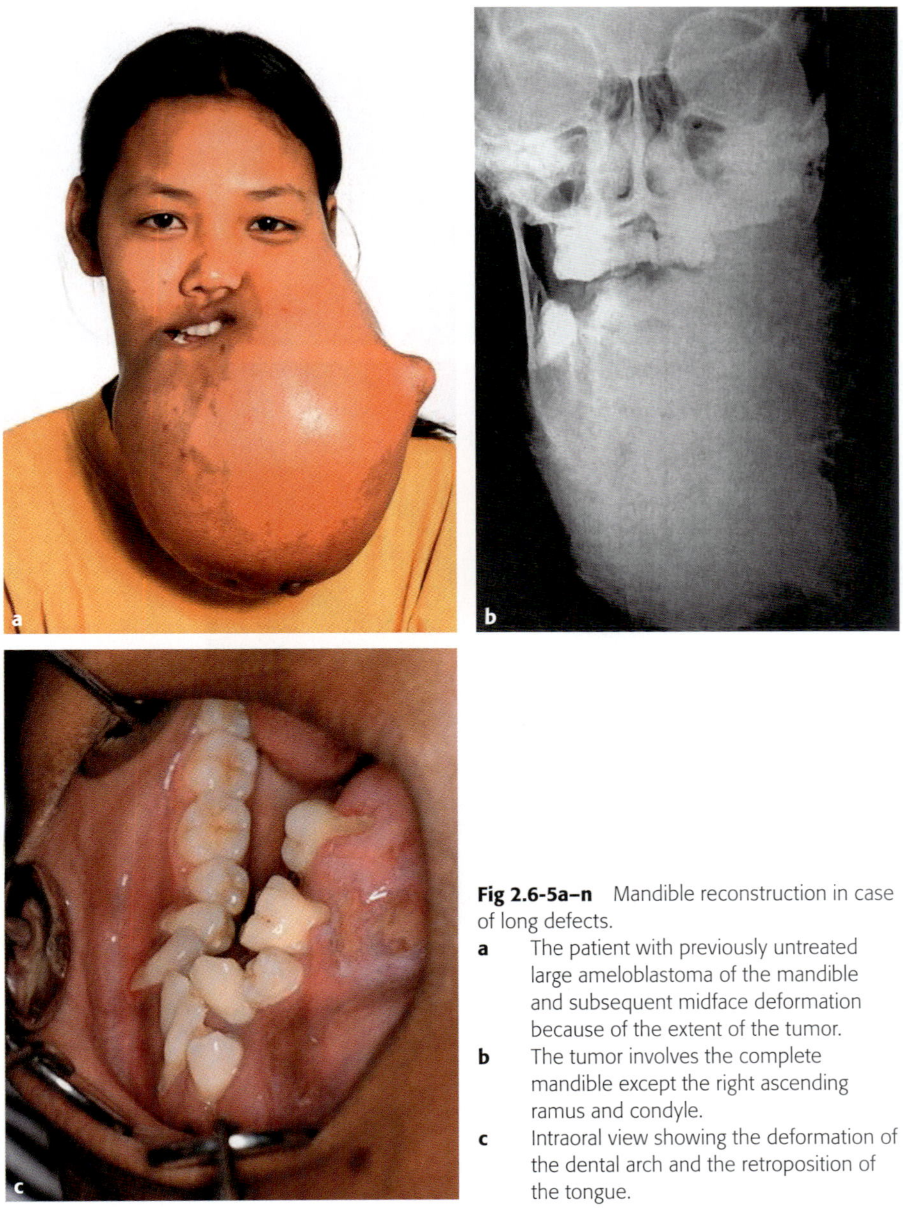

Fig 2.6-5a–n Mandible reconstruction in case of long defects.

- **a** The patient with previously untreated large ameloblastoma of the mandible and subsequent midface deformation because of the extent of the tumor.
- **b** The tumor involves the complete mandible except the right ascending ramus and condyle.
- **c** Intraoral view showing the deformation of the dental arch and the retroposition of the tongue.

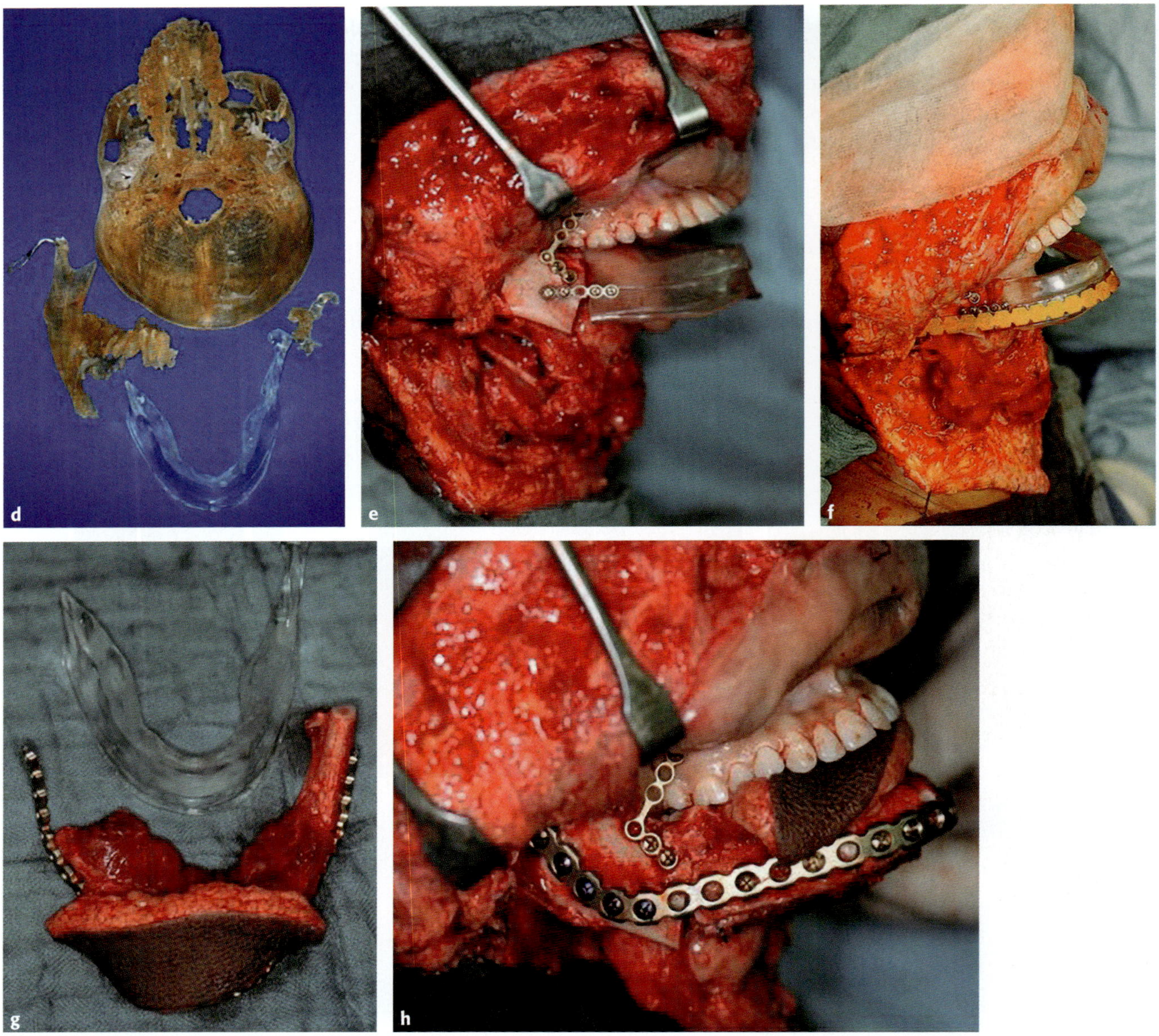

Fig 2.6-5a–n (cont) Mandible reconstruction in case of long defects.

d Reconstruction planning based on a stereolithographic model. The tumor mass does not show because of insufficient ossification. The right ramus and condyle are the only intact areas of the mandible. Note the deformation of the upper dental arch, zygoma, and zygomatic arch on the left side. An acrylic mandible template (blue) fitting to the patient's skeletal anatomy has been manufactured manually in a dental laboratory.

e Before tumor resection the right ascending ramus and condyle were fixed to the maxilla with an L-shaped miniplate. The acrylic mandible template is temporarily fixed to the ascending ramus to control dimensions and fit. The template has a groove on the buccal side for positioning of the reconstruction plate.

f The reconstruction plate template is placed in the groove and contoured to the mandible template. It will serve as a bending template for the reconstruction plate.

g The raised and contoured fibula bone flap is fixed to the reconstruction plate with multiple monocortical screws before flap insert. A skin portion has been harvested for intraoral lining.

h Bone flap is inserted and fixed to the right ascending ramus.

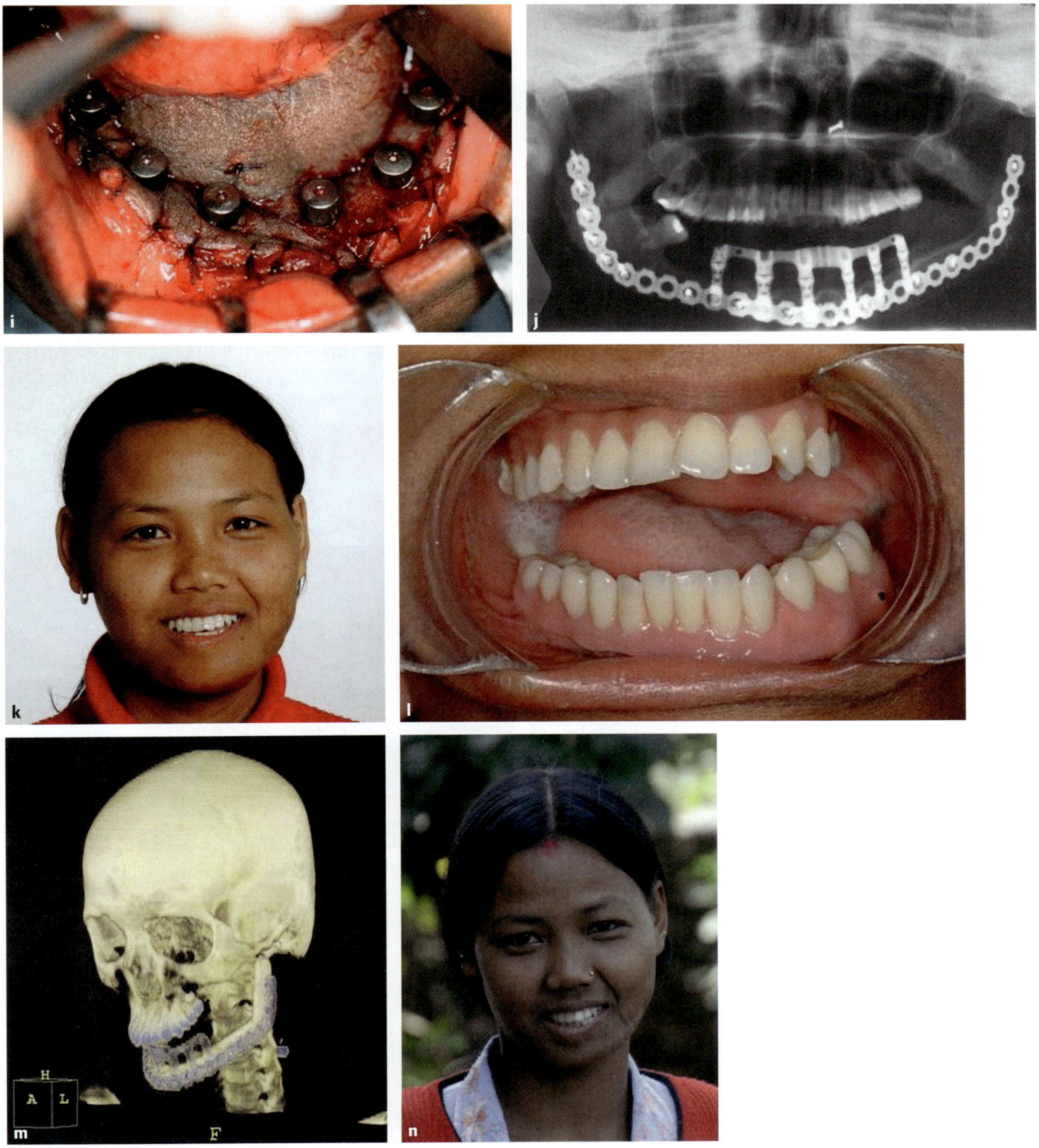

Fig 2.6-5a–n (cont) Mandible reconstruction in case of long defects.

- **i** Secondary dental implant placement 3 months after mandible reconstruction. The skin portion has been thinned out at the same time.
- **j** Postoperative OPT showing bone flap, reconstruction plate, and dental implants.
- **k** The patient after mandible reconstruction and prosthodontic rehabilitation with an implant supported removable denture.
- **l** Intraoral situation.
- **m** Postoperative 3-D CT showing bone flap, reconstruction plate, and dental implants.
- **n** The patient 18 years after surgery, still wearing the initial denture.

If a fibula flap is not available, for example, because of vessel variations or if the patient does not wish a fibula flap to be taken, the alternative for long-spanning defects is the use of two iliac or scapula bone flaps, or the combination of a fibula and a scapula bone flap.

If smaller segments of the mandible need to be reconstructed it is important to understand that each of these subunits possesses different qualities that require special attention to achieve a successful functional and esthetic reconstructive outcome.

The chin has important functional and cosmetic qualities, which must be re-established following ablative surgery or avulsive trauma to obtain a satisfactory result. In addition to its cosmetically conspicuous location, functionally the anterior mandible is the support structure on which the surrounding musculature of the chin, lips, anterior floor of mouth, and tongue rely. Defects involving either bone or soft tissue must be reconstructed accurately to reestablish proper oral competence, mastication, swallowing, speech, and facial expression.

The complex 3-D shape of the chin mandates that the surgeon be able to contour a flap for an appropriate fit. In addition, placement of osteointegrated implants is often necessary for subsequent prosthodontic rehabilitation, as the anterior mandible is the most frequent site of implantation. To sustain these devices, a segment of bone with adequate shape and volume is included in the reconstructive flap.

The fibula flap is a good option for chin reconstruction when used in a double-barrel fashion [Disa et al, 2000; Cordeiro et al, 1999; Hidalgo et al, 1998; Shpitzer et al, 1997; Shpitzer et al, 2000; Takushima et al, 2001; Hidalgo, 1989]. It is ideal for both bone-only and composite defects. The iliac crest flap provides ample bone for chin reconstruction and is still favored by some for anterior replacement (**Fig 2.6-6**).

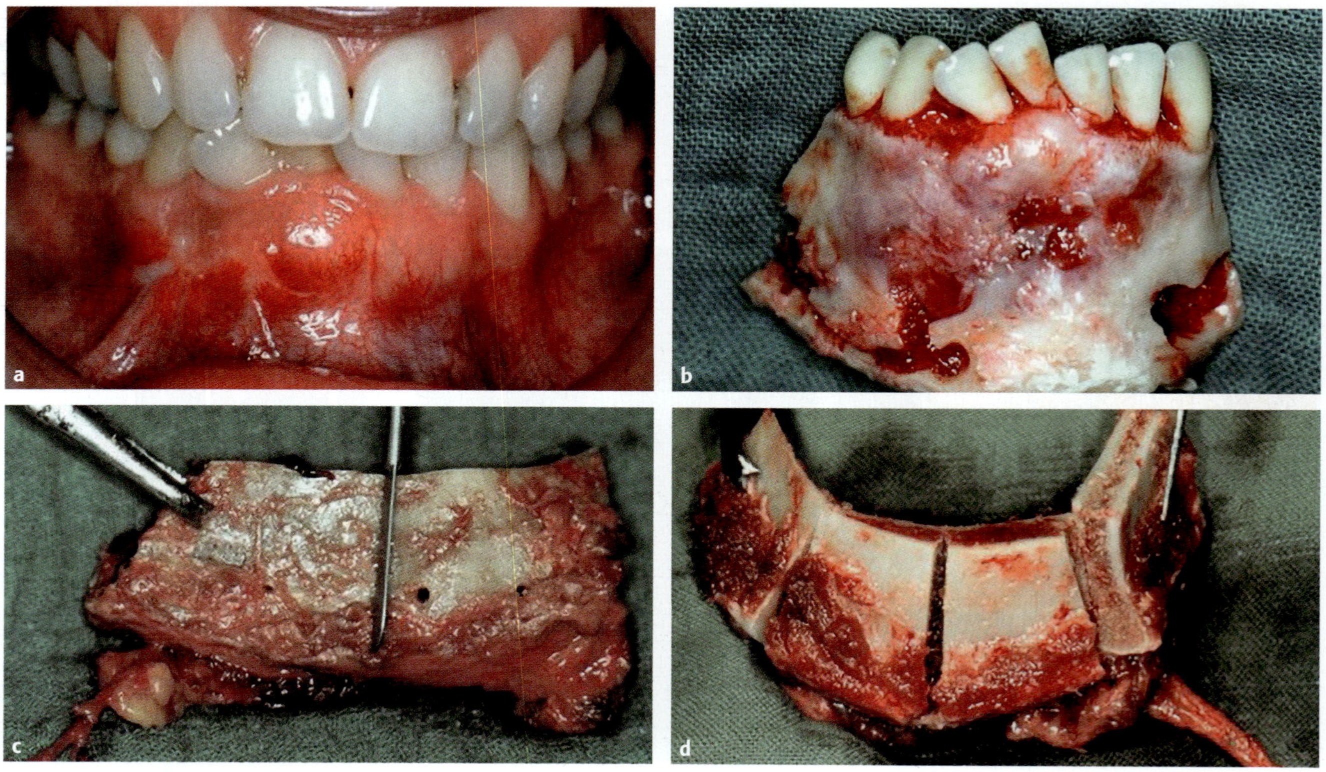

Fig 2.6-6a–n Chin reconstruction in a dentate young patient.

- **a** Odontogenic myxoma in the chin region. Note that surgery has been performed 25 years ago. Today an odontogenic myxoma is not necessarily an indication for segmental mandible resection.
- **b** Specimen with holes after multiple mapping biopsies, which were taken previously.
- **c** Microvascular iliac bone flap with a thin strip of iliacus muscle and muscles of the abdominal wall on the medial side of the ileum. Preparation for an osteotomy of the lateral cortex.
- **d** Bone flap contouring after three monocortical osteotomies designed as opening osteotomies. The osteotomies are made through the lateral cortex of the iliac bone. The medial (inner) cortex is fractured. The vascular pedicle lies medial to the inner cortex.

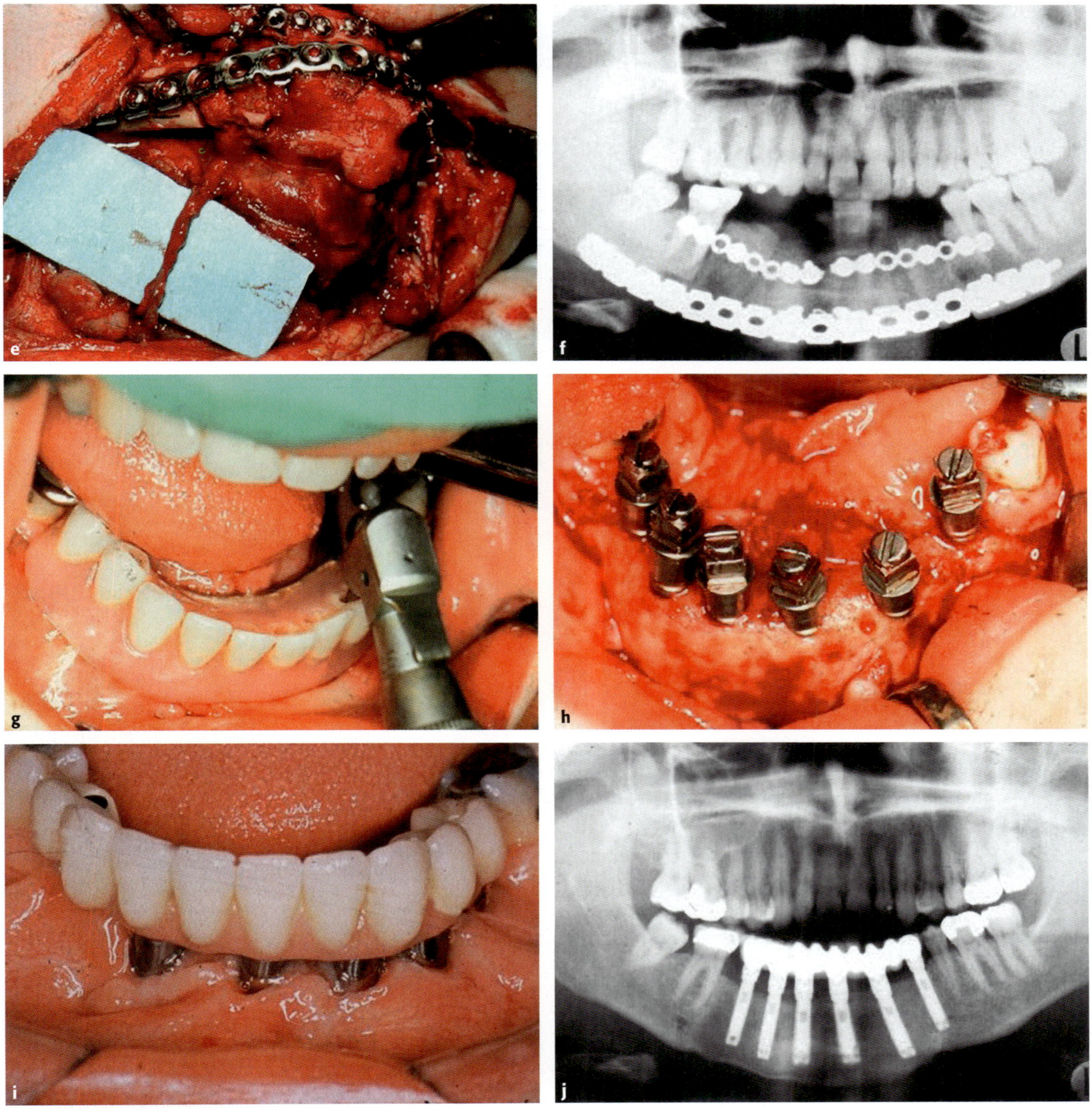

Fig 2.6-6a–n (cont) Chin reconstruction in a dentate young patient.

- **e** Bone flap inserted and fixed to the residual elements of the mandible with a stainless-steel reconstruction plate and miniplates. The bone gaps following the opening osteotomies are filled with cancellous bone and bone marrow harvested from the same site. Microvascular anastomosis has been performed.
- **f** Orthopantomogram (OPT) after bone transplantation.
- **g** Three months after bone transplantation dental implants are inserted. A provisional denture is used as a positioning guide.
- **h** Dental implants are inserted, the bone gaps created by opening osteotomies have completely healed.
- **i** Prosthodontic rehabilitation with a fixed bridge.
- **j** Postoperative OPT after bone transplantation, dental implant placement, and prosthodontic rehabilitation.

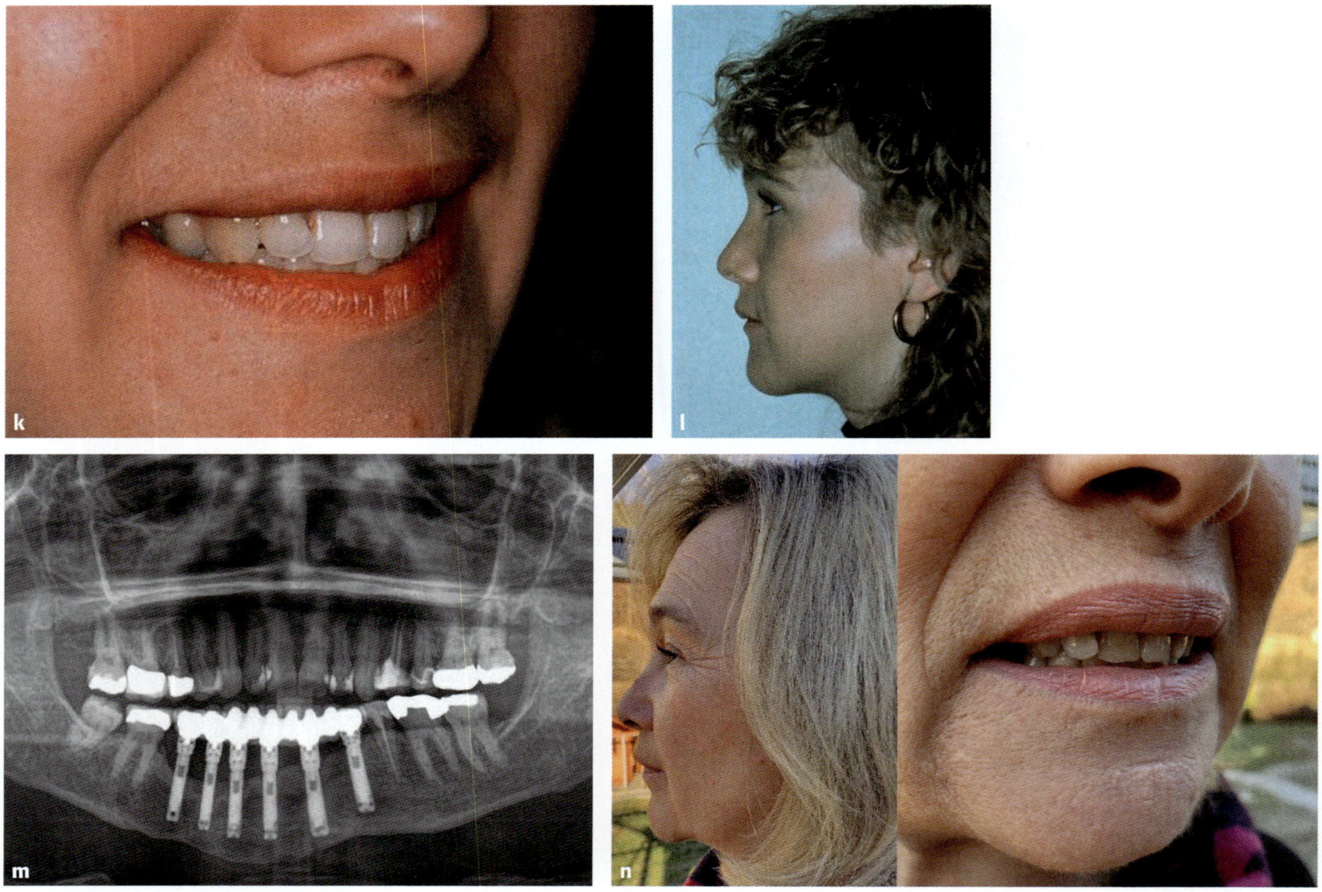

Fig 2.6-6a–n (cont) Chin reconstruction in a dentate young patient.
k Smile of the patient after surgery.
l Lateral view after chin resection and reconstruction. The iliac bone flap provides enough volume for contour reconstruction.
m The OPT 25 years after initial surgery. Some vertical bone loss is present in the right canine region, but the fixed bridge is still in place.
n Clinical result 25 years after mandible reconstruction.

In cases with large mucosa defects an iliac bone flap may be used with the additional internal oblique muscle (**Fig 2.6-7**).

For large through and through defects of the chin region, it is still debatable which flap(s) to use. The amount of bone and soft tissue needed to repair these defects places a high demand on the patient's available donor sites and pushes the technical process of the surgical team. The scapula flap has been argued as the flap of choice for through and through defects of the mandible [Urken et al, 2001; Urken et al, 1998]. Its advantages include the use of only a single donor site and the availability of large independent skin paddles. The drawbacks are the limited available bone and an unfavorable patient position during surgery. A single fibula flap may also be used for small to moderate sized defects by deepithelializing a central strip of the skin paddle, thereby producing two separate skin islands [Christie et al, 1994]. For large skin and mucosal defects, though, this technique may not be adequate. Over-aggressive stretching of the skin paddle to accommodate a large defect could be detrimental to skin perfusion and viability. The iliac crest osteomusculocutaneous flap is another choice. The internal oblique muscle can

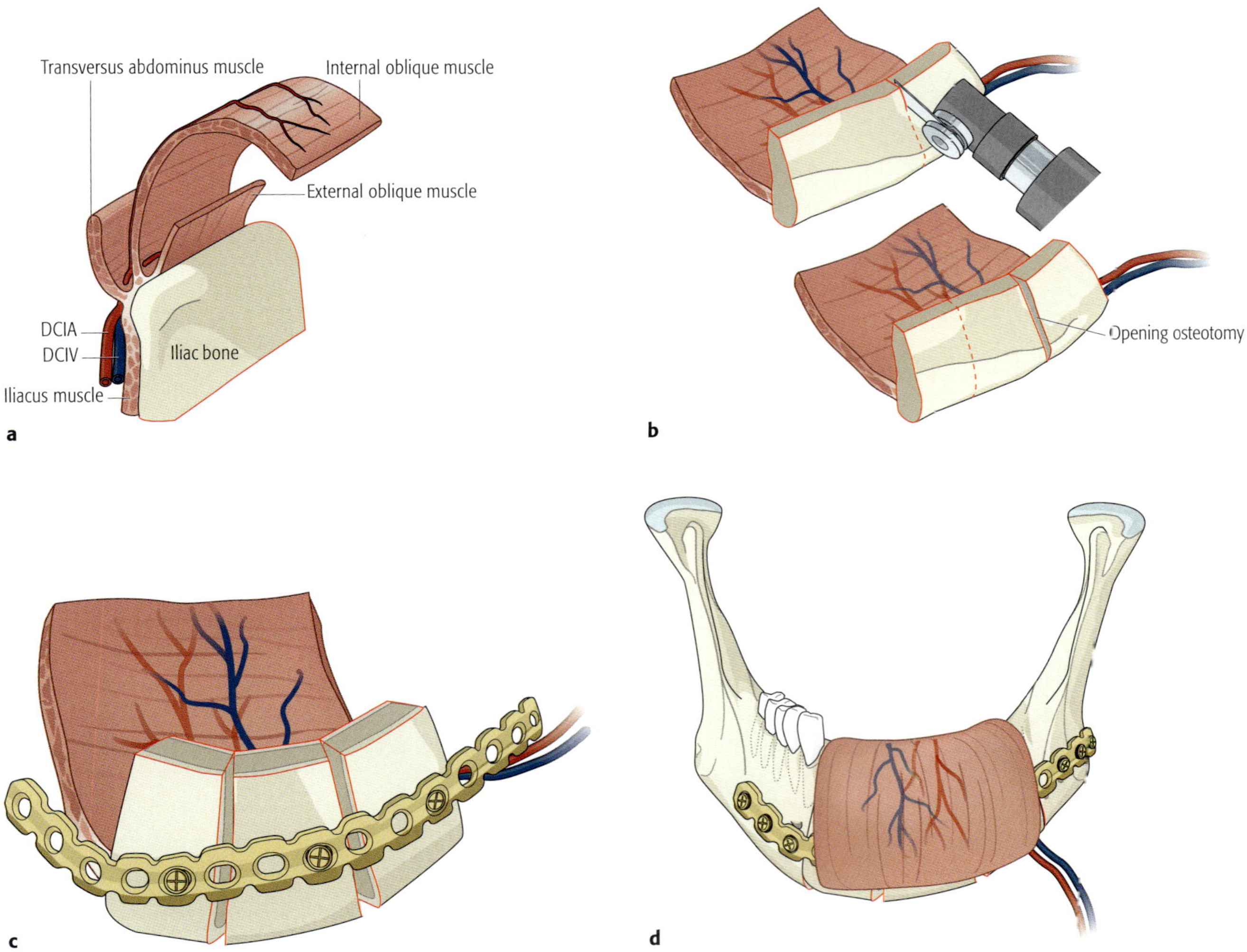

Fig 2.6-7a–d Iliac bone flap with internal oblique muscle.

- **a** Iliac bone flap harvested with an extended internal oblique muscle component.
- **b** The bone is contoured with the help of monocortical opening osteotomies.
- **c** The iliac bone is first fixed to a reconstruction plate. The soft-tissue components of the flap including the vascular pedicle are positioned on the medial side, opposite the plate.
- **d** The internal oblique muscle is used to reconstruct the missing mucosa and is left to secondary granulation and epithelialization.

restore the mucosal defect and the skin paddle the external defect (**Fig 2.6-8**). The bony component remains in between.

The double free flap method has been successfully performed for repair of large through and through defects [Chana et al, 2004; Deschler et al, 2000; Shpitzer et al, 1997; Jones et al, 2003], or extended mucosa or skin defects difficult to reconstruct with one soft-tissue flap component (**Fig 2.6-9**).

This method of reconstruction involves the simultaneous harvest of an osseous flap (such as the fibula or iliac bone flap) and a fasciocutaneous flap (such as the radial or ulnar forearm fasciocutaneous flap). Pairing of these flaps provides abundant soft tissue for lining and adequate bone for shaping of the affected region. When using this double flap method of reconstruction, it is recommended that two independent vascular supplies be used for the anastomosis to potentially avoid double flap compromise [Cordeiro et al, 1999]. This is not always possible in previously irradiated patients and those with extensive neck disease. The major downside to this method of repair is that two free flaps must be harvested at the same sitting. This results in increased operative time, places a higher technical demand on the surgical team, and results in increased donor site morbidity for the patient.

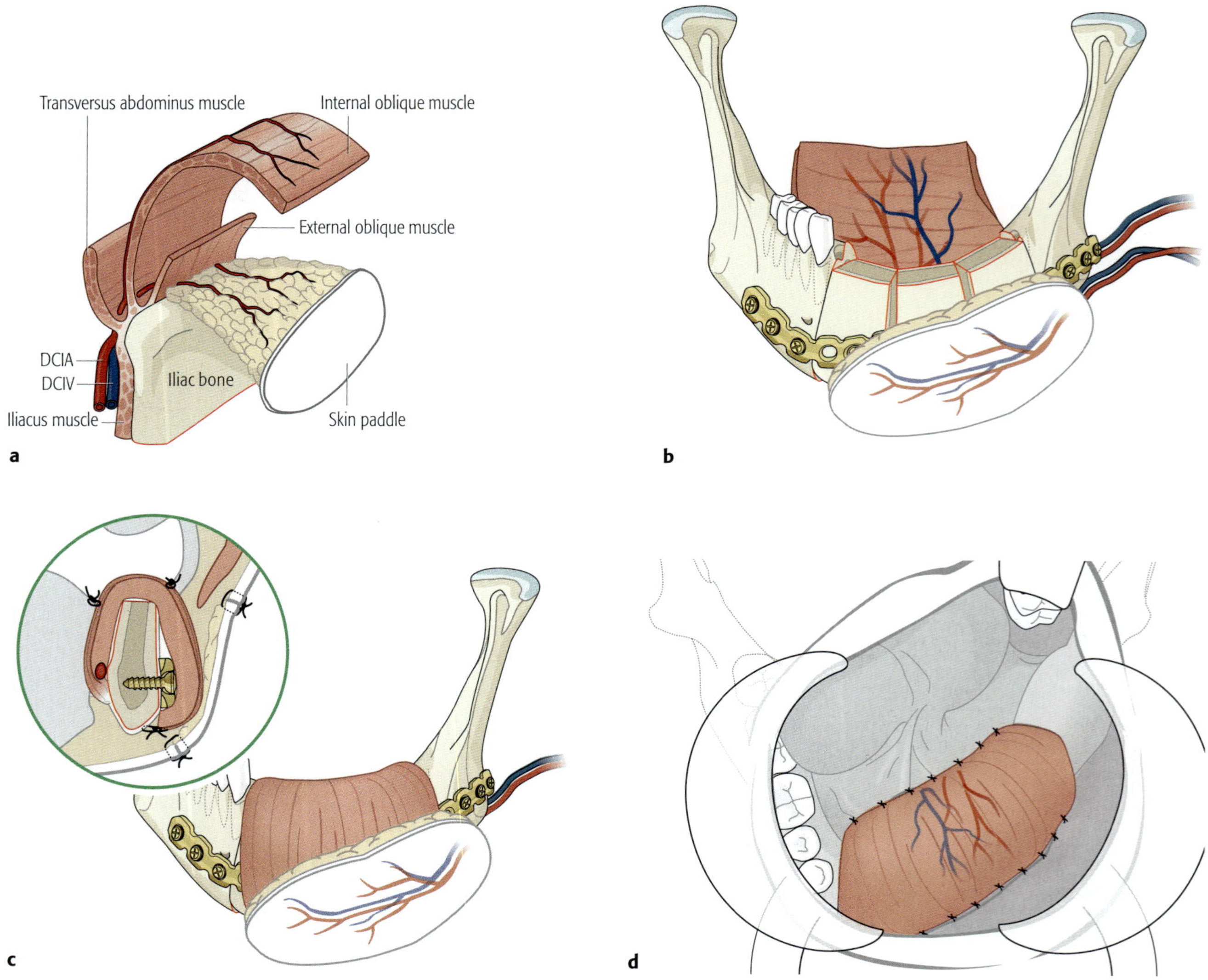

Fig 2.6-8a–d Iliac bone flap with internal oblique muscle and skin island for combined mucosa, bone and skin defects.
a Iliac bone flap harvested with an extended internal oblique muscle and a skin component.
b The bone is first fixed to the reconstruction plate before the two soft-tissue components are inserted (internal oblique muscle and skin). The perforators/tissue bridge to the skin island lies underneath the iliac bone and therefore the neomandible.
c The oblique muscle is used to reconstruct the intraoral mucosa defect, and the skin to reconstruct areas of the cheek or chin.
d Internal oblique muscle sutured in place.

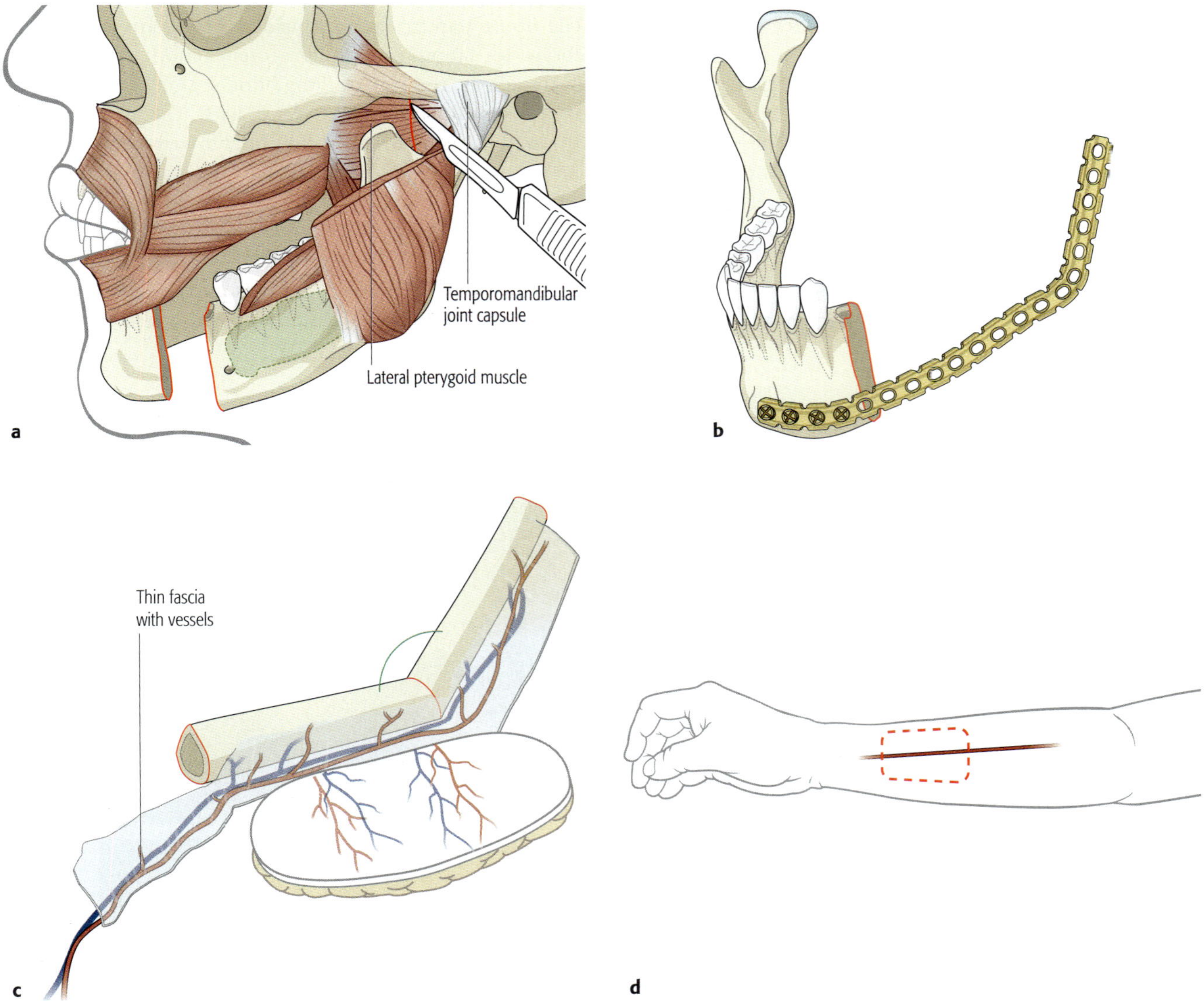

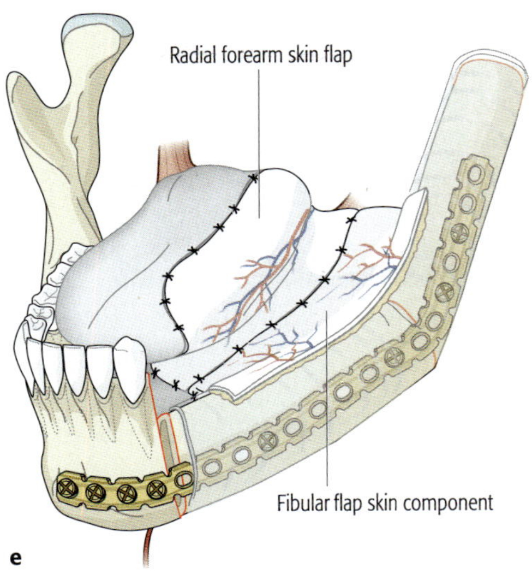

Fig 2.6-9a–e Mandible resection with an extended intraoral soft-tissue defect, and reconstruction with a fibula osteocutaneous flap and a radial forearm flap (two-flap technique).

- **a** Resection of the left mandibular body, angle, ascending ramus and condyle, with an extended intraoral mucosa defect.
- **b** A prebent or patient-specific reconstruction plate is fixed to the mandible to stabilize and provide contour.
- **c** A fibula flap is raised with a skin island and contoured according to the angle of the mandible.
- **d** Additional soft-tissue lining is provided by a radial forearm flap.
- **e** Two flaps inserted. The fibula bone is fixed to the reconstruction plate. The skin island from the fibula is used to cover the alveolus, and the radial forearm flap is used to reconstruct the floor of the mouth and the tongue.

For lateral mandible reconstruction (body and angle) the type of flap or flaps required for repair will again depend on the degree of bone and soft-tissue loss. Lateral defects of the mandible tend to be more forgiving to the reconstructive surgeon compared with anterior defects. The lateral mandible is cosmetically not as conspicuous, and the natural contour of this region requires fewer, if any, osteotomies to the bone flap. In addition, prior studies have shown lower failure rates for reconstructions of the lateral mandible compared with the anterior region [Wei et al, 1999; Boyd, 1994].

The fibula flap is, again, considered by many as the best choice for lateral mandible reconstruction, especially for those defects requiring a long bone segment [Cordeiro et al, 1999; Takushima et al, 2001; Head et al, 2003]. The iliac crest is an alternative, often with an additional internal oblique muscle for intraoral soft-tissue repair. The scapula and radial forearm osteocutaneous flaps can also be used for lateral defect repair [Disa et al, 2000; Cordeiro et al, 1999; Hidalgo et al, 1998; Villaret et al, 2003; Guyot et al, 2004]. Because of their large pliable skin paddles, these flaps may be good choices for defects requiring a small bone segment and a large lining surface (**Fig 2.6-10**).

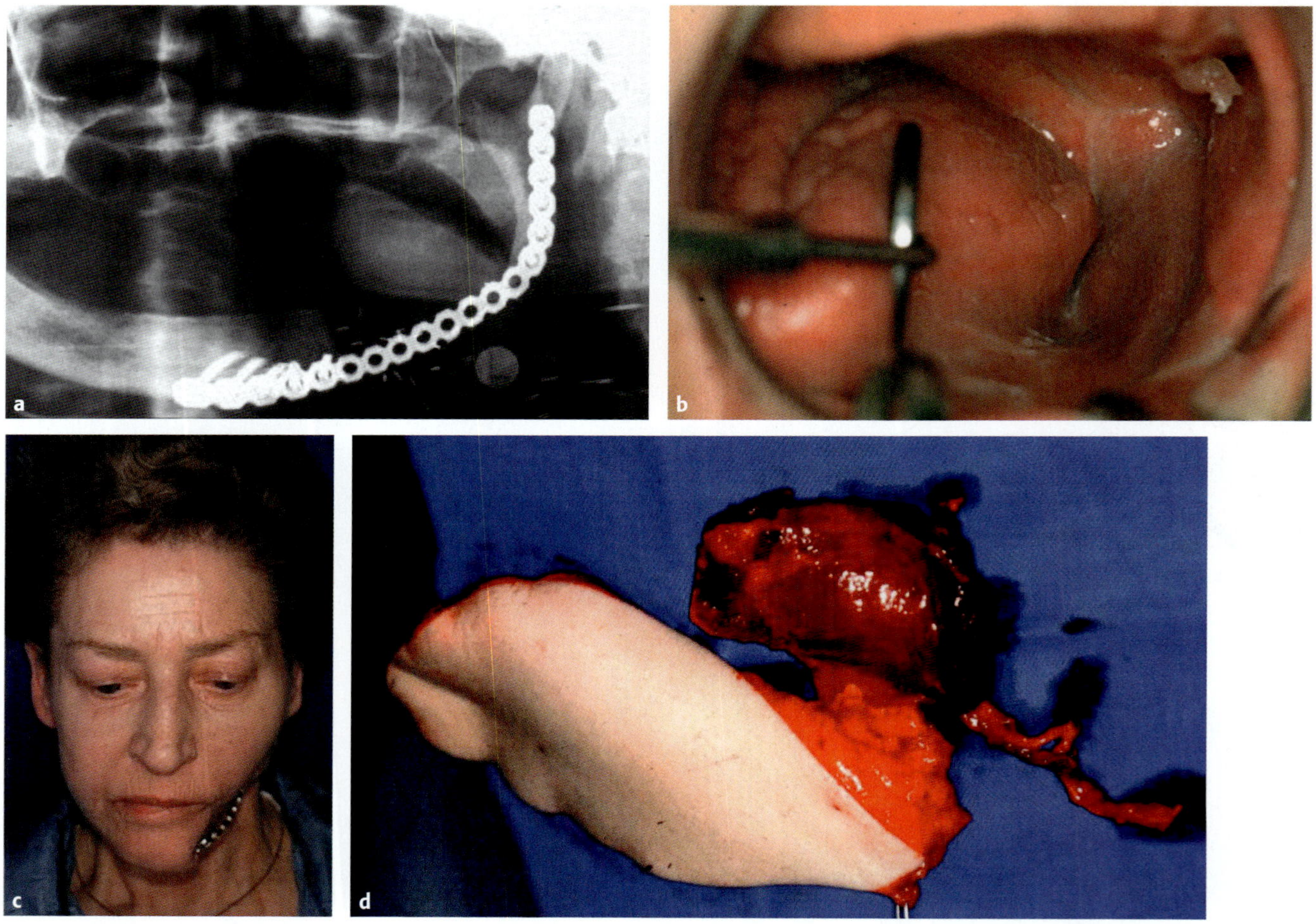

Fig 2.6-10a–h Scapula bone and parascapular soft-tissue flap for segmental mandible defect and soft-tissue deficiency in the cheek and neck.
a Orthopantomogram (OPT) immediately after segmental mandible resection in the left mandibular body.
b Intraoral soft-tissue reconstruction was performed with a radial forearm flap.
c Plate exposure after full-dose postoperative radiation therapy.
d Scapula bone and parascapular soft-tissue flap raised on one vascular pedicle for simultaneous reconstruction of the mandible, the lower cheek, and upper neck.

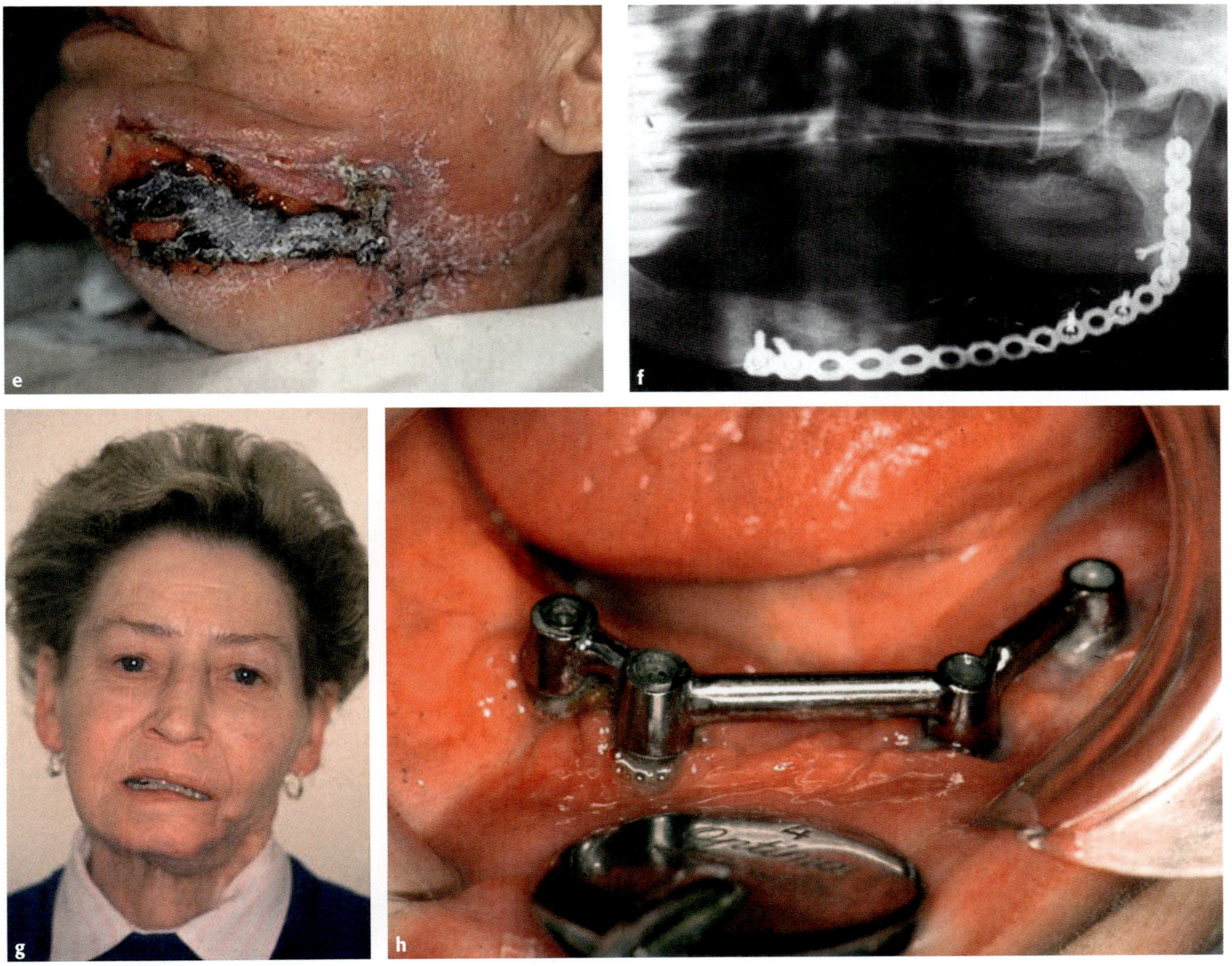

Fig 2.6-10a–h (cont) Scapula bone and parascapular soft-tissue flap for segmental mandible defect and soft-tissue deficiency in the cheek and neck.

- **e** Situation 2 weeks postoperatively with partial necrosis of the irradiated paramandibular skin. The parascapular neck shows no signs of compromise.
- **f** Postoperative OPT showing the reconstructed mandible.
- **g** Appearance after delayed and secondary wound healing in the lower cheek region. An implant supported prosthodontic rehabilitation has been achieved with a removable denture.
- **h** Implant supported bar construction.

Through and through defects of the lateral mandible can be managed similar to the anterior mandible. Smaller defects may be amenable to repair by using the technique of deepithelializing a strip of skin from the paddle of a fibula to create two separate lining surfaces [Christie et al, 1994]. Again, it is important not to overstretch the skin paddle because it can result in ischemia of the flap. Both the iliac crest and fibula free flaps can be used in combination with ulnar and radial forearm fasciocutaneous flaps for effective repair in complex defects [Shpitzer et al, 1997; Deschler et al, 2000; Chana et al, 2004]. For extensive defects, the use of the scapula flap has an advantage since only a single donor site is involved. The patient must be repositioned during surgery; however, postoperatively the patient can be mobilized faster since neither the hip nor lower extremities are involved during surgery.

The posterior aspect of the mandible, including the ascending ramus and condyle, remains challenging. Loss of mandibular height, development of occlusal alignment discrepancies and chronic temporomandibular joint (TMJ) problems are potential outcomes of tumor resections and reconstructions involving this region. The main trunk of the facial nerve lies near this area and is always at risk of damage when operating on this segment of the mandible. Since the ascending ramus contains no teeth, there is no need for dental reconstruction with implants; therefore, volume of the donor bone flap is not of significant concern. If tumor size mandates resection of the condyle, it is recommended that the TMJ disc be preserved to reduce the risk of joint ankyloses [Kroll et al, 1998] (**Fig 2.6-11**).

If this is not feasible, local soft-tissue flaps such as temporalis muscle or temporoparietal fascia can be used for lining of the glenoid fossa when mandible reconstruction is planned. The main disadvantage of using this flap is the creation of an additional donor site defect, which at times can be deforming.

It has been shown that restoration of posterior mandible defects or the temporomandibular condyle is not always necessary, and that satisfactory functional and cosmetic results can be achieved solely with a soft-tissue free flap, provided that the contralateral joint is intact and functional [King et al, 2002; Butler et al, 2004; Patel et al, 2001]. It is believed that loss of soft-tissue bulk is the cause of much of the functional morbidity following tumor resection of the posterior mandible, and that its reestablishment with flaps such as the rectus abdominus musculocutaneous free flap easily satisfies this problem. The use of such a flap obviates the need for tedious reconstruction of the condyle and TMJ, and may be better suited for older patients or those with a poor prognosis who would not necessarily benefit from a complex reconstruction. It may, however, result in a crossbite and malocclusion in the dentate patient.

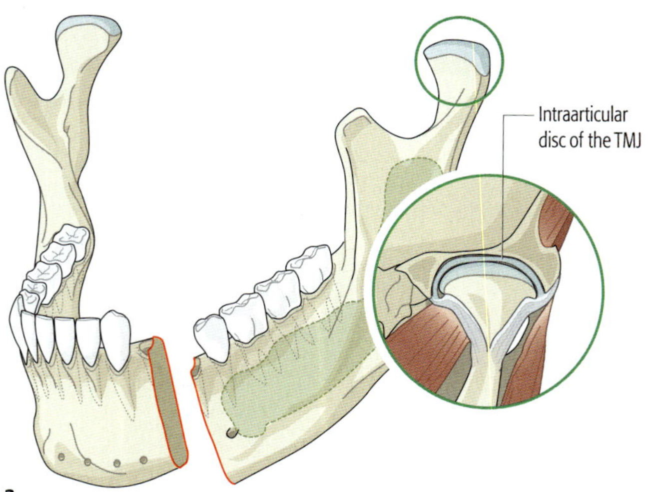

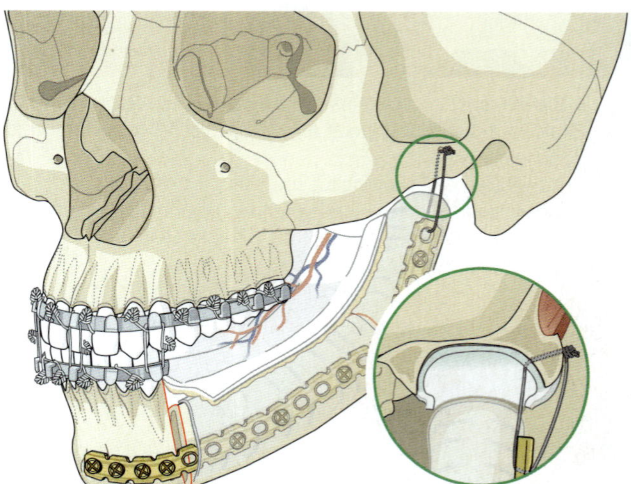

Fig 2.6-11a–b Preserving the temporamandibular disc and use of a free ending fibula flap for reconstruction in the temporomandibular joint (TMJ) area.

a Whenever oncologically sound the temporomandibular disc should be preserved and maintained during mandible resection.

b The fibula flap is contoured as such that it ends in a distance from the fossa. The disc is preserved to avoid bone exposure in the temporal area and to have a separating layer between the bone flap and the fossa. Some surgeons prefer to use an additional layer of temporalis fascia and/or muscle to separate the two areas even better. The free ending fibula is connected to the temporal bone or zygomatic arch with a wire to prevent sagging of the bone.

For young patients and those with large composite defects of the posterior mandible, repair of a bone defect can be performed with the fibula, iliac crest, scapula, or radial bones. As discussed for the other regions of the mandible, the fibula flap remains a valuable option and is considered by some as the flap of choice for reconstruction of the ascending ramus and condyle [Cordeiro et al, 1999; Ung et al, 2002]. The iliac crest is not as commonly used for isolated posterior mandible repair, since bone volume is not as important in this region. The scapula and radial forearm osteocutaneous flaps can be useful for defects which require a small bone segment but have an associated large intraoral mucosal defect as seen with extensive retromolar trigone and tonsillar fossa cancers [Disa et al, 2000; Cordeiro et al, 1999; Hidalgo et al, 1998; Guyot et al, 2004; Hidalgo et al, 1995]. Through and through defects of the posterior mandible can be successfully reconstructed with the methods described for these types of defects in other areas of the mandible.

Fortunately, the condyle region is not frequently the origin of mandibular tumors; however, often it must be resected to achieve adequate tumor-free margins. If condylar reconstruction is undertaken, it is recommended that autogenous tissue be used whenever possible [Disa et al, 2000; Cordeiro et al, 1999; Daniel et al, 2004]. This is especially true for those patients receiving adjuvant radiation therapy whose surrounding soft tissues will be compromised by radiation damage. Although a metallic condylar prosthesis is an available option, it is not recommended that it be used in patients before or after radiation therapy [Daniel et al, 2004].

Autogenous tissue options for reconstruction of the condyle during mandible reconstruction include shaping of the proximal end of a free flap bone to resemble a neo-condyle [Ung et al, 2002; Kroll et al, 1998] (**Fig 2.6-5** and **Fig 2.6-11**), if possible using the native condylar head as an autograft [Hidalgo et al, 2002; Disa et al, 2000; Cordeiro et al, 1999; Perrott et al, 1994] which can be added to the end of a bone flap, or harvesting a separate costochondral rib graft from the patient [Nahabedian et al, 2001]. When deciding to use the native condyle as a free autograft, one must be sure that oncological margins are not compromised. The decision for which option to use for condylar reconstruction will ultimately depend on the reconstructive surgeon. All the above choices have resulted in successful outcomes. Autotransplantation of the condyle and molding of the free flap are probably the two most common methods used today, and both methods have shown good results with minimal changes to the joint complex on postoperative radiographs [Hidalgo et al, 2002; Kroll et al, 1998]. The benefit of using a contoured free flap as the new condyle is that it is vascularized.

Technically, the manufacturing of a patient-specific condylar prosthesis for use together with a microvascular flap is an option (**Fig 2.6-12**) for non-irradiated patients.

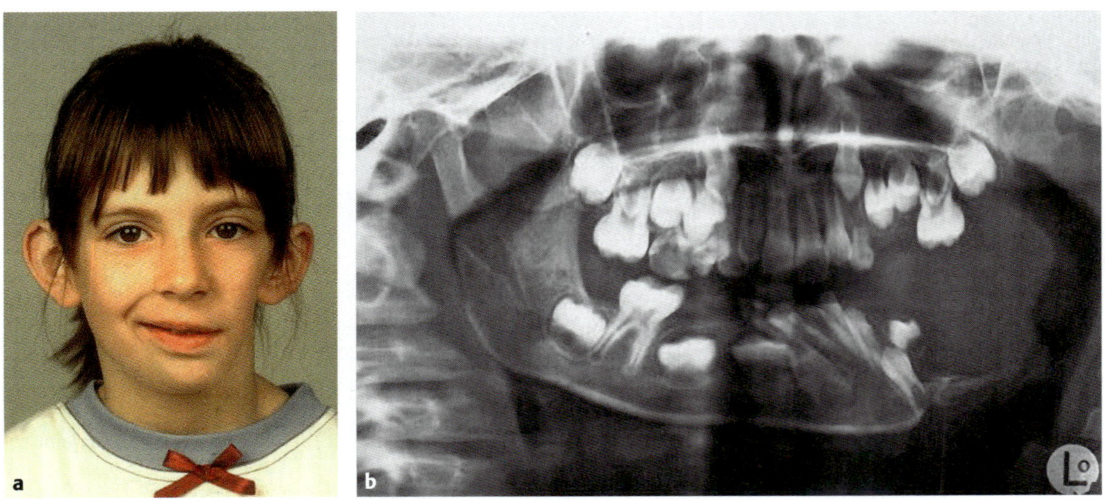

Fig 2.6-12a–l Mandible reconstruction with microvascular iliac bone flap and condylar prosthesis.
a An 8-year-old girl after resection of the left mandibular body, angle, ascending ramus, and condyle.
b Corresponding orthopantomogram (OPT).

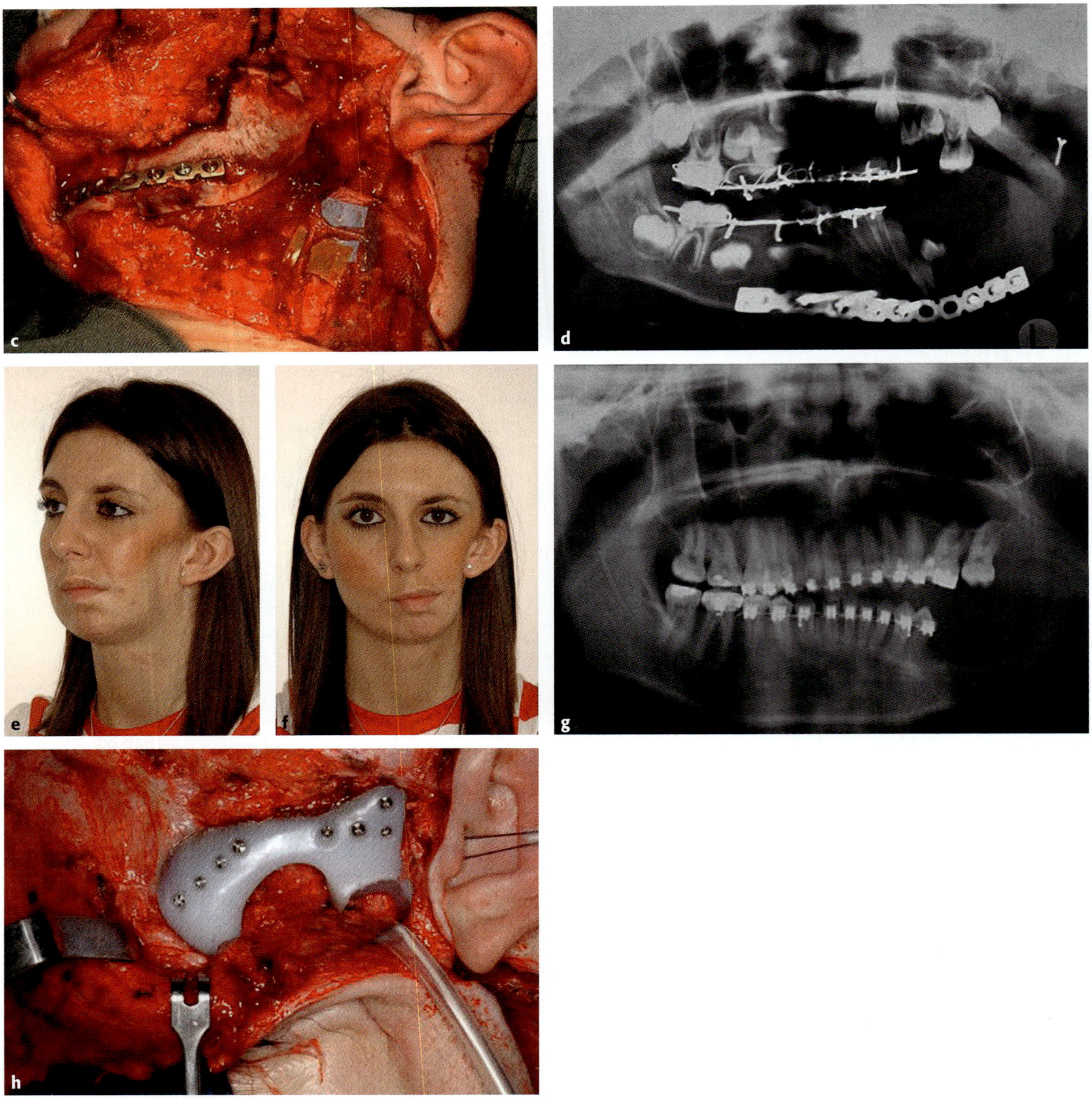

Fig 2.6-12a–l (cont) Mandible reconstruction with microvascular iliac bone flap and condylar prosthesis.

c Microvascular iliac bone flap inserted and fixed with a reconstruction plate. In the region of the coronoid process and the condyle, the bone is lined with slices of cartilage from the iliac crest for ankylosis prevention. Microvascular anastomosis has been performed.

d OPT postoperatively.

e–f The patient's appearance 15 years later.

g The OPT 15 years after initial surgery. The iliac bone flap has not grown adequately, especially in the vertical dimension. The patient had no stable occlusion because of missing support in the left temporomandibular joint (TMJ) area.

h Custom-made TMJ prosthesis (TMJ concepts) to replace the condyle and elongate the left ramus. In addition, an extension into the zygomatic arch and zygoma area has been designed and made to compensate for some of the tissue deficit in the upper cheek. Fossa component fixed to the temporal skull base.

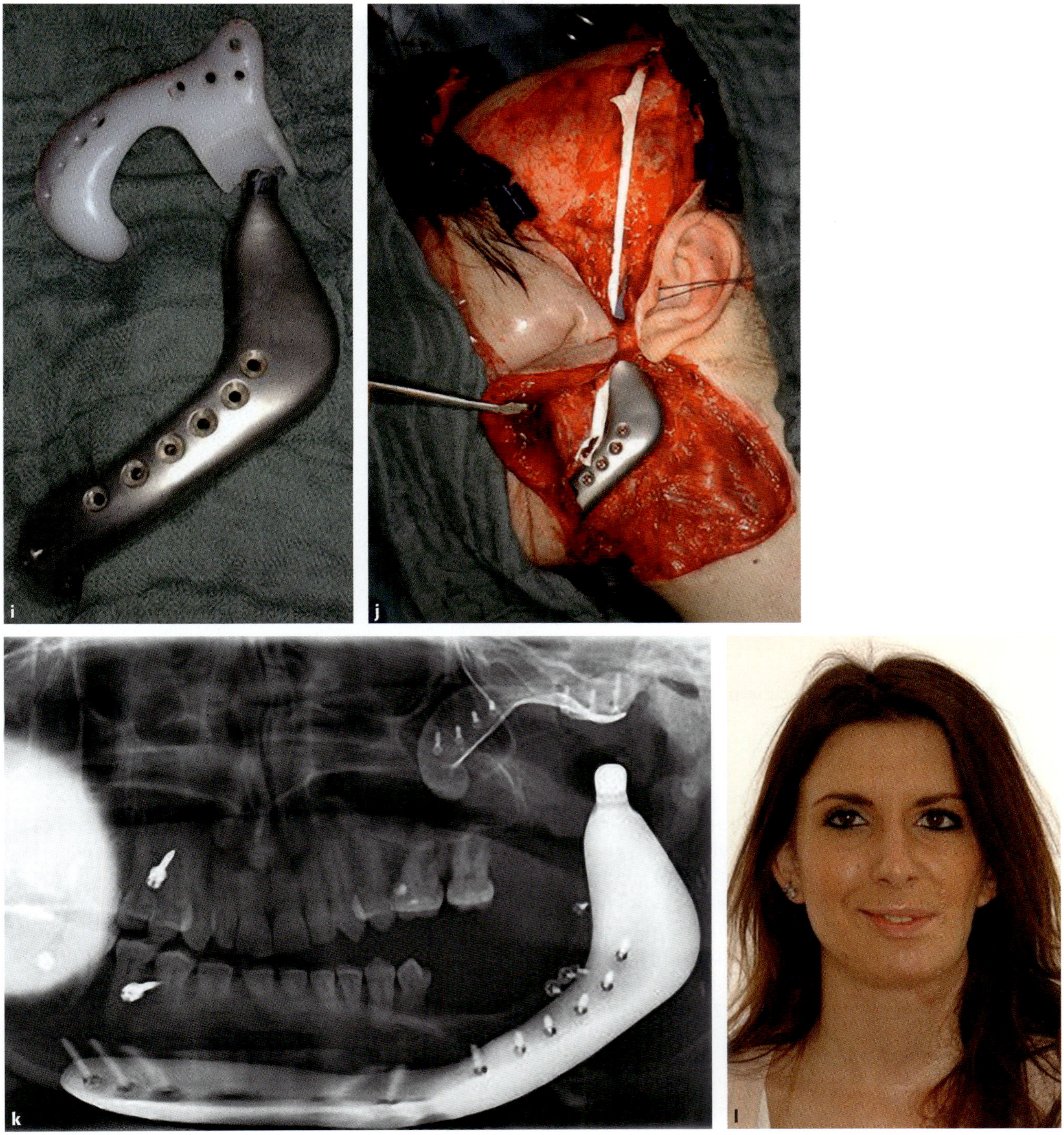

Fig 2.6-12a–l (cont)

- **i** Ascending ramus/condyle and fossa component.
- **j** Condylar head and ascending ramus component fixed to the iliac bone flap. In addition, a Gore Tex strip (white) is attached to the condylar prosthesis and anchored to the temporal skull via a miniplate to prevent sagging of the condylar head.
- **k** The OPT following placement of the extended TMJ prosthesis.
- **l** Patient after placement of the TMJ prosthesis.

4.2 Soft-tissue requirements

In scenarios with relatively small bone and large soft-tissue defects, especially if the soft tissues need to be oriented and inserted independently from the bone, bone and soft-tissue flap combinations from the scapular region have advantages over fibula and iliac bone flaps. These latter flaps provide only soft-tissue components in the immediate vicinity of the bone portion of the flaps.

4.3 Recipient vessels in the neck

Discussion of the presence of recipient vessels in the neck is usually not required in primary mandible reconstruction, but an important aspect not only for flap selection but even more for selection of the best suited donor side in secondary reconstruction. For planning secondary reconstructions in a vessel depleted neck after previous surgery and sometimes irradiation, preoperative CT or MRI angiogram is recommended.

Pedicle length and diameter are always excellent in scapula and radial forearm flaps. The same is true for fibula flaps, as long as the whole fibula is not needed either for long defects or double barrel construct. The vascular pedicle in iliac bone flaps is relatively short (usually 8–10 cm maximum) and tends to be more delicate, which is a point for consideration especially in secondary reconstruction.

4.4 Tissue quality in the recipient site

Tissue quality and quantity (scar formation, soft-tissue deficits, previous irradiation, chronic infection) are important for flap selection. In secondary reconstruction a tight soft-tissue envelope, as it is often the case after previous operations and irradiation, makes placement of a bulky flap, such as the iliac bone flap, more difficult. In such cases the fibula or scapula flap have advantages because of their reduced hard-tissue volume, although the volume of the neomandible will also be reduced. In addition, in those scenarios soft-tissue transplantation especially to replace deficient skin may become necessary because without it soft-tissue closure over a bone flap may not be possible.

4.5 Flap fixation aspects

Flap fixation planning immediately starts with flap selection and especially with donor site selection. During fibula harvest the lateral side of the fibula can be stripped from soft tissues, the same is true for the lateral aspect of the ileum. Fixation material should be placed on the bare bone and on the opposite side of the vascular pedicle, thus avoiding compression or other damage during osteotomies or during the drilling process for fixation holes. In contrast to the fibula and iliac bone flaps the lateral border of the scapula is harvested in a cuff of surrounding musculature, which should not be extensively stripped. Therefore, it is recommended to perform miniplate fixation for short scapular segment fixation, which can be done at the ends of the bone flap without major soft-tissue stripping. If osteotomies of the scapula need to be performed and a reconstruction plate is indicated to provide contour and stability, the surgeon must be careful not to pull the bone segments too tightly to the reconstruction plate and leave some space underneath the plate to accommodate the muscle. To achieve this, locking reconstruction plates are preferred. The sides for both fibula and iliac crest harvest should be chosen in a way that the lateral aspects of the flaps become the lateral (buccal) sides of the neomandible, thus allowing for placement of whatever osteosynthesis material a surgeon prefers to use (for planning aspects see chapter 5.3.12).

Fixation of free vascularized bone flaps to the native mandible can be done using either a single large titanium reconstruction plate or miniplates. Because of the transplantation of vital bone flaps the contact zones between residual mandible segments and bone flap(s), as well as the osteotomy gaps within the flap(s), resemble fracture gaps. Biomechanically they may be considered as load-sharing or load-bearing situations, depending on bone height (cross section) and the amount of bone-to-bone contact. Available variations of reconstruction plates include conventional reconstruction plates, prebent reconstruction plates, and patient-specific reconstruction plates.

When reconstruction plates are used, at least three bicortical screws should be inserted to the native mandible and plate on either side of the defect. When a conventional reconstruction plate is used, the plate should be shaped to the native mandible before segmental mandibulectomy and temporarily secured into place with bicortical screws on either side of the planned resection defect, if the pathology allows for it. The plate and screws are then removed and properly recorded for orientation purposes during the mandibulectomy. In situations where tumor bulk does not allow for contouring of the plate on the native mandible before resection, either mandibulomaxillary fixation (MMF) or an external fixation device can help to maintain position control of the nonresected part of the mandible [Wei et al, 2003]. Today virtual planning software as well as preplanned surgical guides exist to help to define the amount of resection and plan for an anatomically correct reconstruction (see chapter 5.3.12).

Once the plate has been properly contoured and oriented, it can be resterilized and passed to the donor site where attachment of the bone containing free flap to the plate can be performed while the flap is still connected to the vascular pedicle. This limits ischemic time and minimizes flap manipulation once the vascular anastomosis has been completed. Alternatively, adaptation of the bone to the plate can be completed on a back table under ischemic time following ligation of the flap's vascular pedicle.

Monocortical screws should be used to secure the bone flap to the plate since the placement of bicortical screws into a bone flap creates the risk of bone devascularization. Before anastomosis at the recipient site, the flap and plate unit can be secured into place onto the native mandible using the predrilled screw holes. This minimizes excessive motion of the flap during the microvascular anastomosis. Final placement of any remaining screws can be done once the vascular anastomosis has been completed.

For condylar reconstruction, attachment of either a condyle autograft or a costochondral graft to the proximal end of a free flap is done using a single titanium miniplate and screws. Ideally, at least four screws (two in each segment) should be used to secure the condyle graft to the bone flap. When preservation of the condyle in the TMJ complex is possible, attachment of a vascularized bone flap at the condylar neck to the undisrupted joint complex can be completed. This is believed to preserve postoperative TMJ function and prevent some of the complications associated with its reconstruction [Schmelzeisen et al, 2002]. When tumor resection requires removal of the native condyle from the TMJ, stabilization of the neocondyle (shaped free flap, condyle autograft, or costochondral graft) in the glenoid fossa can be accomplished with placement of either permanent suture or wire at the zygomatic arch [Carroll et al, 2000].

Once the vascular anastomosis and final screw placement have been completed, closure of the skin and soft tissue is undertaken. Skin edge closure should be tight for repair of intraoral defects. The skin paddle should never be placed under tension or over stretched. This could result in skin paddle ischemia and exert unnecessary inward pressure on the flap resulting in compromised perfusion. Appropriate drains should be used to prevent fluid accumulation around the flap, which may result in compression of the vascular pedicle.

5 Complications and technical errors

Complications associated with vascularized free tissue transfer for mandible reconstruction have diminished over the years. The perfection of surgical techniques including planning and development of modern osteosynthesis materials have obviously contributed greatly to this decrease. Success rates for free flap transfers in this setting have exceeded 95%. Unfortunately, complications still occur more often than desired. Reconstruction for tumor defects is different from mandible reconstruction after trauma. Patients with malignant tumors are often undernourished due to difficulty with oral feeding and a large percentage are long-standing drinkers and tobacco users. Long-term exposure to tobacco toxins and chronic malnourishment can, in turn, detrimentally affect wound healing and has a negative effect to both intermediate and terminal vessels. In addition, there is a need for adjuvant radiation therapy in a large percentage of these patients, which increases the potential for tissue break down and other postoperative complications.

Complications associated with bone flap transplantation can be subdivided into recipient and donor site complications. The most serious perioperative recipient site complication includes vascular compromise of the transferred flap, which may ultimately result in flap necrosis and flap loss. This can occur via arterial or more commonly venous insufficiency. Arterial compromise will lead to a pale, cold, and nonperfused (white) soft-tissue flap, as well as venous drainage problems, such as venous compression or thrombosis, in a congested (blue) flap (**Fig 2.6-13**).

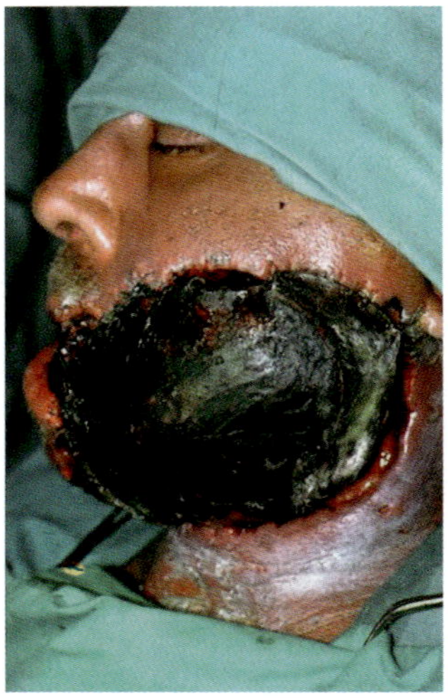

Fig 2.6-13 Complete necrosis of a combined scapula bone flap, parascapular and latissimus dorsi flap in a previously irradiated patient with tumor recurrence. Situation of multiple thrombectomies after recurrent venous thrombosis, before removal of the necrotic latissimus dorsi flap.

The bone portion of a flap and especially a buried bone-only flap is difficult to monitor. Small monitor skin island, which are later removed, are an option to monitor buried bone flaps. Flap loss needs a contingency plan, which for bone defects ideally is another bone flap but as a compromise may also be a bulky soft-tissue flap, such as a pectoralis major flap, often in combination with a bridging reconstruction plate.

To minimize iatrogenic contributions to vascular failure, the surgical team must be attentive to all details. Avoidance of placing intravenous lines in the region of the proposed free flap site will minimize undue trauma and irritation to the donor vessels. Intraoperatively, meticulous dissection and preparation of both the donor and recipient vessels, along with calculated suture placement under microscopic guidance, will reduce the risk of anastomotic site thrombosis. Direct communication with the anesthesia team is important throughout the case. Diligent patient fluid management, both in the operating room and postoperatively, will assist in maintaining optimal perfusion pressures for the flap. Alpha adrenergic pressers and other vasoconstrictive agents are to be avoided. Limitation of the patient's head and neck movements in the immediate postoperative period will help prevent pedicle kinking and undue mechanical stress on the anastomotic site. Routine use of systemic anticoagulants is not recommended; however, local irrigation at the anastomotic site is supported. It is recommended to establish an algorithm for flap monitoring, which is still largely based on clinical controls and judgement.

To minimize the potential for bone flap devascularization during surgery, several important points should be emphasized. First, the surgeon should try to limit the number of osteotomies performed. This is especially true when using the radius, scapula, and iliac crest bone flaps. Although the fibula bone has been reported as having the most robust blood supply, it too carries a risk of devascularization if shaping becomes over aggressive. Subperiosteal dissection of the bone should also be kept to a minimum.

The development of salivary fistulae always remains a possibility in oromandibular reconstruction. Takushima et al noted a 6% rate of major fistula formation in his series of 178 mandible reconstruction cases **[2001]**. More recently, Suh et al reported a 2.8% rate in their review of 400 free flap reconstructions of the head and neck region **[2004]**. Fistulae can arise from partial or total flap failure, infection, or tissue bed breakdown. Standard precautions, such as perioperative intravenous antibiotics and careful flap handling, as discussed above, are always used for these reconstructions. If an orocutaneous fistula develops, a treatment plan for its correction should be undertaken immediately. Management of most fistulae can usually be performed via conservative measures (non-oral alimentation, dressing changes, and antibiotics) and watchful waiting as long as vital structures, such as the carotid artery, are not in the path of the draining saliva. In certain situations, a pectoralis major or latissimus dorsi pedicled flap may be used to solve the problem. Although these flaps are more limited than a free flap due to a pedicle attachment, they are relatively easy to harvest and inset, and save the patient from a more extensive secondary free flap surgery. In situations where a pedicled flap may not reach properly or when there is substantial flap loss (including bone), a new vascularized free flap is the best choice. The choice of which flap to use will depend on the patient's existing comorbidities and the preference of the operating surgeon. Replacement of bone loss, however, can also be performed using a reconstruction plate covered by a soft-tissue free or pedicled flap, depending on the status and overall long-term prognosis of the patient.

Plate exposure is a potential complication of rigid fixation in microvascular bone reconstruction. Exposure in the early postoperative phase is usually due to breakdown and/or necrosis of overlying soft tissue. If the bone flap is viable, a reconstruction plate may be left initially uncovered. Secondary plate coverage with local or distant soft-tissue flaps may be considered. Late exposure after healing of the bone flap may happen in cases with thin and/or low-quality overlying tissues, for instance after radiation. In such a scenario, total or partial plate removal needs to be considered.

Donor site complications are always a possibility with free flap harvest and require adequate handling [Suh et al, 2004]. Delayed wound healing, mostly due to skin graft failure, has been reported as the most frequent type of donor site complication after fibula flap harvest (**Fig 2.6-14**).

Prevention is achieved by performing a meticulous dissection, careful closure, and maintaining a diligent postoperative wound care regimen. In cases in which the skin can only be closed under tension skin grafts are recommended (**Fig 2.6-15**).

The fibula and scapula osteocutaneous flaps both have relatively low incidences of disabling donor site complications. Cases of motor weakness of the great toe, ankle stiffness, and ankle instability have been reported in fibula flap patients [Takushima et al, 2001], however most return to full ambulation without major incident [Gabr et al, 2004]. The iliac crest flap has been associated with chronic pain, gait disturbance, and hernia formation. In rare cases ectopic bone formation may be seen (**Fig 2.6-16**).

At the time of donor site closure, we strongly recommend the placement of support sutures from the abdominal wall fascia to holes drilled directly into the remaining iliac crest to help give abdominal wall support and minimize the risk of postoperative hernia formation. In addition, a resorbable mesh may be used to support the abdominal wall. The radial forearm osteocutaneous flap was initially associated with a relatively high complication rate related to delayed fracture of the remaining radial bone [Villaret et al, 2003]. More recent studies, which involve placing a plate across the donor bone, have shown no evidence of delayed fracture in these patients [Guyot et al, 2004; Jones et al, 2003].

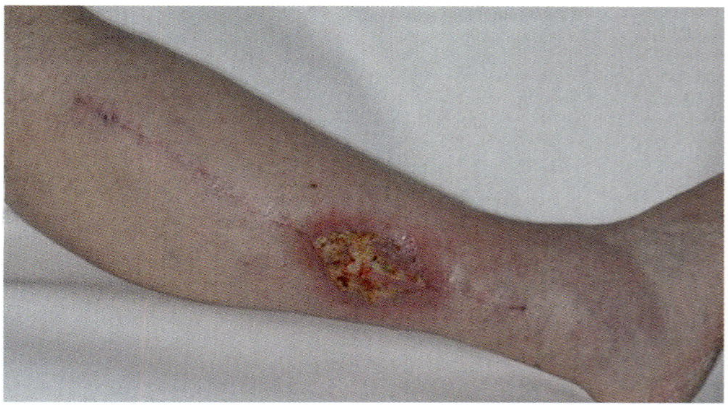

Fig 2.6-14 Secondary healing after fibula flap harvest with skin island.

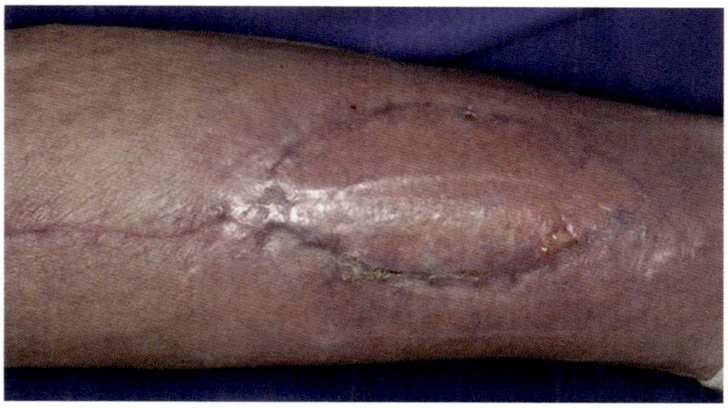

Fig 2.6-15 Fibula donor site after harvest of a skin island and primary closure with a thin full thickness skin graft.

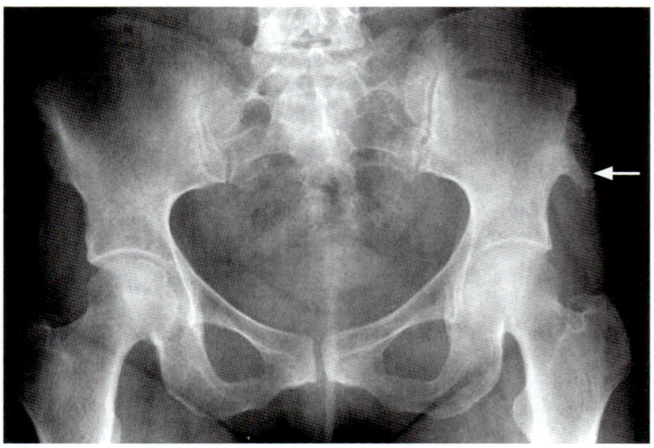

Fig 2.6-16 Ectopic bone formation after iliac bone flap harvest (arrow) on the left side.

6 Summary

The use of free vascularized bone for mandible reconstruction after tumor resection or major bone loss after trauma in combination with modern fixation systems, dental implants and more recently digital planning and CAD/CAM technology has revolutionized mandible reconstruction and has made many of the reconstructions truly functional. The currently available donor sites for reconstruction provide the surgeon with multiple treatment options. The fibula free flap today is the dominant flap for all areas of mandible reconstruction, but a reconstructive CMF surgeon should be able to offer at least fibula, iliac crest, and scapula flaps. The flaps have certain differential indications related to their characteristics, and it may be that the one or other flap harvest is not possible in a specific patient because of anatomical reasons. Patients' wishes also would need to be respected. Careful preoperative planning and execution of surgery are cornerstones to a successful outcome.

7 References and suggested reading

Blackwell KE, Buchbinder D, Urken ML. Lateral mandibular reconstruction using soft-tissue free flaps and plates. *Arch Otolaryngol Head Neck Surg*. 1996 Jun;122(6):672–678.

Blackwell KE, Lacombe V. The bridging lateral mandibular reconstruction plate revisited. *Arch Otolaryngol Head Neck Surg*. 1999 Sep;125(9):988–993.

Boyd JB. Use of reconstruction plates in conjunction with soft-tissue free flaps for oromandibular reconstruction. *Clin Plast Surg*. 1994 Jan;21(1):69–77.

Boyd JB. The place of the iliac crest in vascularized oromandibular reconstruction. *Microsurgery*. 1994;15(4):250–256.

Boyd JB, Gullane, PJ, Rotstein LE, et al. Classification of mandibular defects. *Plast Reconstr Surg*. 1993,92:1266–1275

Butler CE, Lewin JS. Reconstruction of large composite oromandibulomaxillary defects with free vertical rectus abdominis myocutaneous flaps. *Plast Reconstr Surg*. 2004 Feb;113(2):499–507.

Carroll CM, Pathak I, Irish J, et al. Reconstruction of total lower lip and chin defects using the composite radial forearm—palmaris longus tendon free flap. *Arch Facial Plast Surg*. 2000 Jan–Mar;2(1):53–56.

Chana JS, Chang YM, Wei FC, et al. Segmental mandibulectomy and immediate free fibula osteoseptocutaneous flap reconstruction with endosteal implants: an ideal treatment method for mandibular ameloblastoma. *Plast Reconstr Surg*. 2004 Jan;113(1):80–87.

Christie DRH, Duncan GM, Glasson DW. The ulnar artery free flap: the first 7 years. *Plast Reconstr Surg*. 1994;93:547–551.

Ciocca L, Mazzoni S, Fantini M, et al. CAD/CAM guided secondary mandibular reconstruction of a discontinuity defect after cancer ablative surgery. *J Craniomaxillofac Surg*. 2012 Dec;40(8):e511–515.

Cordeiro PG, Disa JJ, Hidalgo DA, et al. Reconstruction of the mandible with osseous free flaps: a 10-year experience with 150 consecutive patients. *Plast Reconstr Surg*. 1999 Oct;104(5):1314–1320.

Daniel E, Browne JD. Minimizing complications in the use of titanium condylar head reconstruction prostheses. *Otolaryngol Head Neck Surg*. 2004 Mar;130(3):344–350.

Deschler DG, Hayden RE. The optimum method for reconstruction of complex lateral oromandibular-cutaneous defects. *Head Neck*. 2000 Oct;22(7):674–679.

Disa JJ, Hidalgo DA, Cordeiro PG, et al. Evaluation of bone height in osseous free flap mandible reconstruction: an indirect measure of bone mass. *Plast Reconstr Surg*. 1999 Apr;103(5):1371–1377.

Disa JJ, Cordeiro PG. Mandible reconstruction with microvascular surgery. *Semin Surg Oncol*. 2000 Oct–Nov;19(3):226–234.

Foster RD, Anthony JP, Sharma A, et al. Vascularized bone flaps versus nonvascularized bone grafts for mandibular reconstruction: an outcome analysis of primary bony union and endosseous implant success. *Head Neck*. 1999 Jan;21(1):66–71.

Gabr E, Kobayashi MR, Salibian AH, et al. Mandibular reconstruction: are two flaps better than one? *Ann Plast Surg*. 2004 Jan;52(1):31–35.

Gabr EM, Kobayashi MR, Salibian AH, et al. Role of ulnar forearm free flap in oromandibular reconstruction. *Microsurgery*. 2004;24(4):285–288.

Gabr EM, Kobayashi MR, Salibian AH, et al. Oromandibular reconstruction with vascularized free flaps: a review of 50 cases. *Microsurgery*. 2004;24(5)374–377.

Guyot L, Richard O, Layoun W, et al. Long-term radiological findings following reconstruction of the condyle with fibular free flaps. *J Craniomaxillofac Surg*. 2004 Apr;32(2):98–102.

Head C, Alam D, Sercarz JA, et al. Microvascular flap reconstruction of the mandible: a comparison of bone grafts and bridging plates for restoration of mandibular continuity. *Otolaryngol Head Neck Surg*. 2003 Jul;129(1):48–54.

Hidalgo DA, Pusic AL. Free-flap mandibular reconstruction: a 10-year follow-up study. *Plast Reconstr Surg*. 2002 Aug;110(2):438–451.

Hidalgo DA, Disa JJ, Cordeiro PG, et al. A review of 716 consecutive free flaps for oncologic surgical defects: refinement in donor-site selection and technique. *Plast Reconstr Surg*. 1998 Sep;102(3):722–734.

Hidalgo DA. Fibula free flap: a new method of mandible reconstruction. *Plast Reconstr Surg*. 1989 Jul;84(1):71–79.

Hidalgo DA. Condyle transplantation in free flap mandible reconstruction. *Plast Reconstr Surg*. 1994 Apr;93(4):770–783.

Hidalgo DA, Rekow A. A review of 60 consecutive fibula free flap mandible reconstructions. *Plast Reconstr Surg*. 1995 Sep;96(3):585–602.

Jewer DD, Boyd JB, Manktelow, RT, et al. Orofacial and mandibular reconstruction with the iliac crest free flap: a review of 60 cases and a new method of classification. *Plast Reconstr Surg*. 1989,84:391–403; discussion 404–405.

Jones NF, Vogelin E, Markowitz BL, et al. Reconstruction of composite through-and-through mandibular defects with a double-skin paddle fibular osteocutaneous flap. *Plast Reconstr Surg*. 2003 Sep;112(3):758–765.

Kildal M, Wei FC, Chang YM, et al. Mandibular reconstruction with fibula osteoseptocutaneous free flap and osseointegrated dental implants. *Clin Plast Surg*. 2001 Apr;28(2):403–410.

King TW, Gallas MT, Robb GL, et al. Aesthetic and functional outcomes using osseous or soft-tissue free flaps. *J Reconstr Microsurg*. 2002 Jul;18(5):365–371.

Kroll SS, Robb GL, Miller MJ, et al. Reconstruction of posterior mandibular defects with soft tissue using the rectus abdominis free flap. *Br J Plast Surg*. 1998 Oct;51(7):503–507.

Kuzon WM, Jejurikar S, Wilkins EG, et al. Double free-flap reconstruction on massive defects involving the lip, chin and mandible. *Microsurgery*. 1998;18:372–378.

Lethaus B, Poort L, Bockmann R, et al. Additive manufacturing for microvascular reconstruction of the mandible in 20 patients. *J Craniomaxillofac Surg*. 2012;40:43–46.

Levine J, Patel A, Saadeh P, et al. Computer-aided design and manufacturing in craniomaxillofacial surgery: the new state of the art. *J Craniofac Surg*. 2012;23:288–293.

Lovie MJ, Duncan GM, Glasson DW. The ulnar artery forearm free flap. *Br J Surg*. 1984;37:486–492.

Mehta RP, Deschler DG. Mandibular reconstruction in 2004: an analysis of different techniques. *Curr Opin Otolaryngol Head Neck Surg*. 2004 Aug;12(4):288–293.

Nahabedian MY, Tufaro A, Manson PN. Improved mandible function after hemimandibulectomy, condylar head preservation, and vascularized fibular reconstruction. *Ann Plast Surg*. 2001 May;46(5):506–510.

Ozdemir R, Ortak T, Kocer U, et al. Total lower lip reconstruction using sensate composite radial forearm flap. *J Craniofac Surg*. 2003 May;14(3):393–405.

Patel A, Maisel R. Condylar prostheses in head and neck cancer reconstruction. *Arch Otolaryngol Head Neck Surg*. 2001 Jul;127(7):842–846.

Perrott DH, Umeda H, Kaban LB. Costochondral graft construction/reconstruction of the ramus/condyle unit: long-term follow-up. *Int J Oral Maxillofac Surg*. 1994 Dec;23(6 Pt 1):321–328.

Poli T, Ferrari S, Bianchi B, et al. Primary oromandibular reconstruction using free flaps and thorp plates in cancer patients: a 5-year experience. *Head Neck*. 2003 Jan;25(1):15–23.

Roser S, Ramachandra S, Blair H, et al. The accuracy of virtual surgical planning in free fibula mandibular reconstruction: comparison of planned and final results. *J Oral Maxillofac Surg*. 2010;68:2824–2832.

Schmelzeisen R, Neukam FW. Microvascular reconstruction of the condyle and the ascending ramus. In: Greenberg A, Prein J, eds. *Craniomaxillofacial Reconstructive and Corrective Bone Surgery*. New York: Springer; 2002:462–477.

Schultz BD, Sosin M, Nam A, et al. Classification of mandible defects and algorithm for microvascular reconstruction. *Plast Reconstr Surg*. 2015;135(4):743e–754e.

Schusterman MA, Reece GP, Kroll SS, et al. Use of the AO plate for immediate mandibular reconstruction in cancer patients. *Plast Reconstr Surg*. 1991 Oct;88(4):588–593.

Shpitzer T, Neligan PC, Gullane PJ, et al. Oromandibular reconstruction with the fibular free flap. Analysis of 50 consecutive flaps. *Arch Otolaryngol Head Neck Surg*. 1997 Sep;123(9):939–944.

Shpitzer T, Neligan PC, Gullane PJ, et al. The free iliac crest and fibula flaps in vascularized oromandibular reconstruction: comparison and long-term evaluation. *Head Neck*. 1999 Oct;21(7):639–647.

Shpitzer T, Gullane PJ, Neligan PC, et al. The free vascularized flap and the flap plate options: comparative results of reconstruction of lateral mandibular defects. *Laryngoscope*. 2000 Dec;110(12):2056–2060.

Suh JD, Sercarz JA, Abemayor E, et al. Analysis of outcome and complications in 400 cases of microvascular head and neck reconstructions. *Arch Otolaryngol Head Neck Surg*. 2004;130:962–966.

Takushima A, Harii K, Asato H, et al. Mandibular reconstruction using microvascular free flaps: a statistical analysis of 178 cases. *Plast Reconstr Surg*. 2001 Nov;108(6):1555–1563.

Thoma A, Khadaroo R, Grigenas O, et al. Oromandibular reconstruction with the radial-forearm osteocutaneous flap: experience with 60 consecutive cases. *Plast Reconstr Surg*. 1999 Aug;104(2):368–380.

Ung F, Rocco JW, Deschler DG. Temporary intraoperative external fixation in mandibular reconstruction. *Laryngoscope*. 2002 Sep;112(9):1569–1573.

Urken ML, Buchbinder D, Costantino PD, et al. Oromandibular reconstruction using microvascular composite flaps: report of 210 cases. *Arch Otolaryngol Head Neck Surg*. 1998 Jan;124(1):46–55.

Urken ML, Bridger AG, Zur KB, et al. The scapular osteofasciocutaneous flap: a 12-year experience. *Arch Otolaryngol Head Neck Surg*. 2001 Jul;127(7):862–869.

Urken ML, Weinberg H, Vickery C, et al. Oromandibular reconstruction using microvascular composite free flaps. *Arch Otolaryngol Head Neck Surg*. 1991;117:733–744.

Villaret DB, Futran NA. The indications and outcomes in the use of osteocutaneous radial forearm free flap. *Head Neck*. 2003 Jun;25(6):475–481.

Wei FC, Demirkan F, Chen HC, et al. Double free flaps in reconstruction of extensive composite mandibular defects in head and neck cancer. *Plast Reconstr Surg*. 1999 Jan;103(1):39–47.

Wei FC, Celik N, Yang WG, et al. Complications after reconstruction by plate and soft-tissue free flap in composite mandibular defects and secondary salvage reconstruction with osteocutaneous flap. *Plast Reconstr Surg*. 2003 Jul;112(1):37–42.

Zenn MR, Hidalgo DA, Cordeiro PG, et al. Current role of the radial forearm free flap in mandibular reconstruction. *Plast Reconstr Surg*. 1997 Apr;99(4):1012–1017.

Zhang C, Zhang Z. Reconstruction of mandible with fibular flap and dental implant distractor: a new approach. *Chinese Med J*. 2002;115(12):1877–1880.

Zheng G, Su Y, Liao G, et al. Mandible reconstruction assisted by preoperative virtual surgical simulation. *Oral Surg Oral Med Oral Pathol Oral Radiol*. 2012;113:604–611.

2.7 Reconstruction with prefabricated flaps

Dennis Rohner, Raquel Guijarro-Martínez, Peter Bucher, Beat Hammer

1 Introduction

Reconstruction of moderate to large craniomaxillofacial defects after tumor resection, trauma, or atrophy is a complex task which requires the replacement of hard and soft tissues as well as the reestablishment of normal function and esthetics. All dimensions and stages of composite craniomaxillofacial reconstruction require precision and excellent multidisciplinary coordination to achieve an optimal anatomical and functional result.

Selection of the ideal tissue transplant(s) depends on the patient's specific hard- and soft-tissue requirements, dental condition of the unresected jaw(s), and condition of the potential donor sites. Small (< 4–6 cm) osseous defects may be reconstructed with nonvascularized bone grafts if there is well-vascularized surrounding soft tissues and appropriate closure can be achieved. Larger or composite defects are best reconstructed with compound vascularized flaps. In the latter cases, where substantial bone deficiency is present, the fibula, scapula, and iliac crest are currently the preferred donor sites. If implant placement and anchorage is required, the fibula and the iliac crest are the most suitable options. The fibula flap is preferred by many surgeons due to its ease of harvest and its versatility.

2 Considerations associated with fibula flap transplantation

2.1 Primary inadequacy of the skin paddle

Intraorally, the skin paddle used in association with the fibular bone in osteoseptocutaneous flaps is often too thick and prone to periimplant inflammation in combination with dental implants. Consequently, flap shaping and debulking, vestibuloplasty, and further soft-tissue grafting procedures are necessary before an adequate implant-borne prosthetic rehabilitation can be installed. This delays the final restoration at an average of 6 months, during which the patient is often functionally and esthetically impaired.

2.2 Limited height of the barrel

Anatomically, although the length of the fibula is usually sufficient to reconstruct most defects in the craniomaxillofacial region, the height of the barrel is limited to approximately 14 mm. To achieve sufficient height to reconstruct a resected mandible, the double-barrel fibula flap may be used.

2.3 Difficulty in performing multiple osteotomies

The definition of the configuration and number of osteotomies on the donor bone that will give the reconstruction its appropriate shape is often a demanding and time-consuming step. This disadvantage is a common drawback in comparison with other flaps as well. Ideally, surgical planning should include the detailed design of the number, shape, and position of the osteotomized donor bone segments.

2.4 Accuracy of the reconstructive process

The key to optimal reconstructive surgery is meticulous planning of the combined surgical and prosthetic stages of the reconstruction. Traditional techniques often lead to suboptimal reconstructions due to inexact planning, poor communication between the resective and reconstructive teams, or surgical difficulties in adjusting a free flap and osteosynthesis plates into a 3-D defect without the help of any templates or surgical guides. However, the incorporation of CAD/CAM technologies has enabled the refinement of surgical and prosthodontic strategies in the context of a multidisciplinary team comprised of the craniomaxillofacial technician, the prosthodontist, and the surgeon. Novel technologies enable meticulous planning of the surgical and prosthetic phases and permit an effective transfer of the preoperative plan to the operating room. This becomes important in complex reconstructions, particularly in the context of the prefabrication technique for the restoration of maxillary and mandibular defects.

3 Dental implants in maxillofacial reconstruction

The patient's quality of life is likely to improve after the insertion of dental implants into the transplanted bone and subsequent prosthodontic rehabilitation. In general, dental implants are inserted after a healing period into the grafted bone and after radiotherapy if administered. If the reconstruction is performed without an interdisciplinary discussion of the prosthetic plan, the transplanted bone may simply be used to bridge the defect but may not be in a position to allow for functional implant-supported prosthodontic rehabilitation. Pretreatment interdisciplinary discussion and the inclusion of prosthodontic concepts in preoperative planning are mandatory for adequate functional implant position and prosthodontic rehabilitation.

3.1 Concept of prefabrication (backward planning)

Craniomaxillofacial reconstruction with prefabricated flaps entails a dramatic conceptual change in the conventional treatment workflow. Starting point is the desired final occlusion and the desired functional-esthetic outcome. Based on this goal, which is patient specific, the entire step-by-step reconstruction is designed and "prefabricated" [Rohner et al, 2013]. This workflow is called "backward planning." Backward planning ensures correct placement of dental implants and accurate positioning of a flap.

The prefabrication treatment algorithm involves two technical and two surgical steps. The first surgical step is the "flap prefabrication" stage. The selected donor site, most often the fibula, is approached. Dental implants are inserted and a split-thickness skin graft is adapted around them to attain a stable and thin epithelial soft-tissue layer. This thin epithelial layer is essential for successful implant integration and stable long-term periimplant conditions. After a healing period of 6–8 weeks to allow for implant osseointegration and for stable revascularization and integration of the epithelial layer, the second surgical step follows to harvest the flap, osteotomize the bone as necessary (using surgical guides and templates) for its adjustment with a prepared prosthesis, and transfer of the flap-prosthesis complex to the defect. The patient regains full function and esthetics within 6–10 weeks.

4 Patient selection

The indication of a staged prefabrication-reconstruction procedure implies careful case selection. Two types of variables (defect specific and patient specific) must be considered.

4.1 Defect-specific variables

4.1.1 Cause of the defect

Regarding the cause that initiated the defect requiring reconstruction, an important distinction must be made between patients with head and neck cancer versus other pathologies.

Noncancer patients: In general, the prefabrication technique is indicated in patients with preexisting maxillary or mandibular defects, severe atrophy, benign bone tumors, osteoradionecrosis or chronic osteomyelitis; in other words, conditions that allow for a staged approach.

Cancer patients: The prefabrication technique is usually not recommended in patients with malignant tumors of the head and neck. The need to urgently perform primary tumor resection and therapeutic or prophylactic neck dissection does not allow for a staged approach. However, cases of secondary reconstruction, after primary cancer surgery with curative intention (accompanied or not by adjuvant therapy) and if the patient is disease-free, are excellent candidates for prefabrication. In the case of maxillary cancer, the defect can temporarily be closed with an obturator during the period between primary resection and reconstruction.

4.1.2 Size of the defect

As with every microvascular free flap transfer, the particular dimensions of the craniomaxillofacial defect to be reconstructed are crucial for the planning of the ideal reconstructive strategy. The size of the defect must be at least 2 cm because vascularization of small microvascular bone flaps below this size is not predictable. Bone defects may be treated with free bone grafts, provided that the peripheral soft tissue is sufficient in quantity and quality (ie, well vascularized), or adequate soft tissue is transferred to the defect by means of local, rotational, or free microvascular flaps. For long-spanning bone and composite bone and soft-tissue defects, microvascular bone and soft-tissue transplantation is state-of-the-art.

4.2 Recipient vessels

In patients who have had a previous neck dissection as part of their treatment, the status of the residual blood vessels in the recipient site must be specifically evaluated with appropriate imaging techniques. The length of the potential flap pedicle must be long enough to reach the recipient vessels, preferably without the need for intermediate vessel grafts.

4.3 Patient-specific variables

Age

In general, chronological age itself should not be considered as an absolute contraindication for microvascular reconstruction. Rather, the specific health status and underlying diseases of the patient are determining factors for the selection of a reconstructive plan.

Vascular anomalies and other comorbidities

Peripheral vascular disease with complete or incomplete occlusion of blood vessels in the donor site is considered a contraindication to microvascular flap transfer. In the case of the fibula flap, the status of the peroneal vessels should be specifically assessed (eg, angiography, digital subtraction angiography, Gadolinium magnetic angioresonance), especially in cases with abnormal pedal pulses or a significant history of leg trauma or surgery. Patients with a hypoplastic anterior tibial artery (with blood supply to the foot derived primarily from the peroneal artery via a perforating branch) must also be excluded for a fibula flap.

Other medical contraindications include any underlying conditions that preclude an extended operative procedure or result in a hypercoagulable state that cannot be medically controlled. Relative contraindications include any disorders that have a potential impact on the patient's coagulation or healing capacity (eg, severe obesity, connective tissue disorders, venous insufficiency, and uncontrolled diabetes mellitus).

5 Workflow

The original technique of prefabrication is demonstrated using stereolithographic models in combination with dental casts. A case of maxillary reconstruction with a prefabricated fibula flap will be used to illustrate in detail each step of the workflow of the backward planning.

5.1 Technical stage one: prosthodontic and surgical planning

The starting point of prosthodontic planning is the desired end occlusion. In partially dentate patients, the ideal outcome is an implant-supported fixed partial denture. Hence, the starting point is the position of the future restored dentition in proper engagement with the opposing remaining dentition. Edentulous patients may be provided with either a fixed prosthesis if sufficient implants are available, or with an implant-supported or implant-assisted overlay denture.

Impressions are taken with a trial denture. Models are fabricated and transferred to a semiadjustable articulator. The model studies are compared with the clinical situation and in addition speech and esthetic parameters are recorded. According to these, the desired position of the restored teeth is established with respect to the residual dentition. At this point, the trial denture is duplicated and processed in resin, including strategically inserted radiopaque markings.

Subsequently, 3-D polyamide stereolithographic models of the donor fibula and the skull are fabricated with the help of rapid prototyping technology. To this effect, high-resolution computed tomographic (CT) scans of the lower limbs and the skull are obtained. In the latter, the patient is scanned with the trial denture in occlusion, and later an additional scan of the prosthesis alone is obtained. In partially dentate patients, a thin splint of radiotransparent material is fabricated to slightly increase the patient's vertical dimension and hence obtain a clear record of the dental contours. This allows the precise superimposition of the scanned portion of the prosthesis within the defect due to the radiopaque markings.

The planned defect shows in the skull model. The desired occlusion is then transferred to the skull model. In partially dentate patients, an occlusal key is highly recommendable and will be advantageous for graft positioning in the final surgical step (**Fig 2.7-1**). The base of the trial prosthesis is reduced to leave enough space for the new alveolar ridge to be reconstructed with the fibular bone. Based on the desired occlusion, the ideal number of implants and the location of the fibular osteotomy(ies) are marked.

In the 3-D model of the donor fibula, the outline of the fibular vessels is represented, for instance, by a red string. Pencil markings are made throughout the length of the bone on its posterior aspect. These markings are subsequently carved with a round burr. A plaster cast is fabricated to monitor the fibular position. Former carvings are etched in the plaster model, thereby maintaining the fibula in the exact same position on the plaster cast. Extra ink markings are drawn on the lateral aspect of the bone and continued on the plaster cast (**Fig 2.7-2**). Hence, two marking systems are used to serve as a double check.

Subsequently, the surgeon designs the number and configuration of the fibular osteotomies and their position in relation to the defect and the fibular vessels (**Fig 2.7-3**).

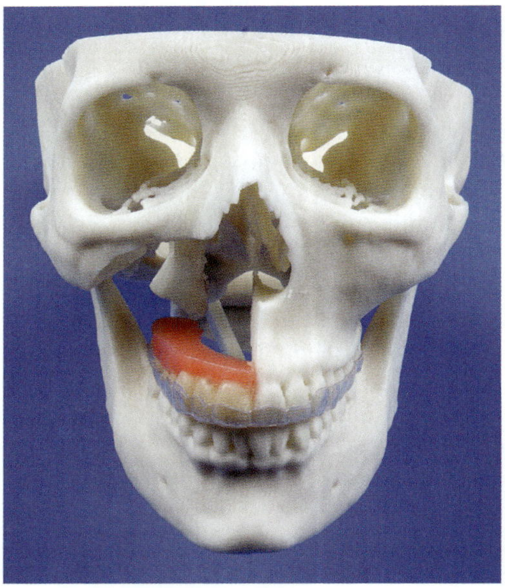

Fig 2.7-1 Trial partial denture setup mounted on the stereolithographic model.

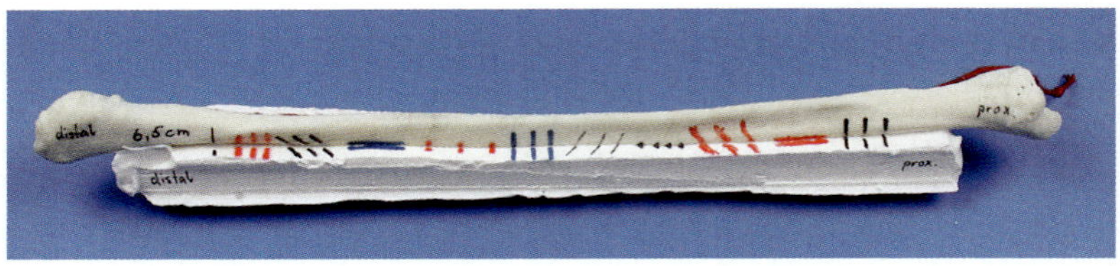

Fig 2.7-2 A plaster cast is fabricated to keep exact control of fibular position. Former carvings are positivized in the plaster model, thereby maintaining the fibula in the exact same position on the plaster cast. Extra ink markings are drawn on the lateral aspect of the bone and continued on the plaster cast. Hence, two marking systems are used to serve as a double check.

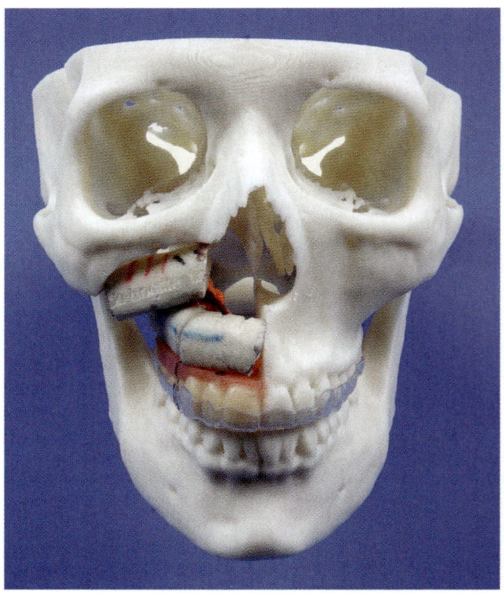

Fig 2.7-3 Planned reconstruction with a 3-segment fibular graft.

After an impression of the whole reconstruction is taken with silicone putty, the occlusal splint together with the denture teeth and planned dentition-bearing bone segments are removed from the skull. A duplication of the fibular bone-dentition construct is fabricated. The construct formed by the splint, the desired dentition, and the dentition-bearing fibular segments is mounted on a plaster cast (**Fig 2.7-4**). This plaster model represents the residual dentition with the stereolithographic fibular segments that will be used to restore the alveolar ridge. Following placement of the drill markings on the occlusal splint, the preplanned implant position is transferred to the fibular bone (**Fig 2.7-5**). The dentition-bearing fibular segments are easily remounted on the fibula plaster shell due to the markings on the bone and cast (**Fig 2.7-6**). The technician then fabricates a surgical template to guide implant placement in the first surgical procedure (defining implant position and angulation) and osteotomy performance in the second surgical step (defining the number, position, and angulation of the fibular osteotomies) (**Fig 2.7-7**) [Rohner et al, 2013].

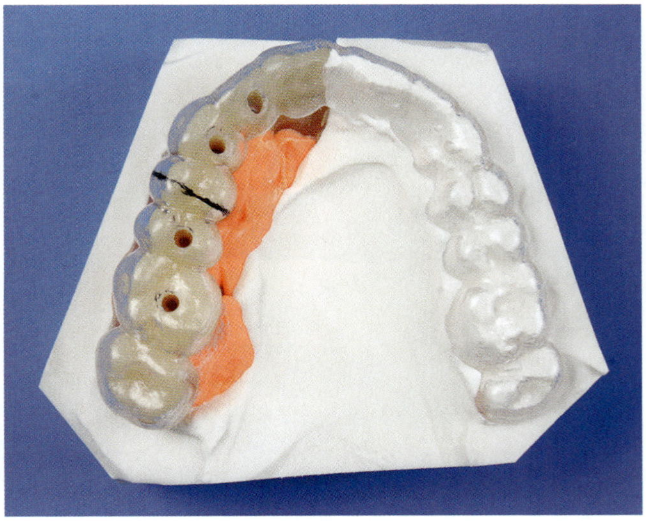

Fig 2.7-4 The construct formed by the splint, the desired dentition, and the dentition-bearing fibular segments is mounted on a plaster cast. The fibular segments are kept in place with the help of silicone material.

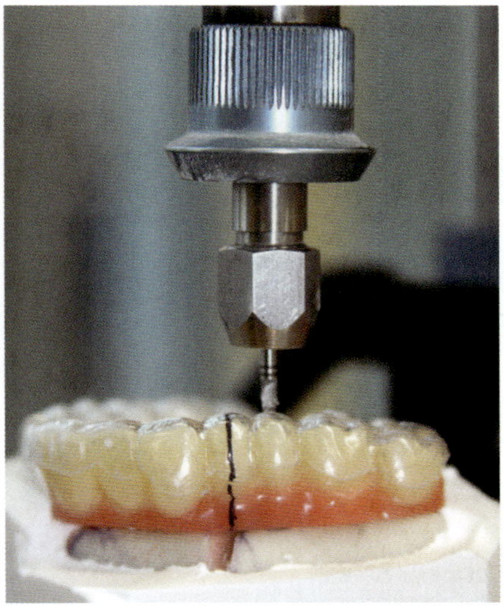

Fig 2.7-5 Transfer of the preplanned implant position to the fibular bone segments following the drill markings.

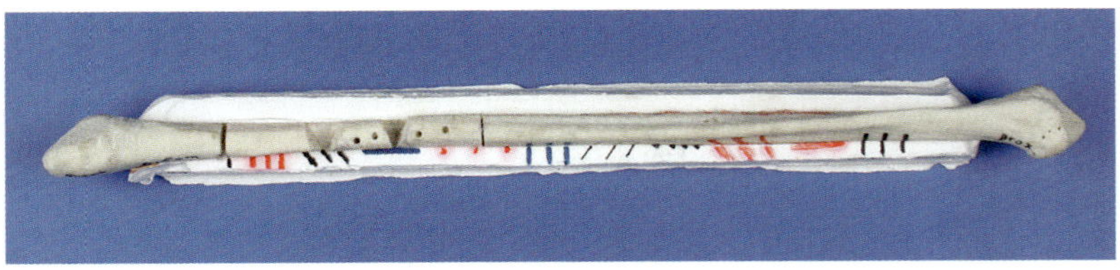

Fig 2.7-6 The dentition-bearing fibular segments are easily remounted on the fibula plaster shell because of the markings on the bone and cast.

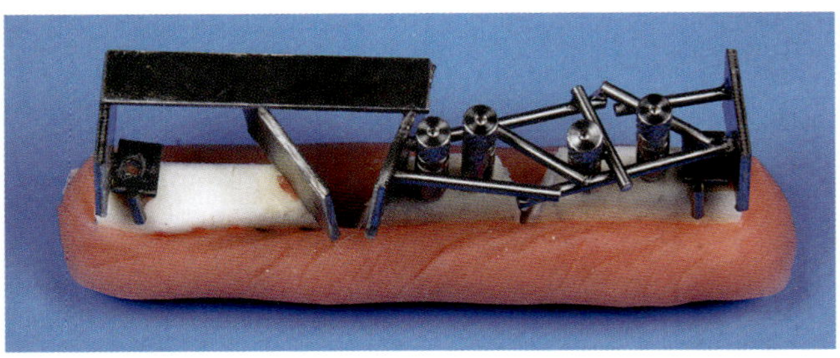

Fig 2.7-7 Fabrication of surgical template to guide implant placement (first surgical step) and osteotomy performance (second surgical step).

5.2 Surgical stage one: flap prefabrication

The lateral aspect of the selected donor fibula is exposed through a standard approach. Particular attention is paid to preservation of the periosteum. The surgical template fabricated in technical stage one is mounted on the fibular bone in the exact preplanned position and fixed to it with the help of miniscrews (**Fig 2.7-8**). Implant sites are prepared according to the drill guides of the template. After removal of the template, the planned implants are inserted. Sterile pickup impression copings are connected, and an impression is taken with silicone material. During this procedure, the bone and implants are protected with a sterile rubber dam. Subsequently, the polymerized impression together with the copings and rubber dam are removed and implants are sealed with healing screws.

Subsequently, a 0.5 mm split-thickness skin graft is harvested, for example, from the anterior thigh. The graft is adapted over the fibular segment containing the implants, which adequately emerge above previously prepared holes (**Fig 2.7-9**). Resorbable 4/0 polyglactin sutures are used to fix the skin graft in place, and the whole fibular segment is covered with an expanded polytetrafluoroethylene membrane (**Fig 2.7-10**), which is safely secured and fixed with miniscrews.

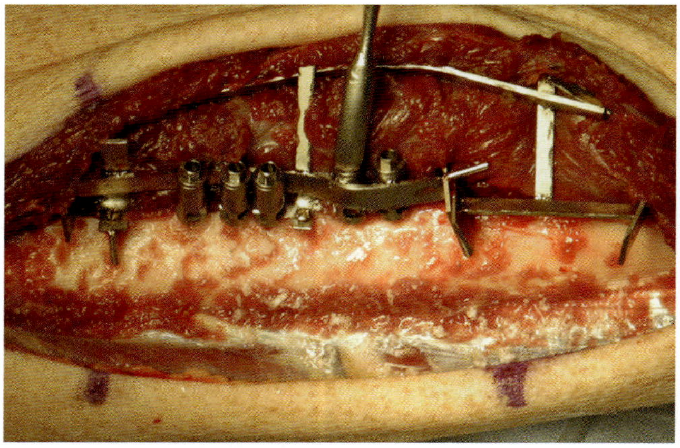

Fig 2.7-8 Surgical template mounted on the planned fibular region and secured in place with four miniscrews.

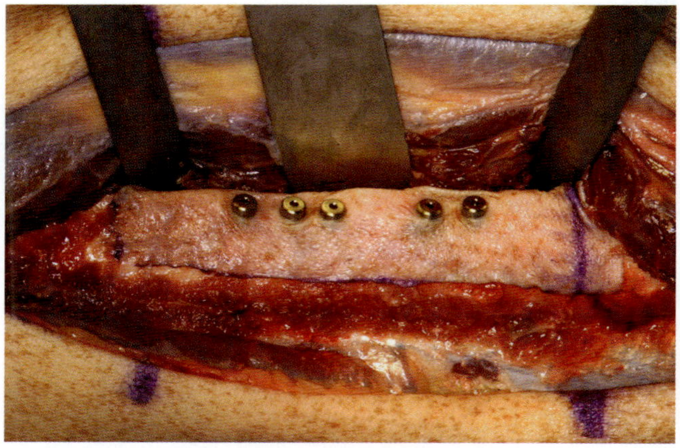

Fig 2.7-9 Split-thickness skin graft placed over the lateral aspect of the fibula containing the implants. Adequate emergence of the caps is achieved by perforating the graft with a rubber dam plier.

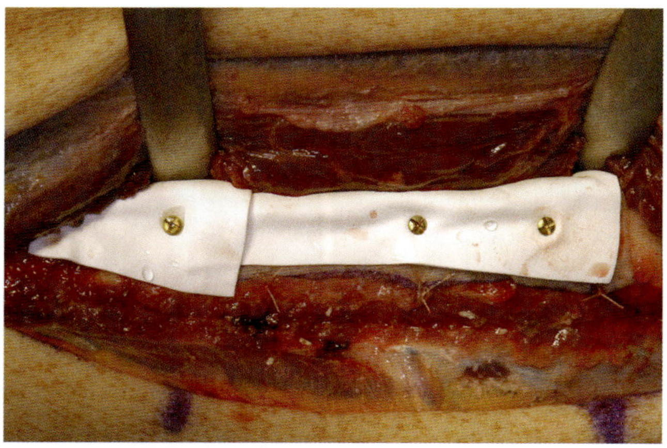

Fig 2.7-10 The whole fibular segment is covered by a polytetrafluoroethylene membrane that is secured in place with the help of three screws.

5.3 Technical stage two: fabrication of the prosthesis

Implant fixture analogs are connected to the copings and a master cast is fabricated (**Fig 2.7-11**). The previously fabricated surgical template is secured to the cast via the implants. Subsequently, the cast is "osteotomized" along the vertical shields of the template just as if it was the fibular bone. The segments are then bent to the planned position to reproduce the contour of the maxilla. A plaster mastercast is obtained from this. The previously prepared prosthesis is then connected to the implant analogs (**Fig 2.7-12**) and a fixed partial denture is fabricated (**Fig 2.7-13**). This new prosthesis is installed on the fibula model and the construct can then be transferred to the defect of the stereolithographic model of the skull in proper occlusion. The surgeon is then able to plan graft fixation to the residual bone and to prebend the fixation plates (**Fig 2.7-14**).

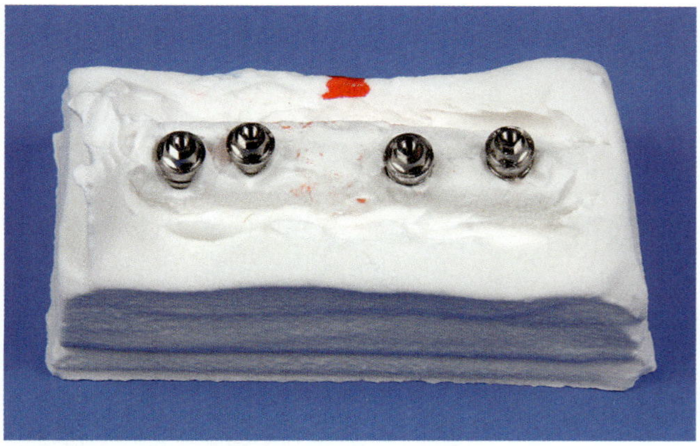

Fig 2.7-11 Plaster cast model fabricated using the impression taken during surgical stage one. Impression copings have been removed. In this case, the impression has been taken on multi-unit level.

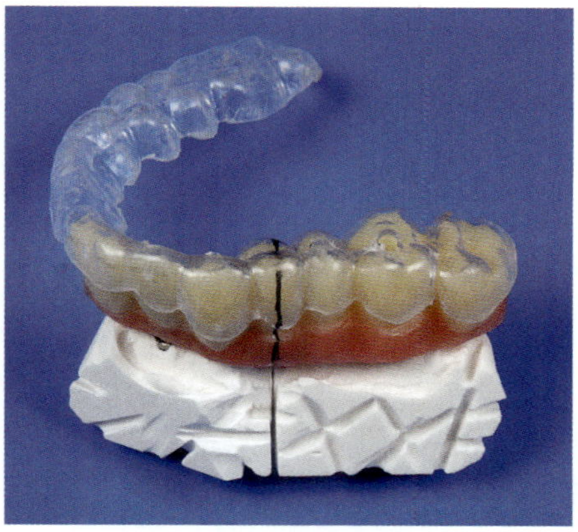

Fig 2.7-12 Plaster cast model separated in two segments according to the plane determined by the surgeon. The two segments are repositioned into the occlusal splint.

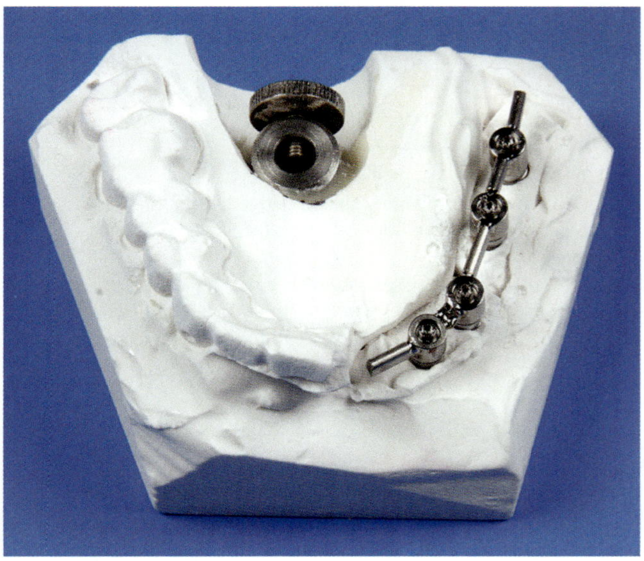

Fig 2.7-13 Using a mini-parallelometer, the segments of the bar construction are placed and fixed in between the bar abutments using the laser welding technique.

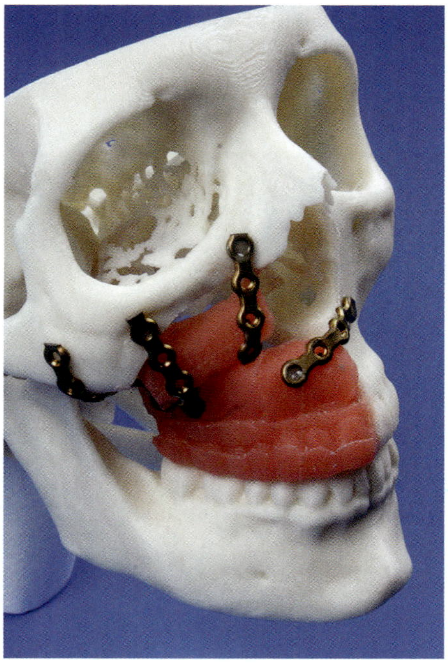

Fig 2.7-14 Plate positioning and prebending on the skull model.

5.4 Surgical stage two: final reconstruction

The fibula is reexposed 6–8 weeks after flap prefabrication. Removal of the barrier membrane reveals a newly formed epithelial lining around the implants and along the lateral sides of the fibula, in other words, along the future alveolar ridge. The healing screws secured to the implants are removed and the fibula is osteotomized distally and proximally. After clipping and releasing the vessels distally, the graft is dissected from distal to proximal. Before proximal vessel release, the surgical template is repositioned on the implants (**Fig 2.7-15**) and the fibula is osteotomized as indicated by the vertical shields [Rohner et al, 2013]. Proper configuration of the bone segments according to the preplanned contour is achieved by mounting the provisional prosthesis onto the bone (**Fig 2.7-16**). The vessels are then clipped proximally and the prosthesis-fibula-muscle-vessel construct is transferred to the recipient site and positioned according to the occlusion dictated by the opposing dentition (**Fig 2.7-17**). Mandibulomaxillary fixation allows for the stabilization of the construct in this position while the prebent plates are used to fix the construct to the adjacent bone. Microvascular anastomoses are then performed.

Six months after the reconstructive procedure, the definitive acrylic prosthesis with a titanium scaffold is fabricated and installed with no need for further preprosthetic soft-tissue procedures.

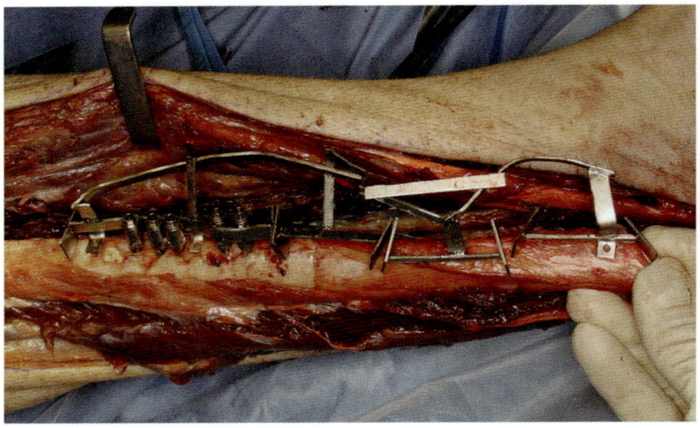

Fig 2.7-15 Repositioning of the surgical guide on the fibula before proximal vessel release.

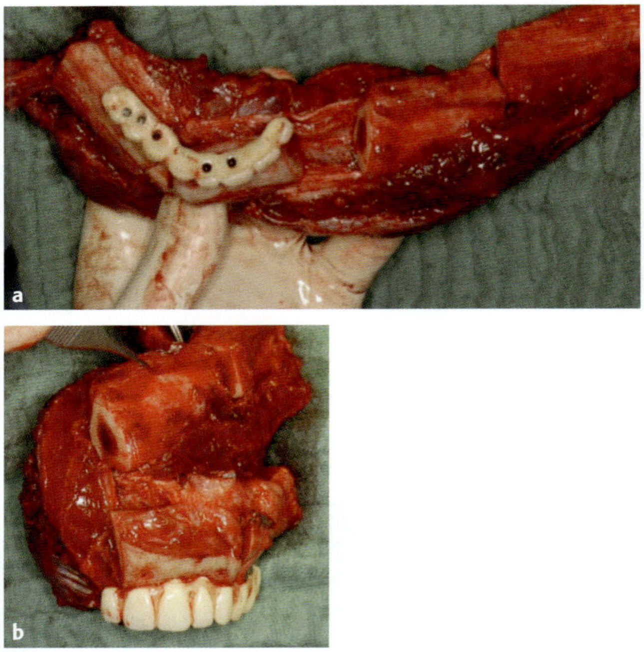

Fig 2.7-16a–b
a Confirmation of the new alveolar ridge by mounting the prosthesis onto the bone while graft vascularity is still maintained.
b After proximal vessel release, the construct is bent to its final configuration and transferred to the defect, where it will be placed according to the occlusion of the opposing dentition.

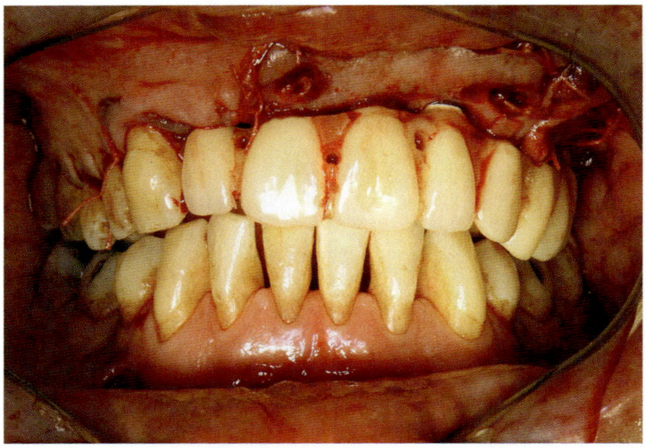

Fig 2.7-17 Flap positioning according to the desired final occlusion.

6 Additional remarks about maxillary defects

When a prefabrication approach is planned in extended maxillary defects, an important distinction must be made between the palate and the alveolar ridge. While the deficient alveolar ridge contour must be reconstructed with fibular bone to allow for adequate implant support, there is no need for a bony reconstruction of the hard palate. The latter, together with the soft palate, may be efficiently restored using an adequate muscle cuff attached to the fibula bone flap. As it happens with the temporalis muscle flap for the closure of oroantral and oronasal fistulae, the muscle cuff will initially develop hypergranulation and then metaplastic epithelization.

The reconstruction of a maxillary defect often requires a long pedicle running along the ascending ramus of the mandible toward the neck. In rare cases, ossification of the pedicle may occur. This calcification process of the vessels is most probably due to the presence of osteoconductive and/or osteoinductive cells around the vessels. These cells "follow" the course of the pedicle supported by the anterograde flow impulse within the pedicle vessels. Ossification of the vascular pedicle may lead to an increasing limitation in the mandible's range of motion, which can require surgical dissection and removal of the calcifications. Therefore, if possible, the use of the temporal vessels as recipient vessels is advantageous.

7 Success and complication rates: authors' statistics

From December 1999 until January 2019, a total of 71 flaps have been transferred following the prefabrication concept shown here. An overview of our personal experience during the last 20 years is summarized in the following chart:

Reconstructed region		**Maxilla**	**Mandible**	**Total**	
				No.	**%**
Microvascularized flap used	Fibula	33	35	68	95.8
	Iliac crest	1	1	2	2.8
	Scapula	0	1	1	1.4
Flap failure	Segmental	2	2	4	5.6
	Total	2	1	3	4.2
Vascular pedicle ossification		3	0	3	4.2
No. of implants placed		137	131	277	-
Implant failure	Early	10	5	15	5.4
	Delayed	11	8	19	6.9

Hence, the following conclusions can be drawn:

- The fibula represents our gold standard as prefabricated flap for the reconstruction of complex maxillofacial defects. This flap was used in 95.8% of our cases.
- Flap survival rate was 90.2% (total and segmental failure). Implant survival rate was 87.7%.
- Segmental flap failure occurred in 5.6% of the cases. Possible related variables were flap over segmentation in two cases, vascular disruption in one and comorbidity with diabetes mellitus in another.
- Total flap failure occurred in 4.2% of the cases and was due to arterial thrombosis in one case and spasm in two. These total failures required another microvascularized flap or an alternative reconstructive method.
- Vascular pedicle ossification occurred in three cases of maxillary reconstruction. These led to limited mandibular mobility and were managed with surgical release of the vessels from the calcified tissue.

8 Advantages of prefabrication

Compared with conventional maxillofacial reconstruction with microvascular bone flaps, prefabrication has the following advantages:

- The starting point of preoperative planning is always the desired position of the restored dentition in adequate occlusion to the opposing healthy dentition or bone (backward planning). This ensures an optimal position of the flap that enables functional and prosthodontically desired implant placement.
- The future gingiva (epithelial layer) is prefabricated and thus incorporated into the flap. This mucosal lining is suitable for successful implant integration under stable long-term periimplant conditions and saves the patient from secondary multistage soft-tissue procedures before prosthodontic rehabilitation.
- Operating room time, ischemia time, and handling trauma to the flap are reduced. This is due to several factors. First, the position and design of the osteotomies are planned and transferred to a surgical guide that will aid the surgeon intraoperatively. Second, plates are prebent according to the stereolithographic simulation to further facilitate and speed up accurate graft fixation. Third, the need for additional hard- or soft-tissue augmentation procedures may be predicted using the 3-D model and hence can be planned. Specifically, leaving no need for intraoperative improvisation.

9 Virtual planning

Currently, the workflow described entails the fabrication of solid models and is dependent on a close collaboration with a dental laboratory and dental technician.

The incorporation of CAD/CAM technology and rapid prototyping to the field of complex craniomaxillofacial reconstruction allows a thorough evaluation of the 3-D complexity of a defect, assists in the design of an accurate anatomical reconstruction plan, and enables optimal prosthodontic rehabilitation. Virtual planning is used in dental implant surgery and is becoming more and more common in reconstructive surgery. There are several software packages available on the market that allow for virtual planning in craniomaxillofacial reconstruction including osteotomies of bone flaps, fabrication of drilling and cutting guides, and even creation of patient-specific implants. On the other hand, virtual planning tools are available for dental implant placement using drilling guides. Commercially available products are being developed to manage this problem (see chapter 5.3.12)

10 References and suggested reading

Bähr W, Stoll P, Wächter R. Use of the "double barrel" free vascularized fibula in mandibular reconstruction. *J Oral Maxillofac Surg*. 1998 Jan;56(1):38–44.

Beumer J, Marunick MT, Garrett N, et al. Rehabilitation of maxillary defects. In: Beumer J, Marunick MT, Esposito SJ, eds. *Maxillofacial Rehabilitation: Prosthodontic and Surgical Management of Cancer-Related, Acquired, and Congenital Defects of the Head and Neck*. 3rd ed. Illinois: Quintessence; 2011:155–212.

Chang YM, Santamaria E, Wei FC, et al. Primary insertion of osseointegrated dental implants into fibula osteoseptocutaneous free flap for mandible reconstruction. *Plast Reconstr Surg*. 1998 Sep;102(3):680–688.

Chang YM, Chan CP, Shen YF, et al. Soft tissue management using palatal mucosa around endosteal implants in vascularized composite grafts in the mandible. *Int J Oral Maxillofac Surg*. 1999 Oct;28(5):341–343.

Chiapasco M, Biglioli F, Autelitano L, et al. Clinical outcome of dental implants placed in fibula-free flaps used for the reconstruction of maxillo-mandibular defects following ablation for tumors or osteoradionecrosis. *Clin Oral Implants Res*. 2006 Apr;17(2):220–228.

Chiapasco M, Brusati R, Galioto S. Distraction osteogenesis of a fibular revascularized flap for improvement of oral implant positioning in a tumor patient: a case report. *J Oral Maxillofac Surg*. 2000 Dec;58(12):1434–1440.

Cordeiro PG, Disa JJ, Hidalgo DA, et al. Reconstruction of the mandible with osseous free flaps: a 10-year experience with 150 consecutive patients. *Plast Reconstr Surg*. 1999 Oct;104(5):1314–1320.

David DJ, Tan E, Katsaros J, et al. Mandibular reconstruction with vascularized iliac crest: a 10-year experience. *Plast Reconstr Surg*. 1988 Nov;82(5):792–803.

Eckardt A, Swennen GR. Virtual planning of composite mandibular reconstruction with free fibula bone graft. *J Craniofac Surg*. 2005 Nov;16(6):1137–1140.

Forrest C, Boyd B, Manktelow R, et al. The free vascularised iliac crest tissue transfer: donor site complications associated with eighty-two cases. *Br J Plast Surg*. 1992 Feb-Mar;45(2):89–93.

Hidalgo DA. Fibula free flap: a new method of mandible reconstruction. *Plast Reconstr Surg*. 1989 Jul;84(1):71–79.

Hidalgo DA, Rekow A. A review of 60 consecutive fibula free flap mandible reconstructions. *Plast Reconstr Surg*. 1995 Sep;96(3):585–596; discussion 597–602.

Hirsch DL, Garfein ES, Christensen AM, et al. Use of computer-aided design and computer-aided manufacturing to produce orthognathically ideal surgical outcomes: a paradigm shift in head and neck reconstruction. *J Oral Maxillofac Surg*. 2009 Oct;67(10):2115–2122.

Jaquiéry C, Rohner D, Kunz C, et al. Reconstruction of maxillary and mandibular defects using prefabricated microvascular fibular grafts and osseointegrated dental implants—a prospective study. *Clin Oral Implants Res*. 2004 Oct;15(5):598–606.

Nakayama B, Matsuura H, Hasegawa Y, et al. New reconstruction for total maxillectomy defect with a fibula osteocutaneous free flap. *Br J Plast Surg*. 1994 Jun;47(4):247–249.

Pogrel MA, Podlesh S, Anthony JP, et al. A comparison of vascularized and nonvascularized bone grafts for reconstruction of mandibular continuity defects. *J Oral Maxillofac Surg*. 1997 Nov;55(11):1200–1206.

Reychler H, Iriarte Ortabe J. Mandibular reconstruction with the free fibula osteocutaneous flap. *Int J Oral Maxillofac Surg*. 1994 Aug;23(4):209–213.

Rohner D, Jaquiery C, Kunz C, et al. Maxillofacial reconstruction with prefabricated osseous free flaps: a 3-year experience with 24 patients. *Plast Reconstr Surg*. 2003 Sep;112(3):748–757.

Rohner D, Kunz C, Bucher P, et al. [New possibilities for reconstructing extensive jaw defects with prefabricated microvascular fibula transplants and ITI implants]. *Mund Kiefer Gesichtschir*. 2000 Nov;4(6):365–372. German.

Rohner D, Bucher P, Kunz C, et al. Treatment of severe atrophy of the maxilla with the prefabricated free vascularized fibula flap. *Clin Oral Implants Res*. 2002 Feb;13(1):44–52.

Rohner D, Bucher P, Hammer B. Prefabricated fibular flaps for reconstruction of defects of the maxillofacial skeleton: planning, technique and long-term experience. *Oral Craniofac Tissue Eng*. 2011;1:11–19.

Rohner D, Guijarro-Martinez R, Bucher P, et al. Importance of patient-specific intraoperative guides in complex maxillofacial reconstruction. *J Craniomaxillofac Surg*. 2013;5:382–390.

Rohner D, Bucher P, Hammer B. Prefabricated fibular flaps for the reconstruction of defects of the maxillofacial skeleton: planning, technique, and long-term experience. *Int J Oral Maxillofac Implants*. 2013;5:221–229.

Roser SM, Ramachandra S, Blair H, et al. The accuracy of virtual surgical planning in free fibula mandibular reconstruction: comparison of planned and final results. *J Oral Maxillofac Surg*. 2010 Nov;68(11): 2824–2832.

Shpitzer T, Neligan PC, Gullane PJ, et al. The free iliac crest and fibula flaps in vascularized oromandibular reconstruction: comparison and long-term evaluation. *Head Neck*. 1999 Oct;21(7):639–647.

Taylor GI, Miller GD, Ham FJ. The free vascularized bone graft. A clinical extension of microvascular techniques. *Plast Reconstr Surg*. 1975 May;55(5):533–544.

Thoma A, Archibald S, Payk I, et al. The free medial scapular osteofasciocutaneous flap for head and neck reconstruction. *Br J Plast Surg*. 1991 Oct;44(7):477–482.

Vinzenz KG, Holle J, Würinger E, et al. Prefabrication of combined scapula flaps for microsurgical reconstruction in oro-maxillofacial defects: a new method. *J Craniomaxillofac Surg*. 1996 Aug;24(4):214–223.

Vinzenz KG, Holle J, Würinger E, et al. Revascularized composite grafts with inserted implants for reconstructing the maxilla—improved flap design and flap prefabrication. *Br J Oral Maxillofac Surg*. 1998 Oct;36(5):346–352.

Wallace CG, Chang YM, Tsai CY, et al. Harnessing the potential of the free fibula osteoseptocutaneous flap in mandible reconstruction. *Plast Reconstr Surg*. 2010 Jan;125(1):305–314.

Warrer K, Buser D, Lang NP, et al. Plaque-induced peri-implantitis in the presence or absence of keratinized mucosa. An experimental study in monkeys. *Clin Oral Implants Res*. 1995 Sep;6(3):131–138.

Yim KK, Wei FC. Fibula osteoseptocutaneous flap for mandible reconstruction. *Microsurgery*. 1994;15(4): 245–249.

Yim KK, Wei FC. Fibula osteoseptocutaneous free flap in maxillary reconstruction. *Microsurgery*. 1994;15(5):353–357.

3.1 Approaches and access osteotomies to the midface

Douglas W Klotch, Nicholas J Panetta

1 Introduction

Disorders involving the midface are numerous including congenital abnormalities, acquired posttraumatic deformities, benign and malignant neoplastic lesions, as well as degenerative and inflammatory processes.

The midface is a fundamental anatomical structure paramount for both the cosmetic and functional properties of the face including orbital support, mastication, airway, and facial appearance. Treatment of the disorders of the midface are complicated because of important structures, such as the orbits and the anterior portion of the skull base, and the need to preserve or reconstruct functional entities like the upper dental arch, airway, and maxillary and ethmoid sinuses. This complexity paired with the diversity of pathologies has historically garnered significant attention from surgeons to both refine existing and develop novel therapeutic approaches. Complete removal of disease remains the most basic mandate of oncological principles, which necessitates the experienced surgeon to master a variety of techniques, both open and endoscopic, in managing disorders involving the midface. From these efforts, a plethora of surgical techniques have been developed to gain access to the different areas of the midface. The goal of these approaches is to provide adequate exposure without compromise to treatment of the disorder with little cosmetic or functional morbidity and optimized reconstructive potential.

2 Diagnostic procedures and imaging

A comprehensive history and physical examination remains the cornerstone of sound preoperative evaluation when approaching diseases of the midface. A thorough examination of the lateral nasal wall, floor, and septum, as well as the nasopharynx and oropharynx should be performed. This is done by both visual examination and palpation of the soft and bony tissues of the nose, oral cavity, oropharynx, upper lip, cheek and canine fossa. Flexible endoscopic evaluation of the nasal cavity, nasopharynx and oropharynx is essential. Careful examination of the neck for the presence of regional adenopathy is critical, as well as a complete assessment of cranial nerve function.

Today high-resolution computed tomography (CT) and magnetic resonance imaging (MRI) are critical in establishing the extent of injury or disease (**Fig 3.1-1**).

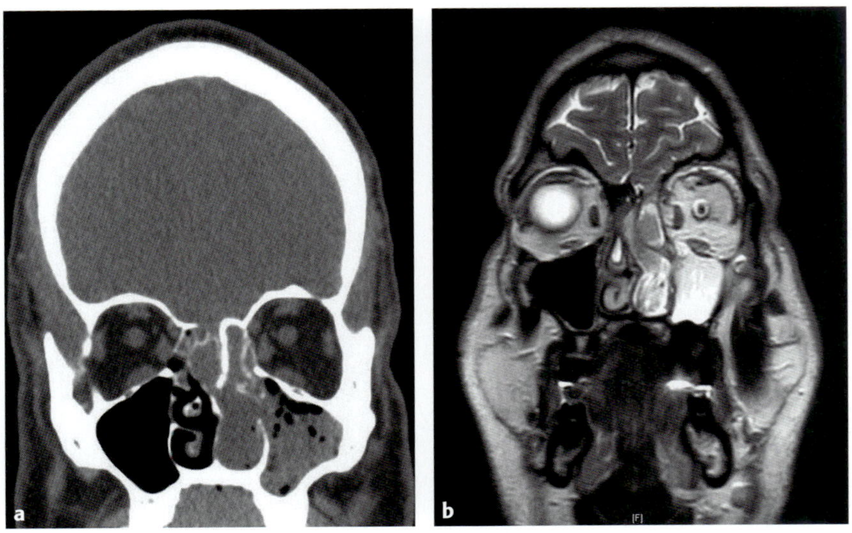

Fig 3.1-1a–b
a Coronal computed tomographic scan showing an erosive right ethmoid mass crossing the midline and encroaching on the skull base.
b Corresponding coronal magnetic resonance image showing that the tumor is confined to the ethmoid and nasal space with fluid within the maxillary sinus.

A CT imaging allows for detailed analysis of regional bone and soft-tissue involvement. An MRI provides important information regarding the extent of invasion into peritumoral soft tissues and more accurately assess intracranial extension. It also differentiates between tumor and sinonasal mucus to show the true extent of the disease. These examination tools have not only improved the accuracy of preoperative clinical staging but also opened the door to increasingly focused surgical approaches to tumors of the midface. When addressing vascular lesions, angiography and/or CT angiography, or MRI angiography should be considered. The use of fusion PET/CT scans have little value in assessing regional disease, but in selected cases may aid in assessing regional and distant metastatic disease.

In tumor surgery, depending on the clinical problem, a biopsy is mandated to allow appropriate diagnosis and planning of a resection. At times when the tumor is inaccessible for biopsy before surgery, the surgeon must rely on an intraoperative biopsy to obtain a diagnosis before planning the extent of resection.

Careful discussion with the patient of all treatment options, in addition to associated risks and benefits of each procedure, is mandated. Considerations of possible adjuvant and/or alternative radiation and/or chemotherapy should be included within this discussion. A multidisciplinary team approach is standard today to ensure optimal outcomes in the treatment of more advanced malignancies.

3 Surgical approaches including osteotomies

Many approaches to the midface have been described, transoral, transnasal, transfacial, and coronal. These can be used alone or in combination depending on the level of access needed.

3.1 Transoral/sublabial approach

For benign lesions of the maxillary sinus, a transoral approach allows for easy access with minimal morbidity. The soft-tissue approach is usually combined with an osteotomy/ostectomy of the anterior maxillary sinus wall. For treatment of benign conditions, the bone is replaced during wound closure. In case of invasive pathologies or conditions which result in erosions of the anterior sinus wall, the wall may be replaced with a titanium mesh (**Fig 3.1-2** and **Fig 3.1-3**).

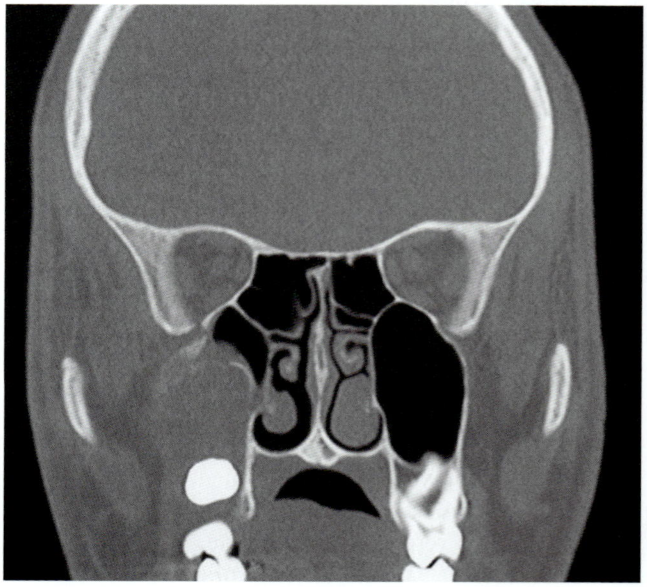

Fig 3.1-2 A computed tomographic scan showing a dentigerous cyst eroding the anterior and lateral maxilla.

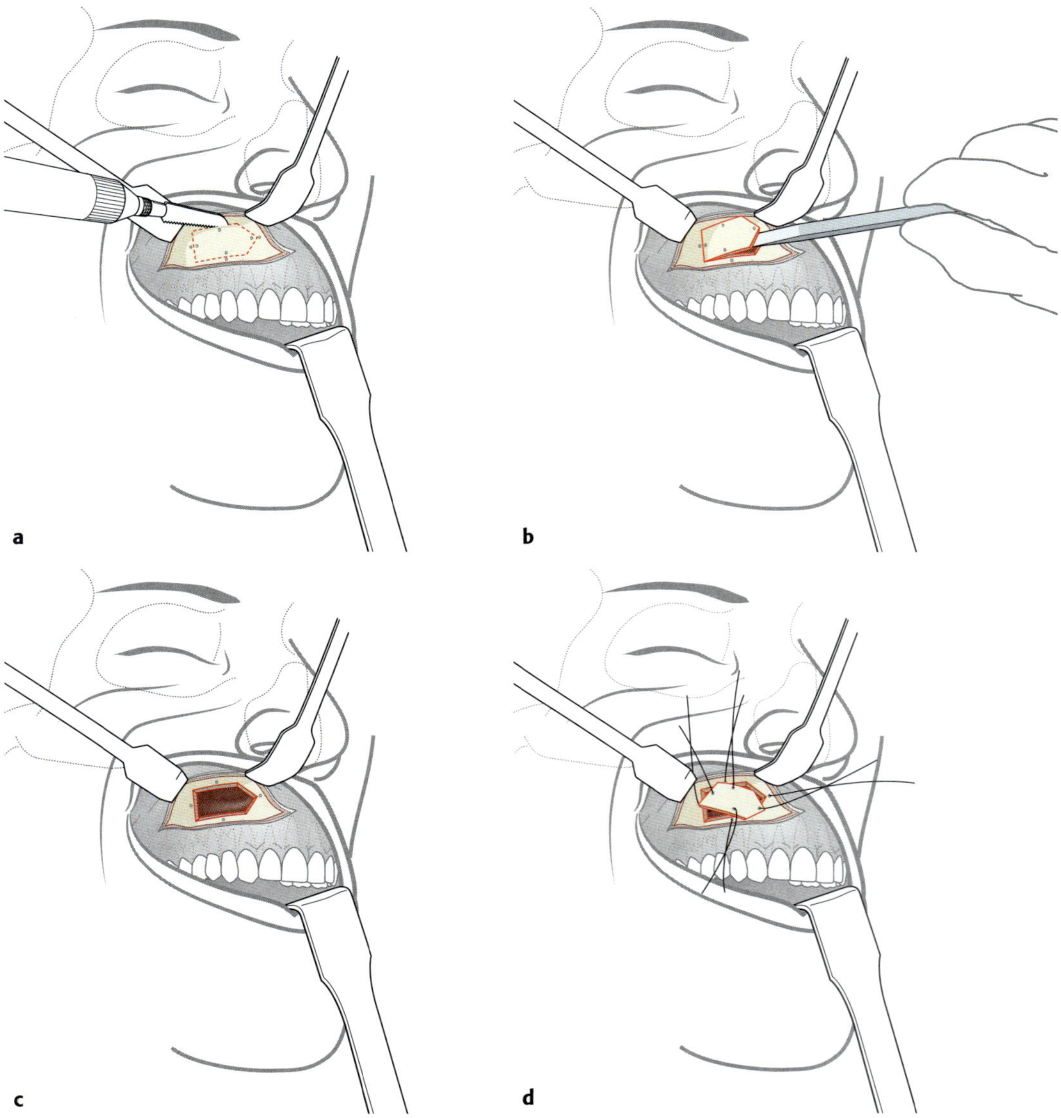

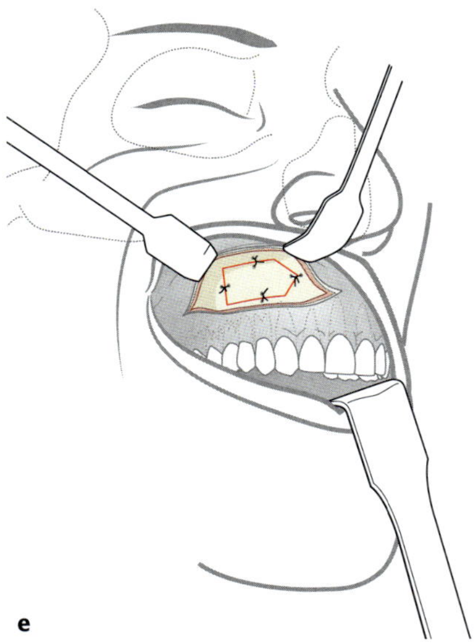

Fig 3.1-3a–e Canine fossa: anterior maxillotomy approach.

- **a** Exposure of anterior maxillary sinus wall, osteotomy lines for a bone window are outlined. The osteotomy is performed with a reciprocating saw.
- **b** Elevation of the bone lid.
- **c** Access to the sinus after removal of bone lid.
- **d** Replacement of bone and fixation with sutures. Plate fixation can be done alternatively.
- **e** Situation after bone replantation.

The sublabial approach provides excellent exposure to tumors of the maxillary alveolus (**Fig 3.1-4**).

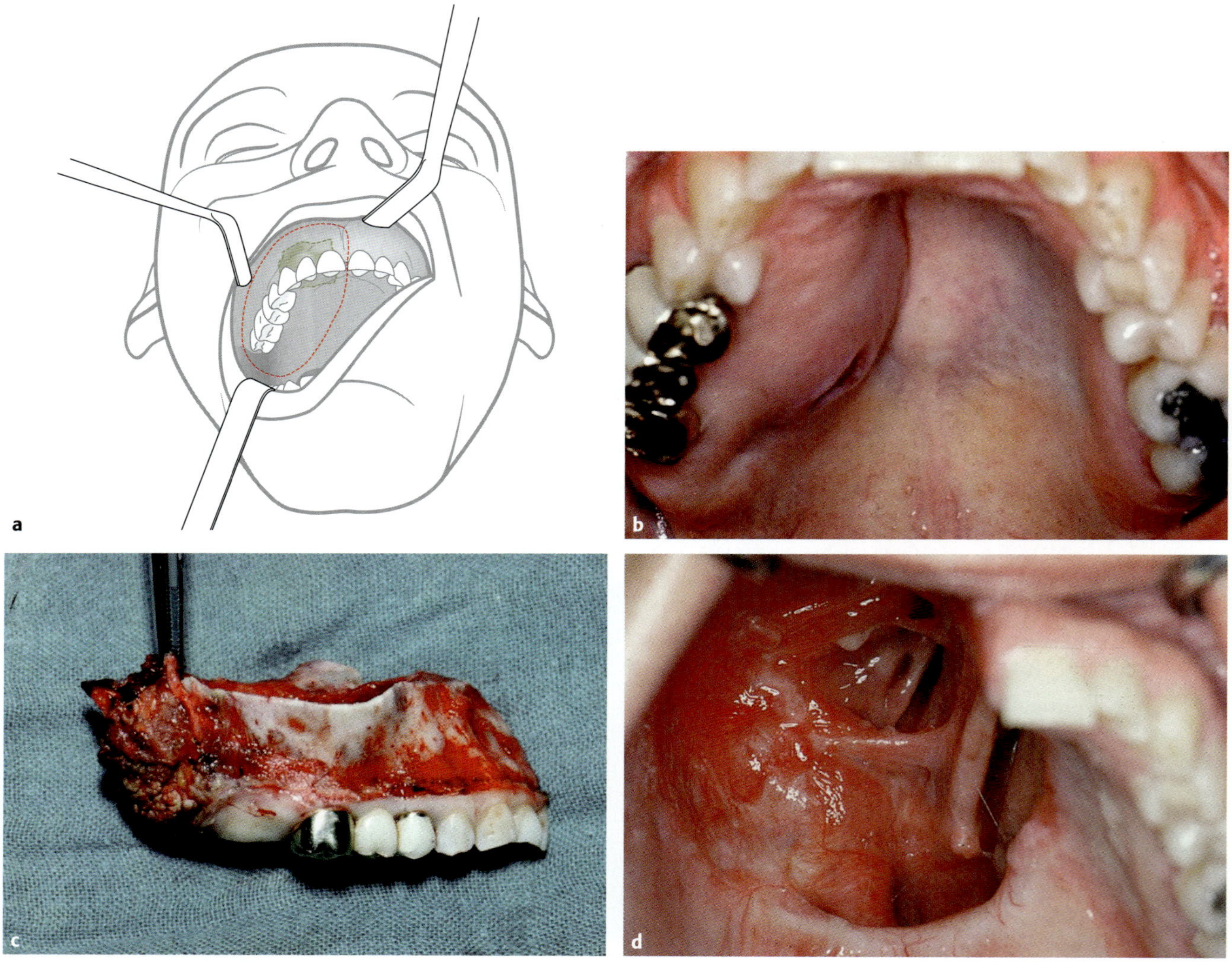

Fig 3.1-4a–h

a Removal of alveolar and palatal malignant lesion with osteotomies involving the alveolus, inferior maxilla and palate.
b Adenoid-cystic carcinoma of the upper right alveolus and palate.
c Resected specimen of the upper right alveolus and palate.
d Defect of the right inferior maxilla and palate after primary healing.

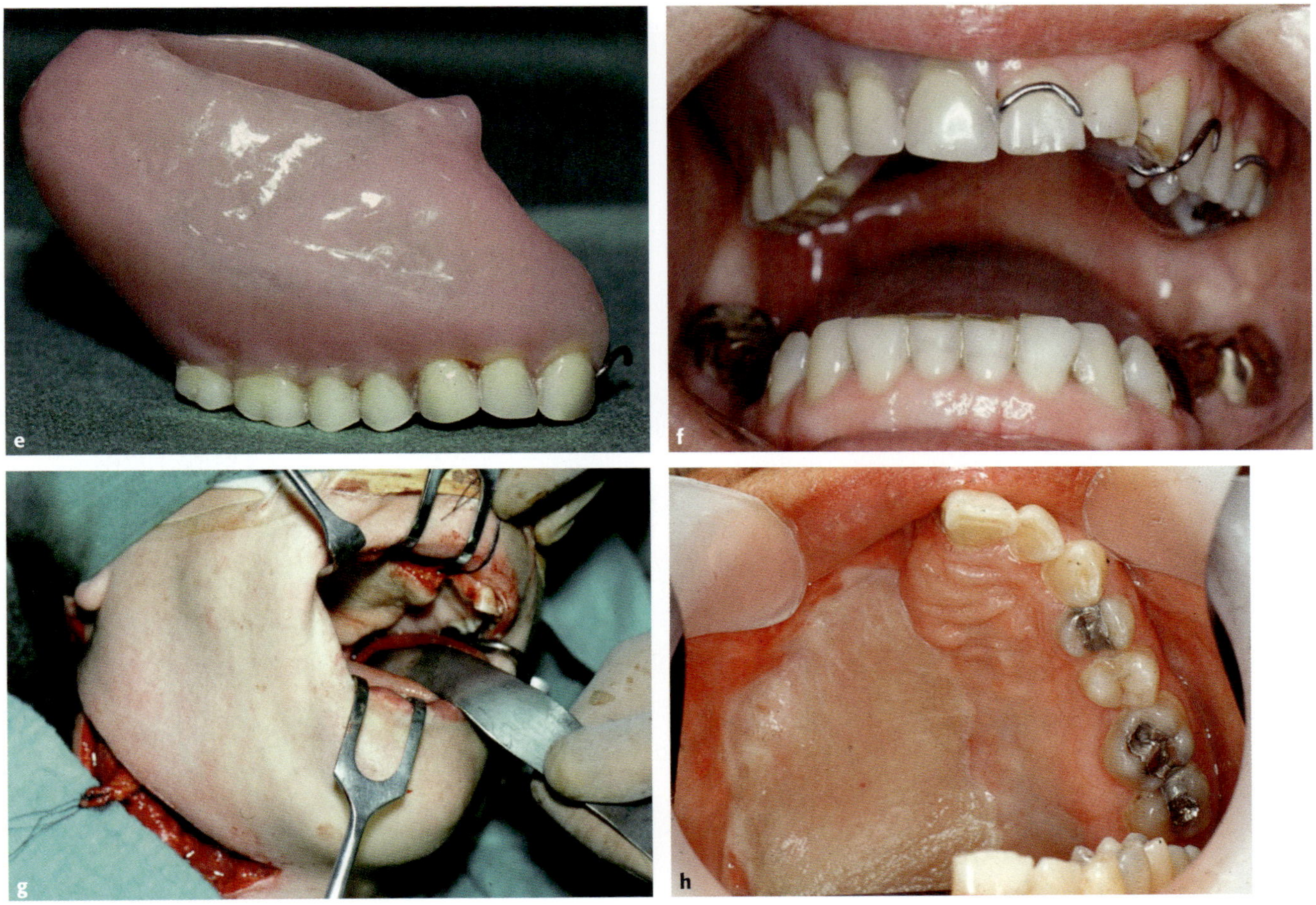

Fig 3.1-4a–h (cont)

e An obturator is used initially to support the soft tissues of the cheek and replace missing parts of the alveolus and palate. The obturator is made hollow to reduce weight.

f Obturator in place.

g Secondary reconstruction with a radial forearm flap. Flap in place before suturing. Vascular pedicle in the submandibular region.

h Flap in place after complete healing (case provided by Prof M Ehrenfeld).

3.2 Midface degloving approach

Many lesions involving the maxilla and central midface can be removed via midfacial degloving approaches. There are some limitations, for example, when the disease extends medially superiorly or wraps around the orbital rim. This approach provides excellent exposure to both sides of the face and nose. It allows access to the pterygomaxillary space and can be enhanced by using endoscopes and image guidance. The addition of these enhancements benefits in the complete removal of lesions involving this region (ie, neurogenic tumors of cranial nerve V or juvenile angiofibromas). This approach also provides access to the pterygoids in the posterior maxilla, so osteotomies can be performed when performing orbit-sparing maxillectomy procedures. These osteotomies are combined with palatal osteotomies and anterior maxillary osteotomies (nasomaxillary and zygomaticomaxillary) and division of the soft palate attachment to the hard palate to allow en bloc removal of the maxilla (**Fig 3.1-5**).

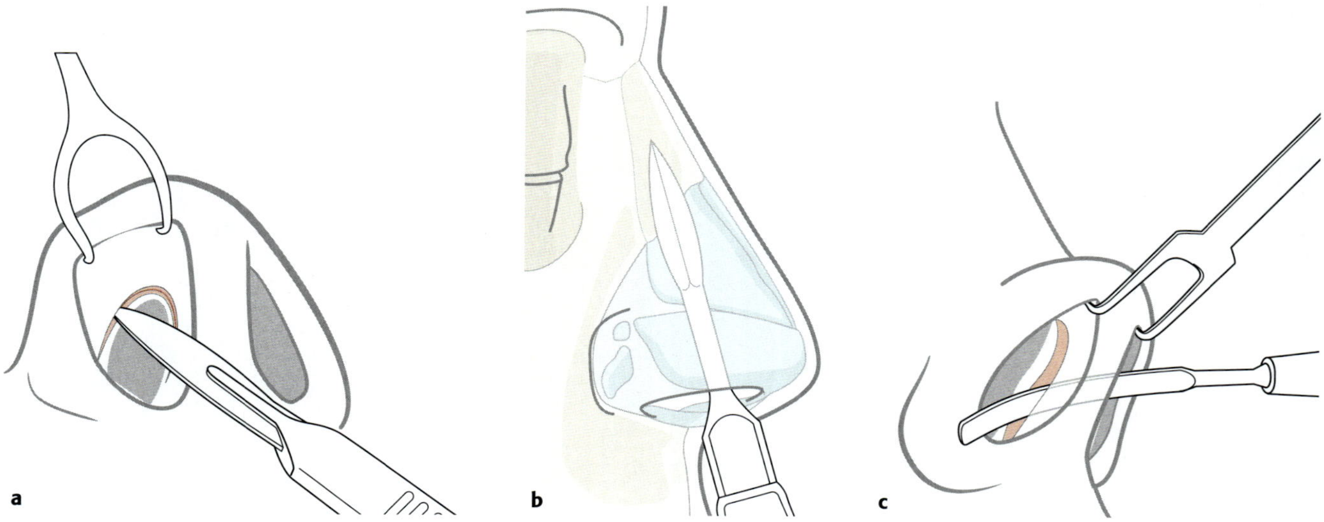

Fig 3.1-5a–h Facial degloving approach to one or both sides of the midface with no facial incisions providing generally acceptable access and good cosmetic results.

- **a** Intranasal mucosal incisions are made between the upper and lower lateral cartilages on both sides of the nose.
- **b** The mucoperichondrium and periosteum are elevated off the cartilaginous and bony nasal septum. Be careful to minimize the risk of perforating of the skin.
- **c** A full thorough incision is made between the caudal end of the septum and columellar portions of the lower lateral cartilages.

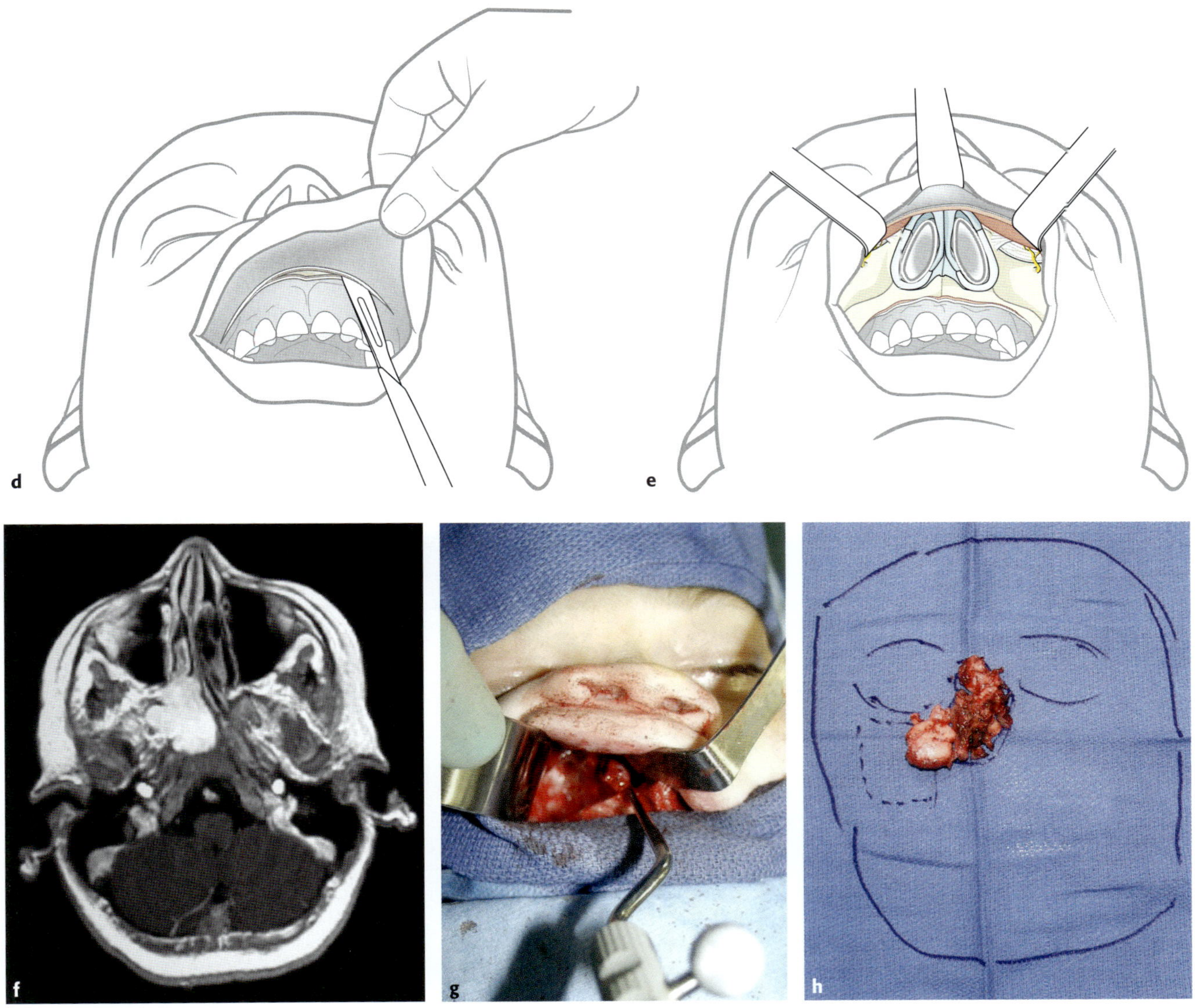

Fig 3.1-5a–h (cont)

d The intraoral sublabial incision is performed and connects with the intranasal incision.
e The maxilla is "degloved", exposing both sides of the maxilla.
f A patient with a juvenile angiofibroma of the nasopharynx and pterygomaxillary space.
g Facial degloving approach provides excellent exposure of the lesion, and when combined with image guidance assures complete removal of the tumor.
h Cartoon of the angiofibroma removal via the sublabial image-guided assisted approach.

3.3 Transpalatal approach

Transpalatal approaches have limited use as stand-alone approaches. They may be combined with resections of the alveolar process for tumors involving the premaxilla, alveolus, and anterior floor of the nose. They may also be combined with osteotomies of the attachments to the septum or maxilla depending on tumor location to release the superior attachments. Obviously, the extent or resection is dependent on the size and location of the tumor.

Transpalatal approaches for the pituitary have also been described, but have mostly been replaced by transnasal microscopic and transnasal endoscopic approaches. Likewise, transpalatal approaches may provide primary or extended access to the nasopharynx as well as to high anterior cervical fusions. Generally, separation of the soft palate with (temporary) resection of the posterior hard palate gives more restricted access than if one separates the soft and hard palate, and then divides the soft palate in the midline. Care must be taken to preserve the vascular supply of the posterior soft palate. Extensive cautery lateral to the midline is not advised and careful retraction of the palate with stay sutures is preferable to overzealous use of self-retaining retractors. This approach is seldom needed and is best performed by an experienced craniomaxillofacial surgeon to minimize morbidity. Most lesions can be removed by other approaches especially when enhanced with endoscopic image guidance.

3.4 Transoral approach in combination with Le Fort I osteotomy

A Le Fort I osteotomy, usually done from an upper buccal/ sublabial incision, with down fracture of the inferior part of the maxilla, provides good access to the posterior nasal cavity and epipharynx, especially for vascular lesions which may require good access for bleeding control. For this approach and osteotomy, the osteotomy line in the maxilla is outlined, the anterior and lateral maxillary pillars are preplated. The miniplates are then removed, the osteotomy and down fracture are performed, and the lesions treated as indicated. After that the inferior portion of the maxilla is repositioned and fixed with typically four miniplates along the anterior and lateral pillars of the midface, as it is done in orthognathic surgery (**Fig 3.1-6**).

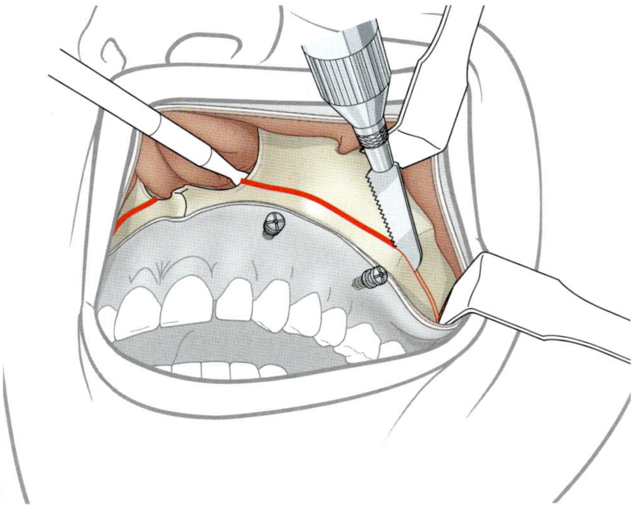
a

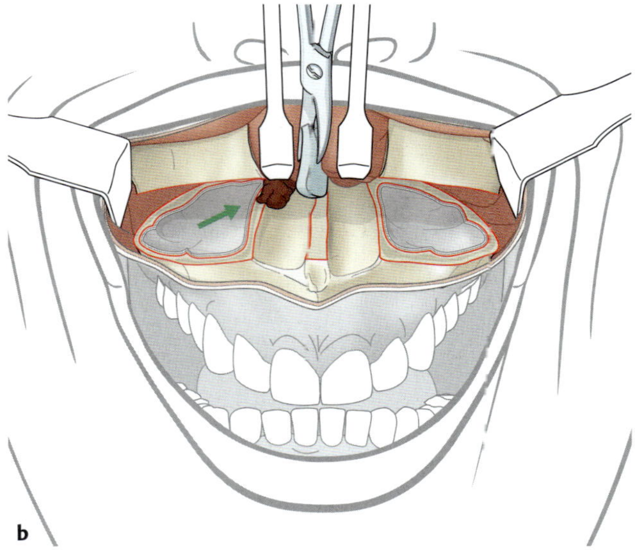
b

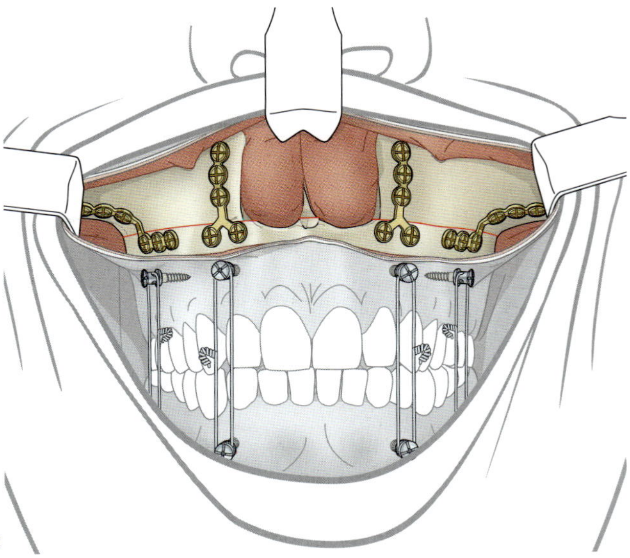
c

Fig 3.1-6a–c

- **a** Le Fort I osteotomy for approach to retromaxillary tumor. MMF screws are placed to align the occlusion during later osteosynthesis.
- **b** After down fracture of the inferior maxilla, good access to the tumor (arrow) is provided.
- **c** After tumor removal and reduction of the lower maxillary segment osteosynthesis along the lower anterior and posterior vertical facial buttresses with four miniplates. Osteosynthesis is performed with the patient in MMF.

3.5 Transfacial approaches

Lateral rhinotomy approach

A transfacial approach combined with a lateral rhinotomy is an excellent approach for tumors involving the nasal cavity. This allows exposure of the entire nasal cavity. Superiorly, this extends to the skull base and inferiorly to the floor of the nose. All three turbinates are also exposed. The lateral rhinotomy is still the preferred approach for tumors involving the mucosa and/or cartilage of the membranous collumella, ala and dome of the nose (**Fig 3.1-7**).

3.6 Weber Ferguson (Dieffenbach Weber) approach

The Weber Ferguson approach is indicated as access for tumors involving the maxilla extending superiorly to the infraorbital nerve and into the orbit. It provides a wide access to all areas of the maxilla, nose, and orbital floor. The incision line is drawn through the vermillion border, along the filtrum of the lip, extending around the base of the nose (or entering the nostril floor for a better esthetic result) and along the facial nasal groove (in the border of both esthetic units). It then extends infraorbitally 3–4 mm below the cilium to the lateral canthus. The incision can be extended laterally or superiorly as necessary for tumor removal (**Fig 3.1-8a–k**).

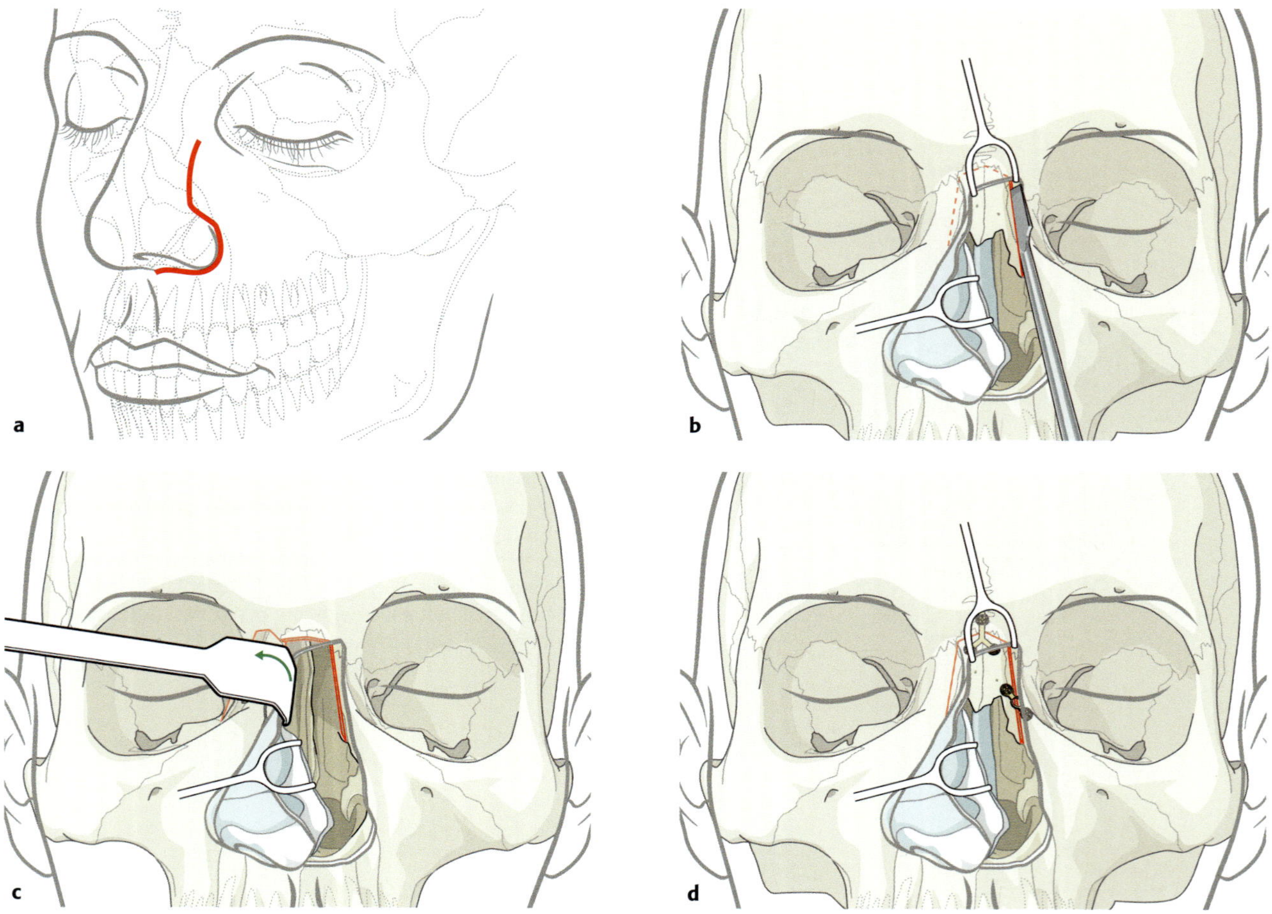

Fig 3.1-7a–d

- **a** The incision is made around the base of the nose (or entering the nostril floor for a better esthetical result) and along the facial nasal groove (in the border of both esthetic units). The dissection goes deep to the subperiosteal plane of the frontal process of the maxilla. Below the nasal bone, the incision is deepened through the nasal mucosa.
- **b** The lateral aspect of the nasal bone is identified. A unilateral nasomaxillary osteotomy is made with a small osteotome, and the two osteotomy lines are joined at the level of the nasofrontal junction.
- **c** The soft tissue and nasal skeleton are elevated and reflected to the contralateral side. This allows the exposure of the nasal cavity. The septum is cut and freed from the mobilized segment according to the resection plan. This cut is usually part of the tumor resection.
- **d** The elevated part of the nasal skeleton is back in the original place and fixed with microplates.

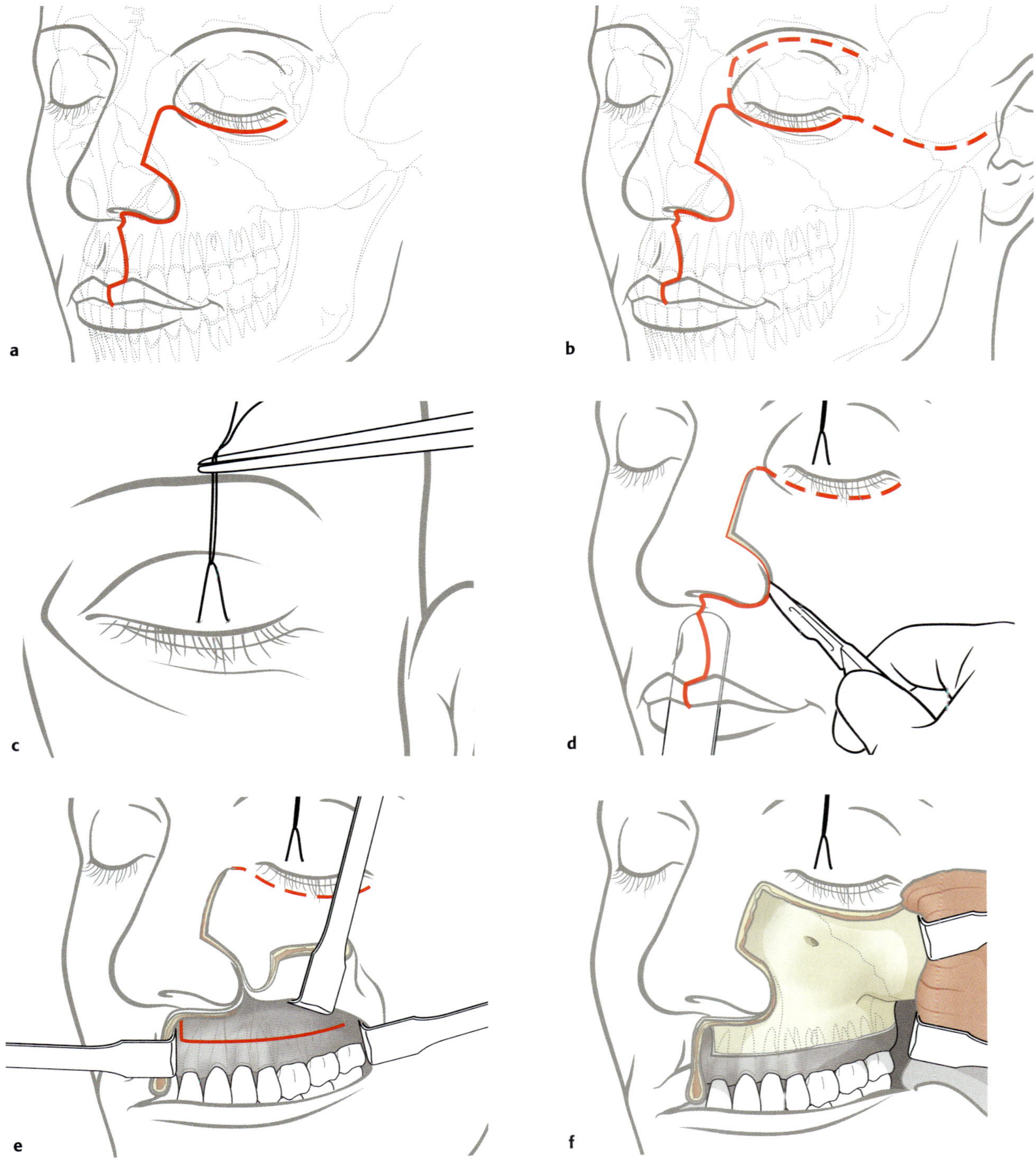

Fig 3.1-8a–n

- **a** The Weber Ferguson approach is indicated as access for tumors involving the maxilla including the nose, extending superiorly to the infraorbital nerve and into or involving the orbit. It provides a wide access to all areas of the maxilla, nose, and orbital floor.
- **b** The incision can be extended laterally or superiorly as necessary for tumor removal.
- **c** Tarsorrhaphy sutures are placed in the eyelids.
- **d** The incision is made through skin and subcutaneous tissue along the nose. The full thickness upper lip is transsected, and the labial artery ligated or coagulated.
- **e** It then extends sublabially along the mucobuccal fold preserving as much mucosa as possible, up to the maxillary tuberosity.
- **f** The cheek flap is elevated off the maxilla to its lateral border in a subperiosteal plane with electrocautery. A supraperiosteal dissection plane will be necessary in the subcutaneous tissues if there is tumor invasion of the anterolateral maxillary wall. In most cases the infraorbital nerve is relinquished to facilitate tumor removal.

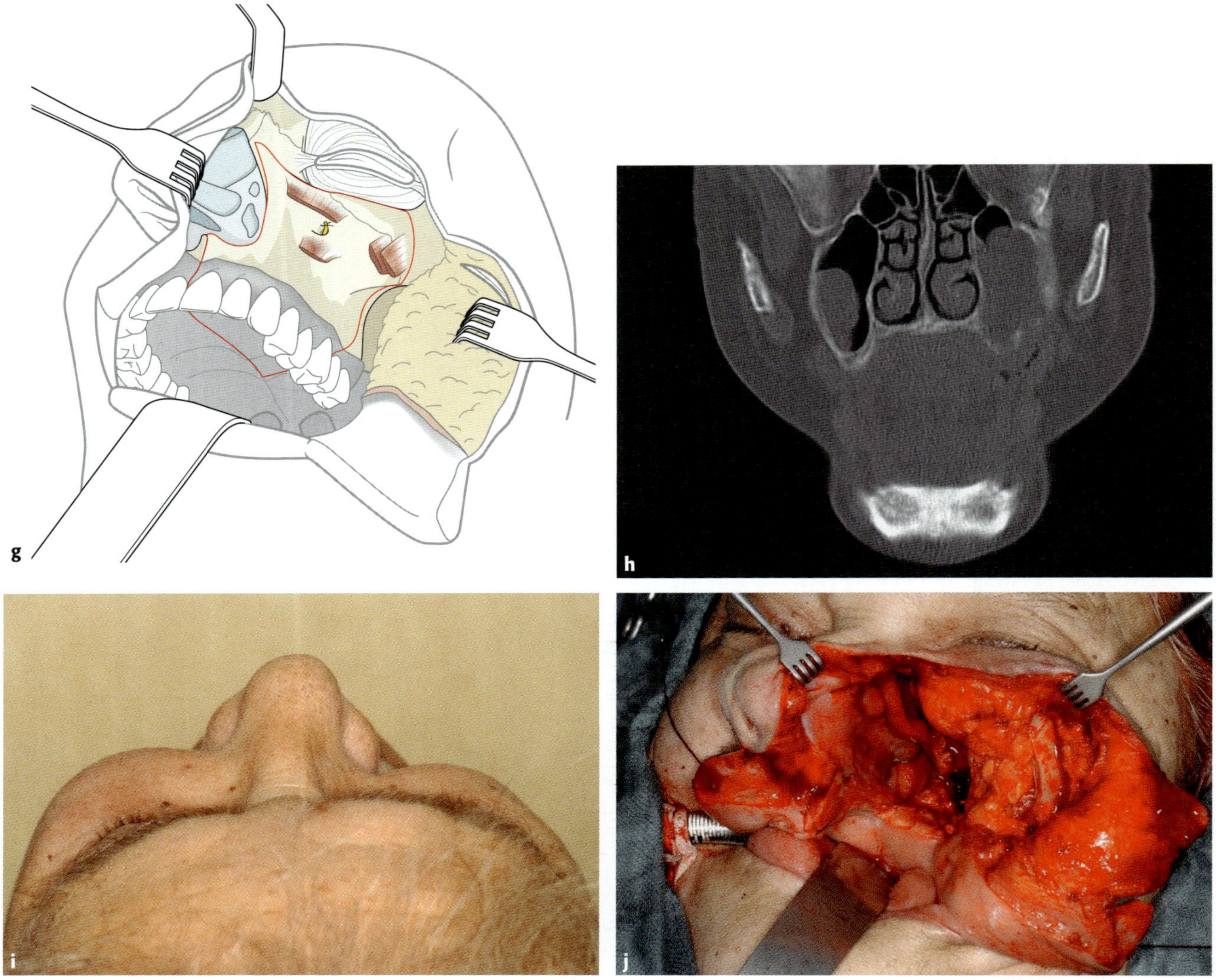

Fig 3.1-8a–n (cont)

g Weber Ferguson approach with an extended bone resection outlined including the left maxilla and parts of the palate.
h Adenocarcinoma of the left maxillary sinus invading the maxilla and the cheek. Mucosal cyst in the right maxillary sinus.
i Forward projection of the left cheek because of tumor invasion/expansion.
j Via a transfacial Weber Ferguson incision, resection of parts of the maxilla, zygoma, left orbital floor, and palate.

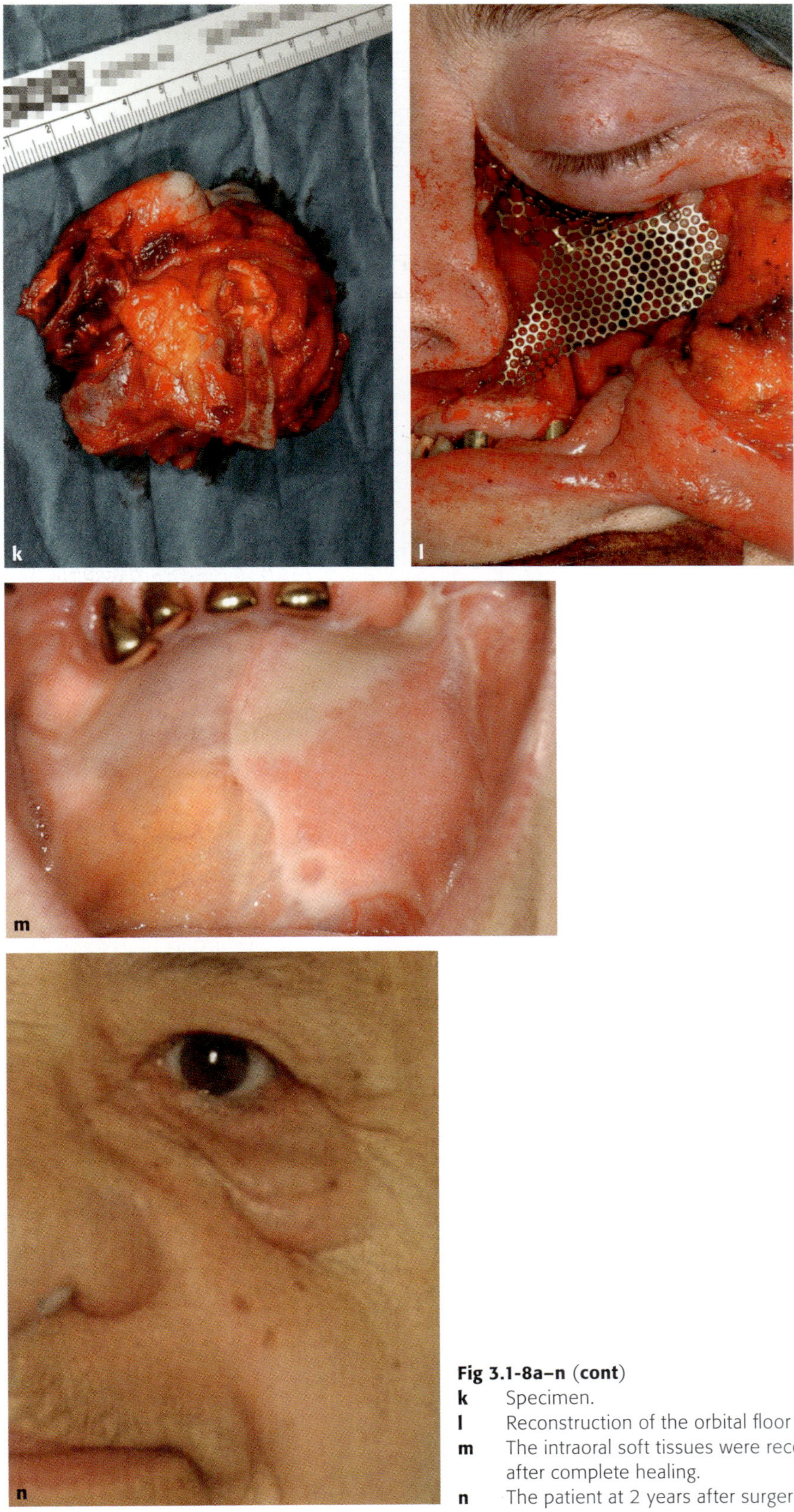

Fig 3.1-8a–n (cont)

k Specimen.

l Reconstruction of the orbital floor and the anterior sinus wall with titanium meshes.

m The intraoral soft tissues were reconstructed with a radial forearm flap; situation after complete healing.

n The patient at 2 years after surgery (case provided by Gerson Mast, MD).

3.7 Access through defects after tumor ablation

Besides the traditional transfacial approaches, in scenarios where skin resection because of tumor invasion is required, this may provide good and direct access to the underlying facial bones and midface cavities such as the sinuses, nasal cavities, and orbits.

3.8 Endoscopic approaches

Open approaches are consistent with the variety of clinical scenarios that patients present to surgeons, but open approaches to the midface in combination with osteotomies can result in substantial morbidity for patients. This has engendered an expanding interest in the development of minimally invasive endoscopic, endoscopically assisted, and image-guided approaches.

Today many midface lesions can be treated via transnasal endoscopic procedures. Extensions of these procedures may also provide access to the skull base, orbit and frontal sinus. Better visualization with potentially less wide and disruptive exposure can facilitate surgical removal with less surgical morbidity. They have enhanced application when coupled with image guidance systems. They can enhance traditional approaches to assess disease extension, provide improved visualization, and provide better assessment of the complete removal of the process being treated (image guided) (**Fig 3.1-9**).

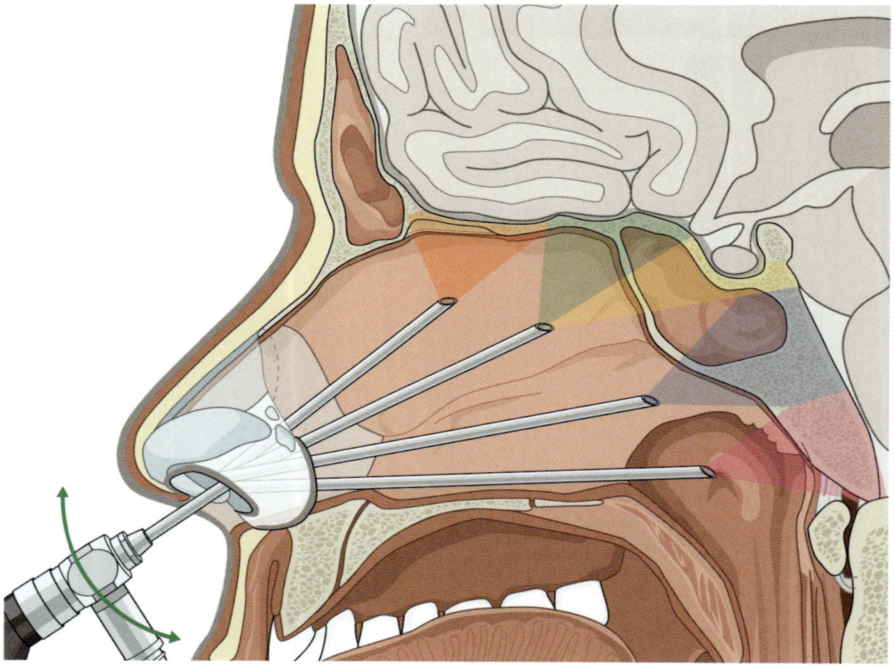

a

Fig 3.1-9a–e

a Possible endoscopic approaches for skull base tumor resections.

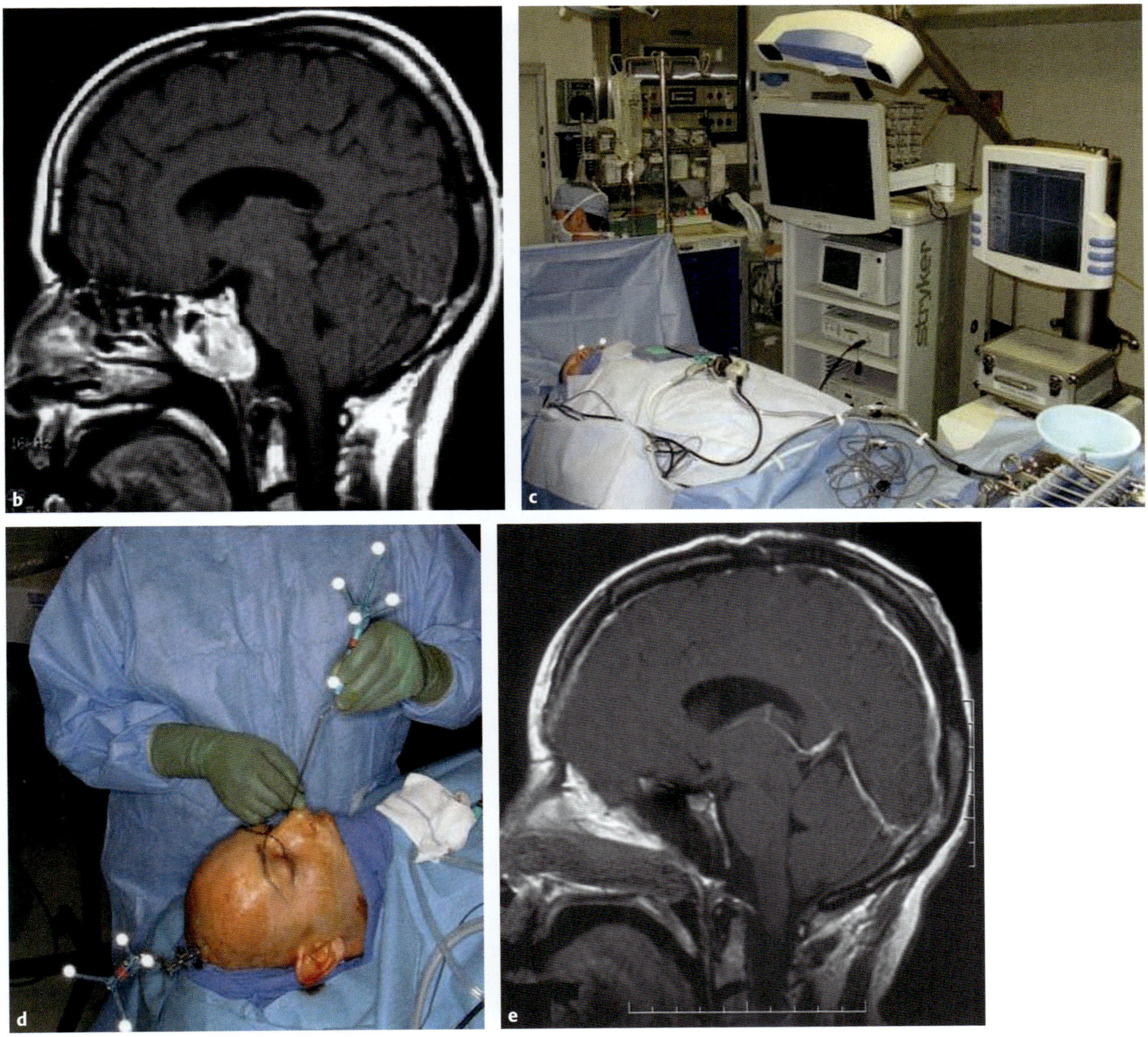

Fig 3.1-9a–e (cont)

b Sagittal magnetic resonance imaging scan of a clival chordoma. Removal planned via intranasal endoscopic approach with image guidance.

c Operative set up of guidance system and patient positioning.

d Use of guidance probe to verify position of instruments at the skull, tumor location, and removal.

e A 12-month postoperative sagittal magnetic resonance imaging scan after complete tumor removal.

Excellent examples of the application of modern image-guided resection techniques to neoplastic processes are being observed especially in the treatment of juvenile angiofibromas, inverted papillomas, and neurogenic tumors. Rates of recurrence and operative complications following endoscopic or endoscopic-assisted resection of juvenile angiofibromas now approximate that observed following traditional open operations. This is also true for removal of inverted papilloma and several other neoplasias involving the maxilla. The older paradigm of en bloc removal appears less rigid. Indeed, what is required is complete removal. Furthermore, the innovation of intraoperative image guidance systems used in endoscopic approaches has offered surgeons improved real time anatomical localization of their resection. This allows for complete endoscopic resection of technically challenging lesions with less potential morbidity resulting from injury of vital structures. Other applications for endoscopic image-guided approaches include medial maxillectomy for inverted papilloma, and maxillary division fifth nerve neuromas. These techniques may also be used to assist in placement of implants for trauma, treatment of exophthalmos, optic nerve decompression and cerebrospinal fluid leak repair. Importantly, it cannot be overstated that the guiding principles of endoscopic intervention should mirror those of traditional approaches to midface pathology; achieving adequate exposure as to allow for the safe and complete excision of all involved tissue is critical.

The nature of the lesion also determines whether endoscopic approaches can be used. Traditional anterior transmaxillary approaches are still required for more extensive malignant processes, which may erode through the posterior or lateral table of the maxilla, floor of orbit, and alveolus. Traditional osteotomies are commonly used in the treatment of malignant tumors and removal of hard tissues (bone tumors, teeth). Transmaxillary approaches may also provide access to lesions or disorders involving the orbit and nasopharynx. Frequently in using transmaxillary approaches for tumors not involving the anterior bony structures, the anterior bone may need to be osteotomized and replaced at the end of the ablative procedures providing better postoperative cosmetic results. The surgeon must use the approach which best addresses the patient's disease without compromise in removal or to function and appearance.

Ultimately, the surgeon's decision regarding whether to implement an endoscopic approach hinges on both their individual technical skill set, as well as whether complete resection can be accomplished using a minimally invasive approach. Cases must be carefully selected, and patients always counseled about the potential need for a more radical approach if their tumor is not amenable to endoscopic resection. To this end, a surgeon must always remain aware of the potential intraoperative discovery of unanticipated disease extension. Such situations may mandate modification of the operative plan, requiring a more extensive resection including for instance orbital exenteration. Likewise, an experienced team is required to provide optimal outcomes, treatment for malignant tumors is best discussed and consented in a tumor board.

4 Complications and pitfalls

Complications resulting from midface approaches and osteotomies have largely been divided into four categories; namely facial, intraorbital, intraoral, and vascular [Lofchy et al, 1998]. In brief, these may include bleeding, ecchymosis, infection, hardware-related complication, infraorbital nerve impairments, epiphora, oroantral fistulae, extraocular muscle weakness/entrapment, anosmia, cerebrospinal fluid leak, and facial scar retraction and more rarely blindness.

Osteotomies performed endoscopically are undertaken with well-defined risk of minor and major complications as well. It is important to remember that with ever increasing use of endoscopic and image-guided approaches to the resection of midface and maxillary tumors, there is no substitute for surgeon experience and excellent operative exposure. As such, the surgeon must always remain cognizant of his/her own level of comfort when operating using these more minimally invasive techniques, and retain a low threshold to convert to a more invasive approach when anatomical clarity is blurred. Furthermore, when treating complex tumors, it is essential to have a team approach. A tumor board is beneficial and should integrate the expertise of multiple disciplines including—the radiologist, surgeon (ablative and reconstructive), prosthodontist, radiation oncologist, medical oncologist, pathologist, speech and swallowing specialists. Well-established multidisciplinary approaches best serve the patient who is faced with a serious disease and a potentially deforming surgery.

5 References and suggested reading

Batra PS, Luong A, Kanowitz SJ, et al. Outcomes of minimally invasive endoscopic resection of anterior skull base neoplasms. *Laryngoscope*. 2010 Jan;120(1):9–16.

Beumer HW, Puscas L. Computer modeling and navigation in maxillofacial surgery. *Curr Opin Otolaryngol Head Neck Surg*. 2009 Aug;17(4):270–273.

Bhattacharyya N, Orlandi RR, Grebner J, et al. Cost burden of chronic rhinosinusitis: a claims-based study. *Otolaryngol Head Neck Surg*. 2011 Mar;144(3):440–445.

Bleier BS, Kennedy DW, Palmer JN, et al. Current management of juvenile nasopharyngeal angiofibroma: a tertiary center experience 1999-2007. *Am J Rhinol Allergy*. 2009 May–Jun;23(3):328–330.

Carrau RL, Snyderman CH, Kassam AB, et al. Endoscopic and endoscopic-assisted surgery for juvenile angiofibroma. *Laryngoscope*. 2001 Mar;111(3):483–487.

Heiland M, Habermann CR, Schmelzle R. Indications and limitations of intraoperative navigation in maxillofacial surgery. *J Oral Maxillofac Surg*. 2004 Sep;62(9):1059–1063.

Herman P, Lot G, Chapot R, et al. Long-term follow-up of juvenile nasopharyngeal angiofibromas: analysis of recurrences. *Laryngoscope*. 1999 Jan;109(1):140–147.

Levine HL. Functional endoscopic sinus surgery: evaluation, surgery, and follow-up of 250 patients. *Laryngoscope*. 1990 Jan;100(1):79–84.

Lofchy NM, Bumsted RM. Revision and open sinus surgery. In: Cummings CW, ed. *Otolaryngology—Head & Neck Surgery*. 3rd ed. St Louis: Mosby; 1998:1173–1188.

Nicolai P, Berlucchi M, Tomenzoli D, et al. Endoscopic surgery for juvenile angiofibroma: when and how. *Laryngoscope*. 2003 May;113(5):775–782.

Nijmeh AD, Goodger NM, Hawkes D, et al. Image-guided navigation in oral and maxillofacial surgery. *Br J Oral Maxillofac Surg*. 2005 Aug;43(4):294–302.

Terrell JE. Primary sinus surgery. In: Cummings CW, ed. *Otolaryngology—Head & Neck Surgery*. 3rd ed. St Louis: Mosby; 1998:1145–1172.

Welch KC, Stankiewicz JA. A contemporary review of endoscopic sinus surgery: techniques, tools, and outcomes. *Laryngoscope*. 2009 Nov;119(11):2258–2268.

3.2 Midface resection and reconstruction

Neal D Futran

1 Introduction

The importance of the central portion of the face, including palate, cheek, maxilla, upper lip, orbit, and nose cannot be underestimated. It is the functional and esthetic cornerstone of the mid-facial unit and includes each of the key mid-facial elements. The maxilla functions as the structural support between the skull base and the occlusal plane, resisting and absorbing the forces of mastication, anchoring the dentition, separating the oral and nasal cavities, supporting the globe and the soft-tissue envelope and its mimetic musculature. The soft tissues of the midface are supported by the maxilla which esthetically provides much of the facial appearance unique to each individual and serving as an icon for the whole person. Due to the disparate shapes and sizes of tumors affecting the maxilla and the complex surgical anatomy, the broad category of "maxillectomy" encompasses a group of diverse defects that range from a small oro-antral or oro-nasal fistula to a large cavity, bounded by the tongue inferiorly and the anterior skull base superiorly. Tumors treated by maxillectomy are rarely confined by the bony walls of the maxilla itself (**Fig 3.2-1**); thus, resection of adjacent tissues in the velum, palate, midface, and orbits is commonly performed simultaneously. The morbidity of maxillectomy defects is rarely trivial. It potentially includes impairment of deglutition and nutrition, ocular function and vision, speech and communication, self-image and mental health, as well as maintenance of hygiene and social acceptability. Clearly, when one or all the functions of the maxilla are lost, a return to good quality of life depends on the degree to which these functions are reconstituted.

The goal of reconstruction is always to replace the form and function of native tissue. Ideal reconstruction in the midface in particular requires the following goals be met. They are in order of importance [Triana et al, 2000; Brown et al, 2000]: (1) healed wound; (2) separation of the oral and nasal cavities; (3) restoration of maxillary buttresses; (4) restoration of functional dentition, mastication, and deglutition; (5) restauration of globe position or cosmetical rehabilitation of an exenterated cavity; (6) maintain a patent nasal airway; (7) support and suspend adynamic facial soft tissues, including avoidance of ectropion; and (8) restore midfacial contour.

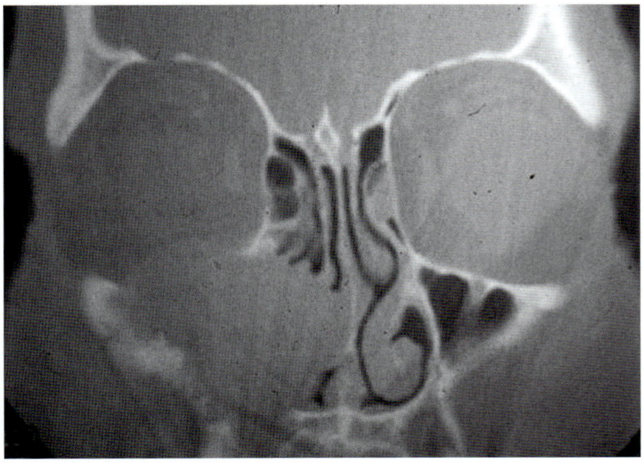

Fig 3.2-1 Coronal computed tomographic scan of a tumor of the maxillary sinus extending beyond the walls of the sinus.

2 Indications and planning

Indications for partial or total maxillectomies mostly come from tumor surgery, primarily from malignant tumors. However, maxillary defects may also be congenital or the result of extensive facial trauma, especially shotgun injuries.

For reconstructive purposes, several midface defect classification systems have been developed. The classification according to Brown and Shaw is shown [Brown et al, 2010] [Brown et al, 2000; Cordeiro et al, 2000] (**Fig 3.2-2**).

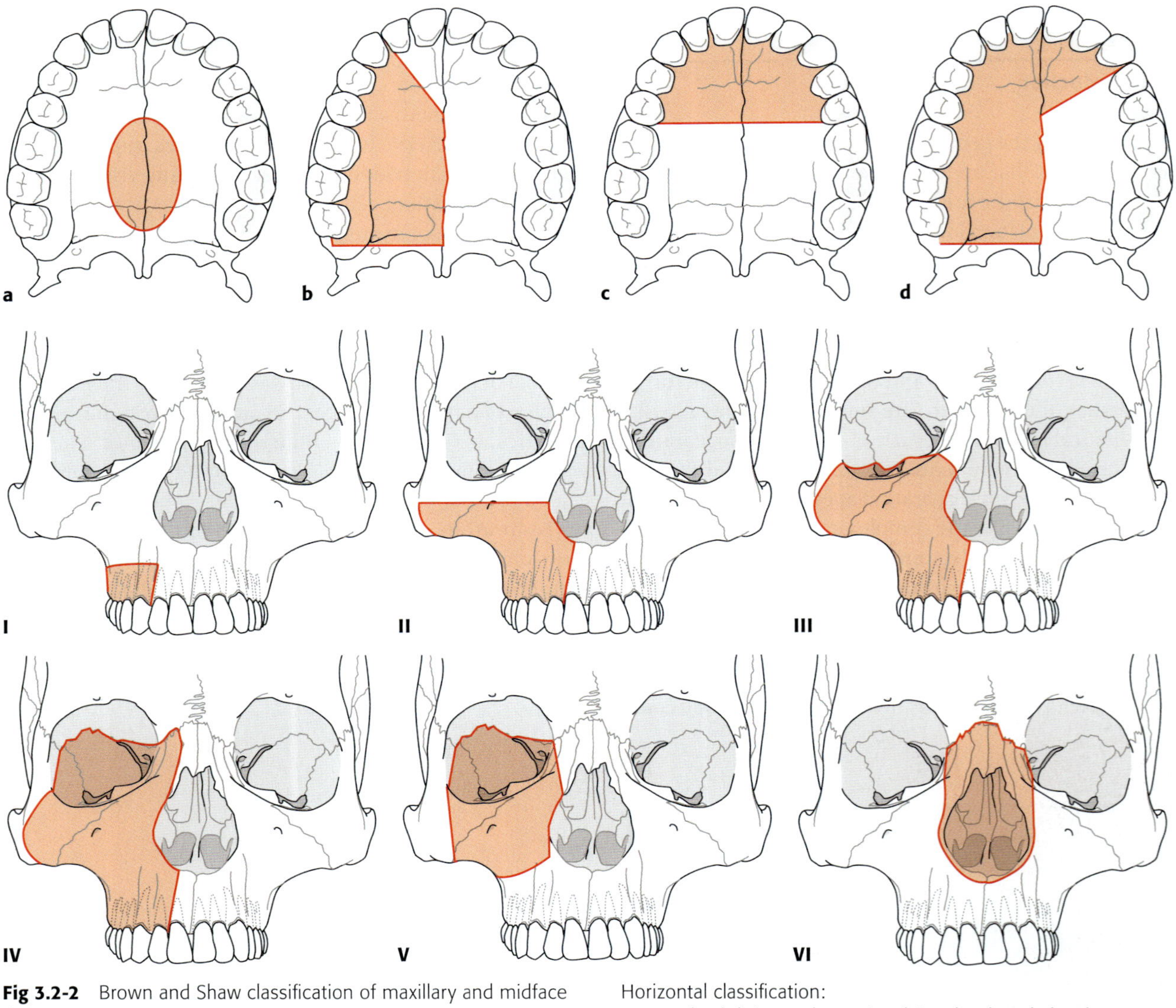

Fig 3.2-2 Brown and Shaw classification of maxillary and midface defects.

Vertical classification:

- **I** Maxillectomy not causing an oronasal fistula.
- **II** Maxillectomy not involving the orbit.
- **III** Maxillectomy involving the orbital adnexae with orbital retention.
- **IV** Maxillectomy with orbital enucleation or exenteration.
- **V** Maxillectomy with orbitomaxillary defect.
- **VI** Maxillectomy with nasomaxillary defect.

Horizontal classification:

- **a** Palatal defect only, not involving the dental alveolus.
- **b** Palatal defect less than or equal to half unilateral.
- **c** Palatal defect less than or equal to half bilateral or transverse anterior.
- **d** Palatal defect greater than half maxillectomy.

3 Diagnosis and imaging

See chapter 3.1, paragraph 2, for details.

4 Resection and reconstruction of the midface

Resection of midface structures imposes significant functional and esthetic consequences on the patient; therefore, they require reconstruction. It is crucial for a surgeon performing ablative surgery in this area to be familiar with the various reconstructive options even though that skill set may be provided by other reconstructive surgeons. Therefore, an overview is given at the beginning of this chapter.

Placement of a maxillary prosthesis is one traditional and reliable method to obturate maxillary defects [McGregor et al, 1986; Wells et al, 1995] (**Fig 3.2-3**). The prosthesis restores the oral/nasal separation, which is a fundamental principle necessary for speaking and swallowing. Dentition can be included for chewing and appearance. The surgical complexity and length of operative procedure is less with obturator compared with tissue reconstructions. A prosthesis may also be fashioned to restore maxillary as well as nasal, orbital, and ocular defects.

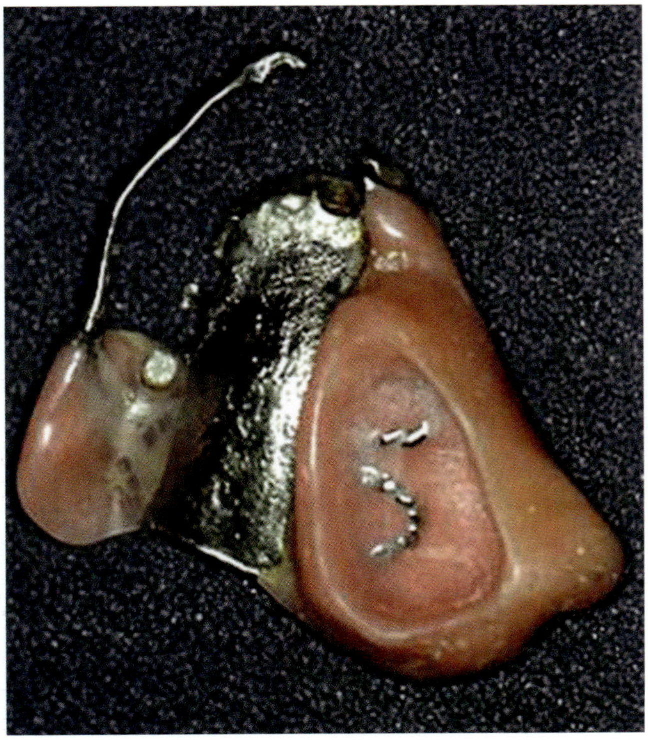

Fig 3.2-3 Removable maxillary obturator (prosthesis).

These larger prostheses depend significantly on support from native tissues, and are compromised when native hard-tissue support is lacking. In particular, the status of the canine and molar teeth is important for the retention of a prosthesis. Depending on the defect, orbitofacial and dental prostheses may be used either alone or in addition to surgical flaps. For individuals reconstructed with a maxillary prosthesis only, a cheek packing is left for 7 days postoperatively and the patient will need to receive appropriate gram-positive antibiotic coverage while the packing is retained. On returning to clinic, he/she is seen by the CMF prosthodontist; the packing is removed, the cavity is cleaned and inspected and after that an obturator is manufactured and the patient is started on frequent nasal saline irrigations and home humidification. Over time, the maxillary prosthesis can be altered to "best fit" the evolving defect.

Nevertheless, prosthetic rehabilitation has significant shortcomings and patients may become dissatisfied for several reasons. Speech and swallowing require use of the device, and the device needs frequent removal and cleaning for hygiene, which may be cumbersome and technically difficult, especially for the elderly or those left with monocular vision. Poor retention due to denture bulkiness, poor residual dentition (both quality and quantity), and poor or deficient retentive surfaces can create leakage and oronasal regurgitation. In addition, as more of the zygomatic prominence is lost, the esthetic success and stability of the prosthesis is decreased. Radiation also has a negative impact on the comfort and retention of the obturator as well as the quality of underlying tissues to support it. Although initial use of a prosthesis does not preclude future tissue reconstruction, performing immediate reconstruction is technically easier than secondary procedures. Additionally, immediate reconstruction of large defects averts significant psychological and emotional distress because of disfigurement during a delay period. The theoretical advantage in tumor surveillance with prostheses compared with flap coverage remains unproved, and this is likely due to the accuracy and availability of modern imaging modalities that allow for accurate assessment of the resection bed without direct inspection [Robb et al, 2001].

In the 1980s, development of microvascular techniques allowed for free tissue transfers, yielding a tremendous improvement in the ability to resect and reconstruct in a single stage without the limitations of reach and orientation of regional pedicled flaps. These techniques allow a wide variety of donor tissue types to be used, permitting the surgeon to customize the reconstruction to match the defect. The various nuances of soft tissue and osseous needs (shape, bulk, and quality) can be incorporated into the reconstructive plan. Various free tissue transfer donor sites have been described for maxillectomy defects, including radial forearm [Marshall et al, 2003], rectus abdominis [Browne et al, 1999], fibula [Yim et al, 1994; Futran et al, 2002], scapular system [Swartz et al, 1986; Uglesic et al, 2000], and iliac crest [Brown, 1996; Genden et al, 2001]. Flap selection should be determined by various factors. The amount, location, and quality of residual bone in the midface, the quality of the existing dentition and/or denture bearing alveolar arch, determine whether a bone-containing flap is necessary. Ideally, skin, soft tissue, mucosa, and bone needs are matched to the characteristics of the appropriate flap before undertaking a reconstructive procedure. Length of the vascular pedicle, thickness or thinness of the skin, muscle, and subcutaneous fat, the volume of the tissues available, the durability and thickness of the bone and donor-site morbidity are all important factors that must be considered.

When only the soft tissues of the alveolus are reconstructed, conventional dentures may provide functional dentition if adequate teeth and/or retentive surfaces are available to provide stability. In many cases, soft-tissue reconstruction alone results in a flatter surface of maxillary arch than in the native condition. Blunted neo-alveolar contours are created and there is loss of the gingival buccal sulcus and palatal arch depth. This results in a 'trampoline-like' surface so that the reconstructed maxilla functions poorly to retain a denture [Funk et al, 1998; Futran, 2001] (**Fig 3.2-4**). If sufficient underlying bone is available, osseointegrated implants may overcome this problem, but reconstruction of a large composite defect with soft tissue alone is done at the expense of dental prosthetic rehabilitative options. Soft-tissue free flap reconstruction of the maxilla should be reserved for patients who retain adequate dentition for mastication and/or patients who do not agree to the rigors of more complex reconstructive procedures [Cordeiro et al, 2000].

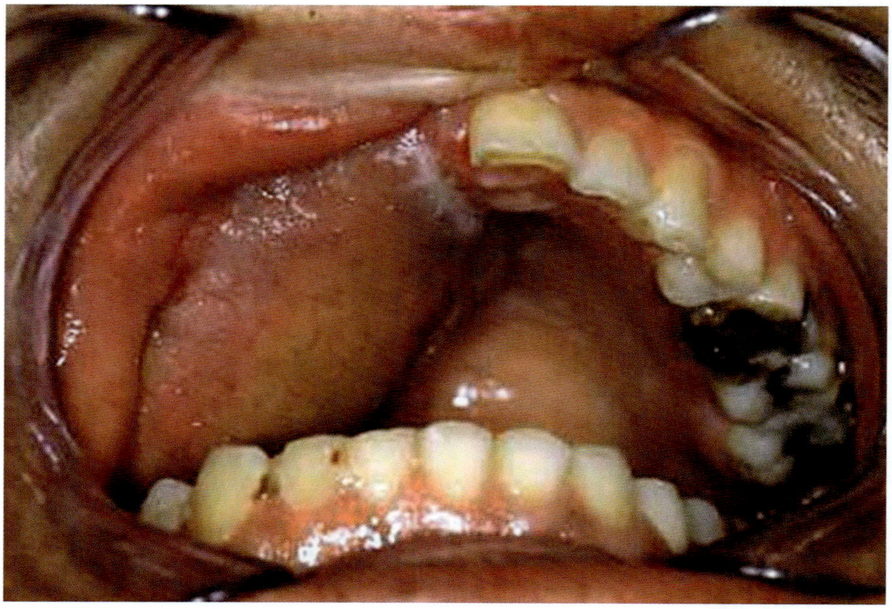

Fig 3.2-4 Soft-tissue free flap obliterating the maxillary sinus and for reconstruction of the alveolus and sealing the palate.

Alternatively, bony reconstruction partly restores the 3-D alveolar ridge and allows use of osseointegrated implants for functional dentition when adequate bone stock is replaced [Triana et al, 2000; Futran et al, 1999] (**Fig 3.2-5**). Free flaps with sufficient bone stock to support osseointegrative implantation include the fibula, iliac crest, and sometimes, the scapula. The radial forearm free flap may be harvested with a bony component but the length and width of the bone available limit its use to small anterior defects not requiring implantation.

4.1 Maxillectomy with orbital preservation

In extended maxillary defects, in addition to the considerable task of restoring oral functions, reconstitution of an inferior orbital wall and zygoma become a paramount consideration (**Fig 3.2-6**). Without adequate support of the orbit, enophthalmos, hypophthalmos, and diplopia may result. Reconstruction of the orbital floor is necessary to prevent dystopia and to preserve eye function postoperatively. The reconstructive tasks for this defect are, therefore, technically more challenging than when the orbital contents have been resected. Soft-tissue pedicled flaps, such as the temporalis flap rotated through the defect from the osteotomized zygomatic arch, are useful in patients unable to undergo free tissue transfer. The addition of vascularized calvarial bone to the temporalis flap may also provide bone for orbital support in these patients but the geometry of getting the bone and soft tissue each into the right place may be difficult to accomplish [Parhiscar et al, 2002]. Access to the orbital floor and infraorbital rim to insert temporalis flaps requires at least a partial resection of the lateral maxilla, which may weaken the important zygomaticomaxillary buttress. However, this flap places the facial nerve at risk, particularly in the upper division, and results in an unnatural appearing temporal depression. This could be an advantage in situations where just thin bony reconstruction is needed with minimal soft-tissue bulk. Given that this is rarely the case in total maxillectomy defects, this option can be combined with other soft-tissue flaps that could then provide bulk and be fashioned independently from the bony reconstruction.

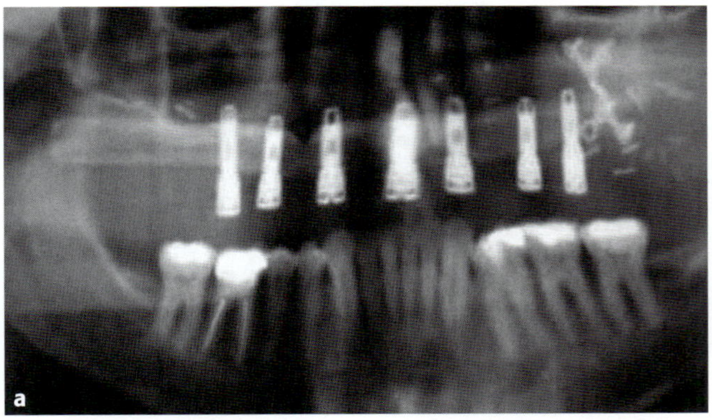

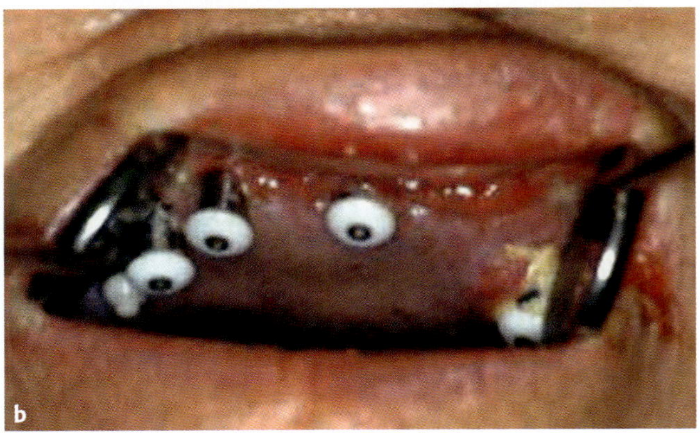

Fig 3.2-5a–b
- **a** Panoramic radiograph of osseointegrated implants in maxillary reconstruction with a fibula.
- **b** Clinical picture of implants in the same patient.

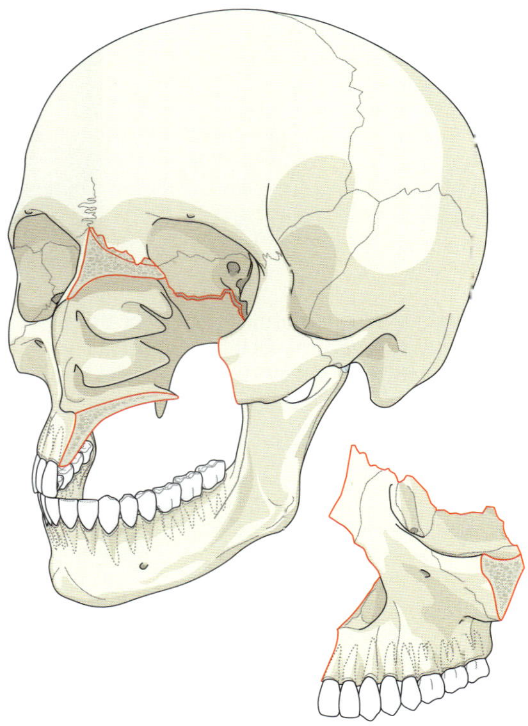

Fig 3.2-6 A maxillectomy in which the palate, orbital floor, and parts of zygoma are removed.

Because of the volume required to fill the midface contours, many authors have recommended soft-tissue free flaps to obtain a sealed palate and achieve an esthetically satisfactory recontouring of the face and cheek soft tissues [Marshall et al, 2003; Browne et al, 1999; Cordeiro et al, 2000; Cordeiro et al, 2000]. Preference for fat, fascia, and skin as donor material limits the unpredictable atrophy (30–90%) associated with denervated muscle-alone. Soft-tissue-alone reconstructions, however, do not address the maxillary bony skeleton, particularly the orbit, zygoma, and alveolus. Nonvascularized bone or alloplasts have been advocated to improve globe position and bone support, but bone may undergo substantial resorption (**Fig 3.2-7a–b**). The remainder of the defect is filled with vascularized free tissues (**Fig 3.2-7c**). Muscle-alone flaps should be avoided as they do not provide a lasting solution because of atrophy.

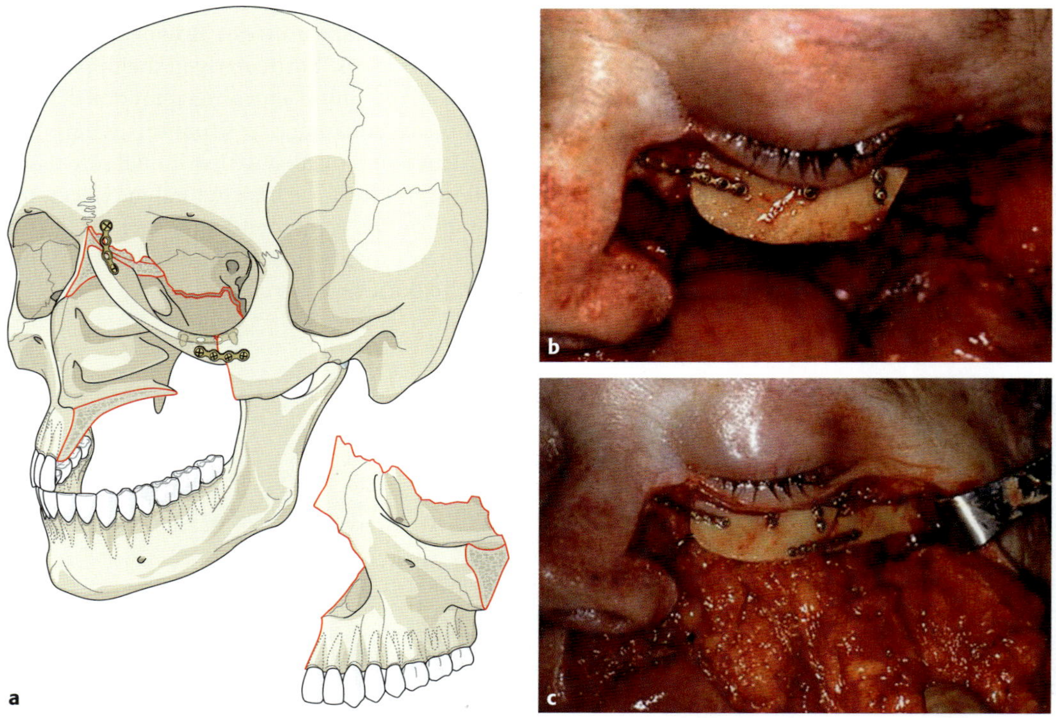

Fig 3.2-7a–c
a Cranial bone grafts used to reconstruct the inferior orbital rim.
b The cranial bone graft to reconstruct the inferior orbital rim in place.
c The bone grafts are surrounded by vascularized soft tissue.

Vascularized osteomusculocutaneous free flaps have the advantage of better infection resistance than nonvascularized bone graft reconstructions and are better able to maintain bony volume. For total maxillectomy defects with orbital preservation, the subscapular system of flaps, while technically more complex, offers perhaps the greatest versatility in flap reconstruction [Swartz et al, 1986; Uglesic et al, 2000]. Replacement of the alveolar arch inferiorly with the lateral scapula (supplied by the circumflex scapular artery) and the orbital floor and rim with the scapular tip (supplied by the angular branch of the thoracodorsal artery) suits this reconstruction need well (**Fig 3.2-8**). The thoracodorsal artery supplies the latissimus dorsi muscle and overlying tissue, which may be harvested partially or completely for a wide range of soft-tissue reconstructive needs. Furthermore, each of the two components of this flap may be rotated independently of each other. In the series by Triana et al [2000], various flaps based on the subscapular system of vessels were used to reconstruct maxillectomy defects in ten patients. Dental and/or orbital restoration was performed in four of these patients with the use of osseointegrated implants. Schliephake [2000] found that it is difficult to tailor the bone in a fashion that simultaneously restores the malar prominence, the infraorbital rim, and the maxillary wall, and at the same time place the lateral border of the scapula in an appropriate position for placement of these implants. Miles et al [2011] have described the use of the vascularized scapular tip flap to restore the palate or the zygomatic contour with the scapular soft tissue (fat, fascia, and skin) filling the remainder of the maxillary defect. The scapular bone may not always be suitable for placement of osseointegrated implants, unless secondary bone augmentation is performed. A relative disadvantage in the use of the subscapular system include challenges to position the patient to harvest the flap simultaneously with the extirpative procedure, difficulty in orienting the bone to provide orbit, zygoma, and alveolar reconstruction and the relatively short pedicle length.

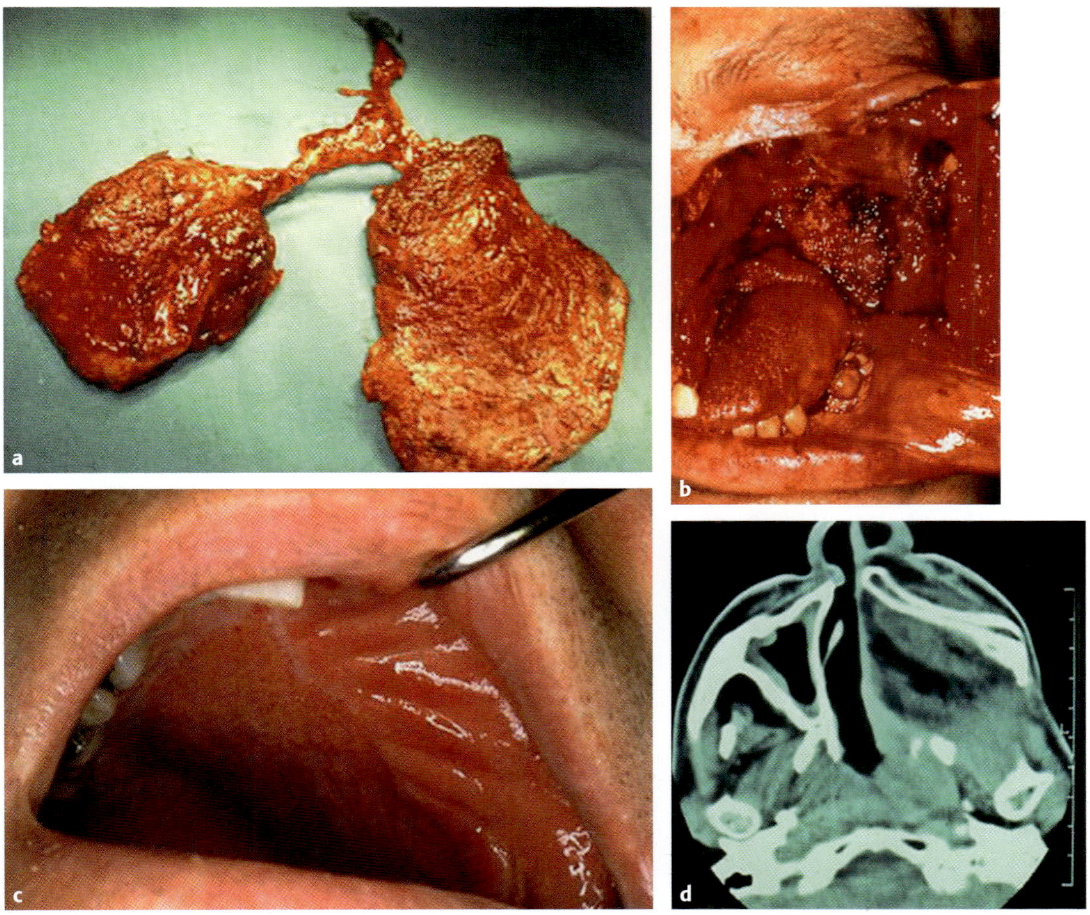

Fig 3.2-8a–d

a Scapula bone and latissimus dorsi osteomusculocutaneous free flap on vascular pedicle.
b Left maxillectomy defect.
c View of reconstructed left palate.
d Axial computed tomographic scan showing scapula bony reconstruction of the zygoma and maxilla.

The fibular flap has sufficient bone stock and a soft pliable skin paddle that can be used for either intraoral and/or cutaneous reconstruction (**Fig 3.2-9**). Futran et al [2002] used the revascularized fibular osteocutaneous free flap in seven patients with total maxillectomies and orbital preservation. Superior and inferior bony support was accomplished, and cosmesis was only considered fair because of flattening in the midface. In comparison one patient in this series whose flap failed and ultimately used a prosthesis, was noted to have poor cosmesis. Osseointegrated implants were placed or planned in this entire group. The fibula bone stock is more reliably implantable than the scapula. This represents an advantage of the fibula over the scapula for this defect, although cosmesis favors the scapula.

The iliac crest free flap provides an excellent bone source for palate and maxillary reconstruction [Brown, 1996; Genden et al, 2001] (**Fig 3.2-10a**). A single block can restore the alveolus, zygomatic prominence, and infraorbital rim. This allows for excellent restoration of structure to support both the globe and a dental prosthesis (**Fig 3.2-10b–e**). It is harvested with the internal oblique muscle that restores the palatal mucosa. The disadvantages of using this flap for the maxilla are its potentially excessive bulk, limited soft-tissue mobility in relationship to the bone and short pedicle length.

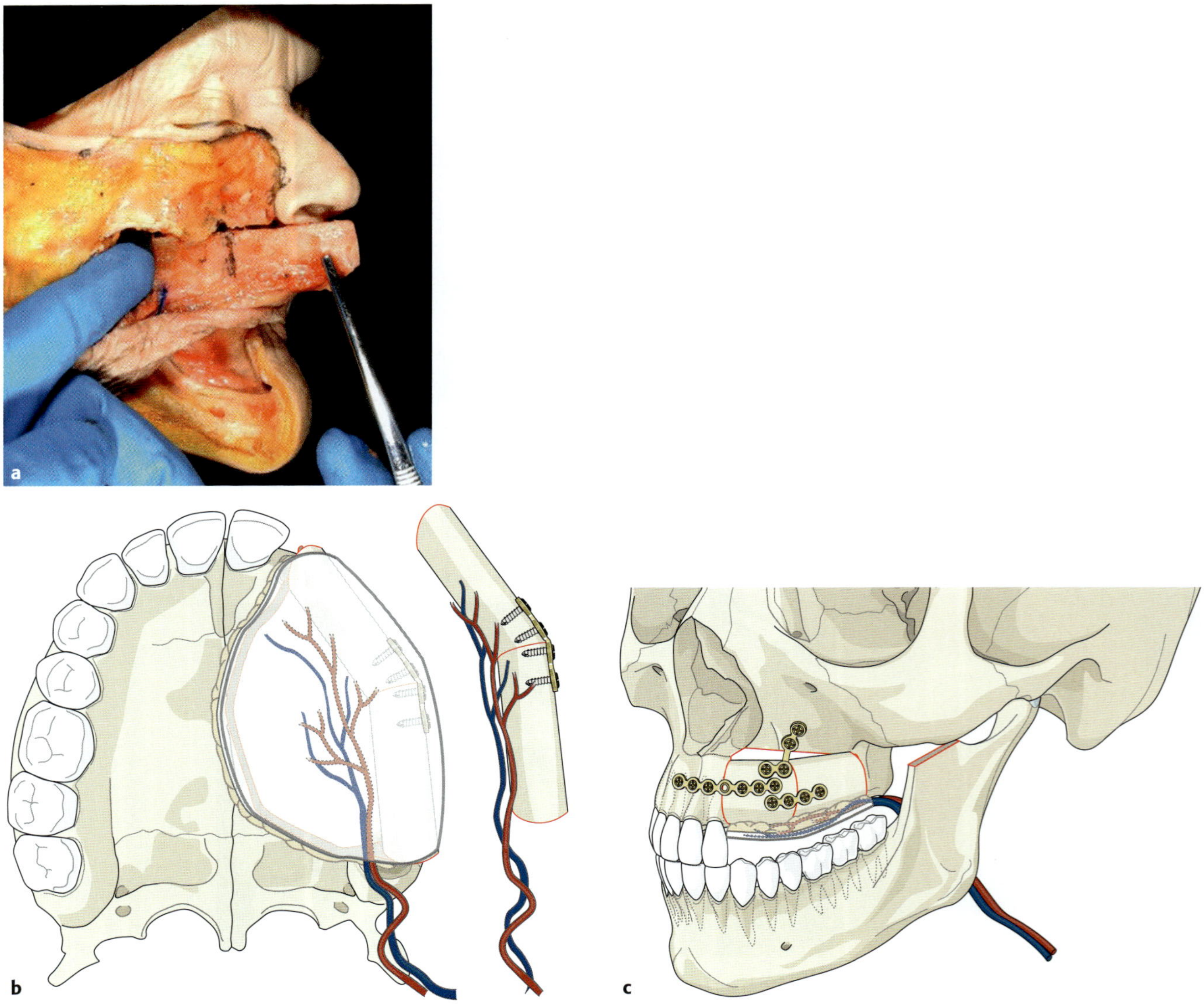

Fig 3.2-9a–c
a Human anatomical model showing placement of the vascularized fibula to reconstruct the inferior maxilla.
b–c Views of the fibula bone and soft-tissue placement with the vessels draped posteriorly to the angle of the mandible.

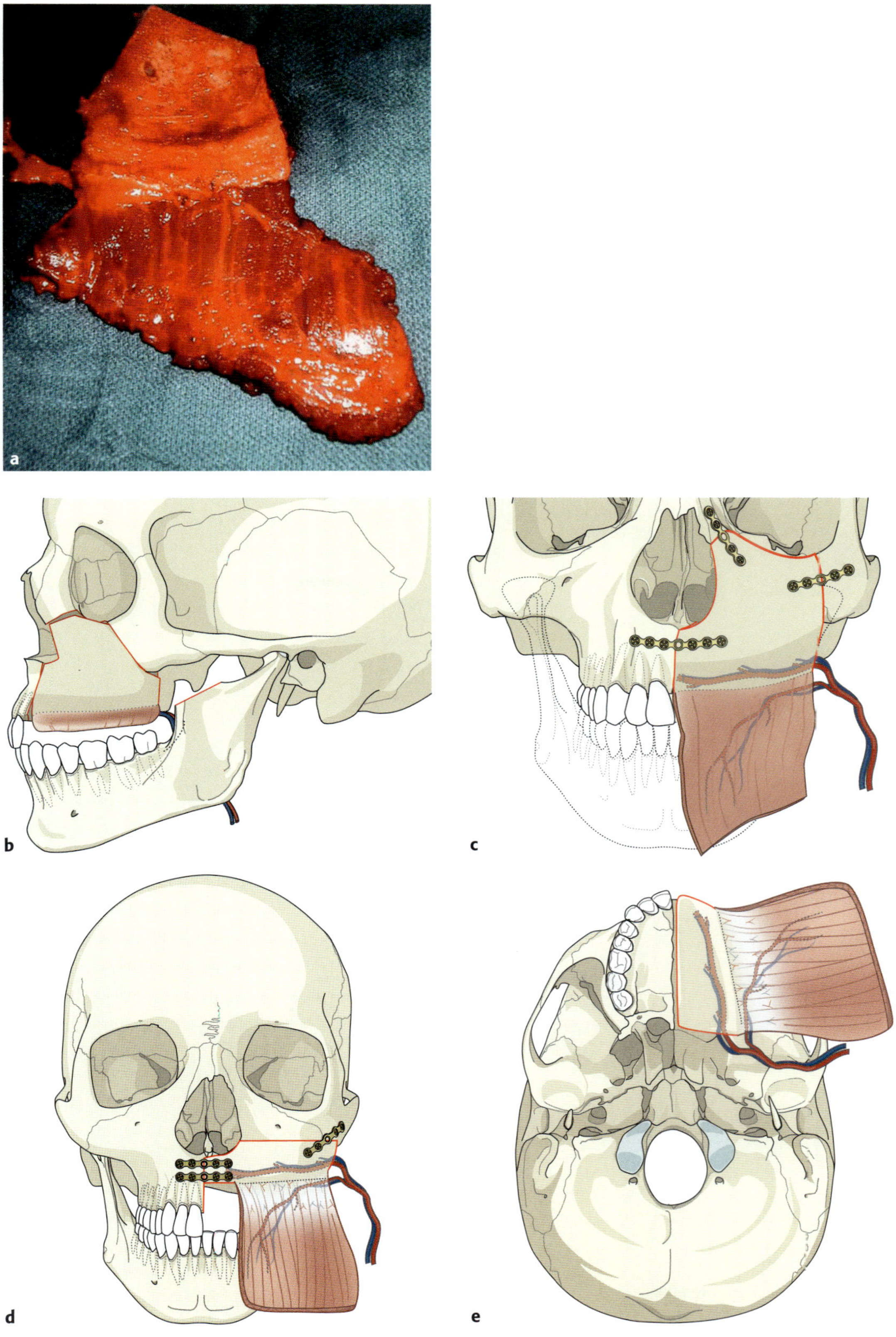

Fig 3.2-10a–e
a Iliac crest free flap with internal oblique muscle.
b–e Placement of flap for full maxillectomy defect.

4.2 Maxillectomy with orbital exenteration

When tumor resection extends from tongue to supraorbital rim, reconstructive options depend on the amount of remaining dentition. If adequate teeth and alveolar arch remain, a prosthesis may be used. The use of a prosthesis that spans the defect from the oral cavity to the orbit is subject to cheek retraction over time and poor fit as well as the distracting appearance of an unblinking, expressionless eye. These defects provide an additional challenge to the prosthodontist because of the large amount of associated dead space that is created. Reconstruction is usually ideally accomplished through the use of a bulky soft-tissue free flap, such as a rectus abdominus, latissimus dorsi or anterolateral thigh flap to fill the midface volume, including the orbit (**Fig 3.2-11a**). These flaps can be supplemented with separate free nonvascularized bone grafts for additional structural support when the zygomaticoorbital complex is removed as part of the resection. This complex reconstruction in one study resulted in a fair cosmetic result in 46% of patients, normal or near-normal speech in 77%, and limitation to a soft diet in 54% [Cordeiro et al, 2000]. To achieve adequate bone volume for the infraorbital and zygomatic region as well as the alveolar arch, any of the bony options described above can be used but adequate soft tissue must be harvested to obliterate and/or line the orbital component of the defect.

In those cases where there is intracranial communication, the skull base must be sealed as well and cranial protection provided. The advantages of autogenous tissue to seal the skull base include its durability and viability.

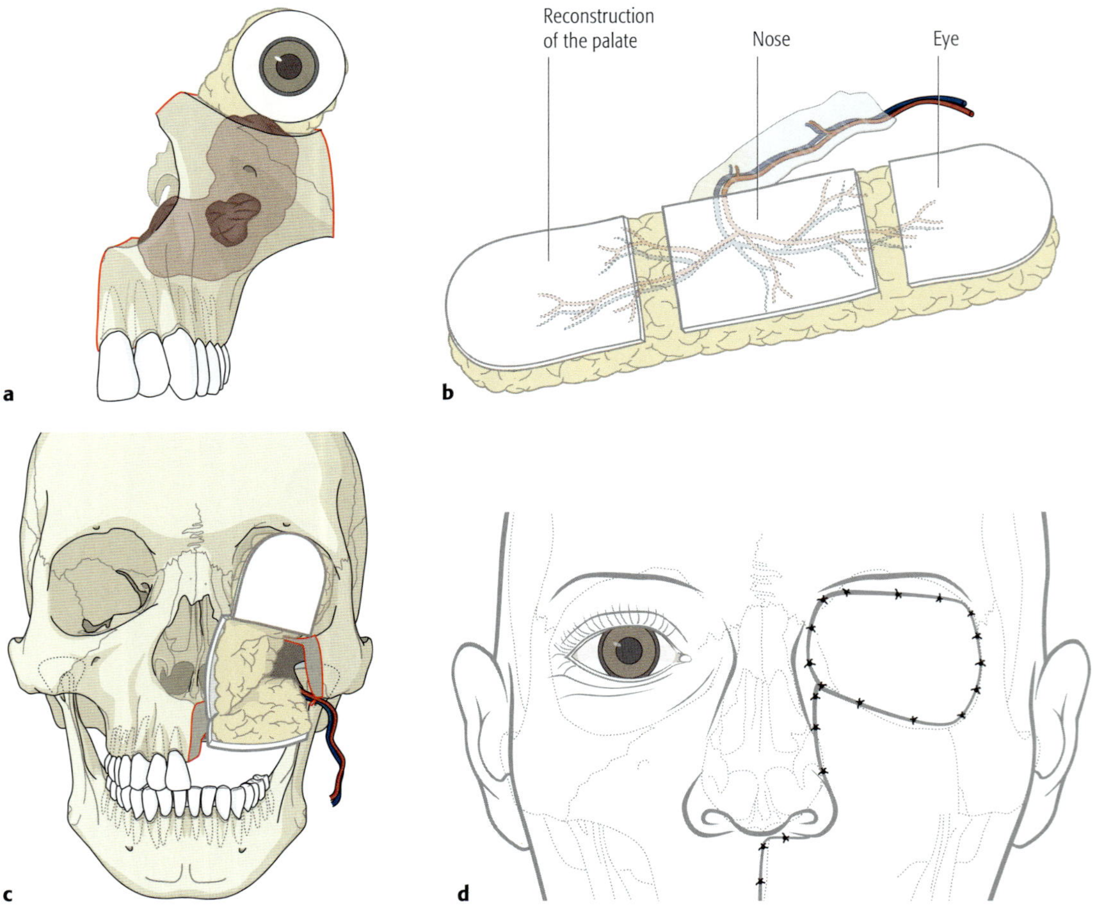

Fig 3.2-11a–d

- **a** Maxillectomy specimen including orbital exenteration.
- **b** Rectus abdominis free flap segmented to reconstruct the different components of the defect.
- **c** The free flap filling the defect with vessels exiting posteriorly. A coronoidectomy is performed to prevent impingement of the free flap vessels with mandibular motion. The distal cutaneous portion of the flap is used to seal the orbit.
- **d** The facial suture line.

4.3 Total maxillectomy

In individuals undergoing total maxillectomy, defects are created with insufficient retentive surfaces and without remaining dentition to support a conventional prosthesis. It is therefore preferable to reconstruct the area with vascularized bone and soft tissue to allow for closure of the palate, and a stable base for osteointegrated dental implants. Ultimately an implant-borne prosthesis will be added. The main determinants of which flap to use are the size of the palate's defect as well as whether there are additional areas that need bony support, such as the orbital floor or the malar eminence. Futran et al [2002] reported a series of 27 consecutive patients receiving a fibula free flap for reconstruction of maxillectomy defects involving the palate that were not amenable to an obturator. In this group, 18 patients received implants with fabrication of prostheses. Four patients had wound complications managed successfully with local wound care and there was one flap loss. All patients had intelligible speech over the telephone and all were able to resume an oral diet, with 14 patients on a regular diet and 13 using soft diet. The fibula free flap has a large amount of available bone, long pedicle length and minimal donor site morbidity and is the most popular choice for total maxilla reconstruction. Scapula flaps can be a versatile option for more complex defects but disadvantages include somewhat thinner bone that does not as reliably accept implants. Simultaneous midface surgery and flap harvest are not feasible. The iliac crest is less frequently used but provides excellent bone stock, though it has excessive bulk and a short vascular pedicle. Nonvascularized free bone grafts when used in combination with soft-tissue flaps can provide structure to the face, improving contour but they have not been shown to reliably accept dental implants and in addition resorb substantially and often almost completely.

An example of a total maxillectomy requiring fibula free flap reconstruction is shown in **Fig 3.2-12a–k**. The maximal length of bone is harvested, and osteotomies are then performed proximally and distally to allow for shaping of the neo-maxilla (**Fig 3.2-12e**). The vascular pedicle is then passed through a tunnel created in the cheek, into the neck for microanastomosis. This tunnel is usually made in a subcutaneous plane superficial to the facial nerve branches and should be able to accommodate at least two fingers to ensure adequate space for the vessels. This is simpler than going beneath the facial musculature and also avoids potential kinking of the vessels. Miniplates are then used to secure the fibula to the medial and lateral buttresses of the remnant midfacial skeleton (**Fig 3.2-12f**). The skin paddle of the fibula is then inset to reconstruct the mucosa of the palate (**Fig 3.2-12g**). Delayed placement of osteointegrated implants, a prosthesis, and a long-lasting stable result is shown in **Fig 3.2-12h–k**.

4.4 Donor site management

Management of each free flap donor site has been previously described in the literature. In short, the radial forearm free flap donor site should be closed with a split thickness skin graft and a bolster placed over the graft. The arm is then casted or placed in a volar splint for 7 days before removal to improve graft take. If bone is taken and the radius plated, arrange an appropriate follow-up with an orthopedic or hand specialist. After a fibula free flap, the donor lower leg should be cast with the ankle at a right angle for 5 days or 7 days if a skin graft is used at the donor site. The patients can then touch-down their body weight as tolerated. After the cast is removed, they can ambulate and work with physical therapy to optimize leg function. A splint should be placed to keep the foot at 90° to the leg when in bed. Flaps from the subscapular system require no particular rehabilitation care but closed suction drains should remain until a minimal output is achieved over several days to avoid seroma formation (minimal output less than 30 cc per day). Rectus abdominus and iliac crest donor sites require that the patient not strain or lift heavy objects for at least 2–4 weeks to avoid hernia formation.

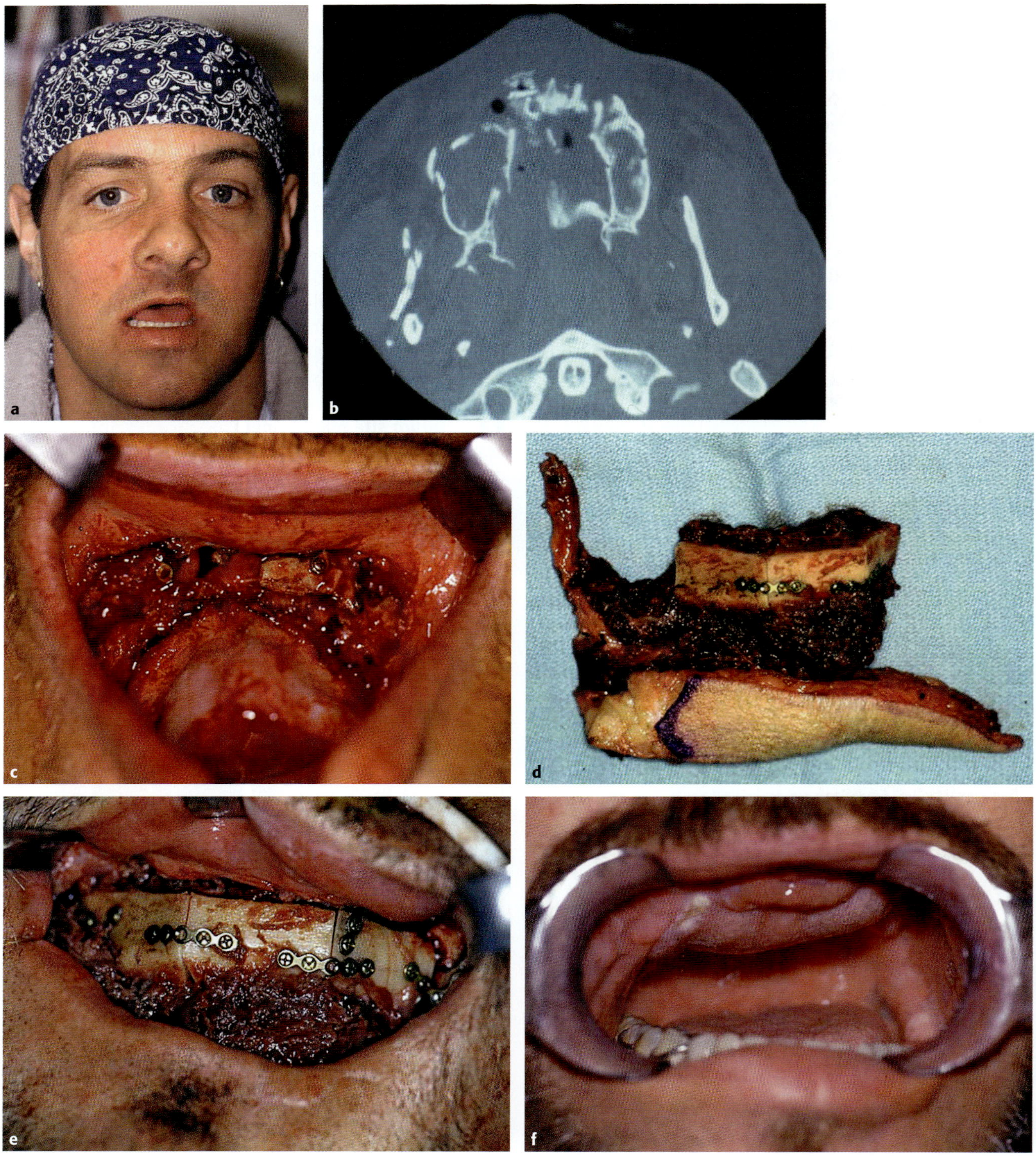

Fig 3.2-12a–k

- **a** A 32-year-old man 8 months after severe midface trauma with osteomyelitis and bone necrosis refractory to antibiotic therapy and requiring a total maxillectomy.
- **b** Axial computed tomographic scan showing loss of midface bone.
- **c** Intraoral defect with exposed maxillary bone and granulation tissue.
- **d** Fibula free flap fashioned for the inferior maxilla and alveolus.
- **e** A fibula flap replacing the inferior maxilla including the soft tissues of the alveolus and palate.
- **f** A 3-month postoperative view of the intraoral result.

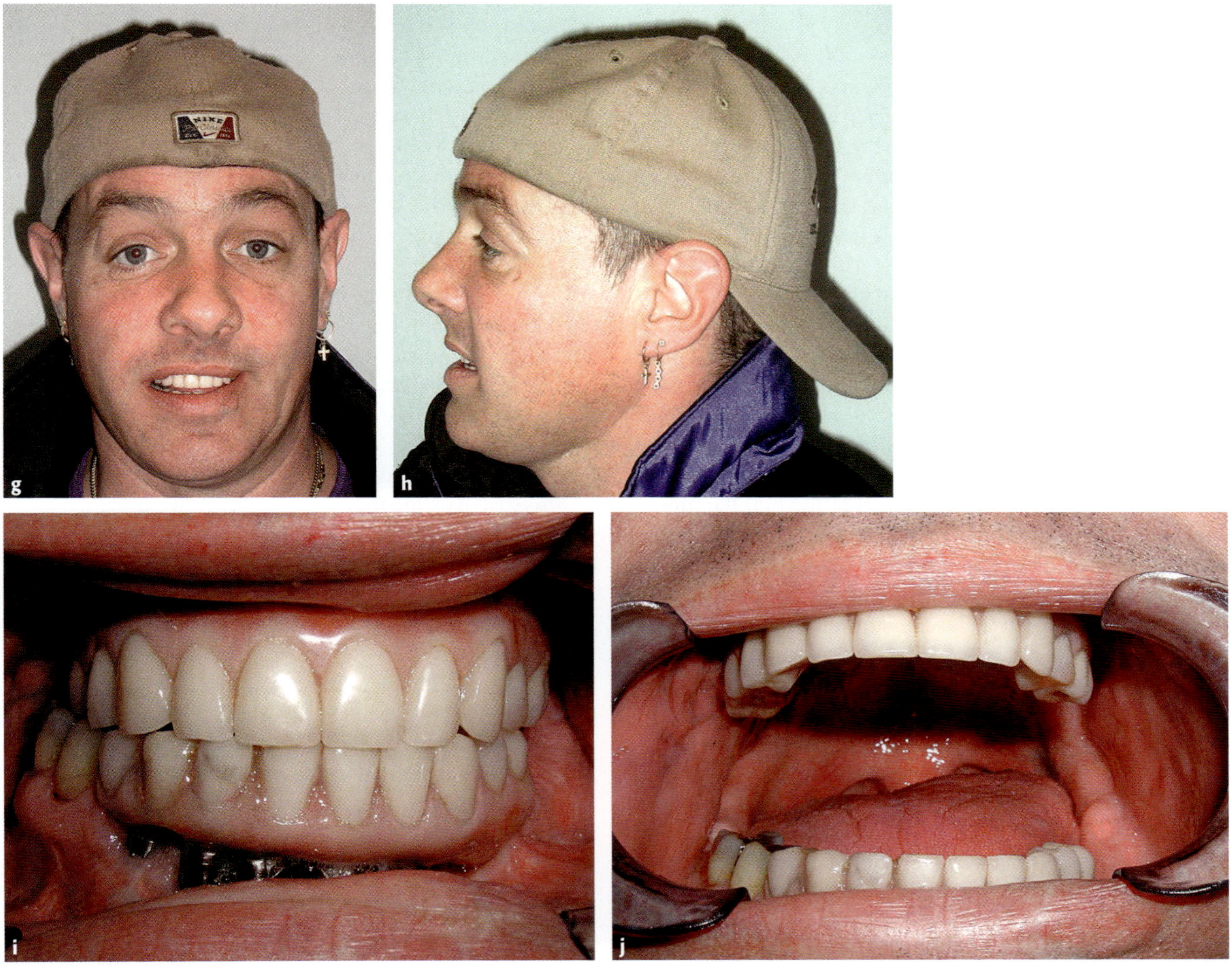

Fig 3.2-12a–k (cont)
g A 2-year postoperative anterior facial view.
h A 2-year postoperative lateral facial view.
i Implant-borne prosthesis in occlusion.
j Implant-borne prosthesis in open view.

5 Complications and pitfalls

Major potential complications from maxillary resection include substantial bleeding, especially from the retromaxillary venous plexus or the maxillary artery. A rare but significant complication is blindness following maxillectomies with preservation of the orbital content. A frequent adverse effect is sensory disturbances in the innervation areas of the infraorbital or/and zygomatic nerves. Those can be dysesthesias ranging from numbness to pain.

As a whole, free tissue transfer is relatively contraindicated in individuals with poor underlying health status or in those with a poor prognosis with expected short-term survival. In such instances, maxillary prostheses can be used in an effort to decrease operative time and morbidity. Specific contraindications also exist for each individual flap donor site. In instances where the morbidity from the flap harvest is unacceptable to the patient, a maxillary prosthesis or alternative simpler reconstructive technique should be considered. Temporoparietal fascial flaps and temporalis flaps are contraindicated in individuals where the superficial and deep temporal arteries have been sacrificed during past or the present surgical interventions. When selecting free tissue transfers, flaps with long pedicles are preferred to minimize the need for vein grafts. Upper neck recipient vessels are preferred for vessel anastomoses. Although the superficial temporal artery is reliable in most cases, the vein caliber and integrity are variable and the geometry is not ideal. A useful technique is to dissect facial vessels over the mandible, as these are excellent recipient vessels for anastomoses to bone flap vascular pedicles that are typically shorter than soft-tissue flap vascular pedicles. The surgeon must be prepared for using vein grafts, as the vascular pedicle of the flap may not always reach recipient neck vessels. A generous subcutaneous tunnel should be established between the maxilla and the neck vessels to allow for unrestricted and unkinked passage of the vascular pedicle. The coronoid process of the mandible can also be resected for additional space (**Fig 3.2-13**). When using bone flaps, the vascular pedicle can be pinched in between the bony segments and also in the pterygoid region. Careful attention to an absence of pedicle compression in these areas is mandatory. Residual maxillary bone for rigid fixation is limited. Miniplates 1.5 or 2.0 are preferred and the zygomatic buttress and piriform aperture areas provide the best anchorage. It is also critical to be totally comfortable with the geometry of the vascular pedicle before plating the bone of the flap because once the bone is secure and/or the soft tissue is inset, any adjustments are difficult. When the eye is preserved, correct orbital position is technically challenging to achieve and a forced duction test should always be done to make sure the globe is not entrapped by the reconstruction.

When a free flap is used, it must be regularly monitored to ensure vascular integrity.

In patients where there is an intraoral mucosal skin suture line, a feeding tube should be placed at the time of surgery allowing the patient to be kept nil per os for 5–7 days. If issues develop with velopharyngeal insufficiency or dysphagia, assessment by a speech and swallowing pathologist may be indicated. When the lateral nasal wall is reconstructed, especially when a bulky soft-tissue flap is used, the nasal airway should be stented with gauze packing or a Merocel sponge for 5 days. An obturator may be necessary thereafter in certain cases.

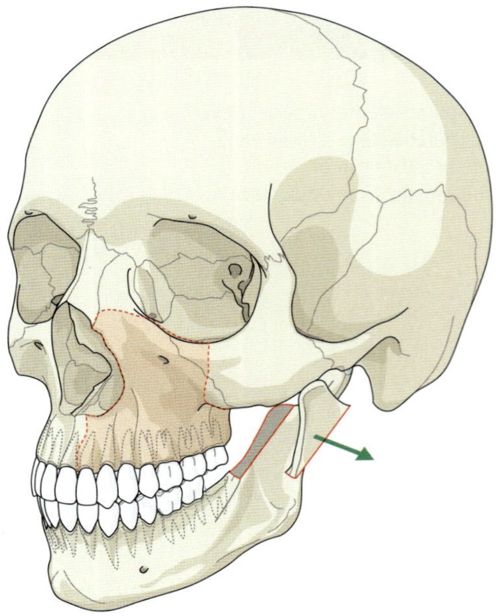

Fig 3.2-13 A coronoidectomy is performed to prevent impingement of the free flap vessels with mandibular motion.

6 References and suggested reading

Brown JS. Deep circumflex iliac artery free flap with internal oblique muscle as a new method of immediate reconstruction of maxillectomy defect. *Head Neck*. 1996 Sep–Oct;18(5):412–421.

Brown JS, Rogers SN, McNally DN, et al. A modified classification for the maxillectomy defect. *Head Neck*. 2000 Jan;22(1):17–26.

Brown JS, Shaw RJ. Reconstruction of the maxilla and midface: introducing a new classification. *Lancet Oncol*. 2010 Oct;11(10):1001–1008.

Browne JD, Burke AJ. Benefits of routine maxillectomy and orbital reconstruction with the rectus abdominis free flap. *Otolaryngol Head Neck Surg*. 1999 Sep;121(3):203–209.

Cordeiro PG, Santamaria E. A classification system and algorithm for reconstruction of maxillectomy and midfacial efects. *Plast Reconstr Surg*. 2000 Jun;105(7):2331–2346.

Cordeiro PG, Disa JJ. Challenges in midface reconstruction. *Semin Surg Oncol*. 2000 Oct–Nov;19(3):218–225.

Funk GF, Arcuri MR, Frodel JL Jr. Functional dental rehabilitation of massive palatomaxillary defects: cases requiring free tissue transfer and osseointegrated implants. *Head Neck*. 1998 Jan;20(1):38–51.

Futran ND, Haller JR. Considerations for free-flap reconstruction of the hard palate. *Arch Otolaryngol Head Neck Surg*. 1999 Jun;125(6):665–669.

Futran ND, Wadsworth JT, Villaret D, et al. Midface reconstruction with the fibula free flap. *Arch Otolaryngol Head Neck Surg*. 2002 Feb;128(2):161–166.

Futran ND. Retrospective case series of primary and secondary microvascular free tisssue transfer reconstruction of midfacial defects. *J Prosthet Dent*. 2001 Oct;86(4):369–376.

Genden EM, Wallace D, Buchbinder D, et al. Iliac crest internal oblique osteomusculocutaneous free flap reconstruction of the postablative palatomaxillary defect. *Arch Otolaryngol Head Neck Surg*. 2001 Jul;127(7):854–861.

Marshall DM, Amjad I, Wolfe SA. Use of the radial forearm flap for deep, central, midfacial defects. *Plast Reconstr Surg*. 2003 Jan;111(1):56–64; discussion 65–66.

McGregor IA, McGregor FM. Cancer of the face and mouth. In: *Pathology and Management for Surgeons*. 1st ed. New York: Churchill Livingstone; 1986:553.

Miles BA, Gilbert RW. Maxillary reconstruction with the scapular angle osteomyogenous free flap. *Arch Otolaryngol Head Neck Surg*. 2011 Nov; 137(11):1130–1135.

Parhiscar A, Har-El G, Turk JB, et al. Temporoparietal osteofascial flap for head and neck reconstruction. *J Oral Maxillofac Surg*. 2002 Jun;60(6):619–622.

Robb GL, Marunick MT, Martin JW, et al. Midface reconstruction: surgical reconstruction versus prosthesis. *Head Neck*. 2001 Jan;23(1):48–58.

Schliephake H. Revascularized tissue transfer for the repair of complex midfacial defects in oncologic patients. *J Oral Maxillofac Surg*. 2000 Nov;58(11):1212–1218.

Swartz WM, Banis JC, Newton ED, et al. The osteocutaneous scapular flap for mandibular and maxillary reconstruction. *Plast Reconstr Surg*. 1986 Apr;77(4):530–545.

Triana RJ, Uglesic V, Virag M, et al. Microvascular free flap reconstructive options in patients with partial and total maxillectomy defects. *Arch Facial Plast Surg*. 2000 Apr–Jun;2(2):91–101.

Uglesic V, Virag M, Varga S, et al. Reconstruction following radical maxillectomy with flaps supplied by the subscapular artery. *J Craniomaxillofac Surg*. 2000 Jun;28(3):153–160.

Wells MD, Luce EA. Reconstruction of midfacial defects after surgical resection of malignancies. *Clin Plast Surg*. 1995 Jan;22(1):79–89.

Yim KK, Wei FC. Fibula osteoseptocutaneous free flap in maxillary reconstruction. *Microsurgery*. 1994;15(5):353–357.

3.3 Ablative and reconstructive surgery of the orbit

Christopher Mohr, Roman P Pförtner, Alexander Metz

1 Introduction

1.1 Introduction and history

In addition to the eyeball, the orbit with its bony walls contains the eye muscles and nerves, fatty tissue and glandular structures of all germ layers. Therefore, various types of tumors can be found in the eye socket that are often associated with complex treatment requirements.

The most common symptom of orbital masses is exophthalmos. In addition to the visible protrusion of the globe, double vision, motility disorders, and a reduction in visual acuity, lateral and/or medial displacement and rotation of the eyeball may indicate an orbital tumor. Until the 19th century, orbital tumors, if they were operated on at all, were almost always treated by exenteration regardless of their pathology.

Advances in anesthesia and the introduction of osteotomy techniques have expanded the options for operations inside the orbit. In 1888, Krönlein was the first to describe the temporary resection of the lateral orbital wall for the removal of a dermoid while maintaining the eyeball. The mobilized piece of bone pedicled on the periosteum healed without any problems after tumor removal [Krönlein, 1888].

In 1941, Dandy could extirpate a meningioma in the optic canal for the first time via a transcranial access route after removing the orbital roof. Dandy subsequently proclaimed that this access route should be used for all orbital tumors [Dandy, 1941]. He even performed the first cranial bone graft, which he used in reconstruction.

Today, if an orbital lesion is suspected, operations can be planned based on computed tomographic (CT) scans and magnetic resonance imaging (MRI) procedures. The localization and size of the tumor and its anatomical link to the adjacent structures determines the most appropriate approach for the operation on a case-by-case basis. The globe is preserved if possible. The use of intraoperative navigation techniques can facilitate the removal of orbital tumors while maintaining function.

1.2 Etiology and epidemiology

The basis for exophthalmos in almost 50% of cases is endocrine orbitopathy, followed by inflammatory orbital pseudotumors. With few exceptions, the disease occurs on both sides. In contrast to this, orbital pseudotumors are responsible for approximately 16% of all one-sided cases of exophthalmos [Jones et al, 1979].

True orbital tumors are rare. The incidence varies between 3 and 20 cases per 1,000,000 people [Eldrup-Jörgensen, 1970; Henderson, 1987].

Epithelial neoplasias may originate from the conjunctiva or the lids but also from the lacrimal glands or the choroid. In terms of numbers, adenomas are the most common epithelial lacrimal gland tumors but carcinomas and other malignancies are also observed. Epidermoid cysts are typically localized in the orbit. Benign neurogenic tumors in the orbit that arise from the outer germ layer are also observed.

Mesenchymal tumors can originate from the extraocular muscles, the fatty tissue, the orbital vessels and more rarely the orbital bones. Here, the diagnostic spectrum ranges from benign cavernous angiomas, lipomas and osteomas to sarcomas and malignant lymphomas.

The most important and largest group of malignant neoplasias during childhood are rhabdomyosarcomas. However, benign orbital diseases and orbital dermoid are even more common in numbers and can make operations during early childhood a necessity.

In adults, endocrine orbitopathy is the most common orbital mass. Malignant lymphomas are observed frequently in patients older than 60 years [Shields et al, 2008].

In addition to this, orbital metastases and various primary tumors are also observed. Extension of sinonasal carcinomas may happen and can penetrate the orbit from the maxillary, ethmoid and/or frontal sinuses. Metastases, for instance from breast carcinomas or melanomas, are also observed and sometimes first occur more than 10 years after the primary treatment as an isolated manifestation.

2 Treatment principles

2.1 Interdisciplinary treatment concepts

The treatment of orbital masses and tumors should be an interdisciplinary task. Ophthalmology is usually the first point of contact for a patient affected by a tumor of the orbit. Frequently, an interdisciplinary treatment concept involves surgical and nonsurgical specialties. Common collaboration partners for orbital surgery includes, neurosurgeons, craniomaxillofacial surgeons, radiation oncologists, and medical oncologists in addition to ophthalmologists.

2.2 Presurgical diagnostics

The clinical symptoms of orbital tumors are often nonspecific and only rarely indicative of the diagnosis. Conclusions can be drawn about the location of the tumor based on a visible displacement of the globe, motility disorders, double vision, ocular pain or a reduction of visual acuity.

A complete ophthalmological evaluation includes assessment of visual acuity, motility and visual field testing. If applicable, it can be expanded by the determination of visually evoked potentials and eye pressure measurements that provide important results relating to the preoperative functional status of the diseased orbit. The patency and function of the lacrimal system should also be evaluated, as should ocular lubrication.

The CT and/or MRI show the exact location of the tumor and are indispensable in most cases.

2.3 Treatment principles

With the aid of modern imaging techniques for preoperative localization, the most gentle and accurate operative access route for each individual case can be determined and the risk of complications significantly reduced. A clear operative field with a wide osteotomy of the orbital walls prevents unnecessary intraoperative compression of the orbital contents, and significantly reduces postoperative dysfunction. It is also necessary to avoid long periods of traction on the globe or orbital muscles during the operation.

3 Surgical techniques

3.1 Biopsy and surgical planning

The confirmation of a diagnosis by means of a biopsy before the planning of a specific treatment is standard of care.

However, in the case of tumors in the retrobulbar area, it can be necessary to use complicated access routes to harvest representative tissue. The surgeon is then faced with the difficult decision of whether to remove the tumor entirely when first accessing the area. The depiction of the lesion in the MRI/CT image performed to plan the operation is also used for guidance. When there is a clear delineation between the tumor and the surrounding structures, an attempt should be made at primary total extirpation. This applies to most cavernous angiomas and many neurofibromas in the orbit.

An initial biopsy is a contraindication in the case of pleomorphic adenomas of the lacrimal gland as a significantly increased rate of recurrence is to be expected in the case of prior sample excision [Front et al, 1978; Henderson, 1987; Wright et al, 1992].

If epidermoid or dermoid cysts are expected because of the clinical presentation and imaging, the mass should be enucleated in total because biopsy may lead to a leakage of the contents of the cystic lesions and subsequent contamination of the orbital tissues. This may result in pronounced orbital inflammation and an increased rate of recurrence despite the subsequent extirpation of the cysts [Bartlett et al, 1993; Shermann et al, 1984].

3.2 Surgical approaches and techniques

3.2.1 Orbitotomies without osteotomy

Anterior orbitotomies with no additional osteotomies are suitable for sample biopsies and for encapsulated tumors in the anterior third of the orbit and with some limitations in the central third. In anterior orbitotomies without osteotomy of bony orbital walls, a distinction is made between transseptal and transperiosteal access routes.

In the transseptal approach, the fibers of the orbicularis oculi muscle are split in the direction of flow via an incision in the natural creases of the lid. Then the orbital septum is examined and opened (**Fig 3.3-1**). This operative technique is particularly suitable for dermoid cysts during childhood that are often localized in front of and behind the orbital septum. Difficulties can arise because benign tumors slide back into the depths of the orbit when an attempt is made to remove them, so it can be difficult to grip them.

Transperiosteal approaches for sample biopsies of undefined tumors are an alternative approach in case the mass is not located close to the skin. With this approach, the contact area between the anterior end of the orbit and the lids remain undisturbed.

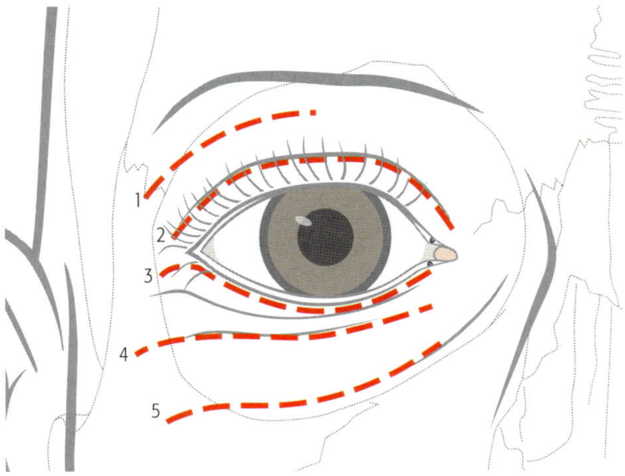

a

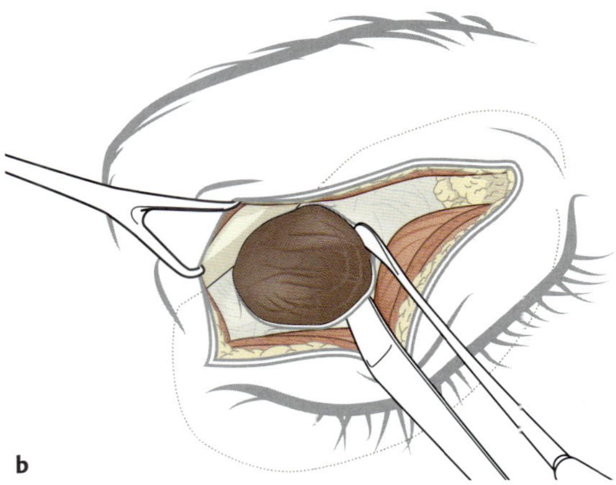

b

Fig 3.3-1a–b Transseptal interior orbitotomy.

a Marking of the skin incision in the natural skin folds of upper and lower lid.
 1 upper eyelid incision
 2 upper blepharoplasty incision
 3 subciliary incision
 4 mid eyelid
 5 infraorbital rim incision

b After splitting of the orbicularis oculi muscle the orbital septum is opened; the tumor is exposed, a biopsy specimen can be taken or the mass can be removed.

The skin incision is either made as an inferiormedial brow, lateral brow, orbital rim, mid eyelid, subciliary, or transconjunctival. The latter can, if necessary, be extended by a lateral canthotomy (**Fig 3.3-2**). The orbital septum remains intact in this process. After the incision of the periosteum, the orbital wall close to the tumor is exposed, the periorbital tissue is split in a sagittal direction and the orbital tumor is exposed. To do this, a sufficiently large incision must be made in the periorbital tissue (normally 90° of the orbital circumference). The subsequent closure of the wound is carried out in all anatomical layers in combination with a deep silicone drain.

Pitfalls

In single sample biopsies, the anterior periorbital area should remain intact to prevent a prolapse of the tumor out of the orbit.

3.2.2 Orbitotomies with osteotomy

Without the temporary removal of one or more orbital walls it is difficult to operate adequately on tumors in the central and posterior third of the orbit, if they are located inside the cone-shaped muscles of the orbit. In principle, all osteotomies should be carried out with fine saw blades or piezoelectric devices. The repositioning and stabilization of the osteotomy segment is then carried out using two single microscrews or microosteosynthesis plates 1.0 or 1.3.

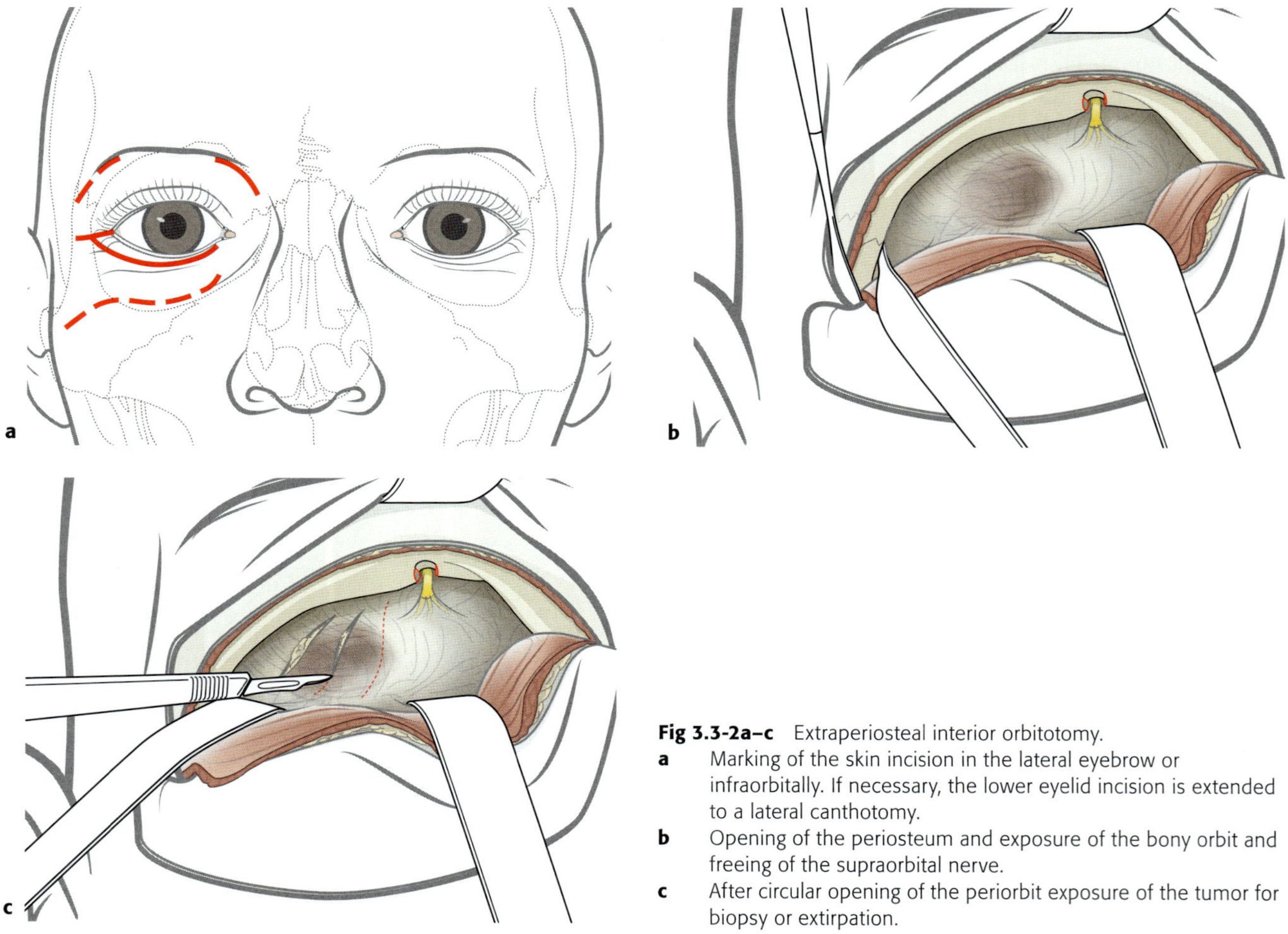

Fig 3.3-2a–c Extraperiosteal interior orbitotomy.

- **a** Marking of the skin incision in the lateral eyebrow or infraorbitally. If necessary, the lower eyelid incision is extended to a lateral canthotomy.
- **b** Opening of the periosteum and exposure of the bony orbit and freeing of the supraorbital nerve.
- **c** After circular opening of the periorbit exposure of the tumor for biopsy or extirpation.

3.2.2.1 Lateral orbitotomy

Since lacrimal gland tumors and most primary orbital tumors are both generally located lateral to the optic nerve, this access route frequently offers ideal conditions for removing tumors while maintaining function. In all orbitotomies with temporary removal of the lateral and/or superior orbital wall, a coronal incision is advantageous. The skin incision is taken down to the preauricular region on the tumor side. A subgaleal/epiperiosteal dissection up to approximately 2 cm above the eyebrow is performed (**Fig 3.3-3a**). At the height of the upper edge of the tragal cartilage, the external temporalis muscle fascia is incised and the incision is extended via the crista temporalis through the frontal periosteum to the contralateral side (**Fig 3.3-3b**).

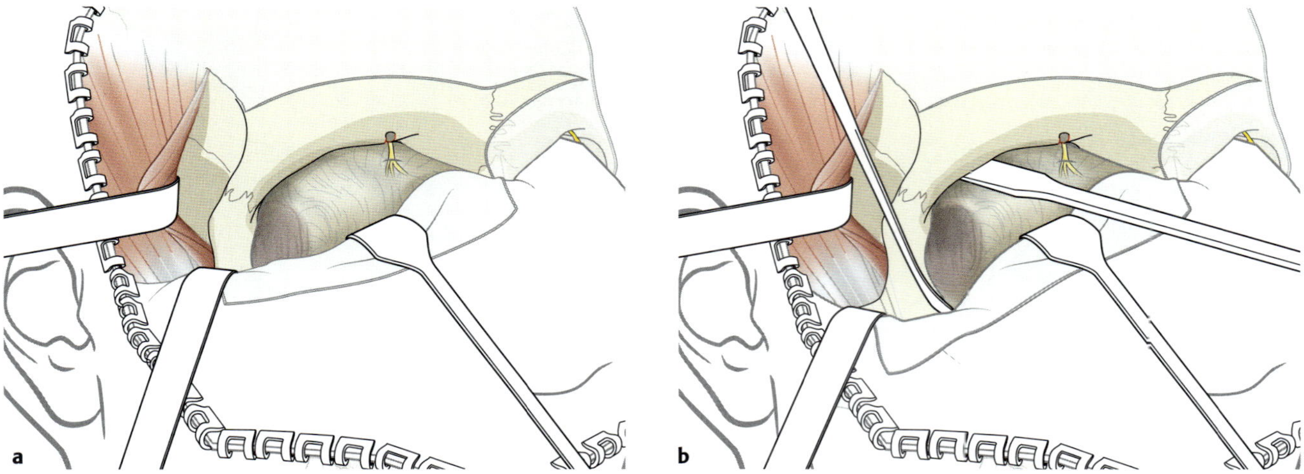

Fig 3.3-3a–b Exposure of the orbit via a coronal incision.
a Subperiostal elevation of the temporalis muscle. The facial nerve is not in the access route.
b 270° detachment of the periosteum. The tumor is well visible.

The course of the frontal branch of the facial nerve is localized using an electrical nerve stimulator. Dissection between the layers of the superficial and deep temporal fascia or under the anterior layer of the deep temporal fascia in the subfascial fat and the subperiostal frontal dissection guarantees reliable protection of this nerve and broad subperiostal exposure of the orbital rim. The frontal branch of the trigeminal nerve is then dissected from or released from the supraorbital foramen by means of chisel osteotomy and shifted into the orbit at the same time as the periorbital periosteum is detached (normally 270° of the orbital circumference). The temporalis muscle is released from the crista temporalis in the anterior third of the muscle and deflected in a dorsal (posterior) direction. It is recommended that a small rim of the muscle be left in the muscle's attachment to the crista temporalis for later suturing of the muscle to its insertion. The temporal fossa is completely exposed including the lateral orbit wall. A slight angular osteotomy is carried out through the lateral orbital rim (**Fig 3.3-4a**) down to the inferior orbital fissure. From there, a separation of the lateral orbital wall as far dorsal as possible in the junction between the lateral orbital wall and the temporal bone is performed. The saw cut runs above the frontozygomatic suture. The osteotomy is completed with osteotomes and the lateral segment of the orbit is temporarily removed (**Fig 3.3-4b**). The surgical assistant controls the orbital penetration depth of the saw blade during the osteotomy and protects the orbital content with a spatula.

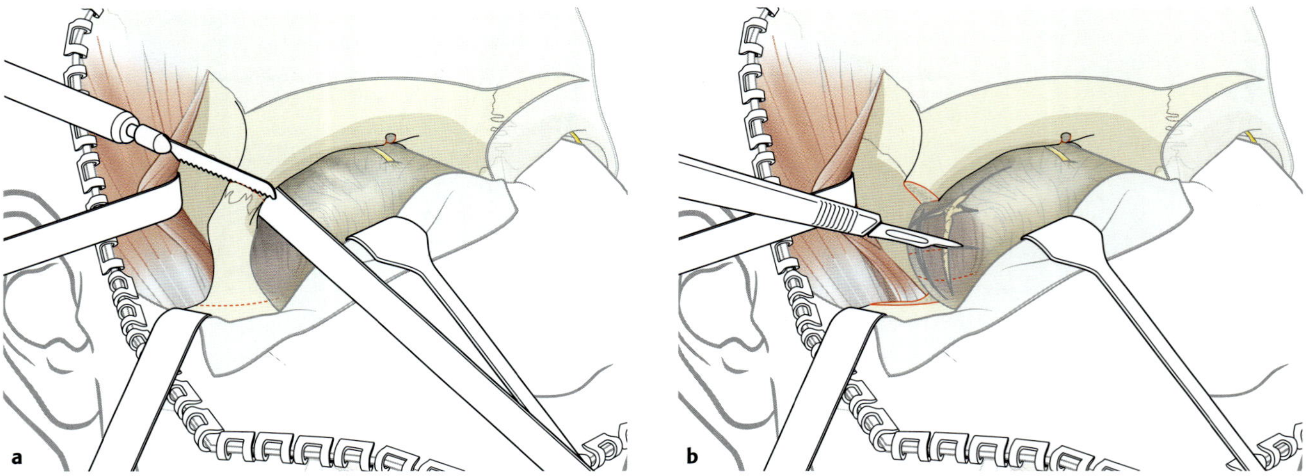

Fig 3.3-4a–b Lateral orbitotomy.
a Osteotomy through the lateral ring of the orbit down to the inferior orbital fissure, dorsally through the lateral orbital wall down to just above the frontozygomatic suture.
b Temporary removal of the bone, which allows complete access to the lacrimal gland and the lateral bulbar space. The periorbit is incised above the tumor.

3.2.2.2 Extended frontolateral orbitotomy

Tumors located in the intraconal and extraconal regions can be removed in a gentle manner via an extended frontolateral orbitotomy. Depending on the need, the lateral orbitotomy can be extended on an individual basis in a supraorbital and caudal lateral direction. The temporary removal of one or more orbital walls, if applicable with the zygoma and/or parts of the supraorbital edge enables clear and expanded access to the retrobulbar region. In doing this, the osteotomy is guided as a V-shape through the zygoma, and the zygomatic arches are detached from the articular tubercle at the temporomandibular joint. In the supraorbital area, the saw placement is supraorbital through the frontal bone.

3.2.2.3 Inferior orbitotomy

A temporary osteotomy of the infraorbital rim is used to expose tumors in the central and posterior thirds of the orbit caudal to the optic nerve. Above the infraorbital nerve, the bone can be mobilized. If a larger access route is needed, the infraorbital nerve, which runs directly through the operative area, must be completely freed from the mobilized segment (**Fig 3.3-5**). If necessary in the case of tumor expansion far into the medial/caudal direction, an inferior orbitotomy can be combined with an extended superolateral orbitotomy.

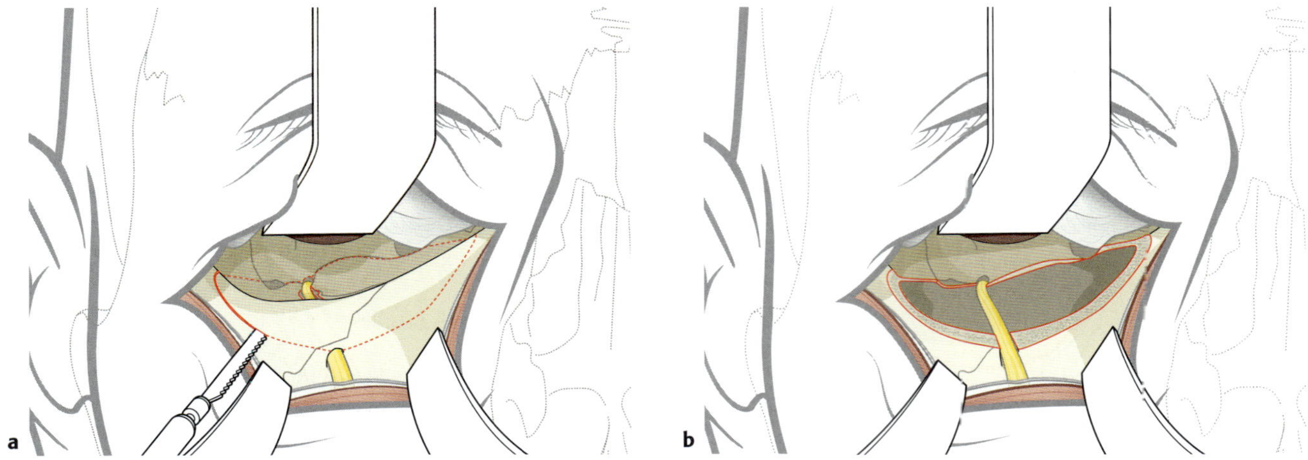

Fig 3.3-5a–b Inferior orbitotomy.

a Osteotomy of the infraorbital rim from the lacrimal duct area to the lateral orbit as well as the anterior floor of the orbit and temporary removal.

b Exposure of the inferior orbital content. Neurolysis of parts of the infraorbital nerve with careful bone resection to avoid nerve damage.

3.2.2.4 Medial orbitotomy

Medial orbitotomies are mostly carried out transnasally or transethmoidally. The operative technique corresponds to that of classic sinus surgery but is always osteoclastic and contains the risk of a postoperative enophthalmos. The indication is therefore present mostly in the case of endocrine orbitopathy, in which the existing exophthalmos should be corrected anyway. An alternative to the transnasal procedure is the transconjunctival/transcaruncular approach. It can be used provided there is strict protection of the nasolacrimal duct and the medial strip attachment (**Fig 3.3-6**). In combination with a lateral canthotomy, the lower lid is rendered free moving by this access route, which is why the operative technique is often referred to as "swinging eyelid approach" [McCord, 1981; Paridaens et al, 2006]. The resection of the lamina papyracea and the removal of the ethmoid mucosa, while maintaining the nasal ethmoid bone wall, can clearly be carried out in this way in endocrine orbitopathy. The connecting line between the anterior and posterior ethmoidal vessels, which are both coagulated and sharply detached from one another, defines the cranial limit of the decompression. If dissection and resection cranial to this line is performed, there is a risk of injury to the fila olfactoria and for a cerebrospinal fluid leak. The posterior ethmoidal foramen is the anatomical landmark to determine the limit of dorsal resection. As a rule the decompression ends here, as the optic nerve will enter the optic foramen 5 mm behind this point.

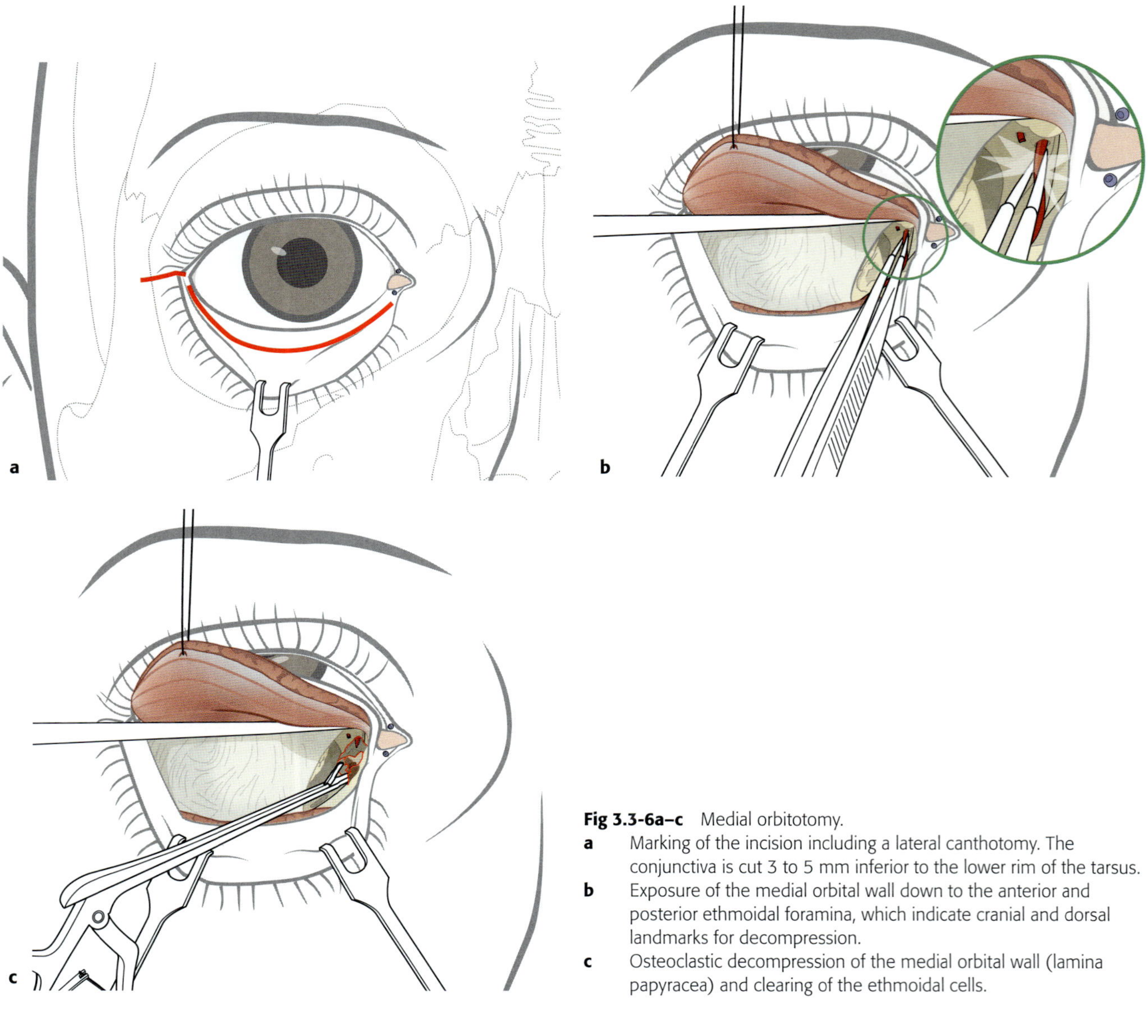

Fig 3.3-6a–c Medial orbitotomy.

- **a** Marking of the incision including a lateral canthotomy. The conjunctiva is cut 3 to 5 mm inferior to the lower rim of the tarsus.
- **b** Exposure of the medial orbital wall down to the anterior and posterior ethmoidal foramina, which indicate cranial and dorsal landmarks for decompression.
- **c** Osteoclastic decompression of the medial orbital wall (lamina papyracea) and clearing of the ethmoidal cells.

3.2.2.5 Superior orbitotomy with craniotomy

Tumors in the orbital apex, on the optic nerve sheath and in the optic canal require a transcranial orbitotomy. Today, as a modification of the original technique, the supraorbital rim is mostly included as part of various modifications of a frontoorbital or frontotemporoorbital osteotomy and is temporarily removed (**Fig 3.3-7**). Neurosurgeons first perform a craniotomy and remove a frontal or a frontotemporal bone flap. The dura is retracted with a brain spatula in the region of the planned orbitotomy and the orbital osteotomy is carried out. The orbital roof is then mobilized as far in the dorsal direction as possible and removed. After the opening of the dura, the optic nerve can be exposed in the intradural and extradural area from the optic nerve chiasm to the posterior aspect of the globe. The temporarily removed bone is later replanted and stabilized wth plates and screws.

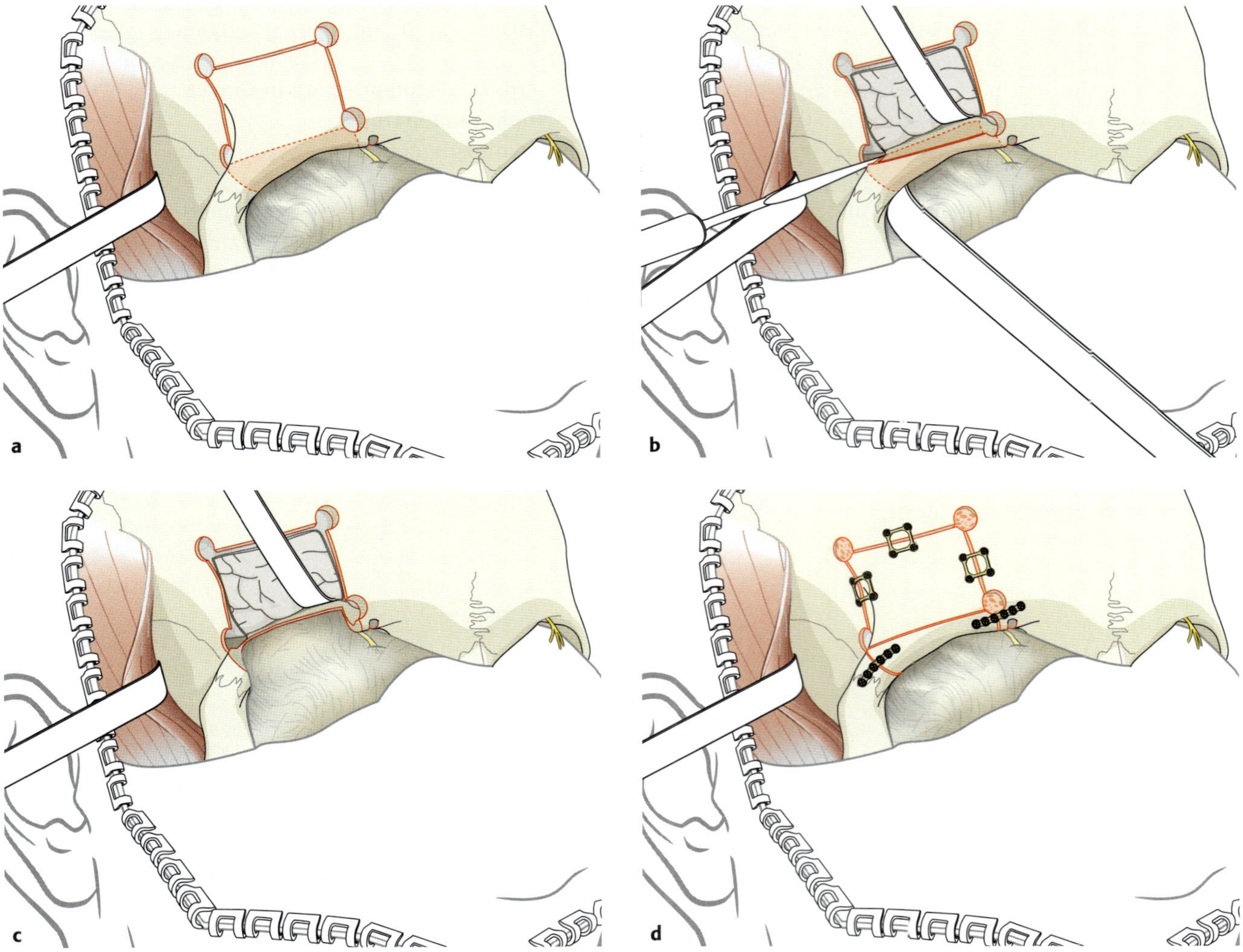

Fig 3.3-7a–d Superior orbitotomy with craniotomy.

a To prevent uncontrolled lacerations of the dura, the frontal or frontotemporal craniotomy is performed first.

b The orbital segment including the roof of the orbit is subsequently osteotomized and temporarily removed, under good visualization and protection of the dura.

c The total content of the orbit is accessible from the cranial aspect down to the foramen of the optic nerve.

d At the end of surgery, the whole bony orbit can be anatomically reconstructed.

3.3 Intraorbital tumor resection

Intraorbital tumor removal must strictly take place microsurgically, with magnifying glasses or microscopes. Initially, the periorbital area is split wide in a circle and in the radial direction with a small, long scalpel (always less than 90°). Using delicate dissecting movements, the orbital fatty tissue is dissected and the rectus eye muscles running through the fatty tissue and if applicable the frontal nerve are displayed. If the tumor is in a mediocranial position, the superior oblique muscle is also exposed in a strictly blunt manner in the region of the trochlea. Between the eye muscles the surgeon reaches the intraconal region. Most orbital tumors can be bluntly removed from the orbital fatty tissue provided they do not originate from the optic nerve, the optic nerve sheath or the muscles (**Fig 3.3-8**). Hemostasis in the orbital fatty tissue is carried out carefully with delicate bipolar forceps. After the extirpation of the tumor, the periorbital area is slightly approximated and sufficient drainage is allowed. The bony orbit is then carefully reconstructed.

Pitfalls

The less pressure and tensile force are exerted on the orbital soft tissue, the lower the risk of permanent losses of function of the orbital muscles and nerves. If there is any doubt, it is better to accept a subtotal removal of a benign tumor than to risk an irreversible loss of function of the orbital cardinal structures. Therefore, wide exposure is recommended (coronal over local).

Direct manipulation on a tumor edge facing the optic nerve is only carried out after the remaining surfaces of the tumor have been completely freed, as the vascular supply to this area via the optic nerve sheath is critical.

Close postoperative examination of pupil reactions and vision are essential to recognize intraorbital bleeding and increases in pressure that require early decompression.

Orbital tumors in the craniolateral area entail risk of complications due to their anatomical proximity to the superior orbital fissure and to the ciliary ganglion.

3.4 Orbital decompression in Graves' ophthalmopathy

In endocrine orbitopathy, there is an increase in volume in orbital muscles and the orbital fatty tissue due to a thyroid disease that causes the activation of lymphocytes, fibroblasts and an agglomeration of aminoglycans and tissue fluid. In addition to the clinically visible exophthalmos, compression of the optic nerve can ultimately lead to an acute or slowly progressing loss of vision.

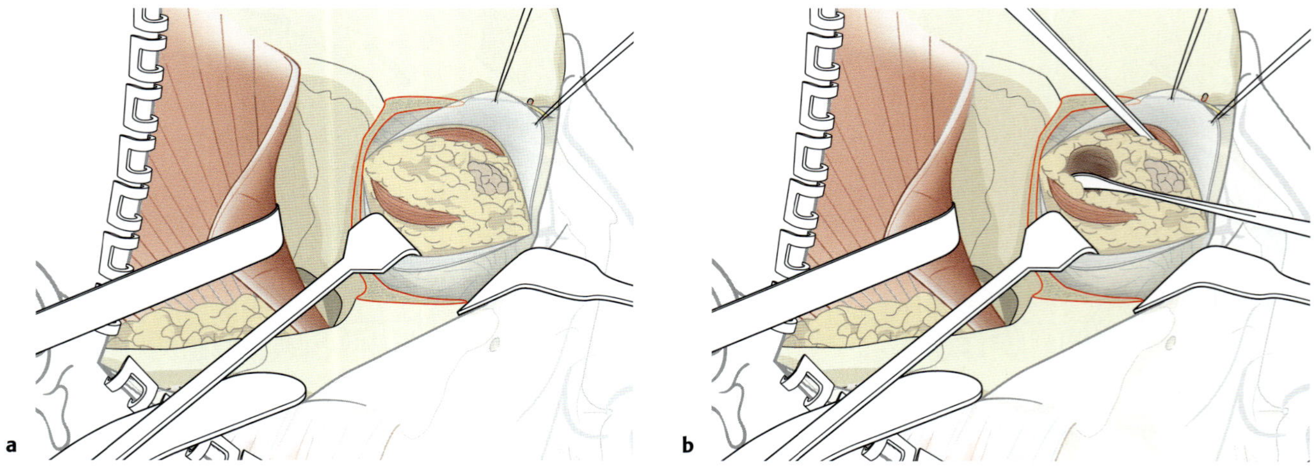

Fig 3.3-8a–b Intraorbital tumor removal.
a Wide opening of the periorbit around the tumor and exposure of the straight eye muscles.
b Blunt dissection of the orbital fatty tissue exposes the tumor and allows mobilization and resection of the tumor.

3.4.1 Bony three-wall decompression and fatty tissue reduction

In the case of endocrine orbitopathy, the principle of the operative procedure involves increasing the orbital volume and simultaneously decreasing the space required. The space available in the orbit can be increased by resecting one or more orbital walls, thereby expanding the orbit in the direction of the maxillary sinus, ethmoid bone cells, temporal fossa or in the direction of the frontal sinus cavity. The three-wall decompression of the caudal, lateral and medial walls is most common for pronounced cases (**Fig 3.3-6** and **Fig 3.3-9**). Diamond-coated ball cutter burs are particularly suitable for the removal of bone as the bone can be removed without any pressure being exerted while simultaneously protecting the infraorbital nerve, the temporalis muscle and the periorbital area. In the medial direction, the ethmoid bone is cleared including the mucosal lining. Among other things, fine bone punches are used for this. The orbital requirement for space is decreased by reducing the orbital fatty tissue. In patients with endocrine orbitopathy, the increase in the volume of the orbital content puts the fatty tissue under so much pressure that it springs up without

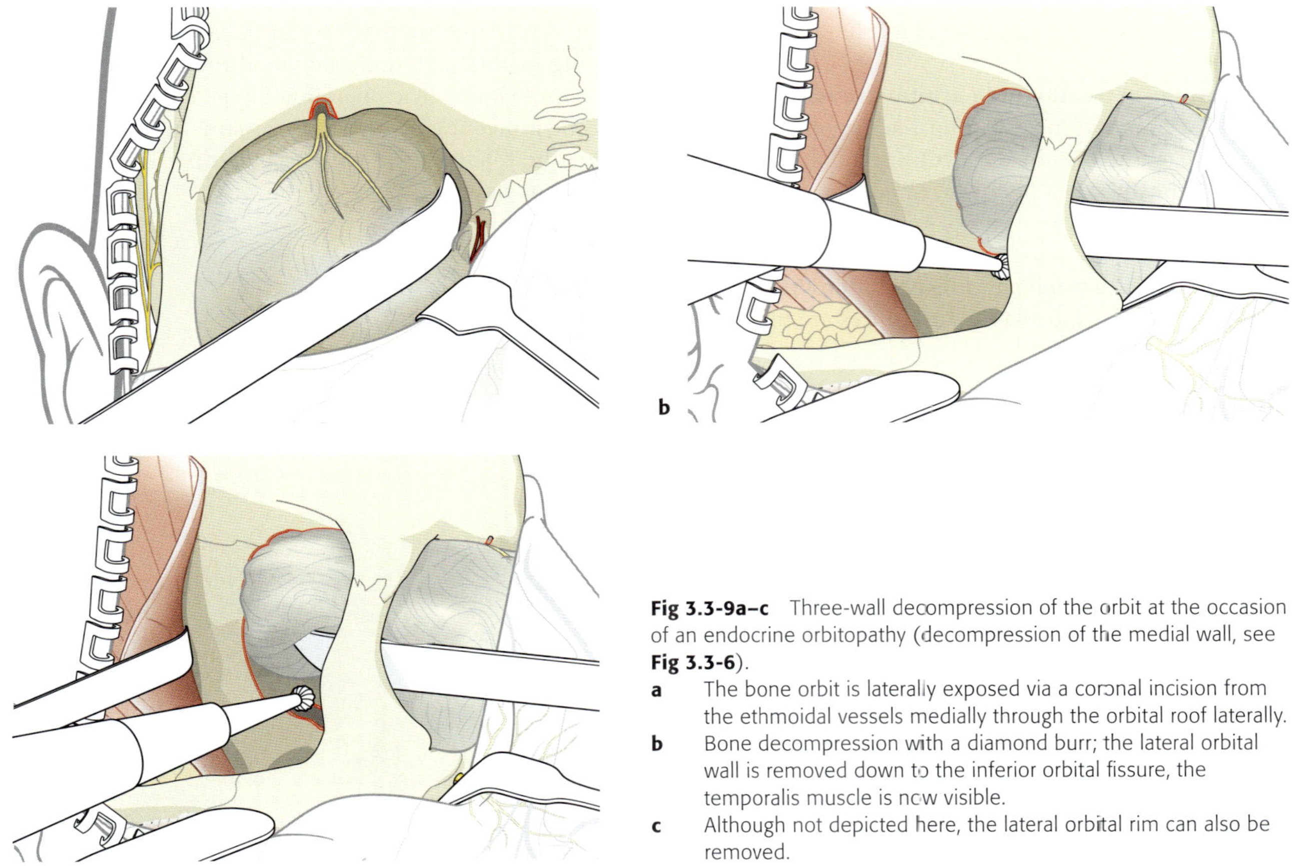

Fig 3.3-9a–c Three-wall decompression of the orbit at the occasion of an endocrine orbitopathy (decompression of the medial wall, see **Fig 3.3-6**).

- **a** The bone orbit is laterally exposed via a coronal incision from the ethmoidal vessels medially through the orbital roof laterally.
- **b** Bone decompression with a diamond burr; the lateral orbital wall is removed down to the inferior orbital fissure, the temporalis muscle is now visible.
- **c** Although not depicted here, the lateral orbital rim can also be removed.

being forced after the radial opening of the periorbital area and can thus be reduced (**Fig 3.3-10**). The infraorbital nerve and the orbital muscles must be identified and protected.

Pitfalls

The bone resection is always performed before the opening of the periorbital area and therefore before the fatty tissue reduction. Otherwise the fatty tissue that springs up significantly disrupts the overview of the operation field and may be the reason for the risk of injury to orbital muscles and nerves.

In the case of long-term endocrine orbitopathy the fatty tissue may be more strongly fibrosed and solid, so its surgical reduction is only achieved gradually and to a limited extent.

3.5 Surgical treatment in orbital pseudotumors

In case of pseudotumors (tumor like lesions), like orbital lymphomas, the task of the CMF surgeon is primarily to establish the diagnosis by means of a biopsy. In the case of treatment refractory progression or a recurrence of the disease, however, the maximum operative reduction of the diseased tissues in combination with antiproliferative/cytostatic and radiotherapy based procedures are indicated.

For surgical procedures, the most extensive exposure of the orbital content must be achieved by means of a maximally extended orbitotomy to be able to reduce or resect poorly delineated, strongly adherent pseudotumors, while maintaining the function of the eye muscles. Like endocrine orbitopathy, the objective of the operation is to decompress the remaining orbital structures. In rare cases, if all attempts to carry out treatment while maintaining the function are unsuccessful, it may be necessary to remove the entire orbital content.

3.6 Enucleation and exenteration of the orbital content

3.6.1 Enucleation of the globe

For ocular tumors that cannot be cured with the eyeball being maintained, the removal of the eyeball is the treatment of choice. The operation aims to remove the eyeball while protecting the eye muscles and the lids. Patients can then be rehabilitated with a conventional eye prosthesis made of glass or plastic.

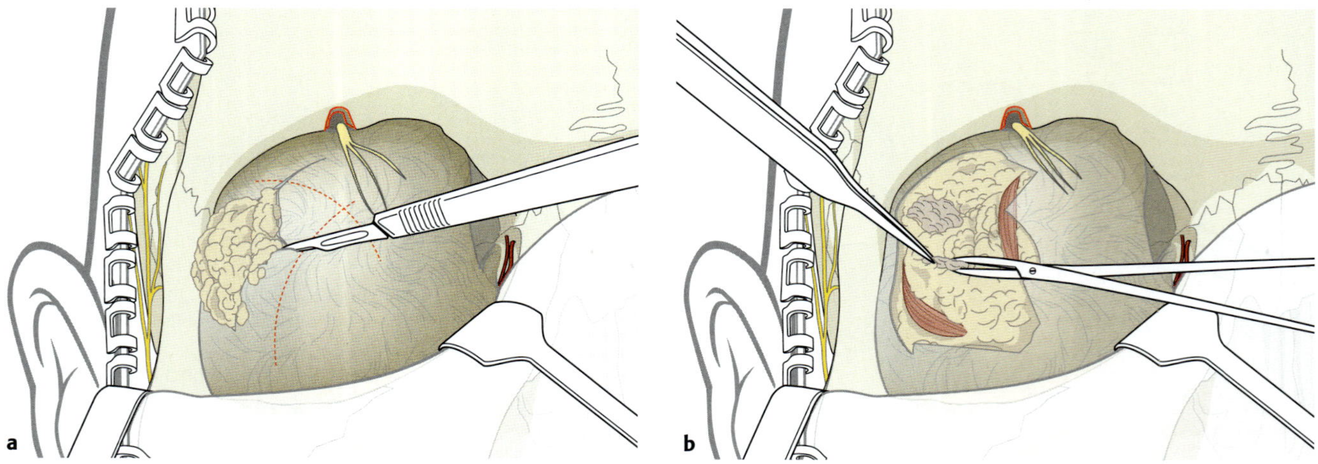

Fig 3.3-10a–b Intraorbital reduction of fatty tissues in the situation of an endocrine orbitopathy.
a Protrusion of the orbital fatty tissue after radial incision of the periorbita following the bony orbital decompression.
b Reduction of fatty tissue in one quadrant. This can continue to all quadrants with protection of orbital muscles and nerves.

3.6.1.1 Operative technique

To be able to remove the eyeball while protecting the rectus eye muscles, the muscle attachments on the globe must first be exposed. To do this, the connective tissue on the globe is subtly split, for example using a small, sharp pair of scissors, from the lateral to the medial angle of the lid, leaving out the corneal limbus, and exposing the sclera. If the connective tissue should also be partially or totally removed because of a tumor, a lateral canthotomy will expand the view significantly. In these cases, the edges of the lid in the lateral canthus are marked using a pinprick and methylene blue, the canthus is opened with a scalpel and the incision is expanded in a lateral direction in a natural fold of the skin as far as the orbital rim. The everted lids are then dissected on the tarsal plate as far as the area above the fornix, and the conjunctiva on the corneal limbus is left pedicled. In doing so, the surgeon reaches the sclera and can then expose the muscle attachments. The muscle attachments of the four rectus eye muscles are marked with blunt nerve retractors. The muscle attachments are then consecutively ligated with 5-0 sutures and divided from the episcleral layer using scissors. The sutures are left primarily uncut in order that all the muscle attachments can later be combined with one another to form a movable muscle stump. This is followed by the retrobulbar blunt preparation of the optic nerve at the location where it enters the eye socket. The optic nerve must then be sharply divided using a curved pair of scissors. Arterial bleeding from the central artery is localized and meticulous hemostasis is accomplished. A decision must be made as to how the loss of orbital volume, which has occurred because of the removal of the globe, can be replaced. Alloplastic spheres may be used for this. In addition to these, dermal fat grafts, for example from the buttock region, have proven particularly effective for autogenous replacement of volume. The extraocular muscles may be sutured to an eyeball prosthesis. Some prostheses have a pin for attachment to a scleral shell for movement.

Pitfalls

In each case, the central positioning of the implant or transplant is crucial to the later esthetics of the eye prosthesis.

In the case of extensive conjunctival resections, however, a lining of the conjunctival sac with mucous membrane or split skin grafts is necessary. The final eye prosthesis can then be manufactured and integrated into the eye socket.

3.6.2 Orbital exenteration

In cases of benign orbital diseases, a radical clearing of the orbital contents can rarely be justified. Exenteration is almost exclusively reserved for malignant tumors [Mohr, 1995].

The extent of the accompanying bone and soft-tissue resections varies significantly depending on the clinical problem, resulting in defects with a wide spectrum of reconstructive challenges.

3.6.2.1 Operative technique

In the classic orbital exenteration procedure, the orbital contents including the lids are removed.

A procedure of this type is typically indicated if the anterior third of the orbit is affected by a malignant orbital tumor. The operation starts with the suturing of the upper and lower lids using 4-0 sutures, which are used as traction threads. The skin is detached above and below the tarsal plate. The lid band attachments are incised in medial and lateral directions (**Fig 3.3.11**). Following the circular separation of the orbicularis oculi muscle, the periosteum of the orbital ring is incised and the lid band attachments are detached from the bony orbit. The periorbital area is then dissected all the way around in a subperiostial plane. This includes a separation of the nasolacrimal duct and a detachment of the inferior oblique muscle from the medial orbital rim. In the cranial direction, the frontal nerve must be coagulated and detached. In the caudal direction, dissection is carried out above the bony floor of the orbit and the infraorbital nerves pushed downward. One small artery and one vein on the nerve at the height of the inferior orbital fissure must be coagulated and detached. The contents of the inferior fissure, which only contains vessels and connective tissue, is then sharply detached. The bands of the connective tissue and the nerves that go through the superior orbital fissure are coagulated and divided. With a pull on the lid traction sutures, the orbital content is now increasingly mobile, so ultimately the optic nerve in the orbital funnel is severed using curved scissors. After the exenteration of the orbital contents, bipolar coagulation is carried out on the arterial bleeding from the central artery of the optic nerve stump, and meticulous hemostasis is accomplished. The exenteration of the orbit conserving the eyelids is shown in **Fig 3.3-12**.

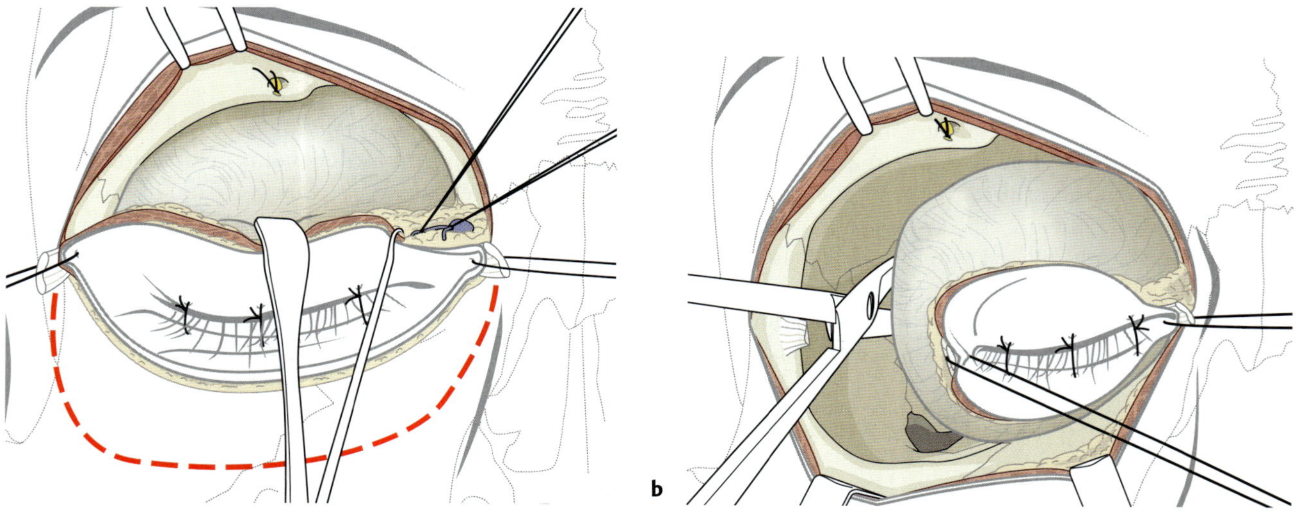

a

b

Fig 3.3-11a–b Exenteration of the orbit.

a The eyelids are closed with 4.0 sutures and skin incisions above and below the tarsal plates are performed. Circular dissection of the orbital ring and 360° freeing of the periorbit and cutting of the ligaments of the eyelids, the frontal nerve, the nasolacrimal duct and the contents of the orbital fissures.

b Transsection of the optic nerve in the orbital cone and removal of the orbital contents. Coagulation of the central artery needs to be performed.

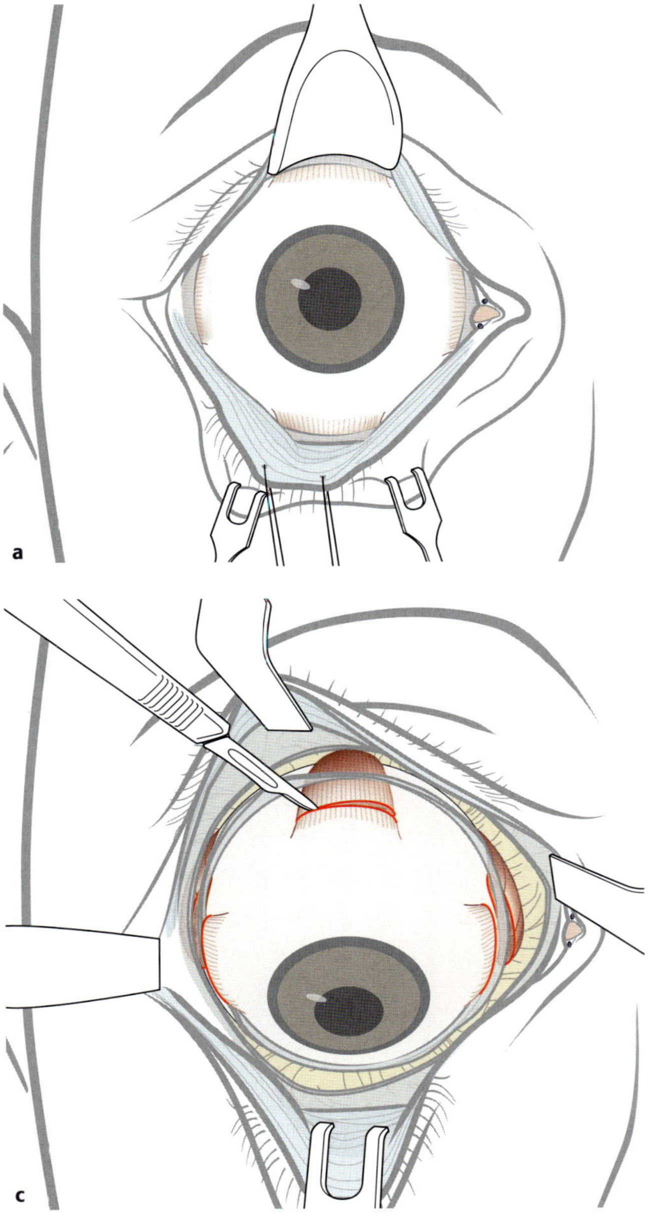

Fig 3.3-12a–c Orbital exenteration conserving the eyelids.
a Incision through the conjunctiva of the globe in a circular manner along the limbus corneae.
b Incision of the periosteum behind the medial insertion of the lid ligament.
c Exenteration of the orbital content conserving the eyelids.

Pitfalls

When dissecting the contents of the orbit, high levels of pressure on the thin orbital walls must be avoided primarily in the medial direction not to risk any orbitonasal connection with subsequent fistula formation.

3.6.2.2 Reconstruction after orbital exenteration

Various methods are indicated for sealing of an orbital exenteration cavity [Levin et al, 1991]. Wherever possible, the eyelids and the conjunctiva should be maintained during resection. In this way, they can partially be used as an epithelial lining of the eye socket in the anterior section. Parts of the temporalis muscle, the frontalis muscle, or galea-periosteum layers from the cranial dissection may be mobilized as vascularized tissue. Free tissue flaps, such as radial forearm flaps, for example, which can be inserted into the eye socket and will be connected via revascularization can be utilized in larger defects. After the orbital exenteration with resection of the eyelids, pedicled flaps from the neighbourhood can be brought into the orbit to cover the bone. Median frontal flaps, lateral frontotemporal skin flaps, retroauricular flaps and cheek rotation flaps are suitable for this. The frontal flap is dissected in the median or paramedian epiperiostal region and embedded as a tunnel flap under the eyebrow.

Osseointegrated implants are particularly suitable for the fixation of an orbital prosthesis. The implants can be anchored in the orbital area as part of the primary operation. After a covered healing phase of 3–6 months, they are exposed in a secondary operation and combined with mechanical or magnetic abutments to which the facial prosthesis is anchored.

Pitfalls

To avoid orbitonasal fistulae that can be associated with nasal drainage under the eye prostheses and nasal speech, the majority of all exenteration cavities are now surgically sealed.

An outflow drainage in the posterior third of the orbit and a gentle pressure bandage are necessary to ensure that a flap attaches to the orbital walls without creating a cavity. This is the only way to ensure that an adequate prosthesis position can be achieved.

4 References and suggested reading

Bartlett SP, Lin KY, Groosman R, et al. The surgical management of orbitofacial dermoids in the pediatric patient. *Plast Reconstr Surg*. 1993 Jun;91(7):1208–1215.

Dandy W. *Orbital Tumors: Results Following the Transcranial Operative Attack*. New York: Oscar Priest; 1941:161–164.

Eldrup-Forgensen P. Primary, histologically confirmed orbital tumours in Denmark 1943–1962: histopathological and prognostic studies. *Acta Ophthalmol (Copenh)*. 1970;48(4):657–661.

Font RL, Gammel JW. Epithelial tumours of the lacrimal gland: an analysis of 265 cases. In: Jakobiec FA, ed. *Ocular and Adnexal Tumours*. Birmingham: Aesculapius; 1978:787–805.

Henderson JW. Adenoid cystic carcinoma of the lacrimal gland, is there a cure? *Trans Am Ophthalmol Soc*. 1987;85:312–319.

Jones IS, Jacobiec FA. *Diseases of the Orbit*. Hagerstown, Md: Harper & Row; 1987:187–261.

Krönlein RU. [Zur Pathologie und operativen Behandlung der Dermoidcysten das Orbita.] *Beitr Klin Chir*. 1988;4:149–163. German.

Levin PS, Ellis DS, Stewart WB, et al. Orbital exenteration: the reconstructive ladder. *Ophthal Plast Reconstr Surg*. 1991;7(2):84–92.

McCord CD Jr. Orbital decompression for Grave's disease: exposure through lateral canthal and inferior fornix incision. *Ophthalmology*. 1981 Jun;88(6):533–541.

Mohr C, Seifert V, Esser J. [Zur Exenteratio orbitae: Individualisierung des operativen und rekonstruktiven Vorgehens.] *Dtsch Z Mund Kiefer GesichtsChir*. 1995;19:55–61. German.

Mohr C. *[Gesichtschirurgischer Beitrag zur Therapie orbitaler Tumoren. Fortschritte der Kiefer- und Gesichts-Chirurgie, Sonderband Orbita.]* Stuttgart: Thieme; 1995:35–44. German.

Paridaens D, Lie A, Grootendorst RJ, et al. Efficacy and side effects of 'swinging eyelid' orbital decompression in Grave's orbitopathy: a proposal for standardized evaluation of diplopia. *Eye (Lond)*. 2006 Feb;20(2):154–162.

Sherman RP, Rootman PJ, Lapointe JS. Orbital dermoids: clinical presentation and management. *Br J Ophthalmol*. 1984 Sep;68(9):642–652.

Shields JA, Shields CL. Eyelid, conjunctival and orbital tumors. In: *An Atlas and Textbook, 2nd ed*. Philadelphia: Lippincott Williams & Wilkins; 2008:745–766.

Wright JE, Rose GE, Garner A. Primary malignant neoplasms of the lacrimal gland. *Br J Ophthalmol*. 1992 Jul;76(7):401–406.

3.4 Secondary frontal sinus surgery

Jeffrey Haller, Neal D Futran

1 Indications and planning

The most common indication for secondary frontal sinus surgery is frontal sinus disease. This includes mucoceles, mucopyoceles, and chronic sinusitis. The disease process most often involves obstruction of the frontal recess. The nasofrontal orifice is the opening from the frontal sinus into the nasal cavity, which drains through the frontal recess (**Fig 3.4-1**). Obstruction anywhere along the outflow system, whether at the nasofrontal orifice or throughout the frontal recess, prevents the outflow of mucus from the sinus resulting in frontal sinus disease. Causes of frontal sinus obstruction include acute or chronic sinusitis. Patients can have polyps blocking the frontal recess or edematous mucosa, which is often associated with allergies. There can be congenital narrowing of the frontal recess or with chronic sinusitis the bone becomes osteitic and the outflow system is narrowed. Additionally, a common cause of frontal sinus obstruction is trauma resulting in a fracture through the nasofrontal orifice or frontal recess (**Fig 3.4-2**) [Stanley et al, 1987].

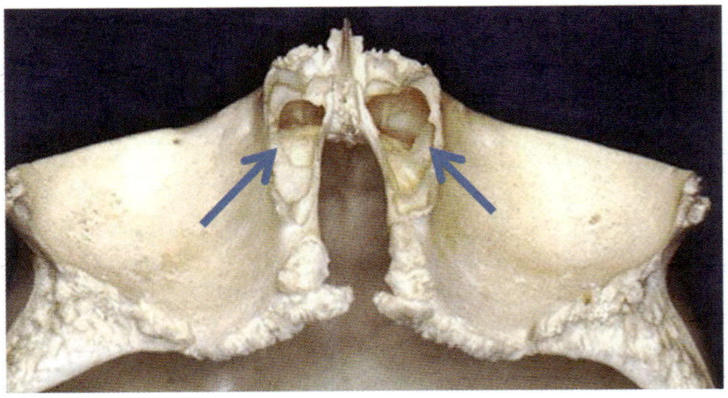

Fig 3.4-1 Submental view of the skull base showing the frontal sinus orifices (arrows).

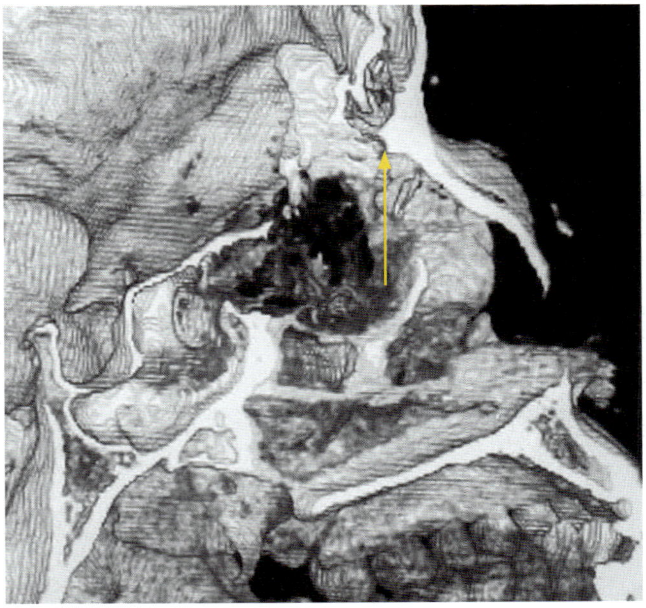

Fig 3.4-2 Sagittal view of the frontal recess (arrow).

In managing trauma to the frontal sinus, most injuries are repaired primarily. However, there are indications for secondary frontal sinus surgery subsequent to trauma. A cerebrospinal fluid (CSF) leak can be caused by frontal sinus fracture with disruption of the dura and the posterior table of the frontal sinus; however, there may be a delay before the leak presents itself. The fistula can be misdiagnosed or delayed secondary to edema associated with the injury, blood clots, or a blood-filled sinus obstructing the outflow. Once the edema subsides or lysis of the blood clot occurs, the fistula can present itself as CSF rhinorrhea. This would be an indication for secondary exploration of the sinus. Additionally, fractures through the posterior table of the frontal sinus can lead to other late complications. These complications include epidural abscess formation or meningitis (**Fig 3.4-3**). Both processes require either decompression or elimination of the frontal sinus disease. Fractures of the anterior table of the frontal sinus that are displaced may result in cosmetic deformities. Because of associated soft-tissue edema, the fractures can be missed or the severity not appreciated with a resultant secondary defect. If the defect is significant, a secondary reconstruction is indicated.

Planning for secondary frontal sinus surgery typically involves a fine-cut computed tomographic (CT) scan, both axial and coronal. While the axial cuts of the CT scan best delineate the anatomy of the anterior and posterior tables of the frontal sinus, the coronal images can be helpful with the nasofrontal recess and the floor of the frontal sinus. Magnetic resonance imaging (MRI) is most often not necessary in imaging frontal sinus disease or trauma. However, large mucoceles or mucopyoceles can destroy the posterior wall of the sinus with a significant intracranial component. An MRI may be helpful in delineating the soft-tissue differences of the mucocele and dura.

When CSF leaks are present, other forms of imaging may be helpful in localizing the leak. In addition to standard fine-cut CT scans, CT scanning with the use of intrathecal nonionic contrast can demonstrate the leak. Radionuclide scans are used with a combination of intranasal pledgets in an attempt to localize the area of the CSF leak. A 6′ Caldwell plain film is often used as a template of the anterior table of the frontal sinus (**Fig 3.4-4**). Care must be taken so the x-ray is not magnified but taken at exact anatomical size. The template is created from the x-ray, sterilized, and brought intraoperatively for precise bone cuts so the sinus is completely opened without intracranial injury. Typically, this is done with an osteoplastic flap leaving the periosteum attached inferiorly, which is one of the most common approaches to the frontal sinus during secondary frontal sinus surgery. Image guidance with an image-guided CT can provide similar guidance to the sinus boundaries allowing for safe osteotomies into the sinus.

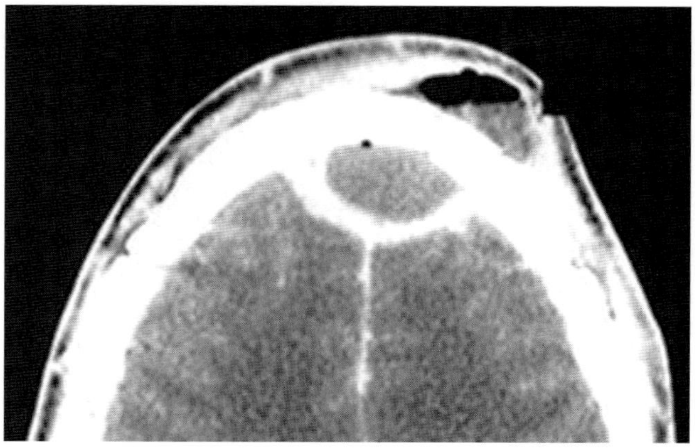

Fig 3.4-3 Axial computed tomographic scan of epidural abscess from frontal sinus disease.

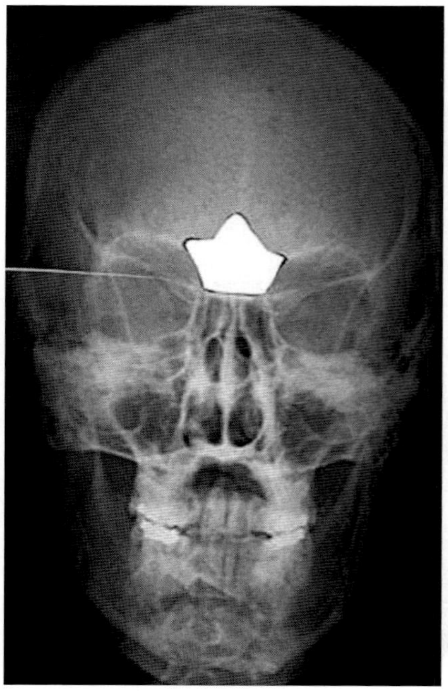

Fig 3.4-4 A 6′ Caldwell plain film is a non-magnified image and can serve as a template of the anterior table of the frontal sinus.

2 Frontal sinus reconstruction

Functional reconstruction of the frontal sinus pertains to reestablishing the frontal sinus flow, which most often relates to the nasofrontal orifices and/or frontal recess. Presently, most functional reconstruction of the frontal sinus is done transnasally and with endoscopes (**Fig 3.4-5**) [Kuhn, 1969].

The initial step in frontal sinus and frontal recess dissection involves identification of the appropriate boundaries and understanding the drainage pathway of the frontal recess [Schaeffer, 1916]. This is examined with fine-cut CT scans and correlated with direct visualization with ridged endoscopes. There are many varieties of telescopes available that visualize at multiple angles. However, 45° or 70° telescopes are particularly useful in frontal sinus recess dissection. Mucosa preservation is of utmost importance when dissecting the frontal recess since removal of the mucosa results in scarring, which can prevent functional outflow of the sinus. Occasionally, in cases of longstanding sinus disease, osteitis will develop and the bone can become markedly thickened. In these cases, the mucosa may need to be denuded in the areas where the bone will need to be reduced. Reduction of the bone is most often performed by drilling. An angled diamond burr is a useful instrument for such cases when performing an extended frontal sinusotomy. Once the ostia are open, irrigation and suction is used to remove thickened mucus [Palmer et al, 2005]. The sinus surgery is precise and meticulous, as is the postoperative care. In-office endoscopy and cleaning can help to prevent excessive scarring and further obstruction of the sinus. This typically gives good results; however, some surgeons elect to place stents through the nasofrontal recess using a soft conformable material, such as silicone [Neel et al, 1976].

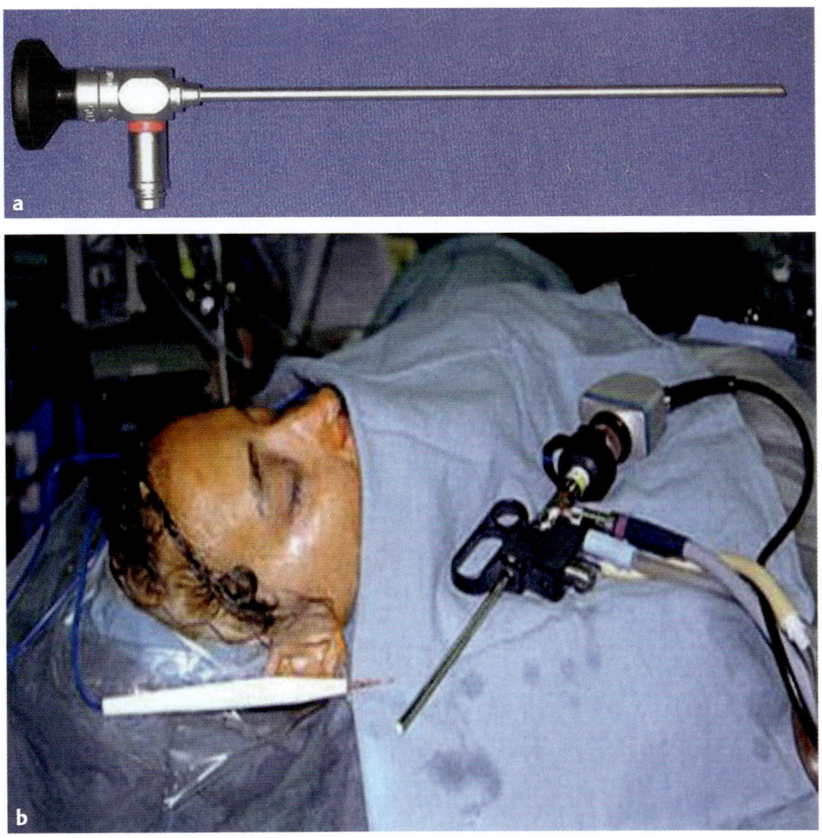

Fig 3.4-5a–b

a A 45° endoscope shows excellent visualization of the frontal sinus and its associated structure.

b Nasal endoscopy is the preferred method to visualize and manipulate the sinuses.

A precise understanding of perinasal sinus anatomy is critical to successful functional frontal sinus reconstruction in establishing outflow through the nasofrontal recess system. The agger nasi sinus cell is present in 70–90% of patients (**Fig 3.4-6**). This sinus air cell is located slightly above and anterior to the middle turbinate. The frontal recess extends superior and anterior to the agger nasi cell. In many patients, the agger nasi cell borders a portion of much of the frontal recess. Removal of the dome of the agger nasi cell may be important in frontal sinus surgery. If it is left and the agger nasi cell becomes edematous or the mucosa is thickened, it will occlude the drainage of the frontal recess [Orlandi et al, 2001]. There are also frontal cells that originate as anterior ethmoidal cells that pneumatize into the frontal recess. These also must be dealt with when performing functional secondary frontal sinus surgery. A pocket called the recessus terminalis is an anatomical variation that is present up to 50% of the time and directs the frontal sinus drainage directly into the middle meatus [Palmer et al, 2005]. This variant can be difficult to dissect resulting in a common cause of failure of endoscopic frontal sinus surgery.

Frontal sinus trephination can be helpful in endoscopic frontal sinus surgery. Trephination of the frontal sinus involves creating a separate opening into the sinus. This is traditionally done through the superior orbit and directly into the floor of the sinus. Trephination can also be done through the anterior wall of the frontal sinus, which can be convenient for placing an endoscope and examining the sinus. Trephination may also be helpful for removing lateral sinus disease, irrigating the sinuses, and help in locating the nasofrontal orifice. Additionally, frontal sinus trephination may be used independently to decompress severe frontal sinus disease that is either acutely symptomatic or resulting in an acute complication such as an epidermal abscess or meningitis.

Wolfgang Draf popularized three endoscopic approaches to the frontal sinus, the Draf I, II, and III [Peltier et al, 2006]. Each progressively involves a wider pathway from the nasal cavity to the frontal sinus to preserve function of the sinus. The most extensive procedure, the Draf III, describes removal of the inferior portion of the interfrontal septum, the superior nasal septum, and frontal sinus floor. The only structures remaining completely intact are the lamina papyracea and the posterior frontal sinus wall. Because of the aggressive exposure, there can be significant postoperative scarring [McLaughlin et al, 1999]. External frontal ethmoidectomy via a small curved (Lynch) incision between the medial canthus and glabella has been used historically in functional reconstruction surgery of the frontal sinuses and frontal recesses. Currently, there is little need for this approach since the same procedure can be performed endoscopically with better access to the natural ostium. The external approach can lead to potential prolapse of the medial orbital contents into the ethmoid sinus. The cosmetic defect associated with the Lynch incision is undesirable.

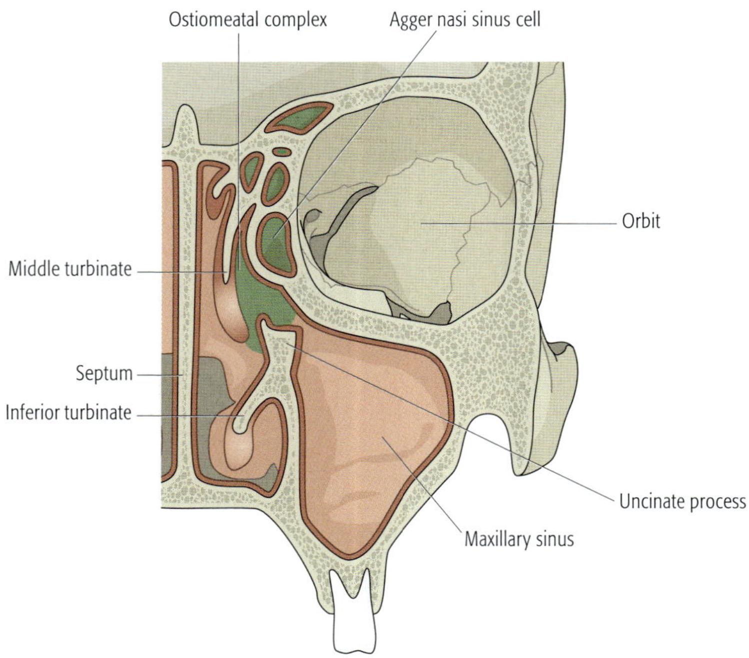

Fig 3.4-6 Coronal diagram of an agger nasi sinus cell that is present in 70–90% of patients.

The most common open procedure still used for functional reconstruction of the final frontal sinus is the osteoplastic flap [Ulualp et al, 2000]. This approach is almost exclusively through a coronal incision (**Fig 3.4-7**).

Brow and mid-forehead incisions are of historical interest but not recommended secondary to cosmetic deformity. The butterfly or brow incision can leave an unsightly scar, which is unnecessary in frontal sinus surgery. There is also often numbing of the forehead by injury to the supraorbital nerves, which can be prevented by using a coronal approach. In acute frontal sinus trauma, existing lacerations can provide exposure to the frontal sinus but this is rarely going to be helpful in secondary frontal sinus surgery.

The osteoplastic flap is elevated by first elevating a cutaneous flap, then elevating the periosteum over the superior and lateral part of the anterior wall of the frontal sinus. The periosteum remains attached inferiorly. A 6′ Caldwell plain film template can then be used to outline the borders of the frontal sinus and make determinations for the bony cuts. Others may prefer an image-guidance CT for localizing the sinus borders. Once the lateral and superior borders of the sinus are cut, it is recommended to make fine drill holes inferiorly so that the inferior portion of the flap is perforated sparingly. This controls the fracture when the bone is elevated and prevents fractures into the orbit. The bone is then elevated as one piece, it may stay attached to the periosteum inferiorly (**Fig 3.4-8**). When the goal is to maintain a functional sinus, the lesion or disease within the sinuses is removed sparing the mucosa. The nasofrontal orifices are opened to reestablish drainage. Endoscopes can also be used from below to aid in this dissection. This approach can be confirmed by visualizing from below thus maximizing exposure and dissection of the frontal recess region. This approach is typically used for small frontal sinus lesions. In most cases, when the frontal sinus is opened from above for sinus disease, the sinus will be obliterated.

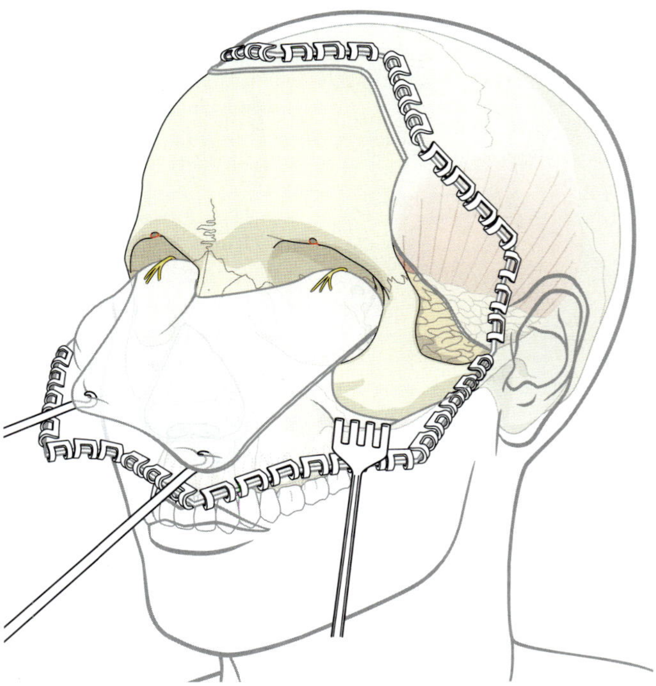

Fig 3.4-7 Coronal incision to approach the frontal sinus.

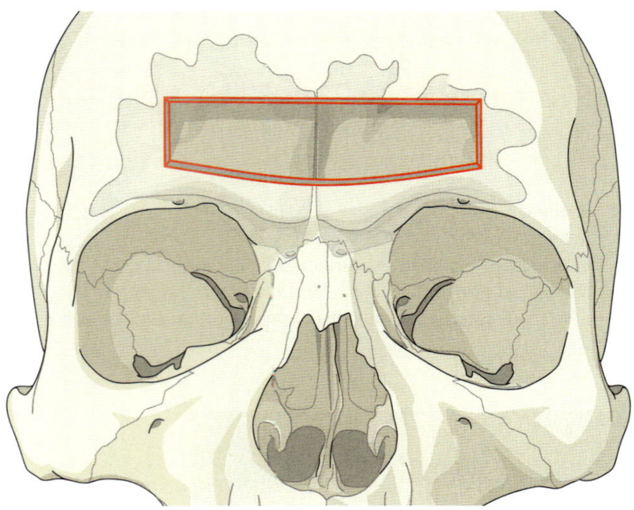

Fig 3.4-8 An osteoplastic frontal sinus flap is created to gain access to the frontal sinus contents.

3 Obliteration

Obliteration of the frontal sinus is a reasonable option when there is diffuse sinus disease or obstruction of the frontal sinus drainage. The authors prefer obliteration when there is question as to functional drainage from the frontal sinus.

Frontal sinus obliteration requires careful removal of all mucosa in the frontal sinus and supraorbital ethmoid cells (**Fig 3.4-9**). This includes careful drilling and often the use of magnification. Any remaining mucosa increases the chances of recurrence. Removing the mucosa over the orbit can be tricky because the bone may be thin or dehiscent. Magnification can be helpful here, especially when separating mucosa from periorbita.

Once all mucosa is removed, the key to frontal sinus obliteration is sealing the nasofrontal orifices. If they are not tightly obliterated, disease and mucosa can migrate retrograde into the frontal sinus. Many materials have been advocated for obliterating the frontal sinuses. A combination of a small bone graft and temporalis fascia can tightly obliterate nasofrontal orifices. Fat can then be placed in the remainder of the sinus. The bone grafts can be obtained from the inner septum of the frontal sinus or a cranial bone graft can be taken. Fat, fascia, and small bone grafts are easily accessible and are met with limited morbidity (**Fig 3.4-10**) [Gonty et al, 1999]. Others have advocated cancellous bone grafts for obliteration of the frontal sinuses. Traditionally, these have been harvested from the hip. While the bone works well in the sinus, the donor site morbidity is real [Rohrich et al, 1992]. Tibial bone grafts may prove a good alternative. Bone substitutes have been used for obliteration of the nasofrontal orifices and frontal recess. Their use is highly cautioned since frontal sinus surgery is often dealing with contaminated areas and these products may cause complications when in contact with any nasal or sinus mucosa [Marthur et al, 2003; Petruzzelli et al, 2002].

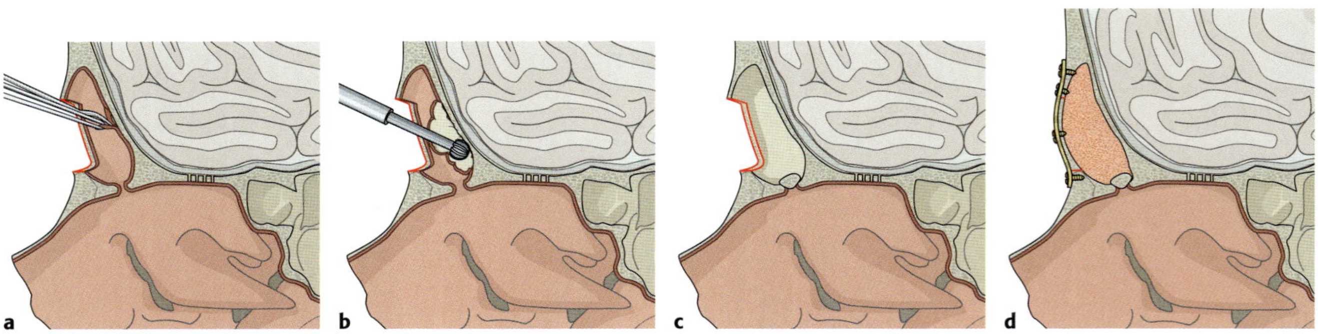

Fig 3.4-9a–d
a Removal of the sinus mucosa.
b Removal of inner sinus bone cortex with a burr.
c The nasal frontal duct is occluded with a bone graft.
d The sinus is fully packed with particulate cancellous bone material. The anterior table is replanted and fixated with plates.

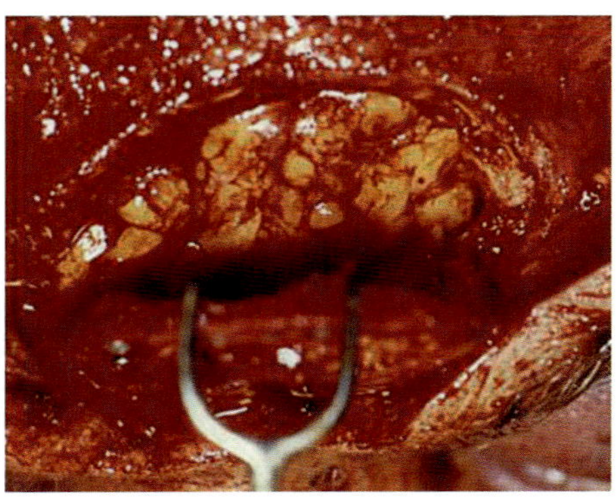

Fig 3.4-10 Alternatively, the frontal sinus can be filled with fat.

4 Cranialization

Cranialization of the frontal sinus may be necessary when there is a loss of structure of the posterior frontal sinus and/or irreparable damage to walls, mucosa or ducts [Donald, 1982; Kellman, 1994]. This may be secondary to trauma or a destructive mass. The most common destructive mass in the frontal sinus is a mucocele or mucopyocele. Malignancies of the frontal sinuses are rare; however, ethmoid sinus tumors can extend superiorly into the frontal sinus causing destruction of the sinus walls. Typically, ethmoid tumors grow into the floor of the sinus but also can destroy the posterior wall. When the posterior wall of the frontal sinus is not suitable for reconstruction, it is removed and the frontal sinus becomes one with the anterior cranial fossa, therefore cranialized (**Fig 3.4-11**). Sealing the nasofrontal orifices remains a critical part in cranialization of the frontal sinus with the techniques described above. Additionally, any remaining mucosa on the anterior table again needs to be completely removed. When there is a disruption of the frontal sinus floor, it will need to be reconstructed to keep the anterior cranial fossa separate from the perinasal sinuses. This can be important in preventing brain herniation or when repairing CSF leaks. When defects are 1 cm or bigger, bone grafting may be an excellent option. Bone grafts can be contoured and plated using microplates. Pericranium can be particularly helpful in sealing the defects of the anterior skull base. These authors prefer to place vascularized or nonvascularized pericranium on the nasal surface of the bone grafts. The bone grafts are then fixed into place creating a watertight seal between the sinuses and the anterior cranial fossa. The pericranium can be split sagittally so a portion can be used for sealing the defect, and a section for repair of dura. Careful reconstruction of this area can aid in preventing pneumocephalus and CSF leaks. In cases where both the anterior and posterior tables of the frontal sinus are severely disrupted, the sinus can be cranialized and bone grafts may be necessary for reconstruction of the anterior table of what becomes the anterior cranial fossa. Free tissue transfer is a viable option for severe cases.

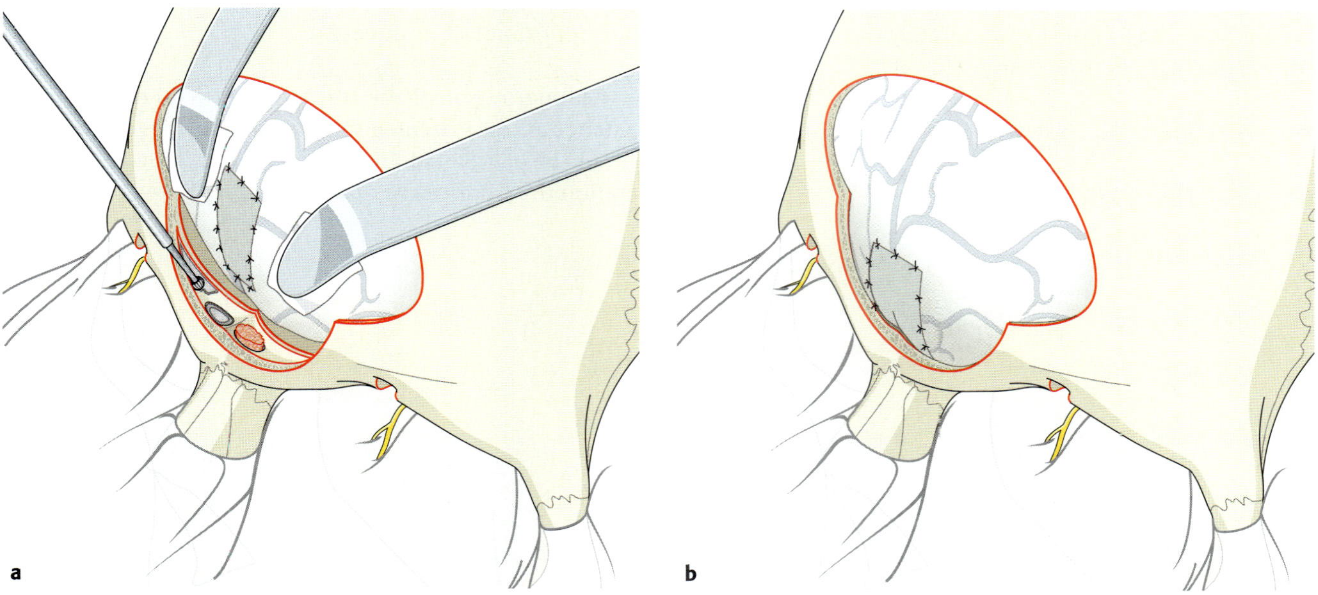

Fig 3.4-11a–b

a The posterior wall of the frontal sinus has been removed. A dural repair with a patch has been performed. One of the frontal recesses is blocked with the bone graft (red); remaining mucosa is removed with a drill.

b The brain falls forward to fill the space.

5 Access and osteosynthesis

As described above, coronal approaches to the frontal sinus are recommended for open frontal sinus procedures. While lacerations can be helpful and can be lengthened, additional scarring in this region can cause cosmetic problems. Midforehead and butterfly or brow incisions are of historical interest. Lynch orbital incision is historical and rarely used today; the most practical use is for control of the anterior and/or posterior ethmoid arteries. Transfacial approaches also can be helpful in cases of orbital abscesses associated with ethmoid sinusitis. Endoscopic approaches to the frontal sinus continue to improve with finer endoscopes and instrumentation. They will continue to play a vital role in functional reconstruction of the frontal sinus.

Bone grafting can be important in frontal sinus reconstruction. In traumatic injuries with extensive bone loss, bone grafting is required for repairing the anterior table (See chapter 1.1 on bone graft harvesting). Bone grafting can also be used for reconstructing the floor of the sinuses and obstructing the nasofrontal orifices. Most of the bone grafts for these specific sites are cortical cranial bone grafts. Cancellous bone can be used for obliterating the sinus and nasofrontal ducts.

6 Complications and pitfalls

The number one complication in frontal sinus surgery is infection. If the mucosa is not completely removed or the nasofrontal orifices are not completely sealed, the sinus is at risk for becoming infected. Additionally, when mucosa remains in the sinus and the sinus is not reconstructed to be functional, the risk of infection is high. In these situations there is the risk of mucocele proliferation, which can become infected and form a mucopyocele. These complications may not become evident for years after the injury. Orbital injury is rare but possible during frontal sinus surgery. This includes injury to the orbital contents and potential, though much less likely, optic nerve injury. Chronic sinus infections can lead to infection in the surrounding bone, ie, an osteomyelitis. In association with osteomyelitis, patients can develop a Potts puffy tumor. This is a swelling of the soft tissue overlying the sinus, which can be difficult to treat and in some cases can require removal of the bone of the anterior table of the sinus resulting in a significant secondary defect. Finally, life-threatening infections can develop when the disease progresses intracranially. Meningitis, epidural, subdural or brain abscesses are all possible secondary complications of frontal sinus disease.

Functional repair of the frontal sinus requires a pristine patent outflow system. If this cannot be achieved, the sinus should be obliterated. If the choice is to proceed with obliteration the sinus needs to be carefully cleaned and sealed.

7 References and suggested reading

Donald PJ. Frontal sinus ablation by cranialization: report of 21 cases. *Arch Otolaryngol.* 1982 Mar;108(3):142–146.

Gonty AA, Marciani RD, Adornato DC. Management of frontal sinus fractures: a review of 33 cases. *J Oral Maxillofac Surg.* 1999 Apr;57(4):372–379; discussion 380–381.

Kellman RM. Safe and dependable harvesting of large outer-table calvarial bone grafts. *Arch Otolaryngol Head Neck Surg.* 1994 Aug;120(8):856–860.

Kuhn FA. Chronic frontal sinusitis: the endoscopic frontal recess approach. *Oper Tech Otolaryngol Head Neck Surg.* 1969;7:222–229.

Marthur KK, Tatum SA, Kellman RM. Carbonated apatite and hydroxyapatite in craniofacial reconstruction. *Arch Facial Plast Surg.* 2003 Sep–Oct;5(5):379–383.

McLaughlin RB, Hwang pH, Lanza DC. Endoscopic trans-septal frontal sinusotomy: the rationale and results of an alternative technique. *Am J Rhinol.* 1999 Jul–Aug;13(4):279–287.

Neel HB, Whicker JH, Lake CF. Thin rubber sheeting in frontal sinus surgery: animal and clinical studies. *Laryngoscope.* 1976 Apr;86(4):524–536.

Orlandi RR, Kennedy DW. Revision endoscopic frontal sinus surgery. *Otolaryngol Clin North Am.* 2001 Feb;34(1):77–90.

Palmer JN, Kennedy DW. *Revision Endoscopic Sinus Surgery: Otolaryngology Head and Neck Surgery.* 4th ed. Cummings: Elsevier Mosby; 2005:1255–1275.

Peltier J, Ryan MW, Quinn FB. *Frontal Sinus Surgery.* Grand Rounds, University of Texas Medical Branch, Dept of Otolaryngology; 2006.

Petruzzelli GJ, Stankiewicz JA. Frontal sinus obliteration with hydroxyapatite cement. *Laryngoscope.* 2002 Jan;112(1):32–36.

Rohrich RJ, Hollier LH. Management of frontal sinus fractures: changing concepts. *Clin Plast Surg.* 1992 Jan;19(1):219–232.

Stanley RB Jr, Becker TS. Injuries of the nasofrontal orifices in frontal sinus fractures. *Laryngoscope.* 1987 Jun;97(6):728–731.

Schaeffer JB. The genesis, development and adult anatomy of the nasofrontal region in man. *Am J Anat.* 1916;20:125–145.

Ulualp SO, Carlson TF, Toohill RJ. Osteoplastic flap versus modified endoscopic Lothrop procedure in patients with frontal sinus disease. *Am J Rhinol.* 2000 Jan–Feb;14(1):21–26.

3.5 Access surgery to the skull base

Neal D Futran

1 Introduction

The skull base is an extremely complex anatomical region in which a variety of heterogeneous pathologies exist with a range of clinical and biological features. These include congenital, inflammatory, and vascular lesions, as well as benign and malignant neoplasms. They may be intradural, extradural or both, but considered together these lesions can be grouped into a common anatomical location that usually requires a multidisciplinary approach to treatment. Malignancies of the skull base represent approximately 3% of neoplasms of the upper respiratory tract.

2 Indications and planning

The cranial base is classically divided into the anterior, middle, and posterior segments. More critical than the specific tumor types, these subdivisions dictate the surgical approaches that can be used to approach pathologies and minimize morbidity (**Fig 3.5-1**).

The anterior base extends from the frontal sinus to the lesser wing of the sphenoid and the planum sphenoidale. The greater wing of the sphenoid forms the anterior wall of the middle skull base while the posterior limit is the clivus. Laterally, it extends to the posterior surface of the petrous bone. Access osteotomies are not used for approaches to the posterior skull base and this area is not discussed in this chapter.

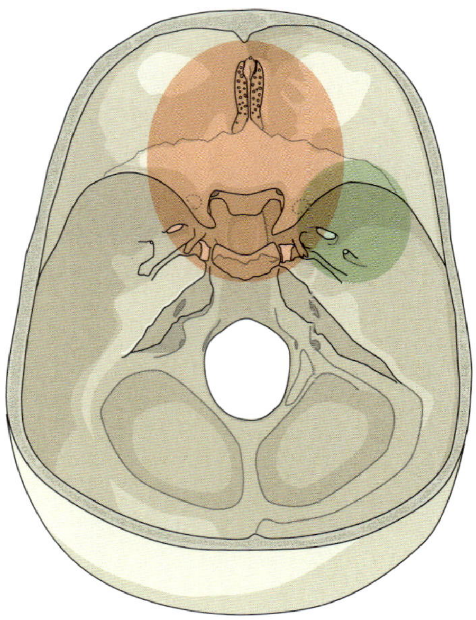

Fig 3.5-1 Skull base territory accessible by calvarial and facial bone osteotomies. Red area is accessible by pure anterior approaches; green area by anterolateral approaches.

3 Diagnosis and imaging

Axial and coronal computed tomographic scans are necessary and useful for delineating the integrity and variations in the bony architecture of the paranasal sinuses and skull base (**Fig 3.5-2**).

Magnetic resonance imaging delineates the soft-tissue planes between tumor and vital adjacent structures, distinguishes tumor from mucus and inflamed mucosa, and is critical in assessing tumor resectability (**Fig 3.5-3**).

Both imaging studies aid in designing a surgical approach to encompass all tumor margins [Osquthorpe et al, 2001].

Tumors that arise from, or extend to, the base of the skull pose a significant management challenge secondary to the proximity to critical neurovascular structures. The surgery of tumors in this area can be difficult because of restrictive access, distortion of normal anatomy, and proximity of vital structures. Anatomical knowledge that allows adequate tumor resection with preservation of vital structures can enable the surgeon to maintain optimal function and cosmesis. Patterns of tumor spread can be predicted if the clinician is familiar with the skull base foramina and preexisting pathways for tumor spread. In general when tumors penetrate the cranial fossa anteriorly (nasal roof, cribriform plate, frontal lobes), fewer vital neurovascular structures are involved and cure rates are higher regardless of the histology than tumors that invade more posteriorly near the cavernous sinus and/or carotid artery [McCattrey et al, 2004].

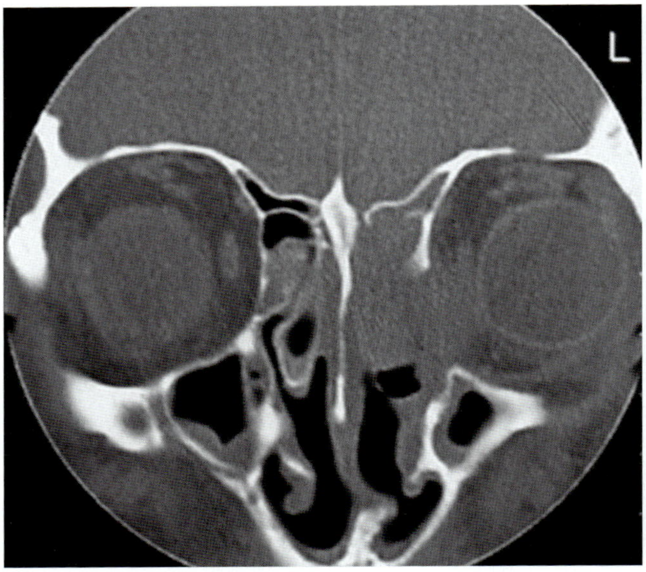

Fig 3.5-2 Computed tomographic scan of an ethmoid carcinoma extending to the skull base.

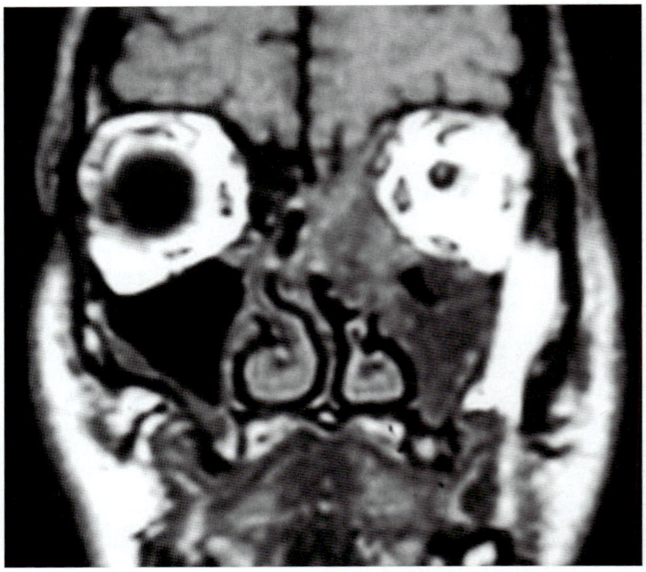

Fig 3.5-3 Corresponding magnetic resonance imaging scan shows tumor in the ethmoid sinus and obstructed mucus in the maxillary sinus.

4 Resection and reconstruction

4.1 Surgical access

The goal of surgical access to the skull base is to offer the simplest technique that will provide optimal exposure, so that the whole tumor pathology can be safely excised with the minimal deformity. When the lesion is malignant, surgery must be designed to excise the entire tumor with a margin of healthy tissue. Anything less guarantees a high incidence of local recurrence even with adjunctive postoperative radiation and/or chemotherapy. In addition to precise imaging, operating microscopes and instrumentation as well as better anesthetic and postoperative care techniques have allowed these tumors to be resected safely. The surgical approach used to obtain adequate exposure of the skull base may be extracranial, transcranial, or in many instances, a combination of both [Raveh et al, 1993, 1995; Al-Mefty, 1992; Nuss et al, 1991].

Optimal surgical access depends on matching the anatomical location and pathological character of the neoplasm to the versatility of the particular approach. In considering exposure, the following general factors are relevant:

- Take the shortest route from the skin to the target, bypassing and/or displacing structures essential for functional survival of the patient.
- Use preexisting or potential 'surgical' avenues if possible.
- Use osteotomies through the facial and skull bones to reduce brain retraction and improve exposure to the lesion (**Fig 3.5-4**).
- Identification and preservation of adjacent vital neurovascular structures.
- Consider previous incisions in relation to vascularity of flaps.
- Control the blood supply to the neoplasm to reduce bleeding.
- Plan access in relation to the reconstruction, so that the dura can be repaired and separation of the intracranial and extracranial cavities can be achieved.
- Respect cosmesis and preserve function.
- Consider the possibility of future surgery.

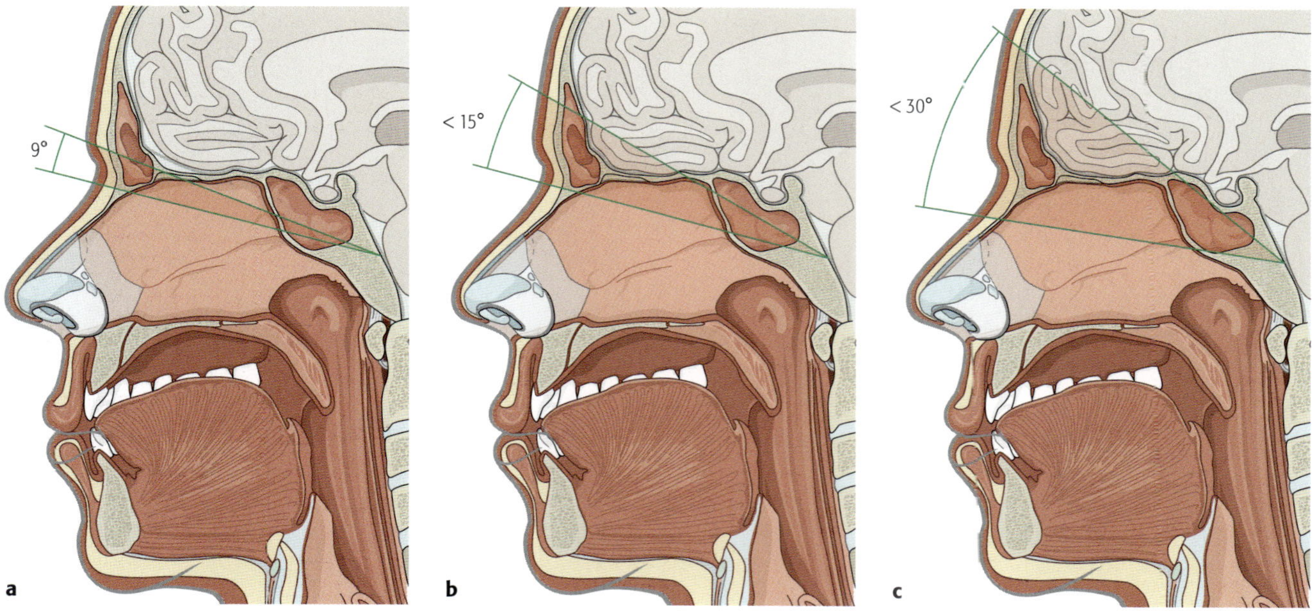

Fig 3.5-4a–c Access achieved by the different anterior access osteotomies:
a Subfrontal.
b Transfrontal.
c Extended transfrontal.

4.2 Osteotomy lines and osteosynthesis

Access to the skull base is achieved via a coronal incision from above and a transfacial and/or transoral incision from below. With the advent of endoscopic techniques in skull base surgery, inferior access can be attained in many cases without the need for facial incisions. Before surgery, in most cases, a lumbar drain is placed in the patient to allow for removal of cerebrospinal fluid during the procedure to minimize brain retraction. For tumors of the anterior cranial fossa, which require an open approach, a coronal incision is preferred [Osquthorpe et al, 2001; Nuss et al, 1991] (**Fig 3.5-5**) from pre-tragal area to pre-tragal area about 15 cm above the nasion instead of following the hairline. This permits a greater length of pericranium to be available for reconstruction and camouflage of the incision in hair-bearing tissue. The scalp is elevated forward to obtain exposure of the orbits, nasal roof, the zygomas and zygomatic arches. Be careful to preserve the frontal branches of the facial nerve as well as the sensory trigeminal branches to the forehead. Two centimeters superior to the zygomatic arch, the superficial temporalis fascia and the adipose tissue are elevated in one layer by establishing a plane between them and the deep temporalis fascia to avoid injury to the frontal branch of the facial nerve. The underlying pericranium is mobilized to the supraorbital foramen (preserving supraorbital blood supply) and is used later to resurface any anterior fossa defect. To reach the planum sphenoidale with this flap, adequate length is achieved by elevating the flap in a subgaleal plane posterior to the coronal incision for 3–4 cm and raising the pericranium anteriorly from there. The periorbita at the roof and upper parts of the medial and lateral walls are elevated in continuity with the pericranium. If present, the supraorbital foramina are converted into notches by fracturing the floor with a small osteotome and the neurovascular bundles are carefully dissected inferiorly with the periorbita. The temporalis muscles are elevated from the anterior portion to the temporal fossa leaving a small cuff for their reattachment. Transfrontal access to tumors penetrating to and through the cribiform plate is established traditionally via a frontal craniotomy alone, or with additional osteotomies. A bifrontal craniotomy can be made in one or two pieces and there are no natural lines of osteosynthesis, as the craniotomy is dictated by the amount of exposure necessary to

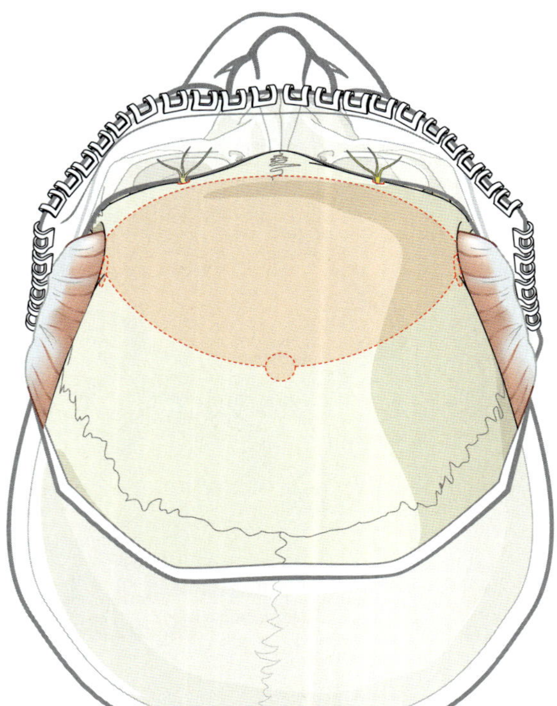

Fig 3.5-5 Coronal approach to the skull base with exposure to the orbital and nasal regions.

remove the tumor. Typically the inferior extent is through the frontal sinus (**Fig 3.5-6a**).

After tumor extirpation, the frontal sinus is cranialized and the frontal bone is fixed with microplates or miniplates.

Frequently to get optimal exposure to the planum sphenoidale and the optic chiasm, an extended frontal approach is used to minimize brain retraction and increase the angle of viewing. In these situations, after the frontal craniotomy has been performed, a second series of osteotomies is made to remove the frontoorbital bar (**Fig 3.5-6b–c**).

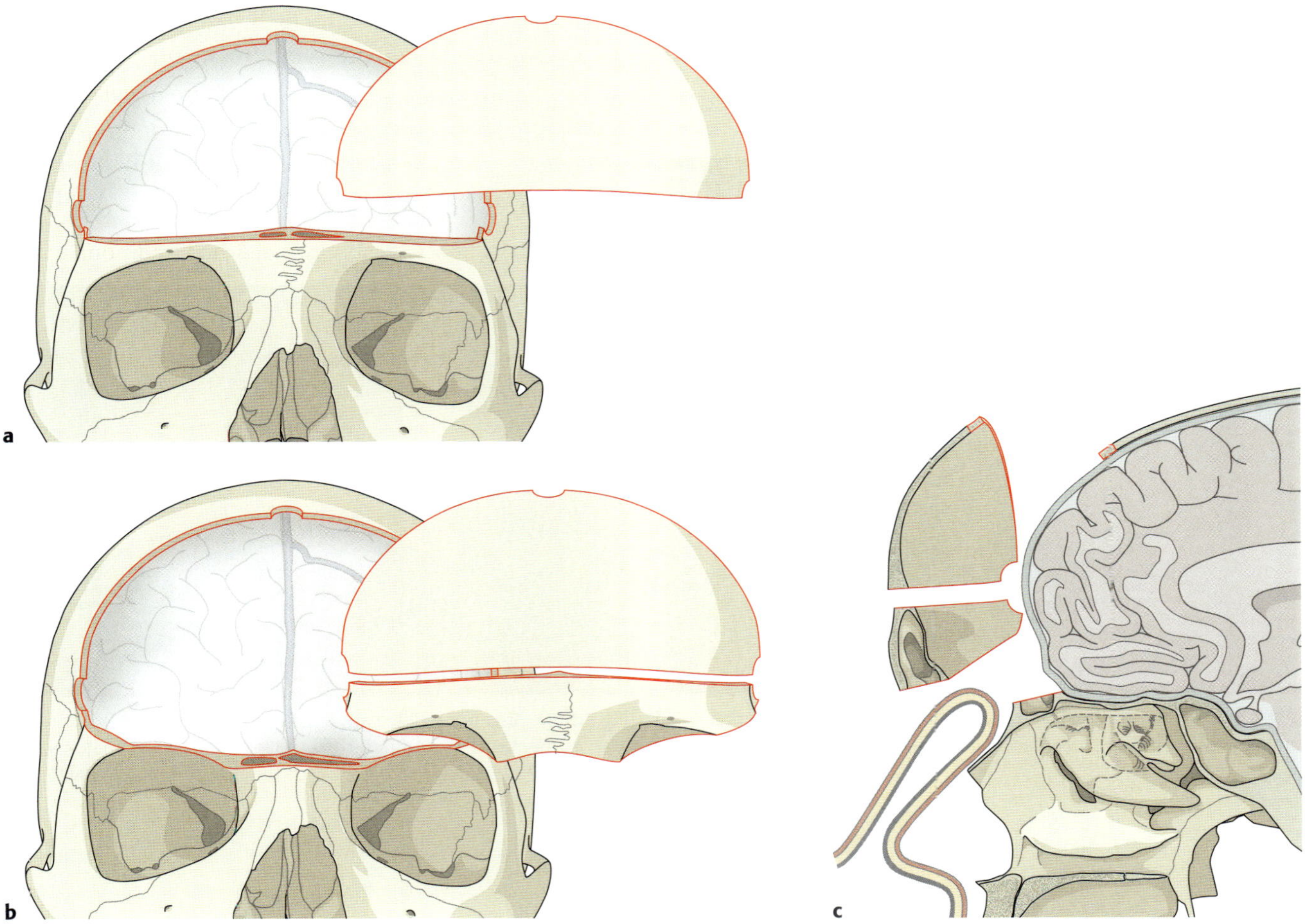

Fig 3.5-6a–c
a Anterior view of the osteotomized frontal bone segment.
b Anterior view of the osteotomized frontal bone segment with separate orbital bar.
c Lateral view of the osteotomized frontal segment with separate orbital bar.

This is designed along the lines of osteosynthesis at the frontozygomatic suture laterally and the nasion medially. Osteotomies are made through these areas and then completed using a drill, saw or piezotome from lateral to medial across the orbital roofs to meet anterior to the cribriform plate. The osteotomy is completed by making a horizontal cut from outside, across the nasion, at the level of the anterior ethmoidal arteries. The entire piece of bone is dislodged and removed with the assistance of a small osteotome. Once the tumor is removed and the skull base is sealed, the frontal orbital bar is replaced and fixated at the nasion and across the frontozygomatic sutures with miniplates. The frontal bone is replaced as described previously (**Fig 3.5-7**).

Although the anterior subcranial approach was initially developed in 1978 for anterior skull base trauma, indications now include access for resection of a variety of skull base tumors [Raveh et al, 1993 and 1995]. It differs significantly from the above-mentioned approaches in that it allows for broad exposure of the anterior skull base from below as opposed to the transfrontal superior route (**Fig 3.5-8**).

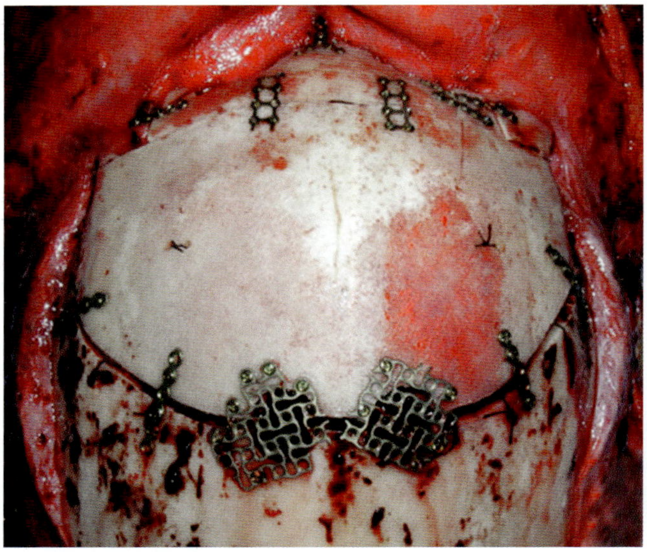

Fig 3.5-7 Plate position for fixation of the extended transfrontal osteotomy segments. Titanium mesh is used to cover the burr hole sites.

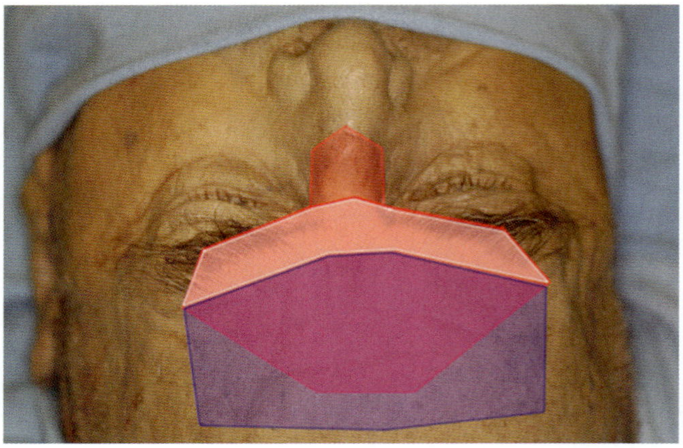

Fig 3.5-8 Area accessible with the subfrontal access osteotomy. The segment is designed based on the individual sinus anatomy. The magenta represents the area in which the frontal sinuses may be developed.

Osteotomy of the frontal-nasal-orbital external skeletal frame provides optimum anterior access to the orbital and sphenoid planes and into the nasal and sinonasal cavities, while avoiding frontal lobe retraction and external facial incisions. Similar to the transfrontal approaches, a coronal flap is raised in the standard fashion. Two types of osteotomy techniques have been described. In the type I technique, an osteotomy of the frontonasal segment leaving the posterior frontal wall intact to be removed in a second step is performed. This procedure is indicated if the tumor involves the posterior frontal sinus wall. The external skeletal frame is removed after dissection of the posterior wall under direct vision, safely and far enough from the tumor borders. In the type II technique, a one-stage removal of the frontonasal segment, including the posterior frontal sinus wall, is done. This is useful when tumors do not involve the posterior frontal sinus wall or have major intracranial extension. The osteotomy borders can be extended cranially and laterally to include segments of the orbital roof as necessary. Prior to making the osteotomies and depending on the size and the extent of both the lesion and the frontal sinus, the outline of the nasofrontal segment is planned. Titanium miniplates for subsequent bone fixation are adapted and drilled to allow for proper adaptation of the bone plate once the tumor is removed (**Fig 3.5-9**).

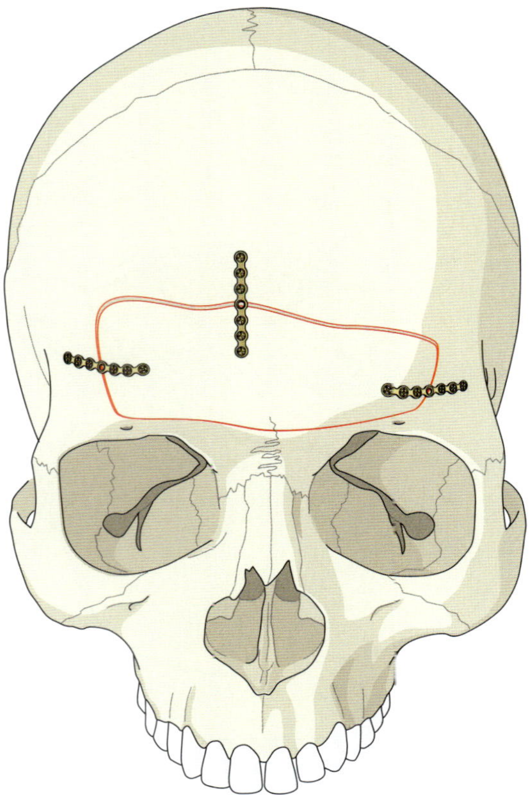

Fig 3.5-9 Plate position for fixation of the anterior table of the frontal sinus segment.

Bilateral ethmoidectomies and sphenoidotomies are performed to permit exposure of the ethmoidal roof and central skull base from below. Accurate delineation of tumor margins and dural excision are facilitated by this exposure and oncological resection takes place. Appropriate dural reconstruction is then performed and closure proceeds as in the previously described approaches.

Another access osteotomy that can be used alone or in combination with approaches from the frontal route is the Le Fort I osteotomy. Although this has been well described for correction of facial deformities, it is particularly useful for clival tumors and juvenile nasal angiofibromas. An upper buccal incision is made from premolar to premolar and dissection continues directly to the maxilla. The anterior face of the maxilla is exposed with particular attention to the lateral margin of the pyriform aperture and the zygomatic buttress region that will provide for the lines of osteosynthesis and fixation. With careful protection of the nasal floor, an osteotomy is made through the anterior face of the maxilla, at least 5 mm above the root apices to the junction of the maxilla and pterygoid plates. Miniplates are applied at the lateral aspect of the pyriform margin and zygomatic buttress on each side (**Fig 3.5-10a**).

The holes are drilled and screws placed. The plates are then removed, kept on a side table for later re-use, and the osteotomies through the medial maxillary wall and pterygoid plates are done to allow for down fracture of the maxilla, exposure of the tumor, and its ultimate removal (**Fig 3.5-10b**).

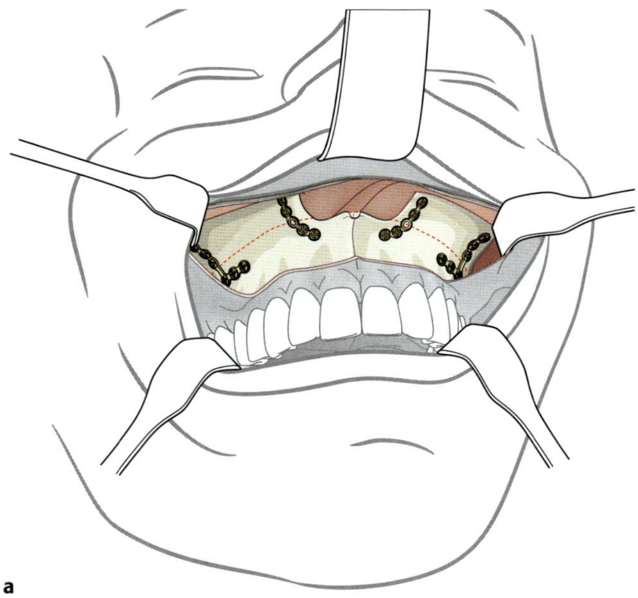

a

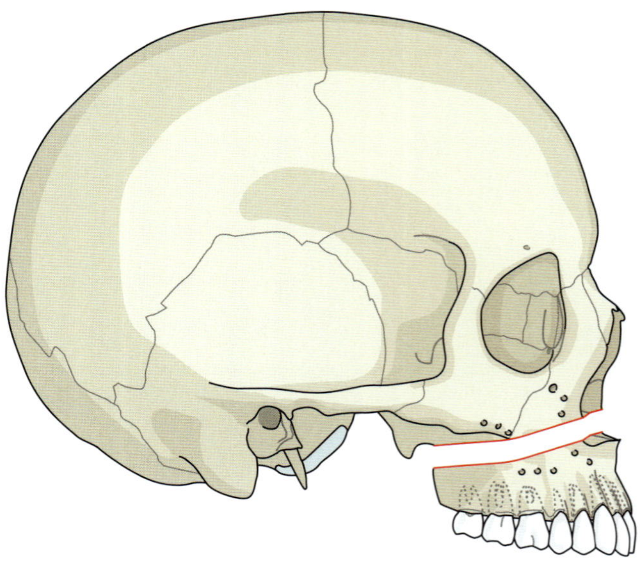

b

Fig 3.5-10a–b
a Plate position for fixation of the Le Fort I osteotomy segment.
b Lateral view of the Le Fort I osteotomy segment.

Once the tumor is resected, the maxilla is replaced and the prebend plates are reapplied to allow for proper fixation of the maxilla and maintenance of proper occlusion. Although transfacial maxillotomy procedures have been described, the advent of minimally invasive techniques has limited their current use.

For more laterally based tumors and those extending to the middle crania fossa (cavernous sinus, parasellar area of the optic chiasm), access via orbitozygomatic osteotomies with a pterygonal craniotomy can be done. These frontolateral approaches incorporate the orbital roof and provide greater access to tumors underneath the frontal and temporal lobes. With modifications of the cranial bone flap (ie, changing the position and size of the flap), incorporation of a posterior orbitotomy and/or zygomatic osteotomy (**Fig 3.5-11**), the cranioorbital approaches can be specifically tailored to optimize the exposure of a given tumor.

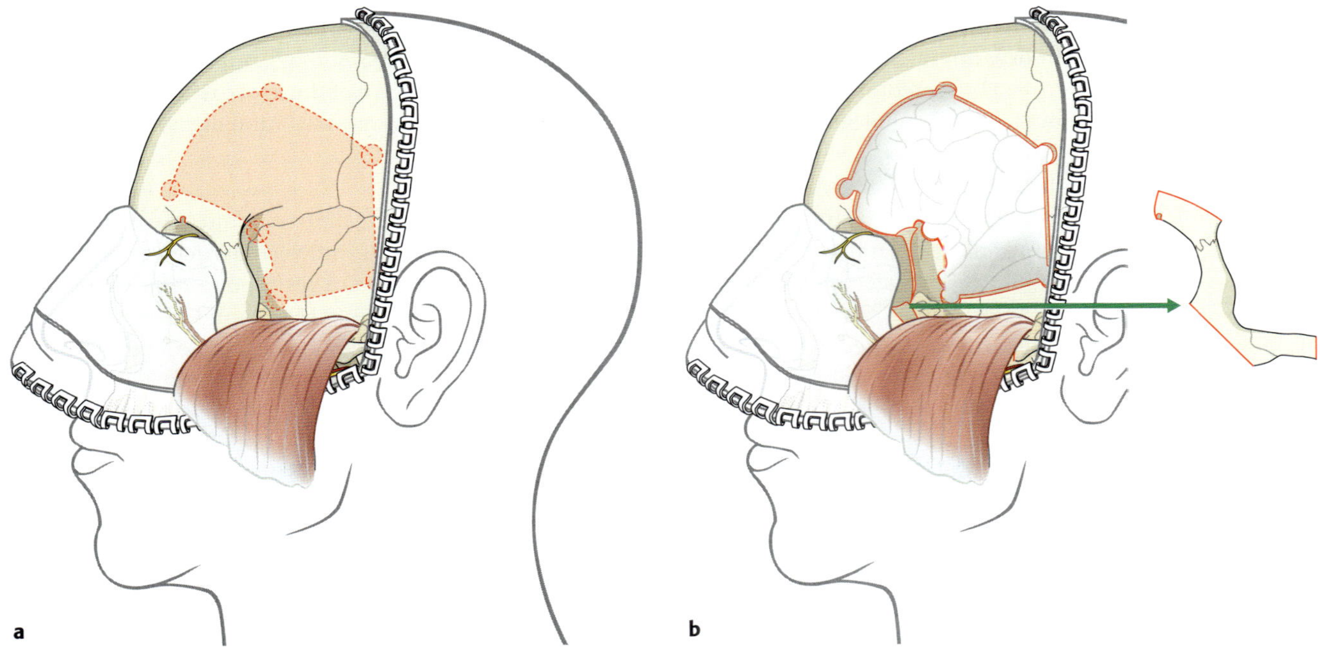

Fig 3.5-11a–b

a The cranial attachment of the temporalis muscle is detached and inferiorly displaced, allowing access for the pterional craniotomy.

b Zygomatico-orbital segment and temporal craniotomy. The zygomatico-orbital segment is preserved and replaced at the end of the procedure.

Depending on the extent of the osteotomy, a coronal or hemicoronal incision can be used. To protect the frontal branch of the facial nerve and expose the zygomatic arch, an incision is made in the superficial temporal fascia 1–2 cm above the zygomatic arch and dissection continues through the deep temporal fascia to the superior border of the zygomatic arch. The periosteum is then elevated to expose both the arch and the body of the zygomatic bone. The zygomatico-mandibular portion of the temporal muscle is incised along the lower border of the zygomatic arch and the arch itself is undermined. The temporalis muscle is then detached from the lateral rim of the orbit and lateral skull, so that it can be retracted inferiorly. Using an oscillating saw in the temporal fossa, an osteotomy is made along the zygomatico-sphenoid suture. This osteotomy begins at the base of the zygomatic process of the frontal bone and extends downward to the inferior orbital suture. A second osteotomy is made at the posterior extension of the zygomatic arch, and finally a third osteotomy is made at the body of the zygomatic bone 1 cm posterior and parallel to the zygomatic maxillary suture. Titanium miniplates are placed across the osteotomy sites and holes drilled again to allow for proper anatomical replacement of the segment after the tumor is removed. Now the infratemporal fossa is completely exposed. The craniotomy can be performed before or after this osteotomy to allow adequate tumor removal. Once the tumor is extirpated and the dura is sealed, the orbitozygomatic and cranial bones can be replaced and the plates applied. The temporalis muscle is then fixed in its proper anatomical position and the wound is closed.

5 Complications and pitfalls

Craniofacial resection of skull-base tumors has a high morbidity that can be related to the approach, resection, and repair, either alone or in combination [Kraus et al, 1994]. The overall morbidity rate is 1.5–3.9% but can be as high as 12% for advanced malignancies that require extended skull base dissection. Central to many of the approaches is dissection of the periorbital tissues, and protection of the orbital contents is paramount. In addition, significant neurovascular structures are encountered, particularly as one approaches the cavernous sinus and absolute knowledge of this anatomy is necessary to protect these structures. Retraction of the frontal and/or temporal lobes is necessary to a degree in every resection. Choice of the approach for each particular tumor can allow for minimization of retraction injuries (**Fig 3.5-4**).

Equally as critical as the approach and resection of skull base tumors is the repair and reconstruction. Specifically the dura must be repaired or restored to reduce the risk of cerebrospinal fluid leak, meningitis, and pneumocephalus (2–14% of patients). In addition, separation of the sinonasal cavity from the intracranial cavity minimizes the risk of meningitis (1–5% of patients). Vascularized tissue in the form of a pericranial flap, pedicled muscle flap, or free-tissue transfer decreases these risks. Accurate fixation of the bone segments allows for accurate anatomical reconstruction of the craniofacial skeleton and maintains proper occlusion when tooth-bearing segments are osteotomized. Proper redraping and suspension of soft tissues is necessary to achieve an optimal esthetic result. Persistent nasal crusting is common and is easily treated with self-administered nasal saline irrigations.

With these approaches, "unresectable" is now a relative term in the management of skull base neoplasms. The surgery must be offered; however, with the clear understanding by the patient of the potential perioperative complications and disability that can occur as well as a realistic assessment of the quality of life that may be achieved.

6 References and suggested reading

Al-Mefty O. The cranio-orbital zygomatic approach for intracranial lesions. *Contemp Neurosurg*. 1992;14:1–6.

Brown DH. The Le Fort I maxillary osteotomy approach to surgery of the skull base. *J Otolaryngol* . 1989 Oct;18(6):286–292.

Kraus DH, Shah JP, Arbit E, et al. Complications of craniofacial resection for tumors involving the anterior skull base. *Head Neck*. 1994 Jul-Aug;16:307–312.

McCattrey TV, Olsen KD, Yohanan JM, et al. Factors affecting survival of patients with tumors of the anterior skull base. *Laryngoscope*. 1994 Aug;104:(8 Pt 1):940–945.

Nuss DW, Janecka IP, Sekhar LN, et al. Craniofacial disassembly in the management of skull-base tumors. *Otolaryngol Clin North Am*. 1991 Dec;24(6):1465–1497.

Osquthorpe JD, Patel S. Craniofacial approaches to tumors of the anterior skull base. *Otolaryngol Clin North Am*. 2001 Dec;34 (6):1123–1142.

Raveh J, Laedrach K, Speiser M, et al. The subcranial approach for fronto-orbital and anteroposterior skull base tumor. *Arch Otolaryngol Head Neck Surg*. 1993 Apr;19:385–393.

Raveh J, Turk JB, Laedrach K, et al. Extended anterior subcranial approach for skull base tumors: long-term results. *J Neurosurg*. 1995 Jun;82(6):1002–1010.

3.6 Reconstruction of the skull base

Patrick J Gullane, Peter C Neligan, Christine B Novak

1 Introduction

The management of neoplasms located in the skull base region presents a challenging problem because of the hidden anatomical location of the tumor and the challenges of reconstruction following extensive resection. Advances in surgery, radiology, anesthesiology and the development of the multidisciplinary surgical team have provided the opportunity for successful treatment of many skull base neoplasms previously thought to be inoperable.

2 Anatomy

The skull base is formed by multiple bones within the anterior, middle and posterior cranial fossae. The intracranial surface of the skull base is formed by the floors of these fossae, the extracranial framework comprises the roof of the orbits, sphenoid sinus, nasopharynx and infratemporal fossa and the occiput. Many vital neural and vascular structures traverse the skull base making this region particularly susceptible to various pathologies and challenging for any surgical intervention.

Several classification systems have been described for the skull base region to assist in the evaluation, classification and management of cranial base tumors. To better understand the surgical reconstructions required following tumor ablation in this region, Jackson et al [1982] recommended separation of the skull base into the anterior and posterior areas; the anterior area represented the anterior cranial fossa and the posterior area was divided into three parts. Jones et al [1987] divided the skull base region into three segments, the anterior, middle and posterior regions, based on the respective cranial fossae. Irish et al [1994] conducted a retrospective clinical review of 77 patients with skull base neoplasms and reported outcome, tumor location and tumor growth patterns. Based on the anatomical boundaries and the tumor growth patterns, the authors developed a classification system [Irish et al, 1994] that divided the skull base into three regions (**Fig 3.6-1**). Region I tumors originated in the anterior skull base and included neoplasms that extended to the clivus as far as the foramen magnum. Region II tumors originated in the lateral skull base, primarily involving the infratemporal and pterygopalatine fossae and continued into the middle cranial fossa. Region III neoplasms derived from the posterior skull base or surrounding region and continued intracranially into the middle or posterior cranial fossae [Irish et al, 1994].

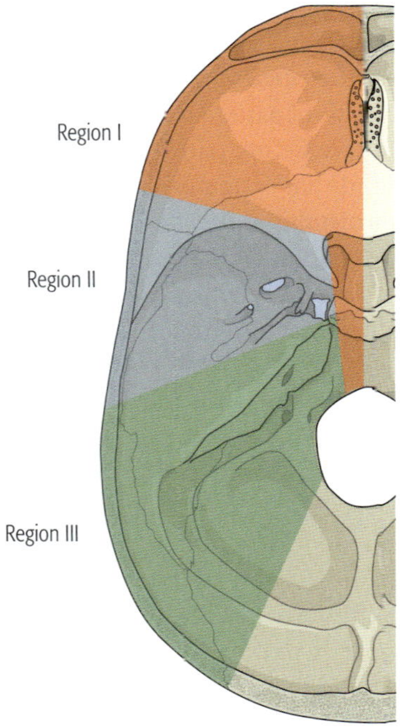

Fig 3.6-1 The skull base may be classified into three regions: region I, region II, and region III.

3 Indications and planning

Tumor pathology and the precise location of the neoplasm within the skull base may vary [Irish et al, 1994; Patel et al, 2003], thus affecting the clinical presentation and patient management. A comprehensive preoperative evaluation can help to determine tumor pathology and to delineate the specific location of the neoplasm. This will assist in the comprehensive management of these complex cases and surgical planning.

3.1 Radiological evaluation

Advances in radiology have provided the opportunity for a more accurate preoperative diagnosis and therefore improved preoperative planning regarding tumor ablation and the subsequent reconstruction. Both computed tomography (CT) and magnetic resonance imaging (MRI) provide valuable information regarding the tumor location, size and involved tissue. Preoperative radiographic evaluation with CT and MRI should be routinely performed for complete assessment of bony and soft-tissue involvement. Standard coronal and axial CT images are used to delineate involvement of the tumor in the surrounding bony structures and MRI provides better detail regarding soft-tissue involvement.

3.2 Tumor pathology

Skull base neoplasms are relatively uncommon [Patel et al, 2003] and with the presentation of heterogeneous tumor pathology, analysis of patient outcome following treatment is complex and predicting patient prognosis difficult. Irish et al [1994] found that squamous cell carcinomas were the most common histology (29%) that occurred in the skull base and were found most frequently involving region III. The next most frequent tumor types were basal cell carcinoma, meningioma, esthesioneuroblastoma, chordoma, and adenocarcinoma [Irish et al, 1994]. Survival analysis at 2 and 4 years following surgery revealed a better prognosis for patients with regions I and III tumors. There were no patients with region II neoplasm who survived for 4 years following surgery [Irish et al, 1994]. Patel et al [2003] in their international collaborative review also reported squamous cell carcinoma and adenocarcinoma as the most frequently occurring malignant tumors in the skull base. They found that the primary tumor pathology, the status of the surgical margins and the extent of intracranial involvement to be vital predictors of outcome.

The heterogeneous pathology of skull base neoplasms makes it complex to select the treatment with the highest probability of survival [Irish et al, 1994; Patel et al, 2003]. Reports of patient outcome with skull base tumors are difficult to compare because various tumors presenting in this region and the degree of intracranial involvement. Better outcomes have been associated with absence of transdural invasion [Feiz-Erfan et al, 2007]. The choice of treatment depends on many factors, including the natural history of the disease, life expectancy, patient symptoms and involved structures. The histological pattern is one of the most important determinants of outcome and a preoperative biopsy of the tumor is usually vital before extensive surgical intervention is planned.

3.3 Multidisciplinary team approach

The use of a multidisciplinary team provides expertise from numerous specialties to optimize preoperative, operative and postoperative care to the patient with skull base pathology. Preoperative evaluation by radiation and medical oncologists is imperative, particularly if adjuvant therapy is necessary postoperatively. Preoperative anesthesia consultation and evaluation provides the anesthesia team with a baseline assessment, which will help with the postoperative management and minimize the risk of perioperative complications. Early inclusion of all necessary medical and surgical specialties makes for efficient use of planning time and allows input from specialty areas of diverse expertise. The CMF surgeon, the neurosurgeon and the CMF surgeon can each contribute unique expertise in the surgical management of skull base neoplasms that were previously inoperable. The use of a two-team approach for tumor ablation and subsequent reconstruction assists in decreasing patient anesthesia time. While one surgical team is proceeding with tumor excision, the other team can begin the reconstruction, particularly if a free tissue transfer is utilized.

4 Tumor ablation and reconstruction of the skull base

The primary goal for treatment of patients with neoplasms in the skull base region is to select a treatment regimen that will result in the highest probability of survival with the least or minimal morbidity [Palme et al, 2009; de Almeida et al, 2012; de Almeida et al, 2013]. Because of the anatomical location of skull base tumors and the complex reconstruction required, surgical intervention for treatment of these patients presents a major challenge. Endoscopic approaches and minimal access surgery have shifted the surgical paradigm and have increased the surgical management options for these patients. Both endoscopic and open approaches must be assessed in the context of outcome, morbidity and mortality [Ganly et al, 2005; Hanna et al, 2009]. Successful outcome necessitates the optimal match and consideration of the factors related to patient comorbidities, tumor biology and surgeon experience. In general, minimal access surgery has changed the surgical paradigm. However, the technical considerations for defect repair remain similar for both approaches.

Following tumor ablation in the head and neck region, the reconstruction must provide a structural foundation and soft-tissue coverage while optimizing patient function and cosmesis. However, the reconstruction after skull base defects is more difficult than for defects in other anatomical locations; the defects are often complex and 3-D, gravity tends to separate the repair away from the skull base, and the dura may have been breached.

The specific operative procedure and surgical approach utilized for safe and complete removal of the neoplasm will be determined by several factors including the tumor size, the location and the tissue involved [de Almeida et al, 2012]. In addition to these tumor-related factors, selection of the reconstructive flap also depends on the integrity of the dura following tumor extirpation. If the dura has been breached, the extent of dural exposure will affect the selection of the reconstructive procedure. To minimize the risk of postoperative complications, it is necessary to establish a watertight dural seal, to support neural structures, to obliterate dead space and to repair the area with well-vascularized tissue. In many patients following resection of skull base tumors, it is also imperative to separate the dural repair from the aerodigestive tract.

This review of the reconstructive options for skull base defects follows a three-region classification system as outlined by Irish et al [1994].

4.1 Skull base region I

Region I [Irish et al, 1994] extends from the anterior skull base to the clivus (**Fig 3.6-1**). Tumors in this region arise from the maxilla, the maxillary sinusses, orbits and midfacial skin and may extend to invade the ethmoid sinuses, the cribriform plate, the dura and the frontal lobes in the anterior fossa of the cranium. Irish et al [1994] reported that the highest percentages of tumors (53%) were in region I and a small percentage of tumors (8%) crossed over regions I and II.

The surgical approach necessary for tumor ablation will vary and depends upon the size, the location and the specific tumor characteristics. However, in most cases a lateral rhinotomy approach provides good surgical access to remove tumors in region I. If the tumor is large, it may be necessary to increase the exposure with a maxillotomy or, in some cases, a partial or total maxillectomy. Depending on the tumor location, a coronal incision and frontal craniotomy may also be necessary for en bloc tumor resection or to provide good visualization of all neural and vascular structures.

Following tumor extirpation, the reconstructive options available will be based on several factors including the size and the position of the defect, the type of tissue required and whether the dura has been breached Several local soft-tissue flaps have been used, including forehead [Ousterhout et al, 1981; Thomson, 1970; Westbury et al, 1975], glabellar [Jackson et al, 1984], the pericranial [Scher et al, 1982; Noone et al, 2002] and the galeal flap [Jackson et al, 1986; Schramm et al, 1979]. The galeal flap and the pericranial flap provide adequate soft-tissue coverage for small midline defects with minimal donor site morbidity. For defects that are located more laterally in the anterior cranial fossa, the temporalis muscle provides well-vascularized tissue for soft-tissue coverage. However, for medial defects, there is an increased risk of flap necrosis because of the decreased vascularity at the distal end of the flap and, therefore, the temporalis flap is less optimal for these repairs. Following transposition of the temporalis flap, a concavity remains in the region of the temporal fossa and this can result in patient dissatisfaction. In some cases, the temporalis muscle may be devascularized during tumor ablation; consequently, this muscle may not always be available for reconstruction.

With more extensive defects, a larger volume of soft tissue is necessary to provide adequate contour and to fill the remaining dead space. Local flaps may not provide enough soft tissue, hence in these cases an alternate source of tissue is necessary. Musculocutaneous pedicle flaps can provide more vascularized soft-tissue bulk than local flaps. The trapezius, the pectoralis major and the latissimus dorsi muscles have been used for the management of skull base defects [Neligan et al, 1996]. However, with the introduction and improvement of the free tissue transfer with excellent outcomes [Neligan et al, 1996], these pedicled flaps are now only used for skull base defects in cases where free tissue transfer is not possible.

Free tissue transfer provides the availability of an abundant source of well-vascularized tissue from numerous anatomical sites and is the best reconstructive option for large skull base defects [Neligan et al, 1996; Califano et al, 2003; Teknos et al, 2002; Weber et al, 2007]. Free flaps can be selected and designed, based on the unique characteristics of the defect and are not restricted by an attachment as occurs with a pedicled flap. Because a free flap can easily be positioned into the recipient site, well-vascularized tissue can be placed where it is needed and thus minimizes the risk of postoperative complications. With appropriate preoperative planning and the use of a free tissue transfer, it may be possible to use a two-team approach for the surgery. With one surgical team performing the tumor ablation and the other team harvesting the tissue for the repair, operative time is decreased and risks to the patient associated with extended time under anesthesia are minimized.

There is an increased likelihood of infection when the dura and aerodigestive tracts have been breached. Musculocutaneous flaps that are well vascularized have a capacity to resist infection, and therefore are usually selected to provide a barrier between these two tracts. Numerous musculocutaneous free flaps have been described for soft-tissue reconstruction [Neligan et al, 1996; Mulholland et al, 1993; Lipa et al, 2004; Neligan, 1999; Urken et al, 1991]. The rectus abdominis and latissimus dorsi muscle flaps and the anterolateral thigh flap are good choices for this area because all provide a large mass of well-vascularized tissue and are an excellent barrier between the aerodigestive tract and the dura [Neligan et al, 1996; Urken et al, 1991]. For reconstruction of small region I defects, local flaps, such as the pericranial or galeo-frontalis flap, are adequate. However, when a large musculocutaneous flap is required, our preferred choice for this reconstruction is the latissimus dorsi or the anterolateral thigh free flap (**Fig 3.6-2**).

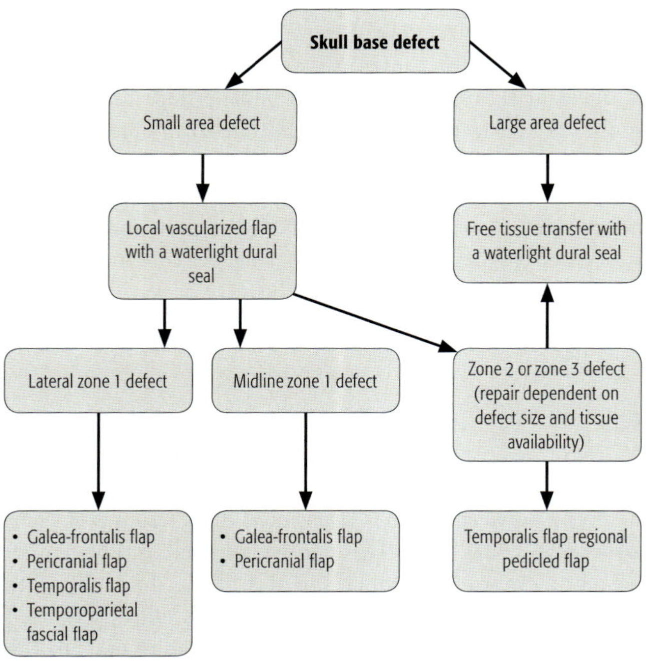

Fig 3.6-2 Management of skull base defects algorithm.

4.2 Skull base region II

The infratemporal and pterygomaxillary fossae and the overlying portion of the middle cranial fossa form region II [Irish et al, 1994] (**Fig 3.6-1**). It extends from the posterior wall of the orbit to the petrous temporal bone. Numerous vascular and neural structures traverse region II enroute through the middle cranial fossa. The internal carotid artery exits through the foramen lacerum (on the inferior surface of the skull) to the carotid groove on the sphenoid. Several cranial nerves pass through this zone including the facial (VII) and auditory (VIII) nerves, and the mandibular and maxillary branches of the trigeminal (V) nerve. Lesions that originate within region II include nasopharyngeal tumors, glomus jugulare tumors, clival chordomas, and meningiomas. However, many neoplasms such as invasive parotid tumors and basal and squamous cell carcinomas of the external and middle ear and the scalp originate outside of this zone and may subsequently invade region II. Neoplasms involving this zone are less common than those in regions I and III, and are associated with a poorer prognosis [Irish et al, 1994].

An infratemporal approach [Sekhar et al, 1986] with a hemicoronal incision and preauricular or postauricular extension may be used to expose neoplasms located in the middle region of the cranial base. This approach provides good exposure of the mandibular condyle and the capability to reflect the parotid gland and facial nerve inferiorly. Combining this approach with either a lateral or anterior mandibulotomy will provide excellent surgical exposure. In rare cases when the tumor involves the mandible, a partial mandibulectomy may be necessary. A transtemporal approach [Fisch et al, 1984] may also be used for ablation of region II tumors and usually necessitates a hemicoronal incision with a postauricular incision and transection of the external auditory canal. Mid-region skull base tumors with an intradural component can be exposed using a frontotemporal craniotomy.

Consideration of the precise location and size of the defect is imperative to determine the available reconstructive options. Historically, region II defects were reconstructed with rotational scalp [Westbury et al, 1975] and deltopectoral flaps [Bakamjian et al, 1971]. For large region II defects, musculocutaneous pedicled flaps including the pectoralis major and the trapezius flap have been described [Ariyan, 1979]. These flaps, however, often fail because of the limitations of flap length, which may leave a communication between the nasopharynx and the dura resulting in an infection and/or a cerebrospinal fluid leak. The use of a free tissue transfer is preferable to a pedicled flap for reconstruction, especially for large defects [Thurnher et al, 2007]. The anterolateral thigh flap (ALT) provides sufficient well-vascularized soft-tissue bulk and can be designed with muscle extensions to cover the sphenoid sinus. When a saphenous vein graft is used to reconstruct the carotid artery, some additional coverage can be provided for the neck region. Like other free flaps, the rectus abdominis or ALT free flaps also have the advantage of permitting a two-team surgical approach.

4.3 Skull base region III

Region III [Irish et al, 1994] is in the posterior cranial fossa (**Fig 3.6-1**). Like the other zones in the skull base, numerous vital neural and vascular structures traverse this area and include the internal jugular vein, the glossopharyngeal, the vagus, the accessory and the hypoglossal nerves. Jones et al [1987] reported the most common neoplasms involving region III were glomus tumors and schwannomas. In the series reported by Irish et al [1994], 14 of 25 patients with neoplasms in region III were diagnosed with squamous cell carcinoma. The reported prevalence of different tumor types in these studies may represent the varying referral patterns of diverse surgical specialties.

A transtemporal surgical approach is routinely used to remove lesions in region III. Bony resection around the carotid artery and sigmoid sinus are occasionally required. Following tumor ablation, local muscle flaps, such as the temporalis and the sternocleidomastoid flap, can be used to fill small defects. However, in cases where a radical neck dissection has been performed, these muscle flaps may be devascularized or included in the resection and so not available for the repair. Historically, pedicled flaps have been used for defects that require more soft tissue than can be provided with a local flap. However, the free tissue transfer has replaced the pedicled flap which provides a large amount of well-vascularized soft tissue for coverage and augmentation in the skull base region [Thurnher et al, 2007] (**Fig 3.6-3**). Currently, for this repair we use the scapular flap or in some cases the latissimus dorsi flap which provide a better color match and we continue to use the anterolateral thigh flap for select cases.

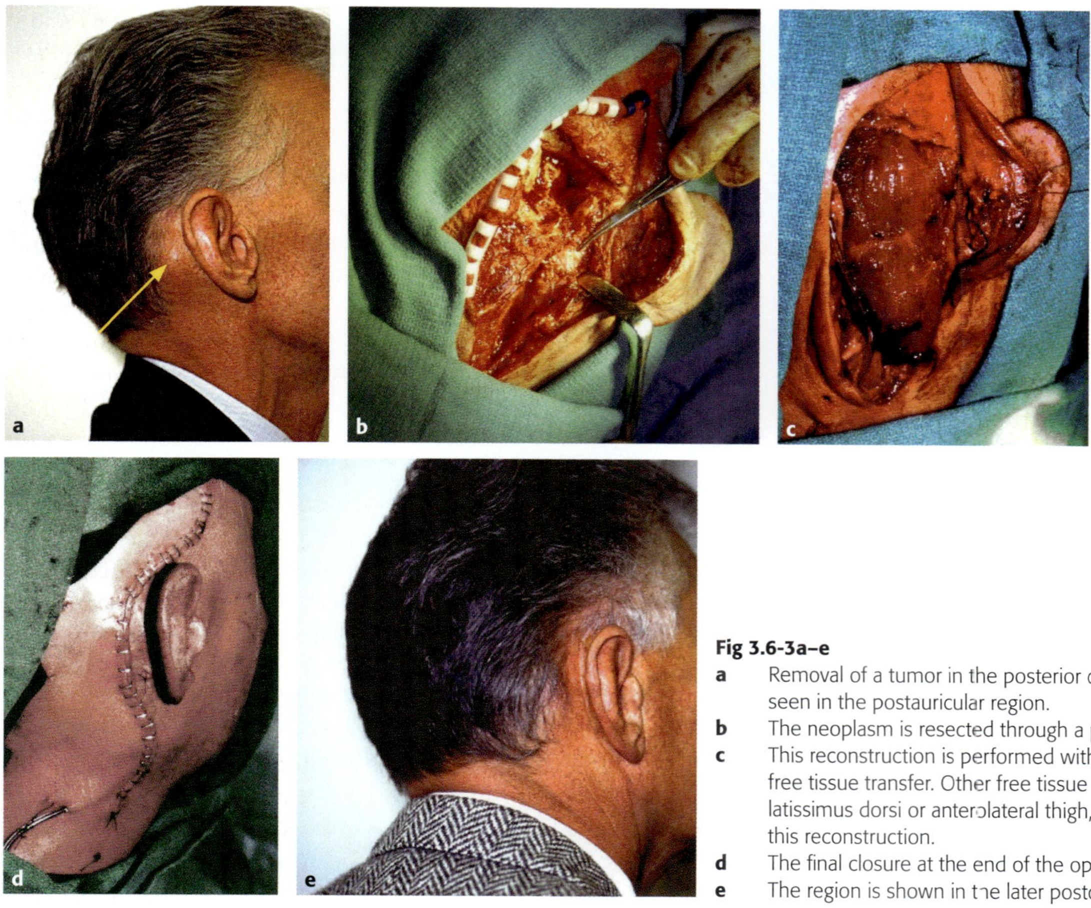

Fig 3.6-3a–e

- **a** Removal of a tumor in the posterior cranial fossa. The tumor is seen in the postauricular region.
- **b** The neoplasm is resected through a postauricular approach.
- **c** This reconstruction is performed with a rectus abdominus free tissue transfer. Other free tissue flaps, such as the latissimus dorsi or anterolateral thigh, may also be used for this reconstruction.
- **d** The final closure at the end of the operative procedure.
- **e** The region is shown in the later postoperative stage.

5 Technical considerations

The reconstruction following either open or endoscopic tumor extirpation must provide a barrier between the sinonasal tract and the cranial cavity to minimize the likelihood of perioperative complications, such as infection, cerebrospinal fluid leaks and meningitis. The use of vascularized flaps has substantially reduced the occurrence of these potentially lethal complications. Successful reconstruction of skull base defects requires the obliteration of dead space and a watertight dural seal. Several technical details require consideration to minimize the risk of perioperative complications. To eliminate dead space, it is necessary to pack the cavity with vascularized tissue such as a muscle or musculo-cutaneous flap and since muscle is flexible, it can easily fill these spaces. To minimize the risk of complications associated with a dural leak, it is imperative that a watertight seal is established. Because of the location of the skull base, there is a gravitational pull on the reconstructive tissue used that acts to separate the flap from the dural repair. This downward force makes it difficult to maintain the dural seal, which subsequently creates more dead space. To minimize this vector of force, the flap is secured to the surrounding bony structures (**Fig 3.6-4**).

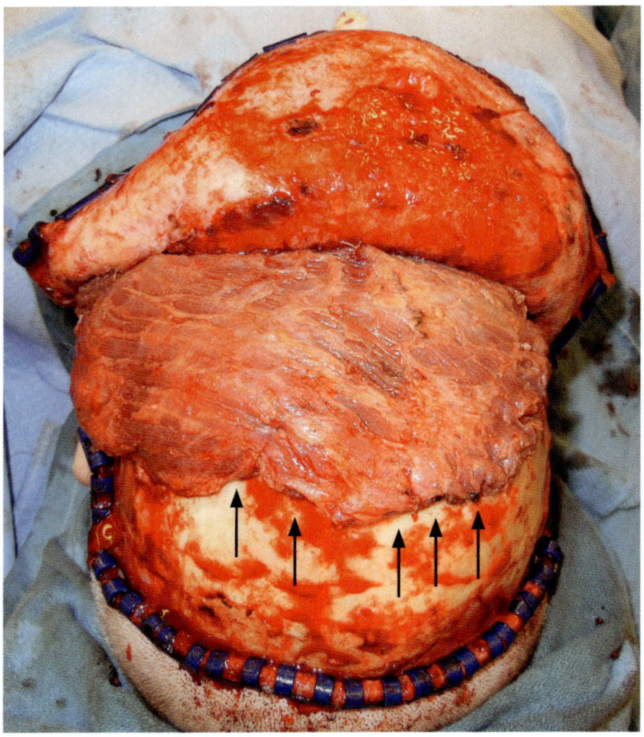

Fig 3.6-4 A microvascular latissimus dorsi flap is secured to the cranial bone with 3-0 sutures through drill holes in the outer table of the calvarium (arrows), thus maintaining the flap in its appropriate position and preserving the dural seal.

This can be achieved either via holes that are drilled into the bone adjacent to a defect, or using devices such as the Mitek anchor. Techniques such as these allow the flap to be pulled up to the defect and secured in that position. Fibrin glue can also be used to reinforce and to provide a seal between the flap and the dural repair. When the rectus abdominis muscle is used for the reconstruction, the suspension sutures are placed in the tendinous intersections that provides a secure attachment to the muscle with minimal risk of dehiscence.

When planning the reconstruction, consider the recipient vessels that will be used to vascularize the flap. The selection of these vessels will depend on several factors including pedicle geometry, pedicle length and vessel diameter. The superficial temporal vein and artery are a reliable vascular source for microvascular reconstruction in the skull base [Nahabedian et al, 2004]; however, when the superficial temporal vessels are not available or appear inadequate, the flap can be brought down into the neck. In the rare situation where pedicle reach is problematic, the use of an arterial venous (AV) loop is advocated. When constructing the AV loop, it is important to use large caliber vessels and our preference is to use a loop between the external carotid artery and the internal jugular vein. A vein graft is sutured end-to-side to the external carotid at one end and the internal jugular at the other end.

In most cases of skull base defects, bony reconstruction is not necessary if the soft-tissue bulk is sufficient. On occasion, some patients will require bony support with rigid fixation. Because of an increased risk of osteoradionecrosis or infection in patients who receive postoperative radiation therapy, vascularized bone, such as the scapula, is preferable. Alloplastic materials, such as titanium mesh or biomaterial bone graft substitute, are available to provide rigid support to the skull base [Badie et al, 2000] and there are no contraindications to postoperative follow-up CT and/or MRI.

When reconstructing zone I defects, we are frequently faced with the problem of not only ensuring a tight dural seal but requiring reconstruction of the nasal lining with or without the palate. Many authors advocate using a flap with multiple skin paddles, which is an acceptable approach [Cordeiro et al, 2000]. Our preference is to avoid multiple skin paddles and rely on mucosalization of the muscle in the nose and mouth. This occurs rapidly and gives a satisfactory and acceptable result.

6 Complications

The reported rates of complications of skull base reconstruction vary from 11.5–63% [Ganly et al, 2005; Imola et al, 2003]. In an international collaborative review by Patel et al [2003], 33% of the patients had a postoperative complication. Significantly more complications were noted in those patients with medical comorbidities, prior radiation treatment and intracranial involvement of the tumor. In the more recent publications, a decrease in the reported complication rate is seen [Imola et al, 2003]. Many factors have likely played a role in this improved outcome including advanced surgical technique, improved postoperative patient care and the increased use of the free tissue transfer for the reconstruction.

6.1 Early complications

Early postoperative complications include local wound infection of the recipient or donor site, exposure of the dura, cerebrospinal fluid leak, cranial nerve dysfunction and ascending meningitis. The most common complication reported by Patel et al [2003] was a local wound infection. However, many of the complications that occur in the early postoperative period are related to inadequate closure of the dura and/or persistent communication between the aerodigestive tract and the intracranial cavity. Since the skull base is near vital neural and vascular structures, postoperative complications can be devastating. These early complications can rapidly progress into life-threatening conditions and therefore it is important that these patients are closely monitored postoperatively and treated promptly and effectively. However, a proactive approach to minimize the risk of complications is recommended with the selection of the appropriate repair based on the surgical defect and patient factors.

6.1.1 Wound infection

Wound infections must be treated aggressively [Brown et al, 2007]. With suitable cultures, the patient is administered the appropriate intravenous antibiotic therapy. If the oral and/or nasal cavities have been exposed, prophylactic antibiotics are indicated and a broad-spectrum cephalosporin combined with an anaerobic pharmacological agent, such as Flagyl, are commonly used.

6.1.2 Flap compromise

Musculocutaneous flaps should be monitored postoperatively for both arterial and venous flow and any compromise in vascular perfusion must be treated with urgency since prolonged compromise can result in flap loss. Early nonoperative intervention, such as the use of leeches, can reverse venous congestion but frequently operative intervention to improve venous and/or arterial flow is required. The success rates for secondary free flaps in head and neck reconstruction is lower than for primary flaps, hence flap monitoring and early treatment of flap compromise are essential [Ross et al, 2012].

6.1.3 Cerebrospinal fluid leak

There is an increased risk of a postoperative cerebrospinal fluid leak as the extent of the resection including dural exposure increases. A watertight dural seal using vascularized tissue is essential to minimize the risk of this complication. Small cerebrospinal fluid leaks may resolve with conservative management including head elevation, lumbar drainage and the avoidance of Valsalva maneuvers. With larger leaks or in those failing to respond to conservative therapy, or where abundant vascularized soft tissue is deficient, a lumbar drain or another operative reconstructive procedure may be necessary.

6.1.4 Intracranial infections

With the advent of free tissue transfer, the prevalence of meningitis has been significantly reduced [Neligan et al, 1996]. On the rare occasion that this complication occurs, broad spectrum or culture-specific antibiotics are used.

6.1.5 Cranial nerve dysfunction

Extensive skull base resection and the need to sacrifice a major cranial nerve may result in significant cranial nerve dysfunction. When they are possible, nerve grafts and repair techniques are used. However, patient education is necessary to minimize further complications, such as corneal ulcer in cases of facial nerve dysfunction. Another major cranial nerve complication occurs in patients who have had sacrifice of the vagus nerve including the sensory and motor components resulting in dysphagia. As the affected vocal cord is paralyzed in the lateral position, an early medialization procedure is recommended to optimize speech and swallowing [Abraham et al, 2001; Spector et al, 2001]. If the nerve was not resected but there is evidence of neural dysfunction, the patient should be monitored for signs of recovery or progression. Appropriate postoperative intervention is required as indicated by patient symptoms in the ongoing assessment.

6.2 Late complications

Late complications following skull base surgery include nasal obstruction, malocclusion, trismus, facial deformity, and diplopia. These complications are usually associated with bony instability, soft-tissue atrophy or postoperative radiation fibrosis. While these complications are not life-threatening, they can negatively affect patient outcome and health-related quality of life.

7 Summary

In recent years, there has been an increased use of vascularized free tissue transfer for reconstruction in the skull base [Neligan et al, 1996]. This has resulted in improved patient outcome and a significant reduction in the complication rate. Ablation of skull base tumors often results in large soft-tissue defects with exposed dura. To ensure a successful reconstruction, it is necessary to create a watertight dural seal that isolates the intracranial contents from the upper aerodigestive tract and minimizes dead space. With the advent of improved surgical techniques including minimal access approaches and ablation, these advancements have diminished patient morbidity and further improve health-related quality of life of patients with skull base tumors.

8 References and suggested reading

Abraham MT, Gonen M, Kraus DH. Complications of type I thyroplasty and arytenoid adduction. *Laryngoscope*. 2001 Aug;111(8):1322–1329.

Ariyan S. The pectoralis major myocutaneous flap. A versatile flap for reconstruction of the head and neck. *Plast Reconstr Surg*. 1979 Jan;63(1):73–81.

Ariyan S. Further experiences with the pectoralis major myocutaneous flap for the immediate repair of defects from excisions of head and neck cancers. *Plast Reconstr Surg*. 1979 Nov;64(5):605–612.

Bakamjian VY, Long M, Rigg B. Experience with the medially based deltopectoral flap in reconstructive surgery of the head and neck. *Br J Plast Surg*. 1971 Apr;24(2):174–183.

Badie B, Preston JK, Hartig GK. Use of titanium mesh for reconstruction of large anterior cranial base defects. *J Neurosurg*. 2000 Oct;93(4):711–714.

Brown SM, Anand VK, Tabaee A, et al. Role of perioperative antibiotics in endoscopic skull base surgery. *Laryngoscope*. 2007 Sep;117(9):1528–1532.

Califano J, Cordeiro PG, Disa JJ, et al. Anterior cranial base reconstruction using free tissue transfer: changing trends. *Head Neck*. 2003 Feb;25(2):89–96.

Cordeiro PG, Disa JJ. Challenges in midface reconstruction. *Semin Surg Oncol*. 2000 Oct–Nov;19(3):218–225.

de Almeida JR, Witterick IJ, Gullane PJ, et al. Physical morbidity by surgical approach and tumor location in skull base surgery. *Head Neck*. 2013 Apr;35(4):493–499.

de Almeida JR, Vescan AD, Gullane PJ, et al. Development of a disease-specific quality-of-life questionnaire for anterior and central skull base pathology—the skull base inventory. *Laryngoscope*. 2012 Sep;122(9):1933–1942.

Feiz-Erfan I, Suki D, Hanna E, et al. Prognostic significance of transdural invasion of cranial base malignancies in patients undergoing craniofacial resection. *Neurosurgery*. 2007 Dec;61(6):1178–1185; discussion 1185.

Fisch U, Fagan P, Valavanis A. The infratemporal fossa approach for the lateral skull base. *Otolaryngol Clin N Am*. 1984 Aug;17(3):513–552.

Ganly I, Patel SG, Singh B, et al. Complications of craniofacial resection for malignant tumors of the skull base: report of an International Collaborative Study. *Head Neck*. 2005 Jun;27(6):445–451.

Hanna E, DeMonte F, Ibrahim S, et al. Endoscopic resection of sinonasal cancers with and without craniotomy: oncologic results. *Arch Otolaryngol Head Neck Surg*. 2009 Dec;135(12):1219–1224.

Imola MJ, Sciarretta V, Schramm VL. Skull base reconstruction. *Curr Opin Otolaryngol Head Neck Surg*. 2003 Aug;11(4):282–290.

Irish J, Gullane PJ, Gentili F, et al. Tumors of the skull base: outcome and survival analysis of 77 cases. *Head Neck*. 1994 Jan–Feb;16(1):3–10.

Jackson IT, Hide TA. A systematic approach to tumours of the base of the skull. *J Maxillofac Surg*. 1982 May;10(2):92–98.

Jackson IT, Adham MN, Marsh WR. Use of the galeal frontalis myofascial flap in craniofacial surgery. *Plast Reconstr Surg*. 1986 Jun;77(6):905–910.

Jackson IT, Marsh WR, Hide TA. Treatment of tumors involving the anterior cranial fossa. *Head Neck Surg*. 1984 May–Jun;6(5):901–913.

Jones NF, Schramm VL, Sekhar LN. Reconstruction of the cranial base following tumour resection. *Br J Plast Surg*. 1987 Mar;40(2):155–162.

Ketcham AS, Hoye RC, Van Buren JM, et al. Complications of intracranial facial resections for tumors of the paranasal sinuses. *Am J Surg*. 1966 Oct;112(4):591–596.

Lipa JE, Butler CE. Enhancing the outcome of free latissimus dorsi muscle flap reconstruction of scalp defects. *Head Neck*. 2004 Jan;26(1):46–53.

Nahabedian MY, Singh N, Deune EG, et al. Recipient vessel analysis for microvascular reconstruction of the head and neck. *Ann Plast Surg*. 2004 Feb;52(2):148–155; discussion 156–157.

Neligan PC, Mulholland S, Irish J, et al. Flap selection in cranial base reconstruction. *Plast Reconstr Surg*. 1996 Dec;98(7):1159–1166.

Neligan PC, Mulholland RS, Boyd JB, et al. Flap selection in cranial base reconstruction: local, pedicled or free? *Plast Surg Forum*. 1993;62:265–266.

Noone MC, Osguthorpe JD, Patel S. Pericranial flap for closure of paramedian anterior skull base defects. *Otolaryngol Head Neck Surg*. 2002 Dec;127(6):494–500.

Ousterhout DK, Tessier P. Closure of large cribriform defects with a forehead flap. *J Maxillofac Surg*. 1981 Feb;9(1):7–9.

Patel SG, Singh B, Polluri A, et al. Craniofacial surgery for malignant skull base tumors. *Cancer*. 2003 Sep 15;98(6):1179–1187.

Palme CE, Irish JC, Gullane PJ, et al. Quality of life analysis in patients with anterior skull base neoplasms. *Head Neck*. 2009 Oct;31(10):1326–1334.

Parson H, Lewis JS. Subtotal resection of the temporal bone for cancer of the ear. *Cancer*. 1954 Sep;7(5):995–1001.

Ross G, Yla-Kotola TM, Goldstein D, et al. Second free flaps in head and neck reconstruction. *J Plast Reconstr Aesthetic Surg*. 2012 Sep;65(9):1165–1168.

Scher RL, Cantrell RW. Anterior skull base reconstruction with the pericranial flap after craniofacial reconstruction. *Ear Nose Throat J.* 1992 May;71(5):210–212, 215–217.

Schramm VL Jr, Myers EN, Maroon JC. Anterior skull base surgery for benign and malignant disease. *Laryngoscope.* 1979 Jul;89(7 Pt 1):1077–1091.

Sekhar LN, Schramm VL, Jones NF. Combined resection of large neoplasms involving the lateral and posterior cranial base. In: Sekhar LN, Schramm VL, eds. *Tumors of the Cranial Base: Diagnosis and Treatment.* New York: Futura Publishers; 1986.

Spector BC, Netterville JL, Billante C, et al. Quality-of-life assessment in patients with unilateral vocal cord paralysis. *Otolaryngol Head Neck Surg.* 2001 Sep;125(3):176–182.

Teknos TN, Smith JC, Day TA, et al. Microvascular free tissue transfer in reconstructing skull base defects: lessons learned. *Laryngoscope.* 2002 Oct;112(10):1871–1876.

Thoma A, Khadaroo R, Grigenas O, et al. Oromandibular reconstruction with the radial-forearm osteocutaneous flap: experience with 60 consecutive cases. *Plast Reconstr Surg.* 1999 Aug;104(2):368–378; 379–380.

Thomson HG. Reconstruction of the orbit after radial exenteration. *Plast Reconstr Surg.* 1970 Feb;45(2):119–123.

Thurnher D, Novak CB, Neligan PC, et al. Reconstruction of lateral skull base defects after tumor ablation. *Skull Base.* 2007 Feb;17(1):79–88.

Urken ML, Turk JB, Weinberg H, et al. The rectus abdominus free flap in head and neck reconstruction. *Arch Otolaryngol Head Neck Surg.* 1991 Aug;117(8):857–866.

Ward GE, Loch WE, Lawrence W Jr. Radical operation for carcinoma of the external auditory canal and middle ear. *Am J Surg.* 1951 Jul;82(1):169–178.

Weber SM, Kim JH, Wax MK. Role of free tissue transfer in skull base reconstruction. *Otolaryngol Head Neck Surg.* 2007 Jun;136(6):914–919.

Westbury G, Wilson JS, Richardson A. Combined craniofacial resection for malignant disease. *Am J Surg.* 1975 Oct;130(4):463–469.

3.7 Reconstruction of the cranial vault

Jesse A Taylor, Navin K Singh

1 Introduction

Indications for reconstruction of the cranial vault result from tumor, infection, neurological symptoms in the face of a cranial defect, and esthetic concerns. Planning for reconstruction is complex, requiring the combined efforts of neurosurgeons, craniomaxillofacial (CMF) surgeons, anesthesiologists, and support staff.

1.1 Indications

Most cranial defects are caused by trauma, tumor including sequelae of tumor therapy (radiation), infection, or present as a deficiency resulting from craniofacial malformations. Penetrating trauma to the cranial vault from low- and high-velocity gunshot wounds creates complex defects in the cranial vault, many of which require both bony and soft-tissue reconstruction. Blunt trauma causes fewer and less complex defects, with scalp lacerations and soft-tissue avulsions dominant among them [Dujovny et al, 1997].

Defects caused by tumor extirpation are the second most common indication for complex reconstruction of the cranial vault. Both cutaneous and intracranial tumors may create significant bone defects that require either single-stage or multistage reconstruction (**Fig 3.7-1**). This may be undertaken acutely to provide brain protection, subacutely after adjuvant therapies, or in the late phase for long-term survivors. A small percentage of patients who have had a craniotomy for tumor extirpation develop "growing" burr holes (skull defects) secondary to a myelomeningocele, a condition also requiring cranial vault reconstruction.

Osteomyelitis is rare in the craniofacial skeleton. It commonly presents as a non-healing ulcer, and is often related to sinus infection, invasive hardware such as intracranial pressure bolts, or osteosynthesis implants. It is more common in patients who are immunosuppressed from chemotherapy after tumor resection or who have been radiated (**Fig 3.7-2**). Osteomyelitis in the craniofacial skeleton requires wide debridement of involved tissues followed by a 6–8 week course of antibiotics and subsequent cranial vault reconstruction. Often, new tissue must be provided.

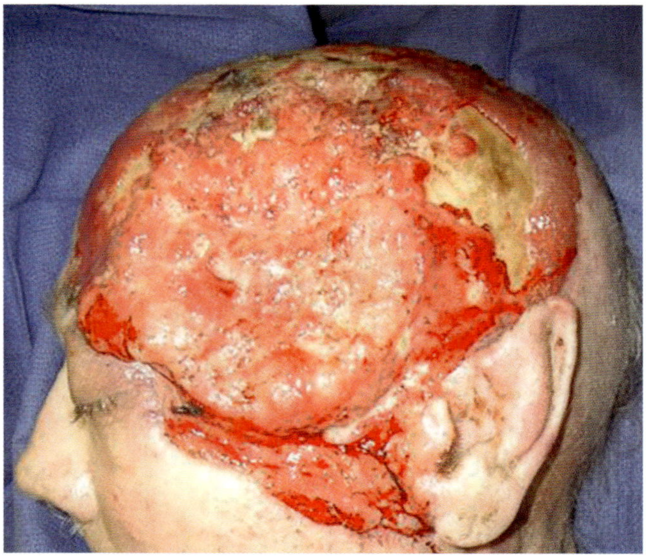

Fig 3.7-1 Cutaneous squamous cell carcinoma of the scalp invading the underlying cranium.

Osteoradionecrosis, sequelae of tumoricidal external beam radiation therapy, presents similarly to osteomyelitis. It, too, requires removal of involved bone, often creating a significant defect. The soft tissues in the area are often of poor vascularity. Immediate reconstruction of the cranial vault is recommended in the setting of osteoradionecrosis, frequently with the need for vascularized soft-tissue coverage.

Some patients develop neurological symptoms from cranial defects. The "syndrome of the trephined" or "sinking skin flap syndrome" consists of a complex set of symptoms involving headache, discomfort, depression, dizziness, and epilepsy. Subcortical gliosis may be caused by compression leading to altered cerebrospinal fluid (CSF) circulation pathways and distortion of the intracranial ventricles. Patients who have undergone soft-tissue reconstruction without a rigid construct may develop neurological deficits related to alterations in intracranial pressure. Relief of neurological symptoms, such as headaches, epilepsy, and previous neurological deficits, has been reported after rigid cranial vault reconstruction, although the mechanism by which this occurs is not proven nor understood.

Abnormalities in the cranial vault are difficult to conceal, and esthetic concerns are a common indication for reconstruction. Frontal craniectomy, delayed reconstruction in a growing child, soft-tissue atrophy post-craniotomy and bony atrophy are all esthetic indications for cranial vault reconstruction.

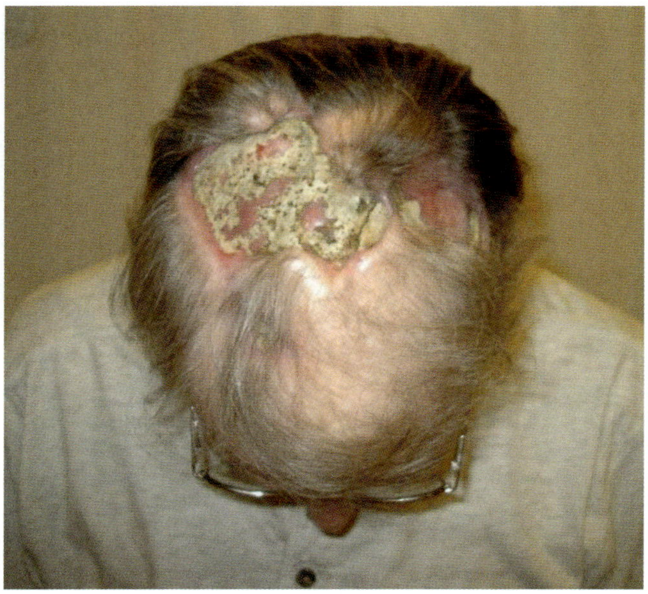

Fig 3.7-2 Osteomyelitis of the cranium with dead exposed bone.

1.2 Planning

Planning for reconstruction of the cranial vault requires a coordinated effort by surgeons, anesthesiologists, and support staff. Planning is guided by a thorough history and physical examination coupled with appropriate radiographic imaging. Plain radiographs are rarely performed but may aid in planning a cephalometrically proportioned reconstruction.

The most widely used imaging technique is a computed tomography (CT) scan of the cranium and face.

The CT scans provide an unmatched high-resolution, cross-sectional image of a defect (or proposed extirpative defect). Axial, coronal, and sagittal images provide enough data to achieve an appropriate reconstruction but the recent decrease in cost and increase in availability of 3-D CT scans is making their use more widespread. Moreover, the datasets from 3-D CT scans can be translated directly into CAD/CAM devices for stereolithography. These datasets can also be transmitted electronically to medical implant companies for fabrication of customized implants made from titanium, polyether-ether-ketone (PEEK), or high-density polyethylene.

Magnetic resonance imaging (MRI) and magnetic resonance angiography are useful adjuncts in cranial vault reconstruction. They aid in diagnosis of infected or necrotic bone, more clearly delineate soft-tissue tumors, confirm patency of the external carotid system, and provide data regarding cerebral perfusion (**Fig 3.7-3**). With the increasing resolution and availability of magnetic resonance angiography, head and neck angiograms are rarely performed.

An important part of the planning process is determining how to arrive at the best possible reconstruction with the fewest stages. A single-staged reconstruction avoids additional procedures, and provides for a single recovery period. Multistaged reconstructions may be used when the completeness of the tumor extirpation is in question, in the face of active infection, or when adjuvant therapies might threaten the reconstruction. Delay of definitive cranial vault reconstruction is indicated in the following circumstances:

- Trauma causing extensive cerebral edema and increased ICP
- Active local infection
- Ongoing sepsis
- Medically unstable patient

When planning a multistage reconstruction, an important consideration is the possible use of tissue expanders before definitive cranial reconstruction. Placement of tissue expanders increases the amount of skin available and effectively "delays" a local skin flap. In children, ports for tissue expanders can be placed remotely for less painful expansion.

2 Techniques

Reconstruction of the cranial vault requires attention to three levels of repair: the dura, the cranium, and the overlying soft tissues. The main objective is to achieve a functional and esthetic reconstruction using reliable methods and materials.

2.1 The dura

Dural reconstruction is a key step in cranial vault reconstruction, as failure to create a water-tight seal may compromise all other layers. Water-tight closure isolates the CSF and brain from the external environment, eliminating the opportunity for seeding implants with infection, or worse, causing meningitis.

Tension-free primary closure of the dura is preferred. When primary closure is unobtainable, various grafts are interposed. Fascial grafts, most commonly from the pericranium or tensor fascia lata, have been reliably used for decades but have the drawback of potential donor site morbidity [Gladstone et al, 1995]. These drawbacks have led to the development of alloplastic graft materials including bovine collagen matrix, bovine pericardial patches, and acellular dermal matrix.

Choice of graft is largely based on surgeon preference. In addition to alloplastic materials, there is a trend toward sutureless repair of the dura by substituting fibrin glue for sutures. Fibrin glue provides an immediate water-tight seal, an advantage over sutures. Patients at high risk for CSF leak, for instance those who have undergone a posterior fossa craniectomy and those who have undergone intraventricular manipulation, are excellent candidates for fibrin glue closure. Supratentorial dural repairs are less likely to develop a CSF leak, and water-tight suture closure is sufficient.

If a water-tight closure is not possible, or if a CSF leak is discovered postoperatively, a lumbar drain is indicated to divert the flow of CSF and its pressure from the wound to allow leaks to seal.

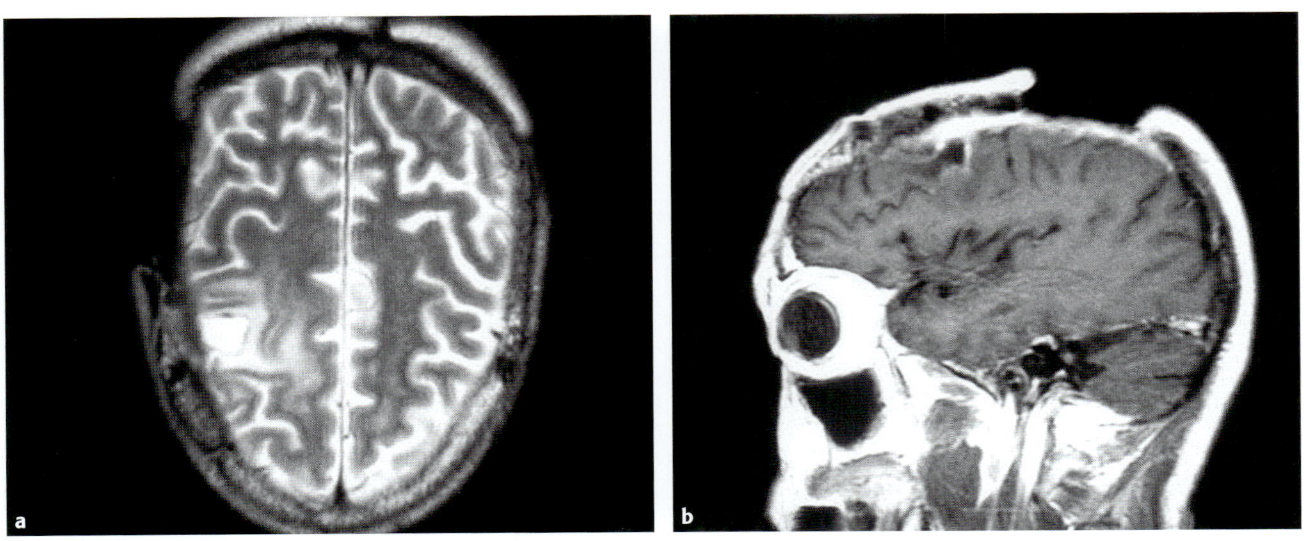

Fig 3.7-3a–b Axial and coronal magnetic resonance imaging of cranial defects.

2.2 The cranium

A cranioplasty, or rigid cranial reconstruction, is interposed between the dural repair and the overlying soft tissues to provide protection to the brain from the mechanically disruptive forces of the external environment. Cranioplasty may be carried out with autogenous bone or alloplastic material. When choosing a technique and biomaterial for cranioplasty, several important factors must be weighed. First is the issue of biocompatibility, or the ability of a material to retain its function without adversely affecting the living tissue into which it is placed [Gladstone et al, 1995]. The stability of the material over time must be such that it does not degrade over time, thus failing its primary goal of replacing or augmenting the cranium. It also must not degrade in such a way as to leach chemicals into surrounding tissues or release toxic or mutagenic chemicals into the system. Furthermore, it must interface with the host to promote stability. The rigid construct must fulfill the role of replacing a section of calvarial bone. Thus, it must behave like calvarial bone, having similar strength characteristics and fracture resistance, resistance to heat conductivity, radiopacity, elastic modulus, and magnetic properties [Gladstone et al, 1995]. Characteristics of common implants used for the rigid construct are listed in **Table 3.7-1**. From the surgeon's standpoint, the material should be easy to prepare, rigidly fixate, and shape.

2.2.1 Bone

Autogenous bone remains a preferred option for cranial vault reconstruction because of its potential for osteoconductive bone formation, its obvious biocompatibility, and its ability to resist infection, its low rates of extrusion, and its readiness for use [Gladstone et al, 1995; Jackson et al, 1987; Manson et al, 1986]. Its drawbacks include variable resorption patterns with obvious cosmetic and strength sequelae, difficulty in molding, and creation of a donor site with concomitant morbidities. Late complications from bone grafts include contour deformities from resorption, often requiring further procedures for correction with materials other than bone [Moreira-Gonzalez et al, 2003].

Bone grafts heal via osteoconductive "creeping substitution". The success of a bone graft depends on vascular supply and osteoblastic migration across a bone gap, thus the condition of the surrounding tissue and the contact between the host and graft is critical. Bone grafts should be rigidly stabilized with good bone-to-bone contact to promote primary bone healing. The most convenient donor site for bone graft is the surgical site, ie, split calvarial bone graft, or a remote donor site including split-rib or iliac crest. Because of the unreliable and variable resorption of autogenous bone grafts, long-term maintenance of contour is not achieved. Further, the additional donor site morbidity makes bone grafts less popular nowadays for reconstructing large defects (> 16 cm²) in the adult cranium.

Material	Density, g/cm²	Elastic modulus, GPa	Yield strength tension, MPa	Ultimate tensile strength, MPa	Poisson's ratio	Elongation, %	Specific heat capacity, J/kg K	Thermal expansion, 1/°C x 10-5
Cortical bone	1.8–2.0	17–24	----	120–133	0.30–0.34	1.4	778	2.4
Titanium (CP4)	4.5	100–120	430–550	400–620	0.36	15–30	---	0.8–1.0
Titanium (Ti-6Al-4V)	4.4	100–124	790–970	896–1020	---	12–15	---	1.2
PMMA	1.1	2.4–3.3	15.8	9.7–32	---	2–7	---	7.0
Hydroxyapatite (40–60% porous)	3.1	7–13	---	1.2–12	0.28	---	439	---
Co-Cr-Mo (Vitallium)	8.3	210	860–1028	1200–1511	---	15–28	----	---
Aluminum (5056)	2.7	69	151	289	0.33	35	895	1.6–2.3
Stainless steel (F56)	7.9	190–210	---	586	0.28	55	490	1.5–2.7
Tantalum	16.6	180–186	140	34–300	0.34	20–50	140	----

Table 3.7-1 Physical properties of cranioplastic implant materials.

2.2.2 Titanium

Titanium has been used in cranioplasty since the end of World War II, but did not gain wide appeal until the development of complex mesh patterns in the early 1980s. The addition of aluminum to make the commercially available alloy TI-6Al-4V (signifying the addition of 6% aluminum and 4% vanadium by weight) both strengthens and stabilizes it. When additional strength and fatigue resistance are required, the titanium is heat processed [Blake et al, 1990]. The result is an alloy that is light, strong, biocompatible, heat resistant, and affordable [Blake et al, 1990]. It does not cause hypersensitivity reactions and is minimally encapsulated by normal wound healing mechanisms. It is neither magnetic nor paramagnetic, and it is fairly radiolucent [Blake et al, 1990]. From the surgical standpoint, it is relatively easy to contour and may be rigidly fixated, usually with monocortical 4 to 6 mm screws. Rigid fixation of titanium mesh into healthy bone minimizes displacement and lifting of the mesh edges. Actually, 1.3 mm or 1.5 mm titanium mesh is sufficient cranial protection for most individuals over the long term (**Fig 3.7-4**).

Despite some adverse experience regarding long-term contour maintenance with titanium mesh in large defects, many surgeons use it in these situations without difficulty. Furthermore, its ease in contouring makes it ideal for complex cranial vault, base and orbital reconstructions (**Fig 3.7-5**).

Titanium mesh is not problematic in case of infection because of titanium's unique ionic bonding to underlying bone and soft tissues, it is minimally encapsulated and thus more accessible to the immune system compared with other materials. Therefore, exposed titanium mesh does not always require implant removal. but often can be treated with local wound care or have skin re-advanced without removing the original implant. Other biomaterials do not exhibit such properties, and would require removal, if exposed.

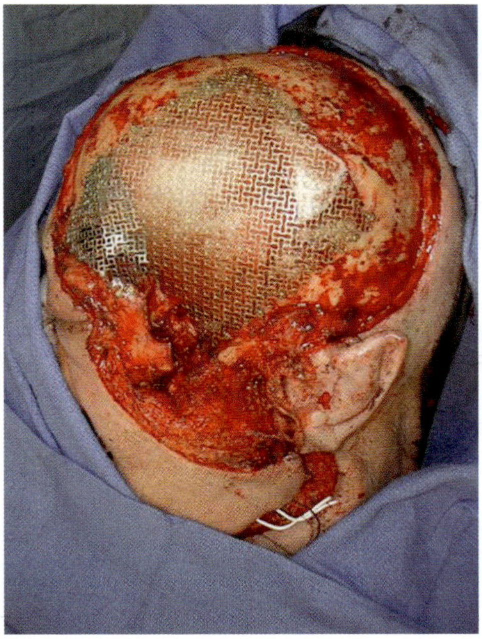

Fig 3.7-4 Frontoparietal titanium mesh cranioplasty (same patient as in Fig 3.7-1).

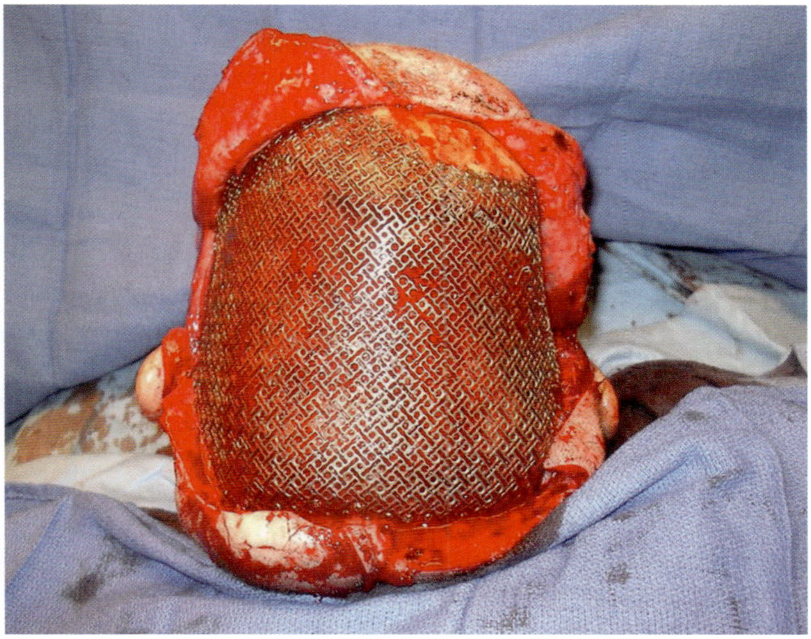

Fig 3.7-5 Titanium mesh cranioplasty in a patient with previous osteomyelitis.

In an effort to enhance cosmetic results and minimize operative time, computer design custom-fitted titanium implants can be made preoperatively based on 3-D CT scans (so-called CAD/CAM technique). At least three fixation devices equivalent to microplates are included in the implant construction so that the custom-fitted implants may be rigidly fixated. Their bone adherent surface is derived from the individual bony contour; their outer surface is designed to blend well with the cranium's outer contours [Eufinger et al, 1998]. Early series using these custom-fitted implants have demonstrated shorter operative times and good esthetic results without increased morbidity [Eufinger et al, 1998]. However, if they do not fit precisely into the defect, these titanium implants cannot be contoured.

2.2.3 Polymethylmethacrylate

Because of its availability, biocompatibility, and ease of use, polymethylmethacrylate (PMMA) is considered by many to be the implant of choice in adult cranioplasty. It is stronger than adjacent cranial bone in compression and torsion testing, and inert with minimal inflammatory reaction [Lara et al, 1998]. It adheres tightly to adjacent bone, is not thermoconductive, and has no magnetic or paramagnetic properties [Lara et al, 1998]. From a radiographic standpoint, PMMA is hypointense on MRI and hyperintense with minimal scatter on CT imaging [Gladstone et al, 1995]. It is easy to contour, providing superior cosmetic results.

Prepared in the operating room, PMMA is a mixture of a powder polymer and a liquid monomer in a 2:1 ratio. Polymerization is an exothermic process, and PMMA can reach temperatures over 60° C, requiring it to be continuously cooled to avoid causing thermal injury to underlying structures. Because it is placed as "dough" and hardens in situ, it is helpful to place it on a scaffold, typically titanium mesh, for added stability and protection. If it is used alone, it is important to ensure immobilization by onlay rigid fixation with screws because fixation can loosen with time [Smith et al, 1999].

Being relatively brittle, PMMA is susceptible to fracture after trauma. In multiple series, PMMA has been demonstrated to have low rates of infection [Manson et al, 1986; Moreira-Gonzalez et al, 2003; Donati et al, 1997], but loosening and fracture of the implant leads to increased rates of long-term problems [Smith et al, 1999]. PMMA is not resistant to infection, and infection is a relative contraindication to PMMA cranioplasty [Manson et al, 1986]. The most common adverse events associated with PMMA are hematoma and seroma, both of which are usually self-limited [Moreira-Gonzalez et al, 2003].

When using paste materials that must "set" in situ, such as PMMA or ceramics, a mesh platform must be created over the dura to prevent dural pulsations from fracturing the setting material before it becomes fully rigid. Fractured material is likely to become a nidus for infection related to micro-motion.

2.2.4 Porous polyethylene

Porous polyethylene has been demonstrated to facilitate reconstruction of small (< 8 cm^2) defects of the cranial vault [Liu et al, 2004]. It is biocompatible, flexible, can easily be contoured, and is non-resorbable. It is porous, allowing for the potential (200 microns only) ingrowth of bone and soft tissues to increase implant strength and resist infection. It provides similar cosmetic results to other alloplastic techniques while generally lowering operative times [Liu et al, 2004]. CAD/CAM technology has been applied to porous polyethylene allowing for custom-milling for complex defects and a renewed enthusiasm of its use. Because it is semirigid, some surgeons are using it for large defects in growing children to provide some degree of cranial protection while allowing for cranial growth. It can also be contoured and trimmed with a rotating burr to achieve the best possible fit. Polyetheretherketone offers similar characteristics, attributes, and indications as porous polyethylene.

2.2.5 Polyetheretherketone

Polyetheretherketone (PEEK) is a colorless organic thermoplastic polymer of the polyacryletherketone family used in engineering applications. Because of its robustness, PEEK is used to fabricate items used in demanding applications, including bone replacement. Using CAD/CAM technologies, individual patient-specific implants can be created for craniofacial application (**Fig 3.7-6**).

3 Future directions in biomaterials

The ideal implant for cranioplasty is biocompatible, malleable yet strong, volumetrically stable over time, resistant to infection, and easy to use. Various strategies to improve on currently available implants include coating them with growth factors to promote ingrowth of adjacent tissues, coating them with antibiotics to resist infection, and using computer-aided design to increase the quality of their fit. Other strategies involve inducing the body's immune system to heal wounds more quickly. New ceramics like calcium phosphate silicates have been shown to induce bony ingrowth not only via osteoconduction and osteoinduction but also by osteoproduction, the process whereby a bioactive

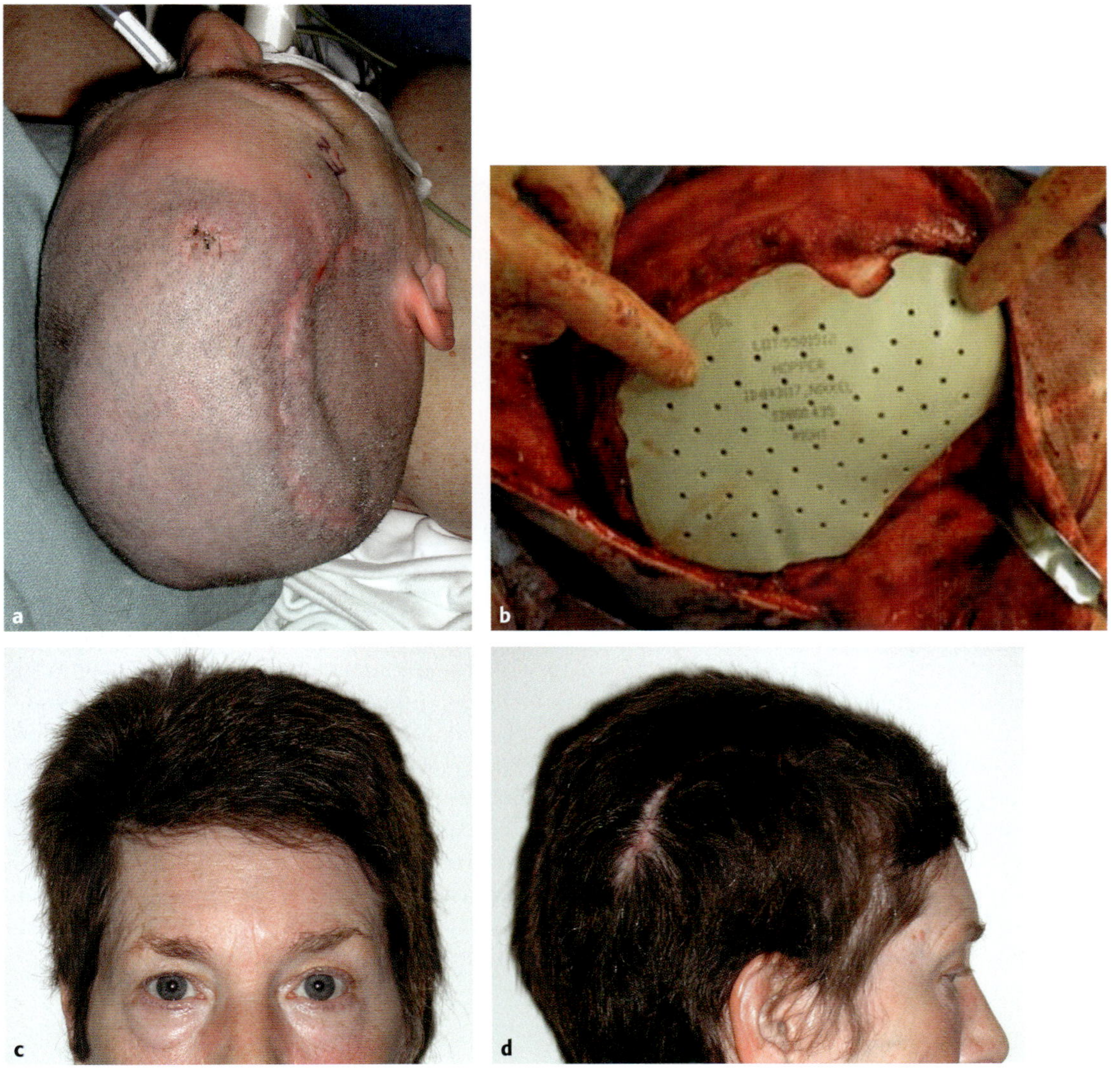

Fig 3.7-6a–d

- **a** A 57-year-woman 5 months after removal of infected cranial bone flap.
- **b** Polyetheretherketone cranioplasty placed.
- **c** Frontal view: 6-month follow-up.
- **d** Lateral view: 6-month follow-up.

substance is colonized by osteogenic stem cells during surgery [Elshahat et al, 2004]. Finally, advances in metallurgy may prove fruitful in achieving better implants.

3.1 Overlying soft tissues

Reconstructing the overlying soft tissues is essential for a successful cranial vault reconstruction. Primary closure is preferred where possible. When a tension-free primary closure is not possible, scalp expansion, local flaps or free-tissue transfer provide protection to the underlying cranioplasty and brain.

Skin grafts provide cutaneous cover with minimal donor site morbidity. They take reliably on dura, pericranium, galea, muscle, and dermis. They take less reliably on healthy, bleeding cortical bone.

Local scalp flaps may be either random pattern flaps or pedicled flaps. They may be enlarged by tissue expansion. The soft tissues of the scalp are richly vascularized, and can be transferred randomly in at least a 2:1 length to width ratio. Local flaps are particularly useful in replacing hair-bearing scalp, especially when coupled with tissue expansion. Multiple advancement and rotational random-pattern flaps have been used, the names and geometry of which are beyond the scope of this chapter.

Pedicled flaps based on the superficial temporal artery or the occipital artery may provide vascularized coverage of defects in all anatomical regions of the cranium. Additionally, local muscle flaps may be rotated and the donor defect covered with a skin graft. Local and regional muscles used commonly in reconstructing the cranial vault include the temporalis muscle, the trapezius muscle, the pectoralis major muscle, and the latissimus dorsi muscle.

When local or regional tissues are not available, free flap reconstruction has been advocated because of the advantages of transporting large amounts of well-vascularized tissue into a recipient site, ease of contour, and good esthetic outcomes [Neligan et al, 1996]. Importing a large volume of healthy soft tissue may help to treat osteomyelitis or protect against exposure. In fact, shorter duration of hospitalization and a higher incidence of primary wound healing have been demonstrated in free flaps for cranial vault reconstruction involving osteomyelitis and radiation [Neligan et al, 1996].

Historically, free muscle flaps, such as a free latissimus dorsi flap or free rectus abdominis flap, have been utilized extensively in cranial vault reconstruction. In the long term, however, a high degree of muscle atrophy of up to 80% has led to an increased interest in fasciocutaneous "perforator" free flaps that maintain their contour and volume more consistently [Lutz et al, 1998] and provide healthy normal skin and subcutaneous tissue as a part of the unit. In addition to lower rates of exposure, fasciocutaneous free flaps satisfy the reconstructive tenet to replace tissues in a "like with like" fashion. Examples of free fasciocutaneous flaps include the anterolateral thigh flap, the deep inferior epigastric perforator flap, and the radial forearm flap (**Fig 3.7-7**).

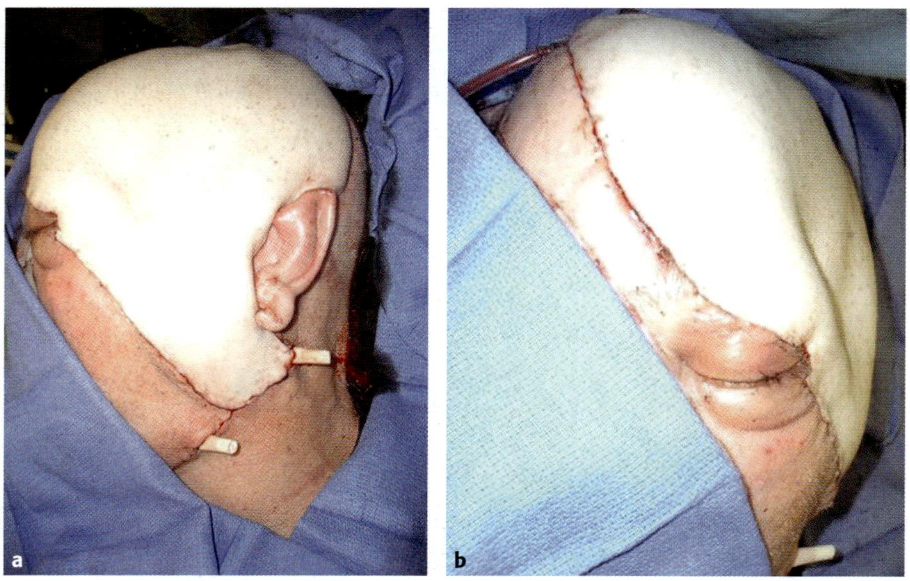

Fig 3.7-7a–b Free anterolateral thigh flap for reconstructing the overlying soft tissues.

4 Complications and pitfalls

4.1 CSF leaks and fistulae

Cerebrospinal fluid leaks and fistulae are rare complications of cranial vault reconstruction that place the brain at risk for infection. If a leak is discovered postoperatively, a lumbar drain may be indicated to divert the flow of CSF from the wound to allow leaks to seal. If a leak does not seal within a reasonable period, operative intervention is indicated to close the leak.

The development of a postoperative myelomeningocele is another indication for reoperation, indicating a failure of the first two layers of the cranial vault reconstruction.

4.2 Infection

The cranial vault has a rich vascularity, and is thus relatively resistant to infection. When infection occurs, the stakes are high, especially when there is communication with the meninges and brain. Overall, the incidence of postoperative infection following cranioplasty is approximately 5% [Manson et al, 1986; Moreira-Gonzalez et al, 2003]. The incidence of infection is higher in those who have undergone frontal cranioplasty, presumably because of proximity to the sinuses. It is highest in those who have been reconstructed with HA, and much lower in those who have had autogenous bone grafts [Moreira-Gonzalez et al, 2003]. It is higher in those who have evidence of loosening or fracture of their implant. Infection of the overlying soft tissues is rare, a fact that is likely related to rich vascularity and good hygiene in the head and neck.

If infection develops, prophylactic antibiotics should be converted to therapeutic antibiotics based on culture-specific data and operative debridement should be considered. Intraoperative biopsy results should be sent for pathology as well as culture and sensitivity for bacteria, mycobacteria, and fungi. An infectious disease consult and long-term intravenous antibiotics are indicated for osteoradionecrosis and osteomyelitis. Hyperbaric oxygen, which facilitates the oxidative burst of polymorphonuclear cells and increases oxygen tension within the wound, can be used along with surgical debridement and intravenous antibiotics to facilitate wound healing.

In malignancy cases infection may be linked to tumor recurrence, which should be ruled out.

4.3 Exposure

Overall, the rate of exposure of cranioplasty implants is under 5%. Exposure of autogenous bone grafts is much less than that of titanium and PMMA, while HA has an exposure rate about twice as high as other alloplasts [Moreira-Gonzalez et al, 2003]. Exposure rates for frontal implants are about twice as high as those of temporal and parietal implants [Moreira-Gonzalez et al, 2003] (**Fig 3.7-8**).

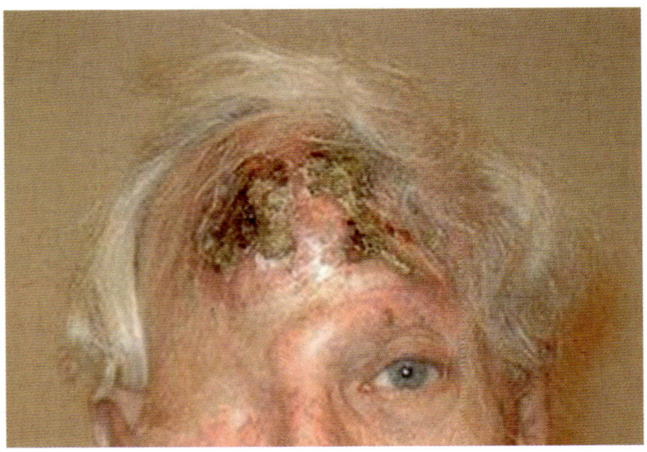

Fig 3.7-8 Exposure of titanium mesh cranioplasty.

Management of exposure usually requires operative debridement, use of intravenous antibiotics, and potential re-advancement of overlying soft tissues or flap reconstruction. Local flaps can be advanced to cover the wound, with split thickness skin grafts placed into the scalp donor site to provide donor site coverage. If these options are not available, a free flap transfer may be indicated. Furthermore, in the event of free flap failure, another free flap may be attempted. There may be a role for negative pressure dressing in problem wounds.

4.4 Hematoma and seroma

Inadequate hemostasis or coagulopathy may lead to a hematoma in any layer of a cranial vault reconstruction. Symptomatic epidural hematomas are surgically drained. Small subcutaneous hematomas will resorb without intervention. Large subcutaneous hematomas may require drainage to prevent pressure necrosis of the overlying soft tissues. Similarly, subcutaneous seromas may be self-limited or require drainage to prevent infection.

4.5 Contour irregularities

Contour irregularities caused by partial resorption of bone may be seen with autogenous bone grafts [Manson et al, 1986; Moreira-Gonzalez et al, 2003]. These contour irregularities may require primary or secondary reconstruction, often with alloplastic materials. Titanium and PMMA have low rates of contour irregularity while HA has a high rate of fracture with subsequent contour irregularity. Several small cranioplasty series using CAD/CAM methods with titanium, PMMA, and porous polyethylene claim low rates of contour irregularity.

4.6 Other

Although biomaterials used routinely in cranioplasty maybe metallic, titanium implants offer great compatibility with MRI and minimize CT scan artifacts for postoperative surveillance of tumor recurrence. The theoretical limitation of creation of radiation scatter or "hot-spots" associated with radiotherapy for tumor remains a concern, but has not been reported to be clinically significant.

5 References and suggested reading

Afifi AM, Gordon CR, Pryor LS, et al. Calcium phosphate cements in skull reconstruction: a meta-analysis. *Plast Reconstr Surg*. 2010 Oct;126(4):1300–1309.

Blake GB, MacFarlane MR, Hinton JW. Titanium in reconstructive surgery of the skull and face. *Br J Plast Surg*. 1990 Sep;43(5):528–535.

Donati L, Baruffaldi-Preis FW, Di Leo A, et al. Ten-year experience with craniofacial implants: clinical and experimental results. *Int Surg*. 1997 Oct–Dec;82(4):325–331.

Dujovny M, Aviles A, Agner C, et al. Cranioplasty: cosmetic or therapeutic? *Surg Neurol*. 1997 Mar;47(3):238–241.

Eufinger H, Wehmoller M. Individual prefabricated titanium implants in reconstructive craniofacial surgery: clinical and technical aspects of the first 22 cases. *Plast Reconstr Surg*. 1998;102(2):300–308.

Elshahat A, Shermak MA, Inoue N, et al. The use of Novabone and Norian in cranioplasty: a comparative study. *J Craniofac Surg*. 2004 May;15(3):483–489.

Gladstone HB, McDermott MW, Cooke DD. Implants for cranioplasty. *Otolaryngol Clin North Am*. 1995 Apr;28(2):381–400.

Jackson IT, Adham M, Bite U, et al. Update on cranial bone grafts in craniofacial surgery. *Ann Plast Surg*. 1987 Jan;18(1):37–40.

Lara WC, Schweitzer J, Lewis RP, et al. Technical considerations in the use of polymethylmethacrylate in cranioplasty. *J Long Term Eff Med Implants*. 1998;8(1):43–53.

Lin AY, Kinsella CR Jr, Rottgers SA, et al. Custom porous polyethylene implants for large-scale pediatric skull reconstruction: early outcomes. *J Craniofac Surg*. 2012 Jan;23(1):67–70.

Liu JK, Gottfried ON, Cole CD, et al. Porous polyethylene implant for cranioplasty and skull base reconstruction. *Neurosurg Focus*. 2004 Mar 15;16(3):ECP1.

Lutz BS, Wei FC, Chen HC, et al. Reconstruction of scalp defects with free flaps in 30 cases. *Br J Plast Surg*. 1998 Apr;51(3):186–190.

Manson PN, Crawley WA, Hoopes J. Frontal cranioplasty: risk factors and choice of cranial vault reconstructive material. *Plast Reconstr Surg*. 1986 Jun;77(6):888–904.

Moreira-Gonzalez A, Jackson IT, Miyawaki T, et al. Clinical outcome in cranioplasty: critical review in long-term follow-up. *J Craniofac Surg*. 2003 Mar;14(2):144–153.

Neligan PC, Mulholland S, Irish J, et al. Flap selection in cranial base reconstruction. *Plast Reconst Surg*. 1996 Dec;98(7):1159–1166.

Sahoo NK, Rangan M. Role of split calvarial graft in reconstruction of craniofacial defects. *J Craniofac Surg*. 2012 Jul;23(4):e326–331.

Smith AW, Jackson IT, Yousefi J. The use of screw fixation of methylmethacrylate to reconstruct large craniofacial contour defects. *Eur J Plast Surg*. 1999;22:17–21.

3.8 Secondary corrections after orbital/nasoethmoidal fractures

Beat Hammer

1 Introduction

Correction of established posttraumatic deformities of the orbital and nasoethmoid skeleton is one of the most difficult problems in facial reconstructive surgery.

The time frame for primary repair of a facial injury is about 2 weeks. If the fractures are reduced and stabilized within this period, the contused soft tissues essentially regain their normal shape and contour. Scarring occurs in a controlled fashion, and even after the most severe injuries a normal or acceptable appearance can be restored in most cases.

When fractures are not or inadequately repositioned and stabilized, unfavorable changes including resorption, pseudarthrosis, and infection may occur. The soft tissues over such a deformed and sometimes unstable skeletal base cannot undergo a regular healing process. Shrinking and distortion of the tissues occur. Within the periorbital region, scarring may limit ocular motility and changes in globe position may occur that may result in diplopia.

The most frequent posttraumatic deformity is enophthalmos, a deformity limited to the internal orbit. More severe injuries may result in displacement of the entire orbital skeleton.

2 Principles of corrective surgery

The basis of corrective surgery requires restoration of normal skeletal anatomy. Skeletal correction is achieved using osteotomies, contouring with burrs, grafting with bone and nonautogenous material, and adequate bony fixation. Other than in primary repair the soft-tissue deformity is often not adequately corrected by normalizing the bony anatomy. Correction of the soft-tissue deformity becomes an important separate part of corrective surgery, requiring repositioning of landmarks, releasing of scars, and augmentation of deficient soft tissue as well as reduction of thickened soft tissue and resection of scar tissue.

2.1 Exposure

Using the subperiosteal facelift technique, the entire soft-tissue mask over the injured area must be undermined. In all but a few cases a coronal approach is necessary, combined with an anterior orbital (author's preference: mid-eyelid), as well as an upper buccal sulcus approach. Dissection is carried down to the zygomatic arch over the deep temporal fascia to expose the arch in the subperiosteal plane.

2.2 Key element: zygoma

The zygoma is a key element of the face, defining the width and anterior projection of the cheek as well as the vertical position of the orbit (**Fig 3.8-1**). Therefore, as a first step in reestablishing the normal orbital anatomy, the position of the zygoma is assessed and, if necessary, corrected.

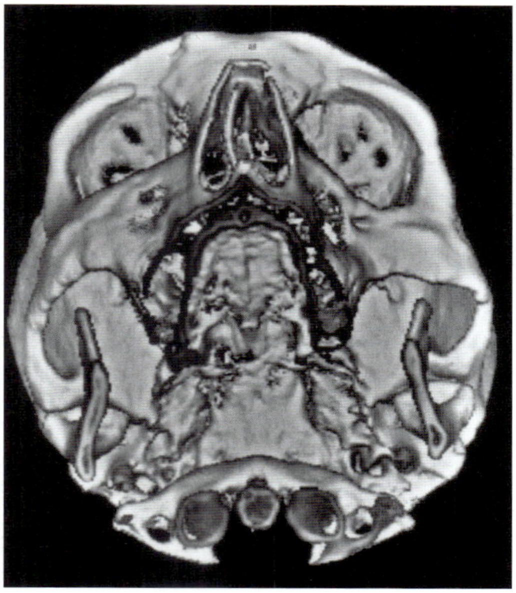

Fig 3.8-1 An unrepaired, severely displaced left zygoma. This led to a shortening and increased width of the left hemiface. The infraorbital rim is caudally displaced, clinically associated with an ectropion due to loss of bony lid support.

There is a conceptual difference between repositioning the zygoma in primary fracture repair and in correcting an established posttraumatic deformity. In primary fracture repair the fragments can be assembled like a puzzle. In late repair it is often not suitable to exactly recreate the initial fracture pattern, which is sometimes not recognizable. Instead, osteotomies are designed individually.

Positioning can best be achieved by aligning the zygoma along the zygomatico-sphenoid suture in the lateral orbital wall, which is also one of the biomechanically most reliable sites for alignment and stabilization (**Fig 3.8-2**) [Hammer, 1995].

2.3 Nasoethmoid region: telecanthus correction

Blunt trauma to the nasoethmoid region causes a disruption of the nasal pyramid, with subsequent widening; thereby, creating the typical aspect of posttraumatic telecanthus (**Fig 3.8-3**).

In primary repair, reduction of the displaced nasoethmoid skeleton restores the medial canthal area in all but the most complex injuries. Correction of an established telecanthus, however, almost always requires a separate direct canthopexy.

For correction a coronal flap is reflected and the deformed nasoethmoid region is widely undermined, thereby completely detaching the medial canthal ligament from its bony insertions. The widened nasoethmoid skeleton is then osteotomized and repositioned (**Fig 3.8-4**).

Before undertaking direct canthopexy, mobilization of the soft tissues again must be evaluated, and if required completed until it is possible to reposition the canthal ligament without any tension. It may be necessary to thin-out scarred tissue medial to the ligament.

Direct canthopexy can be achieved in different ways. A modification of our own technique has been described in detail by Engelstad et al [2012].

It involves two steps: securing the ligament and transnasal fixation.

Securing the ligament can be accomplished using a titanium wire with a tissue anchor, which is inserted directly through the caruncula. Transnasal fixation is performed with a plate providing a hypomochlion (**Fig 3.8-5**).

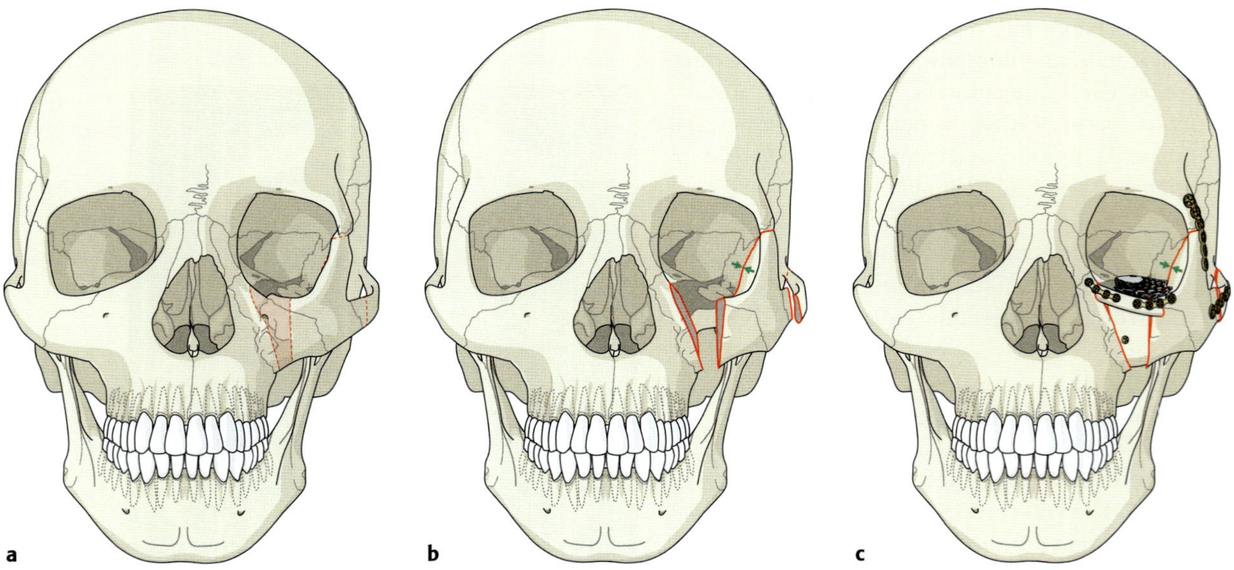

Fig 3.8-2a–c

a In secondary corrections, it is difficult and usually not feasible to exactly reproduce the initial fracture pattern. Instead osteotomies are designed individually.

b The key bony element is repositioned. In most cases the lateral orbital wall is at least partially intact, serving as a guide for positioning. The other osteotomy sites may show gaps or overlapping.

c Stabilization is achieved with plates. Gaps are bridged with bone grafts and/or alloplast.

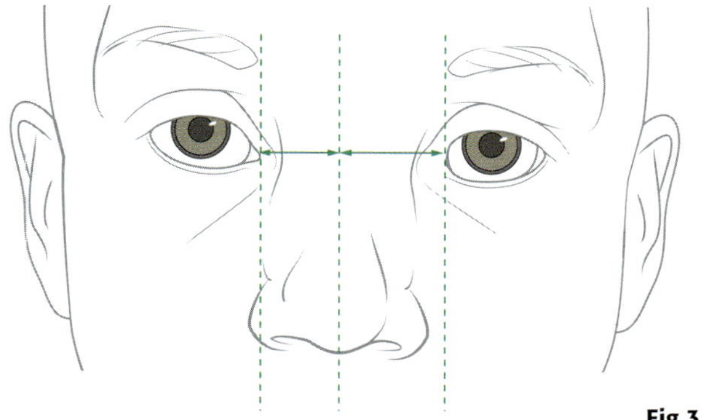

Fig 3.8-3 Telecanthus: increased intercanthal distance and rounding of the medial palpebral angle.

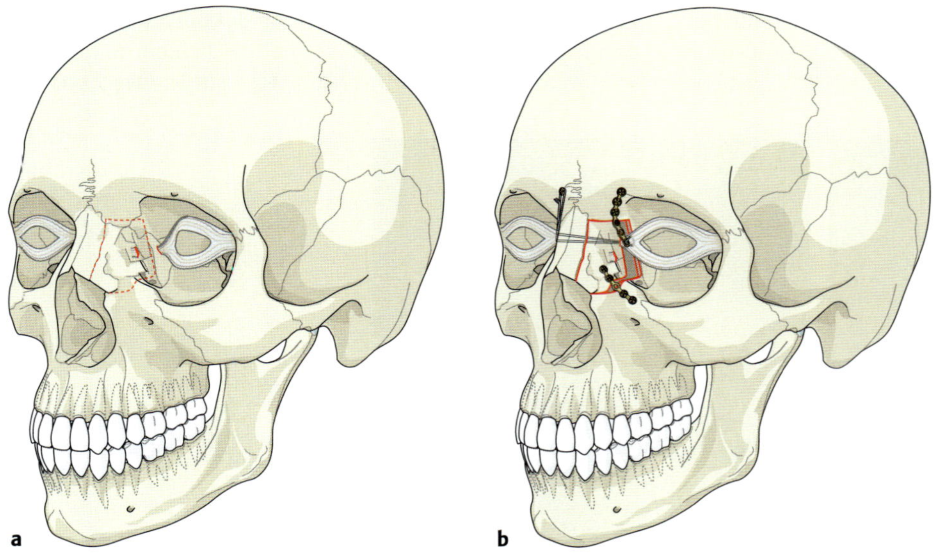

Fig 3.8-4a–b

a For telecanthus correction wide undermining and mobilization of the soft tissues, including detachment of the malpositioned medial canthal ligament from the bone is necessary. The osteotomy does not necessarily reproduce the initial fracture pattern.

b Telecanthus correction is completed. The displaced bone has been medially repositioned and stabilized. Transnasal canthopexy (**Fig 3.8-5**) has been performed.

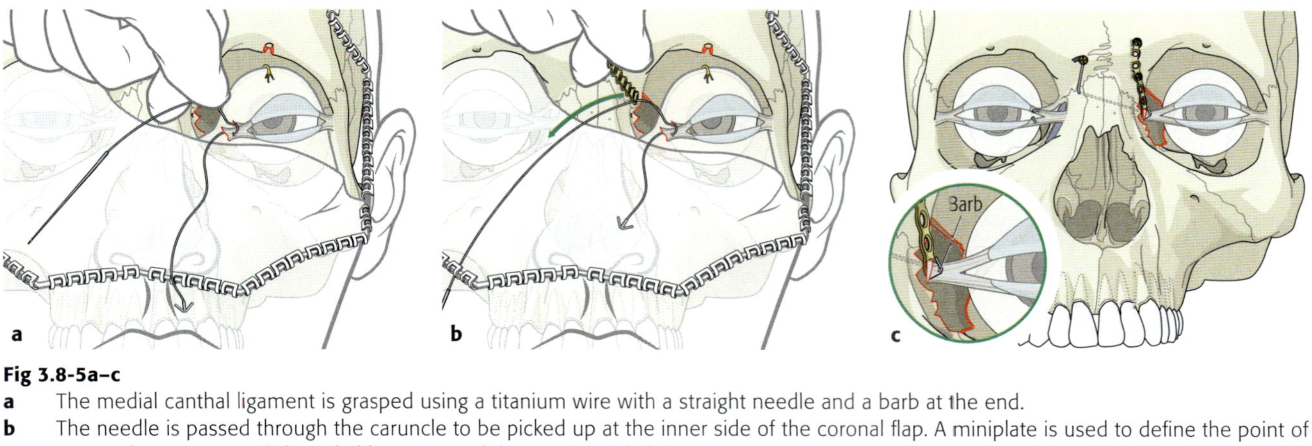

Fig 3.8-5a–c

a The medial canthal ligament is grasped using a titanium wire with a straight needle and a barb at the end.

b The needle is passed through the caruncle to be picked up at the inner side of the coronal flap. A miniplate is used to define the point of contact betweeen medial canthal ligament and the craniofacial skeleton.

c The wire is passed through the last plate hole and transnasally to the contralateral side. Tightening of the wire stabilizes the ligament in the desired position, which is slightly elevated compared with the unaffected side. Inset shows placement of the medial ligament detailed.

2.4 Internal orbit/enophthalmos

Enophthalmos may be a cosmetic and/or a functional problem. When the internal orbit is not adequately restored, the eye loses its support and sinks posteriorly and inferiorly.

The clinical deformity is characterized by a rounded shape of the eye and a deepening of the supratarsal sulcus. With regard to pathogenesis, the main contributing factor for enophthalmos is enlargement of the internal orbit [Manson et al, 1986], usually at the transition from the posterior floor to the medial wall.

For correction, subperiosteal dissection of the orbital contents is necessary, thereby liberating incarcerated tissues and permitting the eye to be repositioned in its normal position. Dissection usually starts from the lateral wall. To expose the uninjured posterior ledge it is necessary to transect the contents of the inferior orbital fissure. The infraorbital nerve needs to be freed from the periorbita by transecting adhesions and small vessels, thereby connecting the lateral wall to the floor of the orbit.

Exposure of the medial wall requires ligation of the anterior ethmoid artery, either from the coronal or a combination of conjunctival-transcaruncular incision. In the more severe cases, a 360° dissection of the orbit is necessary.

Once the entire defect has been exposed it is reconstructed either with bone or allogenic grafts. To detect/avoid incarceration of the periorbita, a forced duction test for medial and inferior restriction is done before dissection, after dissection and after graft insertion (**Fig 3.8-6** and **Fig 3.8-7**).

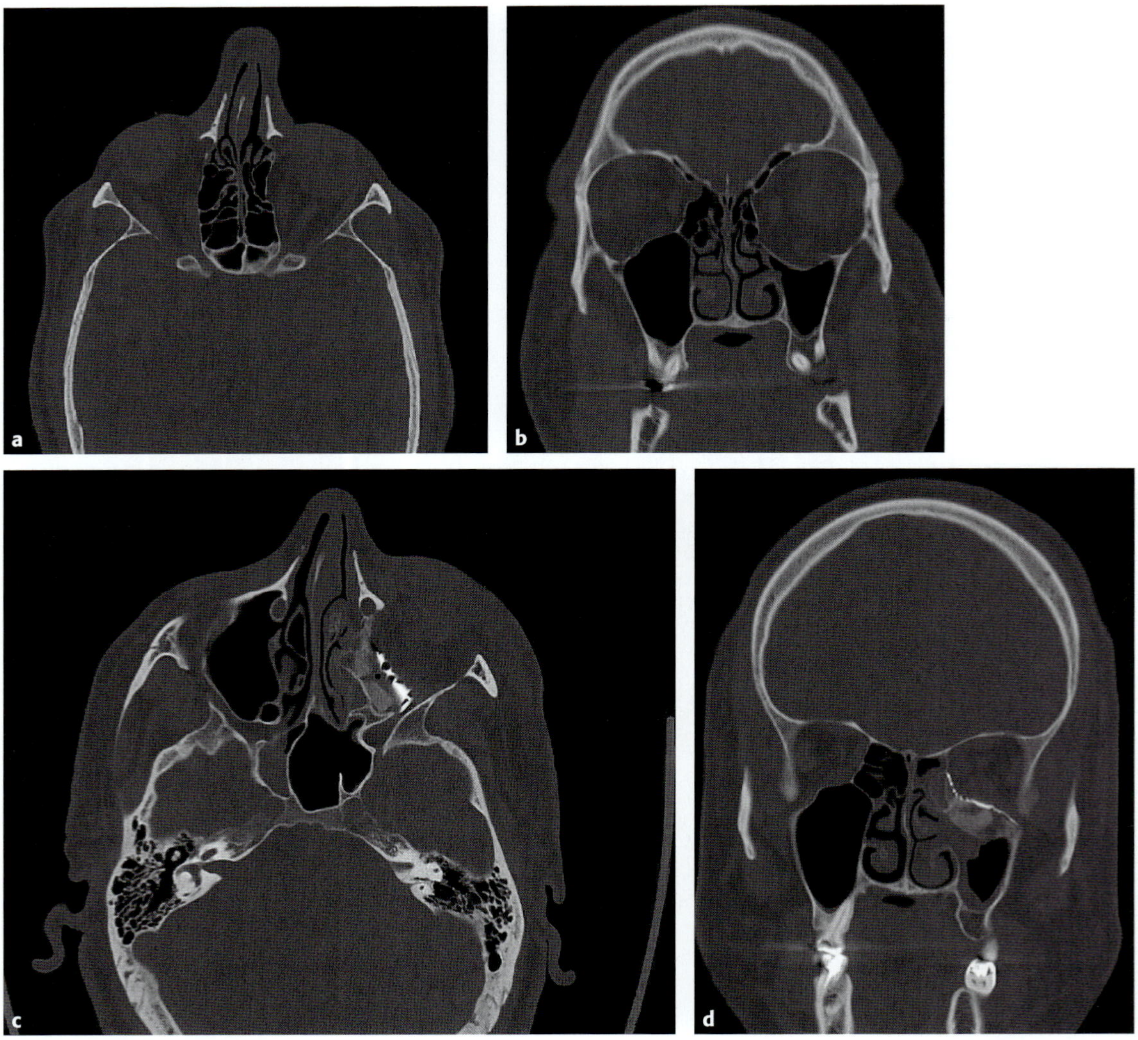

Fig 3.8-6a–d
a–b Enophthalmos (left) after an unrepaired blow out fracture of the orbital floor and medial wall. A concaved enlargement of the orbit has occurred.
c–d Reconstruction with a prefabricated titanium mesh.

3 Risks

When planning enophthalmos correction, the associated risks must be taken into consideration. Scarring makes dissection much more difficult than in primary repair. However, without radical exposure of the intact posterior orbit, mobilization of the eye is not possible.

Reduction of the orbital volume is associated with an increase in orbital and globe pressure [Forrest et al, 1999]. Due to intraperiorbital scarring normalization of pressure occurs more slowly in secondary cases. Globe pressure can be assessed clinically by digital palpation, comparing the operated with the healthy eye. An important warning sign is a decrease in motility ("stiff" globe). Increased intraorbital pressure may limit the amount of enophthalmos correction that can be achieved in one step. In the more severe cases, stepwise correction is necessary. Enophthalmos correction may potentially create double vision (see below).

3.1 Functional aspects, diplopia correction

Potentially there are two mechanisms: release of restricting tissue incarcerations or shift of the field of binocular vision from an unfavorable into a more favorable position.

Mechanical restriction of eye motility is in most cases caused by scarring within the periorbita and is therefore not influenced by enophthalmos surgery. Bringing the globe forward can cause rotation of the globe caused by an injured, shortened extraocular muscle. However, there are sporadic cases of an isolated incarceration where release improves motility.

In most cases, correction of the eye position moves the field of binocular vision from an unfavorable into a more favorable position. However, enophthalmos correction may also have a negative effect on binocular vision because of injury or scar induced by surgery [Iliff, 1991], and the patient must be informed about this possibility.

4 Complex deformities

Complex injuries may not only involve the zygomatico-orbital complex but also the supraorbital bar with or without the frontal sinus, and the frontal bone.

Repair of late sequelae in these cases includes a craniotomy as an indispensable part of supraorbital bar repositioning. Correction rarely can be completed in a single step, and despite all efforts the esthetic and functional results are far behind primary repair.

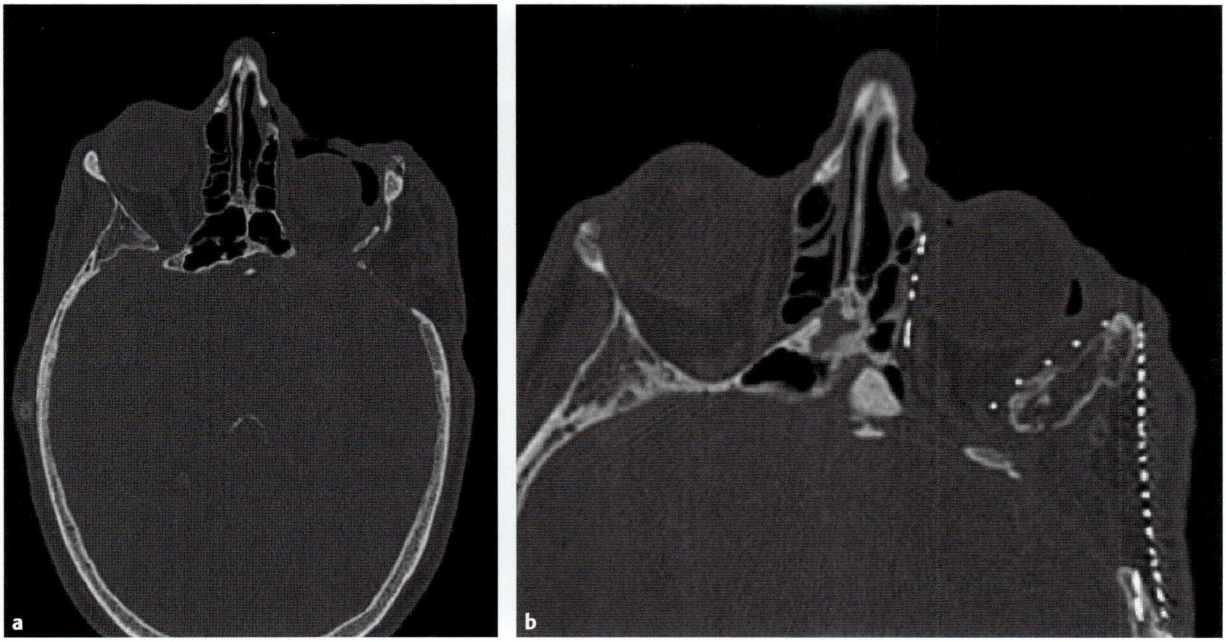

Fig 3.8-7a–b

a Severe residual enophthalmos after multiple corrections of a complex injury of the left orbit. The greater wing of the sphenoid is not visible in the plane of this image.

b Reconstruction was done in two stages, starting with an iliac bone graft that was lined with a titanium reinforced polyethylene sheet 6 months later.

4.1 Case report

A 48-year-old patient was involved in a car crash, resulting in a complex orbitocranial injury. Due to life-threatening cranial and thoracic injuries, repair of the facial injuries was delayed and could only be started several weeks after the injury. Several attempts to restore the normal globe position failed. The patient was seen after more than ten reconstructive procedures with the predominant symptom of a severe left enophthalmos of a seeing eye (**Fig 3.8-8a–b**).

The orbital roof and parts of the lateral orbital wall were missing as well as most of the orbital floor (**Fig 3.8-8c**).

A 3-D model was obtained for visualization and planning of surgery. The supraorbital bar and lateral orbital rim were reconstructed with full thickness cranial bone grafts.

Positioning of the bone grafts is shown in **Fig 3.8-8d–f**.

In a first operation, mobilization of the globe by complete circular dissection of the orbit was done, including separation of the periorbit from the dura of the anterior cranial fossa. The orbital frame was reconstructed with full thickness cranial bone grafts, whereas iliac bone was used for reconstruction of the internal orbit. Positioning of the bone grafts was done by trial and error, with most of the added volume in the superior lateral region of the orbit (**Fig 3.8-8g–h**).

Decreased ocular motility and increased intraorbital pressure indicated the limits of enophthalmos correction in this first procedure.

In a second step, reconstruction of the internal orbit was completed with titanium reinforced polyethylene sheets (**Fig 3.8-8i–j**). At the same time, contouring of the left frontal bone was done using titanium mesh (**Fig 3.8-8k**).

During the crash, rupture of the levator aponeurosis had occurred, resulting in a complete ptosis of the upper lid. Partial lid opening was obtained with a static suspension, limited however by the need to preserve corneal protection (**Fig 3.8-8l–m**).

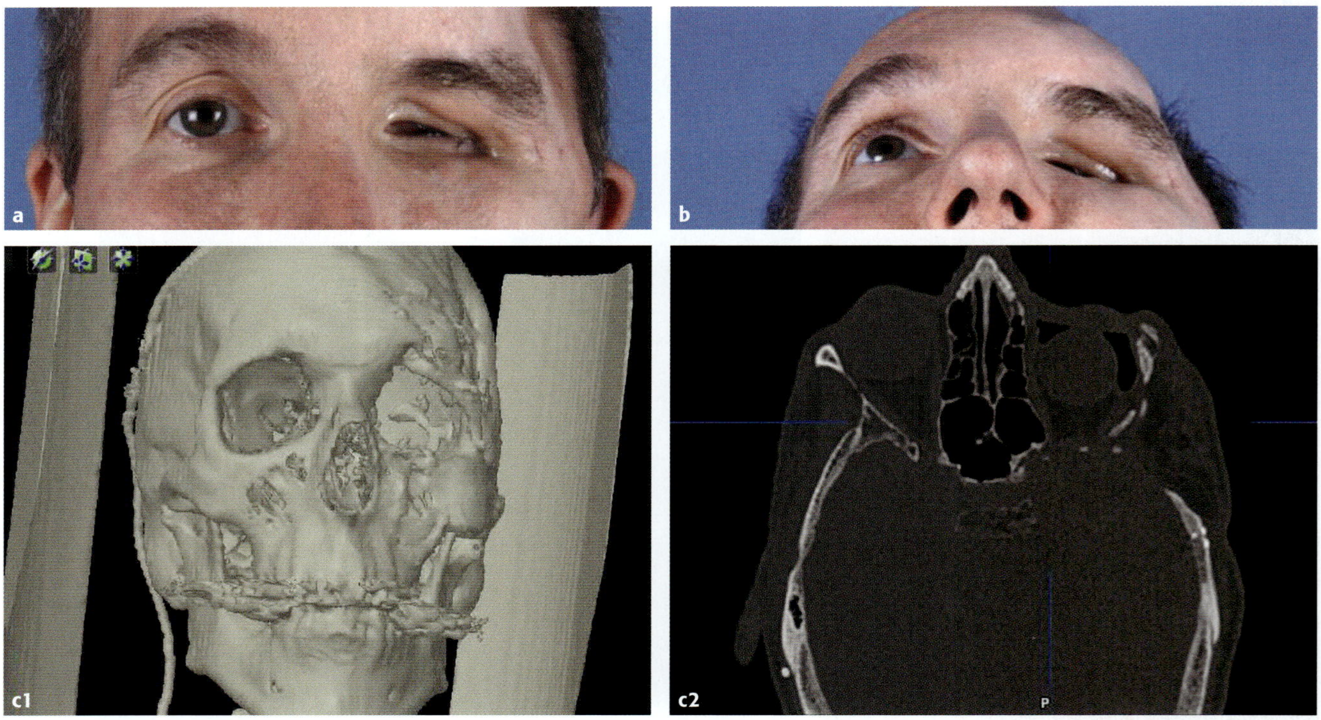

Fig 3.8-8a–m
a–b Orbital deformity with severe enophthalmos after unsuccessful repair of a complex injury.
c The supraorbital bar and lateral orbital rim are missing, as well as major parts of the orbital roof and lateral wall.
c1 3-D reconstruction.
c2 Axial view.

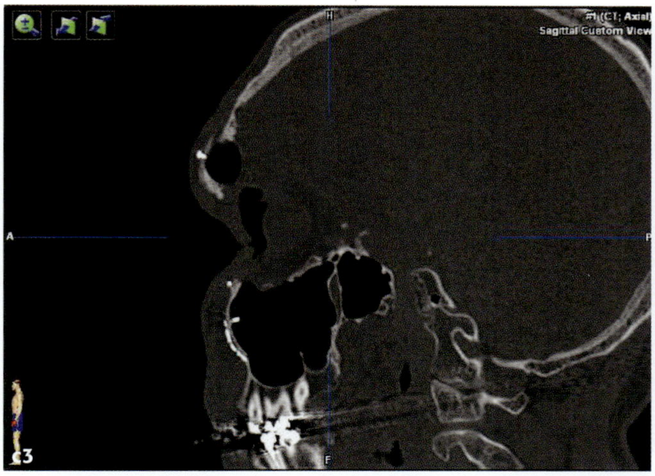

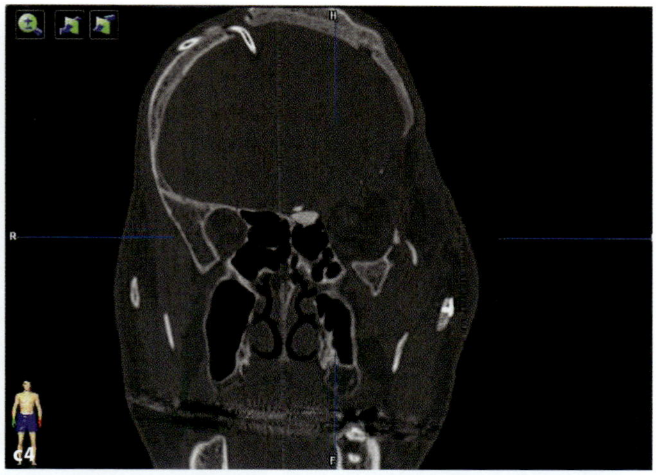

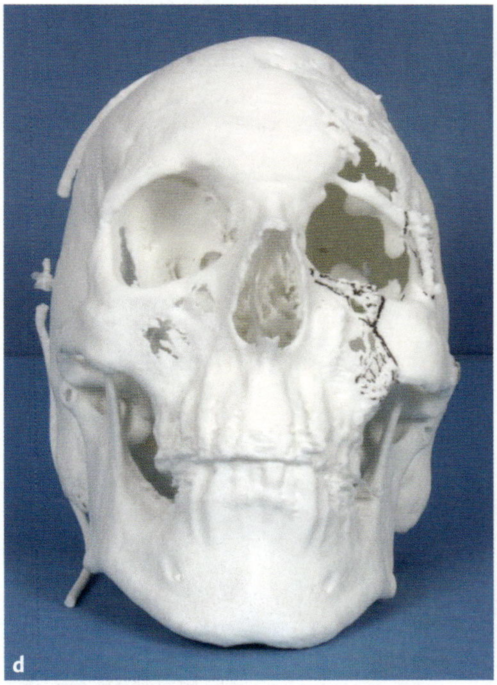

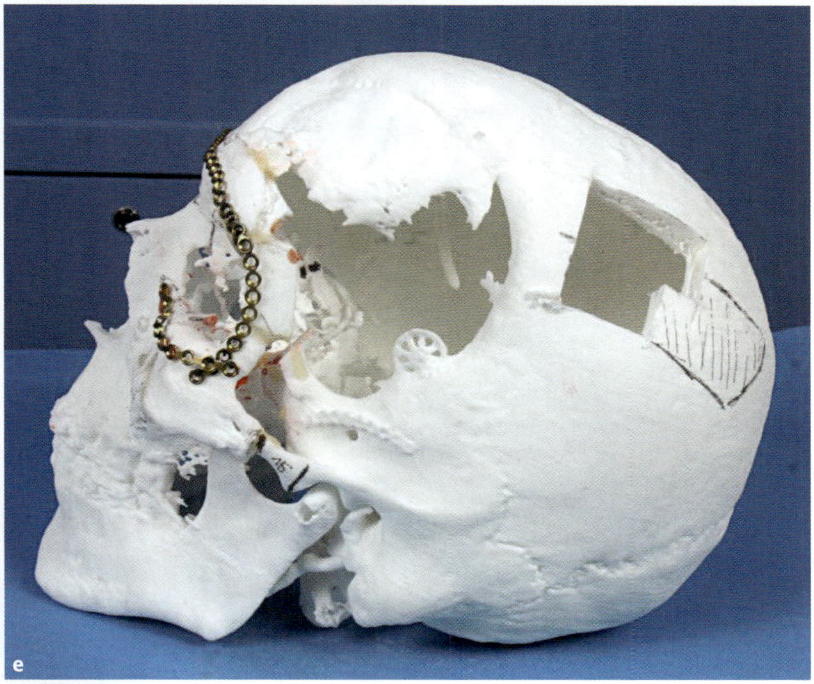

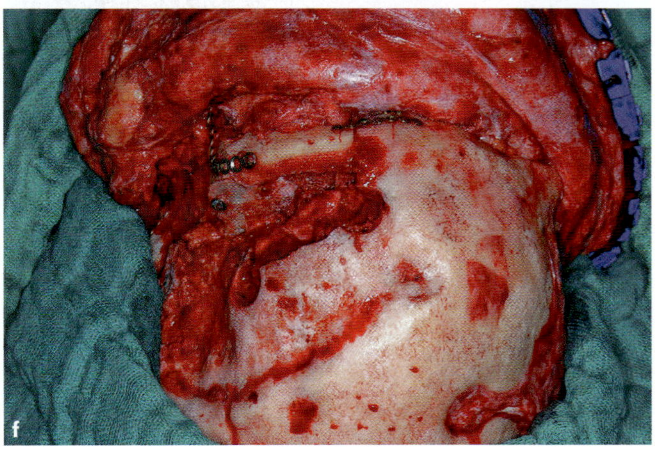

Fig 3.8-8a–m (cont)

c3 Sagittal view.

c4 Coronal view.

d–e 3-D model for visualization and planning. Reconstruction of the orbital frame with cranial bone. A plate serves as a template for positioning of the bone grafts.

f Reconstruction of the orbit with cranial bone. ntraoperative aspect after fixation of the bone grafts.

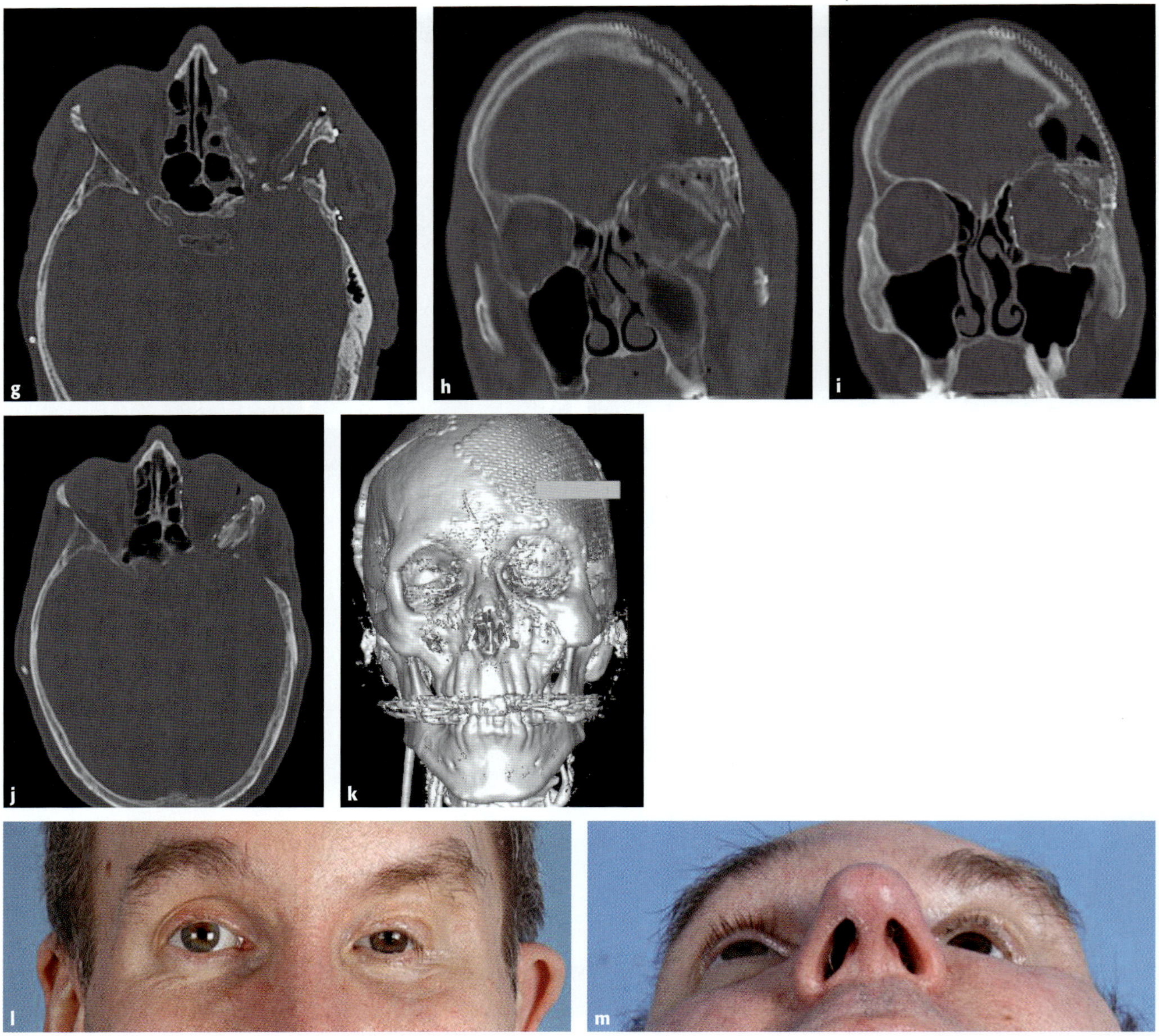

Fig 3.8-8a–m (cont)
g–h First step of internal orbital reconstruction with iliac bone.
i–j Second step of internal orbital repair with titanium reinforced polyethylene.
k Contouring of the frontal bone with titanium mesh.
l–m Partial lid opening by static suspension of the upper lid.

5 Summary

The basic step in correction of secondary posttraumatic facial deformities is to correct the skeletal deformity. Displaced fragments are osteotomized and repositioned into their correct place. Minor displacements can be corrected by contouring, defects are treated with bone grafts or alloplastic implants.

More difficult and usually limiting the result is the soft-tissue deformity, characterized by scarring, displaced landmarks and sometimes missing tissue. Correction requires extensive mobilization, excision of scars, and repositioning the soft-tissue mask in its original position using composite facelift techniques.

6 References and suggested reading

Engelstad ME, Bastodkar P, Markiewicz MR. Medial canthopexy using transcaruncular barb and miniplate: technique and cadaver study. *Int J Oral Maxillofac Surg*. 2012;41:1176–1185.

Forrest CR, Khairallah E, Kuzon WM Jr. Intraocular and intraorbital compartment pressure changes following orbital bone grafting: a clinical and laboratory study. *Plast Reconstr Surg*. 1999 Jul;104(1):48–54.

Hammer B. *Orbital Fractures: Diagnosis, Operative Treatment, Secondary Corrections*. Seattle: Hogrefe & Huber; 1995.

Iliff NT. The ophthalmic implications of the correction of late enophthalmos following severe midfacial trauma. *Trans Am Ophthalmol Soc*. 1991;89:477–548.

Manson PN, Clifford CM, Su CT, et al. Mechanisms of global support and posttraumatic enophthalmos: I. *Plast Reconstr Surg*. 1986 Feb;77(2):193–202.

4.1 Treatment of gunshot injuries

Warren Schubert

1 Introduction

Gunshot wounds and in particular self-inflicted wounds can represent some of the most difficult reconstructive challenges for the craniomaxillofacial (CMF) surgeon. The CMF surgeon needs to take a leadership role in working with other trauma surgeons, as it is often easy for even the experienced surgeon to be distracted by the horror of the injury and forget the basic ABCs of resuscitation. Emphasis must be placed on the workup and evaluation for brain injury, cervical spine, and major vessel injury. The CMF surgeon is often in the best position to coordinate and prioritize the necessary emergent radiographic evaluation and need for the appropriate consultation with neurosurgical, ophthalmological, and orthopedic services.

A fine cut axial and coronal computed tomography (CT) with reformatted views where required is essential. Coronal reconstructions and oblique parasagittal cuts through the orbit, with the possibility of 3-D reconstructions for complex or avulsive injuries are helpful. Modalities for clearing the cervical spine vary and are dependent also on the patient's level of pain and the degree of patient cooperation. A CT scan of the brain and spine are routine. Emergency angiography may be required.

2 Review of ballistics and its relevance

Wounds from projectiles can be divided into three groups including penetrating, perforating, and avulsive injuries. Penetrating refers to wounds where the projectile remains within the body, resulting in the dissipation of all the kinetic energy of the missile within the body. Perforating refers to wounds from projectiles that pass through the body. The amount of energy dissipated in the body may be highly variable. Usually the entrance wounds are smaller than the exit wounds. The amount of damage is related to the structures in the path, and to the degree of bullet fragmentation, the tumble of the projectile, the mass and velocity of the projectile, and the amount of temporary and permanent cavitation. Avulsive wounds refer to injuries where the projectile tears apart significant segments of hard or soft tissue. Often these result in the most complex reconstructive challenges. Although a low-velocity gunshot wound to the face that passes through the cheek or maxillary sinuses requires vigilance on the part of the surgeon to perform a thorough workup, in some cases they may not require any surgical intervention. Most low-velocity gunshot wounds can be managed as fractures with overlying lacerations. This chapter mostly covers the more serious avulsive injuries that often require a series of reconstructive procedures.

The degree of trauma to a structure is in part related to the total kinetic energy (KE) that a projectile imparts. Kinetic energy from a projectile is defined by the following formula:

$$KE = \text{Mass} \times \text{Velocity}^2$$

The amount of damage caused by a projectile can be increased by proportionately increasing the mass. The damage produced is logarithmically increased by increasing the velocity. The desire to decrease the weight of each bullet and therefore increase the amount of ammunition that infantry can carry, fostered the trend to decrease the mass and increase the velocity.

In the case of a bullet that has exited the victim the damage is theoretically proportional to the energy that has been dissipated in the patient. This can be expressed by the formula:

$$\text{Power Expended} = \text{Mass} \times (\text{Velocity at impact} - \text{Velocity at the exit})^2$$

Most publications extensively discussed the mass and velocity of the various projectiles, the nature of the firearm, and the amount of damage that can be caused. Although the discussion is fascinating, for many surgeons this information is not particularly useful in the management of specific injuries. In the acute phase of treatment of nonmilitary injuries, the surgeon often does not know the nature or the exact range of the weapon that was used. Often the most important issue is not the weapon that was used but the trajectory and structures that were affected. A projectile passing through the cheeks may cause minimal damage and may not require any skeletal work. In contrast, a projectile that hits the mandible or teeth may cause these structures to become secondary projectiles causing an extensive avulsive and exit injury.

3 Airway, breathing, circulation

Projectile injuries to the face may be associated with various injury patterns depending on the type of projectile, the weapon, and distance between the weapon and the person. A self-inflicted gunshot to the face is a close range, high-power injury, frequently causing an avulsive defect. It can be challenging to initially identify normal anatomy (**Fig 4.1-1**). Many patients who survive the blast have their brain spared. The unique nature of the projectile trajectory results from the gun being held below the mandible, with the projectile passing through the mandible and palate with an exit through the nose, globe, or low frontal sinus. The force of the rush of air from the barrel abruptly forces the head backward, taking the brain out of the injury path. The lower face is the principal target. It is not uncommon for these patients to have an avulsion of the symphysis of their mandible and lips, as well as their midface structures. Often before the arrival of the ambulance these patients have been able to maintain their airway by remaining erect and coughing and spitting out blood and secretions. Following the arrival of the ambulance they are commonly transported in a supine position. Lacking symphyseal support, the remnants of the tongue fall to the back of the throat, and the airway fills up with blood and secretions. When such patients do not have other injuries, it may be desirable to keep them in an upright position until better control of the airway can be obtained.

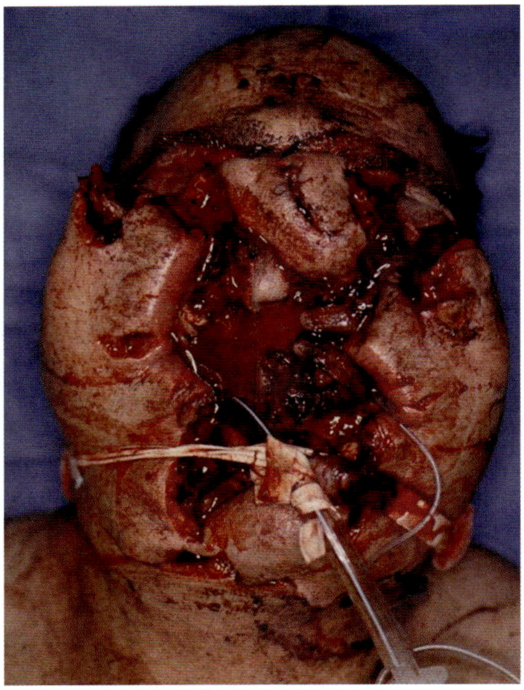

Fig 4.1-1 Patient 1 was an example of a horrific self-inflicted injury where initially few normal structures could be identified.

If airway obstruction is acute, an emergency cricothyroidotomy or tracheotomy must be performed. With good suction and retraction of the tongue, these patients can be easily orally intubated, as the mandible, if divided, can be pushed to the side. Later in the operating room a controlled tracheotomy can be performed.

Condition of the C-spine, possible injuries to the great vessels of the neck, and other severe injuries to the body need to be addressed and if necessary treated. A modern imaging modality to address C-spine, vessels of the neck, and craniofacial skeleton is a CT angiography. Interventional radiology may be necessary for uncontrolled bleeding. Blood loss via the soft tissue and bone injuries in the craniofacial area to some extent is often better controlled with a reduction of the fractures. Determination of brain injury, facial nerve injury, and whether the patient's vision is present is a high priority with initial and follow-up serial examinations.

4 Management of CMF injuries

4.1 Bone and soft-tissue considerations

Principles of bone and soft-tissue reconstruction are the same as for any other facial trauma. The goal (when possible) is to achieve early reestablishment of a skeletal and soft-tissue framework before there is a chance for soft-tissue scarring and retraction. This includes the reconstruction of facial height, width, and projection.

When there has been extensive soft-tissue loss from an avulsive injury, a judgmental decision has to be made whether to initially compromise one of these key dimensions to achieve primary soft-tissue closure. A common example is when the mandibular symphysis or anterior midface has been destroyed and it is not possible to obtain primary skin closure without compromising the AP projection (**Fig 4.1-2** and **Fig 4.1-3**). Skin to mucosa closure is also an option. The other two problems to consider include the 'dimension' of facial movement, and the 'dimension' of time on scarring and retraction.

Many authors have emphasized the need for initial conservative debridement and thorough irrigation, followed by a more delayed reconstruction. Assuming that the patient is stable, it is hard to understand the advantage of a debridement with a delayed closure leaving exposed bony fragments and soft-tissue bathing in saliva. Soft tissue rapidly contracts, resulting in critical loss of soft-tissue volume. As the face has a good blood supply, good judgment can usually determine what is going to survive, and if not, serial debridement every 48 hours will permit early definitive preparation of the wound.

4.2 Sequencing

For comminuted nonavulsive fractures, the sequencing is similar to that of other panfacial trauma. The wounds themselves are often the incisions necessary. There must be an emphasis on reestablishing the mandibulomaxillary unit and proper occlusion. Some surgeons prefer to perform this as the first step, and then work from the "top down". Some start from the calvarium and work their way down paying special attention to the mandibulomaxillary unit after the height and width of the midface have been established. Generally, after establishing the facial framework and reconstruction of the orbital aperture, orbital blowout fractures are addressed toward the end of the upper midface reconstruction. A forced duction test is often the last maneuver to make sure that the extraocular muscles and orbital soft tissues have not become entrapped during the orbital floor or orbital wall reconstruction.

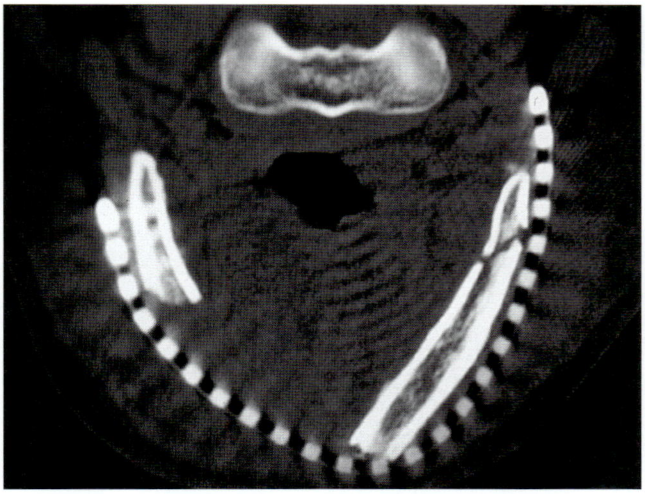

Fig 4.1-2 A reconstruction plate has been used to span Patient 1's mandibular defect. A significant compromise in the AP projection had to be made to have enough soft tissue to close the defect.

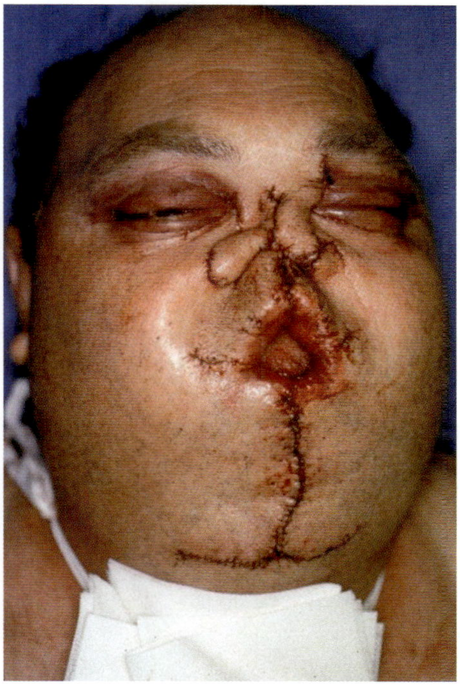

Fig 4.1-3 Despite the nature of Patient 1's avulsive defect, a primary closure was achieved. This required an extensive debridement. Orbits and the central midface were reconstructed with titanium mesh.

In the case of an avulsive injury, the sequencing may have to be radically adjusted to adequately address the reconstruction of avulsed segments. As an example, with self-inflicted wounds the surgeon may be left with all orbital walls destroyed (**Fig 4.1-4**). In these cases, whether one chooses to use molded extensive pieces of titanium mesh, bone graft, or other substances, it may be beneficial to address the orbital reconstruction early in the case while the midface is an 'open book' (**Fig 4.1-5**).

4.3 Principles of internal fixation

The same basic principles are applied that are used for other forms of panfacial trauma. It is important to expose as many of the fractures as possible to have a good exposure and understanding of the puzzle before beginning the placement of temporary or permanent fixation with plates and screws. This will help facilitate a proper reduction and help prevent an open internal fixation with malposition of the segments.

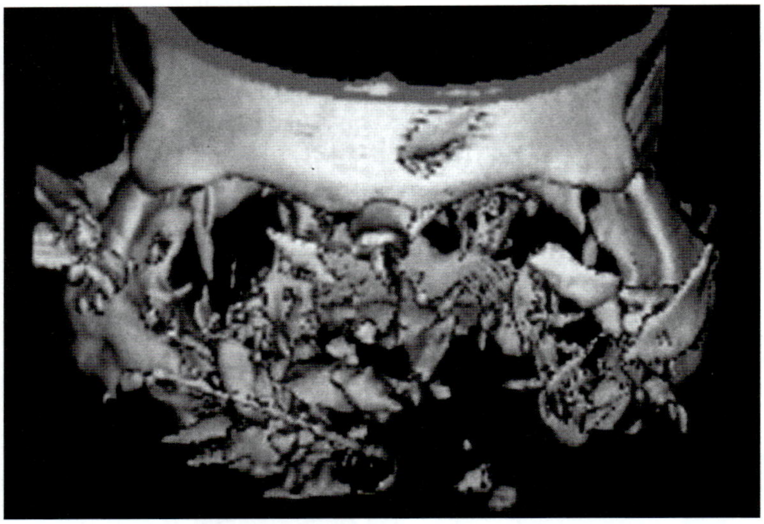

Fig 4.1-4 3-D computed tomography of Patient 1 showing destruction of all orbital walls except the orbital roof.

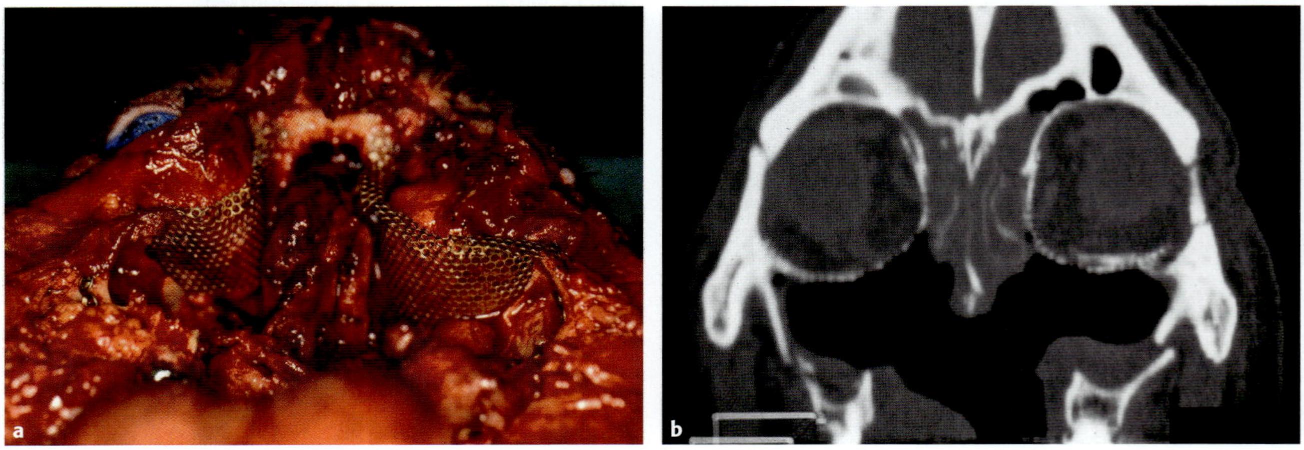

Fig 4.1-5a–b

a Worms eye view of Patient 1 after the placement of extensive titanium meshes to reconstruct the orbital floors and medial orbital walls. With an open book injury of this nature and the need to use large pieces of titanium mesh to position the globes, reconstruction of the orbit is performed early.

b Postoperative coronal computed tomography of the orbits showing the reconstruction was accomplished using titanium mesh.

Avulsive defect injuries of the mandible should be treated like other mandibular 'defect' injuries, using large reconstruction or locking screw plates to span the defect with the remaining mandible in anatomical position (**Fig 4.1-6** and **Fig 4.1-7**). Similarly, comminuted mandibular fractures do not allow for 'load sharing' and structurally behave like "defect" injuries, requiring large plates and screws that span across all segments from one stable segment to another. With the advent of reconstruction plates, the indications for an external fixator are increasingly uncommon.

4.4 Bone and soft-tissue reconstruction

The goal is to restore the skeletal frame needed to support the "canvas" of the skin and other soft tissues, and offer the best long-term esthetic and functional result. While opinions vary regarding the need for bone grafting versus the increased use of titanium mesh and other substances for the acute reconstruction of the skeletal framework. the gold standard is vascularized bone grafting. The acute use of bone grafts, with a special emphasis on the use of split calvarial bone has also proven to be an effective method of reconstruction for limited defects. The use of bone grafting revolutionized management of complex craniofacial trauma and major gunshot wounds. Advantages include availability, cost, and the advantage of replacing missing tissue with a similar substance. Disadvantages of bone grafts include donor morbidity, additional time to harvest, variable bone resorption, excessive thickness when used for orbital reconstruction, and problems if part of the bone is exposed to an open body cavity. Studies have shown titanium mesh to be safe when used for limited orbital reconstruction, but the long-term stability of large segments of orbital mesh is not known. It has also been

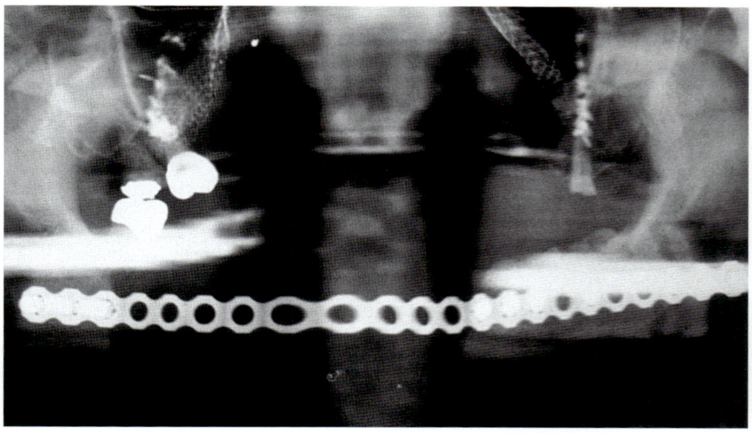

Fig 4.1-6 Orthopantomogram of a large mandibular defect spanned with a long reconstruction plate.

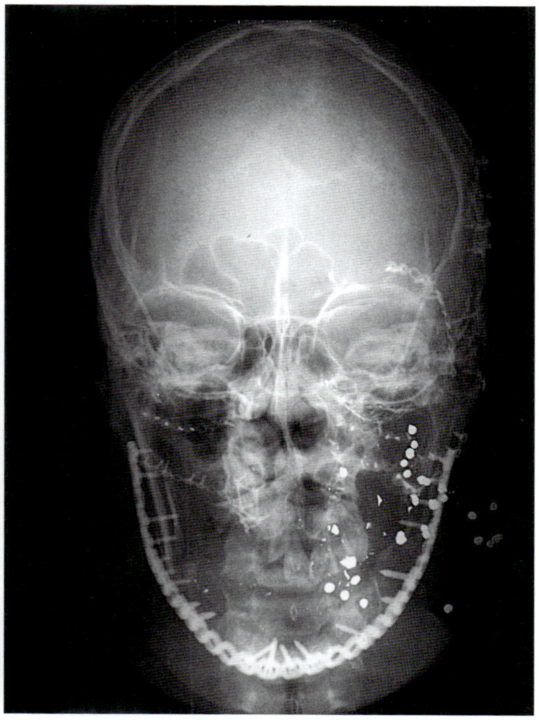

Fig 4.1-7 Gunshot wound of the mandible has initially been spanned by a locking screw plate and later bone grafted.

used to span other midface defects (**Fig 4.1-8** and **Fig 4.1-9**). When exposed to the sinus or nasopharyngeal area, mesh sometimes incorporates in soft tissue which can then become covered with normal nasopharyngeal mucosa (**Fig 4.1-10**).

When the mandible is destroyed, most surgeons primarily plate the defect to length. If there is a significant segmental bone loss, close the soft tissue across the defect and return at a later date to consider vascularized bone grafting and free tissue transfer for mandibular reconstruction when the patient is more hemodynamically and psychologically stable. This provides time to address various medical concerns, and to better determine the need to replace or augment the soft-tissue envelope. In the event that a bone graft is used

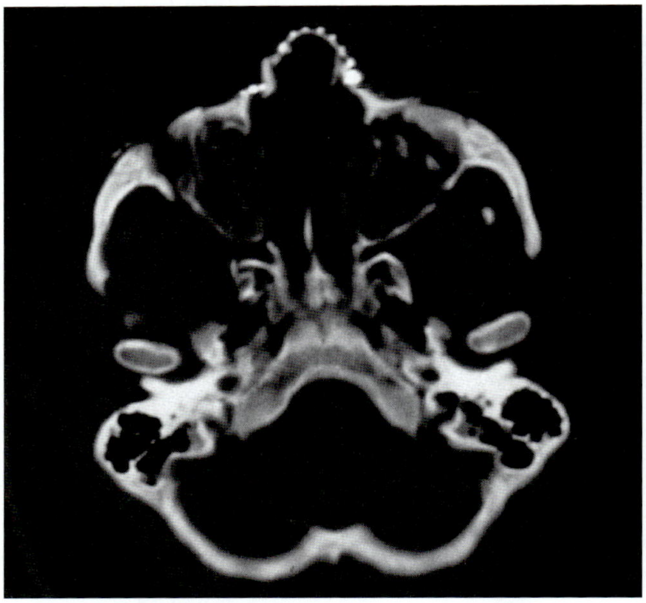

Fig 4.1-8 Nasal bridge defect spanned by a piece of titanium mesh.

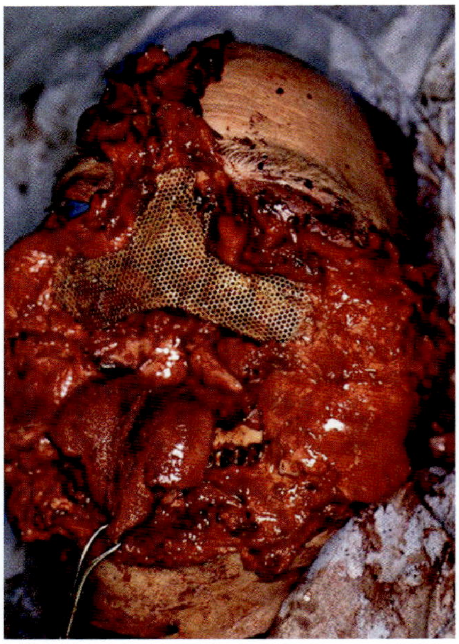

Fig 4.1-9 Patient 1's extensive midface defect was spanned with a large piece of titanium after the reconstruction of the orbits.

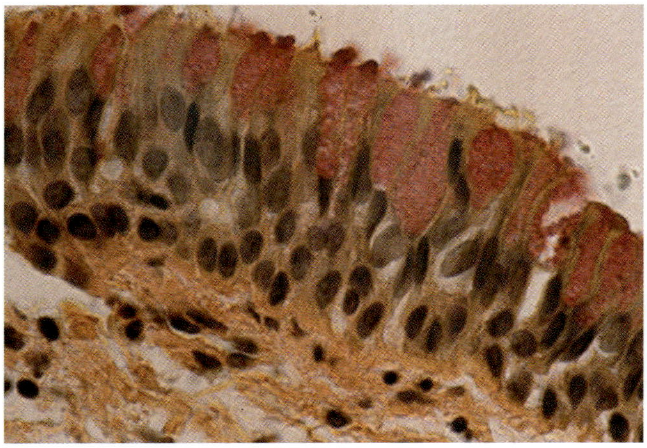

Fig 4.1-10 Normal-appearing respiratory ciliated pseudostratified epithelium with goblet cells. This epithelium resurfaced the soft tissue that has incorporated the titanium mesh used to reconstruct the orbital floors of Patient 1.

the delay can better assure that the grafted area is not exposed to the oral contents. The length of the defect and the quality of the soft-tissue envelope are key determinants as to whether a nonvascularized bone graft or a bone containing free flap is indicated (**Figs 4.1-11–4.1-13**).

Palatal defects may be closed in various ways including obturators, cheek flaps, temporalis flaps, and free flaps. Osseointegrated implants provide a versatile armamentarium for late dental restoration and for the attachment of various reconstructive prostheses.

When the forehead has been spared, it can offer an excellent option for nasal reconstruction. Key principles require the need to address the inner and outer lining as well as the skeletal support and overlying skin.

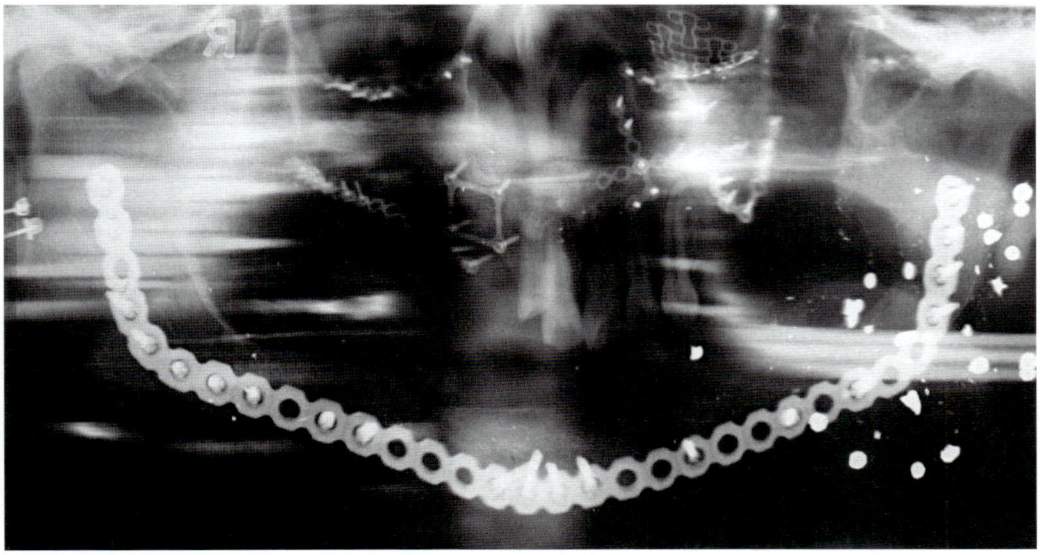

Fig 4.1-11 Accidental gunshot wound with entrance from right and exit on left, where both mandibular bodies were destroyed but the symphysis was left intact.

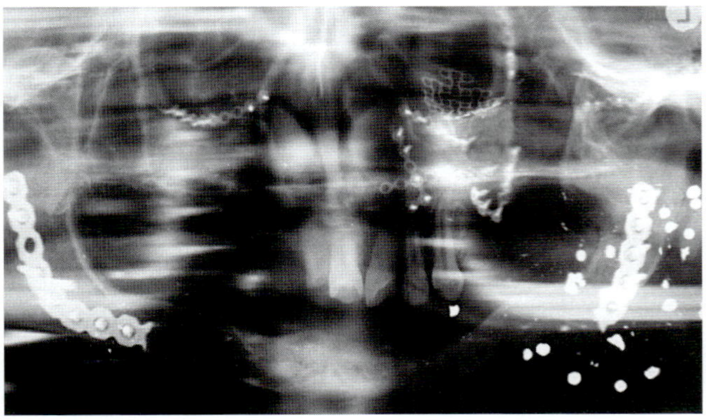

Fig 4.1-12 Patient 1 had an intact symphysis. Here the surgeons choice was between use of a free flap and discard the symphysis, or keep the symphysis and use two free flaps (one for each mandibular body), or simply nonvascularized bone graft the defects. Since the patient had a healthy soft-tissue envelope, posterior iliac bone graft was used to successfully reconstruct both mandibular bodies.

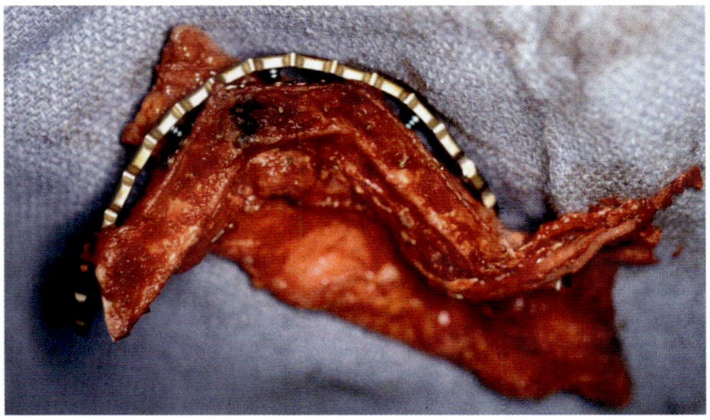

Fig 4.1-13 A fibular free flap is a good alternative for mandibular reconstruction. In this case two osteotomies were used and a locking screw plate was used to span the segments. A skin paddle from the lateral leg was designed to perform reconstruction of parts of the floor of the mouth.

5 Complications and pitfalls

It is easy for the novice to see a patient with extensive mutilation of the face from a gunshot, and be hesitant about whether to proceed with the resuscitation process and the eventual lengthy reconstruction. This is more challenging when the patient has a self-inflicted wound and the family (and sometimes the patient) is telling the caregivers to not pursue resuscitation. Importantly, the suicidal recidivism rate following these mutilating injuries is low, especially if the reconstruction is good. Young patients are usually males, often under the influence of alcohol and/or drugs. The incident often follows an argument or breakup with a significant partner in the patient's life. Most of these patients end up being extremely grateful for the care they have received, and many return to productive lives in society, which is dependent on a good reconstruction. Those who have attempted to take their life because of a chronic illness or malignancy do not have that favorable prognosis.

Issues such as a balance between esthetics and function can offer a special challenge. In many cases the two are inseparable. Lower lip continence can be important from the standpoint of public acceptance and nutrition. In some cases, the patients have undergone various intraoral reconstructions with the hope that they are able to better propel a bolus of food posteriorly and swallow, without any functional improvement. Many patients with mutilating oral wounds are not able to achieve adequate oral nutrition for long periods. Assistance from therapists to help the patient relearn how to swallow and propel food may be useful. The patient may need temporary (or permanent) supplementation from a gastrostomy feeding tube. In an attempt to save the patient's life and climb the reconstructive ladder, the patient's important nutritional needs are often overlooked from the start. Those who have suffered from significant injuries of this nature should have a feeding tube or gastrostomy from the beginning of treatment.

Issues such as the balance between the practical and the impractical can also be a challenge. In an attempt to recreate the proper AP projection, width and height, the surgeon may have inadequate soft tissue to cover the necessary bone graft or hardware. Immediate or delayed exposure of hardware can also be challenging and should prompt consideration for free tissue transfer.

In severely deformed patients it is important to be attentive to the patients' concerns. The surgeon's concern for what should be the highest reconstructive goal may not be a major concern for the patients and their families. At the same time if the patient has certain priorities for reconstruction, it is important to approach the reconstruction in a logical manner. Patients may look in the mirror and may only want a nasal reconstruction. It may be hard to convince them that it may be desirable to first address the deficit in the AP projection of the midface before, for instance, a forehead flap is used for a nasal reconstruction.

On many occasions a member of one specialty has embarked on a reconstructive path to reconstruct the mandible or maxilla with the hope of eventually including osseointegrated dental implants, without including the early involvement of the specialist who would be involved in the patient's dental restoration. The patient has often had an extensive early reconstruction only to find that structures are maligned for implants, or equally disappointing, the patient does not have the financial means to obtain the implants.

Often the most difficult decision for the surgeon and the patient is to determine at what point to terminate the reconstruction and accept, camouflage, or cover up the defect. A classic example is a patient who has an avulsive destruction of his/her orbit, globe, and eyelids. From an esthetic standpoint a judgment has to be made whether a patient is better off having a static prosthesis or wearing an eyepatch (**Fig 4.1-14**). Guiding the patient in these decisions can be most challenging. Encouraging the patient to live with the easy and noninvasive option before embarking on a complex reconstructive option may placate the patient, or make him/her all the more satisfied and appreciative once the complex reconstruction is completed. Our institution's long-term compliance with wearing a prosthetic nose has been poor (**Fig 4.1-15**). At the same time, many patients do well and seem satisfied using a palatal obturator.

Finally, no one can be a world expert at all of the possible different reconstructive options available to a patient with a severely mutilated face. These patients can often benefit from the use of multidisciplinary experts using the expertise and skills of multiple specialties.

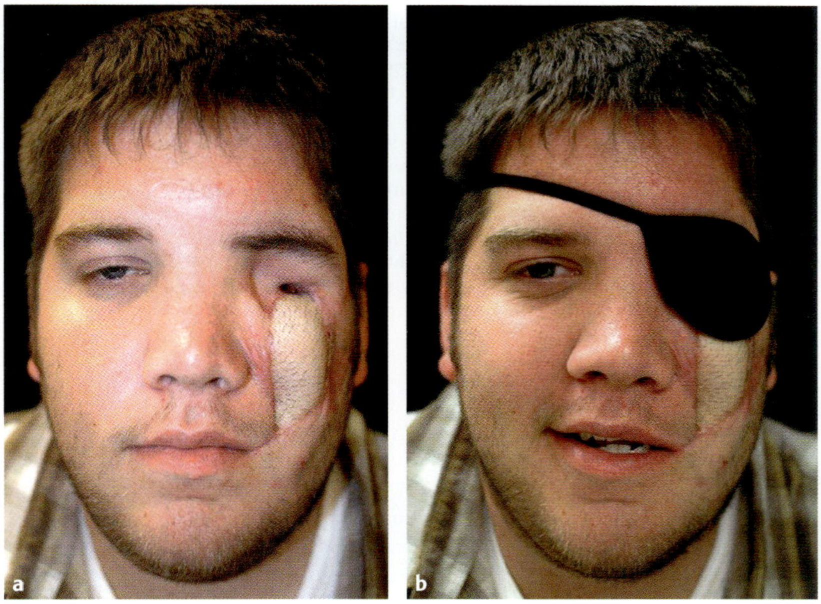

Fig 4.1-14a–b

a Patient 2 has had a fibular free flap with a skin paddle as part of his reconstruction to close an oral-antral-orbital fistula and reconstruct his left midface and zygomatic deficiency.

b He had to choose between a prosthesis to mimic his eyelids and globe, or simply wear an eyepatch. At this stage the patient did not opt for further reconstruction of his periorbit and orbit with a facial prosthesis, and chose to wear an eyepatch.

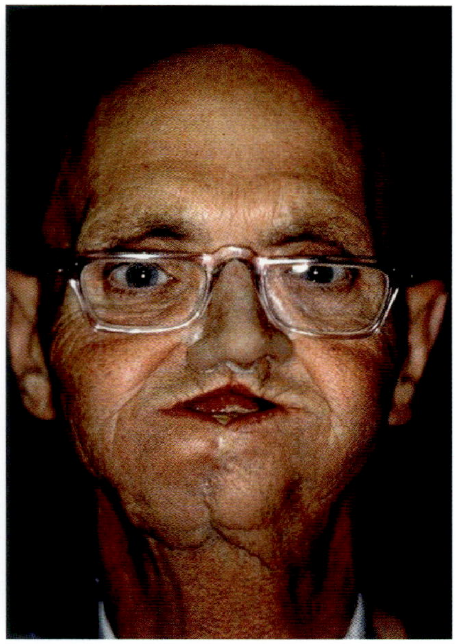

Fig 4.1-15 Patient 1 decided not to have a nasal reconstruction. Here he is wearing a nasal prosthesis that he later discarded. He does not have any significant diplopia and returned to gainful employment.

6 References and suggested reading

Alper M, Totan S, Cankayali R, et al. Gunshot wounds of the face in attempted suicide patients. *J Oral Maxillofac Surg.* 1998 Aug;56(8):930–933; discussion 933–934.

Bowen TE, Bellamy RF, eds. Missile-caused wounds. In: *Second United States Revision Emergency War Surgery NATO Handbook.* Washington, DC: United States Government Printing Office; 1988:13–34.

Clark N, Birely B, Manson PN, et al. High-energy ballistic and avulsive facial injuries: classification, patterns, and an algorithm for primary reconstruction. *J Plast Reconstr Surg.* 1996 Sep;98(4):583–601.

Cusick TE, Chang FC, Woodson TL, et al. Is resuscitation after traumatic suicide attempt a futile effort? A five-year review at a level I trauma center. *Am Surg.* 1999 Jul;65(7):643–646.

Demetriades D, Chahwan S, Gomez H, et al. Initial evaluation and management of gunshot wounds to the face. *J Trauma.* 1998 Jul;45(1):39–41.

Dolin J, Scalea T, Mannor L, et al. The management of gunshot wounds to the face. *J Trauma.* 1992 Oct;33(4):508–514.

Dufresne CR. The use of immediate grafting in facial fracture management: indications and clinical considerations. *Clin Plast Surg.* 1992 Jan;19(1):207–217.

Gear AJL, Lokeh A, Aldridge JH, et al. Safety of titanium mesh for orbital reconstruction. *Ann Plast Surg.* 2002 Jan;48(1):1–7.

Gruss JS, Antonyshyn O, Phillips JH. Early definitive bone and soft-tissue reconstruction of major gunshot wounds of the face. *Plast Reconstr Surg.* 1991 Mar;87(3):436–450.

Gruss JS, Mackinnon SE, Kassel EE, et al. The role of primary bone grafting in complex craniomaxillofacial trauma. *Plast Reconstr Surg.* 1985 Jan;75(1):17–24.

Hollier L, Grantcharova EP, Kattash M. Facial gunshot wounds: a 4-year experience. *J Oral Maxillofac Surg.* 2001 Mar;59(3):277–282.

Holms JD. Gunshot injuries. In: Miloro M, Ghali GE, Larsen PE, et al, eds. *Principles of Oral and Maxillofacial Surgery.* 2nd ed. Hamilton: BC Decker Inc; 2004:509–526.

Jussim E. *Stopping Time: The Photographs of Harold Edgerton.* New York: Harry N Abrams Inc; 1987.

Kelly JF, ed. *Management of War Injuries to the Jaws and Related Structures.* Washington, DC: US Government Printing Office; 1977.

Kihtir T, Ivatury RR, Simon RJ, et al. Early management of civilian gunshot wounds to the face. *J Trauma.* 1993 Oct;35(4):569–575.

Lindsey D. The idolatry of velocity, or lies, damn lies, and ballistics. *J Trauma.* 1980 Dec;20(12):1068–1069.

Newlands SD, Samudrala S, Katzenmeyer WK. Surgical treatment of gunshot injuries to the mandible. *Otolaryngol Head Neck Surg.* 2003 Sep;129(3):239–244.

Rake PA, Rake SA, Swift JQ, et al. A single reformatted oblique sagittal view as an adjunct to coronal computed tomography for the evaluation of orbital floor fractures. *J Oral Maxillofac Surg.* 2004 Apr;62(4):456–459.

Schubert W, Gear AJL, Lee C, et al. Incorporation of titanium mesh in orbital and midface reconstruction. *Plast Reconstr Surg.* 2002 Sep 15;110(4):1022–1030.

Suominen E, Tukiainen E. Close-range shotgun and rifle injuries to the face. *Clin Plast Surg.* 2001 Apr;28(2):323–337.

Thorne CH. Gunshot wounds to the face: current concepts. *Clin Plast Surg.* 1992 Jan;19(1):233–244.

4.2 Treatment of malalignment and incorrect occlusion

Daniel Buchbinder

1 Introduction

The goal of the repair of a facial fracture is the restoration of preinjury form and function. Despite the somewhat routine nature of the intervention, posttreatment complications are common [Alpert, 1998]. A CMF surgeon should know about the etiology of frequent adverse effects and complications as well as certain pitfalls related to the treatment of mandibular fractures and ways to avoid them.

2 Reasons for treatment failures

Treatment failures after mandibular fracture repair may be classified into three broad categories: (1) operator error; (2) patient compliance with treatment; and (3) healing disturbances.

Errors in diagnosis of the injury are usually because the clinician misses a fracture (for instance, in the condylar region or midface) or does not fully appreciate the extent of fracture comminution or, for instance, an oblique nature of the fracture. In some cases, the malocclusion might not be evident immediately at the time of the fracture treatment but will develop some time later when the hardware fails, as in the case of an undiagnosed comminution, or when the mandibulomaxillary fixation (MMF) is released after the application of the internal fixation hardware. Malocclusion may become evident when a distracted condylar head returns to the fossa after release of MMF.

During treatment the basic principles of healing and biomechanics must be respected. Teeth in the line of fracture, devitalized bone fragments and any other possible source of infection must be addressed based on well-described guidelines. Selection of the best surgical approach considering previous incisions and scar formation will decrease the incidence of postoperative complications. Anatomical planes may be disrupted from previous surgeries putting vital structures, such as motor and sensory nerves, at additional risk of injury.

Malunion of the mandible and malocclusion often begins with improper initial reduction using MMF; another reason is inappropriate internal fixation technique including hardware selection at the time of the initial treatment. Before the application of rigid internal fixation, the patient should be placed in secure MMF and the fractured segments aligned anatomically to restore the preinjury occlusion. Loose or ineffective MMF, malreduction, improper plate selection or adaptation can all lead to the development of a posttreatment malocclusion. It has been reported [Moulton-Barrett et al, 1998] that up to 19% of cases will present with a transient malocclusion after open reduction. Further, 4%–8% will require correction with an occlusal adjustment, and 0.5%–3% require secondary revision surgery [Fordyce et al, 1999; Renton et al, 1996].

Errors in the selection of the appropriate treatment apply to both operative and nonoperative treatments [Ellis, 1996]. For example, the use of MMF of unstable, comminuted mandibular segments may lead to overtightening and rotation of the flail segment and result in malocclusion with associated facial asymmetry (**Fig 4.2-1**). In the case of operative treatment, the use of inadequate internal fixation hardware [Ellis, 1996] (load sharing vs load bearing) (**Fig 4.2-2**) may invariably lead to failure of the hardware, an infected fracture, and ultimately a nonunion. The imprecise adaptation of heavier plates will displace the fractured segments leading to a malocclusion and eventually a malunited fracture [Alpert, 1998] (**Fig 4.2-3**).

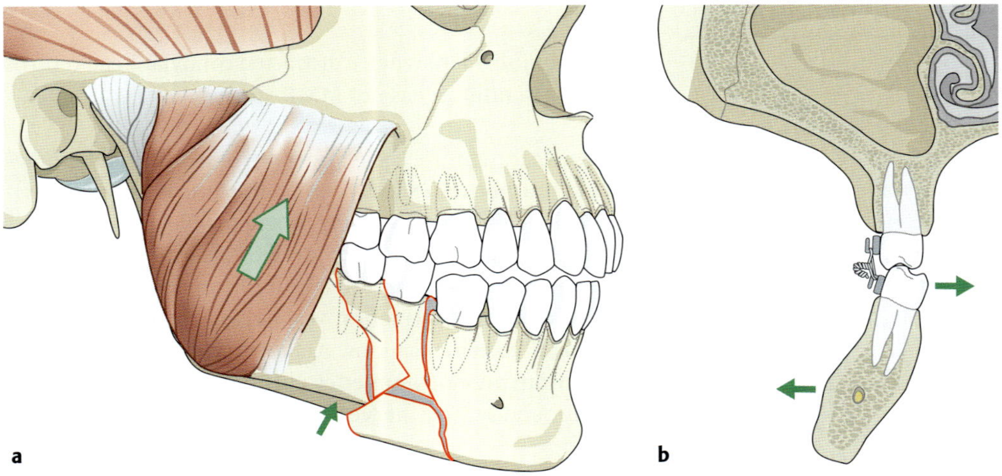

Fig 4.2-1a–b
a Comminuted mandibular body fracture with dislocation due to the pull of the masseter muscle.
b Coronal view of mandibulomaxillary fixation (MMF) of the comminuted body fracture. Overtightening of the MMF results in clockwise rotation of the fractured segments and malocclusion (noncontact of the lingual cusps).

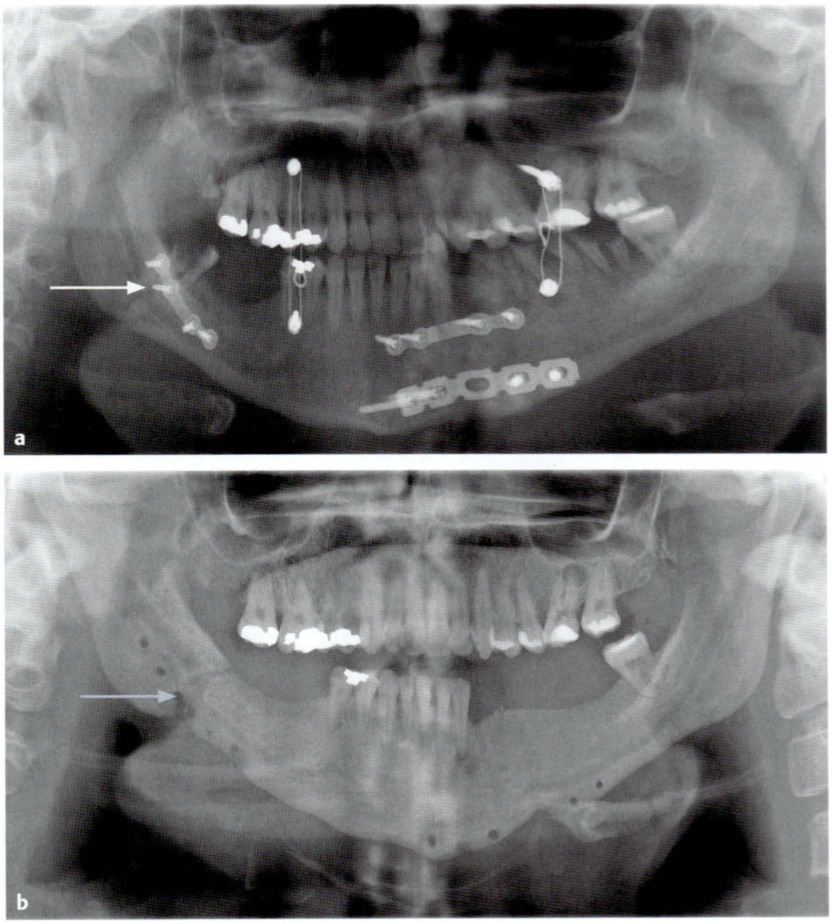

Fig 4.2-2a–b

a The use of inadequate internal fixation hardware (white arrow) invariably leads to failure of the hardware.

b An infected fracture and ultimately a nonunion (blue arrow) is visible in the former fracture area.

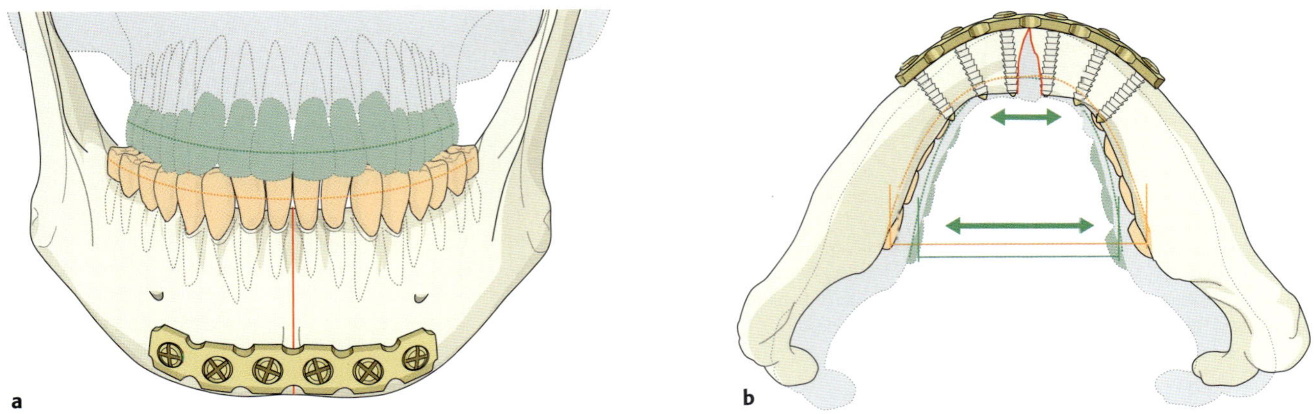

Fig 4.2-3a–b An imprecise adaptation of heavier plates will displace the fractured segments (short arrow) leading to a much bigger posterior widening (long arrow) with malocclusion and finally a malunited fracture.

Condylar and subcondylar mandibular fractures are the most common fractures that can lead to a malocclusion [Spitzer et al, 1997]. Moderately displaced and dislocated fractures often lead to shortening of the height of the ramus on the affected side resulting in premature occlusal contacts on the side of the injury, and a varying degree of open bite anteriorly on the contralateral side (**Fig 4.2-4**). Condylar fractures in the growing individual may also lead to the development of mandibular asymmetries. Bilateral condylar fractures, unless treated appropriately, can result in the presence of a significant anterior open bite and mandibular retrusion.

Patient compliance with the treatment also is important to the success of the intervention [Passeri et al, 1993; Serena-Gomez et al, 2008]. Poor oral hygiene, consumption of alcoholic beverages, smoking, malnutrition, and failure to follow the postoperative instructions (diet, maintaining the MMF, etc) may also lead to complications. Even though the clinician has little control over patient compliance [Alpert, 1998], identification of a patient at risk should alert the clinician to use a treatment method that minimizes the patient's need for compliance [Alpert, 1998].

Healing disorders that will affect the treatment outcome can be the result of a posttreatment infection or conditions, such as long-term steroid use, diabetes and other immunosuppressive conditions, long-term malnutrition (such as alcoholism) and underlying systemic metabolic disorders that affect bone metabolism and healing [Senel et al, 2007].

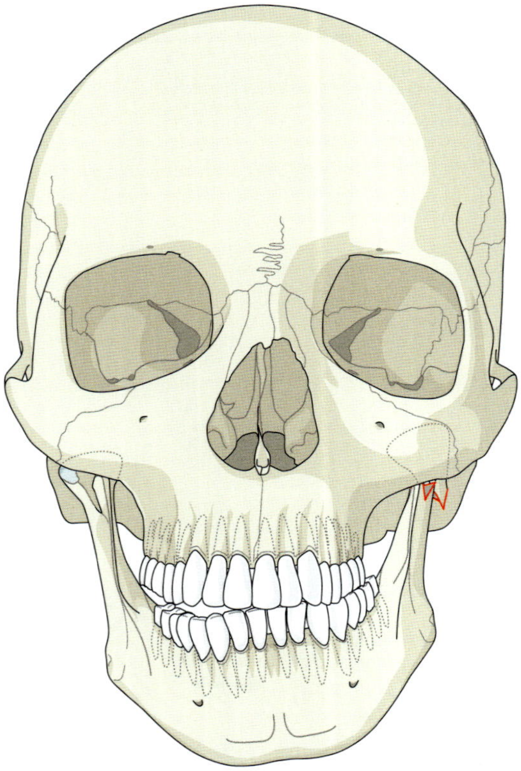

Fig 4.2-4 Displaced and dislocated unilateral condylar fractures lead to shortening of the height of the ramus on the affected side, resulting in premature occlusal contacts on the side of the injury and a varying degree of open bite on the contralateral side.

3 Planning and execution of the revision treatment

The ability to formulate the correct diagnosis is important to the success of the revision treatment. The first step in establishing the etiology of the residual deformity is the collection of information with a thorough clinical examination. A problem-oriented physical examination must include the evaluation of the height and width of the patient's face and examination of preinjury photos when available. Following a thorough clinical evaluation, radiographs are obtained and may be used to generate 3-D virtual models to completely assess the deformity resulting from fracture treatment. Dental casts are useful in planning the revision surgery in cases where osteotomies are considered for the revision of the fracture treatment. Osteotomies are usually designed at the site of the previous fractures unless more traditional osteotomies will address the problem better. The fabrication of acrylic occlusal splints based on the model surgery ensure precise transfer of the planned surgery to the operating room [Vega, 2011] (**Fig 4.2-5**).

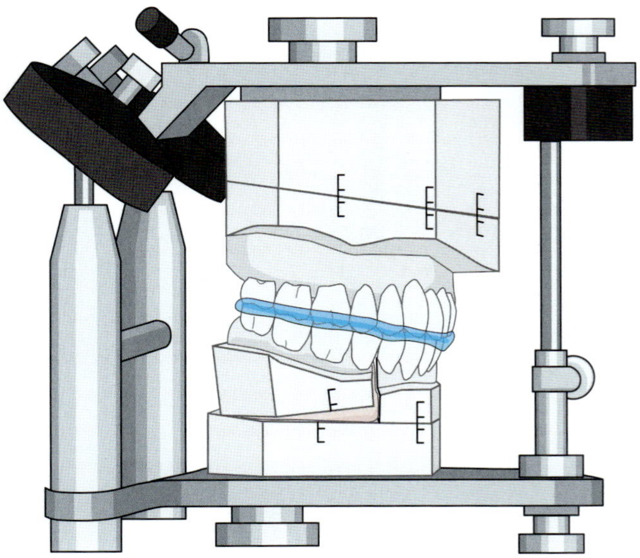

Fig 4.2-5 Occlusal splint (blue) based on the model surgery ensure precise transfer of the planned surgery to the operating room.

Following completion of the osteotomies, the surgical splint can then help reposition the dentition to the desired occlusion. Depending on the amount of interfragmentary contact, load-bearing hardware plus bone grafting to ensure complete healing of the repositioned fragments, should be considered [Alpert, 1998].

Finally, the clinician must also consider the patient's general condition including preexisting comorbidities, leading to the consideration of camouflage procedures to "mask" the deformity. This may include either stock or patient-specific implants manufactured according to the computed tomographic scan data [Goldsmith et al, 2012].

Once a posttreatment malocclusion is identified, the clinician must then determine the possible etiology of the complication to determine the best treatment options [Koury, 1997] (**Table 4.2-1**). Minor malocclusions can be addressed with occlusal adjustment (ameloplasty), orthodontic care, or in some cases prosthodontic treatment [Park et al, 2010]. More severe malocclusions will require an operation at the source of the problem in cases of early diagnosis before a bone union has resulted, or osteotomies to correct the occlusion in cases of a malunited fracture [Spitzer et al, 1997].

The treatment of the malocclusion can be as minor as performing occlusal adjustments, orthodontics, prosthetic reconstruction or might require more extensive corrective jaw surgery to restore an acceptable occlusion.

• Errors in diagnosis
• Errors in surgical technique
– Inadequate fracture reduction
– Inadequate fracture fixation
• Postoperative infection
• Metabolic bone disorders

Table 4.2-1 Etiology of posttraumatic occlusal disturbances.

Late surgical correction of posttraumatic malocclusion resulting from a malunion of the fractured mandible will require osteotomies, repositioning of segments and internal fixation at the site of the injury when it is located within the dentate arch (body or symphyseal region) [Becking et al, 1998] (**Fig 4.2-6**). Some patients with bone loss will also need bone transplantation. Gold standard is the use of fresh autogenous bone. A nonunion will also require repositioning of segments, rigid internal fixation, and sometimes bone transplantation. Unilateral or bilateral ramus osteotomies can be used to treat malocclusions that develop after condylar fractures [Ellis et al, 2009] or fractures beyond the dentate segment (**Fig 4.2-7a–c**). Occasionally, the surgeon may choose to perform a maxillary osteotomy to treat the malocclusion [Zachariades et al, 1993] (**Fig 4.2-7d**).

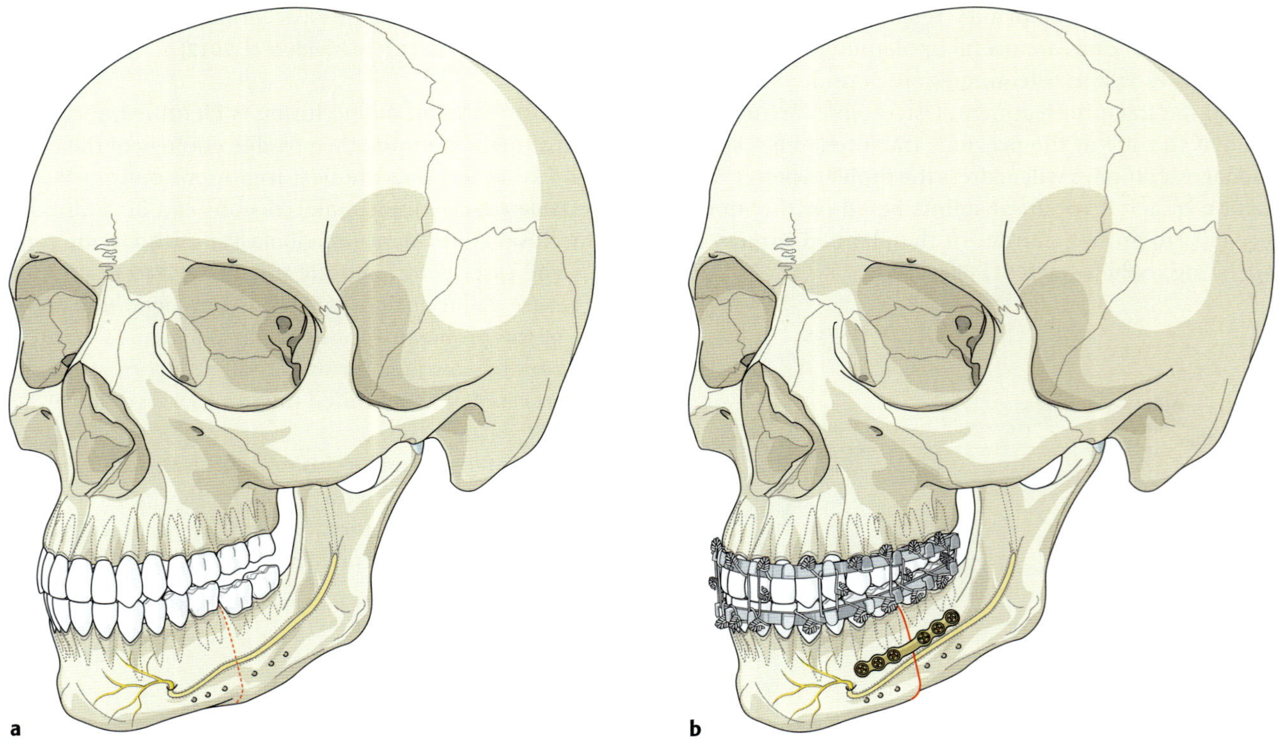

Fig 4.2-6a–b
a Posttraumatic malocclusion resulting from a malunion or nonunion of the left mandible.
b Osteotomy performed at the site of the previous fracture to achieve a normal occlusion.

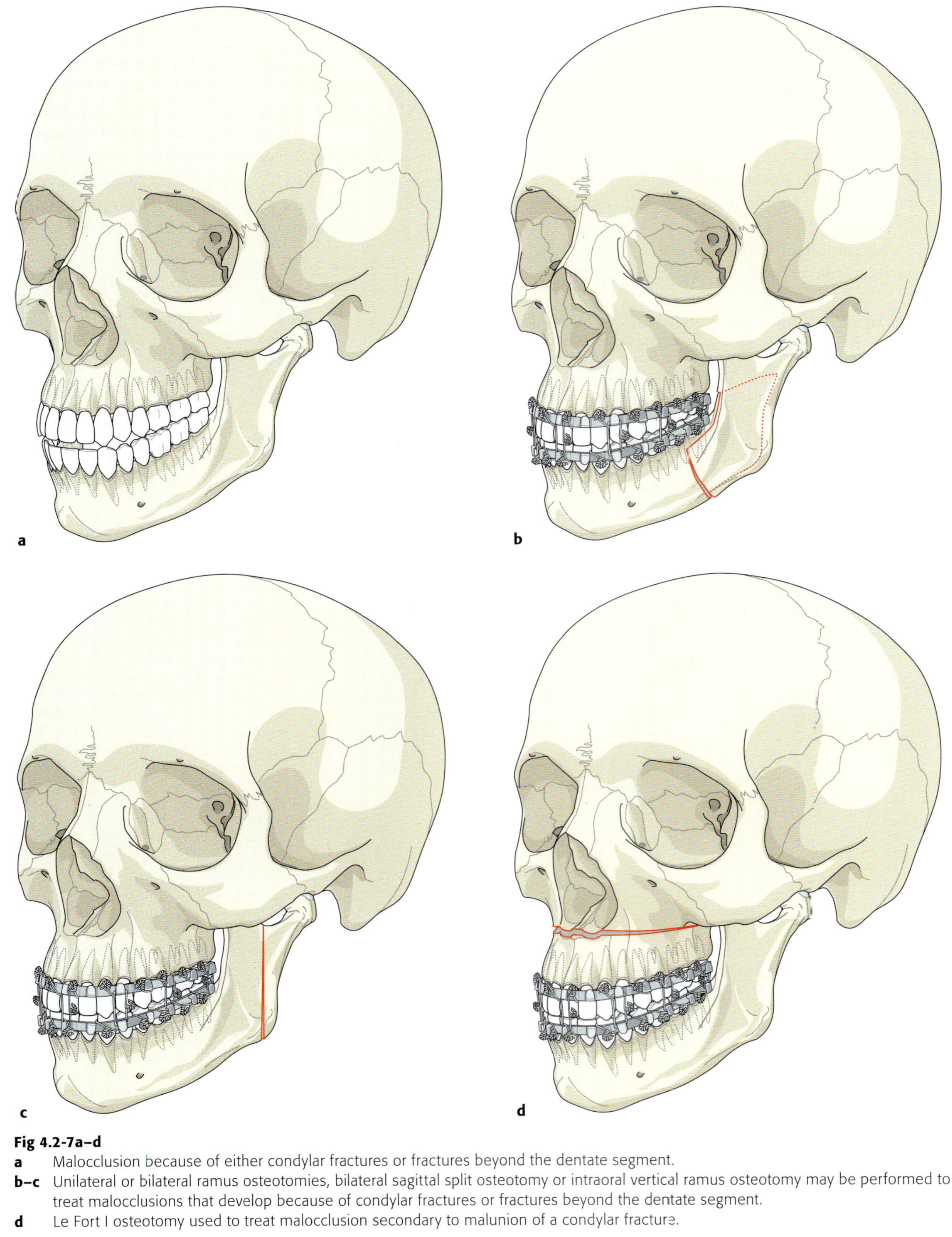

Fig 4.2-7a–d

a Malocclusion because of either condylar fractures or fractures beyond the dentate segment.

b–c Unilateral or bilateral ramus osteotomies, bilateral sagittal split osteotomy or intraoral vertical ramus osteotomy may be performed to treat malocclusions that develop because of condylar fractures or fractures beyond the dentate segment.

d Le Fort I osteotomy used to treat malocclusion secondary to malunion of a condylar fracture.

4 Complications and pitfalls

Correction of a malocclusion through occlusal adjustments, orthodontics and/or prosthetic reconstruction is usually associated with minor complications, if any. Those procedures may be associated with substance losses of the teeth due to occlusal adjustments or prosthodontic procedures, such as the rehabilitation with crowns and bridges, or from demineralization and caries formation during orthodontic treatment. All this may lead to either hypersensitivity of the teeth involved, and finally a devitalization that may create a need for root canal treatment or tooth extractions.

Corrective jaw surgery after malocclusion or nonunion may present with all surgical complications known for orthognathic surgery, such as bleeding, swelling, and swelling-related airway obstruction, nerve damage, tooth injuries, bad splits with irregular fractures, instrument fractures associated with foreign bodies, wound-healing disturbances, such as soft-tissue and/or bone infections, relapse, scar formation, temporomandibular joint disorders, condylar resorption, hardware-related fractures, such as plate fractures or loose screws, nasal and sinus problems, eye complications and bone necrosis because of impaired blood supply [Ehrenfeld et al, 2011].

5 Summary

Even with best treatment efforts, unsatisfactory results, such as nonunion, malunion, malocclusion, and facial asymmetry [Ellis et al, 1992], occur during the management of mandibular fractures. A clear understanding of the etiology of these resulting deformities is essential for the success of the revision surgery. Furthermore, the clinician should be familiar with the reoperative techniques used for the management of these events and deformities [Laine et al, 2004].

6 References and suggested reading

Alpert B. Management of the complications of mandibular fracture treatment. *Operat Tech Plast Reconstr Surg.* 1998;5(4):325–333.

Becking AG, Zijderveld SA, Tuinzing DB. Management of post-traumatic malocclusion caused by condylar process fractures. *J Oral Maxillofac Surg.* 1998 Dec;56(12):1370–1374.

Ehrenfeld M, Manson PN, Prein J. *Principles of Internal Fixation of the Craniomaxillofacial Skeleton.* Stuttgart: Thieme; 2011.

Ellis E 3rd. Complications of rigid internal fixation for mandibular fractures. *J Craniomaxillofac Trauma.* 1996 Summer;2(2):32–39.

Ellis E 3rd, Walker R. Treatment of malocclusion and TMJ dysfunction secondary to condylar fractures. *Craniomaxillofac Trauma Reconstr.* 2009 Mar;2(1):1–18.

Ellis E 3rd, Tharanon W. Facial width problems associated with rigid fixation of mandibular fractures: case reports. *J Oral Maxillofac Surg.* 1992 Jan;50(1):87–94.

Fordyce AM, Lalani Z, Songra AK, et al. Intermaxillary fixation is not usually necessary to reduce mandibular fractures. *Br J Oral Maxillofac Surg.* 1999 Feb;37(1):52–57.

Goldsmith D, Horowitz A, Orentlicher G. Facial skeletal augmentation using custom facial implants. *Atlas Oral Maxillofac Surg Clin North Am.* 2012 Mar;20(1):119–134.

Koury M. Complications of mandibular fractures. In: Kaban L, Pogrel A, Perrott D, eds. *Complications.* 1st ed. Philadelphia: WB Saunders; 1997:121–145.

Laine P, Kontio R, Salo A, et al. Secondary correction of malocclusion after treatment of maxillofacial trauma. *J Oral Maxillofac Surg.* 2004 Oct;62(10):1312–1320.

Moulton-Barrett R, Rubinstein AJ, Salzhauer MA, et al. Complications of mandibular fractures. *Ann Plast Surg.* 1998 Sep:41(3):258–263.

Park IP, Heo SJ, Koak JY, et al. Post traumatic malocclusion and its prosthetic treatment. *J Adv Prosthodont.* 2010 Sep;2(3):88–91.

Passeri LA, Ellis E 3rd, Sinn DP. Relationship of substance abuse to complications with mandibular fractures. *J Oral Maxillofac Surg.* 1993 Jan;51(1):22–25.

Renton TF, Wiesenfeld D. Mandibular fracture osteosynthesis: a comparison of three techniques. *Br J Oral Maxillofac Surg.* 1996 Apr;34(2):166–173.

Spitzer WJ, Vanderborght G, Dumbach J. Surgical management of mandibular malposition after malunited condylar fractures in adults. *J Craniomaxillofac Surg.* 1997 Apr;25(2):91–96

Serena-Gomez E, Passeri LA. Complications of mandible fractures related to substance abuse. *J Oral Maxillofac Surg.* 2008 Oct;66(10):2028–2034.

Senel FC, Jessen GS, Melo MD, et al. Infection following treatment of mandible fractures: the role of immunosuppression and polysubstance abuse. *Oral Surg Oral Med Oral Pathol Oral Radiol Endod.* 2007 Jan;103(1):38–42.

Vega L. Re-operative mandibular trauma: management of posttraumatic mandibular deformities. *Oral Maxillofac Surg Clin North Am.* 2011 Feb;23(1):47–61.

Zachariades N, Mezitis M, Michelis A. Posttraumatic osteotomies of the jaws. *Int J Oral Maxillofac Surg.* 1993;22:328.

4.3 Treatment of ankylosis

Risto Kontio

1 Introduction

Ankylosis of the temporomandibular joint (TMJ) is characterized by bony and/or fibrous adhesions of the articulating structures. It can be categorized depending on location, type of tissue involvement, and extent of fusion of the joint structures. It is important to distinguish true ankylosis (intraarticular) from false ankylosis (extraarticular). In true ankyloses, fibrous or calcified connective tissue bands fuse the mandible to the glenoid fossa or articular eminence (**Fig 4.3-1**). Extraarticular ankylosis (hypomobility) is caused by pathological conditions involving the ligaments, muscles, and/or certain cranial nerves.

Multiple etiological factors may lead to ankylosis, such as trauma, infection, autoimmune disease, and surgical procedures. The most common cause is trauma, comprising 70–90% of cases [Long, 2012]. It is more frequent in children than adults because children have more growth potential in the TMJ region that may cause excessive bone formation associated with trauma. Condylar head fracture is most prone to lead to ankylosis. The immature, thinly covered, and highly vascular condyle tends to spill into the intracapsular space after a traumatic injury. The result is a hemarthrosis containing multiple comminuted fragments of bone with high osteogenic potential. If ankylosis occurs during the growth period of the patient, significant alteration in mandibular development may occur.

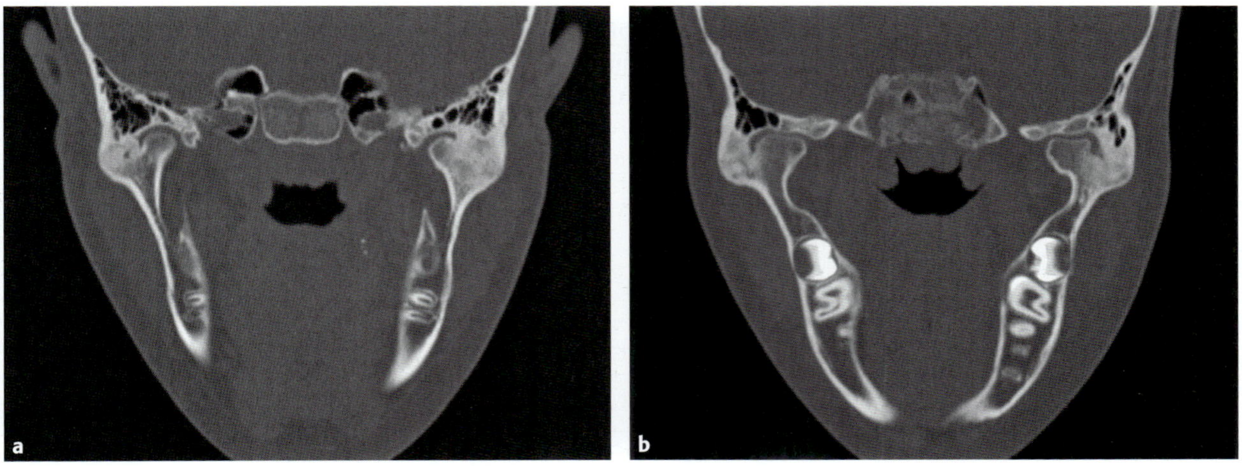

Fig 4.3-1a–b True ankylosis of the condyle.

2 Diagnosis and imaging

After obtaining the patient history, the clinical examination focuses on functional information, such as range of motion and facial deformities. Radiologically, orthopantomogram can be used for screening. High-resolution computed tomographic (CT) scan is the gold standard for evaluation of TMJ ankylosis.

3 Treatment

The aim of therapy is to restore mobility and function of the mandible, and finally to restore the esthetic dimensions of the face. There are different protocols classifying the nature of ankylosis. Sawhney [1986] introduced a classification system that was based on plane radiographs and was divided into four categories. The classification distinguishes only different types of ankylosis, without any inclusion to treatment. Recently, He et al [2011] published a classification protocol based on CT images that combined type and nature of ankylosis with treatment (**Table 4.3-1**) and which has been slightly modified.

Surgical treatment must include the following procedures: removal of ankylotic tissue, repair or reconstruction of the joint surfaces and disc, and correction of jaw deformities. There are three main surgical approaches used for treatment of TMJ ankylosis: "gap arthroplasty" with or without interpositional graft, condyle reconstruction with autogenous tissues or alloplastic materials, and joint reconstruction with alloplastic materials.

Katsnelson et al [2012] performed a systematic review and metaanalysis of two of the above-mentioned treatment approaches. "Gap arthroplasty" was compared with reconstruction using costochondral grafts (CCG). The results suggest that "gap arthroplasty" is associated with better mandible range of motion and significantly larger maximal interincisal opening, although the difference in millimeters was small. The authors suggest considering other factors when deciding on the treatment options, such as age or the patient's ability to tolerate harvesting of a costochondral graft.

3.1 "Gap arthroplasty"

The term "gap arthroplasty" is a misnomer because the procedure has nothing to do with a plastic and reconstructive joint preserving/reconstructing operation. Resection of the ankylotic bone and connective tissue and repair with interpositional material is the principle procedure used in "gap arthroplasty". A modified preauricular incision is the preferable approach to the TMJ region because it leaves an inconspicuous scar at the junction of the ear and the preauricular skin, and it allows direct access to the joint area retracting the preauricular vessels and facial nerve anteriorly. After removal of the ankylotic mass, interpositional material should be placed into the joint space to wall off bony surfaces and to prevent reankylosis. Frequently, a simultaneous coronoidectomy is carried out to improve range of motion. Stripping of the masseter attachments to the ramus may also be considered. Intensive, long-term physical therapy is always necessary. Active opening exercises and physical therapy is appropriate postoperatively to stretch the shortened muscles to a normal functional length and to prevent reankylosis.

A1	A2	A3	A4
Fibrous ankylosis without bony fusion of the joint	Ankylosis with bony fusion on the lateral side of joint	Ankylosis with bony fusion on the lateral side of joint	Ankylosis with complete bony fusion of the joint
	Residual condyle fragment > 50% of the condylar head on medial side	Residual condyle fragment < 50% of the condylar head on medial side	

Treatment	Treatment	Treatment	Treatment
Fibrous tissue release	Resection of lateral bony fusion	Resection of lateral bony fusion and medially displaced condyle, if too small to bear load	Complete removal of bony fusion
TMJ disc reposition or TMF as interpositional material	TMF or MMF sutured to disc laterally as barrier	Reconstruction CCG and TMF or MMF	Reconstruction with CCG and TMF or MMF
If condyle head is severely destroyed: resection and reconstruction with CCG and TMF or MMF	TMJ prosthesis as ultimo ratio	TMJ prosthesis as ultimo ratio	TMJ prosthesis

Table 4.3-1 Classification and treatment protocol of traumatic ankylosis by He et al [2011]*.
* TMJ indicates temporomandibular joint; TMF, temporalis musculofascial flap; MMF, masseter muscle flap; and CCG, costochondral graft.

3.1.1 Interpositional materials in "gap arthroplasty"

The necessity for using interpositional material for correction of ankylosis with "gap arthroplasty" has been widely debated. Topazian [1966] demonstrated less reankylosis after placing interpositional material.

Many interpositional materials have been used, such as autografts, including dermis, cartilage, fascia lata, and alloplast, such as teflon and silastic. Recently, numerous reports have demonstrated that alloplastic materials elicit a significant destructive foreign body response not reported with autogenous grafts [Valentini et al, 2002; Fricton et al, 2002; Abbas et al, 2005; Dimitroulis, 2011].

3.1.1.1 Autogenous material

3.1.1.1.1 Temporalis fascia flap

The main advantage of the temporalis fascia flap is that it is autogenous, resilient, and close to the joint, allowing pedicled transfer of vascularized tissue into the gap joint area. Fascia alone should only be used as interposition material because muscle has the potential for ossification and may facilitate reankylosis.

Balaji [2003] and Brusati et al [1990] have described its use, and stated that the viability of temporalis fascia graft or flap is a critical issue. Guruprasad et al [2010] studied the use of temporalis fascia flap in treatment of TMJ ankylosis. A good success rate was achieved. The average interincisal opening increased from 11 mm (mean) to 38 mm (mean). The results indicated that the temporalis fascia flap is an effective component in treatment of TMJ ankylosis.

3.1.1.1.2 Dermal graft

A nonvascularized dermal graft is another option to fill the space created by "gap arthroplasty". The dermal graft is placed in such a manner that all areas with the potential for reossification are covered. The graft is sutured to the surrounding tissues. Interpositional arthroplasty for TMJ ankylosis using the dermal graft was first reported by Georgiade et al [1957]. Successful results using dermis as an interpositional material in arthroplasty for TMJ ankylosis have been reported [Chossegros et al, 1999; Topazian, 1966].

3.1.1.1.3 Buccal fat pad

The buccal fat pad has also proven to be a safe and effective interpositional material for reducing the danger of reankylosis. One disadvantage is the small risk for facial contour loss in the region of the buccal fat. The fat graft has a higher risk of atrophy than other autogeneous tissues.

3.1.1.2 Alloplastic materials

Alloplastic materials, such as silicone and polytetrafluoroethylene-aluminum oxide, whether secured to the glenoid fossa or over the superior surface of the mandibular condyle are another option to cover the exposed bone after "gap arthroplasty". However, they may fragment, migrate, and create a foreign body reaction when subjected to repeated shear forces. An inflammatory reaction provoked by the alloplast may necessitate its removal.

3.2 Condyle and joint reconstruction

The TMJ ankylosis is released by resecting the ankylotic mass widely. Only the condyle or the whole TMJ complex should be reconstructed. The reconstruction may be performed with autogenous grafts, a condyle prosthesis, or a total joint prosthesis (**Table 4.3-2**). Condyle reconstruction with costochondral grafts (CCGs) provides functional articulation and permits adaptive growth or remodeling. Total joint replacement (TJR) is done with alloplastic materials and will not grow or remodel.

Autogenous graft/flap		**Alloplastic materials**	**Other methods**
Distant sites	Local sites		
Costochondral	Coronoid process	Separate condyle prosthesis, titanium, stainless steel	Distraction osteogenesis
Metatarsal	Posterior ramus	Total joint replacement	
Iliac crest	Ankylotic mass		
Fibula			

Table 4.3-2. Materials and methods for temporomandibular joint reconstruction.

3.2.1 Autogenous materials

3.2.1.1 Costochondral graft

There are several benefits and drawbacks for nonvascularized costochondral grafting for condyle reconstruction (**Table 4.3-3**).

The use of CCGs is based on the assumption that autogenous tissue is better tolerated at the host site and that an interface between cartilage and bone is thought to provide a more freely moving articulation compared to osseous tissues alone. Poswillo [1987] has emphasized the similarity of the condyle to human rib regarding the anatomical cartilage-bone interface in TMJ.

The fourth to eighth ribs are the preferable donors for condylar reconstruction. The graft should include the required length of bone (3 cm) and cartilage (3 mm). A short cartilage portion helps to avoid unwanted overgrowth, while a longer portion of cartilage may produce undesired torsion at the costochondral interface. The ligaments attaching the bone to the cartilage cap must not be detached.

A study by Lindqvist [1986] showed that in most patients (67%) the postoperative function of the mandible was considered to be good or excellent, and nearly all patients were pain free (**Fig 4.3-2**).

There were no postoperative chest infections and only one case of pneumothorax. Zhang et al [2012] used a combination of costochondral grafting and distraction osteogenesis in unilateral ankylosis with mandible retrognathia. Their results indicate that the combination of costochondral grafting and distraction osteogenesis is a safe and effective method to treat TMJ ankyloses.

Some clinicians have advocated adaptation of the costochondral segment along the posterior border of the ramus to bring the full width of the cartilaginous cap into wider contact within the fossa mediolaterally. This option often necessitates significant recontouring of the posterior border of the ramus and makes fixation more difficult compared with a lateral onlay position. Masticatory forces directed transversely to the costochondral junction make it more liable to fracture.

	Benefits	**Drawbacks**
Costochondral graft	Consists of bone and cartilage	Risk of separation of bone and cartilage
	Resembles mandible condyle anatomically	Bone quality poor
	Has growth potential	Growth unpredictable
	Easy approach to raise graft	Risk of donor site complication
Fibula flap	Survival rate good	No cartilage, only bone tissue
	Allows large and wide reconstructions	Risk of severe donor site complications
	Cortical bone dense	
Iliac crest graft	Consists of bone and cartilage (in children)	Risk of severe donor site complications
	Has growth potential	
	Allows large and wide reconstructions	
	Can be used as free graft or vascularized flap	

Table 4.3-3. Bone grafts/flaps used in temporomandibular joint reconstruction: benefits and drawbacks.

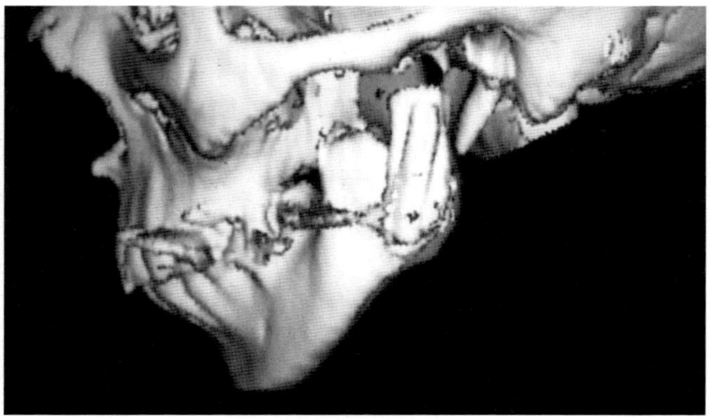

Fig 4.3-2 Costochondal graft fixed onto lateral surface of ascending ramus.

The disadvantages of costochondral grafting include unexpected overgrowth, reankylosis, poor bone quality, and possible donor site complications. It is suggested that costochondral grafting is not a method of choice if the patient has developed recurrent ankylosis. Despite the disadvantages it is the preferred method of TMJ reconstruction in growing children and as an initial reconstruction in adults.

3.2.1.2 Fibula

A fibula free flap can be used to replace the condylar region. For this the fibula flap may be positioned with its bony end into the TMJ region in a distance to the fossa, like a "gap arthroplasty" (see chapter 2.6). Alternatively, the fibula can be fixated with a condylar head bearing reconstruction plate, or a true TMJ prosthesis can be used together with a fibula flap, either simultaneously with the bone transplantation, or in a secondary procedure.

3.2.1.3 Iliac crest

An osseochondral iliac crest graft is only possible during a patient's growth phase; the cartilage on top of the iliac crest no longer exists in adults. The graft consists of full thickness bone containing the overlying cartilage layer as a cap (**Table 4.3-3**). The cartilage cap of the iliac crest may be placed into the glenoid fossa to prevent recurrence of TMJ ankylosis. No creeping substitution of the cartilage columns by bone occurs, and no cases of reankylosis were noticed during the follow-up study of Kummoona et al [2013].

3.2.1.4 Coronoid process

The coronoid process has been used for condyle reconstruction. If the coronoid process is not part of the ankylosis it is suitable as donor material. In addition, coronoidectomy is often performed in connection with ankylosis release. Often the size, shape, and thickness of the coronoid process are suitable for TMJ reconstruction. It can also resist heavier forces compared with costochondral grafts because of its stiffer bone quality. The main limitation is that the ankylotic tissue often involves the coronoid area.

3.2.2 Alloplastic material

3.2.2.1 Prosthetic condylar heads

Condylar head replacement can be done with condylar head add-ons to reconstruction plates. This technique should be only used temporarily because in the long term the heads may penetrate into the middle cranial fossa unless a stable (metallic) fossa component is additionally used. Using only metal condyle prostheses, a clinical and radiological follow-up study showed heterotopic bone formation in 52% of cases and glenoid fossa resorption in 43%. In one patient with rheumatoid arthritis the condyle eroded through the skull base 10 months after surgery (**Fig 4.3-3**) [Lindqvist et al, 1992].

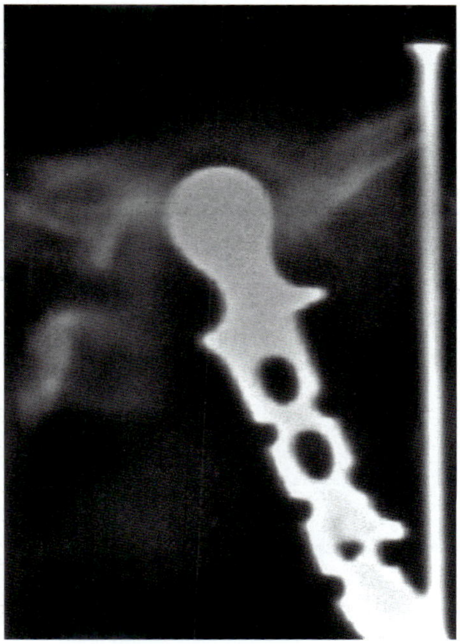

Fig 4.3-3 Metalic condylar head penetrating into the middle cranial fossa.

3.2.2.2 TMJ prosthesis

The goal of TJR is the restoration of TMJ function and reduction of pain and discomfort as a secondary benefit. Since 1992 major developments in material science have taken place. Furthermore, the TJR operation technique has adopted principles from orthopedic joint replacement surgery. Total joint replacement seems to be promising in the treatment of TMJ ankyloses (**Fig 4.3-4**).

A TMJ prosthesis includes both alloplastic fossa and condyle parts (**Fig 4.3-5**). This eliminates the need for a donor site operation and potential complications associated with it. In addition, TJR reduces the total operative time and allows immediate postoperative physical therapy.

Machon et al [2012] published their results of 38 TJR in 27 patients. The most common indication was ankylosis. Interincisal opening increased from a mean of 17 mm to a mean of 29 mm during the follow up. Minor complications were reported but no infections, implant or material failure were detected. Furthermore, no reankylosis was seen during the follow up. They concluded that the TJR appears to be a safe and effective choice for increasing jaw function. The study by Giannakopoulos et al [2012] supports the conclusions drawn by Machon et al [2012]. During a 10-year multicenter clinical trial 442 TJR operations were performed for 288 patients. More than half of the patients were operated on because of TMJ ankylosis. They concluded that TMJ alloplastic replacement, based on sound orthopedic and biomedical principles, is a safe and efficient option.

However, the expected lifetime of such devices, the reliability of the implantation procedure, and the reliability of TMJ prostheses require further evaluation.

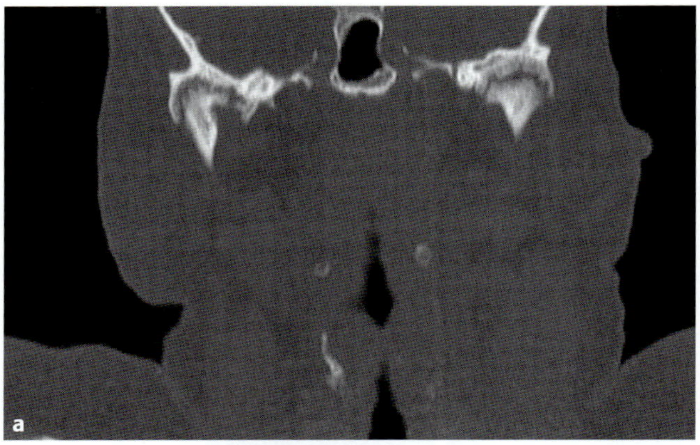

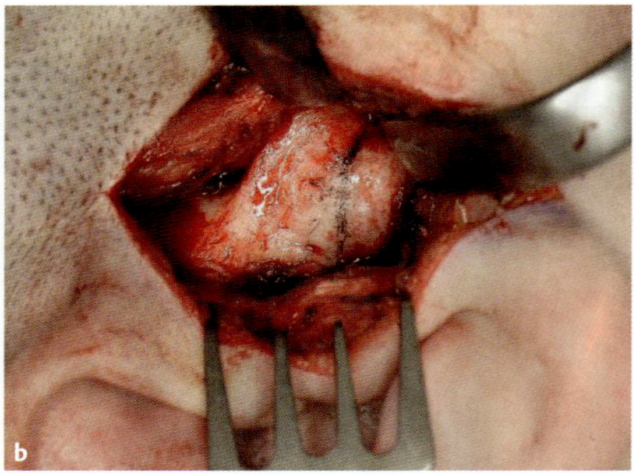

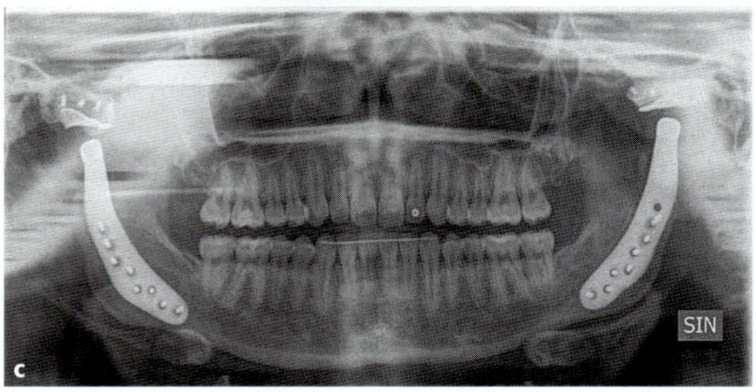

Fig 4.3-4a–c
- **a** Intraarticular ankylosis of temporomandibular joint, bony ankylosis on right and fibrotic/bony ankylosis on left joint (courtesy J Tornwall).
- **b** Intraoperative image of bony ankylosis, pencil drawing marking the first resection line (courtesy J Tornwall).
- **c** Postoperative OPT; 1 year after total joint replacement surgery (courtesy J Tornwall).

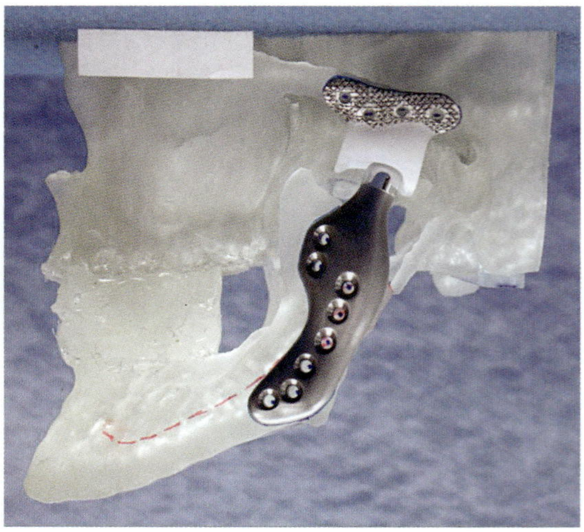

Fig 4.3-5 Total joint replacement prosthesis, note separate fossa and condyle parts.

4 Treatment of children

There are multiple treatment protocols related to TMJ ankylosis in children. One of the treatment protocols is the removal of bone mass as soon as possible after diagnosis, and primary reconstruction with autogenous grafts. Growth may take place by local remodeling in response to function. A costochondral graft is preferred over a prosthetic joint to replace the condylar growth area. Temporalis fascia is used to line the glenoid fossa. A TMJ arthroplasty with temporal fascial interposition and mandibular distraction vertically is a secondary choice in severe TMJ ankylosis in children.

5 Complications and pitfalls

The resection and management of the ankylosis including placement of grafts or alloplastic devices demands utmost care in dissection and tissue handling. The proximity to the retromandibular vein, the maxillary artery or even the internal carotid artery and jugular vein, and ankylotic growth spreading to the temporal bone region mandates careful surgical vigilance. Navigation-aided resection of ankylotic bone and tissue may be a valuable additional technique in this potentially complicated procedure.

The most common difficulty with costochondral grafting is unpredictable growth of the graft. This is a problem largely confined to pediatric patients.

One problem after ankylosis release is reankylosis. To minimize the risk of reankylosis wide exposure of the TMJ region is strongly recommended. In reankylosis following costochondral grafting, it is recommended to perform a "gap arthroplasty" only and postpone reconstructive joint surgery until mobility is stable. In these situations closure of the gap by mandibular distraction secondarily gradually achieves function and symmetry.

In treating malocclusion secondary to ankylosis, the initial step is to manage the joint ankylosis. Pediatric malocclusions secondary to joint injury may be favorably modified over time using functional orthodontic appliances. Early and late complications after TMJ reconstruction are presented in **Table 4.3-4**.

Indications	Contraindications, relative	Complications, intraoperative	Complications, postoperative
• Ankylosis • Failed autogenous graft for TMJ reconstruction • Condylar hypoplasia • Severe inflammatory arthritic disease • Severe degenerative joint changes • Conditions after condylar fracture or condylectomy • Recurrent ankylosis/heterotopic bone formation • Failed previous alloplastic reconstruction	• Immature facial skeleton • Allergy to prosthetic material • Chronic infection • Compromising systemic disease • Uncontrolled parafunctional mandible habits	• Facial nerve injury • Hemorrhage • Mandible nerve injury • Perforation into the oral cavity • Poor adaptations of device components	• Infection • Heterotopic bone formation • Foreign body reaction • Implant failure

Table 4.3-4 Indications, contraindications, and complications in total joint replacement surgery (total joint prosthesis).

6 References and suggested reading

Abbas I, Jamil M, Jehanzeb M, et al. Temporomandibular joint ankylosis: experience with interpositional gap arthroplasty at Ayub Medical College Abbottabad. *J Ayub Med Coll Abbottabad.* 2005 Oct-Dec;17(4):67–69.

Balaji SM. Modified temporalis anchorage in craniomandibular reankylosis. *Int J Oral Maxillofac Surg.* 2003 Oct;32(5):480–485.

Brusati R, Raffaini M, Sesenna E, et al. The temporalis muscle flap in temporo-mandibular joint surgery. *J Craniomaxillofac Surg.* 1990 Nov;18(8):352–358.

Chossegros C, Guyot L, Cheynet F, et al. Full-thickness skin graft interposition after temporomandibular joint ankylosis surgery. A study of 31 cases. *Int J Oral Maxillofac Surg.* 1999 Oct;28(5):330–334.

Clauser L, Curioni C, Spanio S. The use of the temporalis muscle flap in facial and craniofacial reconstructive surgery. A review of 182 cases. *J Craniomaxillofac Surg.* 1995 Aug;23(4):203–214.

Dimitroulis G. A critical review of interpositional grafts following temporomandibular joint discectomy with an overview of the dermis-fat graft. *Int J Oral Maxillofac Surg.* 2011 Jun;40(6):561–568.

Fricton JR, Look JO, Schiffman E, et al. Long-term study of temporomandibular joint surgery with alloplastic implants compared with nonimplant surgery and nonsurgical rehabilitation for painful temporomandibular joint disc displacement. *J Oral Maxillofac Surg.* 2002 Dec;60(12):1400–1411; discussion 1411–1412.

Gaba S, Sharma RK, Rattan V, et al. The long-term fate of pedicled buccal pad fat used for interpositional arthroplasty in TMJ ankylosis. *J Plast Reconstr Aesthet Surg.* 2012 Nov;65(11):1468–1473.

Georgiade N, Altany F, Pickrell K. An experimental and clinical evaluation of autogenous dermal grafts used in the treatment of temporomandibular joint ankylosis. *Plast Reconstr Surg (1946).* 1957 Apr;19(4):321–336.

Giannakopoulos HE, Sinn DP, Quinn PD. Biomet microfixation temporomandibular joint replacement system: a 3-year follow-up study of patients treated during 1995 to 2005. *J Oral Maxillofac Surg.* 2012 Apr;70(4):787–794; discussion 795–796.

Guruprasad Y, Chauhan DS, Cariappa KM. A retrospective study of temporalis muscle and fascia flap in treatment of TMJ ankylosis. *J Maxillofac Oral Surg.* 2010 Dec;9(4):363–368.

Güven O. Treatment of temporomandibular joint ankylosis by a modified fossa prosthesis. *J Craniomaxillofac Surg.* 2004 Aug;32(4):236–242.

He D, Yang C, Chen M, et al. Traumatic temporomandibular joint ankylosis: our classification and treatment experience. *J Oral Maxillofac Surg.* 2011 Jun;69(6):1600–1607.

Katsnelson A, Markiewicz MR, Keith DA, et al. Operative management of temporomandibular joint ankylosis: a systematic review and meta-analysis. *J Oral Maxillofac Surg.* 2012 Mar;70(3):531–536.

Khadka A, Hu J. Autogenous grafts for condylar reconstruction in treatment of TMJ ankylosis: current concepts. *Int J Oral Maxillofac Surg.* 2012;Jan;41(1):94–102.

Kummoona RK. Biological reconstruction of the temporomandibular joint by chondro-osseous graft: clinical and experimental study. *J Craniofac Surg.* 2013 May;24(3):792–796.

Lata J, Kapila BK. Overgrowth of a costochondral graft in temporomandibular joint reconstructive surgery: an uncommon complication. *Quintessence Int.* 2000 Jun;31(6):412–414.

Lindqvist C, Pihakari A, Tasanen A, et al. Autogenous costochondral grafts in temporo-mandibular joint arthroplasty. A survey of 66 arthroplasties in 60 patients. *J Maxillofac Surg.* 1986 Jun;14(3):143–149.

Lindqvist C, Söderholm AL, Hallikainen D, et al. Erosion and heterotopic bone formation after alloplastic temporomandibular joint reconstruction. *J Oral Maxillofac Surg.* 1992 Sep;50(9):942–949; discussion 950.

Long X. The relationship between temporomandibular joint ankylosis and condylar fractures. *Chin J Dent Res.* 2012;15(1):17–20.

Lopez EN, Dogliotti PL. Treatment of temporomandibular joint ankylosis in children: is it necessary to perform mandibular distraction simultaneously? *J Craniofac Surg.* 2004 Sep;15(5):879–885.

van Loon JP, de Bont LG, Stegenga B, et al. Groningen temporomandibular joint prosthesis. Development and first clinical application. *Int J Oral Maxillofac Surg.* 2002 Feb;31(1):44–52.

Machon V, Hirjak D, Beno M, et al. Total alloplastic temporomandibular joint replacement: the Czech-Slovak initial experience. *Int J Oral Maxillofac Surg.* 2012 Apr;41(4):514–517.

Poswillo DE. Biological reconstruction of the mandibular condyle. *Br J Oral Maxillofac Surg.* 1987 Apr;25(2):100–104.

Rémi M, Christine MC, Gael P, et al. Mandibular fractures in children: long term results. *Int J Pediatr Otorhinolaryngol.* 2003 Jan;67(1):25–30.

Sawhney CP. Bony ankylosis of the temporomandibular joint: follow-up of 70 patients treated with arthroplasty and acrylic spacer interposition. *Plast Reconstr Surg.* 1986 Jan;77(1):29–40.

Topazian RG. Comparison of gap and interposition arthroplasty in the treatment of temporomandibular joint ankylosis. *J Oral Surg.* 1966 Sep;24(5):405–409.

Trumpy IG, Roald B, Lyberg T. Morphologic and immunohistochemical observation of explanted Proplast-Teflon temporomandibular joint interpositional implants. *J Oral Maxillofac Surg.* 1996 Jan;54(1):63–70.

Verma A, Yadav S, Singh V. Overgrowth of costochondral graft in temporomandibular joint ankylosis: An unusual case. *Natl J Maxillofac Surg.* 2011 Jul;2(2):172–174.

Valentini V, Vetrano S, Agrillo A, et al. Surgical treatment of TMJ ankylosis: our experience (60 cases). *J Craniofac Surg.* 2002 Jan;13(1):59–67.

Zhang XH, Yang C, Fang B, et al. Simultaneous costochondral graft and distraction osteogenesis in unilateral TMJ ankylosis associated with mandibular retrognathia and asymmetry. *J Craniofac Surg.* 2012 May;23(3):682–684.

4.4 Ridge augmentation of the atrophic maxilla and mandible

Dieter Weingart, Rolf Bublitz, Michael Ehrenfeld

1 Introduction

Atrophy of the mandible or maxilla is in most cases a result of a partial or total edentulism. This is usually an acquired situation after tooth loss for various reasons or due to congenital hypodontia. The lack of functional stimuli by loaded tooth roots to the jaw bone leads to the typical resorption patterns in the edentulous maxilla or mandible [Tallgren, 1972; Atwood, 1971]. Several classification systems have been described, such as that by Cawood and Howell [1988] (**Fig 4.4-1**). Atrophy may also result from trauma and other conditions, such as irradiation.

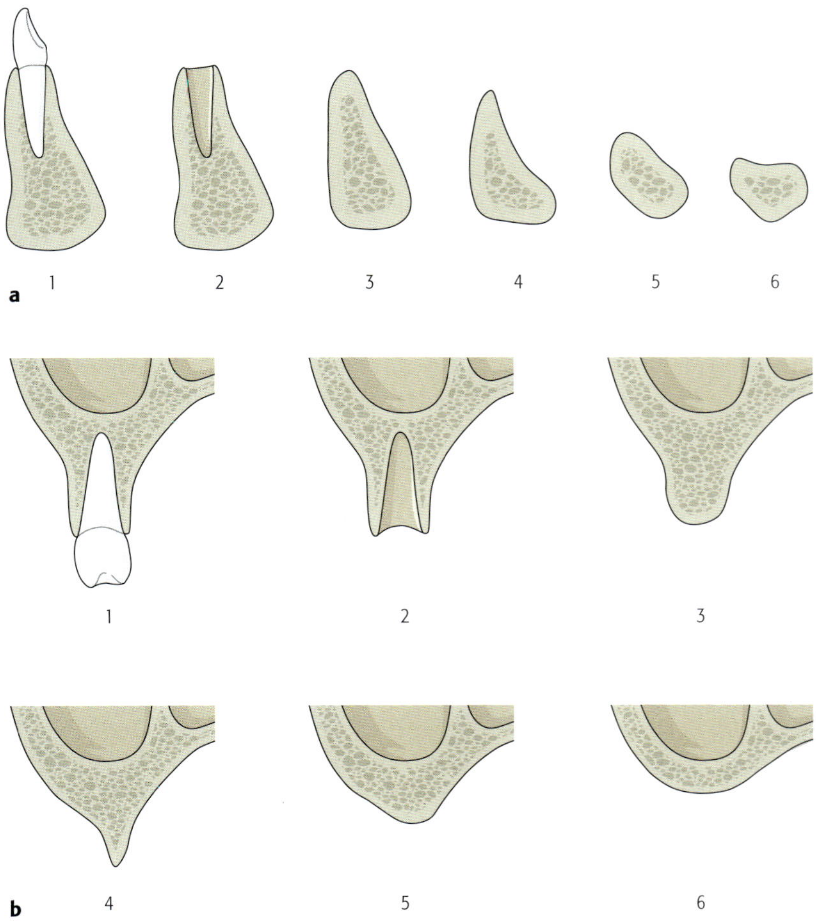

Fig 4.4-1a–b
a Atrophy of the mandible according to the Cawood and Howell classification.
b Atrophy of the maxilla according to the Cawood and Howell classification.

Class I: dentate mandible
Class II: mandible immediately after tooth extraction
Class III: well preserved ridge with sufficient height and width
Class IV: alveolar ridge with adequate height and inadequate width
Class V: atrophic ridge with inadequate height and width
Class VI: highly atrophic ridges, sometimes negative ridges in the mandible

Bone atrophy is always associated with soft-tissue changes, typically atrophy of the attached soft tissues. Intraorally, this is associated with a total or subtotal loss of attached gingiva. Bone atrophy of the facial skeleton and relative excess of lax skin create the impression of an aging face.

Today the main reason to perform ridge augmentation is to prepare alveoli with limited bone stock for dental implant placement. Augmentation procedures alone without implant placement have shown a high degree of resorption if performed with autogenous bone, or insufficient results if done with bone replacement material, such as hydroxyapatite. Dental implant placement in augmented jaws will lead to a functional loading of the bone via the implants and will prevent a quick and early atrophy of bone used for jaw augmentation. The introduction of modern osseointegrated dental implants was key for the treatment of extreme jaw atrophies with good long-term success rates. Solid titanium screw implants are the implants of choice, ceramic implants may be an alternative.

2 Diagnosis and planning

2.1 Examination of the face

Considerations of facial aspects are important, not only from a functional but also from an esthetic point of view. Edentulism leads to typical changes of the facial profile, with pseudoprognathism and soft-tissue changes in the mentolabial and nasolabial regions resulting in premature aging of the face [Tallgren, 1972; Atwood, 1971; Cawood et al, 1988]. This has implications for prosthetic considerations (lip support) as well as for augmentation surgery planning. In severe cases there may be a need for additional surgical procedures (osteotomies) besides augmentation.

2.2 Intraoral examination

Intraoral examination is performed to evaluate quality and quantity of the soft tissues on and close to the alveoli, the form and shape of the alveolar ridges, the bone-soft-tissue relation and, in partially dentate patients, the condition of the remaining teeth. In addition, the vertical distance between the alveolar processes is investigated.

The most frequent finding in jaw atrophy is soft-tissue loss, particularly of the attached gingiva, with a flattening of the vestibule and a high position of the floor of the mouth. Nonetheless the vestibule may also exhibit fibromata, muscle attachments, and frenulae, which may interfere with a proper fit of a denture and therefore may require treatment. In patients with a high position of the floor of the mouth, painful pressure ulcers may be observed after dental implant placement and manufacturing of an implant-retained prosthesis. Those ulcers are caused during swallowing when the oral floor is raised and pressed against the prosthesis. In addition, patients with dental implants and high floors of the mouth often find oral hygiene difficult. Augmentation procedures should be considered in these situations.

The necessity for keratinized crestal mucosa around dental implants is still debated in the literature. Clinical experience has shown that periimplant soft tissues can be maintained in a healthy state for a long period with meticulous oral hygiene, even if the implants are in the mobile mucosa [Krekeler, 1985]. Nevertheless, it is certainly advantageous to have the implants in firmly attached keratinized ridge mucosa because hygiene measures tend to be easier. In the absence of keratinized mucosa, the transplantation of palatal mucosa can be considered [ten Bruggenkate et al, 1991]. If a skin graft has been performed in earlier preprosthetic procedures and the implant will be situated in contact with this graft, a split mucosa transplantation from the hard palate to the alveolar crest after (partial) removal of the skin graft is recommended because otherwise periimplant problems (granulation tissue formation, periimplantitis) may appear or persist.

The quantity and quality of the local bone is obviously vital in an implant-based treatment concept. As dental implants must be inserted in a sufficient bone quantity with at least a 1 mm bone cuff around an implant, the clinical evaluation of the shape of the alveolar ridge, with determination of its height and width, is important in preimplant diagnostics. The thickness of the overlying mucosa can be measured with a pin-prick test with the patient under local anesthesia.

The vertical and sagittal relations between mandible and maxilla are also evaluated because severe jaw atrophy may lead to a maxillary hypoplasia and a relative prognathism of the mandible, according to the centripetal resorption pattern of the maxilla and the centrifugal resorption pattern of the mandible (**Fig 4.4-1**).

2.3 Radiological evaluation

Routine radiology in edentulous patients to screen for bone stock and associated dental pathologies (eg, retained teeth, cysts) should be done with an orthopantomogram (OPT) (**Fig 4.4-2**) [Weingart et al, 2000]. In addition, an OPT will provide the clinician with information about the inferior alveolar canal. It must be emphasized, however, that OPTs have an amplification factor and are not totally reliable for distance accuracy. Another reason for this inaccuracy is because it is a summation picture and not a sectional image. Precise bone height measurement at a desired implant site, however, is possible. For this, a diagnostic wax set-up on plaster-of-Paris models is recommended. After production of an acrylic template, the desired implant positions can be defined with radiopaque markers. An OPT is then taken with the acrylic template inside the patient's mouth and the bone height can be measured in relation to the known height of the markers (**Fig 4.4-6c**).

A lateral cephalometric radiograph is indicated when clinical examination reveals a discrepancy in sagittal positions of mandibular and maxillary alveolar crests. Thus, the mandibulomaxillary relationship can be measured, the bone configuration and the positions of the crests can be determined. Yet, the mandibular shape in the cuspid or premolar region may be totally different from the chin. A lateral cephalometric radiograph is used to determine if an augmentation procedure should be combined with a change of sagittal jaw relations through orthognathic surgery.

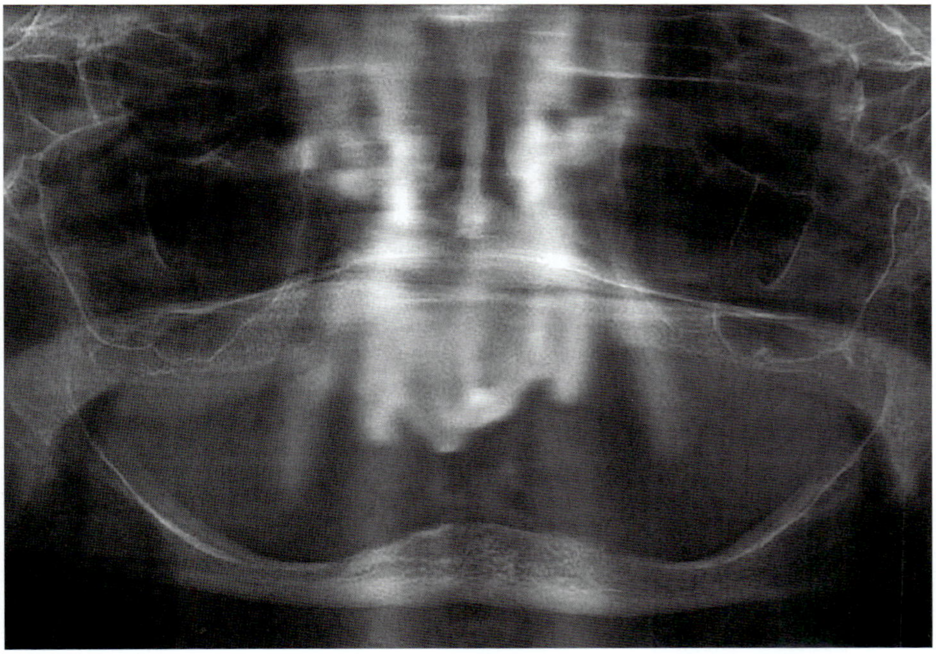

Fig 4.4-2 Orthopantomogram of a patient with advanced maxillary and mandible atrophy.

Today 3-D radiological imaging using cone beam computed tomography (CBCT) or dental CT is a diagnostic tool to precisely determine the amount of bone present in the alveolar processes. The 3-D imaging is especially indicated in patients with a severe atrophy of the maxilla because it not only allows precise measurement of bone volume but also allows for evaluation of the condition of the maxillary sinuses, important especially if sinus augmentation procedures are considered (**Fig 4.4-3**).

Above that anatomical details are easily detected, such as lingual concavities in the mandible because penetration into lingual cavities during implant placement can lead to severe bleeding. Fatal outcomes have been reported. Anatomical variations and the typical resorption patterns of edentulous maxillae and mandibles may result in angulation problems for dental implant placement as well as in unfavorable sagittal and transversal mandibulomaxillary relationships. This is paramount when a fixed implant suprastructure, such as a bridge, is planned. A prominent genial tubercle (lingual mental spine) can easily be detected with 3-D imaging. Even in extremely atrophic mandibles, the genioglossus attachment to the lingual cortex of the mandible remains intact due to its function. When implants are inserted in the interforaminal region, a subsequently manufactured overdenture may come to rest on the prominent genial tubercle and cause pressure ulcers.

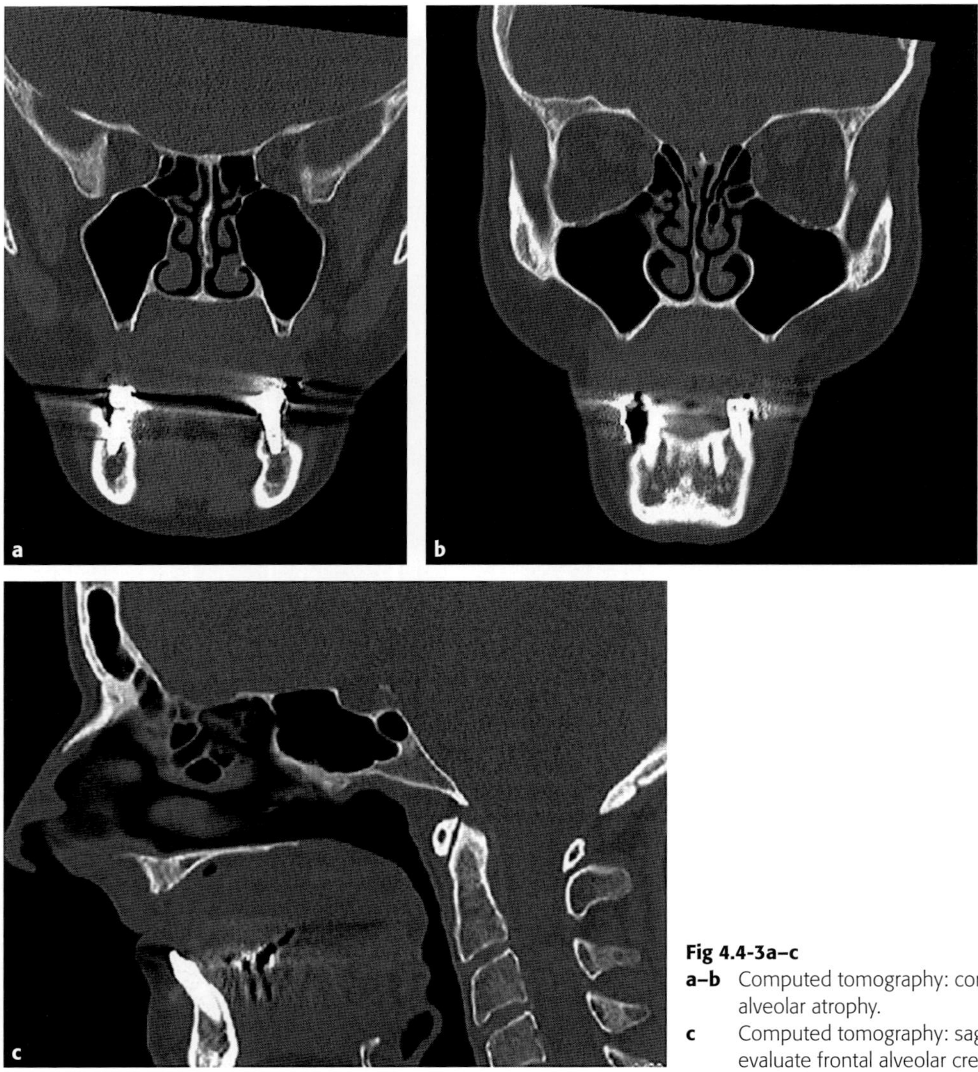

Fig 4.4-3a–c
a–b Computed tomography: coronal cuts with extreme maxillary alveolar atrophy.
c Computed tomography: sagittal cut of alveolar atrophy to evaluate frontal alveolar crest positions of mandible and maxilla.

3 Augmentation techniques and bone graft fixation

Jaw augmentation procedures are performed and indicated both in partially edentulous or completely edentulous jaws with bone atrophy. The goal of the augmentation procedure is to allow placement of dental implants of the appropriate length and in the desired and planned position. It is important to establish a complete treatment plan including the subsequent prosthodontic rehabilitation before the first surgical steps are performed. It is crucial to define the prosthodontic goal of this combined treatment, which can range from a completely fixed prosthodontic rehabilitation with fixed implant or implant and tooth-retained bridges, removable bridges, to implant or implant and tooth-retained removable prosthesis. This means the planning should start with the definition of the desired prosthodontic goal, and based on this the appropriate augmentation technique as well as the number, position, and type of implants should be selected. This procedure is known as backward planning. Today the planning can be done virtually using special planning software.

However, it must be noted that mild degrees of atrophy with sufficient bone stock for dental implant insertion can be treated by implant placement only. These are commonly placed in the anterior maxilla or in the interforaminal area of the mandible. Implant supported and retained overdentures require at least two interforaminal implants in the mandible and four well-spaced implants of at least 8 mm length in the maxilla. The variation in implant number relates to the differences in bone density between mandible and maxilla [Weingart et al, 2000].

Treatment concepts for advanced atrophies generally include bone augmentations and endosseous dental implants. Autogenous bone grafts are considered as gold standard for augmentation procedures in such cases. Alloplastic or allogenic bone substitutes cannot, at this point, fully replace autogenous bone as they do not contain the osteoinductive and osteogenetic properties of autogenous bone [Weingart et al, 2005; Kim et al, 2011]. However they may be used for certain procedures, sometimes in combination and mixed with autogenous bone, for example for sinus augmentation surgeries.

Bone grafts can be harvested from the jaws, the skull, the tibia, or from the iliac crest, which provides almost "unlimited" bone for complex augmentation procedures as well as cortical and cancellous bone (see chapter 1.1). Bone grafts can be used as onlay grafts or as inlay grafts following an osteotomy or a sinus augmentation procedure. The bone grafts need to replace missing bone in all required dimensions to allow to place dental implants into the desired location. Implants may be placed immediately together with jaw augmentation or in a second stage procedure. As a rule, a one-stage concept can be realized if at least 50% of the implant length can be inserted into local bone, and not more than 50% into a bone graft. If this cannot be realized, two-stage procedures are generally preferred and safer. Submerged implants are primarily covered by mucosa and are exposed secondarily after successful implant osseointegration. In combination with bone augmentation, this procedure is safer than a primarily exposed, nonsubmerged implant insertion.

In extreme cases of jaw atrophy, augmentation procedures with microvascular bone flaps have been described.

3.1 Augmentation of the maxillary alveolar process

Augmentation procedures of the maxillary alveolus can be performed circumferentially encompassing the complete edentulous alveolus, or partially, in edentulous or partially dentate patients. They may be combined with orthognathic operations in those cases with profound sagittal discrepancies of the alveoli, which cannot be sufficiently corrected with augmentation procedures or a prosthesis. The technique selected for an individual patient depends on the amount and type of atrophy and above that on the desired prosthodontic outcome [Weingart et al, 2005; Kleinheinz et al, 2005]. All augmentation techniques require adapted strategies for soft-tissue handling because bone atrophy, as stated before, is always associated with soft-tissue atrophy that may require special techniques for recipient-site preparation as well as wound closure.

3.1.1 Exposure

In the edentulous maxilla mucoperiosteal incisions are placed along the alveolar ridge, either along the entire arch from molar to molar regions, or encompassing only one segment of the crest if a limited procedure is planned (**Fig 4.4-4**) [Stephen et al, 2012].

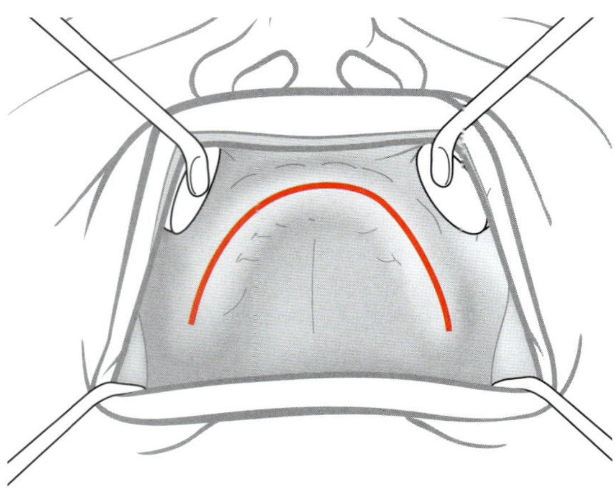

Fig 4.4-4 Incision along the alveolar ridge of the maxilla.

3.1.2 Vertical maxillary augmentation through sinus grafting

Sinus augmentation procedures ("sinus lifts") are used to augment the lateral alveolus of the maxilla by grafting the sinus floor. This technique increases bone volume to allow for dental implant placement, it does not change the mandibulomaxillary relation. Existing vertical deficits need to be compensated by the prosthodontic suprastructure, unless the sinus augmentation is combined with an onlay augmentation of the alveolus. With a round burr, a diamond burr, or a piezoelectric device, a trapdoor bone lid is prepared in the anterior maxillary sinus wall (**Fig 4.4-5a**) [Tatum, 1986].

This must be executed carefully not to injure the sinus mucosa. The sinus mucosa is then elevated from the sinus floor, instruments specifically designed for this purpose may be helpful. In extreme atrophies the mucosa can easily rupture, especially if maxillary sinus septums (Underwood septums) are present. After sinus floor elevation, bone grafts are harvested, for instance, from the iliac crest. Corticocancellous blocks as well as particulate bone and marrow may be used. Some surgeons prefer a mixture of autogenous bone and alloplastic material, such as hydroxyapatite or β-tricalcium phosphate.

The newly created space in the maxillary sinus is filled with augmentation material (**Fig 4.4-5b**). If block grafts are used, they should be fixed by one to three lag screws until primary stability is achieved. Sinus augmentation procedures can be combined with lateral or crestal augmentations (**Fig 4.4-5c–d**). Sharp edges are smoothened with a diamond burr and cancellous bone, or bone replacement material is used to fill remaining spaces. In cases that require only a mild augmentation, some surgeons use bone substitutes alone. In selected cases with mild atrophies, implant placement can be done simultaneously with a sinus augmentation procedure. In cases with severe bone atrophy secondary implant placement is standard (**Fig 4.4-6**). The guided bone regeneration (GBR) technique may be used by placing a resorbable collagen membrane to cover the augmented area, it needs to extend well under the palatal mucosa [Weingart et al, 1992].

A tension-free wound closure may require a periosteal-releasing incision and is performed for instance with single atraumatic sutures. A dental impression can be taken to construct a protective acrylic splint for the early postoperative period.

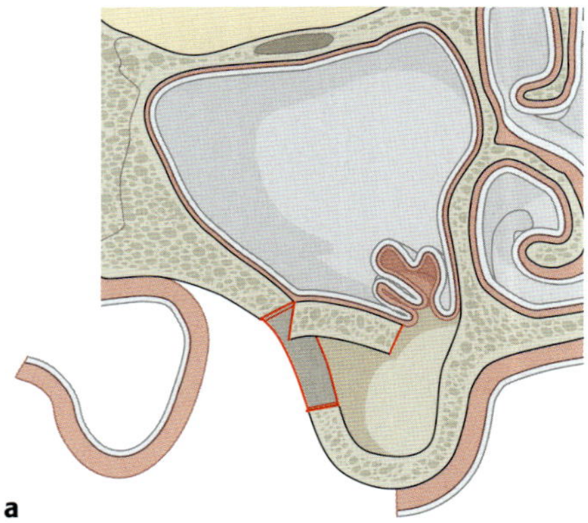

a

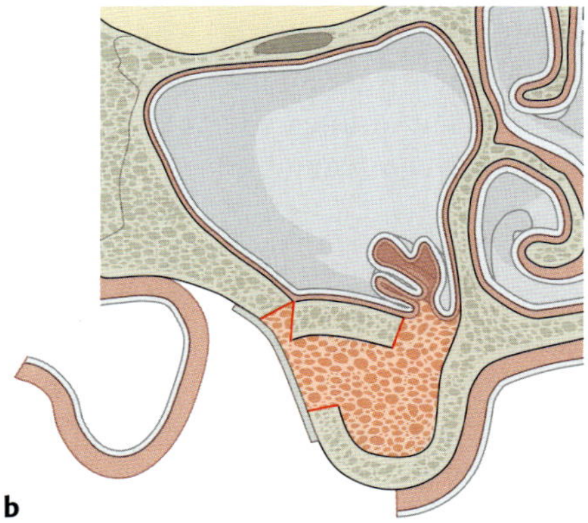

b

Fig 4.4-5a–d

a Preparation of a bone lid into the maxillary sinus wall.

b Placement of cancellous bone after careful elevation of the sinus mucosa from the sinus floor including the bone lid.

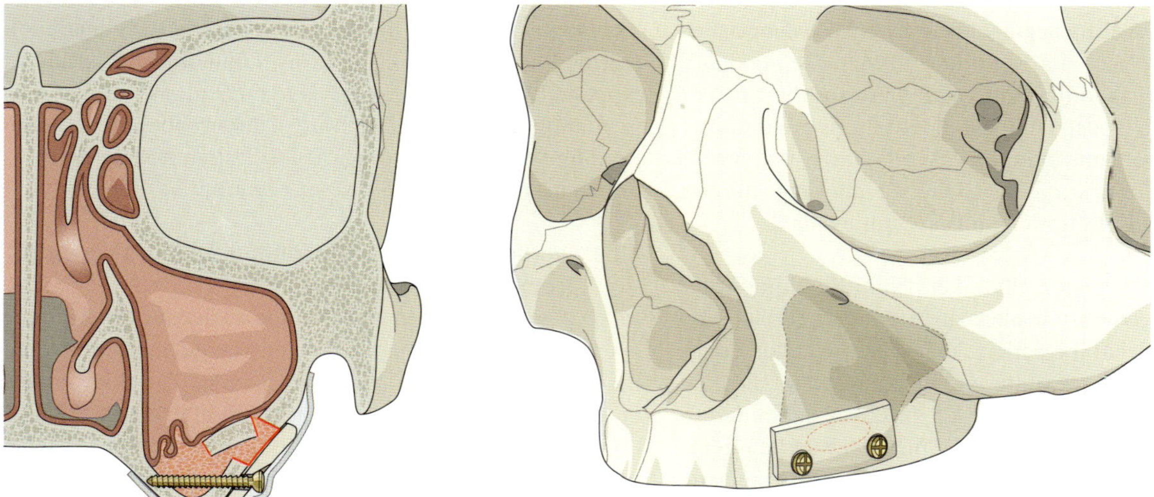

c d

Fig 4.4-5a–d (**cont**)

c Sinus floor augmentation in combination with lateral onlay augmentation of an atrophic maxilla. Screw fixation of the bone block.

d Situation after sinus floor augmentation and lateral augmentation of the maxilla.

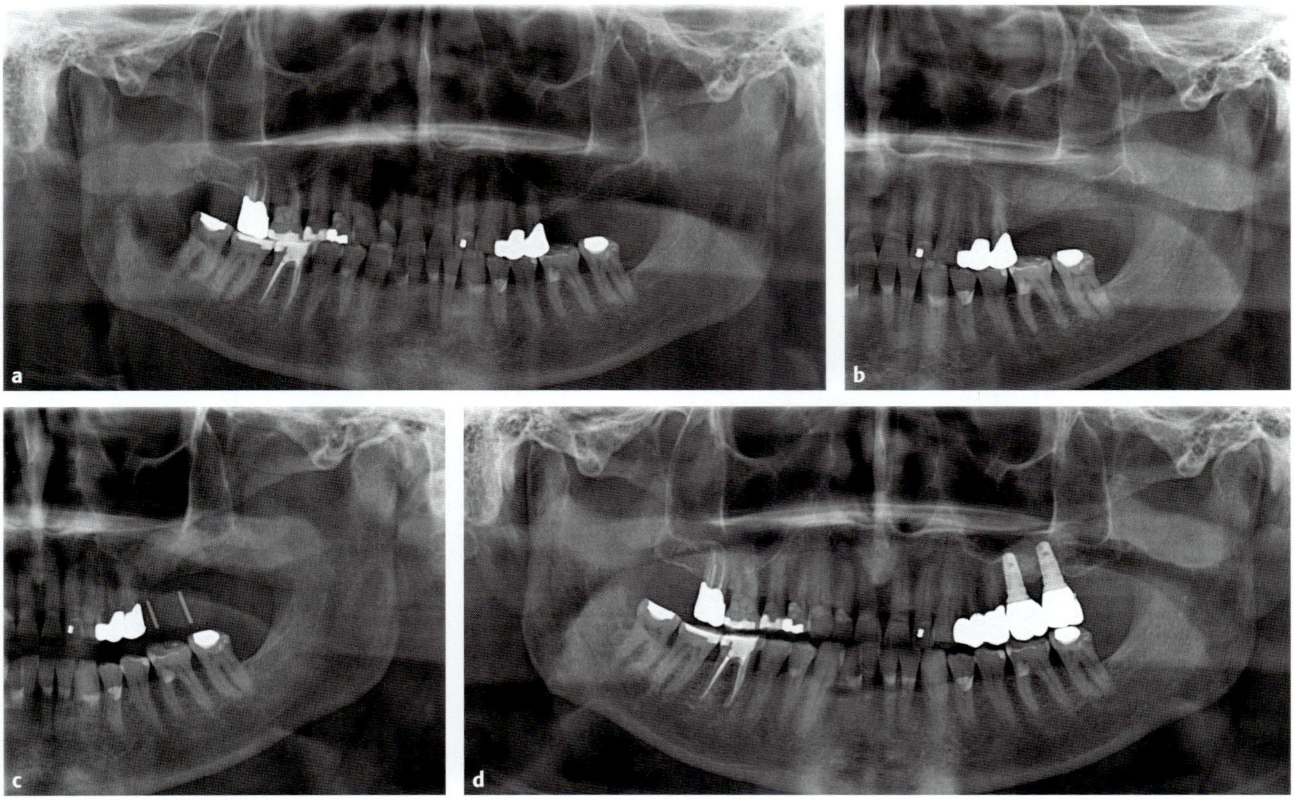

Fig 4.4-6a–d

a Edentitions lateral posterior maxilla with missing teeth 26 and 27 and severe bone atrophy.

b Situation after sinus floor augmentation with cancellous iliac bone.

c Three months after bone augmentation planning for implantation of two dental implants. Implant positions are planned with the help of a positioning template. X-ray is taken with the positioning template in the mouth; radiopaque markers show the planned implant positions and axes.

d Situation after implant placement. Dental rehabilitation with two-implant supported crowns had been performed 3 months after dental implantation.

3.1.3 Vertical maxillary augmentation by onlay osteoplasties

An onlay osteoplasty is a procedure to increase maxillary height by placing an onlay bone graft on top of the alveolar crest [Nyström et al, 2004]. Onlay augmentations are typically done with autogenous bone blocks, alloplastic material is not indicated. Some surgeons today use allogenic human donor bone, but long-term results are not available.

The bone blocks are normally taken from the ilium, outer table (calvarial) grafts are an alternative. For surgical planning either a jaw model of the patient, manufactured after a dental impression, and made of sterilizable plastic material, or an individual model printed after a CT or CBCT examination using sterilizable material, is useful. The models serve as templates for bone graft harvest, and are used to contour the bone graft to the alveolus on a side table before transplantation. This allows for two team surgeries.

The contoured bone block(s) are fixed to the alveolus with a number of lag screws. Good contact between bone graft and recipient site and immobility of the bone graft are key factors for a successful transplantation (**Fig 4.4-7**). Wound closure is typically a challenge in those operations, and requires extensive vestibular soft-tissue mobilization including periosteal release incisions. Some surgeons prefer to cover bone augmentates with collagen membranes to prevent early resorption and to create a second soft-tissue layer underneath the patients mucosa. Even if done properly and meticulously, onlay augmentations will show a high rate of dehiscence and often the need for secondary suturing. A close patient follow-up is essential to manage such a case successfully.

3.1.4 Vertical maxillary augmentation with inlay grafts in combination with osteotomies

Inlay augmentations in combination with osteotomies have been used to increase vertical alveolar height and at the same time change position of the lower maxilla. To achieve this a modified Le Fort I osteotomy is performed, in which the mucosa on the nasal floor and also the sinus mucosa needs to be preserved. Laterally this is achieved by first creating windows in the anterior sinus wall, like a sinus augmentation procedure. After dissection of the sinus mucosa on both sides as well as the mucosa overlying the nasal floor, a Le Fort I osteotomy with down fracture is performed. The maxilla is mobilized into the desired position, which can be defined with a positioning splint, which in edentulous patient needs to be fixed with screws to the palate. Then the maxilla is bone grafted with bone blocks to increase vertical height and bone stock. Fixation is performed with four miniplates along the four lower anterior vertical buttresses (**Fig 4.4-8**).

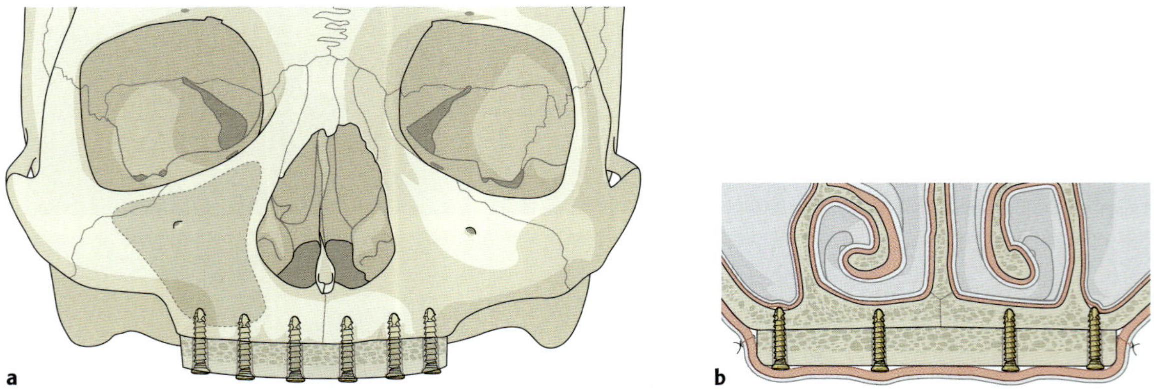

Fig 4.4-7a–b Vertical maxillary augmentation with an onlay bone block.

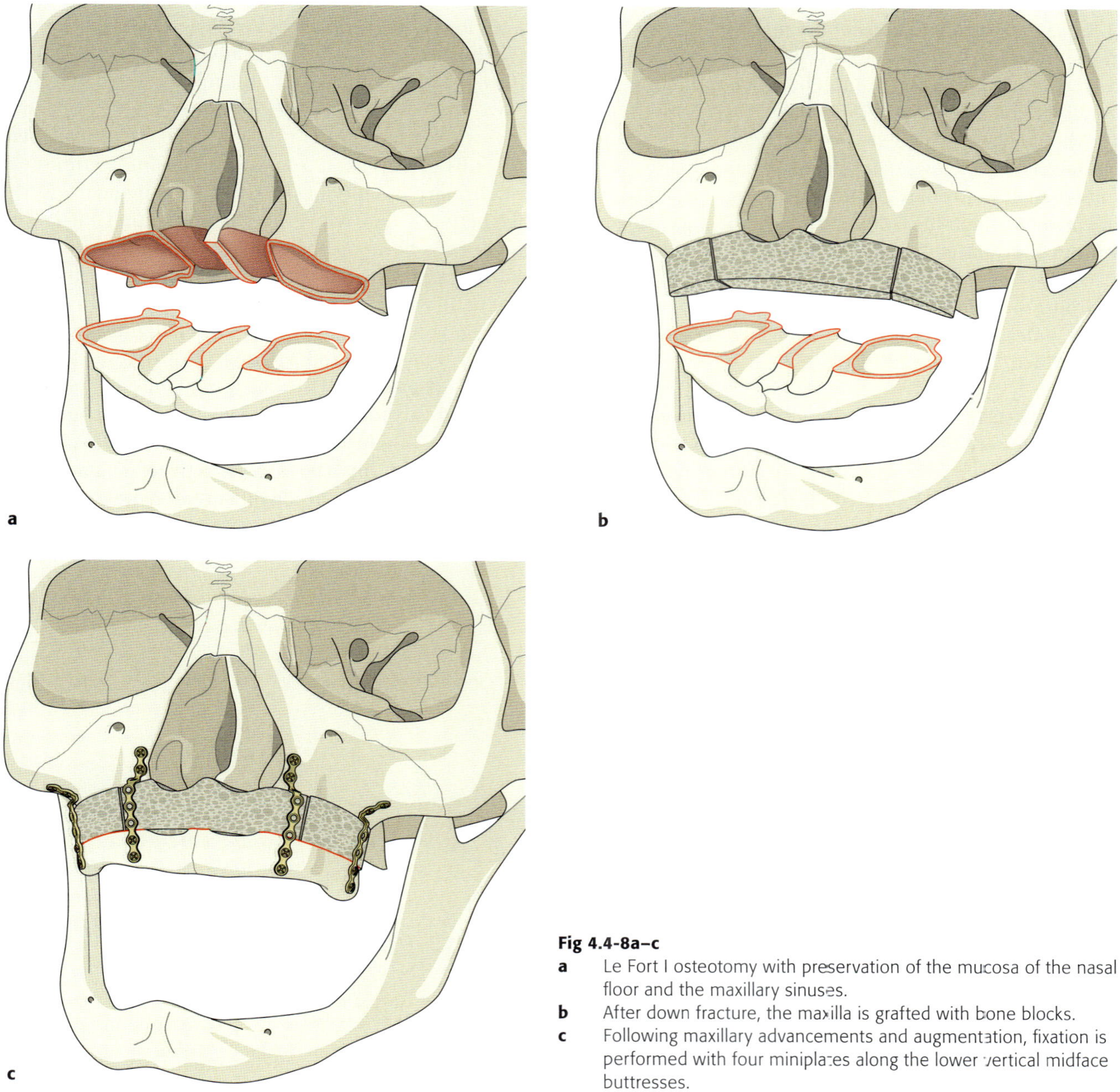

a

b

c

Fig 4.4-8a–c

- **a** Le Fort I osteotomy with preservation of the mucosa of the nasal floor and the maxillary sinuses.
- **b** After down fracture, the maxilla is grafted with bone blocks.
- **c** Following maxillary advancements and augmentation, fixation is performed with four miniplates along the lower vertical midface buttresses.

3.1.5 Lateral augmentations of the maxilla

Lateral maxillary augmentations are done to increase alveolar width. Usually corticocancellous bone grafts are placed laterally to the alveolus after they have been contoured to fit to the underlying bone (**Fig 4.4-9**). Fixation is performed with multiple lag screws. For soft-tissue handling, the same remarks apply as to onlay grafting; however, the dehiscence rates are not as high since the sutures are not placed directly over the bone grafts.

According to a patient's individual situation sinus augmentations, onlay osteoplasties, and lateral augmentations may be combined.

3.1.6 Bone splitting procedures to increase alveolar width

Bone splitting techniques are an alternative to lateral augmentations. Both techniques aim at increasing alveolar width. A bone split is indicated for narrow alveolar ridges with no or only moderate reduction of alveolar height. The alveolar crest is exposed via a crestal incision. The labial and palatinal periosteum is only stripped as much as it is needed for crestal bone exposure. A vertical/sagittal cut is made through the cortical bone along the crest with a microsaw or piezotome. Next a thin chisel is introduced and the two cortices are spread. The planned number of dental implants are inserted after preparation of the implant beds with drills or chisels, if a bone condensing technique is used. Primary stability of the implants is mandatory. The space between the two cortices is then either filled with autogeneous bone or bone replacement material. If the cortices have only been spread moderately, the space can be left to fill with blood and may be covered with a (resorbable) membrane, such as a collagen membrane. Finally, the mucosa is mobilized and a primary soft-tissue closure is performed (**Fig 4.4-10**). If a primary implant stability cannot be obtained only the bone spread with augmentation of the created space should be performed, and the implants should be placed secondarily. The interval between augmentation and implant insertion should be around 3 months if autogeneous material is used, and approximately 6 months if alloplastic material is used.

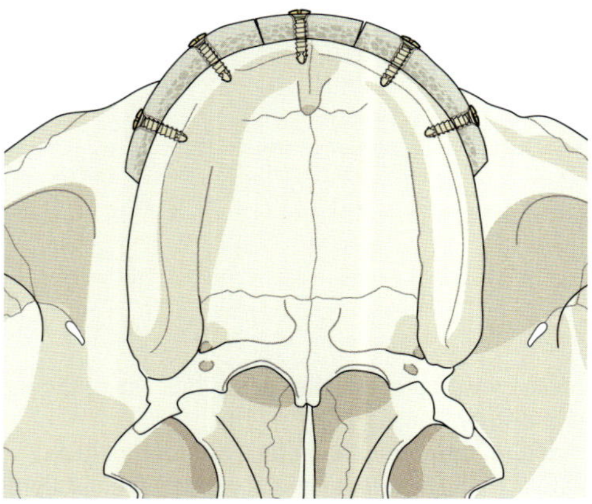
a

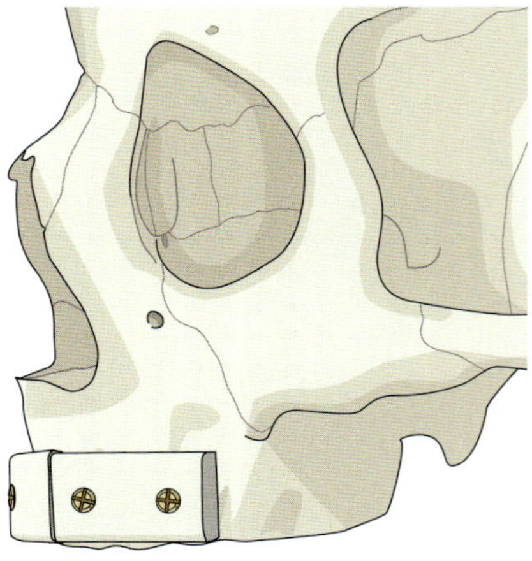
b

Fig 4.4-9a–b Lateral maxillary augmentations.

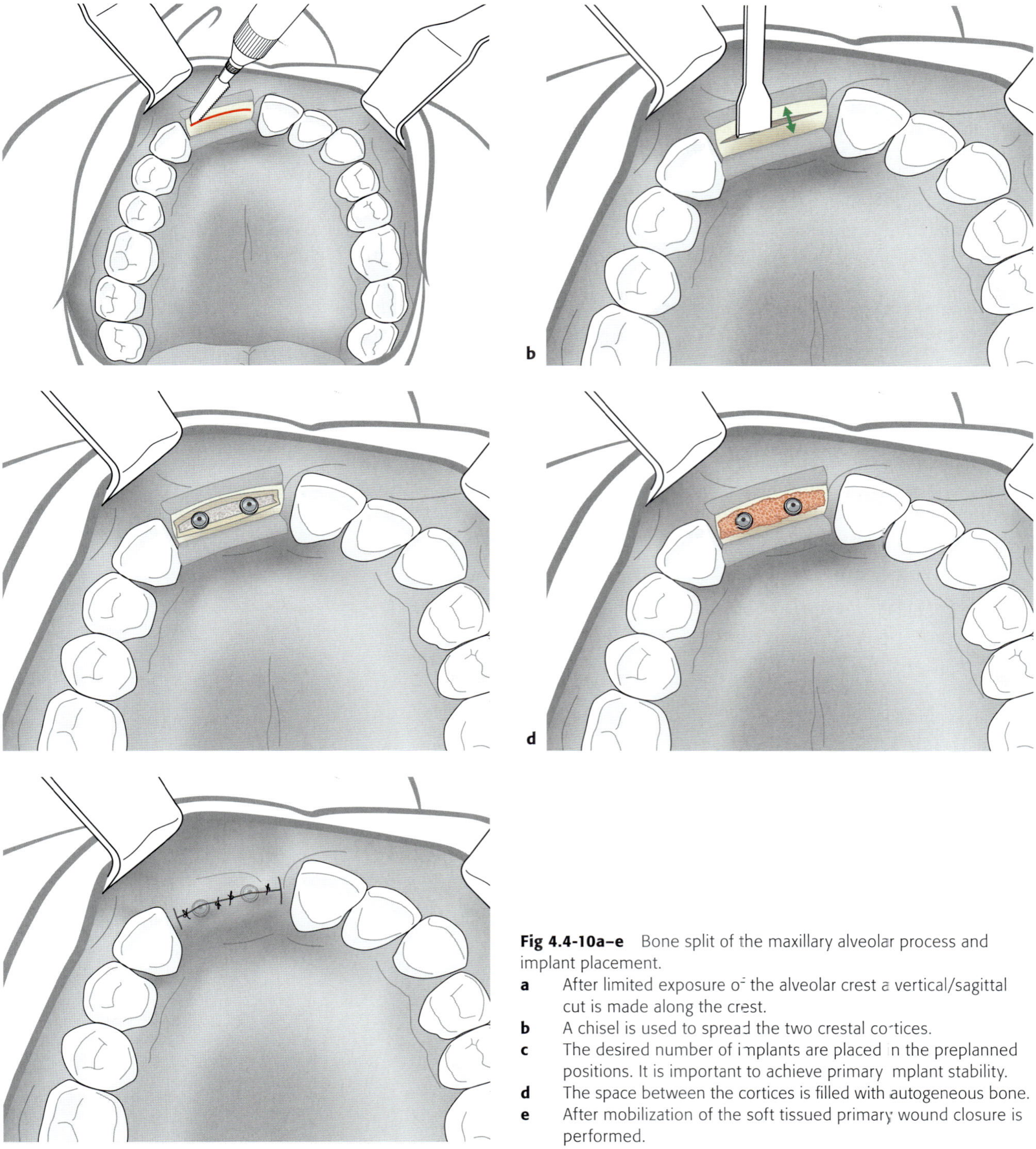

Fig 4.4-10a–e Bone split of the maxillary alveolar process and implant placement.

- **a** After limited exposure of the alveolar crest a vertical/sagittal cut is made along the crest.
- **b** A chisel is used to spread the two crestal cortices.
- **c** The desired number of implants are placed in the preplanned positions. It is important to achieve primary implant stability.
- **d** The space between the cortices is filled with autogeneous bone.
- **e** After mobilization of the soft tissued primary wound closure is performed.

3.1.7 Maxillary augmentation with microvascular bone flaps

Microvascular bone flaps have been described for patients with severe maxillary atrophy. They can be used to augment the maxilla vertically, above that they may be positioned anteriorly to the original atrophic alveolar crest and therefore may be used to correct sagittal discrepancies as well. The fibula flap today is the microvascular flap of choice. It is recommended to plan such a case with virtual planning software and surgical guides because segmentation and placement of the flap segments is challenging [Jaquiéry et al, 2004].

3.2 Augmentation of the alveolar process in the mandible

3.2.1 Exposure

In edentulous patients a mid-crestal incision is made through the remaining keratinized attached mucosa (**Fig 4.4-11**). The mental foramina are identified after careful subperiosteal dissection. In highly atrophic mandibles the inferior alveolar nerve may run on top of the atrophic alveolar ridge. In those cases, the incision should be started anteriorly and the nerve should be identified after subperiosteal dissection toward the lateral aspect of the crest. Only after exposure and identification of the nerve should the lateral mucoperiosteum be divided in full length.

3.2.2 Onlay augmentation

The occlusal aspect of the alveolar crest is smoothened with a round burr. The dense cortical bone is perforated to enable endosseous vessels to grow into the grafts. A surgical stent can be placed to identify the need for bone augmentation in all necessary dimensions at the planned implantation sites. A model from the atrophic mandible, as in the maxillary procedure described above, may be helpful for both graft harvest and for graft contouring. As many cortico-cancellous grafts as necessary are planned, usually three for a complete mandible augmentation, and individually adapted to the local bone to ensure a tight contact. The bone grafts are placed on top of the remaining ridge and fixed with lag screws. The inferior alveolar nerve may need dissection and lateralization to be able to safely augment including graft fixation.

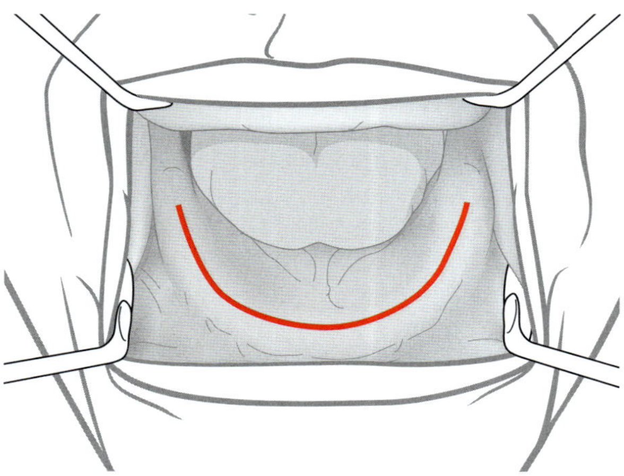

Fig 4.4-11 Mid-crestal incision on alveolar crest of the mandible.

In cases in which the prosthodontic goal is a prosthesis retained on two or four interforaminal implants, an anterior augmentation is usually sufficient. The bone grafts can be covered by collagen membranes, as described earlier. After extensive mobilization, including periosteal release, the mucosa is sutured with single atraumatic sutures.

3.2.3 Lateral augmentation of the mandible

Especially in cases with severe horizontal atrophy, a lateral augmentation may be indicated. The procedure is like a lateral augmentation of the maxilla.

3.2.4 Bone splitting procedures to increase alveolar width of the mandible

The indication and technique for bone splitting procedures in the mandible is identical to what has been described in section 3.1.6 for the maxilla. Because of the often increased density of the mandibular bone, care must be taken not to fracture the lamellae. In the lateral aspect of the mandible the inferior alveolar nerve needs to be respected.

3.2.5 Microvascular augmentation of the mandible

This may be indicated in cases with severe bone and soft-tissue atrophy. Planning and execution is like microvascular maxillary augmentation.

Perioperative medication and aftercare

Patients receive prophylactic perioperative antibiotic treatment. A nasogastric feeding tube can be placed in patients with challenging soft-tissue situations.

3.2.6 Second stage implant placement

Second stage surgery is performed 3–6 months after initial augmentation surgery, often with the patient under local anesthesia. After exposing the augmented areas, the osteosynthesis material is removed. Dental implants are placed usually with the help of a surgical stent according to the predetermined and strictly prosthodontically defined locations, or with the help of navigation (**Fig 4.4-12**). The implants are mostly covered by mucosa in a submerged technique.

Implant uncovering and soft-tissue surgery

The osseointegrated implants are usually exposed after 3 months under local anesthesia. If necessary, a vestibuloplasty is performed with a palatal mucosal graft. Prosthodontic rehabilitation can begin after removal of the sutures and when peri-implant conditions are free of inflammation and stable. Telescoping as well as bar-retained removable dentures or fixed suprastructures are possible technical solutions (**Fig 4.4-13**). Patients need to be kept on a regular recall program.

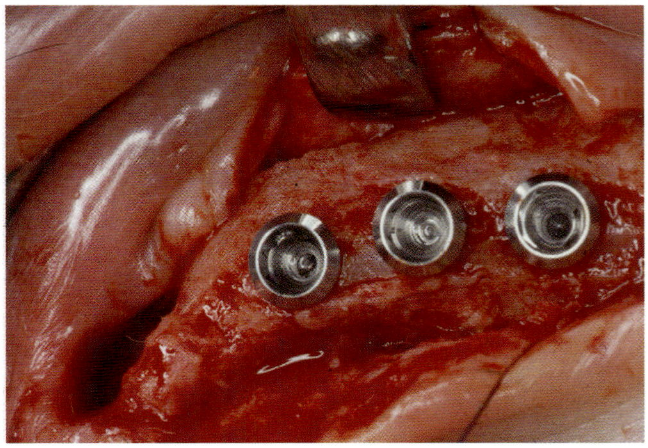

Fig 4.4-12 Six months after lateral and sinus floor augmentation three implants are inserted in a submerged technique.

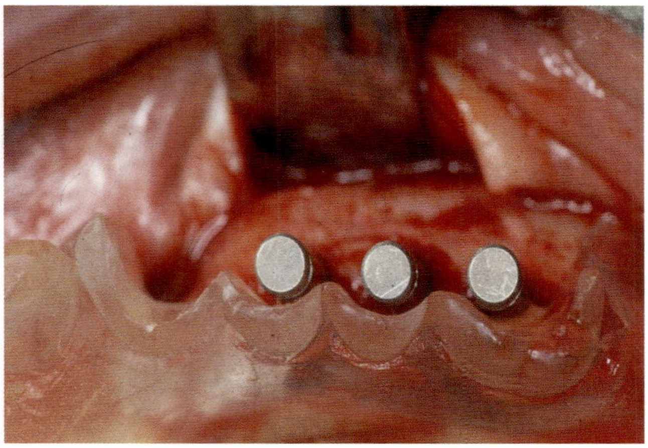

Fig 4.4-13 Implants are exposed 3 months after insertion and are osseointegrated; augmented bone shows sufficient transversal dimensions.

4 Complications and pitfalls

In mandible augmentation procedures loss of attachment of the genioglossus muscles must be avoided, since it may cause swallowing and speech problems.

In case of sinus augmentation procedures, the maxillary sinuses need to be free of inflammation or pathological conditions. They may require treatment before a sinus floor augmentation is performed. Maxillary sinus septae should be identified before sinus augmentations. They make sinus floor elevations difficult and may easily lead to a rupture of the sinus mucosa. Smaller defects in the mucosa do not need special treatment if the perforation closes automatically by pushing up the trap door and folding of the mucosa. Larger defects need to be covered by a resorbable collagen membrane, or should additionally be sutured with resorbable sutures under magnification. An extrusion of grafts or augmentation material into the maxillary sinus must be avoided. It typically leads to sinus complications, such as infection.

Buried submerged implants and second stage exposure of implants is a safer procedure when implants are used simultaneously with bone grafts compared with primarily exposed non-submerged implants. Extreme atrophies are characterized by thin residual local bone or even a lack of any bone because of prior surgery. In these cases, lag screw fixation of the bone grafts might not be possible. Miniplates can be used instead for fixation of bone grafts [Weingart et al, 2002].

Exposure of membranes can be treated by meticulous dental hygiene and application of chlorhexidine digluconate. The mucosa can heal over resorbable collagen membranes and a removal is rarely necessary.

Exposed bone grafts need meticulous hygiene as well. They may need secondary interventions and secondary sutures and have a high risk of infection and uncontrollable bone graft resorption. Bone exposure is prevented by tension-free sutures, sufficient periosteal release and the strict adherence of patients to a denture-free period during the primary healing phase. Dental splints may be used for protection of the underlying tissues and should be carefully adjusted to avoid pressure ulcers.

Intermediate dentures should be designed for esthetic purposes only and must not create load onto the bone grafts or not yet osseointegrated implants. Regular follow-ups in the healing phase are necessary to detect wound-healing complications, especially bone exposure that may need interventions such as re-suturing.

5 Summary

Augmentation surgery for maxilla and mandible are today usually performed with the aim to place dental implants for implant-retained prosthodontic rehabilitation. Dental implants are not only part of the rehabilitation concept but will also provide functional load to bone grafts to prevent and avoid bone resorption. Gold standard for extended augmentation procedures still is the use of autogenous bone. Smaller alveolar ridge deficiencies can also be treated with alloplastic bone replacement materials, provided that the implant(s) can be firmly anchored in local bone, and only parts of the alveolus are augmented.

A variety of techniques are available for maxillary and mandible augmentation, which need to be selected according to the type and extend of the bone deficiency, patients wishes, and last but not least the overall treatment concept including the prosthodontic part. Therefore an interdisciplinary treatment planning is standard, in which the treatment goal is defined first (for instance, fixed bridge versus implant-retained removable prosthesis), and then the necessary treatment steps are determined. This process is called backward planning.

Depending on the bone deficiency and the amount of augmentation needed, the dental implants can be placed immediately during the augmentation procedure (one-stage concept), or secondarily in a separate operation (two-stage concept). A two-stage concept is recommended for patients with extended augmentations, where most of the implant surface will be anchored within the augmented bone.

6 References and suggested reading

Atwood DA. Reduction of residual ridges: a major oral disease entity. *J Prosthet Dent.* 1971 Sep;26(3):266–279.

Cawood JI, Howell RA. A classification of the edentulous jaws. *Int J Oral Maxillofac Surg.* 1988 Aug;17(4):232–236.

Ivanoff CJ, Gröndahl K, Bergström C, et al. Influence of bicortical or monocortical anchorage on maxillary implant stability: a 15-year retrospective study of Branemark System implants. *Int J Oral Maxillofac Implants.* 2000 Jan-Feb;15(1):103–110.

Isaaksson S, Ekfelt A, Alberius P, et al. Early results from reconstruction of severely atrophic (class VI) maxillae by immediate endosseous implants in conjunction with bone grafting and Le Fort 1 osteotomy. *Int J Maxillofac Implant.* 1993;10:303–311.

Jaquiéry C, Rohner D, Kunz C, et al. Reconstruction of maxillary and mandibular defects using prefabricated microvascular fibular grafts and osseointegrated dental implants: a prospective study. *Clin Oral Implants Res.* 2004 Oct;15(5):598–606.

Kim Y, Nowzari H, Rich SK. Risk of prion disease transmission through bovine-derived bone substitutes: a systematic review. *Clin Implant Dent Relat Res.* 2013 Oct;15(5):645-653.

Kleinheinz J, Büchter A, Kruse-Lösler B, et al. Incision design in implant dentistry based on vascularization of the mucosa. *Clin Oral Implants Res.* 2005 Oct;16(5):518–523.

Krekeler G. [Periodontal problems with the implant abutmnent.] *Schweiz Monatsschr Zahnmed.* 1985 Oct;95 Spec No:847–852. German.

Nyström E, Legrell PE, Forsell A, et al. Combined use of bone grafts and implants in the severely resorbed maxilla. *Int J Oral Maxillofac Surg.* 1995 Feb;24(Pt 1):20–25.

Nyström E, Ahlquist J, Gunne J, et al. 10-year follow-up of onlay bone grafts and implants in severely resorbed maxillae. *Int J Oral Maxillofac Surg.* 2004 Apr;33(3):258–262.

Pierrisnard, L, Renouard F, Renault P, et al. Influence of implant length and bicortical anchorage on implant stress distribution. *Clin Implant Dent Relat Res.* 2003;5(4):254–262.

Sutter F, Weingart D, Mundwiler U, et al. ITI implants in combination with bone grafts: design and biomechanical aspects. *Clin Oral Implants Res.* 1994 Sep;5(3):164–172.

Stephen S, Wallace, Dennis P, et al. Maxillary sinus elevation by lateral window approach: evolution of technology and technique. *J Evidence-Based Dent Pract.* 2012 Sep;12(3):161–171.

ten Bruggenkate CM, van der Kwast WAM, Oosterbeek HS. Patient selection in oral implantology: a review. *Int J Oral Implantol.* 1991;7(2):53–60.

ten Bruggenkate CM, Krekeler G, Kraaijenhagen HA, et al. Hemorrhage of the floor of the mouth resulting from lingual perforation during implant placement: a clinical report. *Int J Oral Maxillofac Implants.* 1993;8(3):329–334.

Tallgren A. The continuing reduction of the residual alveolar ridges in complete denture wearers: a mixed longitudinal study covering 25 years. *J Prosthet Dentist.* 1972 Feb;27(2):120–132.

Tatum H Jr. Maxillary and sinus implant reconstructions. *Dent Clin North Am.* 1986 Apr;30(2):207–229.

Weingart D, Joos U, Hürzeler M. Class III correction of alveolar ridge atrophy in edentulous patients using Le Fort I osteotomy with simultaneous endosseous implant placement. *Intern J Oral Maxillofac Implants.* 1992;7:529–534.

Weingart D, Werkmeister R, Joos U, et al. [Korrektur der sagittalen Diskrepanz bei starker Atrophie des Oberkieferalveolarkammes.] *Deutsche Zahnärzt Zeitschrift.* 1995;51:46–49. German.

Weingart D, ten Bruggenkate CM. Treatment of fully edentulous patients with ITI implants. *Clin Oral Implant Res.* 2000;11(Suppl):69–82.

Weingart D, Bublitz R, Petrin G, et al. [Kombination der Sinusliftoperation mit der lateralen Kieferkammaugmentation – ein neues Behandlungskonzept zur die chirurgisch-prothetischen Rehabilitation der extremen Oberkieferalveolarkammatrophie.] *Mund Kiefer GesichtsChir.* 2005;9(5):317–323. German.

Weingart D, Biggel A. [Lokale periimplantäre Augmentation des anterioren Unterkiefer-Alveolarforsatzes nach dem Prinzip der gesteuerten Geweberegeneration.] *Quintessenz.* 1992;43:403–416. German.

Weingart D, Buser DA, Weber HP. The ITI dental system in maxillofacial applications in craniomaxillofacial reconstructive surgery and corrective bone surgery. In: Greenberg AM, Prein J eds. *Principles of Internal Fixation AO/ASIF Techniques.* Berlin: Springer; 2002:164–175.

4.5 Hemifacial microsomia—diagnosis, classification, and management

Adrian Sugar

1 Introduction

Hemifacial microsomia (HFM) is the most common craniofacial birth defect after cleft lip and palate. It is essentially an abnormality of development of the embryonic first and second branchial arches but is also associated with many other congenital abnormalities in other parts of the body. It is usually unilateral and always asymmetrical (**Fig 4.5-1** and **Fig 4.5-2**).

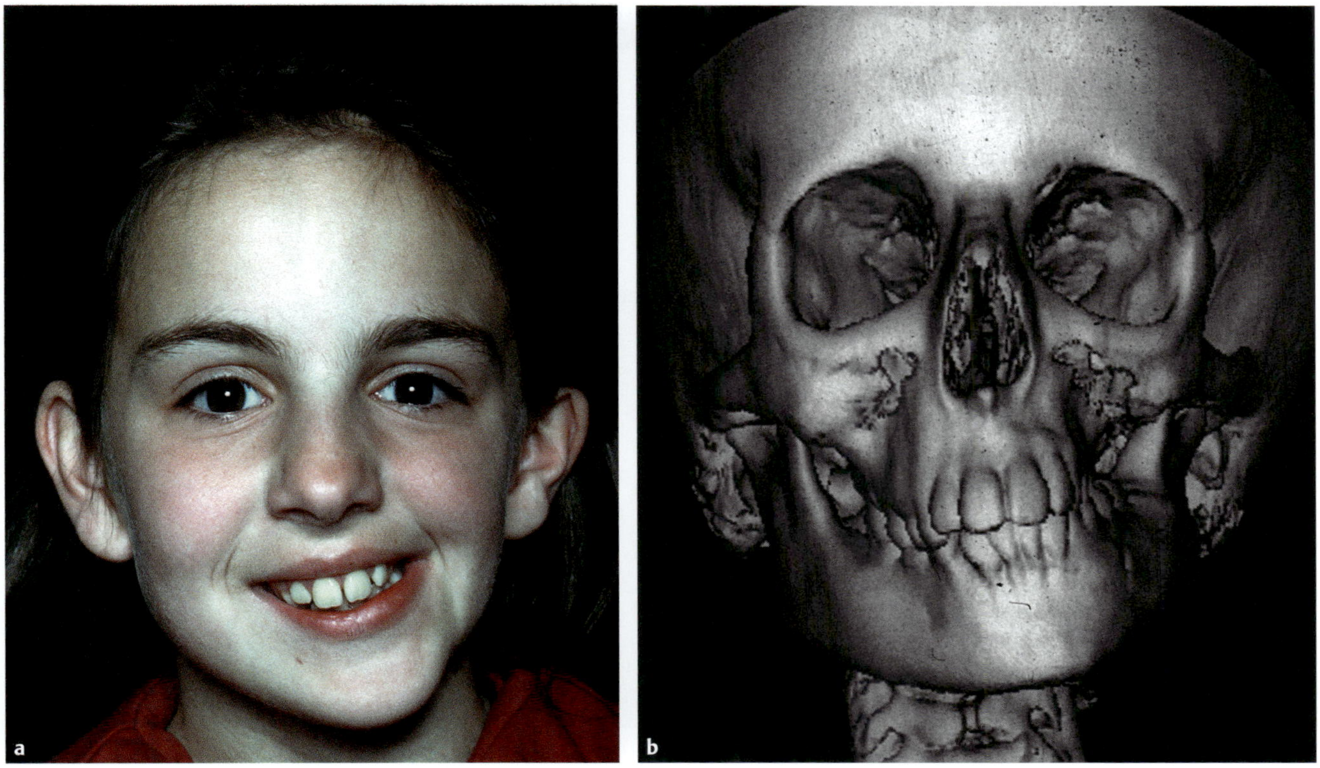

Fig 4.5-1a–b
a A patient with a moderate "Pruzansky IIa" deformity.
b Same patient's 3-D computed tomography.

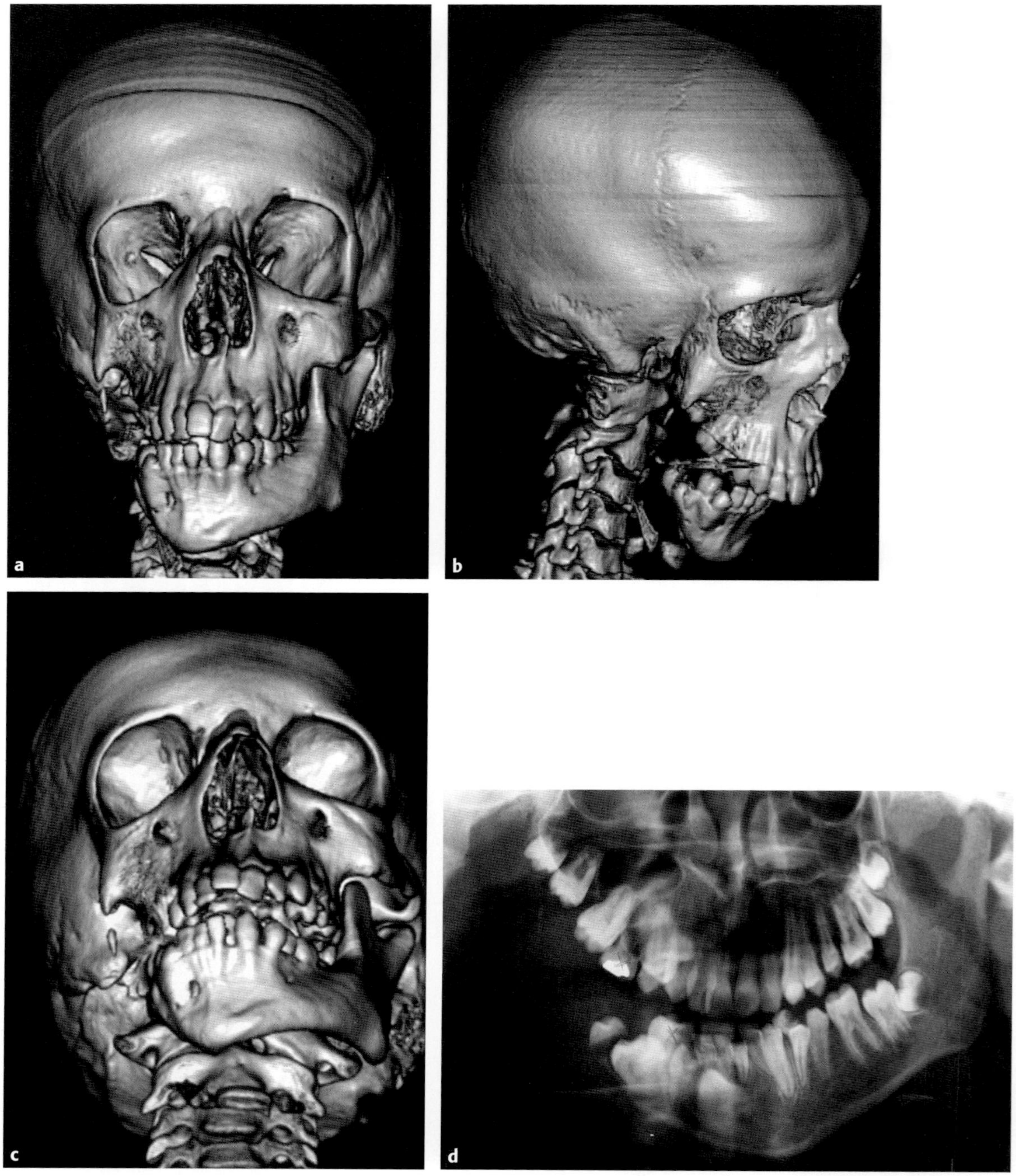

Fig 4.5-2a–d A severe (Pruzansky III) deformity.
a AP 3-D CT view.
b Lateral 3-D CT view.
c Submental 3-D CT view.
d Panoramic radiograph view.

Hemifacial microsomia occurs in approximately 1:5000 to 1:6000 live births and displays a wide spectrum of abnormalities.

Synonyms that are also in common usage are craniofacial microsomia, oculo-auriculo-vertebral-dysplasia and facial-oculo-auriculo-vertebral dysplasia. Goldenhar syndrome is a much overused term liked by pediatricians but only really refers to a small subgroup of patients with HFM who have significant spinal anomalies and epibulbar dermoid cysts.

1.1 Etiology

The etiology of HFM is not known. There does not appear to be a clearly inherited gene. Poswillo [1988] in animal experiments could induce a similar condition by creating a hematoma in the embryonic stapedial artery system. Similar but bilateral examples have also occurred following the use of retinoids in humans during pregnancy (eg, thalidomide) and this has been repeated experimentally in animals.

1.2 Growth

It is not clear whether the facial deformity of HFM gets worse with age and growth or not. A longitudinal study of the mandible by Kaban et al [1984] suggested that the deformity got worse with age, and a further study by Polley et al [1997] suggested that the deformity did not get worse with growth. Our patient below (**Fig 4.5-3** and **Fig 4.5-4**) shows significant worsening of the deformity with growth and we have observed considerable variability in development across our cohort of patients.

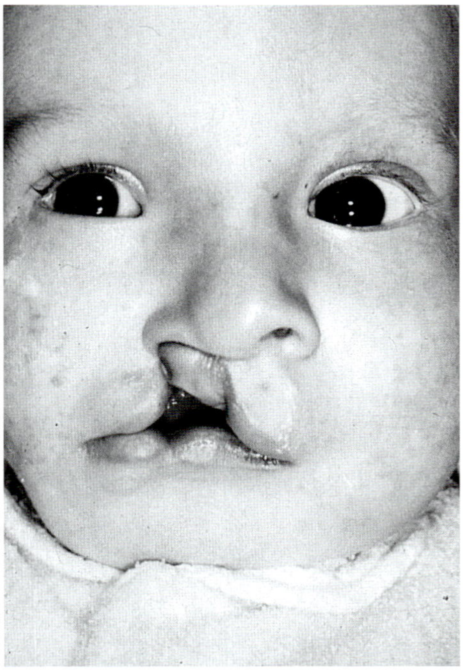

Fig 4.5-3 Baby aged 3 months with Pruzansky III hemifacial macrosomia and right unilateral complete cleft lip and palate.

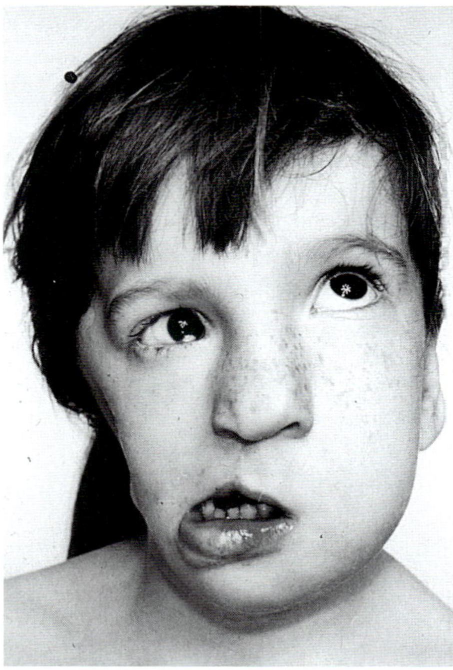

Fig 4.5-4 Same child aged 11 years. The only surgery has been repair of lip and palate.

2 Evaluation of patients with HFM

2.1 Clinical evaluation

Clinical examination is the first and foremost investigation and should always include testing of hearing, vision, and spinal anomalies. Because the incidence of spinal anomalies is high in HFM, all children with HFM should be screened by a pediatric orthopedic surgeon. Generally, this involves clinical examination and plain spinal radiographs. Only those children with significant anomalies are referred to a pediatric spine surgeon and only a small percentage of them will require spine surgery.

Occasionally, there may be problems with respiration because of airway abnormalities. The priorities in the early evaluation of the young child should focus on respiratory problems, spinal anomalies, hearing, vision, cardiac anomalies, and a cleft if they are present. The spectrum of abnormalities is so large that the pediatric investigations should cover almost all organ systems.

Patients with HFM may demonstrate aplasia, hypoplasia, reduced function, or malposition of the following:

- Mandible (especially the ramus)
- Occlusion (which can be canted up on the affected side)
- Teeth (missing, ectopic and/or crowded)
- Ear (microtia/anotia, accessory ear tags)
- Hearing (the outer and/or middle ear may be missing or abnormally formed although the inner ear and the cochlea normally works well)
- Conduction hearing loss, in 75% of cases
- Sensorineural hearing loss, in 11% of cases
- Maxilla
- Malar/zygomatic bone
- Temporal bone, especially the glenoid fossa
- Frontal bone
- Vertebrae/spine (40–60% of cases)
- Facial nerve (22% of cases)
- Macrostomia
- Dermoid cysts (especially epibulbar)
- Muscles (of mastication)
- Fat
- Temporal fascia
- Parotid gland
- Microphthalmia/anophthalmia
- Colobomas
- Lateral facial cleft
- Rarely occipital encephalocele
- Rarely developmental delay
- Clefts of the lip and/or palate (but usually of the palate alone)

Other systemic findings include congenital cardiac abnormalities such as:

- Ventriculo-septal defect (VSD)
- Patent ductus arteriosus
- Fallot's tetralogy (VSD, pulmonary stenosis, right ventricular hypertrophy and overriding aorta)
- Tracheo-oesophageal fistula (TOF)
- Renal/ureteric abnormalities

2.2 Radiological evaluation

To avoid unnecessary radiation, it is advisable to delay radiological investigation on the young child until it will have an impact on treatment. An orthopantomogram (OPT) should be delayed until the child is able to cooperate.

Definitive radiographic evaluation of the head and neck abnormalities of HFM is by high-resolution computed tomography (CT) especially 3-D CT and a panoramic x-ray (OPT). Very young children sometimes require sedation or even general anesthesia for CT acquisition. The current generation of multi-slice CT scanners acquires the relevant high-quality data in less than 1 second.

2.3 Diagnosis and differential diagnosis of HFM

Other conditions that show facial asymmetry and that can sometimes be mistaken for HFM are torticollis and plagiocephaly. By contrast Treacher Collins syndrome (TCS) is a genuine deformity of the first and second branchial arches but is essentially symmetrical and the autosomal dominant gene has been identified. Diagnosis of TCS can, however, sometimes be difficult because 65% of births are new mutations.

Lateral facial clefting (**Fig 4.5-5**) is effectively one extreme of HFM [Tessier, 1976]. Most cases are incomplete and show macrostomia and involvement of the ear and mandible on the affected side.

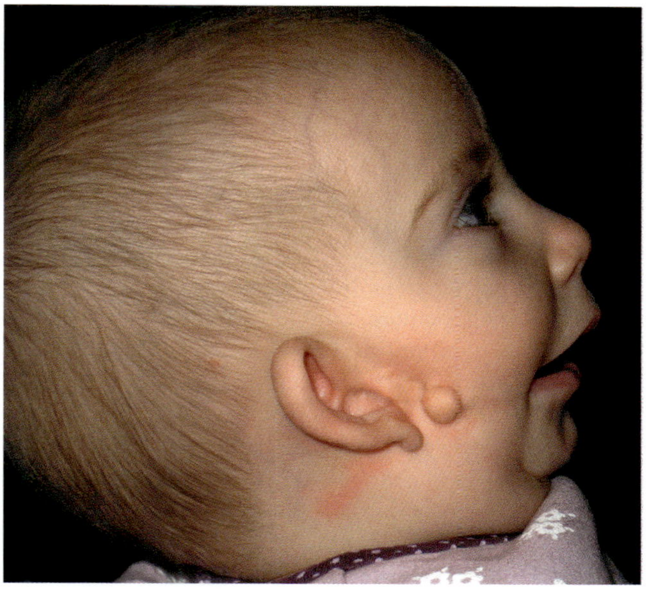

Fig 4.5-5 Incomplete Tessier No. 7 lateral facial clefting. Macrostomia, ear deformity, and preauricular ear tag along the line of the cleft on right side.

3 Classification of HFM

Several classification systems have been proposed especially by Pruzansky [1982], Lauritzen et al [1985], David [1987], Vento et al [1991], and Horgan et al [1995]. The most comprehensive classification system is OMENS+ as described by Horgan et al [1995]. However, surgeons find the classification of the skeletal deformity by Pruzansky, as modified by Kaban (which is incorporated in OMENS+), to be the most useful in practice (**Fig 4.5-6**).

OMENS+
OMENS+ subdivides and grades each of the principal deformities. These are:

O = Orbit
M = Mandible
E = Ear
N = Nerves
S = Soft tissues
+ = Extracraniofacial features

Pruzansky
Pruzansky [1969] subdivided the mandible deformities.

Mandible
I: a small ramus with identifiable anatomy
II: a functioning temporomandibular joint (TMJ) but with an abnormal shape and glenoid fossa
(IIa and IIb as modified by Kaban)
IIa: the glenoid fossa is in an acceptable functional position
IIb: the TMJ is abnormally placed and cannot be incorporated in the surgical construction
III: an absent ramus and nonexistent glenoid fossa

This system has two weaknesses: First, it is possible to have a Pruzansky II with a functioning TMJ but with or without a zygomatic arch and glenoid fossa. Second, it is possible to have a Pruzansky III with no condyle or ramus and no functioning TMJ but with or without a zygomatic arch and a glenoid fossa.

Kaban's modification and the two comments above together with the Pruzansky classification are a clear guide to reconstructive surgery of the mandible and TMJ in HFM. A 3-D CT is essential for classification of this condition and for treatment.

3.1 Use of the classification as an aid to overall diagnosis

3.1.1 Pruzansky I

Pruzansky I is the most minor example of HFM characterized by:

Mandible: A small mandibular ramus but with all the anatomy of the ramus easily distinguishable.

TMJ: Present and intact.

Dental occlusion: The occlusion is generally class I without an occlusal cant.

In addition to the above, the following may be found:
Ear: Every range of ear presentation is possible from a completely normally shaped and positioned external ear with normal middle ear and inner ear structures and normal hearing all the way through to complete anotia with conduction hearing loss.

Orbit: The position of the orbit and the eye on the affected side can be normal but varying degrees of vertical and horizontal dystopia can occur. Microphthalmia and anophthalmia can also occur.

Soft tissues: It is rare for the soft tissues to be significantly deficient in Pruzansky I cases.

Facial nerve: It is rare for the facial nerve to be significantly affected in Pruzansky I cases.

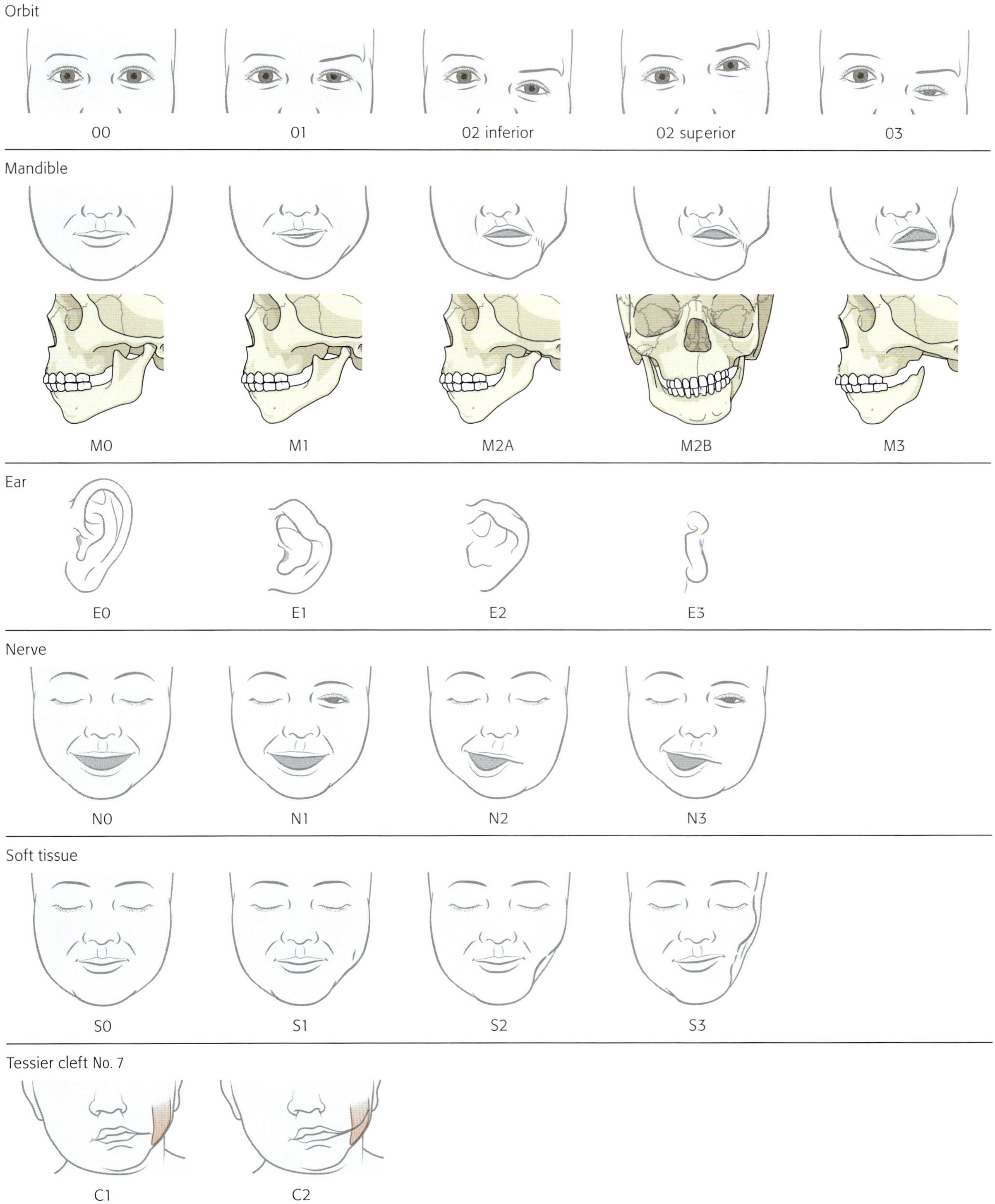

Fig 4.5-6 Pictographic illustration of the OMENS+ classification. (Modified from Gougoutas AJ, Singh DJ, Low DW, et al. Hemifacial microsomia: clinical features and pictographic representations of the OMENS classification system. *Plast Reconstr Surg*. 2007 Dec;120(7): 112e–120e. Used with permission.) It should be noted that M1, M2A, M2B and M3 are Kaban's modification of Pruzansky classification.

3.1.2 Pruzansky IIa

Pruzansky IIa is a more severe subtype characterized by the following (**Fig 4.5-7** and **Fig 4.5-1**):

Mandible: A small deformed hemi-mandible with a small ramus, pronounced antegonial notch and asymmetry of the chin (displaced to the affected side).

TMJ: A hypoplastic TMJ with the glenoid fossa in an acceptable functional and anatomical position, which is approximately equidistant from the midline as the normal side but generally at a lower level.

Dental occlusion: Occlusal cant upward on the affected side. Varying degrees of severity will be observed. The occlusion may be class I, II, or III but the class II pattern predominates.

In addition to the above, the following may be found:
Ear: Every range of ear presentation is possible from a completely normally shaped and positioned external ear with normal middle ear and inner ear structures and normal hearing all the way through to complete anotia with conduction hearing loss.

Orbit: The position of the orbit and the eye on the affected side can be normal but varying degrees of vertical and horizontal dystopia can occur. Microphthalmia and anophthalmia can also occur.

Soft tissues: The soft tissues on the affected side of the face can exhibit a range of severity from effectively normal to severely hypoplastic. Soft-tissue structures, such as the parotid gland, may be absent.

Facial nerve: The branches of the facial nerve on the affected side can function completely normally but can also show a varying range of reduced function (palsy) from mild to severe and affecting one or more of the nerve branches.

3.1.3 Pruzansky IIb

Pruzansky IIb is a more severe subtype characterized in **Fig 4.5-8**.

Mandible: A small deformed hemi-mandible with a small ramus, pronounced antegonial notch and asymmetry of the chin (displaced to the affected side). The key point is that the mandibular ramus and condyle on the affected side are positioned medially.

TMJ: A hypoplastic TMJ with the glenoid fossa abnormally placed medially. The distance between the TMJ and the midline is substantially less than on the unaffected side. Hence, the TMJ cannot be incorporated into the surgical construction. Generally, the TMJ is not at the same vertical level as the normal side.

Dental occlusion: Occlusal cant upward on the affected side. Varying degrees of severity will be observed. The occlusion may be class I, II, or III, but the class II pattern predominates.

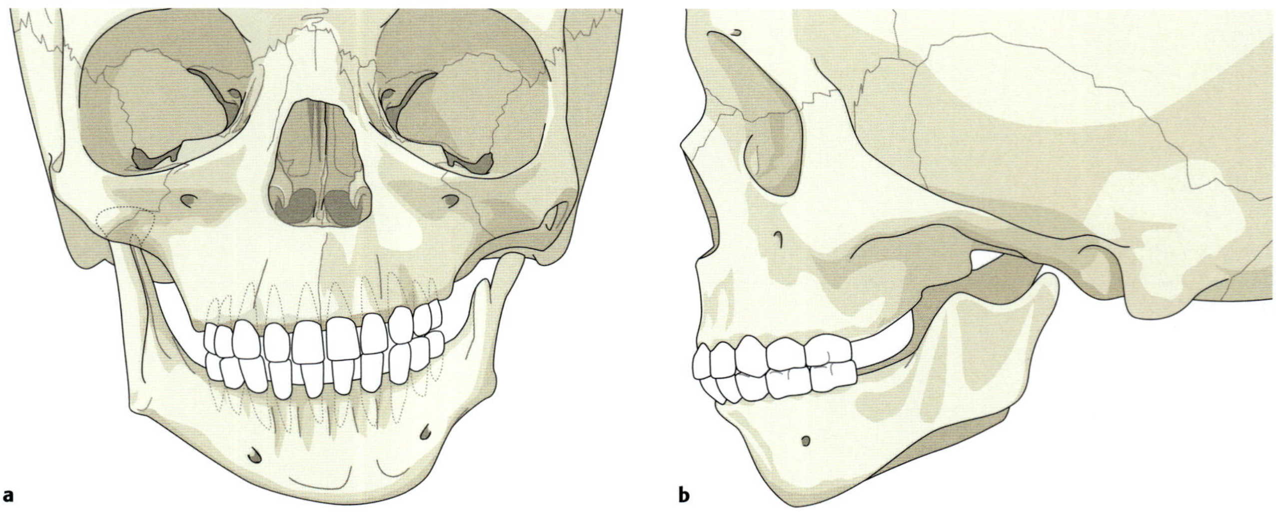

a b

Fig 4.5-7a–b Pruzansky IIa skeletal deformity.

Note: The Pruzansky IIa/IIb classification does not consider those cases where, in addition, part of or all the zygomatic arch is missing. There may be an indication for constructing the arch before any surgery is carried out to the mandible.

In addition to the above, the following may be found:
Ear: Every range of ear presentation is possible from a completely normally shaped and positioned external ear with normal middle ear and inner ear structures and normal hearing all the way through to complete anotia with conduction hearing loss.

Orbit: The position of the orbit and the eye on the affected side can be normal but varying degrees of vertical and horizontal dystopia can occur. Microphthalmia and anophthalmia can also occur.

Soft tissues: The soft tissues on the affected side of the face can exhibit a range of severity from effectively normal to severely hypoplastic or absent.

Facial nerve: The branches of the facial nerve on the affected side can function completely normally but can also show a varying range of reduced function (palsy) from mild to severe and affecting one or more of the nerve branches.

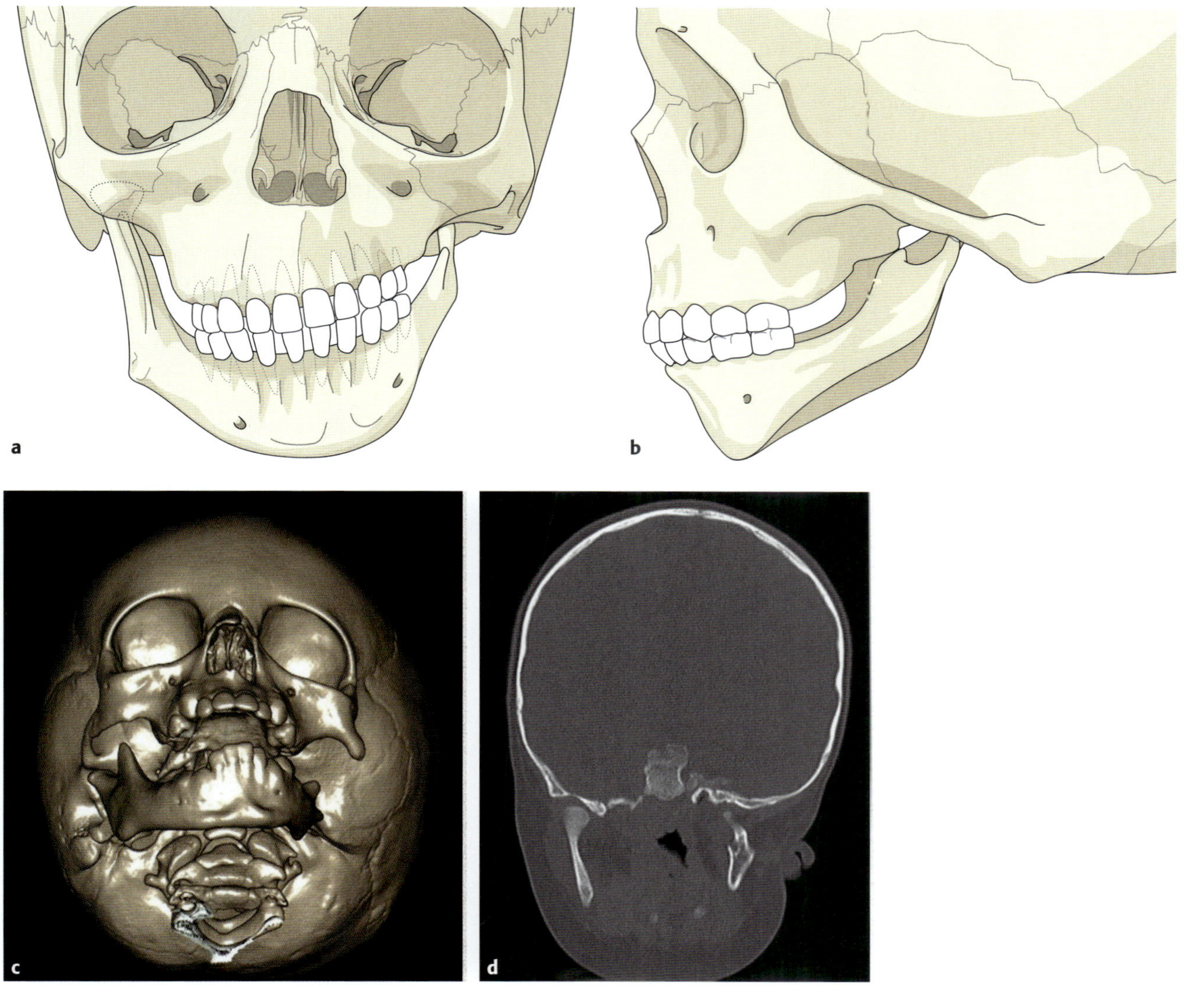

Fig 4.5-8a–d Pruzansky IIb skeletal deformity.
a AP view.
b Lateral view.
c Submental 3-D CT view.
d Coronal CT scan with medially placed condyle and temporomandibular joint.

3.1.4 Pruzansky III

Pruzansky III is the most severe subtype characterized by the following (**Fig 4.5-9**):

Mandible: The affected hemi-mandible is severely deformed. At its mildest only the upper part of the mandibular ramus is missing. At its most severe the whole of the ramus and part of the body are missing.

TMJ: Absent.
Note: It is possible to have a Pruzansky III mandible with no condyle or functional TMJ but with a rudimentary zygomatic arch and apparent glenoid fossa.

Dental occlusion: Severe occlusal cant upward on the affected side. Various degrees of severity are observed. The class II pattern of malocclusion predominates.

In addition to the above, the following may be found:
Ear: Every range of ear presentation is possible from a completely normally shaped and positioned external ear with normal middle ear and inner ear structures and normal hearing all the way through to complete anotia with conduction hearing loss.

Orbit: The position of the orbit and the eye on the affected side can be normal but varying degrees of vertical and horizontal dystopia can occur. Microphthalmia and anophthalmia can also occur.

Soft tissues: The soft tissues on the affected side of the face can exhibit a range of severity from effectively normal to severely hypoplastic. Soft-tissue structures, such as parotid gland, may be absent.

Facial nerve: The branches of the facial nerve on the affected side can function completely normally but can also show a varying range of reduced function (palsy) from mild to severe and affecting one or more of the nerve branches.

4 Treatment algorithm for HFM

Treatment for HFM depends on the clinical severity of the deformity, the age of the patient, the wishes of the patient and their family, and the classification of the deformity. While most surgeons working in this field carry out treatment during growth when clinically indicated based on the complexity and individual features of the deformity, some surgeons prefer to delay all treatment until maturity.

4.1 Mandible and TMJ

4.1.1 Pruzansky I

It is rarely necessary to consider any surgery for the Pruzansky I mandible in childhood as the "deformity" is usually mild. From the age of about 16 years, some patients will benefit from a genioplasty or conventional orthognathic surgery.

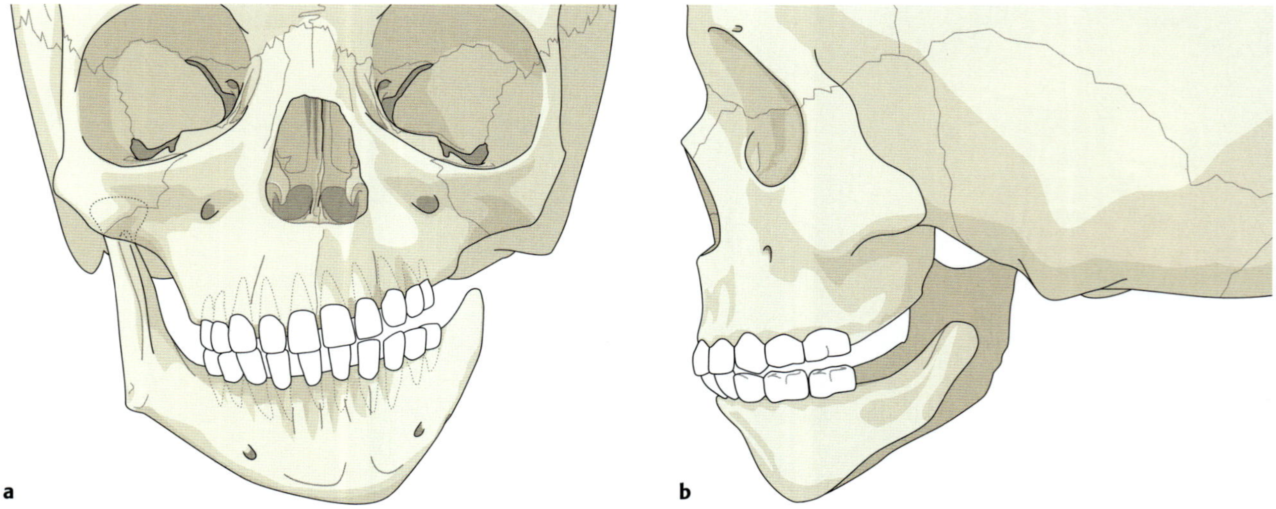

a b

Fig 4.5-9a–b Pruzansky III skeletal deformity.
a AP view.
b Lateral view.

Treatment of the deformity is usually going to be deferred to maturity. In maturity, therefore, this is likely to consist of either:

(1) No surgery

or

(2) Genioplasty

or

(3) Conventional orthognathic surgery

4.1.2 Pruzansky IIa and IIb

There are cases of Pruzansky IIa and IIb in which the zygomatic arch or part of it is missing. Consider whether reconstruction of the arch with a rib graft is beneficial.

Cases of IIb may benefit from repositioning of the glenoid fossa and later the condyle into a more lateral position before lengthening of the ramus is considered. This permits a more lateral reconstruction and, therefore, a better facial contour. Sometimes the position of the TMJ is so severely displaced that it is better to create a new glenoid fossa, condyle, and TMJ (in two stages) in a more lateral position using rib and costochondral grafts as in a Pruzansky III.

Depending on the severity of the deformity and the wishes of the family, Pruzansky IIa (and sometimes IIb cases after repositioning of the TMJ if indicated) can be considered for distraction osteogenesis to lengthen the mandibular ramus from the age of about 3 or 4 years. Some children have such a mild clinical asymmetry that they do not need this. Any young child who receives such lengthening during growth is likely to need further intervention over time because the operated side of the mandible does not usually grow as much as the normal side and the deformity tends to reestablish itself. Parents should always be warned about this possibility, although we have cases in which the correction performed at 3 or 4 years of age has been maintained to maturity.

From the age of 12 years, treated Pruzansky II cases with a persistent deformity (or cases presenting de novo) may be candidates for bimaxillary distraction osteogenesis provided that the occlusion can be managed by orthodontics. From this age onward, lengthening of the mandible alone and the creation of a lateral open bite will not always allow the maxillary teeth to erupt further and the lateral open bite to close.

Some HFM cases may require management of residual skeletal deformity from the age of 16 years onward (end stage). This is mostly performed using orthognathic surgery and usually requires bimaxillary rotational osteotomies. Sometimes on-lay bone grafting is also necessary.

Some cases will have such severe deficiency of the soft tissues that correction of the bony deformity alone is not adequate to correct the facial contours. There are several options to address this problem:

(1) Lateral augmentation of the mandibular angle by distraction osteogenesis (DO) or osteotomy.

(2) Augmentation of the lateral mandible with onlay bone grafting or alloplastic material.

(3) Augmentation of the facial contours with dermis fat grafts and/or fat injections.

(4) Augmentation of the facial contours with soft-tissue vascularized flaps.

4.1.3 Pruzansky III

Pruzansky III cases present with not only severe hypoplasia of the ramus/condyle unit but also with missing bone, especially in the area of the zygomatic arch and glenoid fossa and the mandibular condyle, ramus, and body. Correction is usually achieved by constructing missing parts with a combination of rib and costochondral grafts. These procedures can be started as early as 2–3 years of age. The Pruzansky III case is thus converted to a Pruzansky IIa and can then be treated as described earlier.

Costochondral grafting used alone to lengthen the ramus is rarely effective because there are physical limits to the length that can be achieved and because length alone is rarely sufficient to correct the deformity. For this reason, it is generally better if it is clinically indicated to lengthen again by DO at least 6 months after costochondral grafting.

In some cases, the costochondral graft produces sufficient improvement in appearance and growth, thus further intervention is not needed. Overgrowth can occur but in this author's experience, it is rare in HFM.

5 Treatment procedures for the ear, soft tissues, orbit, and facial nerve

Preauricular skin tags are common and often bilateral. Parents often want these removed as early as possible because they are unsightly. This can be done any time. The author usually offers this from 1 year of age or at the same time as other procedures.

5.1 The ear

Well-formed ears require no treatment although sometimes they are not in a good position. It can be extremely difficult to move them. Sometimes the ear is abnormally formed but most of the tissues are present. Those cases can be managed by correcting the ear deformity rather than by more complete reconstructive surgery.

The options for treatment of severe microtia or anotia are:
(1) Do nothing (unless the child or parents request intervention).
(2) Autogenous construction with skin and cartilage by one of the recognized techniques (eg, Brent [2002], Nagata [1993]) from around 8 years old when the ear is normally fully grown.
(3) A bone-anchored ear prosthesis attached to titanium craniofacial implants placed in the temporal bone can be considered from 3 years old.

5.2 Facial soft tissues

In general, management of the facial soft tissues is carried out late, after completion of the skeletal constructions. Exceptions to this "rule" are:

- Correction of macrostomia, which should be carried out during the first year of life as it is analogous to a cleft lip. The same principle applies to a complete lateral facial cleft. It is important to carry out a definitive muscle repair and to incorporate z-plasties into the closure design.
- Soft-tissue augmentation is sometimes carried out early as part of a composite vascularized free tissue transfer in severe Pruzansky III cases.

Also in Pruzansky III cases when the soft tissues are extremely thin and most of the underlying soft-tissue structures are missing, eg, the parotid gland, the masticatory muscles, skeletal construction can make the face look gaunt and the underlying bone contours can be visible through the skin. Early soft-tissue augmentation may then be advisable and could involve a deepithelialized free flap, a perforator free flap, dermis fat grafts, and/or fat injections. The same techniques apply to later soft-tissue augmentation if indicated. In this author's observation [Coleman, 2004; Coleman et al, 2009], fat transfer can produce wonderful sculpted soft-tissue contours albeit at the expense of multiple episodes and considerable tolerance by both patient and surgeon.

Facial nerve palsy is common in HFM. However, it is rarely severe enough to obtain significant benefits from facial reanimation. Free flaps such as pectoralis minor or gracilis for formal reanimation can be carried out or various sling soft-tissue suspension procedures.

When the facial nerve is affected, the condition needs to be severe and affecting the second and/or third branches of the nerve for surgery to be considered. Various procedures for facial reanimation can be considered although palsy affecting the first branch of the facial nerve is usually managed by the insertion of a gold weight into the upper eyelid to facilitate lid closure.

5.3 The orbit

Orbital dystopia can occur. If mild, no intervention is advisable. If severe (> 1 cm), the principles of correction are the same as for hypertelorism and vertical dystopia (craniofacial four-wall box osteotomy). This is normally performed after the age of 13 years when the teeth in the midface have erupted and are out of the way. Correction involves a major intracranial procedure to move the orbit and eye upward. The dystopia should be severe to justify this procedure.

6 Treatment procedures for HFM in the growing child

6.1 Correction of macrostomia

Correction of macrostomia is based on the principles of cleft lip repair (**Fig 4.5-10**). The commissure of the mouth (the corner of the mouth) is recreated at the same distance from the midline as the normal side. The scar is broken up with z-plasties and the muscle repaired to provide good function.

6.2 Excision of accessory ear tags

Small skin tags and bobbles commonly occur in the immediate preauricular area in the presence of microtia and even sometimes when a completely normal looking ear is present. For reasons not understood, preauricular skin tags are often bilateral. Parents and children often request their removal and this can be done usually by simple surgical excision and primary closure. Some tags contain cartilage that needs to be excised more completely in a deeper plane.

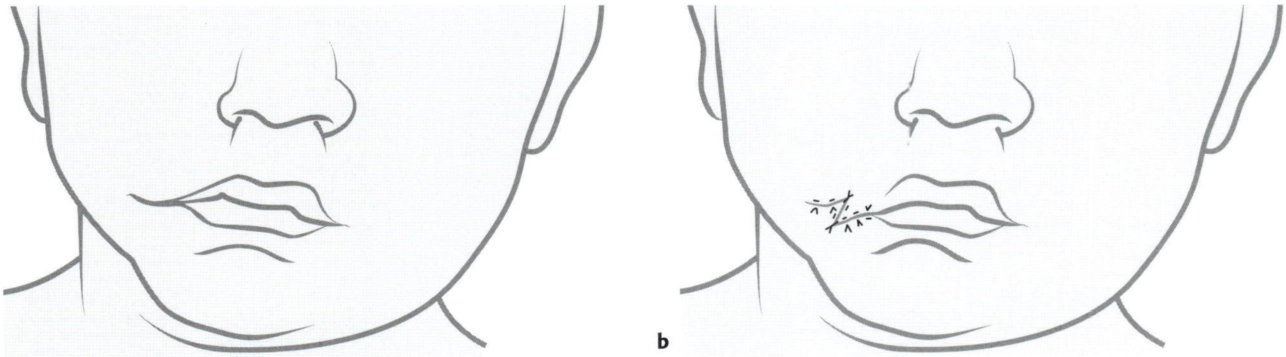

a b

Fig 4.5-10a–b Correction of macrostomia.
a Macrostomia on the child's right side.
b Macrostomia correction.

6.3 Construction of zygomatic arch

When the zygomatic arch is missing (in whole or in part) and the glenoid fossa is present, the arch should be constructed as symmetrically as possible. Mirror imaging of the normal side to the abnormal side using 3-D CT software can provide a guide to the shape and position of the graft required.

The construction of the zygomatic arch is generally carried out during childhood although the same principles apply when a patient presents as an adult. The surgical approach is via a hemicoronal or an extended preauricular incision (**Fig 4.5-11a**). This enables exposure of the posterior part of the arch extending forward to the body of the zygomatic bone.

It is generally possible to construct the zygomatic arch using autogenous rib grafts (**Fig 4.5-11b**). Usually one rib graft is sufficient. The rib is molded using rib benders to the required shape (**Fig 4.5-11c**).

The construct is then stabilized with two screws (eg, 1.5 mm diameter), one anteriorly and one posteriorly. Screw fixation is generally into the body of the zygomatic bone anteriorly and the mastoid process of the temporal bone posteriorly (**Fig 4.5-11d–e**).

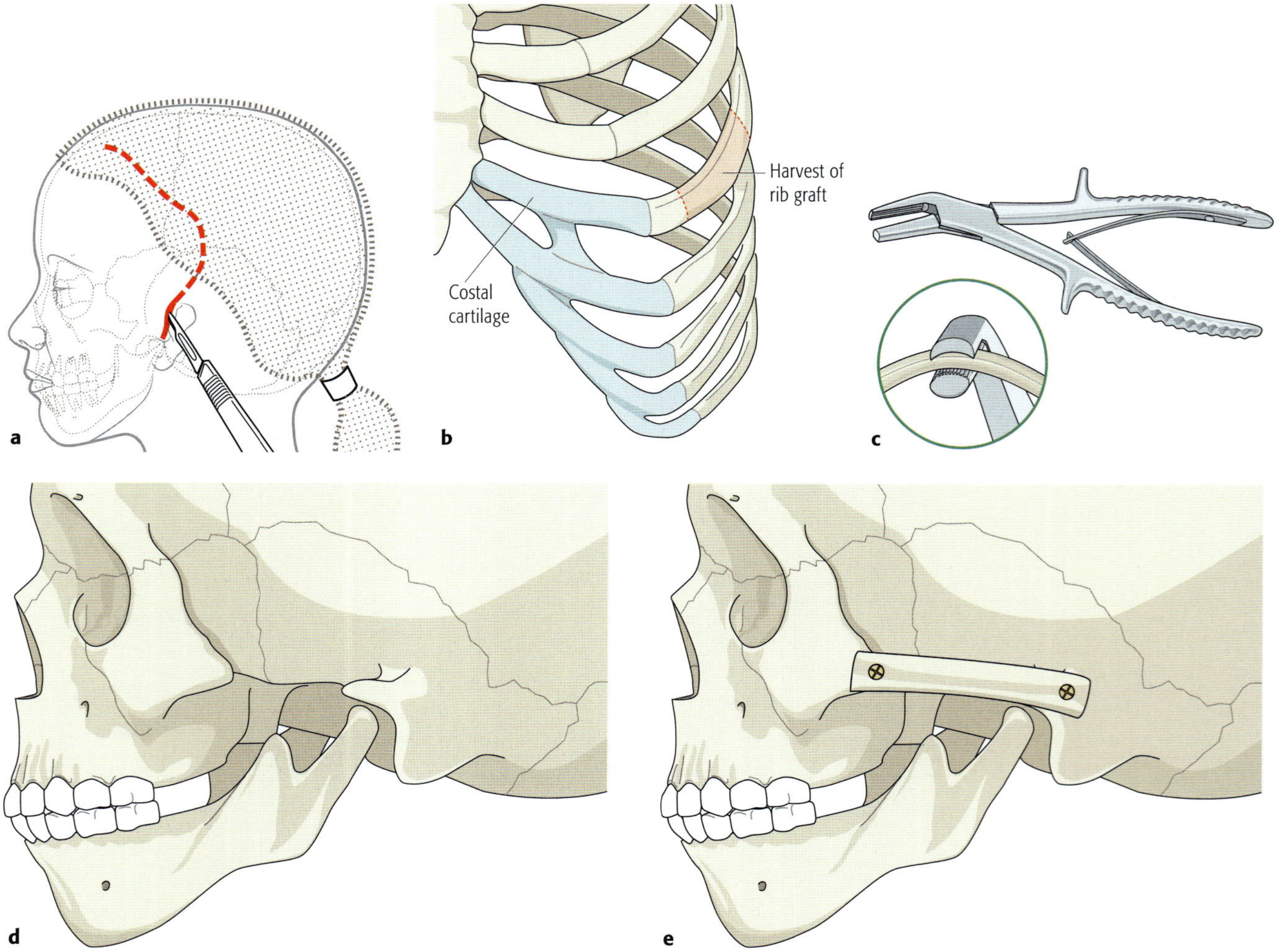

Fig 4.5-11a–e Construction of missing part of the zygomatic arch with a rib graft.
- **a** Hemicoronal/extended preauricular incision.
- **b** Harvest of rib graft.
- **c** Rib bending.
- **d** Zygomatic arch defect preoperatively.
- **e** Zygomatic arch reconstructed with a rib graft.

6.4 Construction of zygomatic arch and glenoid fossa

When the zygomatic arch and the glenoid fossa are missing in whole or in part, they should be constructed as symmetrically as possible. The key is to try to place the glenoid fossa in as similar a position and distance as possible from the midline in all three dimensions. It is rarely possible to achieve this, in this surgeon's experience, in the vertical dimension. Mirror imaging of the normal side to the abnormal side using 3-D CT software can provide a guide to the shape and position of the graft required.

The construction of the zygomatic arch and the glenoid fossa is usually performed during childhood although the same principles apply when a patient presents as an adult. The surgical approach is via a hemicoronal or an extended preauricular incision. This enables exposure of the TMJ area, including the: (1) mastoid bone posteriorly; (2) body of the zygomatic bone anteriorly; and (3) lateral orbital rim.

It is normally possible to construct the zygomatic arch and glenoid fossa using autogenous rib grafts. Usually one long rib graft (10–12 cm) is sufficient but sometimes two should be harvested. The rib is molded using rib benders to the required shape. In the region of the glenoid fossa, multiple layers of rib are assembled with screws and the fossa is carved out of the ribs with a drill. The construct is then fixed in place with two screws (eg, 1.5 mm diameter), one anteriorly and one posteriorly. Screw fixation is usually into the body of the zygomatic bone anteriorly and the mastoid process of the temporal bone posteriorly (**Fig 4.5-12**).

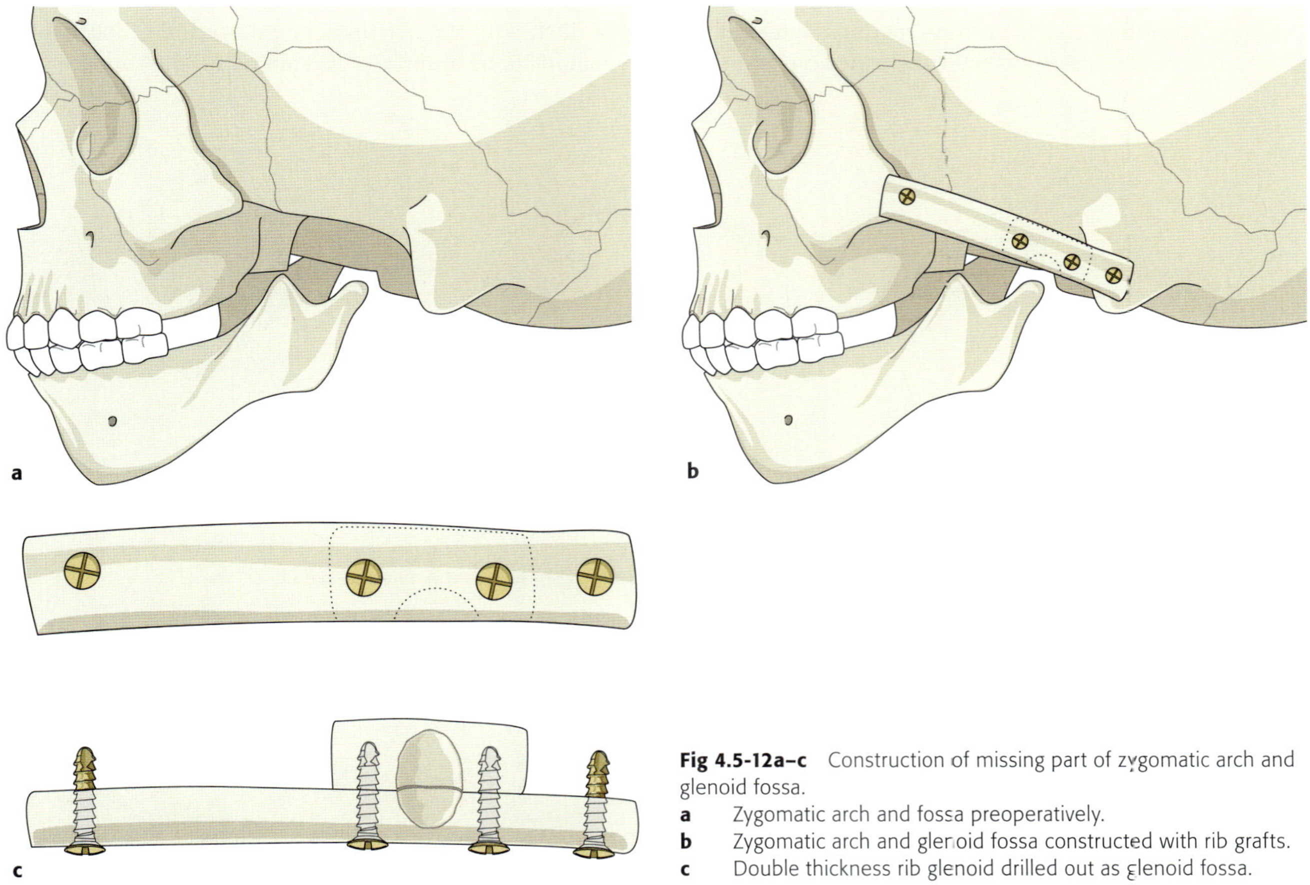

Fig 4.5-12a–c Construction of missing part of zygomatic arch and glenoid fossa.
a Zygomatic arch and fossa preoperatively.
b Zygomatic arch and glenoid fossa constructed with rib grafts.
c Double thickness rib glenoid drilled out as glenoid fossa.

It is important to ensure that the bony construct, especially of the glenoid fossa, is covered with soft tissue to prevent TMJ ankylosis. This can either be carried out during this procedure or at the time of mandibular condyle construction. The best material to cover the fossa is fascia. Sometimes temporal fascia is available and can be turned over the construct as a pedicle flap. Sometimes it needs to be used as a free graft. In the absence of suitable local tissue (muscle should be avoided because it has the potential to ossify) fascia lata can be harvested from the lateral aspect of the thigh. These bone grafts can resorb. Sometimes it is necessary to augment them with further rib grafts later or in conjunction with other surgical procedures.

6.5 Zygomatic arch and glenoid fossa osteotomy

Occasionally, the zygomatic arch and glenoid fossa are present but abnormally positioned. If the position is not acceptable (ie, if the glenoid fossa is placed too far medially to obtain good symmetry when reconstructing the mandible) the alternatives are either to reconstruct the arch and fossa with rib grafts (**Fig 4.5-12**) or to osteotomize the arch and fossa and move them into a new position (**Fig 4.5-13** and **Fig 4.5-14**).

The ideal position of the arch and glenoid fossa on the affected side should be determined by mirror imaging the normal side using CT planning software (**Fig 4.5-13b–c**). The arch and glenoid fossa can be virtually osteotomized and repositioned as close as possible to the ideal mirrored image as shown in the illustration. An osteotomy guide can be constructed, which allows the accurate positioning of the osteotomies and repositioning of the osteotomized segment. Intraoperative navigation can also be used for this purpose.

Careful assessment of planar CT images especially in the coronal plane is essential to check the bone thickness before performing the osteotomies. The surgical approach is via a partial coronal incision. This enables exposure of the TMJ area, including the mastoid bone posteriorly, body of the zygomatic bone anteriorly and lateral orbital rim.

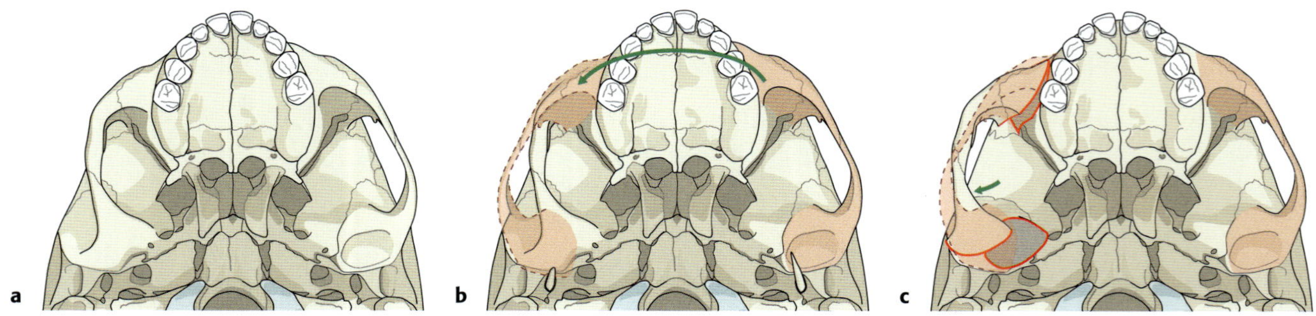

Fig 4.5-13a–c Zygomatic arch and glenoid fossa osteotomy.
a A medially displaced right glenoid fossa and zygomatic arch.
b Normal left zygomatic arch and glenoid fossa mirror imaged to right side.
c After osteotomy the arch and fossa moved laterally to conform as closely as possible to the mirror imaged position.

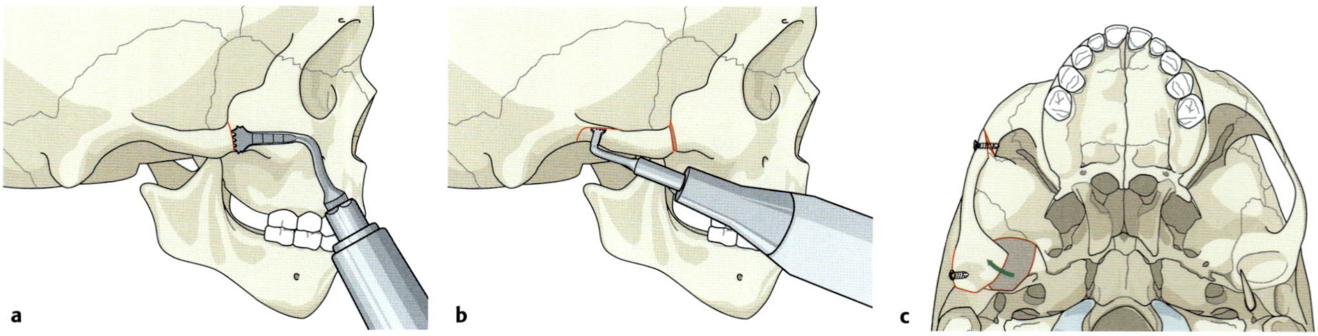

Fig 4.5-14a–c Osteotomies of the zygomatic arch and fossa and their repositioning.
a Anterior osteotomy of the zygomatic arch.
b Posterior osteotomy of the glenoid fossa.
c Arch fossa unit repositioned and fixed with screws.

Osteotomies are performed as dictated by the planning. The anterior osteotomy is made sagittal at the junction between the arch and the body of the zygomatic bone. Posteriorly two osteotomies are needed. One is made vertically at the root of the zygoma just anterior to the external auditory meatus. The second osteotomy is made extracranially horizontally above the glenoid fossa and below the middle cranial fossa.

To minimize the risk of perforation into the cranial cavity and to avoid injury to the dura of the temporal lobe, it is helpful to perform this procedure with a piezoelectric saw. Care is still required but in theory the piezoelectric saw should not damage soft tissues. Once osteotomized, the zygomatic arch and the fossa are mobilized gently and moved into the predetermined position. A surgical guide constructed from the planned virtual model can help with the positioning, or navigation can be used. In the new position the mobilized complex needs to be stabilized, usually with screws.

It is important to ensure that the mobilized arch-fossa-segment is covered with soft tissue to prevent TMJ ankyloses. The same principles as in fossa reconstruction with rib grafts apply.

7 Construction of mandibular ramus and condyle

Construction of the missing mandibular condyle and/or ramus/body presupposes that the glenoid fossa is either present, or has been constructed or repositioned into approximately the correct place compared with the normal side. The assumption is made that the glenoid fossa is lined with soft tissue. If this is not the case, the glenoid fossa must be relined with soft tissue before constructing the condyle as described above. Although many materials have been used for condylar construction in this situation, most surgeons' first choice remains a costochondral graft, especially in children. In adults, microvascular flaps and/or TMJ prosthesis may be considered an option.

Sometimes a costochondral graft needs to be supplemented by additional rib grafts. The surgical approach is usually from a preauricular incision (**Fig 4.5-15**) supplemented by a submandibular approach. Occasionally, these incisions may be joined as a parotid or facelift (**Fig 4.5-16** and **Fig 4.5-19**) approach when the missing bone tissue from the mandible is so extensive that it is impossible to determine the bone plane for the ramus-condyle construction without first dissecting out the branches of the facial nerve.

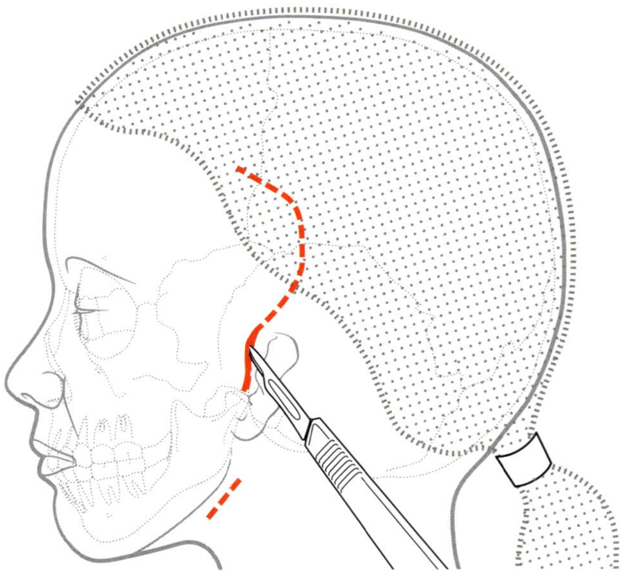

Fig 4.5-15 Preauricular and submandibular incisions.

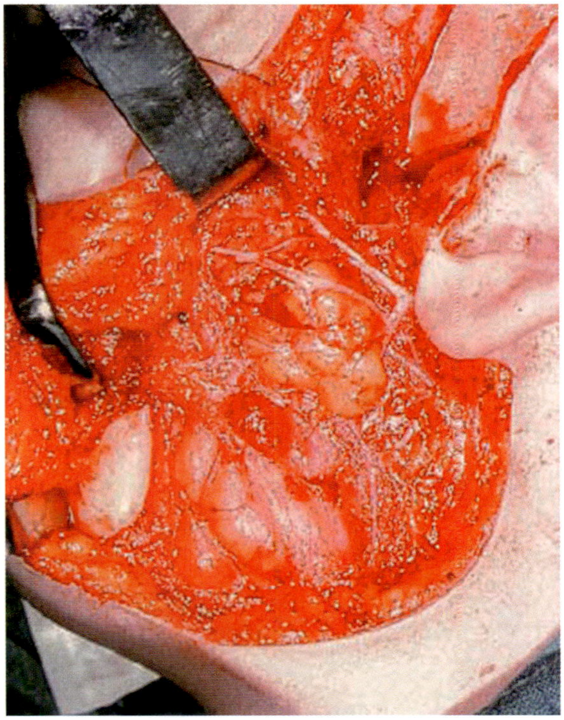

Fig 4.5-16 Parotid or facelift approach.

To harvest the costochondral graft (**Fig 4.5-17**), an incision is made in the anterior chest wall over the sixth or seventh rib in the inframammary fold in girls. This can be challenging in young girls before breast development, and an educated guess is required. In boys, the positioning of the incision is less critical and can focus on the graft required. Remember that the costochondral junction is well lateral in young children.

The following are important considerations:

- Choice of sides: in general, if a long costochondral graft is required for the left side it is harvested from the right side of the chest and vice versa because of the bone curvature required.
- Incision of the periosteum over the bony portion of the rib to be harvested
- Retention of a rectangle of periosteum over the costochondral junction to reduce the risk of bone separation from the cartilage.
- Raising of the periosteum with a periosteal elevator and a Doyen rib raspatory. Be careful when carrying this out beneath the cartilage, as there is an increased risk of perforating the pleura.
- Ensuring the harvesting of a sufficient length of rib
- Division of the cartilage with a knife
- Avoiding damage to the underlying periosteum and the pleura
- Division of the rib laterally with rib sheers or a piezotome
- Accurate repair of the periosteum with sutures
- Sometimes it is necessary to harvest a second rib.

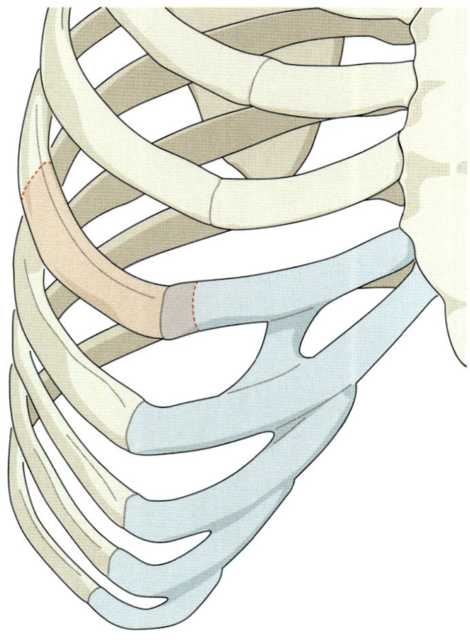

Fig 4.5-17 Harvest site for the costochondral graft.

If the periosteum and/or the pleura are damaged, it is sometimes possible to repair them with simple sutures having the anesthetist fully inflate the lung before completing suturing provided that the lungs continue to expand normally. If they do not do so, the insertion of a chest tube connected to water seal becomes necessary.

The type of the ramus-condyle construction will be determined by the amount of bone that is missing and by the availability of bone in the recipient stump of the mandible for fixation of the rib graft without damaging unerupted teeth.

7.1 Positioning relative to the facial nerve

Where most of the ramus is missing, or when all the ramus and some of the body of the mandible are missing, it can be difficult to determine the plane of dissection in relation to the facial nerve. In such cases a formal facial nerve dissection may be required. It can sometimes be difficult to find the trunk of the nerve because of the abnormal anatomy, and then a peripheral branch needs to be identified and followed back to the trunk.

In theory, an anatomical construction would place the ramus-condyle construction deep to the nerve branches. In practice, this does not usually allow sufficient lateral contour of the mandible for symmetry without risking damage to the facial nerve. Consequently, we tend to perform construction of these severe cases superficial to the facial nerve branches (**Fig 4.5-18** and **Fig 4.5-19**).

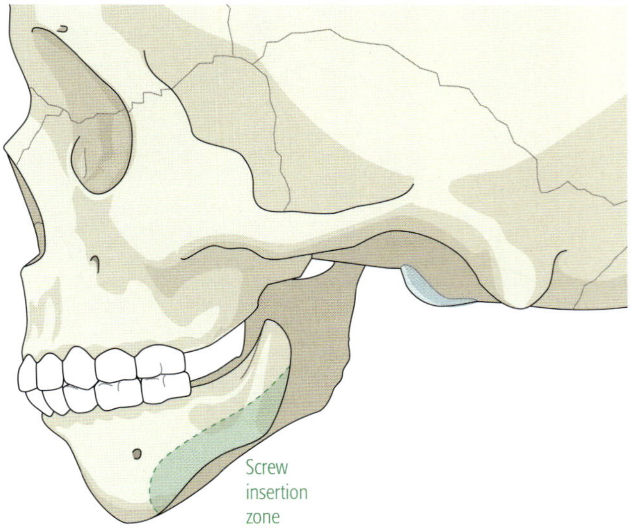

Fig 4.5-18 A Pruzansky III mandible with large defect of body, ramus and condyle.

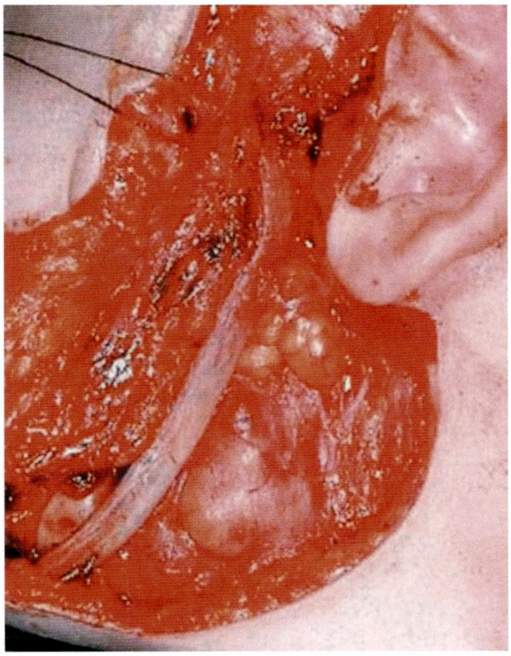

Fig 4.5-19 Extended parotid approach with dissection of the facial nerve and placement of a long costochondral graft lateral to the nerve.

7.2 Shaping of the rib graft

The cartilaginous cap of the rib graft is shaped with a knife to approximate the condyle morphology (**Fig 4.5-20**). Some surgeons believe that the amount of growth produced by the costochondral graft is related to the size of the cartilage portion (ie, the more cartilage the more growth there will be) but there is no strong evidence to support this. The rib may need to be bent to produce the right shape and to adapt it to the native mandible.

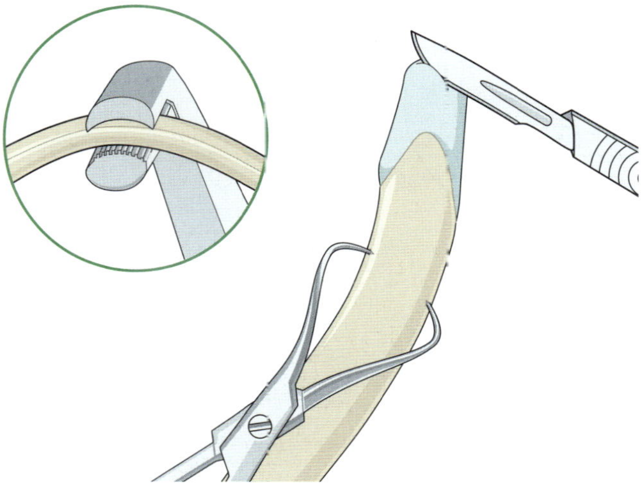

Fig 4.5-20 Bending the rib graft and shaping the cartilaginous cap.

7.3 Positioning and fixation

The chondral part of the rib is then positioned in the glenoid fossa under direct vision. Sometimes it is helpful to use a suture to hold it in position. It is important to ensure that it does not displace laterally. Inferiorly, it is fixed to the underlying mandible with at least two screws avoiding essential structures, such as developing unerupted tooth germs and the inferior dental nerve. Sometimes that fixation should be taken as far forward as the chin to avoid developing tooth buds. One plate eyelet (a single plate hole cut from a long plate) can be used as a washer (**Fig 4.5-21**) to distribute the load of the head of the screw, as the screw is tightened and thus avoid splitting of the bone graft.

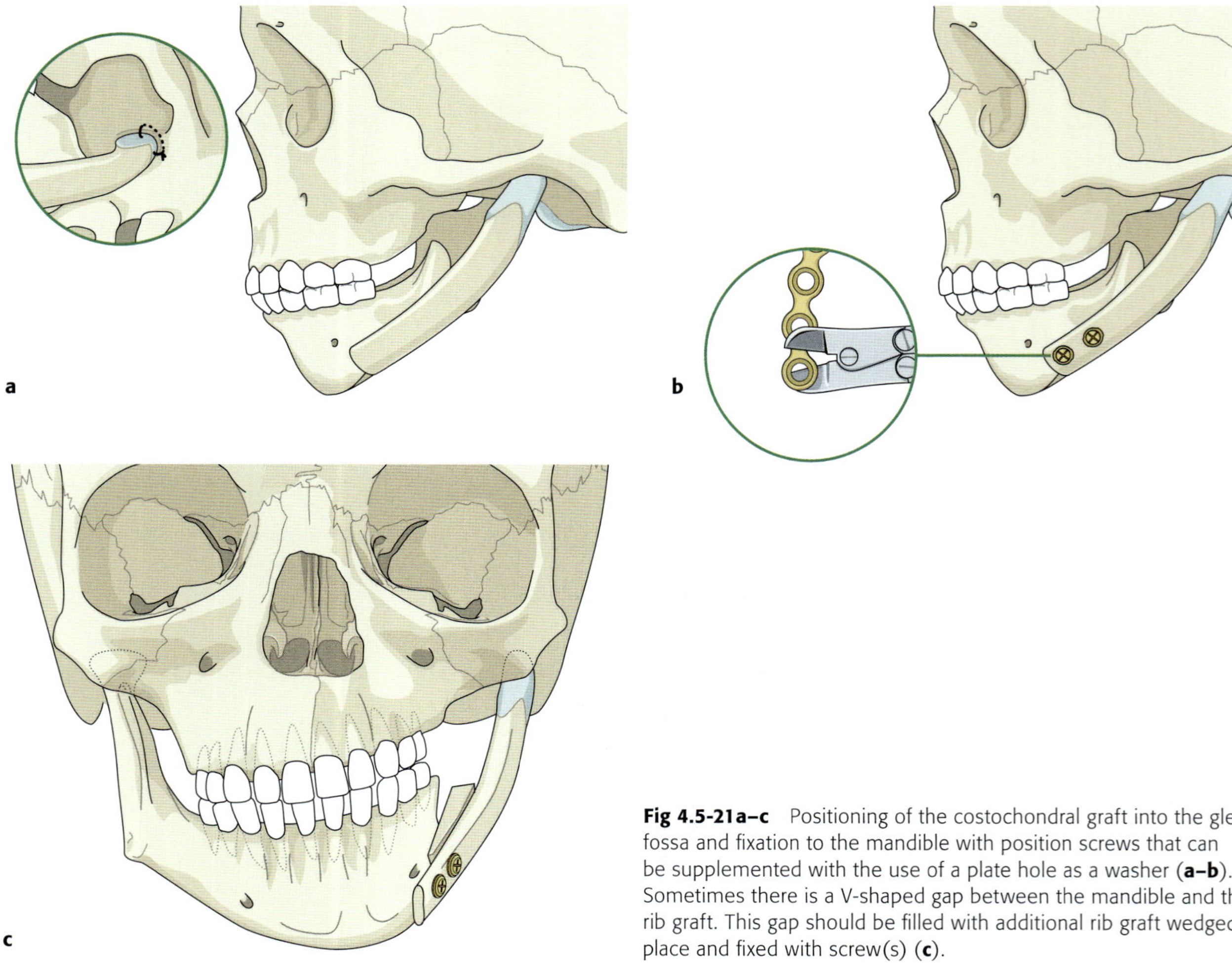

a b c

Fig 4.5-21a–c Positioning of the costochondral graft into the glenoid fossa and fixation to the mandible with position screws that can be supplemented with the use of a plate hole as a washer (**a–b**). Sometimes there is a V-shaped gap between the mandible and the rib graft. This gap should be filled with additional rib graft wedged into place and fixed with screw(s) (**c**).

We have long abandoned the fixation of bone grafts with plates and screws whenever possible because of the scar tissue that develops around them and the difficulty encountered in their removal. By contrast, screws alone produce little peripheral scar tissue, later demonstrate clearly the amount of graft resorption below the screw head and can easily be removed if they become prominent either at the same time as future procedures or through small cutaneous incisions.

8 Distraction osteogenesis of mandibular ramus

The principle of lengthening the mandibular ramus with DO is that the positioning of the distractor and the vector of distraction in most cases should ensure that the force is vertical and passes through the condylar process. In effect this lengthens the ramus, creates a new position for the mandibular angle, creates a lateral open bite, and corrects chin asymmetry.

8.1 Planning

Distractors can be placed free-hand without any guides but the results can be unpredictable and sometimes unsatisfactory. This section, therefore, describes a more predictable approach using computer-assisted planning. Planning is carried out in virtual reality on a 3-D CT scan using appropriate software. An estimate can then be made of the amount of distraction required and the bone stock available. This is helpful in deciding which distractor to use.

The greater the deformity, the smaller will be the mandibular ramus and the greater will be the distraction distance required. This is problematic because there is less space available for an internal distractor. This problem can be solved using either an external distractor or an internal distractor that uses an external activation rod (a semi-submerged distractor). External pin distraction has the disadvantage of leaving unsightly facial scars, especially as the bone pins are distracted through the soft tissues. Consequently, we prefer whenever possible to use a semi-submerged distractor that is fixed internally but with an externally accessible activation rod.

The virtual distractor is selected and placed on the mandibular ramus avoiding damage whenever possible to developing tooth buds (**Fig 4.5-22**). A horizontal osteotomy is marked above the lingula. The virtual osteotomy is completed and the distractor virtually activated. If the movement is not satisfactory, the virtual distractor position can be adjusted until the desired vector is achieved.

A guide can be constructed (**Fig 4.5-23**) that allows the accurate positioning of the distractor and the osteotomy. Intraoperative navigation can achieve a similar result.

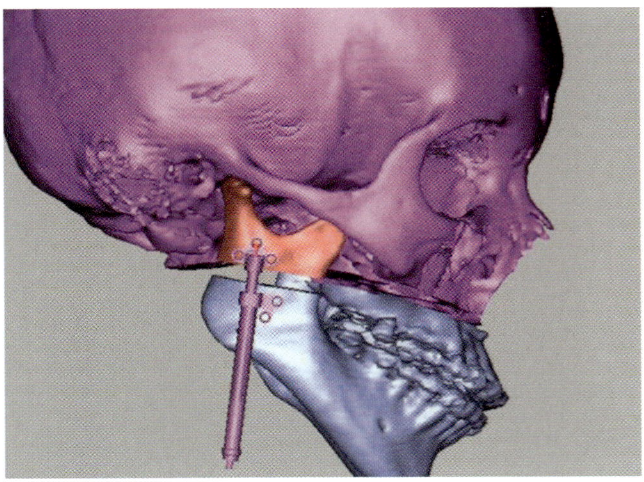

Fig 4.5-22 Distractor chosen and placed on virtual model, bone cut, and distractor activated to simulate the actual process.

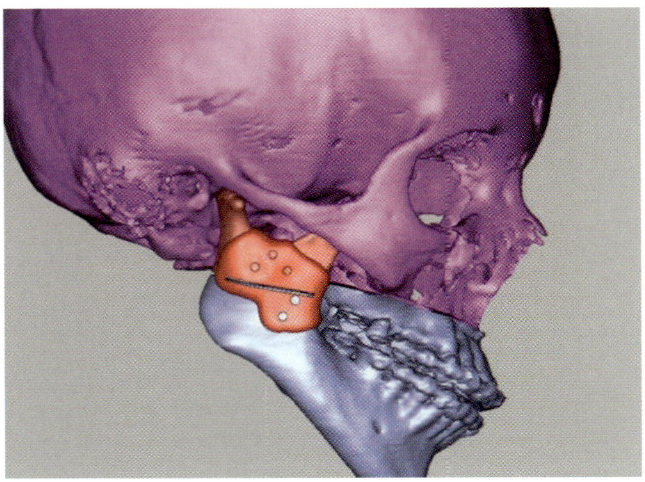

Fig 4.5-23 A guide made on the virtual model to enable precise osteotomy and distractor positioning.

The surgical approach depends to some extent on the age of the patient and the severity of the deformity. The type of distractor used is also a factor. Provided the ramus of the mandible is flared, a transoral approach (**Fig 4.5-24**) can be used but with a few modifications:

- The ramus is exposed subperiosteally up to the condylar neck and the sigmoid notch, and down to the mandibular angle and the posterior border.
- A small incision in the submandibular region is placed to allow for the exit of the activation rod.
- A transbuccal approach is used for screw insertion.

In very young children when the deformity is severe and in older children when the ramus is not flared (so that intraoral vision is extremely difficult), a purely external approach (**Fig 4.5-25**) should be considered usually from a submandibular approach to the mandibular angle and ramus. The whole lateral aspect of the mandibular ramus is exposed. Virtually no periosteal stripping is required medially.

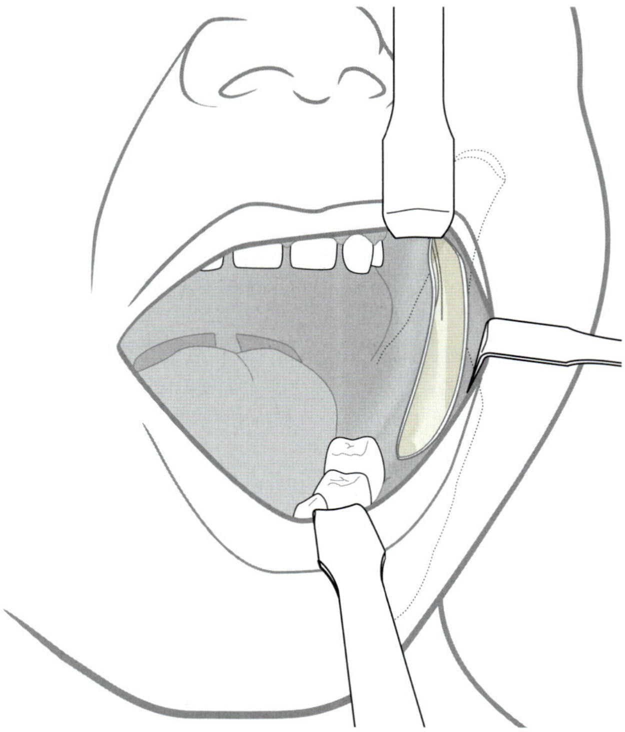

Fig 4.5-24 Transoral approach to the angle and ramus of the mandible.

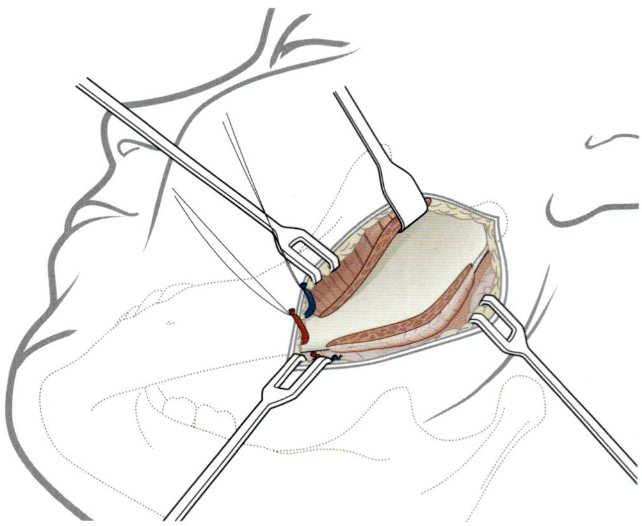

Fig 4.5-25 The angle and ramus of the mandible exposed from an external submandibular skin approach.

The surgical guide is positioned and stabilized with a screw (**Fig 4.5-26**). The holes for the distractor screws are drilled and the osteotomy line marked on the bone. The guide is removed and the osteotomy completed with a saw and osteotome.

The distractor is placed and a small submandibular incision is required to exteriorize the activation rod (**Fig 4.5-27**). If an external skin approach has been used, a separate skin incision for the distractor emergence is usually better esthetically than bringing it through the skin approach. The distractor is stabilized in position using screws in the previously made screw holes. The distractor is activated to ensure that it is working properly and is then deactivated (returned to starting position). The wounds are then closed with a dressing applied to the external port.

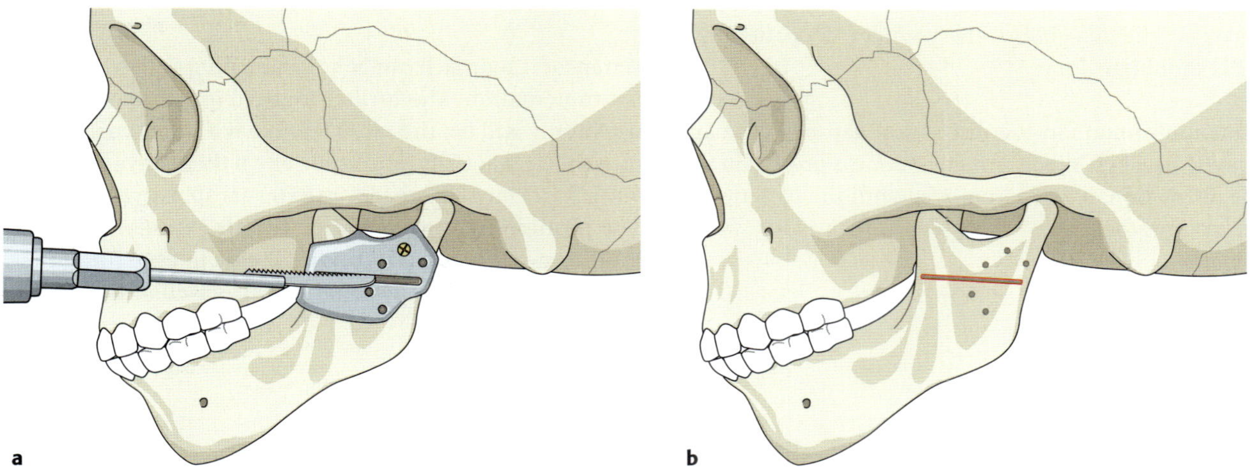

Fig 4.5-26a–b The guide fixed in position with a screw and the osteotomy cut being made with a saw. A reciprocating saw is shown, which is ideal for an oral (anterior) approach. For an external submandibular approach, an oscillating saw is preferable. After removal of the guide the osteotomy is completed.

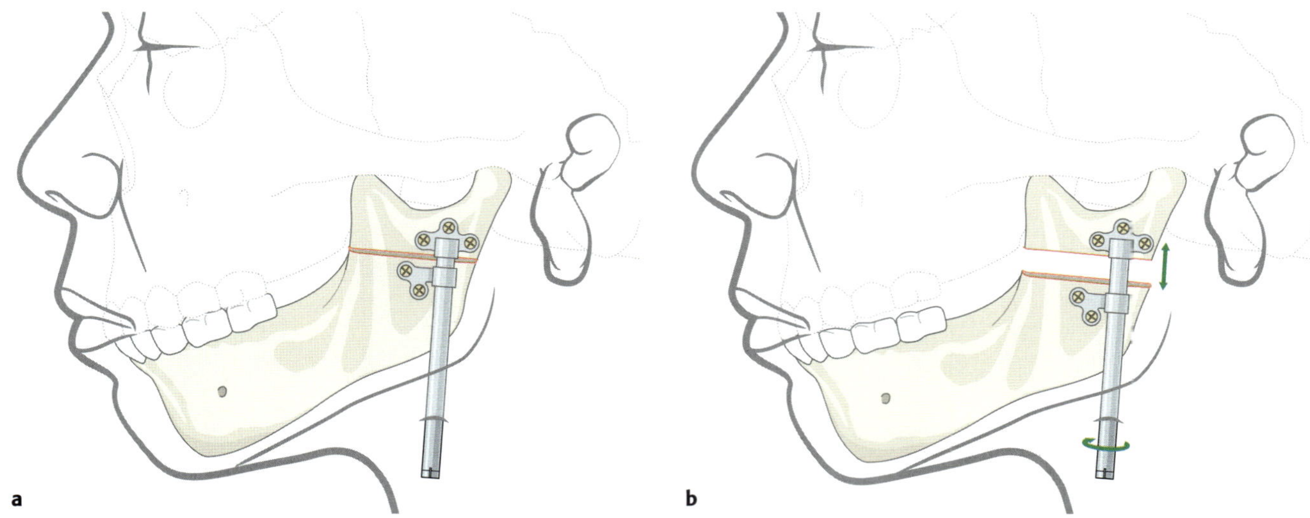

Fig 4.5-27a–b The distractor placed, fixed, and activated.

After a suitable latency period (3–5 days), the ramus is distracted usually at a rate of 1.0 mm per day and generally by the parents (**Fig 4.5-28**). Weekly review of the patient is required until the planned distraction has been achieved. The device is then left in place to retain the distraction and to allow for bone consolidation.

It is valuable to check periodically with radiographs that distraction is progressing well. An occasional PA mandible view or OPT will confirm that the distraction gap is opening and later that bone infill is taking place. It is useful to slightly overcorrect the deformity—the younger the patient the more this should be done.

Consolidation of bone in the distraction gap will take approximately 8 weeks. When sufficient bone is present in the gap, the distraction device is removed with the patient under general anesthesia.

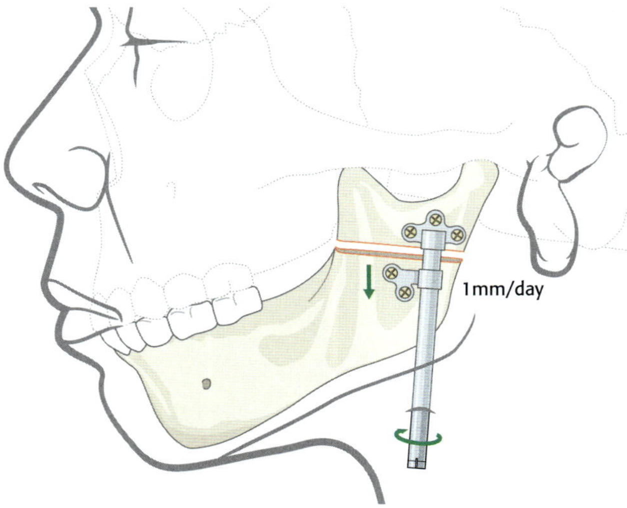

Fig 4.5-28 Distractor now in place and being activated at 1 mm per day.

9 Mandibular advancement by distraction osteogenesis

If mandibular advancement is necessary in the growing child, it is best to use distraction osteogenesis. The amount of mandibular advancement is rarely symmetric, especially in patients with HFM. However, it is generally necessary to perform bilateral distraction. The approach depends on the age of the child, the severity of the deformity, and the part of the mandible in which the distraction is going to be performed.

A transoral approach can be supplemented with transbuccal instrumentation. The further forward in the mandible the osteotomy will be, the more feasible is a pure transoral approach. Occasionally, and especially if there have been previous facial incisions made, an external approach is chosen. The positioning of the incision for an external approach must respect the natural (future) crease lines of the patient and the branches of the facial nerve as well as the area to be exposed.

9.1 Planning

Planning is carried out in virtual reality on a 3-D CT scan (**Fig 4.5-29**) using appropriate software. Semi-submerged distractors are generally preferred as described above especially when the barrel and activation rod/port exit either into the oral cavity or externally through the skin posteriorly.

The virtual distractors are selected and virtually placed on the left and right mandibular body (**Fig 4.5-30**). The virtual osteotomies are marked and completed. The distractors are virtually activated (**Fig 4.5-31**). If the movement is not satisfactory, the virtual distractor positions can be adjusted until the desired vector is achieved.

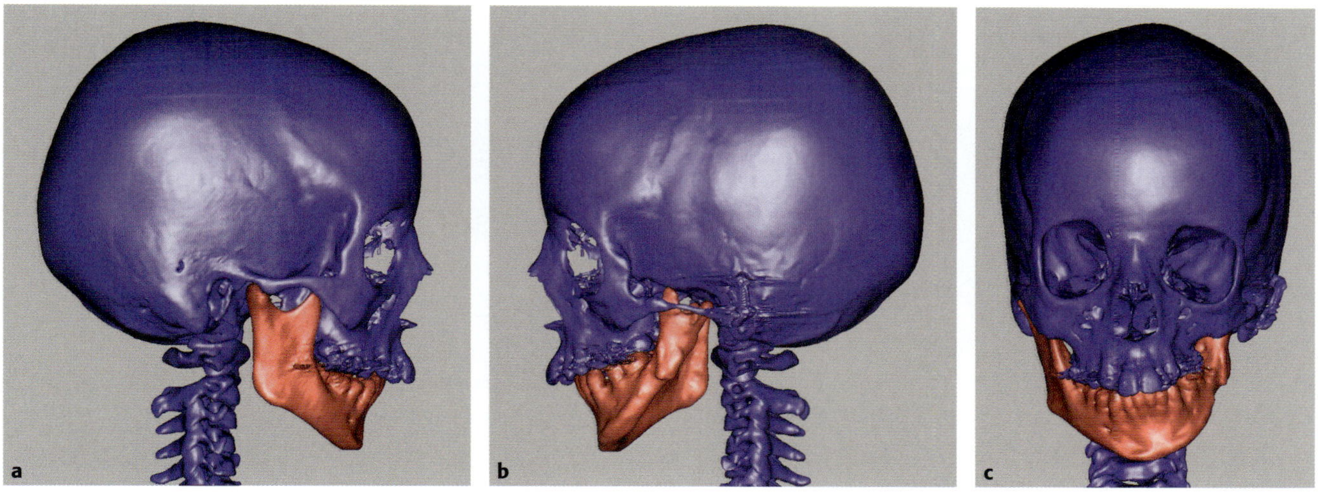

Fig 4.5-29a–c Virtual models from 3-D CT scans showing a patient with hemifacial microsomia on the left side and significant mandibular retrognathia and asymmetry.

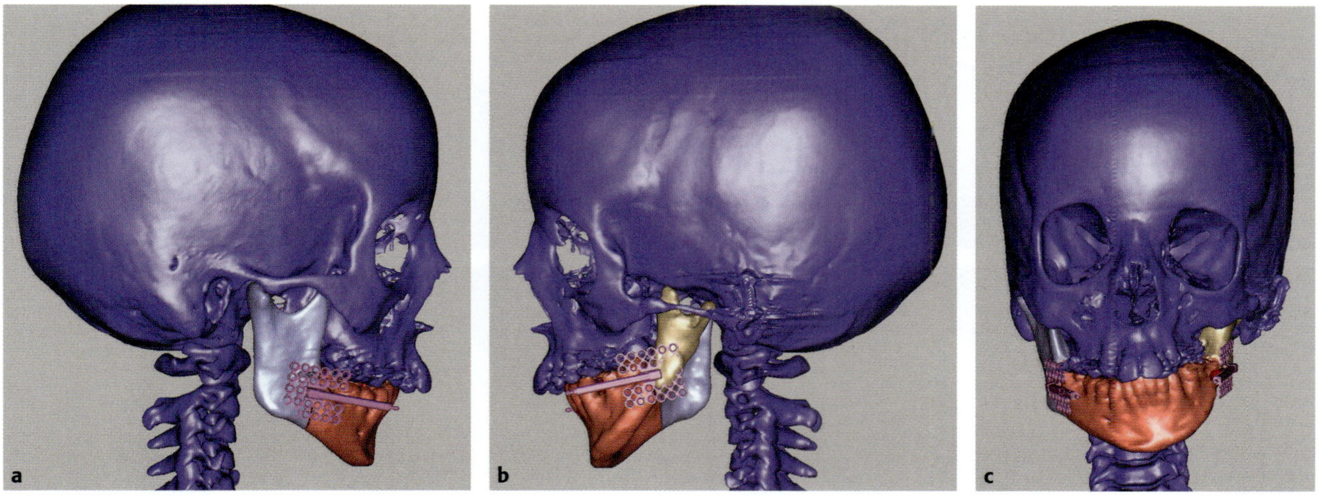

Fig 4.5-30a–c Placement of virtual distractors on virtual models on a computer screen in preparation for distraction osteogenesis.

A virtual guide can then be manufactured (**Fig 4.5-23**). Alternatively, a physical model of the mandible can be produced using stereolithography (**Fig 4.5-32**). The distractors are adapted to the mandible in the planned positions. Guides are constructed that allow the accurate positioning of the distractors and the osteotomies. Intraoperative navigation can achieve a similar result. Consequently, the distractors and the distraction vector should be exactly as planned.

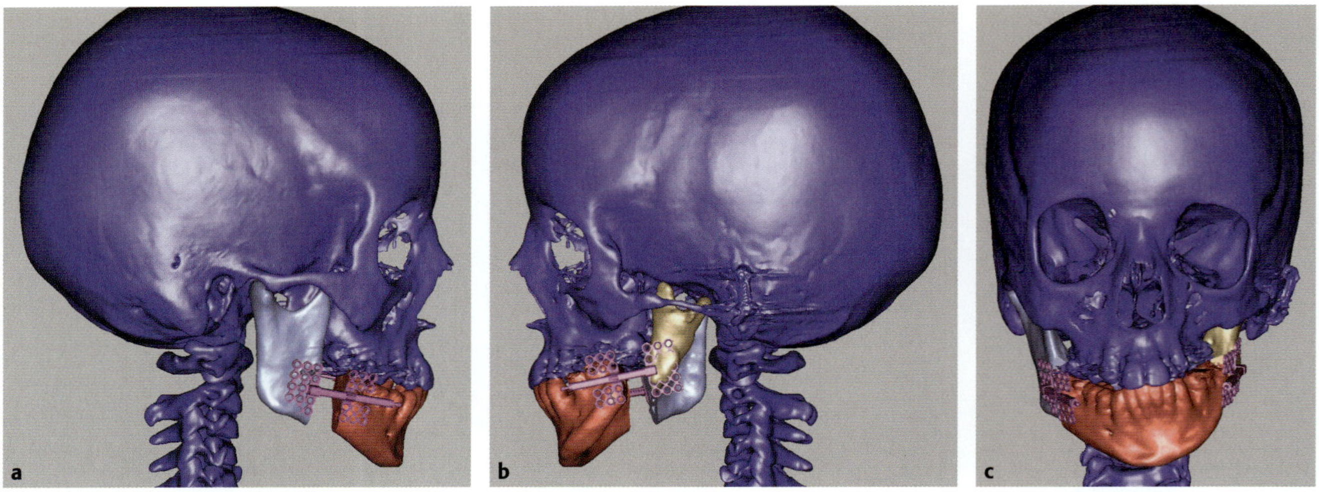

Fig 4.5-31a–c The virtual distractors are activated on the virtual model to simulate advancement of the mandible.

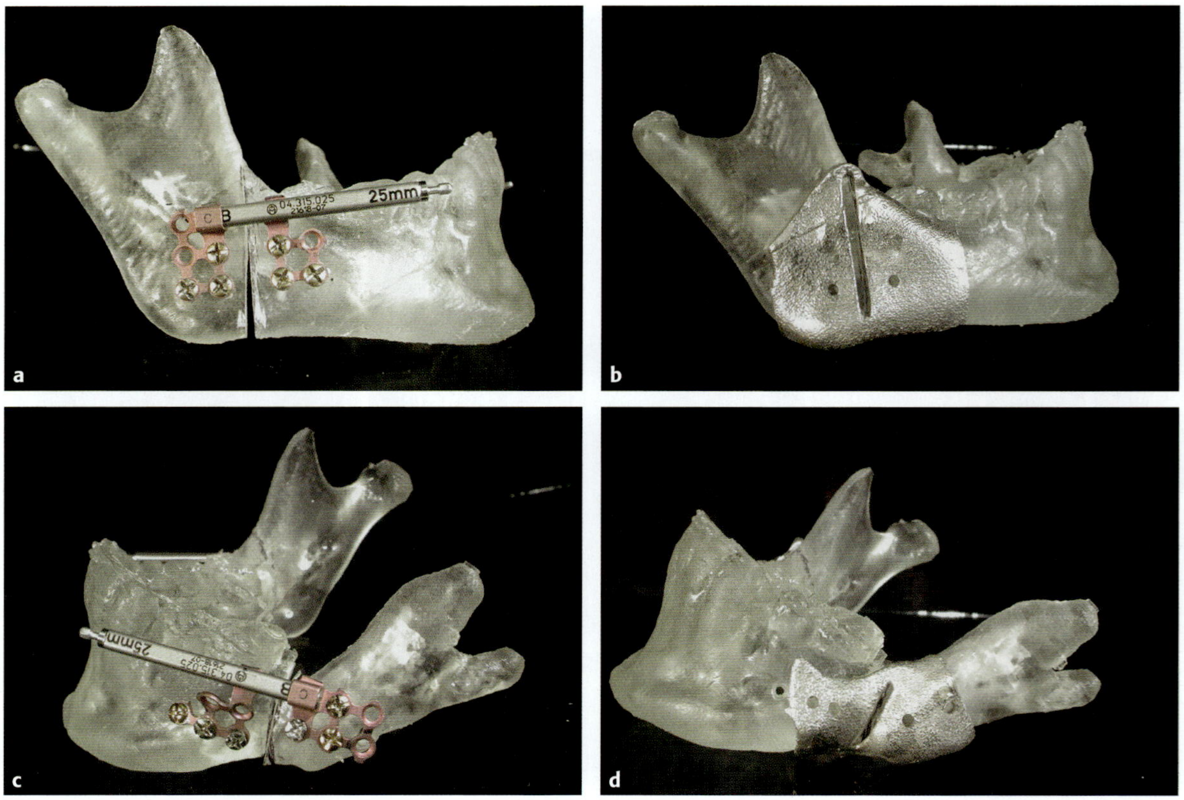

Fig 4.5-32a–d Physical 3-D printed stereolithographic model of the mandible showing guides and distractor positioning.

9.2 Osteotomies and placement of distractors

The surgical guides are positioned and stabilized with at least one screw (**Fig 4.5-33**).

The holes for the distractor screws are drilled and the osteotomy lines marked on the bone. The guides are then removed. The osteotomies are completed through the outer cortex. Fine osteotomes are then used to complete the osteotomies avoiding the area of the inferior alveolar nerve. Twisting an osteotome in the osteotomy (a Smillie menisectomy knife is ideal for this purpose) is performed to assure complete mobilization. The distractors are then placed using the predrilled screw holes. The distractor is activated to ensure that it is working properly and is then deactivated (returned to the starting position) (**Fig 4.5-34**).

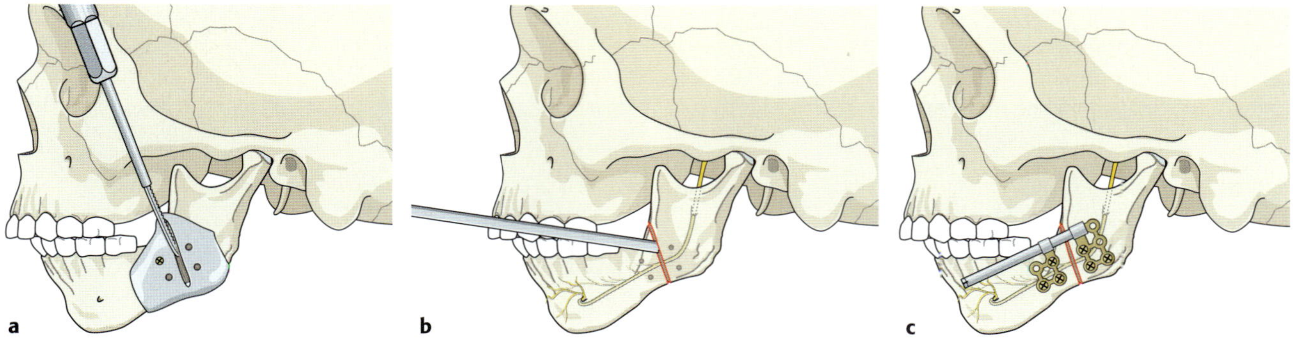

Fig 4.5-33a–c Guide in position, screw holes drilled, osteotomy cut made, and distractors positioned and fixed.

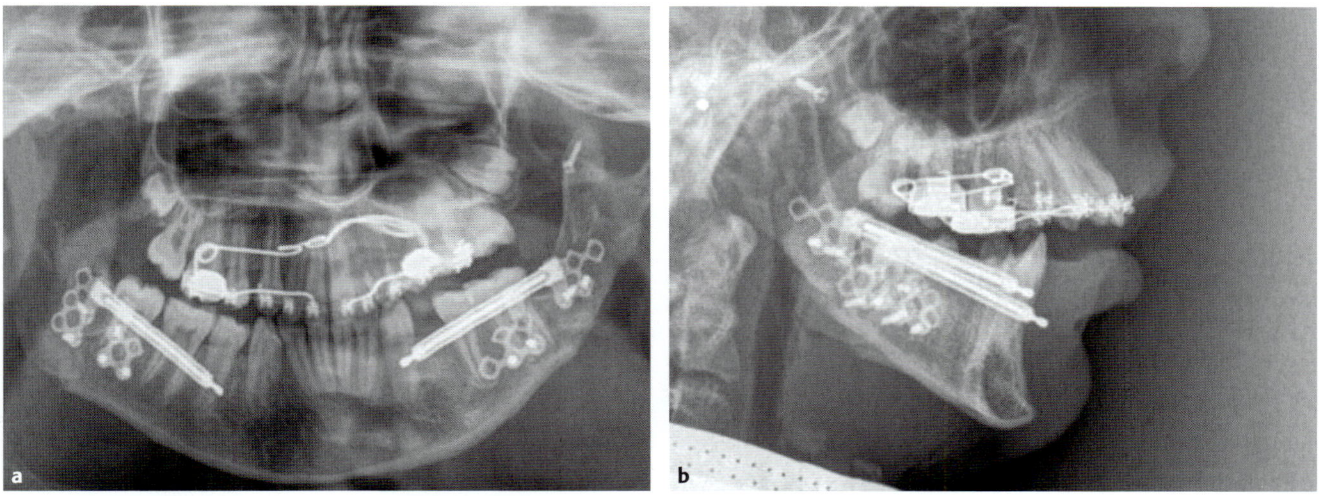

Fig 4.5-34a–b Radiographs showing distractors in position before commencing distraction.

9.3 Distraction

After a suitable latency period, the ramus is distracted daily by the parents with weekly review by the surgeon until the required distraction has been achieved. Occasional plain radiographs are taken to check progress. It is useful to slightly overcorrect the deformity—the younger the patient the more this should be done. The device is then left in place to retain the distraction and to allow for bone consolidation which will take approximately 8 weeks and the regeneration of bone into the distraction gap can also be verified with radiographs (**Fig 4.5-35**).

When sufficient bone is present in the gap, the distractors are removed. Precise positioning of the occlusion can be carried out using fixed orthodontic appliances and mandibulomaxillary elastics.

The radiograph (**Fig 4.5-36**) shows bone formation after removal of the distractors. The lateral radiographs of the face in (**Fig 4.5-34** and **Fig 4.5-36**) demonstrate the mandibular advancement achieved.

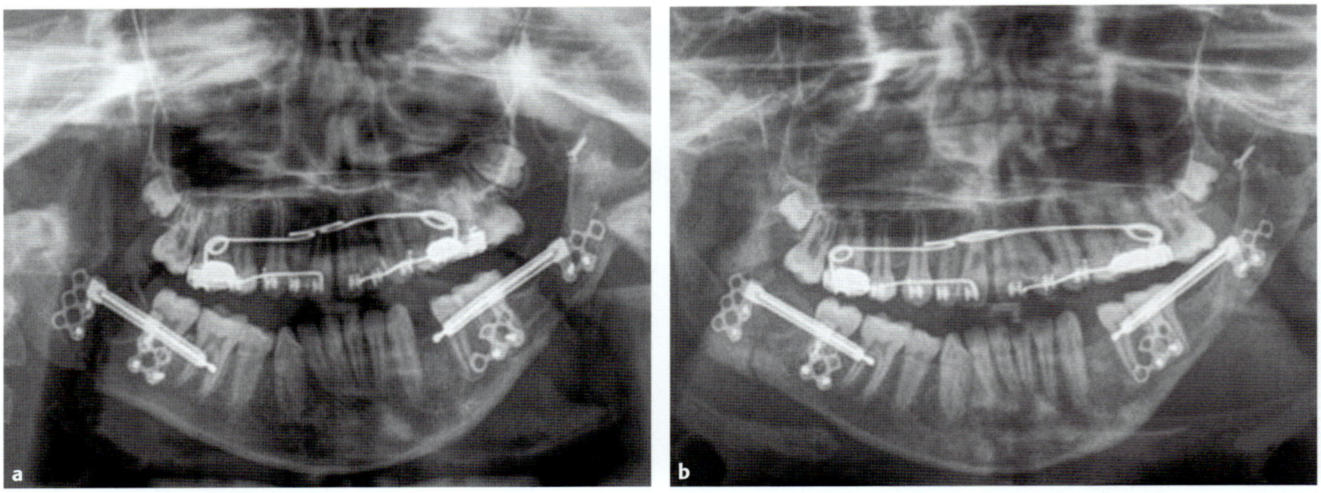

Fig 4.5-35a–b Radiographs showing during (**a**) and at the end of distraction and consolidation (**b**).

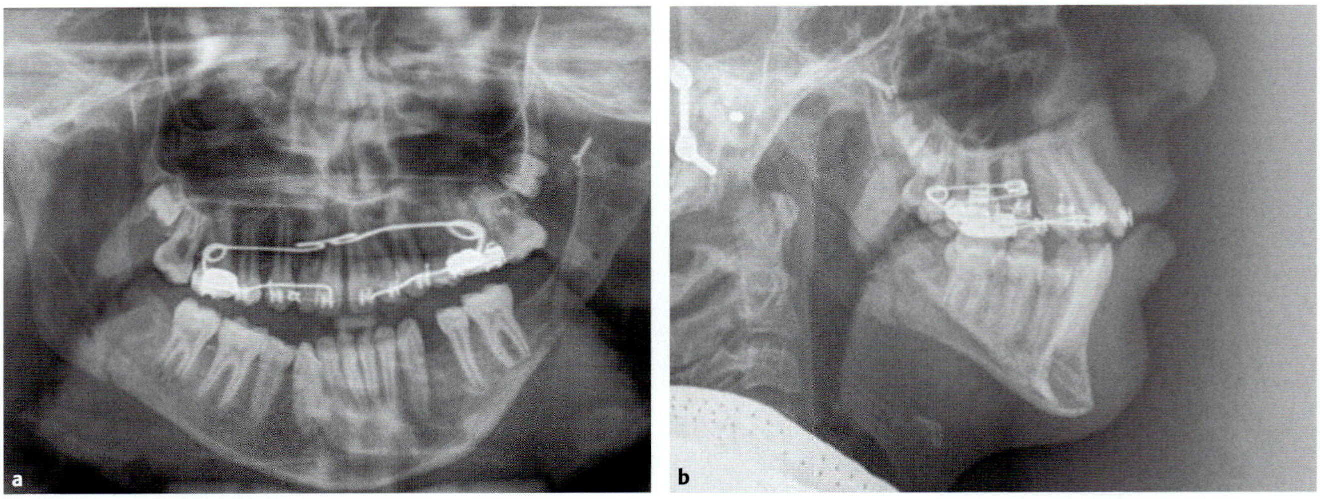

Fig 4.5-36a–b Radiographs taken after removal of the distractors.

We have occasionally encountered bilateral HFM cases which are asymmetrical but with bilaterally small rami, anteroposterior mandibular deficiency, and an anterior open bite. Correction of such deformities is analogous to the treatment of the mandibular deformity of Treacher Collins syndrome. Advancement of the mandibular body alone does not address the short rami or the anterior open bite. The rami can be lengthened by DO and then the distractors removed a little early and the "regenerate" bone bent to close the anterior open bite (at surgery and midway during the consolidation phase) and the jaws held in mandibulomaxillary fixation for a period (**Fig 4.5-37**).

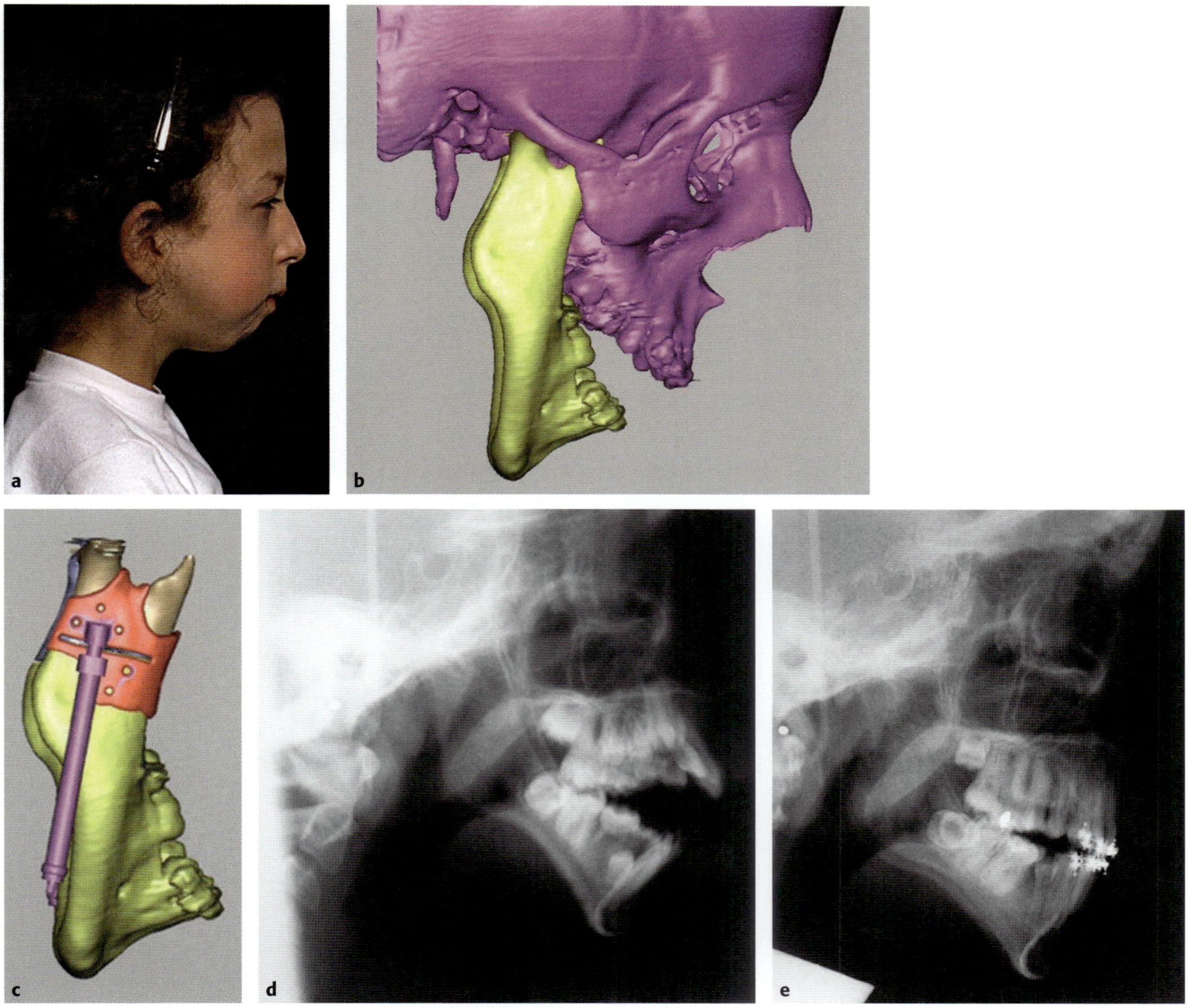

Fig 4.5-37a–e Lengthening of the mandibular rami bilaterally and then closing of the anterior open bite by bending the regenerate.
a–b Situation before lengthening of the ascending ramus.
c–d Vertical lengthening of the ascending ramus.
e Situation after bending the regenerate.

However, an alternative (and arguably better) approach is offered by curvilinear DO bilaterally which lengthens the rami, advances the body and closes the anterior open bite. It is highly desirable to plan such procedures in 3-D (**Fig 4.5-38**) to ensure the correct choice and positioning of these distractors.

10 Ear construction

In HFM, ear deformity is common varying from a nearly normal ear to complete anotia (**Fig 4.5-39**).

10.1 Autogenous ear construction

In anotia or severe microtia, total autogenous ear construction using carved cartilage may be indicated. This is typically performed at 8 years or older but some experienced surgeons believe that better results can be obtained if surgery is delayed until the child is 10–12 years old.

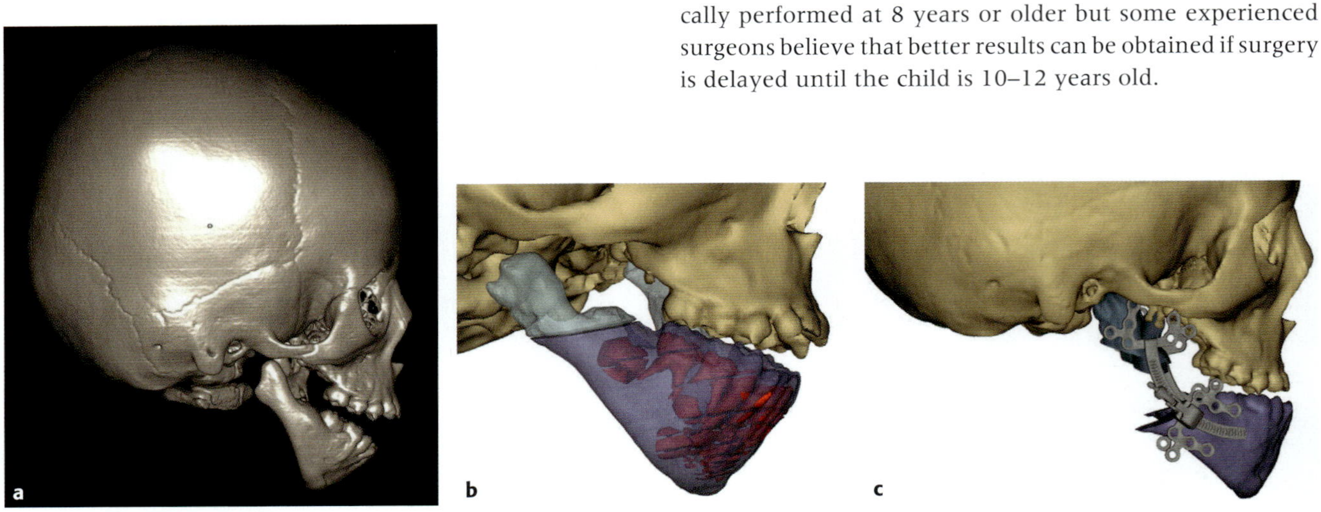

Fig 4.5-38a–c Planning on a virtual model of bilateral curvilinear distraction of the mandible.

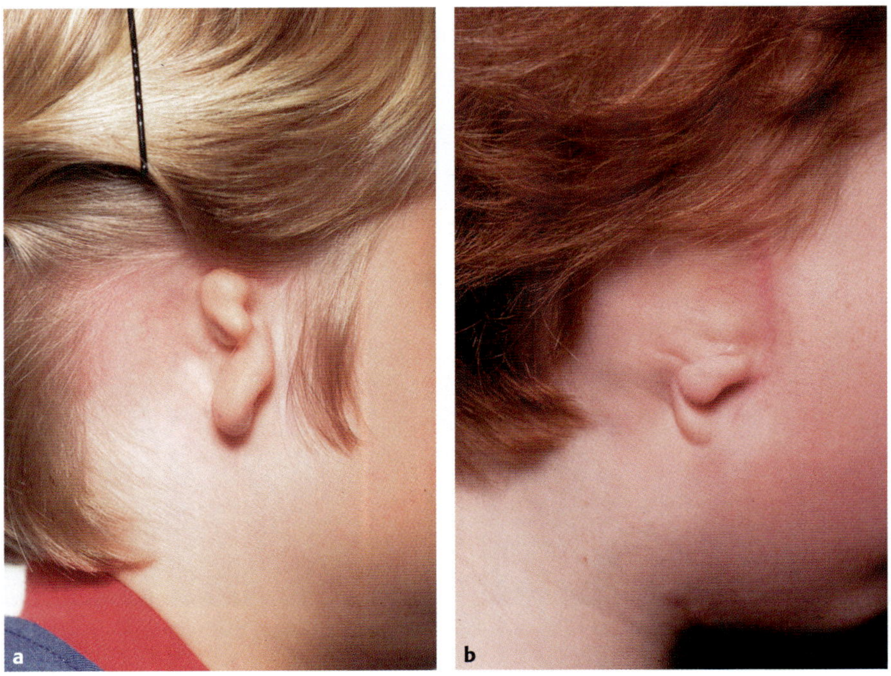

Fig 4.5-39a–b Typical different microtic ears.

A template is traced of the unaffected ear using clear plastic film (**Fig 4.5-40a**). The template is reversed and positioned on the affected side in the most satisfactory position based on the opposite side ear position, the hair line, and the microtic remnants which may be used to construct the ear lobe (**Fig 4.5-40b**). Costal cartilage is harvested from ribs 6–10 (**Fig 4.5-40c**). The cartilage framework is carved to include the base and helical rim (**Fig 4.5-40d**). The recipient site is prepared by undermining the skin with or without transposition of the lobe (**Fig 4.5-40e**). The cartilage construct is placed subcutaneously together with suction drain (**Fig 4.5-40f**).

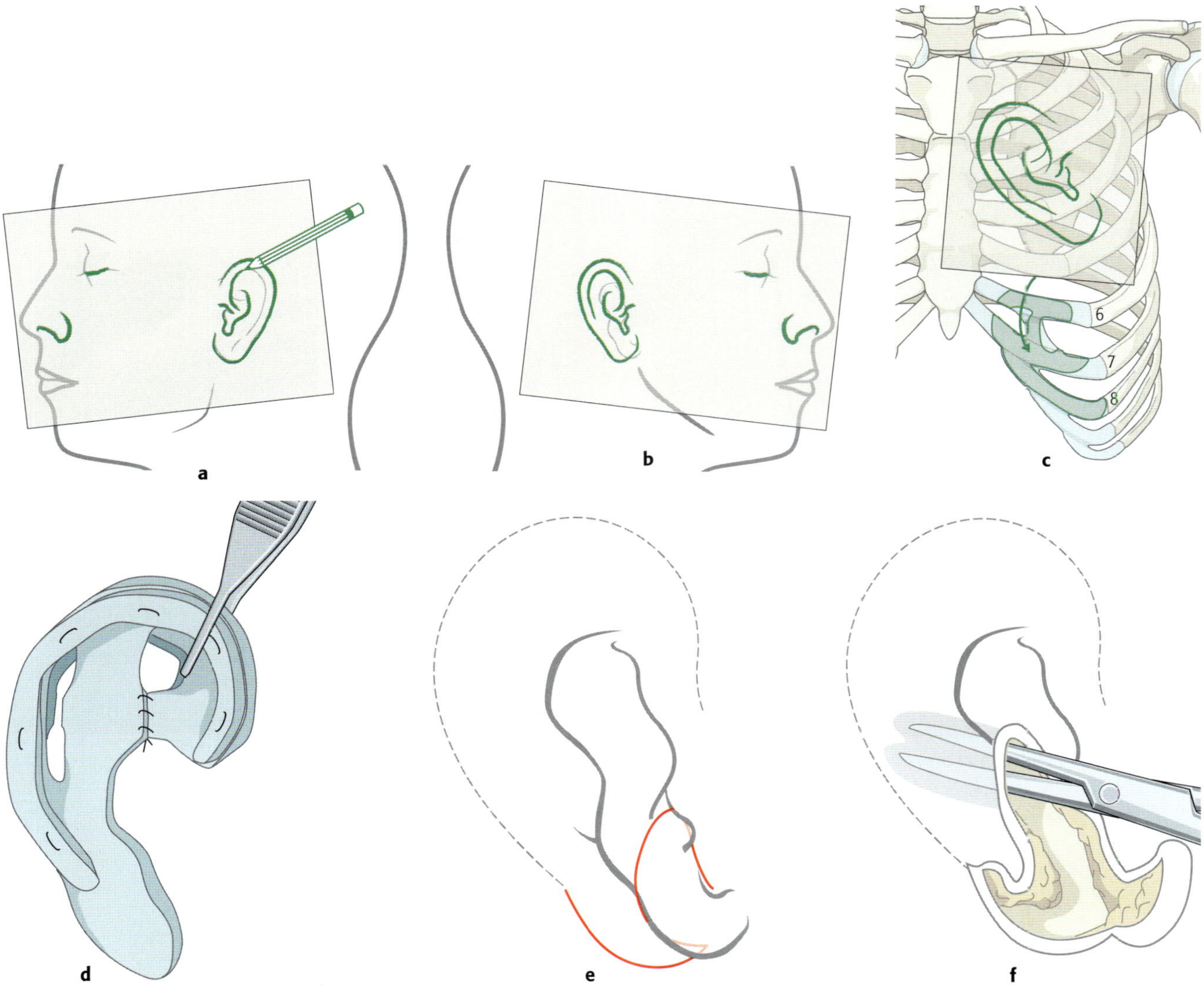

Fig 4.5-40a–f Planning of autogenous external ear construction and preparation of cartilaginous framework.

After stage one healing is complete (**Fig 4.5-41a**), and if the lobule has been moved in stage one, the ear is elevated and additional cartilage is used to project the ear. This creates a soft-tissue deficiency which is closed with a turnover mastoid flap or temporal parietal flap and a skin graft (**Fig 4.5-41b**). Additional soft-tissue rearrangements are performed in the lobule area if needed (**Fig 4.5-41c**).

10.2 Bone anchored ear prosthesis

The management of microtia in HFM is complicated by the need for reconstructive surgery for the surrounding facial anomalies. It is, therefore, sometimes difficult to decide which to do first. There is no clear rule. Often the decision will be made according to the individual case and the wishes of the parents and child.

The microtic ear in HFM is commonly in an abnormal position. In general, this can be managed by the excision of such remnants usually with primary repair and the construction of a prosthetic ear in an ideal position relative to the contralateral unaffected side. Sometimes attention should be given to the augmentation of the surrounding soft tissues to achieve a good result. The presence of a malpositioned ear canal makes prosthetic rehabilitation much more difficult and needs to be managed in consultation with and with the assistance of the relevant CMF surgeon.

10.2.1 Planning for a bone anchored ear prosthesis

The ideal position for titanium implants in relation to the prosthetic ear is seen in **Fig 4.5-42**. Two options are described for planning the procedure.

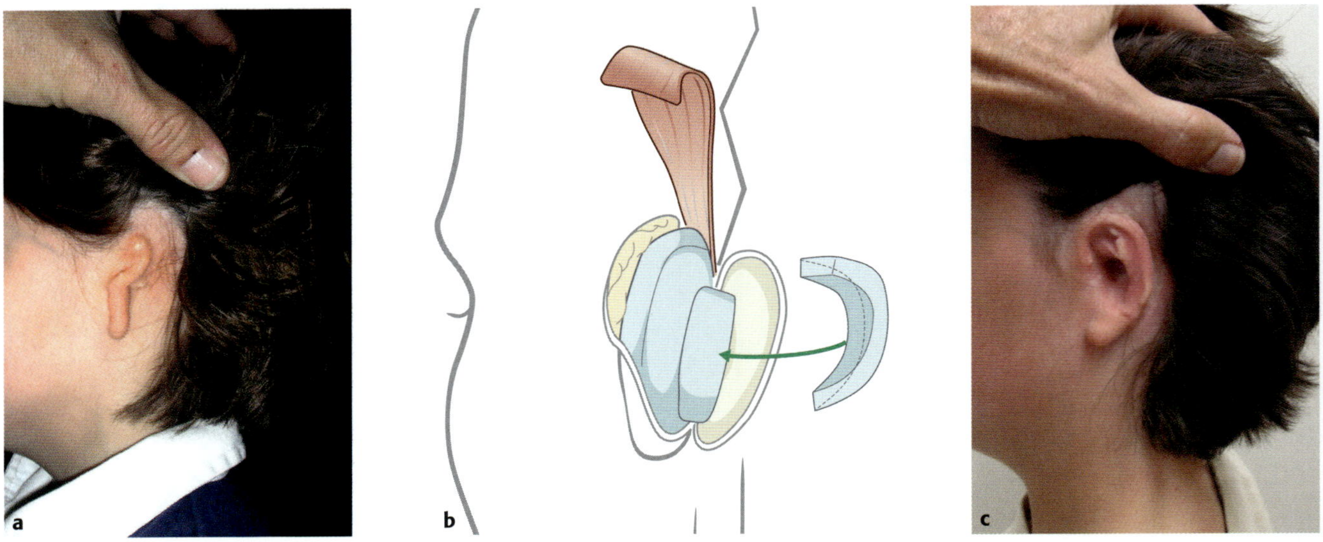

Fig 4.5-41a–c Projection of the ear construction and clinical outcome.

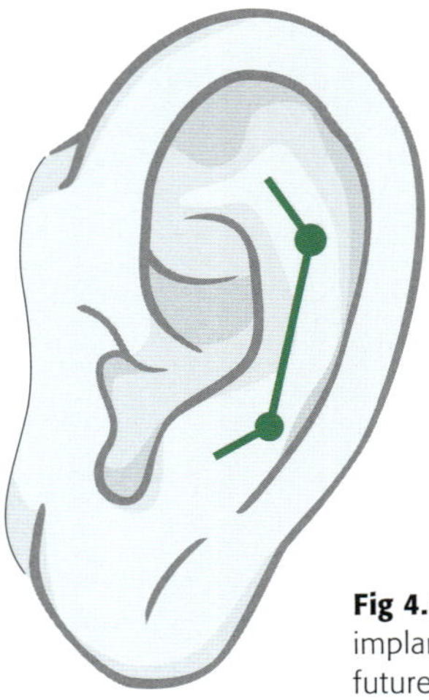

Fig 4.5-42 Ideal position of implants and bar relative to the future prosthesis.

10.2.2 Conventional noncomputerized planning

An impression is taken with dental impression material of the unaffected ear and a plaster model made. A wax ear is sculpted as a mirror image of the ear model. Holes are made in the wax ear in the ideal position for the placement of two implants. The ear is positioned on the affected side and moved around until its position is ideal and symmetric (**Fig 4.5-43a–c**). The ideal sites for implant placement are marked on the skin with a pen using the wax template (this works well provided those sites also have sufficient bone) (**Fig 4.5-43d**). An impression is made of the affected side, a plaster model made and the implant positions marked on that model. A plastic template (surgical drilling guide) is made on the model for use at the time of surgery (**Fig 4.5-43e**). After implant placement and osseointegration, the implants are uncovered in a second stage surgery, approximately 4 months after placement. Impressions are made and a bar is constructed to retain the ear prosthesis (**Fig 4.5-43e–g**).

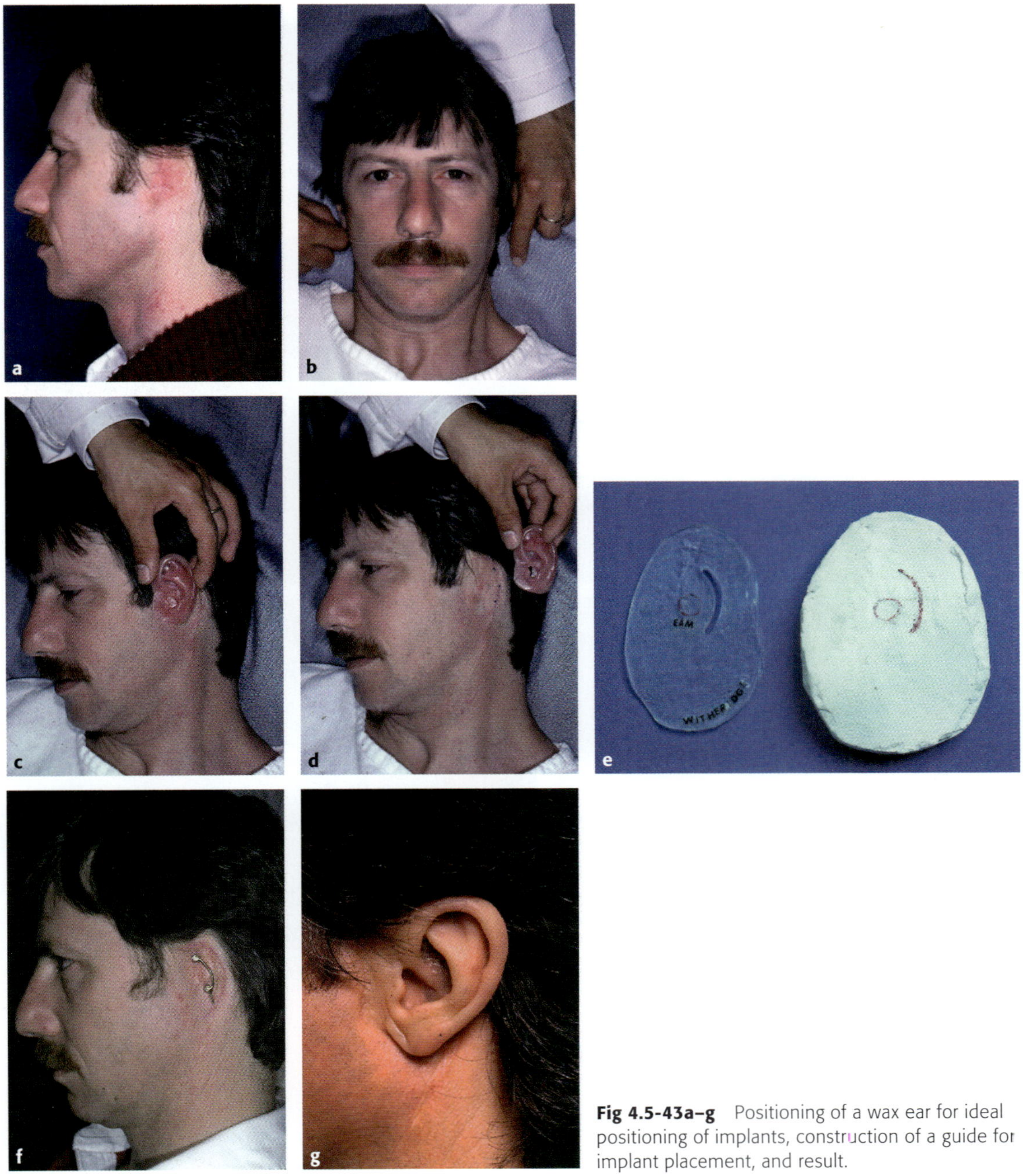

Fig 4.5-43a–g Positioning of a wax ear for ideal positioning of implants, construction of a guide for implant placement, and result.

10.2.3 Digital computed planning

A high-definition CT scan is obtained of the patient's whole head and face including both hard and soft tissues in three planes as well as 3-D (**Fig 4.5-44a–f**). Planning is then carried out using computer-assisted planning software using the following steps:

Step 1: A mirror image of the unaffected ear is produced (**Fig 4.5-44a**).

Step 2: The mirrored ear is overlaid on the affected side and moved until its position is ideal and symmetric (**Fig 4.5-44b–c**).

Step 3: The ideal position for the virtual implants in relation to the mirrored normal ear is noted on the CT scan and the virtual implants are inserted in the 3-D virtual model (**Fig 4.5-44d–f**).

Step 4: The soft-tissues are removed (**Fig 4.5-44g–h**) and a cross-section is made through the implant holes and surrounding bone in the virtual model to check the quantity and quality of the surrounding bone (shown in red) (**Fig 4.5-44i**). If the bone is not of adequate thickness or of poor quality, other implant positions must be considered.

Step 5: When the implant positions and the bone stock around them are acceptable, a template or surgical drilling guide is designed as a bone-borne guide. This is done on the virtual model, and then manufactured by 3-D printing (**Fig 4.5-44j**).

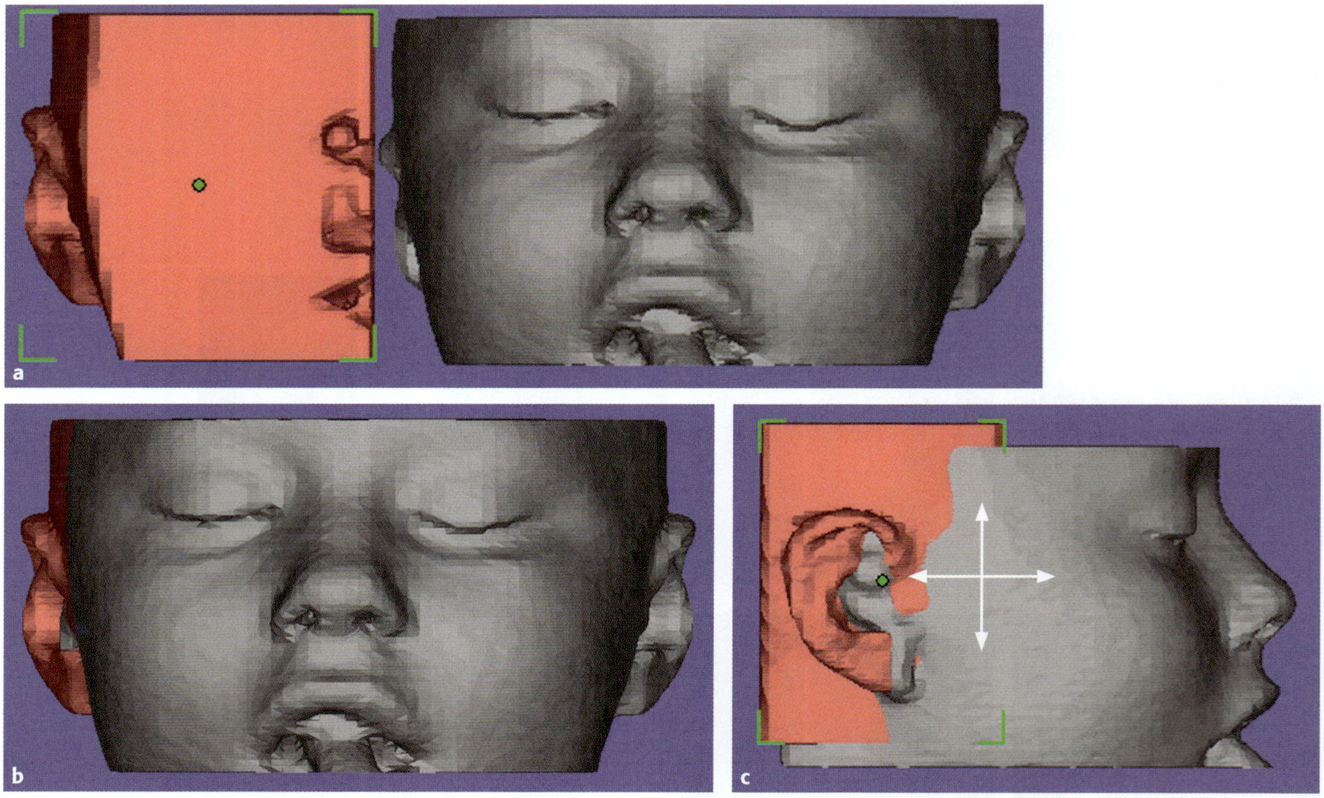

Fig 4.5-44a–j On screen virtual modeling from 3-D CT allowing mirror imaging of the normal ear and selection of the ideal implant sites. A physical guide (bone borne) can then be manufactured by 3-D printing (**j**).

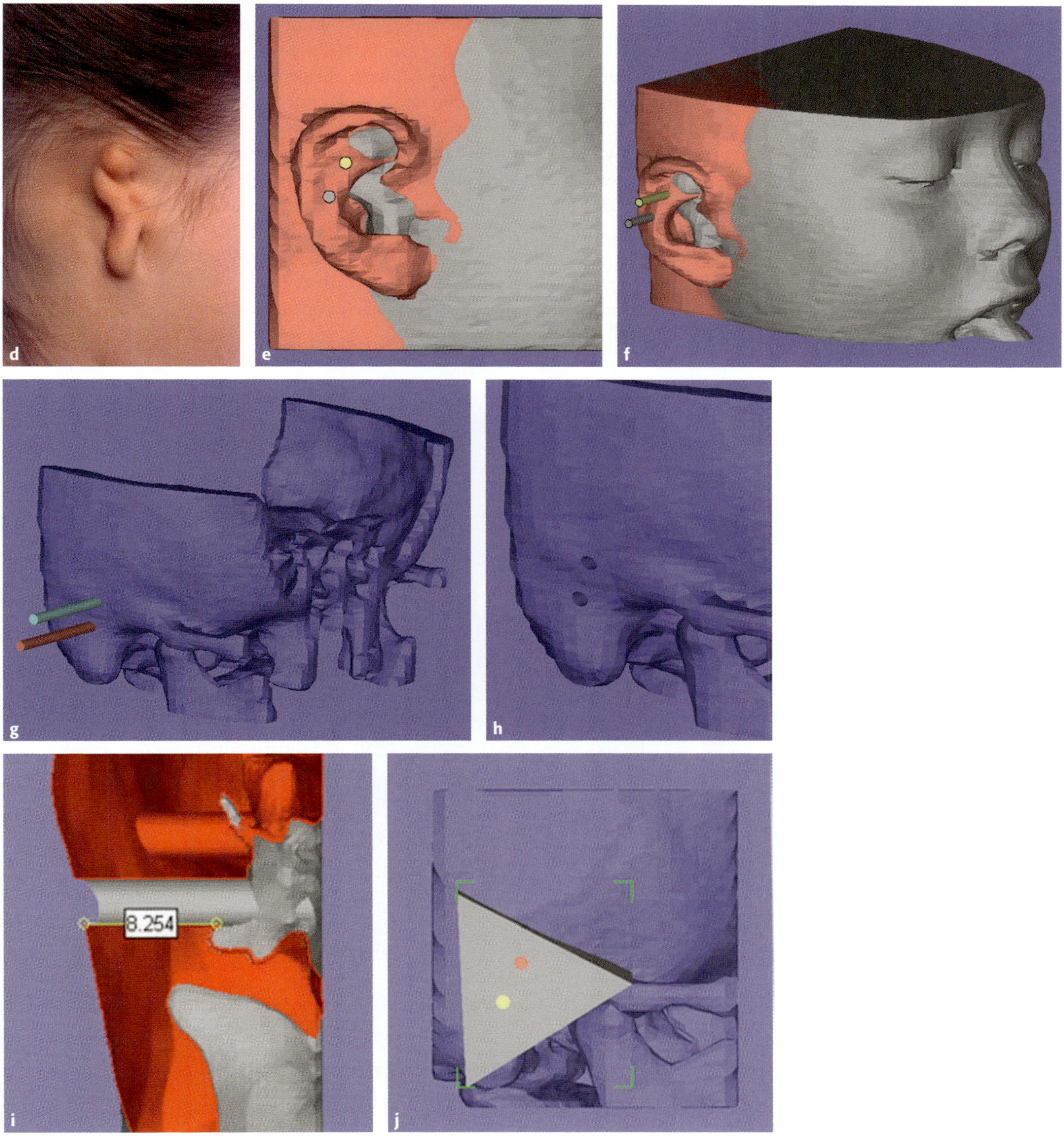

Fig 4.5-44a–j (cont) On screen virtual modeling from 3-D CT allowing mirror imaging of the normal ear and selection of the ideal implant sites. A physical guide (bone borne) can then be manufactured by 3-D printing (**j**).

10.2.4 Surgery

Surgery to insert the implants is performed in two stages in children but generally in one stage in adults. The rationale for this is that the bone in children is soft and immediate loading of the implant should not be attempted. Usually, one should allow 4 months to elapse between the two stages to ensure adequate osseointegration of the implants. The implants used are craniofacial-flanged fixtures which are made of commercially pure titanium.

First stage surgery and one stage surgery

If an external guide is being used, the sites for the implants are marked on the skin and tattooed to the subcutaneous tissue using a long needle and ink. An incision is made through the skin and down to the periosteum posterior to the proposed site of the implant placement. A flap of skin and subcutaneous tissue is raised exposing the underlying periosteum. If a bone-fitting guide has been constructed (**Fig 4.5-45**), this is then placed on the surface of the bone (although sometimes it can be placed over the periosteum instead). The implant sites are marked on the bone with ink. If an external guide has been used, the ink markings are identified. If the periosteum has been left on the bone, a circle of periosteum is excised around each implant site.

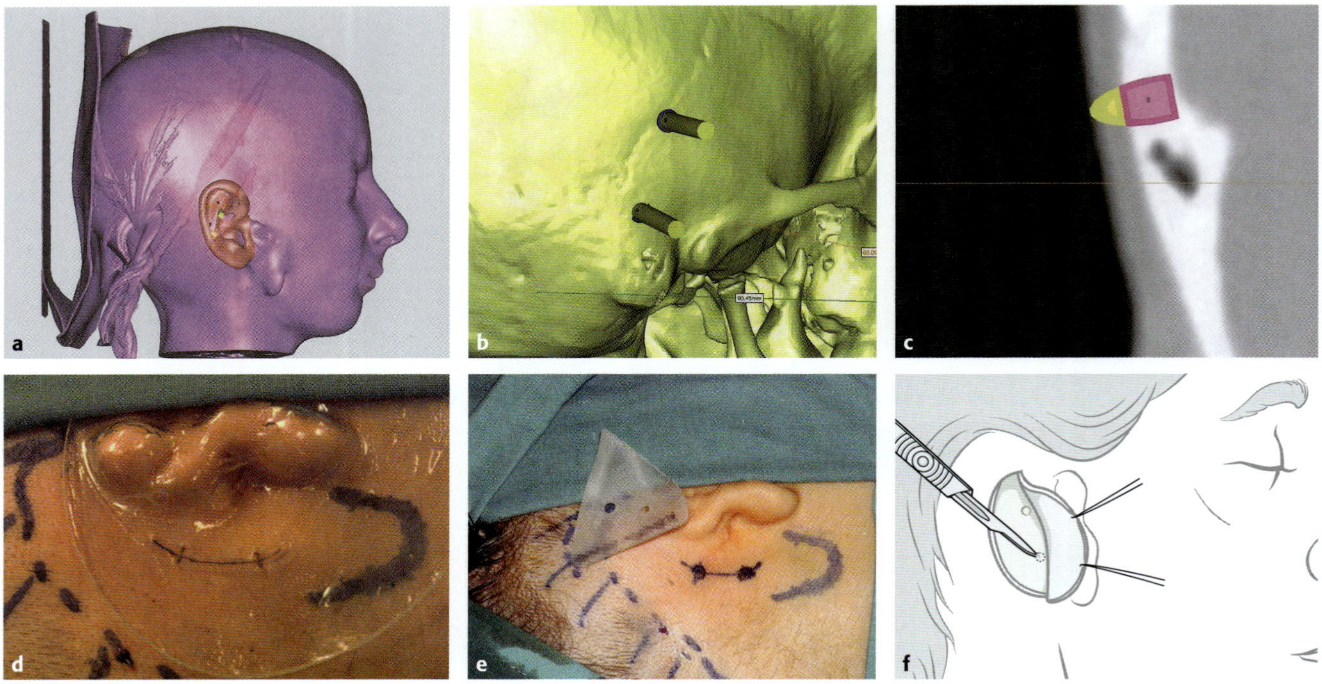

Fig 4.5-45a–f

a Computer planning of a prosthetic ear reconstruction by mirror imaging the ear from the unaffected side to the affected side and defining the position of two bone-anchored implants.
b Previously defined implant positions are marked on the skull.
c Bone thickness at the implant sites is measured and thus the appropriate implant length is selected.
d An implant guide fitting over the soft tissues.
e A guide to fit on the bone.
f For approach a curved incision is made to expose the temporal bone.

The drilling sequence starts with a pilot hole using a round burr (**Fig 4.5-46a**) and is then followed by preparation of the implant cavity (**Fig 4.5-46b**). The bone is prepared using a drill at low speed; chilled saline irrigation is used to minimize the risk of bone injury due to overheating. The flanged fixtures are inserted typically with a torque controlled wrench by hand (**Fig 4.5-46c–d**). Cover screws are placed to avoid tissue ingrowth (**Fig 4.5-46e**).

If a two-stage procedure is performed, the incision is closed in layers and the implants are left to osseointegrate undisturbed for approximately 4 months. Skin tags and/or skin/ear remnants are not normally removed until the second stage.

If a one-stage procedure is performed, the residual ear tags and ear remnants are normally excised. The skin flap is thinned with excision of substantial amounts of subcutaneous tissue to ensure that the skin around the implant abutments is thin and tightly bound to the bone. Abutments are inserted as described below.

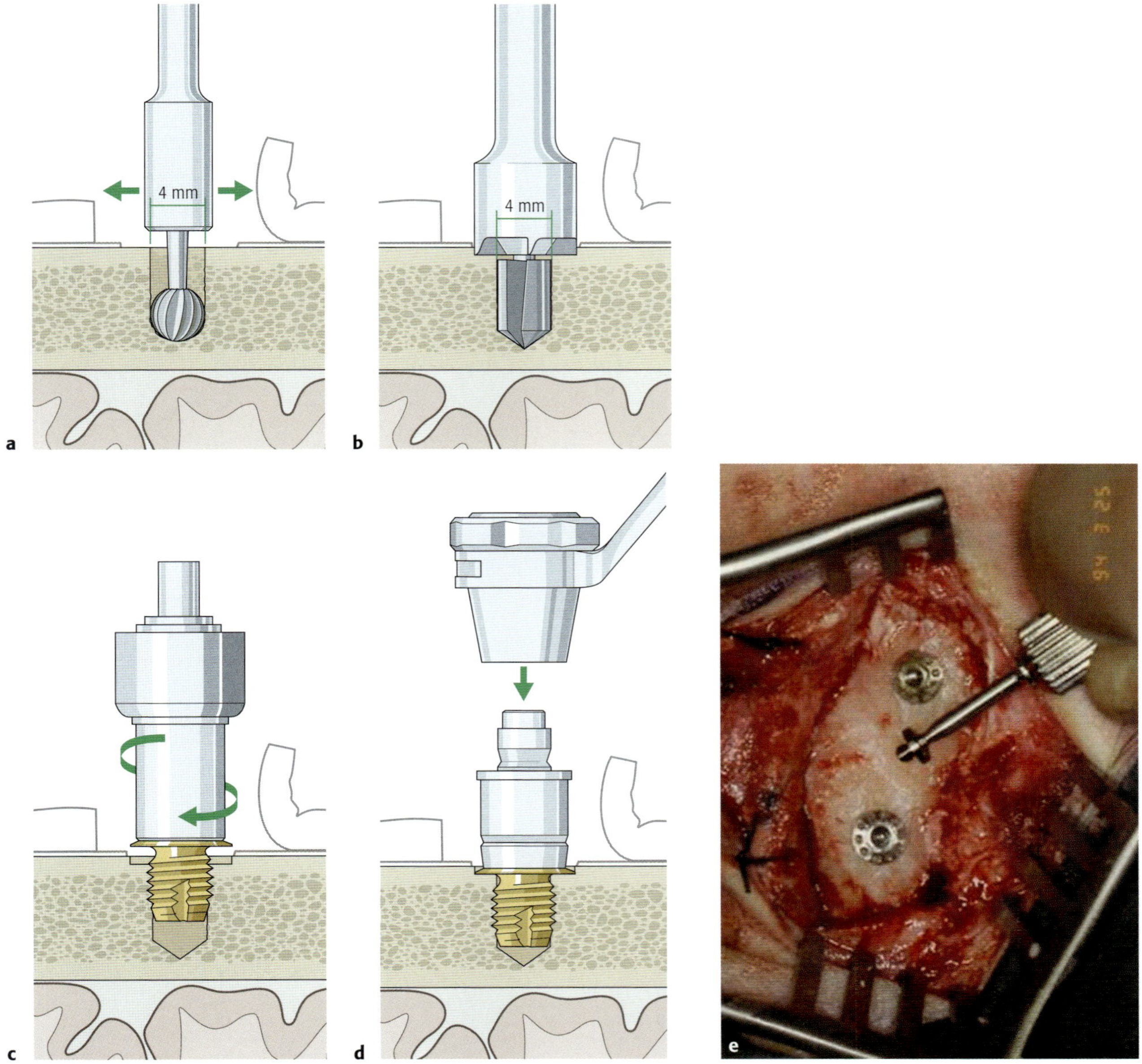

Fig 4.5-46a–e Drill sequence and implant placement.

Second stage surgery

If a two-stage procedure is performed, the ear tags and ear remnants are excised at the second stage (**Fig 4.5-47a**). A skin flap is raised over the site of the implants and the implants are identified and checked for osseointegration (**Fig 4.5-47b**). The cover screws are removed. The skin flap is thinned, replaced and sutured. Thinning out of the skin is important to avoid mobile skin around the implants, which may lead to local complications such as infection. The skin overlaying the implants is removed with a biopsy punch or scalpel. Titanium abutments are screwed into the implants (**Fig 4.5-47c**). It is sometimes preferable to replace the skin and subcutaneous tissues over the implant site with a split skin graft to ensure that the soft tissue covering the implants is thin and bound down to the bone minimizing the risk of chronic inflammation around the fixtures. Healing caps are then screwed into the abutments to help retain the dressing. The standard dressing now consists of ribbon gauze soaked in antibacterial solution wound around the abutments and under the healing caps. When a split skin graft is used, it is better to use multiple layers of Vaseline gauze as a first dressing as this places less pressure on the skin graft; thus, preventing it necrosing. If this is a one-stage procedure, a tie over dressing of flavine wool covers this or alternatively a thick layer of sponge stapled in situ. Dressings are repeated at weekly intervals until the wounds are fully healed and the abutments well exposed (approximately 4 weeks) (**Fig 4.5-47d–e**). The in-surgical sequence for both stages can be seen in **Fig 4.5-48**.

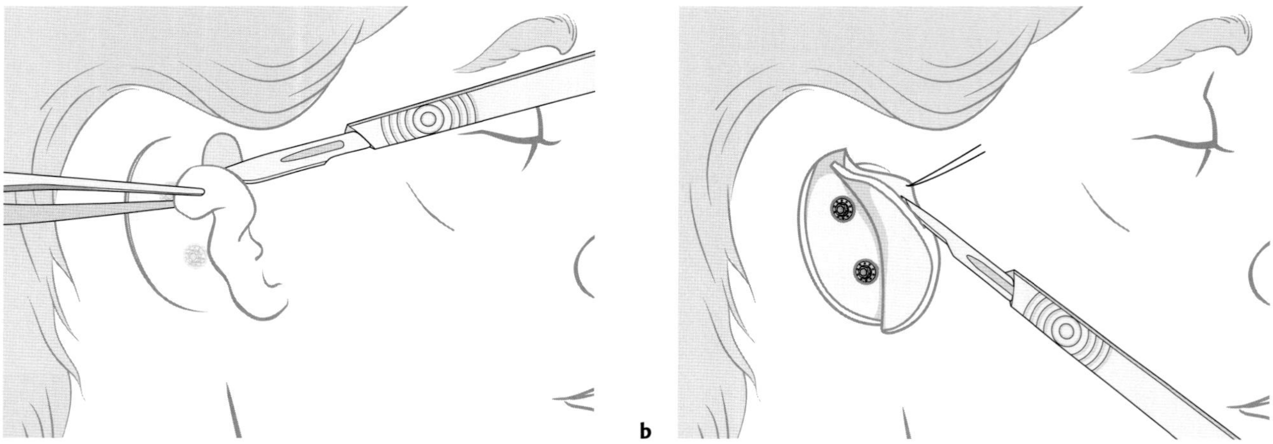

a b

Fig 4.5-47a–e Sequence for second stage removal of ear remnants, thinning of subcutaneous tissue, and placement of abutments.

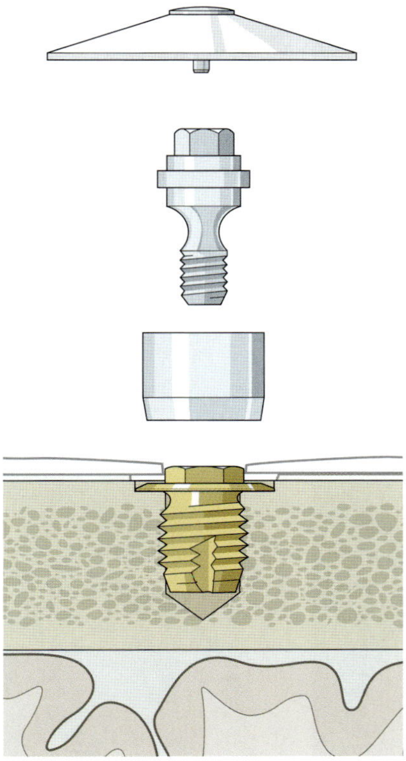

c

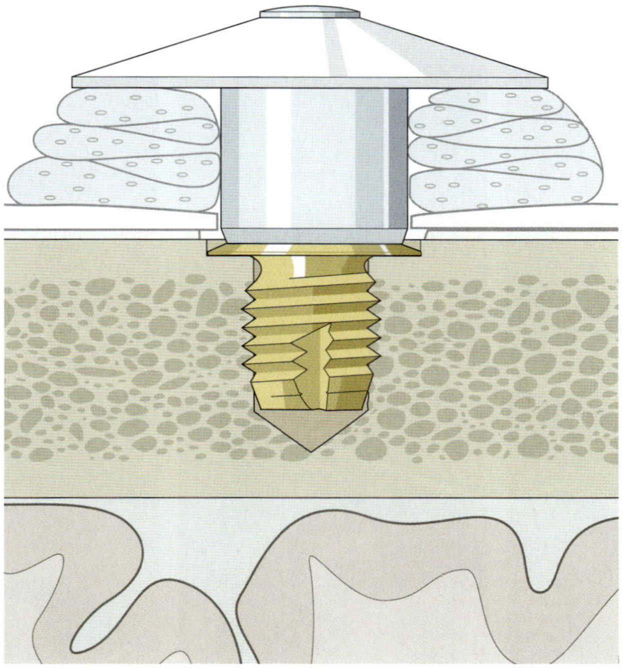

d

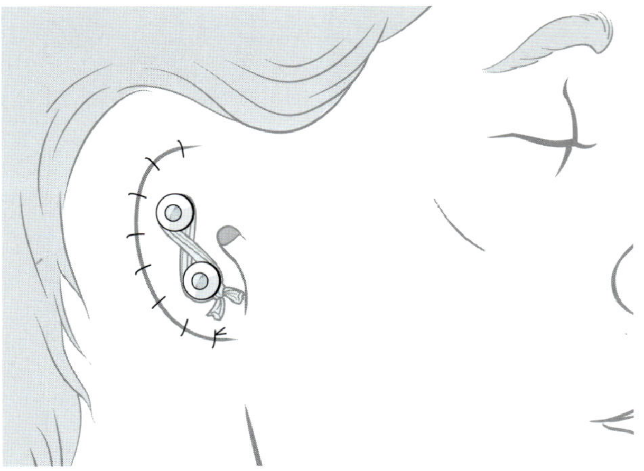

e

Fig 4.5-47a–e (cont) Sequence for second stage removal of ear remnants, thinning of subcutaneous tissue, and placement of abutments.

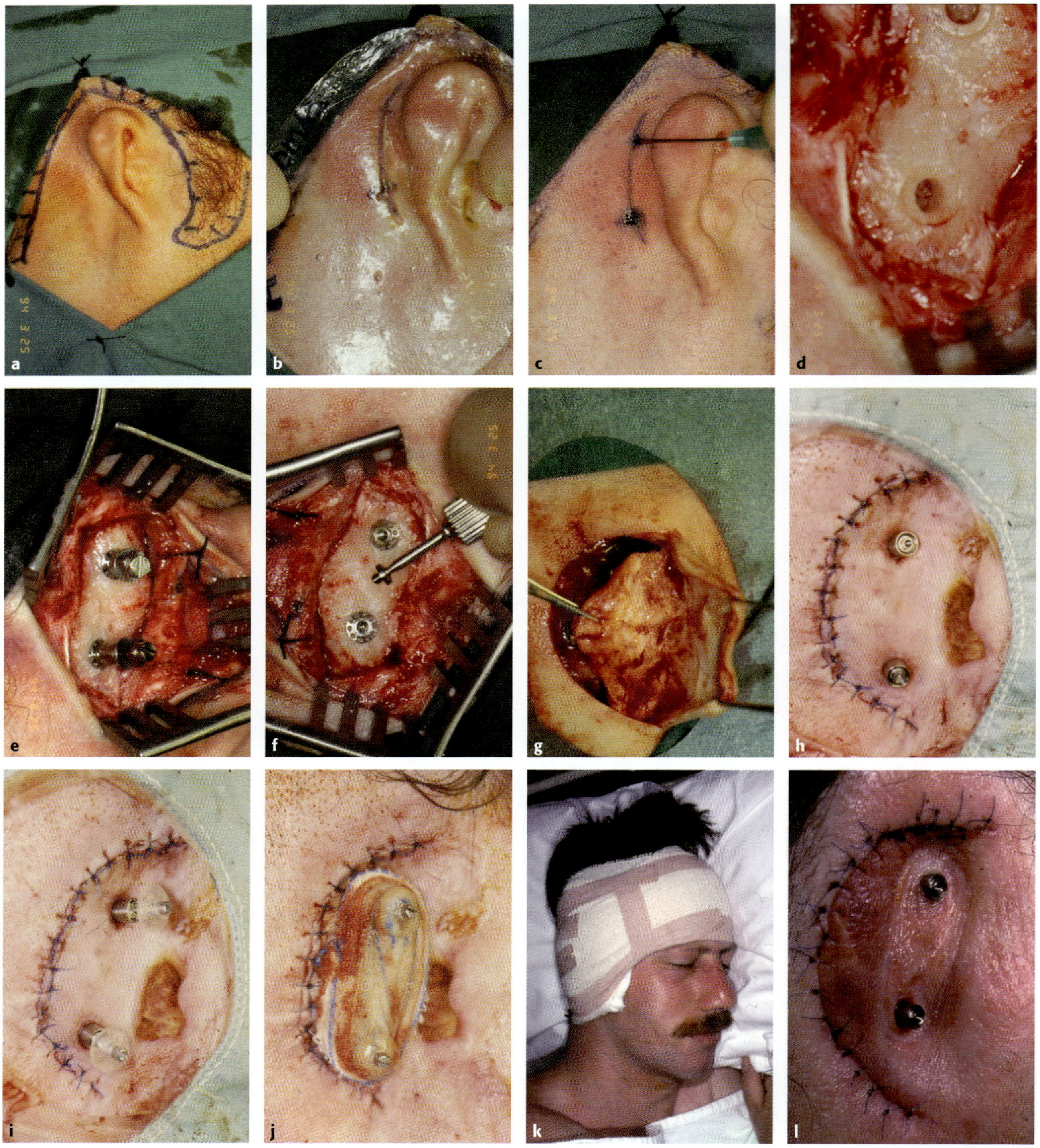

Fig 4.5-48a–l In-surgical sequence, both stages of implant insertion.

10.2.5 Prosthetic construction

Prosthetic treatment usually starts 4–6 weeks after the second (or first) stage. Construction takes 2–3 days and the patient is present while the prosthetist carves, fits and characterizes the prosthesis.

The first stage is to construct a custom-cast gold bar (**Fig 4.5-49a**). The bar is screwed into the abutments with gold screws.

With the bar in place, the next step is construction of the substructure (**Fig 4.5-49b**). This is made from hard plastic and holds the gold clips that attach to the bar. This substructure is bonded into the silicone prosthesis.

The ear prosthesis is initially carved in wax (**Fig 4.5-50a**) to enable adjustments to the shape and fit to be made. With a 3-D virtual digital image of the normal ear (this can be from 3-D photographic data or CT data), a virtual mirror image of that normal ear can be constructed and a wax model produced by rapid prototyping. This then becomes the starting pointing for the hand carving, saving many hours of challenging manual work and improving the accuracy of the anatomical replication.

Once the position and shape are satisfactory, the edge of the wax prosthesis is closely adapted to the patients' skin. The wax pattern is then flasked (**Fig 4.5-50b**) to allow to produce the silicone prosthesis. The flask can be used to produce several duplicates of the prosthesis if needed.

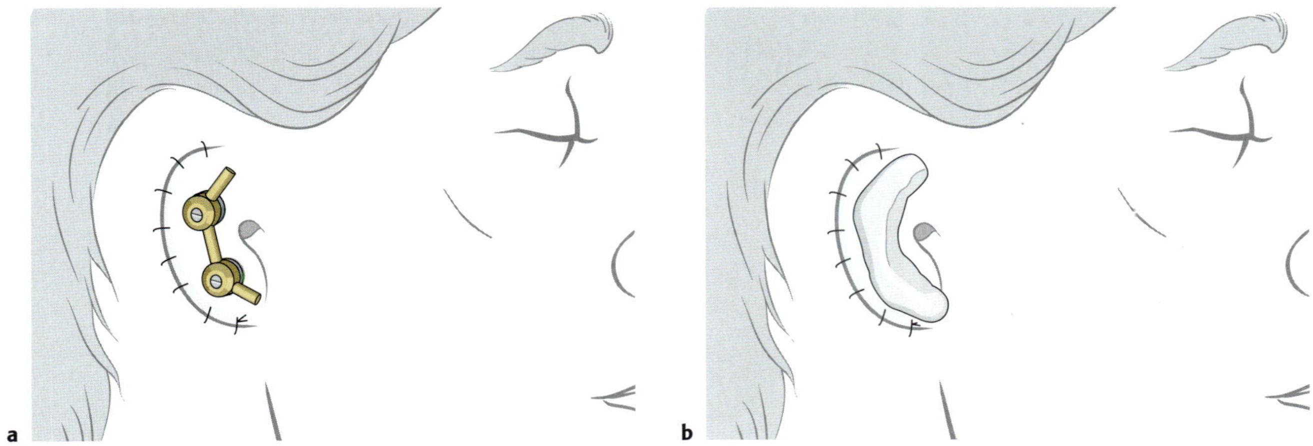

Fig 4.5-49a–b Custom-cast gold bar and substructure.

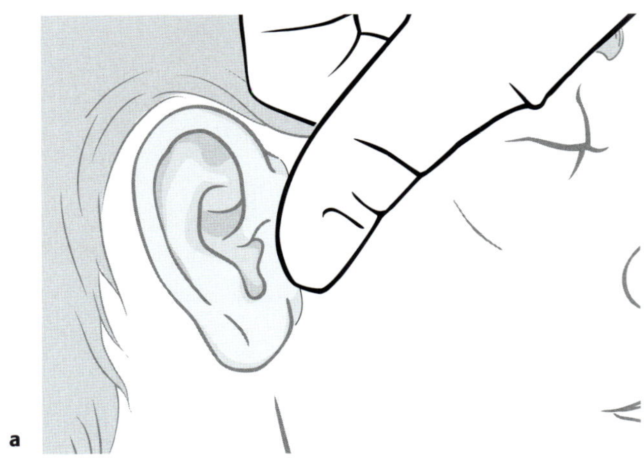

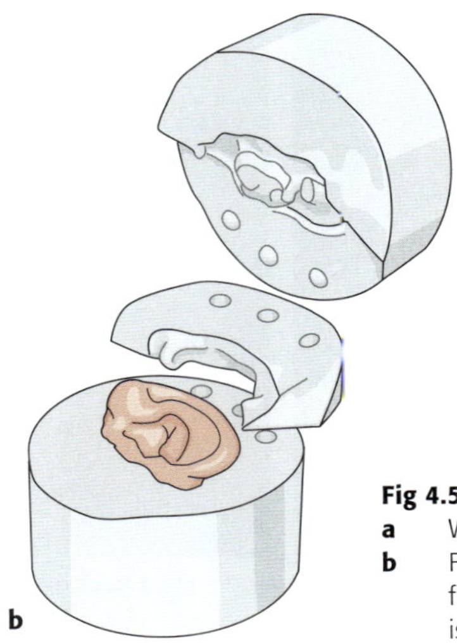

Fig 4.5-50a–b
a Wax ear carving.
b Flasked carved wax ear from which a silicone ear is produced.

One the technician has fabricated the silicone prosthesis, it is fitted to the patient and any minor color adjustments are made. The patient is shown how to attach and remove the prosthesis. Magnets can also be used instead of a bar and clip arrangement to maintain the prosthesis. These are typically bonded directly into the body of the prosthesis (**Fig. 4.5-51**).

11 Treatment procedures for HFM in the adult

11.1 Lateral augmentation by distraction osteogenesis

This procedure provides lateral augmentation to the face by using a sagittal split osteotomy with lateral distraction of the proximal segment. Careful patient selection is necessary to ensure that this is a good option for the individual patient and his or her deformity.

The surgical approach is transoral to the angle as for a sagittal split mandibular osteotomy. Minimal planning is required. It is only necessary to determine that there is sufficient bone stock to perform the osteotomies and place the distraction device. Neither orthodontic appliances nor arch bars are necessary to control the occlusion during distraction. However, it is necessary to hold the teeth in occlusion while the distractor is being tightened in position. If any screws or other fixation devices are present in this part of the mandible from previous surgery, these should be removed at the start of the procedure.

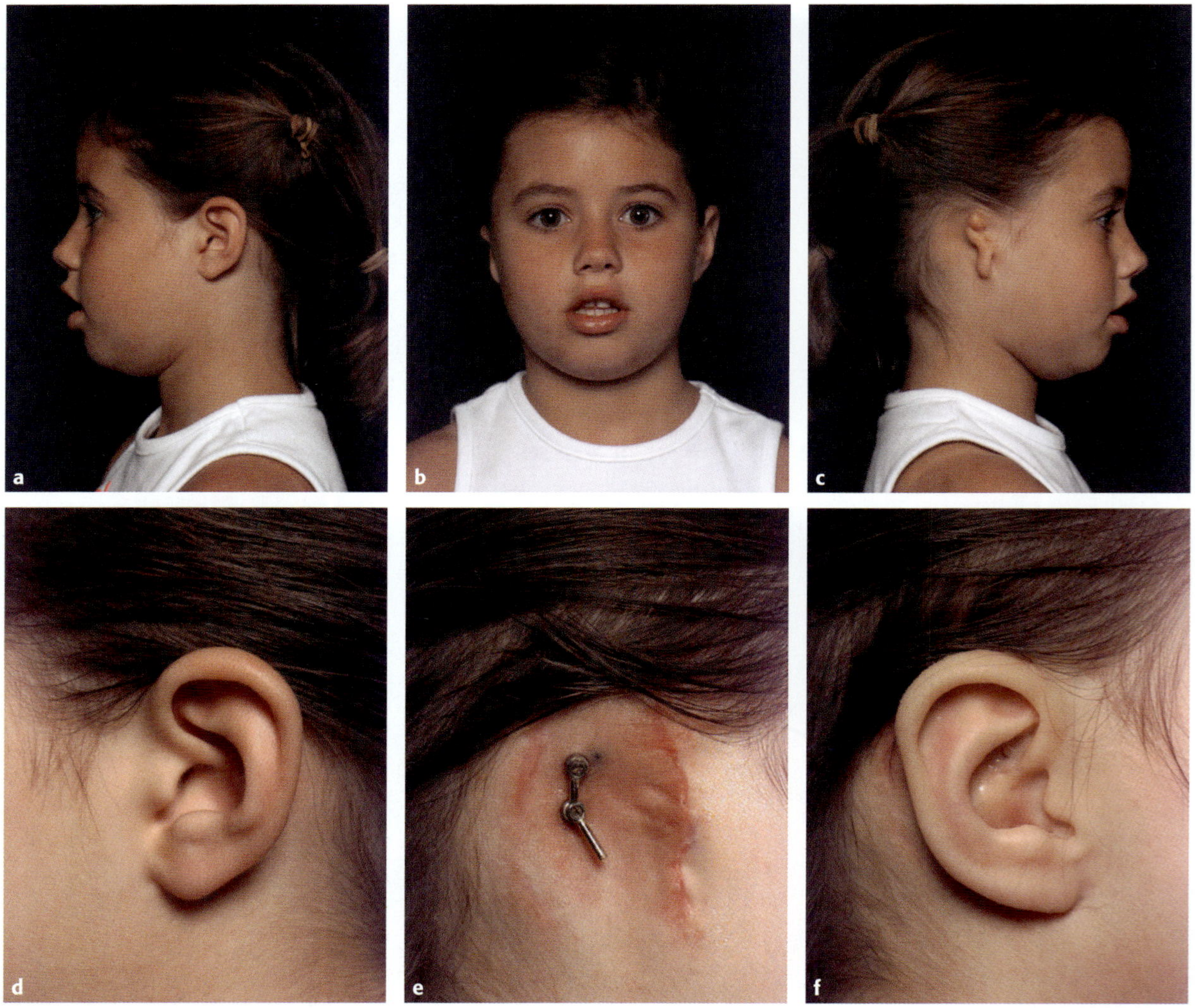

Fig 4.5-51a–f Same girl with microtia planned in **Fig 4.5-44**. Here with the clinical preoperative and postoperative appearance with bone-anchored ear prosthesis in place.

An Obwegeser-Dal Pont type sagittal split osteotomy (**Fig 4.5-52**) is performed. Remember that previous surgery has been performed in this area and the bone quality and quantity may be deficient.

The procedure starts in the same way as for a sagittal split with three corticotomies. The first cut is made horizontally through the lingual cortex just above the mandibular foramen parallel to the occlusion with a long reciprocating saw blade from the anterior to the posterior borders of the ramus. The second corticotomy is made vertically with the same saw blade through the buccal cortex adjacent to the first or second molar. The third corticotomy uses a sagittal saw blade to connect the first two osteotomy lines along the anterior border of the ascending ramus. The final split is completed with fine osteotomes, splitting the entire ascending ramus from the anterior to the posterior border and separating the lateral from the medial part of the ramus.

One pair of pins is then inserted transcutaneously and bicortically in the main body of the mandible anterior to the vertical osteotomy, through the lower border of the mandible (**Fig 4.5-53**).

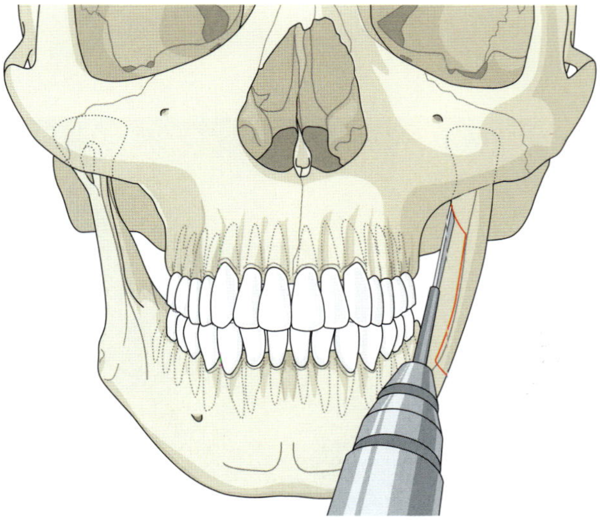

Fig 4.5-52 Osteotomy cuts being made for sagittal split of the left mandibular ramus.

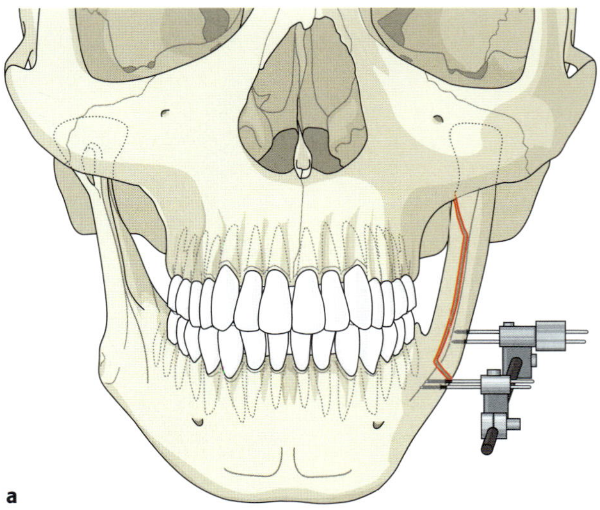

a

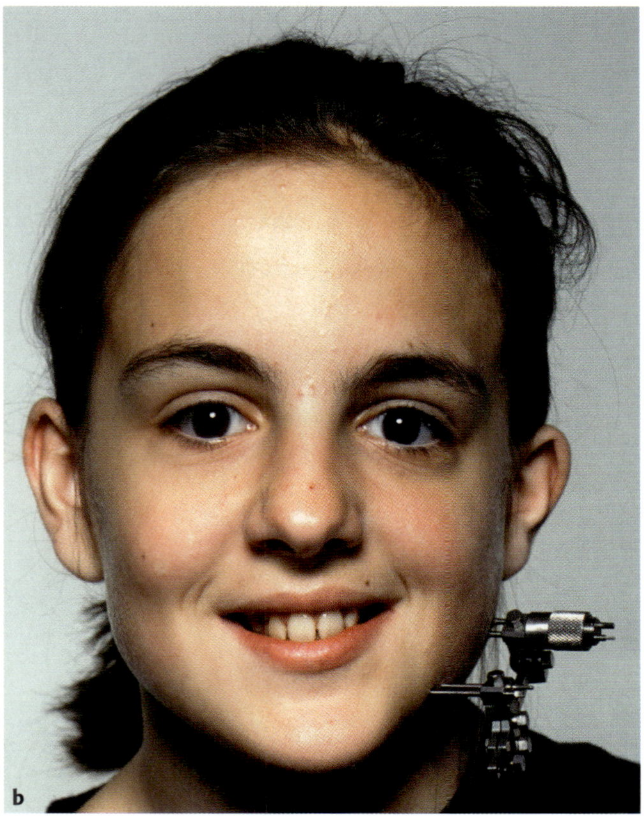

b

Fig 4.5-53a–b Lateral external distractor placed for the same patient shown in **Fig 4.5-1**.

The distance between the pins is determined by the distraction device. The pins are placed using a special drill guide. A second pair of pins is inserted also transcutaneously but monocortically into the lower border of the proximal condylar fragment. The distance between the pins is again determined by the distraction device. The pins are attached to an external distractor that functions by drawing the pins attached to the proximal fragment laterally (**Fig 4.5-54a**). The teeth are held together in centric occlusion before the distractor is tightened in place. The teeth are also held together while the distractor is tested to ensure it is working.

After a suitable latency period, the ramus is distracted at a rate of 1 mm per day (**Fig 4.5-54b**). The patient is advised to keep the teeth together while the device is activated. Frequent review of the patient is valuable until the required distraction has been achieved.

The end point for distraction can be difficult to determine because the patient will inevitably be a little swollen following surgery. In addition, it is not known how far the ramus can be lateralized before the patient will experience problems with the TMJ. Our own experience with just a few patients suggests that approximately 1 cm of lateralization can be produced without causing any sequelae.

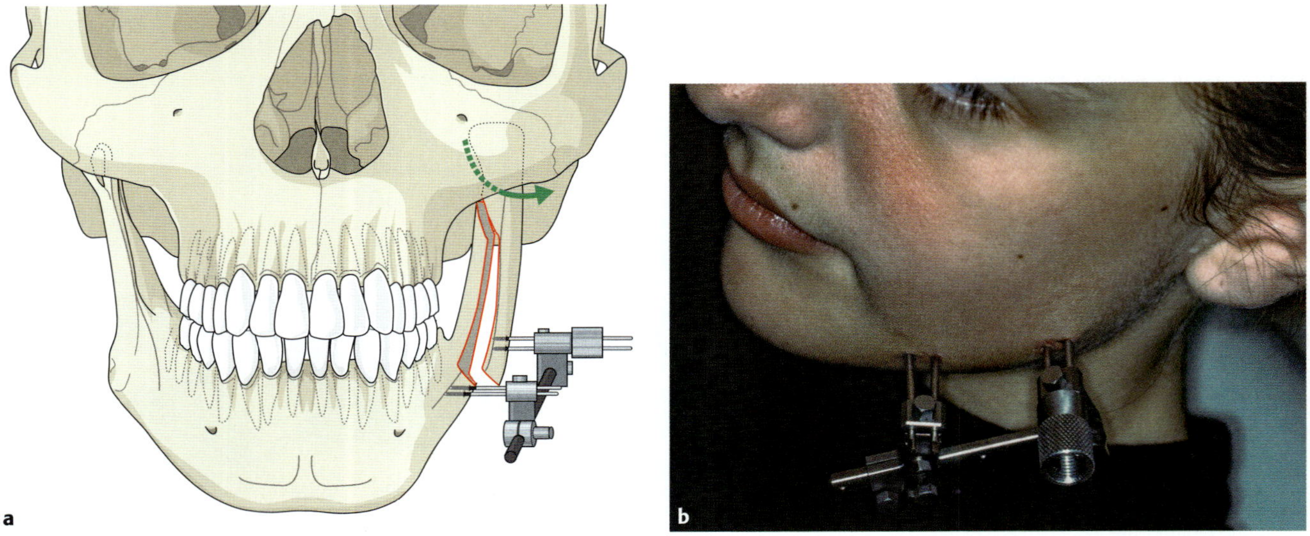

Fig 4.5-54a–b Distractor in place and activated.

After reaching the desired end point the distractor is left in place to allow for bone consolidation. This takes approximately 8 weeks and the regeneration of bone into the distraction gap can be verified with radiographs. When sufficient bone is present in the gap, the distractor is removed (**Fig 4.5-55**).

11.2 Lateral augmentation by osteotomy

Similar correction of lateral contour can be achieved as a fixed correction by performing a sagittal split osteotomy as described above but with the insertion of an interpositional corticocancellous bone graft within the split (**Fig 4.5-56**). Fixation is usually with bicortical screws which help to hold the graft in position.

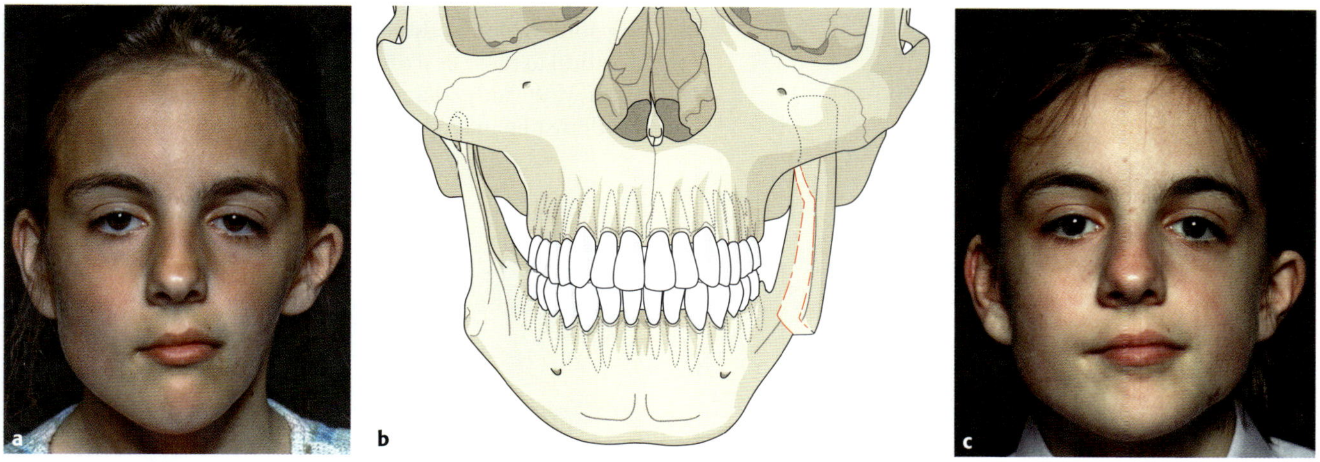

Fig 4.5-55a–c Before and after lateral distraction osteogenesis.

- **a** The patient shown in **Fig 4.5-1** with a Pruzansky IIa HFM after distraction to lengthen the ramus but with a lateral contour deficiency.
- **b** The result after lateral distraction.
- **c** The clinical outcome after lateral distraction.

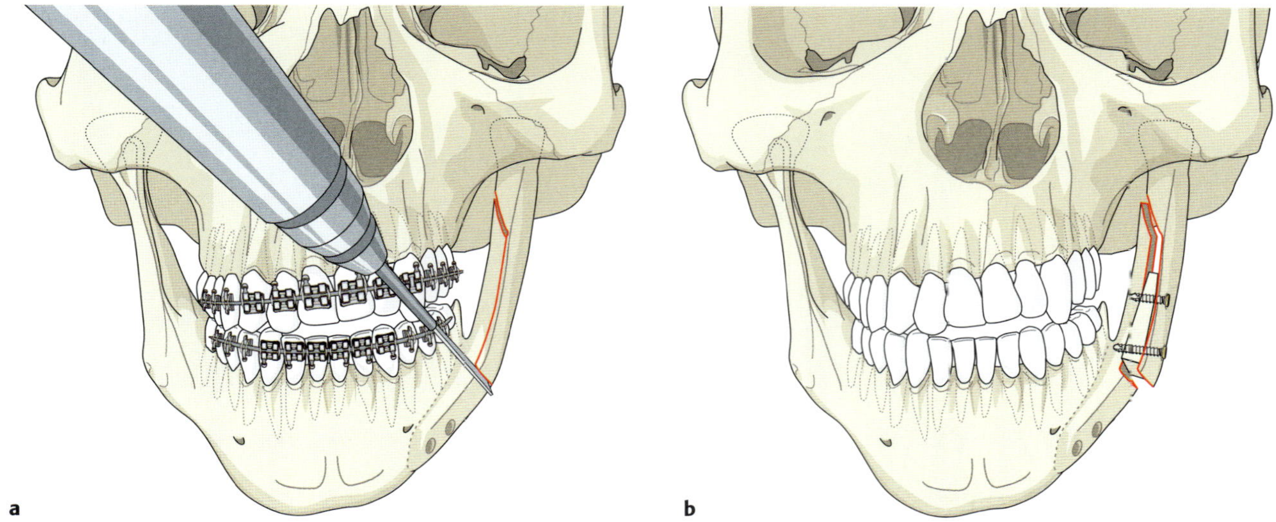

Fig 4.5-56a–b Sagittal split of the left mandibular ramus being made and fixed by screws with interposition of a bone graft to ensure lateral positioning of the ramus.

If further widening is required as part of a definitive orthognathic correction, the above procedure can be combined with bilateral sagittal split mandibular ramus osteotomies as well as a midline body osteotomy to allow widening of the affected side of the mandible as illustrated. The occlusion can be maintained by a two-piece Le Fort I maxillary osteotomy with widening of the affected side of the maxilla (**Fig 4.5-57**).

11.3 Rotational bimaxillary osteotomies including inverted-L ramus osteotomy and genioplasty

Most end-stage reconstructions in HFM require rotational bimaxillary orthognathic surgery. Of course, there are exceptions which can be managed with more limited procedures. The challenges are surgery on a patient with often severely deformed asymmetric bone structures who may have undergone operations many times previously with consequent presence of scar tissue. In addition, the rotational movements required commonly stretch the enveloping soft tissues to their limit. Most of the techniques are identical to those described under conventional orthognathic surgery. We only comment here on the special considerations that must be made for HFM cases.

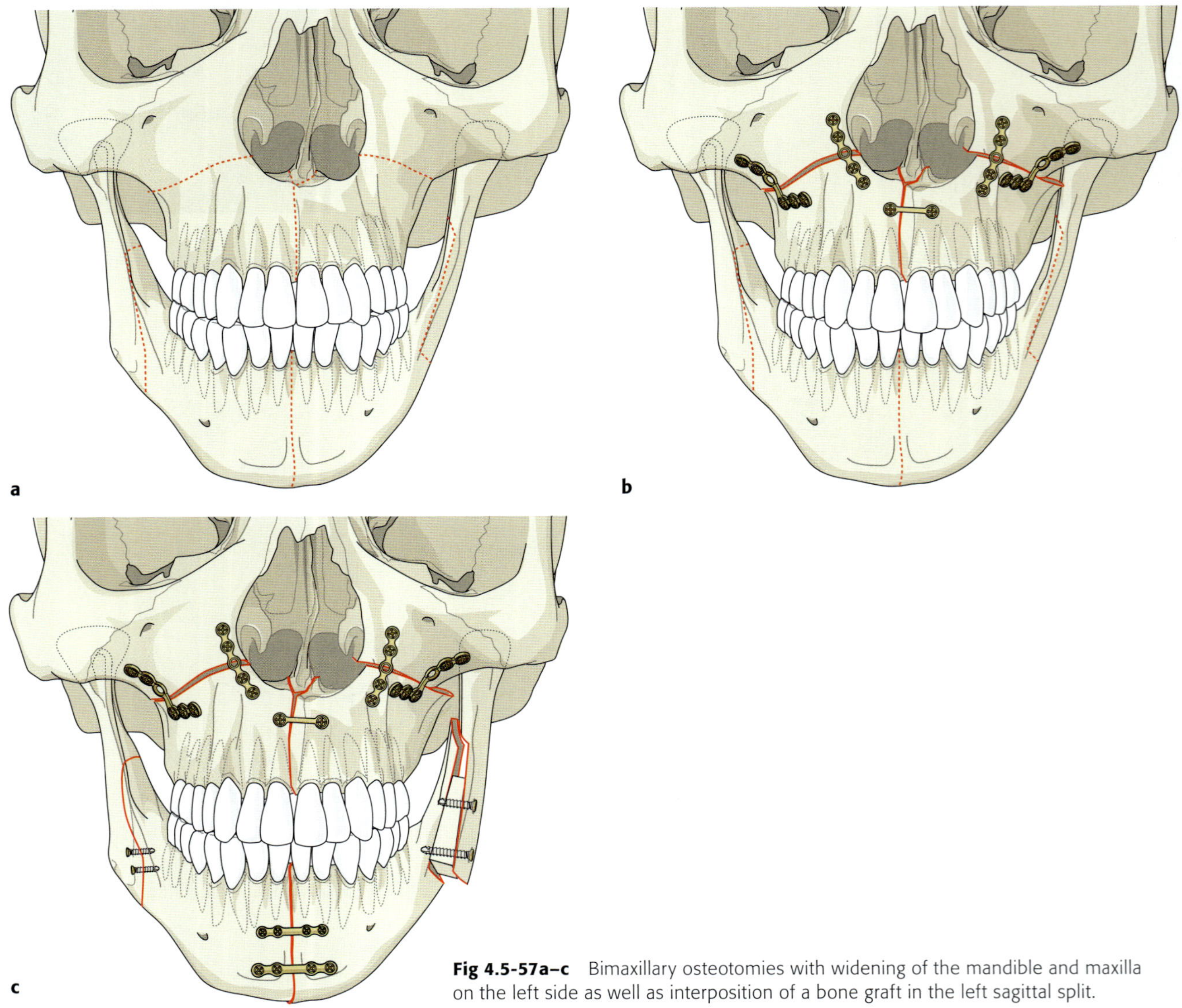

Fig 4.5-57a–c Bimaxillary osteotomies with widening of the mandible and maxilla on the left side as well as interposition of a bone graft in the left sagittal split.

Planning of these cases is best carried out in 3-D using a combination of proprietary software into which a CT scan is imported; virtual model planning of procedures and commonly physical model planning (**Fig 4.5-58**); and using a stereolithographic rapid prototyped skeletal model.

Typically surgery starts in the maxilla. The maxillary surgical technique is usually as for a conventional Le Fort I osteotomy. The osteotomized maxilla is rotated to place the dental center on the facial midline, level the occlusal plane and move about the midline to achieve the rotational movement required for the correction of the maxillary and mandibular deformities. The maxilla is then stabilized to the upper facial skeleton with miniplates. Corticocancellous bone grafts, ideally harvested from the iliac crest, can be used to fill any gaps resulting from any inferior repositioning of the maxillary segment and for anterior augmentation.

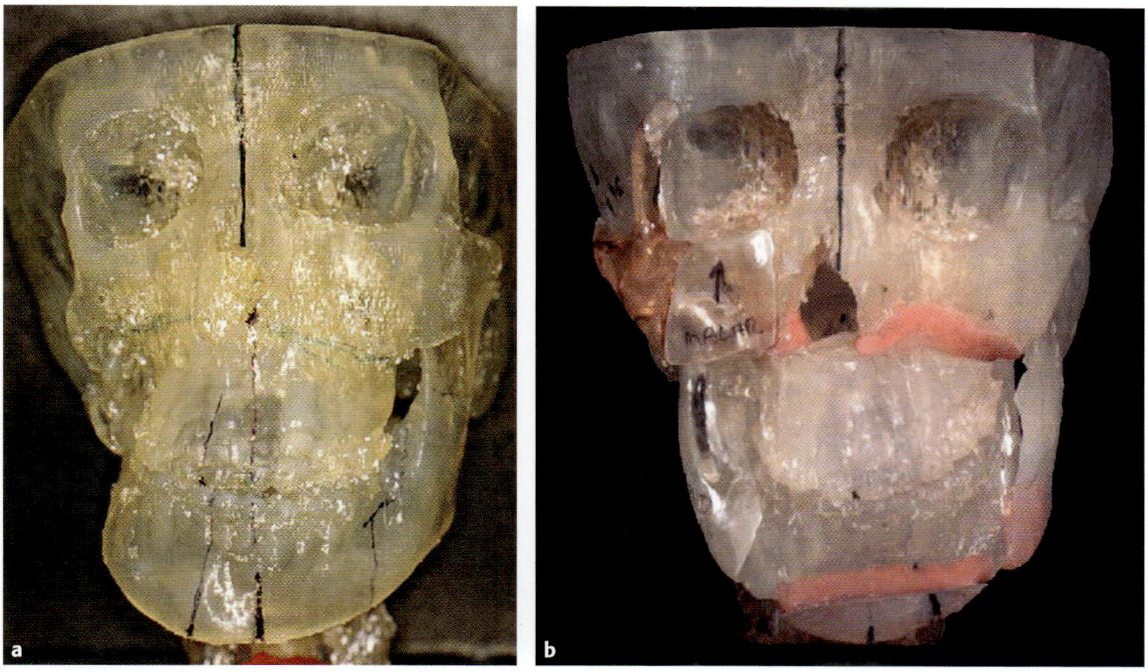

Fig 4.5-58a–b Stereolithographic model of an 18-year-old man with Pruzansky III HFM who underwent reconstruction of the right mandible and zygomatic arch with a vascularized free flap 10 years earlier. Model on the right after planning of rotational Le Fort I, right inverted-L mandibular and left sagittal split osteotomies, genioplasty and augmentation bone grafting have been performed.

Bilateral sagittal split osteotomies in HFM can sometimes be used to correct the mandibular deformity if the affected side ramus does not need to be lengthened. When the surgical planning results in significant lengthening of the ramus or when a sagittal split osteotomy is challenging due to previous surgery, as is often the case on the affected side of HFM cases, it is better to perform an inverted-L osteotomy with internal plate fixation and interpositional bone grafts on the affected side. A sliding genioplasty is often also indicated (**Fig 4.5-59**).

Any residual fixation material from previous operations should be removed first. It is unusual for the mandibular ramus to require lengthening on the nonaffected side, so it is almost always possible to carry out a sagittal split osteotomy on that side. Although an inverted L-osteotomy can be carried out transorally, its adequate fixation and bone grafting from a transoral approach are challenging and a transcutaneous approach is desirable.

In some cases, delaying the genioplasty is possible to allow for the true evaluation of the chin symmetry once the major rotational osteotomies have been performed. However, on the other hand, of all these procedures the genioplasty is the one most easily revised later.

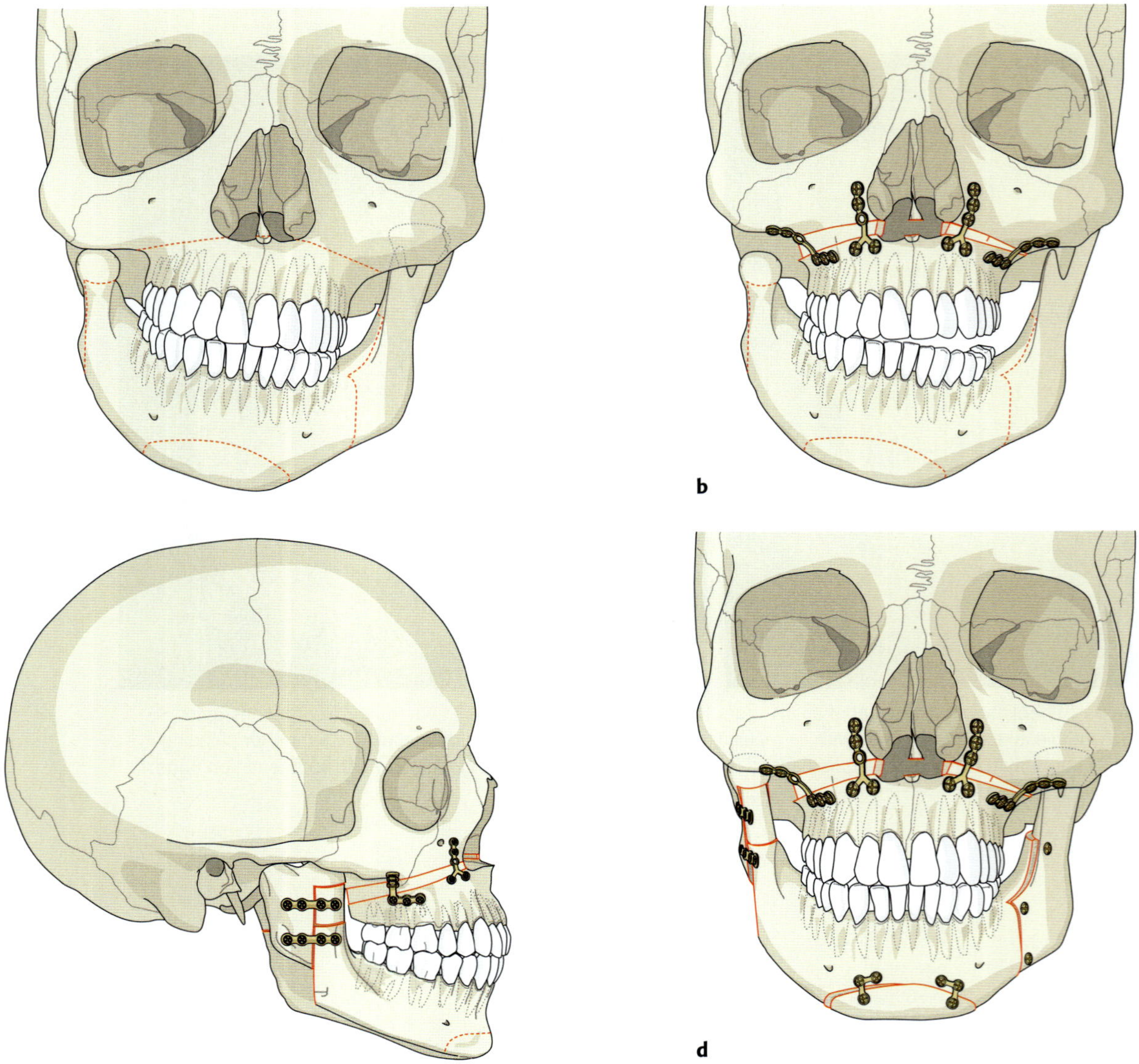

a b c d

Fig 4.5-59a–d Rational osteotomies of the maxilla (Le Fort I) with bone grafting, the mandible (sagittal split on the normal side and inverted L with bone grafting on the affected short-deformed side), and genioplasty to complete centralizing of the chin and correction of the facial skeletal asymmetry.

11.4 Orbital four-wall osteotomy for dystopia

A coronal approach is used but, unlike in craniosynostosis, only the anterior portion of the temporalis muscle is elevated. Additional exposure through transconjunctival and transoral approaches are performed so that the orbit can be degloved 360° leaving the medial canthal ligament attached (some surgeons detach the medial canthal tendon and reattach it at the end of the procedure).

The interorbital distance and the vertical discrepancy between the orbits are measured with a caliper. For vertical repositioning, a wedge of supraorbital bone must be removed (**Fig 4.5-60**). For horizontal discrepancy, bone needs to be removed medially to allow the orbit to be repositioned.

Note: This surgery should not be performed until after the maxillary teeth have erupted sufficiently that they will not be damaged by the osteotomy cuts.

After the exposure of the forehead and the orbits, a unilateral frontal craniotomy beginning 1 cm above the superior orbital rim and extending from the midline to behind the coronal suture is outlined (**Fig 4.5-61**).

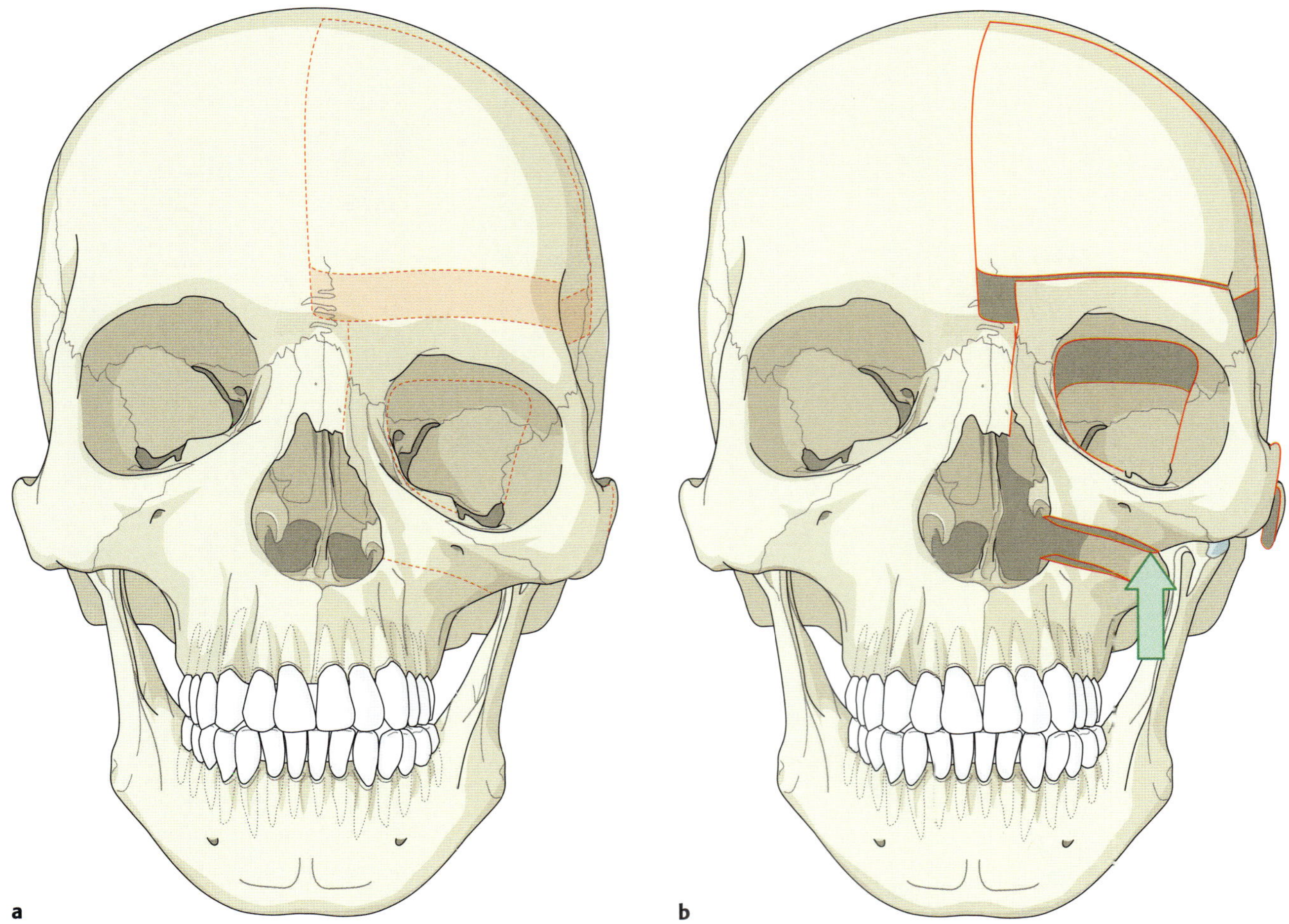

a b

Fig 4.5-60a–b Correction of vertical orbital dystopia.

Burr holes are first placed at the vertex and nasal frontal region as well as temporally an epidural dissection between these points is made. The neurosurgeon then completes the osteotomies using a craniotome. After the bone flap is removed, the brain is freed from the anterior and middle fossa in the extradural plane. The surface of the brain is protected by neurosurgical swabs. Malleable retractors are used intracranially to protect the brain and intraorbitally to protect the orbital contents. With retractors in the orbit and anterior cranial fossa, an osteotomy just posterior to the lateral orbital rim and through the lateral orbital wall is made (**Fig 4.5-61**).

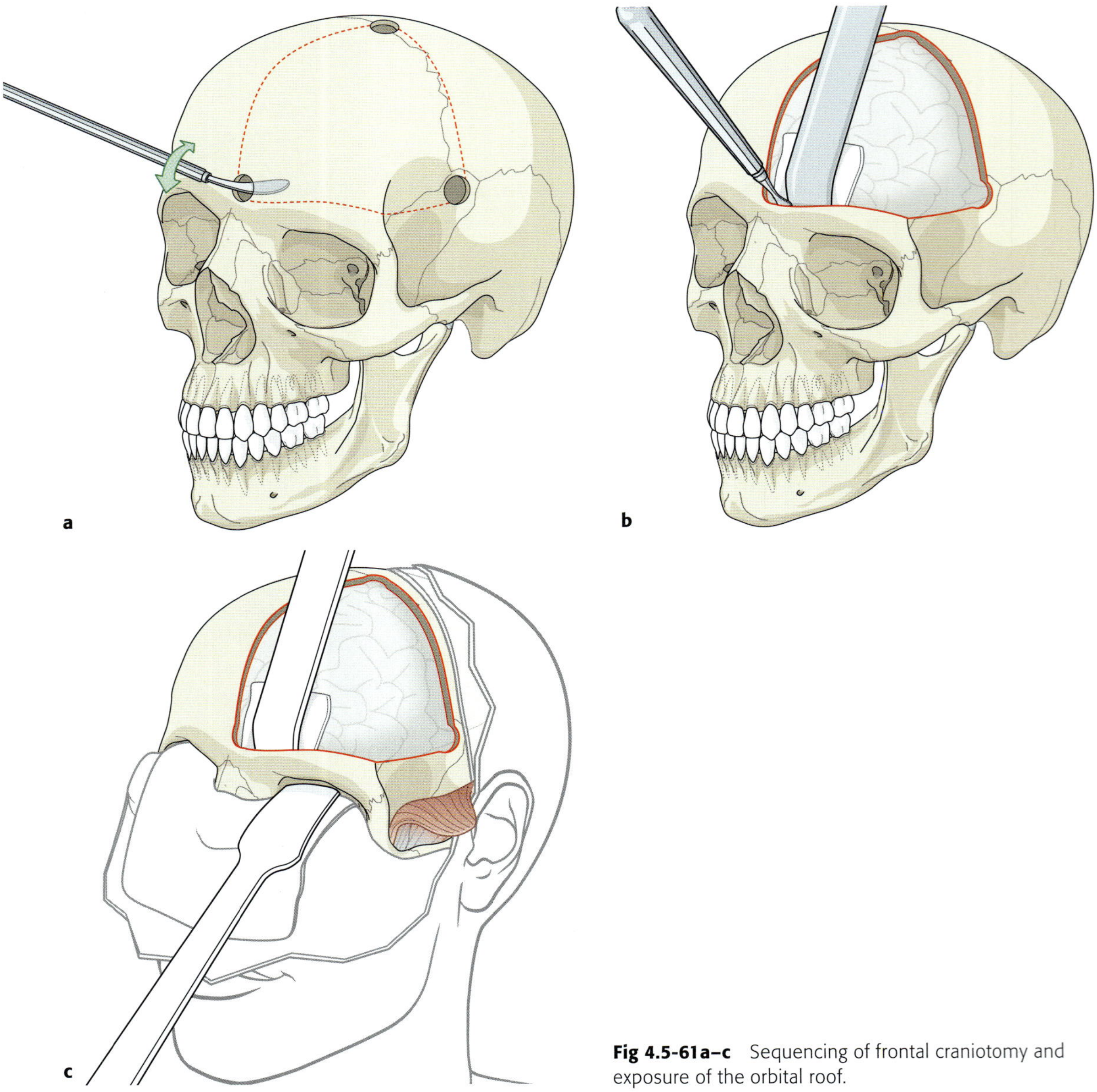

Fig 4.5-61a–c Sequencing of frontal craniotomy and exposure of the orbital roof.

A vertical osteotomy (**Fig 4.5-62**) is performed at the junction of the zygomatic arch and zygomatic eminence. An osteotome is introduced from the temporal fossa and a cut is made along the deep orbital floor to the level of the posterior portion of the inferior orbital fissure.

The lateral orbital floor is cut with an osteotome placed just behind the lateral wall at the level of the zygoma and courses medially to join the osteotomy of the medial orbit.

Note: The inner orbital osteotomies of the floor, medial and lateral walls and roof must be behind the equator of the orbit to ensure that when the orbit is moved it takes the globe of the eye with it.

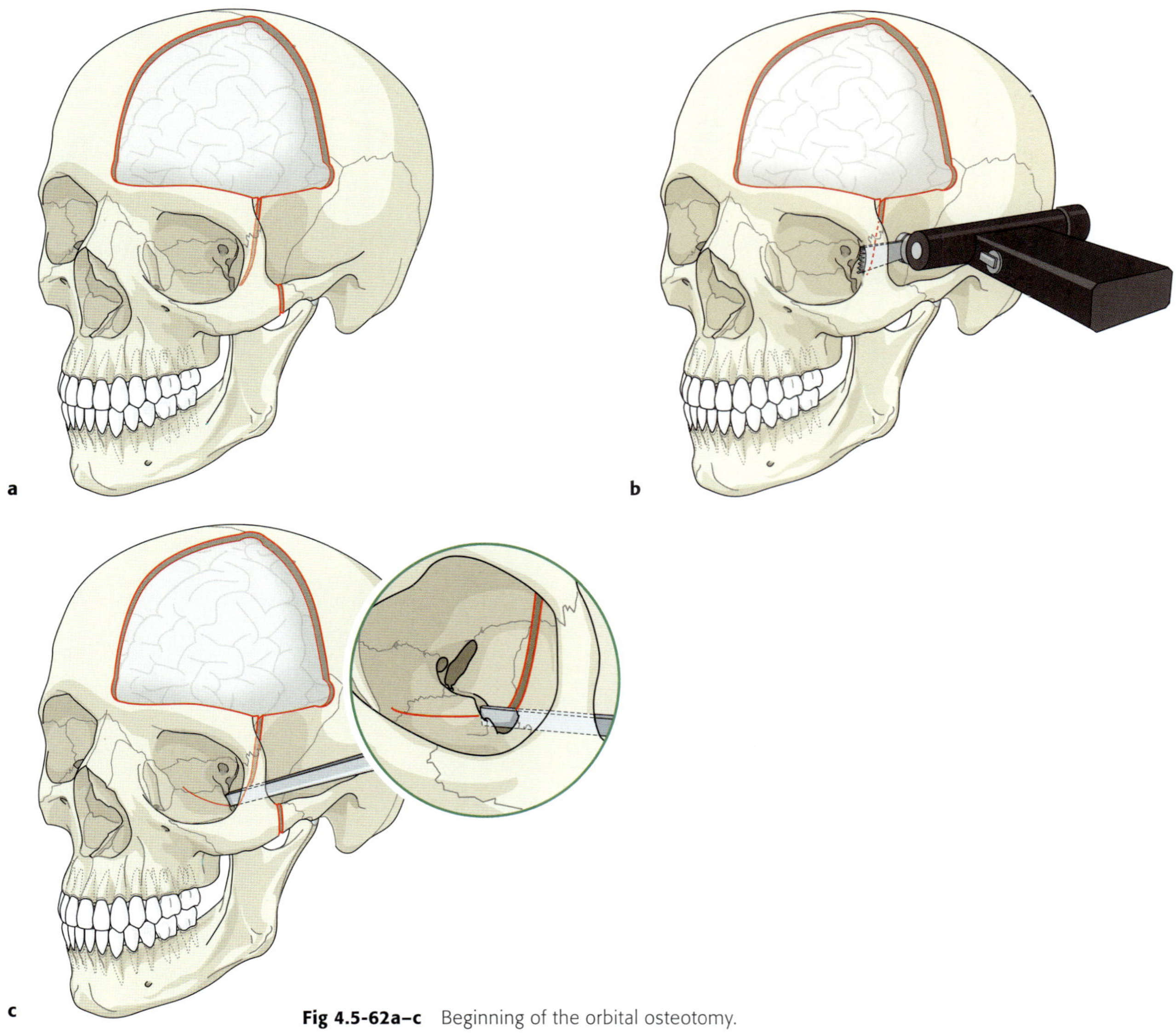

Fig 4.5-62a–c Beginning of the orbital osteotomy.

A right-angled saw is then turned intracranially and the orbital roof is cut beginning at the pterion laterally and ending at the cribriform plate. An osteotome is then inserted at the pterion and the lateral orbital wall cut completed. An osteotome is then inserted from intracranially and the medial orbit is cut posterior to the canthus and on to the medial floor. Using the upper buccal sulcus or lid incision, a saw is used to cut from the zygomatic eminence below the infraorbital nerve to the pyriform buttress. A single cut is then made from the anterior cranium down the affected side of the nasal bone to the bone cartilage junction. The orbit should now be completely mobile and able to be translocated superiorly (**Fig 4.5-63**).

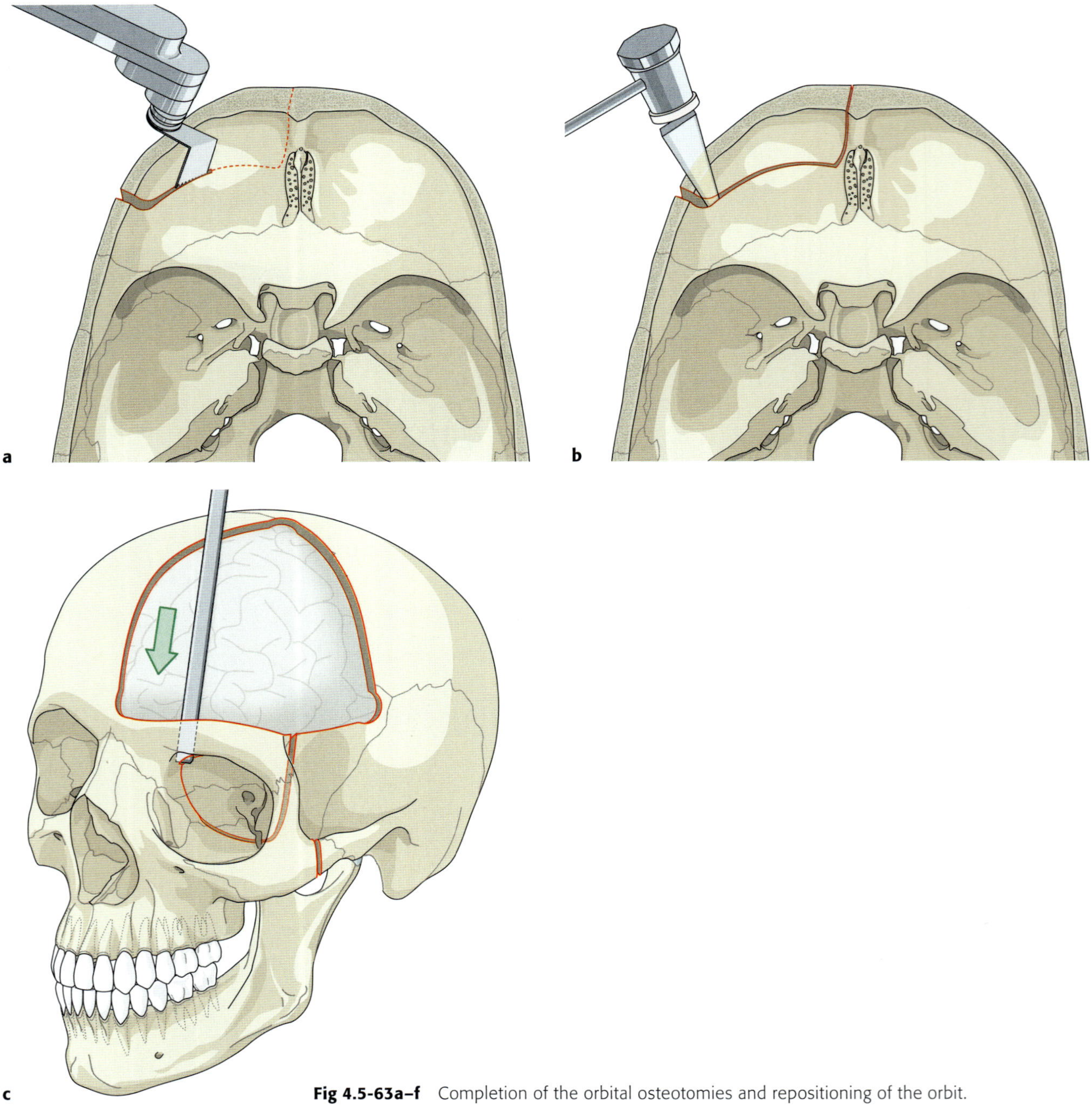
a b c

Fig 4.5-63a–f Completion of the orbital osteotomies and repositioning of the orbit.

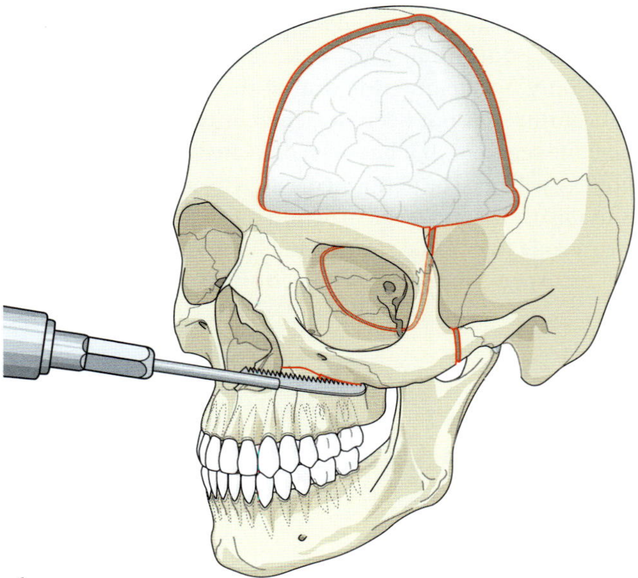

d

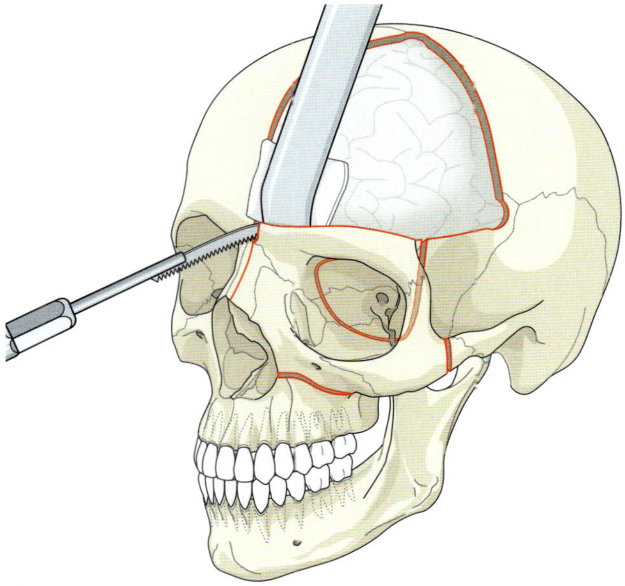

e

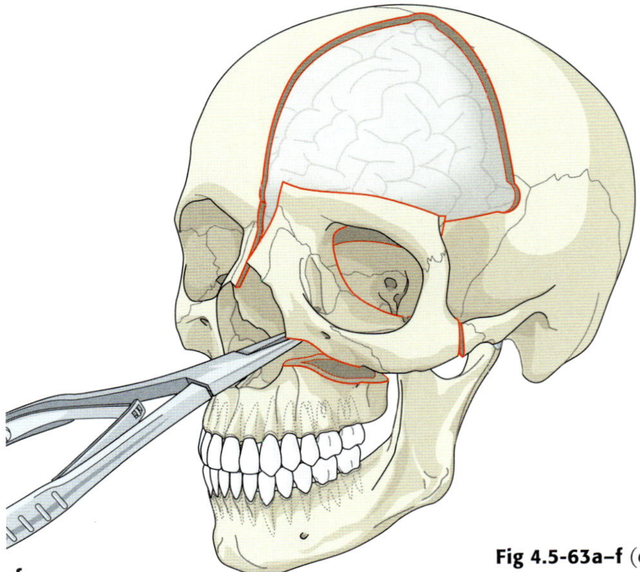

f

Fig 4.5-63a–f (cont) Completion of the orbital osteotomies and repositioning of the orbit.

Any interference with bone spicules or ethmoid sinus tissue may need to be removed with a rongeur. There may be interference at the pyriform level as well requiring bone removal. The orbit may also need to be rotated a little and possibly advanced laterally. Temporary fixation can be secured with one or two wires superiorly. The definitive new position of the orbit is then fixed with 1.5 titanium plates and screws (**Fig 4.5-64**). The frontal bone segment should be reduced before it is replaced and fixed with miniplates and screws. This reduction provides bone-grafting material which is then used to fill in gaps, especially below the inferior osteotomy on the anterior wall of the maxilla. If the medial canthus has not been detached, it will be moved with the bone segment. If it has been detached, a transnasal canthopexy will need be performed with wire and metallic plates as in posttraumatic reconstruction, with a bone anchor, or with strong transnasal sutures and bone grafts. Lateral canthal resuspension may also be performed.

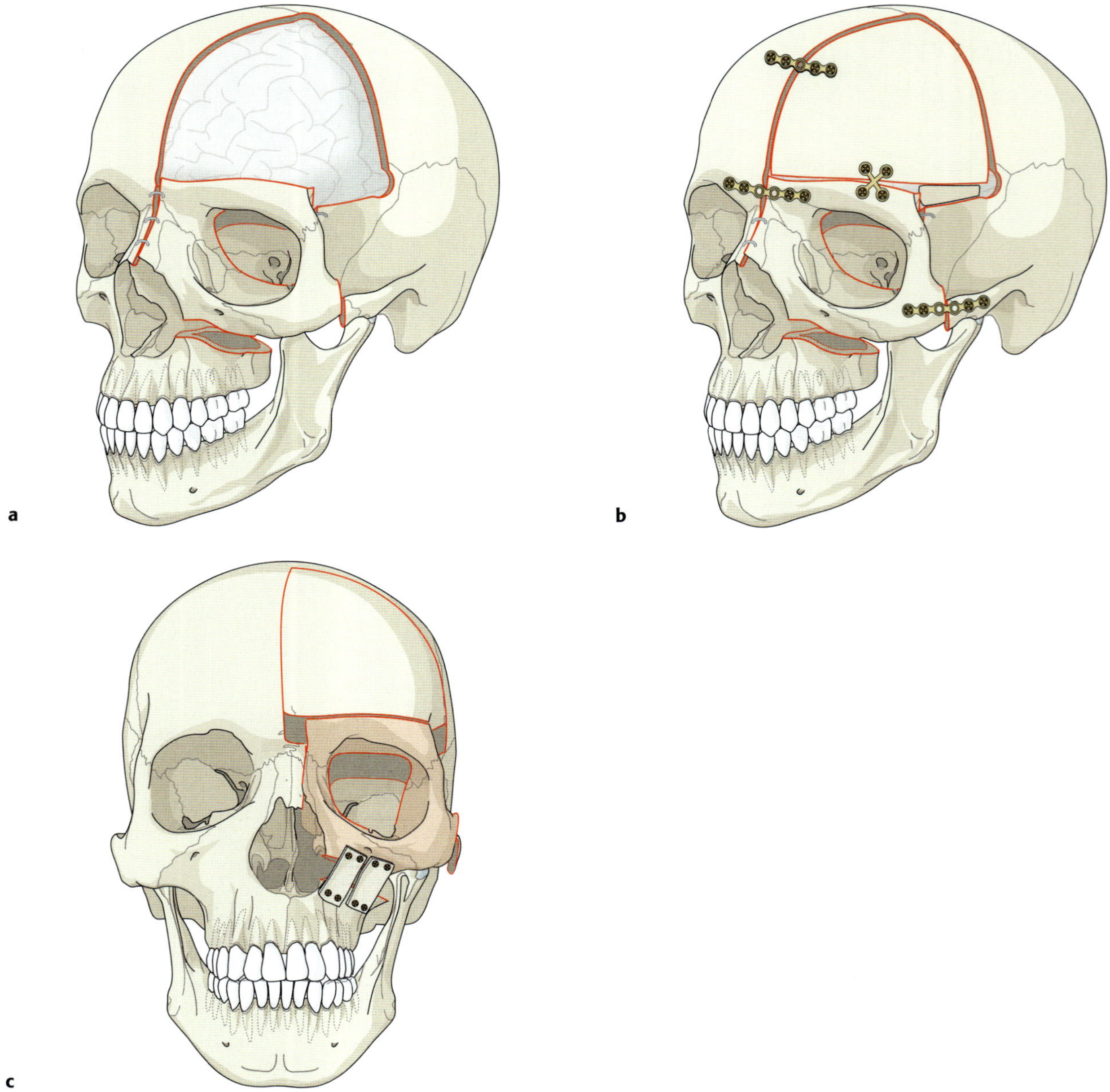

Fig 4.5-64a–c Fixation of the orbital osteotomies and bone grafting.

Some surgeons will also place transnasal sutures tied over gauze to help the soft tissues adhere to the new nasal bone position. Some surgeons continue to use percutaneous bolsters to ensure adaptation of the skin to the underlying bone. However, these should be applied with great caution to avoid underlying skin necrosis.

11.5 Soft-tissue augmentation

Correction of the skeletal deformity in these children and adults frequently improves the appearance of the face. However, some cases will have deficiency of the soft tissues and correction of the bony deformity alone is not sufficient to correct the facial contours. There are several options to address this problem but they are generally delayed until after skeletal surgery. There are occasions where soft-tissue augmentation needs to be considered earlier. For example, in a severe Pruzansky III where there is almost no soft tissue below the skin (eg, no masticatory muscles, no parotid gland).

The choice of augmentation procedures depends very much on the precise nature of the deformity, its precise location and the wishes of the surgeon and patient. The options are:

- Augmentation of facial contours with dermis fat grafts and/or fat injections
- Augmentation of facial contours with soft-tissue vascularized flaps, eg, parascapular, various perforator flaps, etc (see chapter 5.3.12).

11.6 Facial reanimation

Facial nerve palsy is common in HFM. However, it is rarely severe enough to obtain significant benefit from nerve transplantation for facial reanimation. Sling procedures can be performed as well as free tissue transfer. Generally, severe palsy of the upper branch of the nerve is managed by a gold weight in the upper eyelid to facilitate closure of the eyelid. If severe and better eye protection is required, it may be necessary to perform a lateral canthopexy.

12 Summary

Hemifacial microsomia is a complex but fascinating condition with a large variety of manifestations of so many anatomical structures with hugely varying severity. For this author, it has been a professional lifetime of discovery, challenge and effort to help the children and adults affected. This chapter is dedicated to those patients.

13 Acknowledgments

My thanks to Scott Bartlett, MD, craniomaxillofacial surgeon, Philadelphia Children's Hospital, USA, for his contribution to this chapter, in particular the sections on autogenous ear construction and correction of vertical orbital dystopia. My thanks also to my colleague, Steve Key, with whom I have shared the surgery of these patients for some years and with whom a multidisciplinary clinic dedicated to the management of children and adults with hemifacial microsomia was established and continues and a clinic with Mark Cooper, plastic surgeon, for the treatment of microtia patients.

We also acknowledge the contribution to the management of these patients of the Maxillofacial Prosthetists at Morriston Hospital, Peter Evans, Alan Bocca, Lawrence Dovgalski and Steven Hollisey-McLean, the unique 3-D planning skills of Heather Goodrum, the orthodontic support from Malcolm Jones, Charlotte Eckhardt and Helen Taylor and the clinical psychology support to the children in particular of Vanessa Hammond.

14 References and suggested reading

Baluch N, Nagata S, Park C, et al. Auricular reconstruction for microtia: a review of available methods. *Plast Surg.* 2014 Spring;22(1):39–43.

Bibb R, Bocca A, Sugar A, et al. Planning osseointegrated implant sites using computer aided design and rapid prototyping. *J Maxillofac Prosthetics Technol.* 2003;6:1–4.

Brent B. Microtia repair with rib cartilage grafts: a review of personal experience with 1000 cases. *Clin Plast Surg.* 2002 Apr;29(2):257–271.

Clark RN, Sugar AW, Evans PLl, et al. One stage surgery for bone anchored facial prostheses. *Br J Oral Maxillofac Surg.* 1997;35(3):209.

Coleman S. *Structural Fat Grafting.* New York: Thieme; 2004.

Coleman S, Mazozola R. *Fat Injection: From Filling to Regeneration.* New York: Thieme; 2009.

David DJ, Mahatumarat C, Cooter RD. Hemifacial microsomia: a multisystem classification. *Plast Reconstr Surg.* 1987 Oct;80:(4):525–535.

Grabb WC. *Plastic Surgery.* 3rd ed. Boston: Little, Brown & Co; 1979.

Hodder SC, Sugar AW, Taylor H, et al. Distraction osteogenesis for congenital mandibular deformity. *Br J Oral Maxillofac Surg.* 1997;35(3):203.

Horgan JE, Padwa BL, LaBrie RA, et al. OMENS-Plus: analysis of craniofacial and extracraniofacial anomalies in hemifacial macrosomia. *Cleft Palate Craniofacial J.* 1995 Sep;32(5):405–412.

Jacobsson C, Granstrom G. Clinical appearance of spontaneous and induced first and second branchial arch syndromes. *Scand J Plast Reconstruct Surg Hand Surg.* 1997;31(2):125–136.

Kaban LB, Mulliken JB, Murray JE. Three-dimensional approach to analysis and treatment of hemifacial microsomia. *Cleft Palate J.* 1981 Apr;18(2):90–99.

Kaban LB, Moses MH, Mulliken JB. Surgical correction of hemifacial microsomia in the growing child. *Plast Reconstr Surg.* 1988 Jul;81(1):9–19.

Kaban LB, West B, Conover M, et al. Midface position after Le Fort III advancement. *Plast Reconstr Surg.* 1984;73:758–767.

Lauritzen C, Munro IR, Ross RB. Classification and treatment of hemifacial microsomia. *Scand J Plast Reconstr Surg.* 1985;19(1):33–39.

McCarthy J. The role of distraction osteogenesis in the construction of the mandible in unilateral craniofacial microsomia. *Clin Plast Surg.* 1994 Oct;21(4):625–631.

Meazzini MC, Mazzoleni F, Bozzetti A, et al. Brusati R. Comparison of mandibular vertical growth in hemifacial microsomia patients treated with early distraction or not treated: follow up till the completion of growth. *J Craniomaxillofac Surg.* 2012 Feb;40(2):105–111.

Murray JE, Kaban LB, Mulliken JB. Analysis and treatment of hemifacial microsomia. *Plast Reconstr Surg.* 1984 Aug;74(2):186–199.

Nagata S. A new method of total reconstruction of the auricle for microtia. *Plast Reconstr Surg.* 1993 Aug;92(2):187–201.

Ortiz Monasterio F, Molina F, Andrade L, et al. Simultaneous mandibular and maxillary distraction in hemifacial microsomia in adults: avoiding occlusal disasters. *Plast Reconstr Surg.* 1997 Sep;100(4):852–861.

Padwa BL, Kearns GJ, Todd R, et al. Simultaneous maxillary and mandibular distraction osteogenesis with a semiburied device. *Int J Oral Maxillofac Surg.* 1999 Feb;28(1):2–8.

Polley JW, Figueroa AA, Liou EJ, et al. Longitudinal analysis of mandibular asymmetry in hemifacial macrosomia. *Plast Reconstr Surg.* 1997 Feb;99(2):328–339.

Poswillo D. The aetiology and pathogenesis of craniofacial deformity. *Development.* 1988;103 Suppl:207–212.

Pruzansky S. Craniofacial surgery: the experiment on nature's experiment. Review of three patients operated by Paul Tessier. *Eur J Orthod.* 1982;4:151–171.

Pruzansky S. Not all dwarfed mandibles are alike. *Birth Defects.* 1969;1:120–129.

Tahiri Y, Chang CS, Tuin J, et al. Costochondral grafting in craniofacial microsomia. *Plast Reconstr Surg.* 2015 Feb;135(2):530–541.

Tessier P. Anatomical classification facial, cranio-facial and latero-facial clefts. *J Maxillofac Surg.* 1976 Jun;4(2):69–92.

Tjellström A. Osseointegrated implants for replacement of absent or defective ears. *Clin Plast Surg.* 1990 Apr;17(2):355–366.

Sugar AW. The management of syndromic mandibular asymmetry, especially hemifacial microsomia. *Br J Oral Maxillofac Surg.* 2009 Sep;47(6):503–504.

Sugar AW. Congenital deformities: cleft deformities and hemifacial microsomia teaching websites. Available at: http://www.aocmf.org. AOCMF Surgery Reference; 2012.

Sugar AW, Pradhan R. Temporo-mandibular joint ankylosis in the growing child: costo-chondral grafting as an approach to management. *Indian J Surg.* 1984;46:352–362.

Sugar AW, Beumer III J. Reconstructive prosthetic methods for facial defects. *Oral Maxillofac Surg Clin N Am.* 1994;6(4):755–764.

Vento AR, LaBrie RA, Mulliken JB. The O.M.E.N.S. classification of hemifacial microsomia. *Cleft Palate Craniofac J.* 1991 Jan;28(1):68–76; discussion 77.

Whyte AM, Hourihan MD, Earley MJ, et al. Radiological assessment of hemifacial microsomia by three-dimensional computed tomography. *Dentomaxillofac Radiol.* 1990 Aug;19(3):119–125.

4.6 Cleft bone grafting and management of the alveolar ridge defect

Jeffrey C Posnick

1 Introduction

A child born with a cleft lip and palate may undergo successful soft-tissue closure of the lip and palate, but bone defects of the alveolar process, floor of the nose, and hard palate will remain. Despite appropriate initial cleft repair the full rehabilitation of the maxilla, alveolar ridge, base of the nose, intraoral soft tissues, and dentition will require further skeletal and soft-tissue reconstruction carried out in conjunction with orthodontic alignment of the teeth.

2 Current standard of care

Reconstruction of the alveolar process in patients with unilateral cleft lip and palate (UCLP) and bilateral cleft lip and palate (BCLP) is an essential part of cleft care. Accomplishing this goal provides support for the base of the nose, the teeth in the cleft region, and the periodontium of those teeth. There are three basic methods described for closure of the cleft alveolus. The surgical options include primary bone grafting, secondary bone grafting, and gingival periosteoplasty (GPP). The method of primary bone grafting is now generally recognized to result in severe midface growth disturbance and has therefore been almost universally abandoned throughout the world. The use of secondary (mixed dentition) bone grafting is generally recognized as an effective method to avoid the problem of any additional midface growth disturbance and to successfully achieve support to the nasal base, bone for eruption of the lateral incisor or canine through the cleft site, and effective periodontal support. The technique of GPP was first described by Skoog in 1965 as a method to achieve fusion across the cleft alveolus at the time of lip repair. The goal was to "remove" the cleft in infancy with the hope that no harm would result. Millard [1990] combined the "Latham device" to position the alveolar ridges close to one another before going forward with the GPP procedure at the time of cleft lip repair. Grayson and Cutting [2001] later proposed the use of a nasoalveolar molding (NAM) device before GPP and primary lip repair to accomplish the same alveolar ridge fusion. Since the late 1970s, clinical studies have been carried out to assess the long-term effects of GPP on midfacial growth in cleft patients. Many studies [Millard et al, 1999; Berkowitz et al, 2004; Matic et al, 2008; Henkel et al, 1997] have found that patients treated with GPP had poor occlusal relationships with a higher than expected need for orthognathic surgery in the teenage years. More recently, Hsieh and colleagues [2010] completed a retrospective clinical study to specifically evaluate the effects of GPP on facial growth of patients with UCLP. This was a detailed clinical study of a consecutive series of patients who were placed in two study groups. The study groups included those receiving NAM treatment with GPP and those receiving NAM treatment without GPP. The use of gingival periosteoplasty at the time of lip repair was found to have significant negative effects on the maxillary position (SNA), intermaxillary position (ANB), maxillary length (PMP-ANS), and maxillary alveolar length (PMP-AN) at the age of 5 years. The authors concluded that in patients with an alveolar cleft, the sagittal growth of the maxilla was significantly adversely affected by GPP procedure.

Most cleft lip and palate centers currently agree with the benefits of placing autogenous cancellous bone graft in the palatal, alveolar, and nasal floor skeletal defects with simultaneous closure of residual oronasal fistulae in the mixed dentition before eruption of the permanent maxillary canine tooth through the cleft site. This treatment protocol of "early-secondary" grafting is now considered an essential element of the cleft patient's rehabilitation.

3 Orthodontic treatment before alveolar grafting

Interceptive orthodontic treatment is carried out in the mixed dentition and coordinated with the surgical objectives to achieve an intact "noncleft" maxilla, without fistulae and with adequate arch form and dental alignment.

In the patient with UCLP the preoperative interceptive orthodontic goals are: (1) to re-expand the maxillary arch width to a normal dimension; (2) to avoid tipping the cleft adjacent teeth into the cleft as this would result in loss of periodontal support, and (3) to make a decision about which cleft adjacent, erupted, or impacted primary and supernumerary or rudimentary lateral incisor teeth are not of long-term value and best extracted. For the patient with BCLP the preoperative interceptive orthodontic goals are the same but, in addition, the position of the mobile premaxilla should be considered. Positioning of the premaxilla to establish an improved dental midline to the facial midline and, if feasible, to correct any anterior or posterior malalignment are also objectives.

Achieving these limited orthodontic objectives just before grafting is the goal. We do not suggest beginning the interceptive orthodontic phase of treatment until the permanent maxillary first molars have fully erupted. This allows for adequate transverse growth of the maxilla before bone grafting. Waiting until the permanent first molars have erupted provides efficient (first molar) anchorage for the rapid orthodontic expansion of any arch width collapse. This is completed with the use of a palatal appliance (eg, a Hyrax or Quadhelix appliance). Treatment is generally initiated just 2–6 months before the planned date of surgery.

The age at which bone grafting is planned should be based on dental development rather than chronological age. It is important to remember that patients with cleft palate will often have delayed dental eruption. The maxillary first molars and central incisors may not erupt until 7 or 8 years of age. The permanent maxillary canine at the cleft site may not erupt until 13 years of age. Occasionally, extraction of retained primary teeth is carried out to expedite the process. In any case, the graft should be placed well in advance of the eruption of the permanent canine tooth at the cleft site.

4 Surgical technique

The patient undergoes intubation, and a degree of hypotensive anesthesia is preferred to limit blood loss (the need for transfusion is rare). The anterior iliac crest on one side and the head and neck are prepared and draped in the usual sterile fashion. Intravenous antibiotics are given for prophylaxis before making an incision.

4.1 Bone graft harvesting

Attention is first turned to the hip region. A 3–4 cm incision is made parallel and lateral to the iliac crest and just posterior to the anterior superior iliac spine. The incision is carried through skin and subcutaneous tissue and then followed down to the iliac crest. Care is taken to avoid cutting through or contusing either the gluteus medius muscles laterally or the external or internal abdominal oblique or transverse abdominis muscle medially. Bruising either of these muscle groups when approaching the iliac crest is the source of postoperative hip or abdomen discomfort, respectively, with negative impact on ambulation (see chapter 1.1).

If a cartilaginous cap remains over the crest (before approximately 12 years of age), it is split down the center directly over the crest with perpendicular relaxing incisions in the cartilage at either end. This will allow easy lifting of each half of the cap from the underlying marrow space. Cartilage lifting is accomplished with a periosteal elevator. Cancellous bone is then harvested with curettes. After adequate bone is obtained, a thin layer of bone wax may be used in the marrow cavity for hemostasis. The cartilaginous cap is then repositioned and sutured back in place. The fascia and skin are closed in layers with resorbable suture. Steri-Strips and an occlusive dressing are placed. A drain is usually neither necessary nor advantageous.

If the ilium is mature (after approximately 12 years of age) and no cartilaginous cap remains, then a window of cortical bone is removed from the medial aspect of the crest and down the medial cortex for several centimeters. This is efficiently accomplished with the use of a sagittal and oscillating saw. With the window of cortical bone removed, cancellous bone is harvested with curettes. The small cortical bone segment does not need to be replaced, as the integrity of the crest is not violated and a bone defect will not be palpable or detectable through the closed skin wound. Interestingly, regeneration of the harvested bone is anticipated to the extent that reharvesting from the same location is the rule at the time of orthognathic surgery if a graft is required [Posnick, 2015].

4.2 Maxillary reconstruction

Attention is next turned to the head and neck. The pharynx is suctioned, a throat pack is placed, and the mouth is cleansed. To adequately elevate the palatal flaps and achieve fistula closure at surgery the palatal placed orthodontic appliance is removed either by the orthodontist just before the surgical procedure or by the surgeon in the operating room. Significant differences exist in the technique of flap elevation, graft placement, and wound closure for the patient with UCLP and the BCLP.

4.2.1 For the UCLP patient

Labial mucogingival flaps are developed on either side of the alveolar cleft. The lesser segment labial flap is elevated (on the cleft side) by making an incision that splits the attached (keratinized) gingiva obliquely, generally adjacent to the permanent first molar. The incision continues forward to the cervical margin of the mesial aspect of the first molar and then continues anteriorly through the gingival sulci until the mesial papilla of the primary canine is reached (**Fig 4.6-1a**). The incision continues superiorly along the mesial line angle of the canine and then through the upper most rim of mucosa, further separating the oral and nasal fistula. The incision continues down the distal line angle of the central incisor tooth. The incision continues with elevation of the contralateral greater segment labial flap (on the non-cleft side) through the gingival sulci of both central incisors. With a periosteal elevator, each labial mucogingival flap is elevated superiorly in the subperiosteal plane exposing the anterior maxilla up toward the infraorbital nerve (**Fig 4.6-1a–b**).

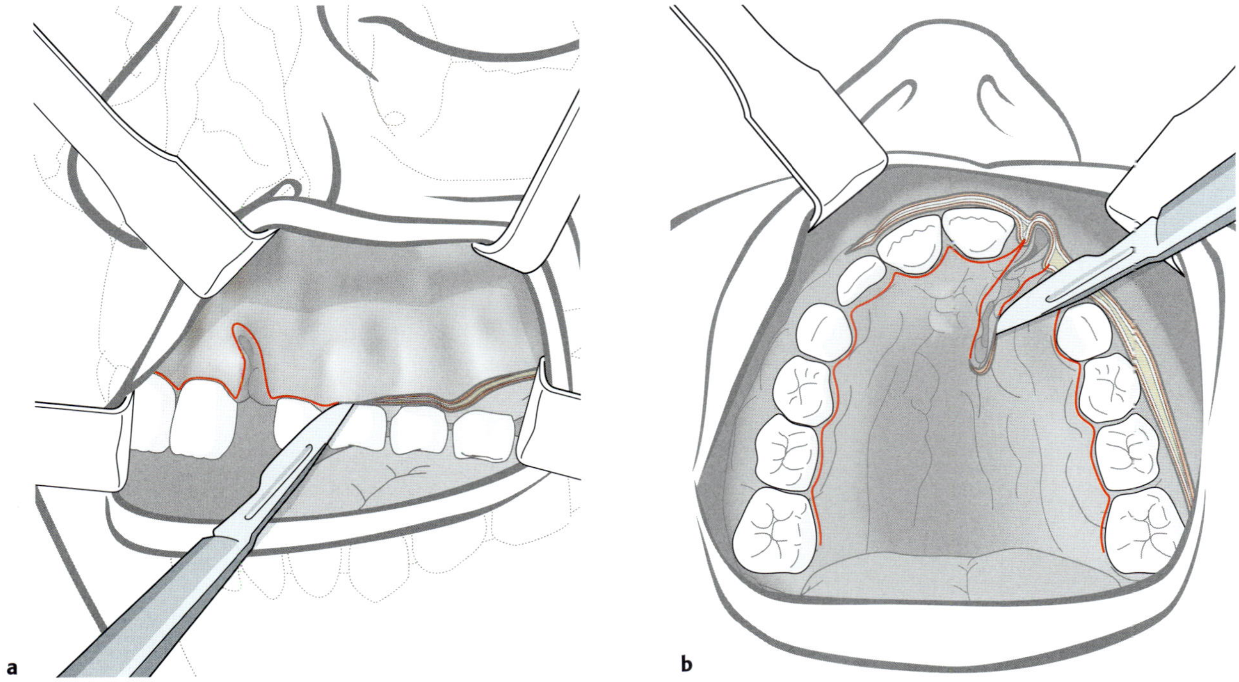

Fig 4.6-1a–g Techniques for bone grafting and management of residual oronasal fistula in a 9-year-old patient with unilateral cleft lip and palate. The lip and palate were repaired in infancy and early childhood.

a View of the left labial mucogingival incision in progress.

b Attention is turned to the palate for elevation of the palatal flaps and separation of the oral and nasal mucosa at site of fistula.

Bilateral full-thickness mucoperiosteal palatal flaps are then elevated beginning posteriorly at each first molar with an incision through the gingival sulci and continuing anteriorly (from each side) until the fistula site is approached at the alveolar cleft (**Fig 4.6-1b**). Bilateral, parallel incisions are begun at the alveolar ridge and continued posteriorly, separating the oral and nasal mucosa of the fistula. The incisions continue to the most posterior aspect of the fistula. Therefore, this may extend only as far back as the incisal foramen or more posteriorly into the soft palate. Each full-thickness mucoperiosteal palatal flap is elevated off the hard palate. Maintaining the integrity of an intact greater palatine vessel within each flap improves its circulation (**Fig 4.6-1c–d**).

The nasal mucosa flaps are completely separated from the oral mucosa of both the labial and palatal flaps and from the alveolar ridge and hard palate. The separated nasal mucosa is swept back up into the floor of the nose. Generally, there is an enlarged bulbous inferior turbinate and this is reduced in size with scissors to make room for the bone graft and to improve nasal breathing. The nasal mucosa wound edges are freshened of scar and granulation tissue and then sutured to achieve closure with resorbable sutures. It is difficult and unnecessary to gain complete closure of the most posterior aspect of the nasal flaps (**Fig 4.6-1e**).

The elevated palatal flaps are freshened along the previous fistula tract with removal of scar and granulation tissue. Resorbable sutures are placed to achieve palate closure.

The harvested cancellous bone is then packed into the skeletal defects throughout the hard palate, floor of the nose, alveolar cleft, and anterior surface of the hypoplastic maxilla (**Fig 4.6-1f**).

The previously elevated lesser segment labial mucogingival flap is scored at the periosteum to allow for advancement anteriorly to the fistula site. The two labial flaps are sutured to each other along the previous fistula tract and then to the palatal flaps over the alveolar ridge. Further suturing of the labial flaps to the palatal flaps is completed through the interdental papillae as far back as the flaps were elevated (**Fig 4.6-1g**).

This technique of "four" flap elevation, and "three" layered wound closure (ie, nasal layer, bone graft layer, oral layer) ensures both fistula closure and placement of keratinized gingiva in the region of eruption of the permanent canine tooth while still maintaining adequate attached gingiva in the more molar region.

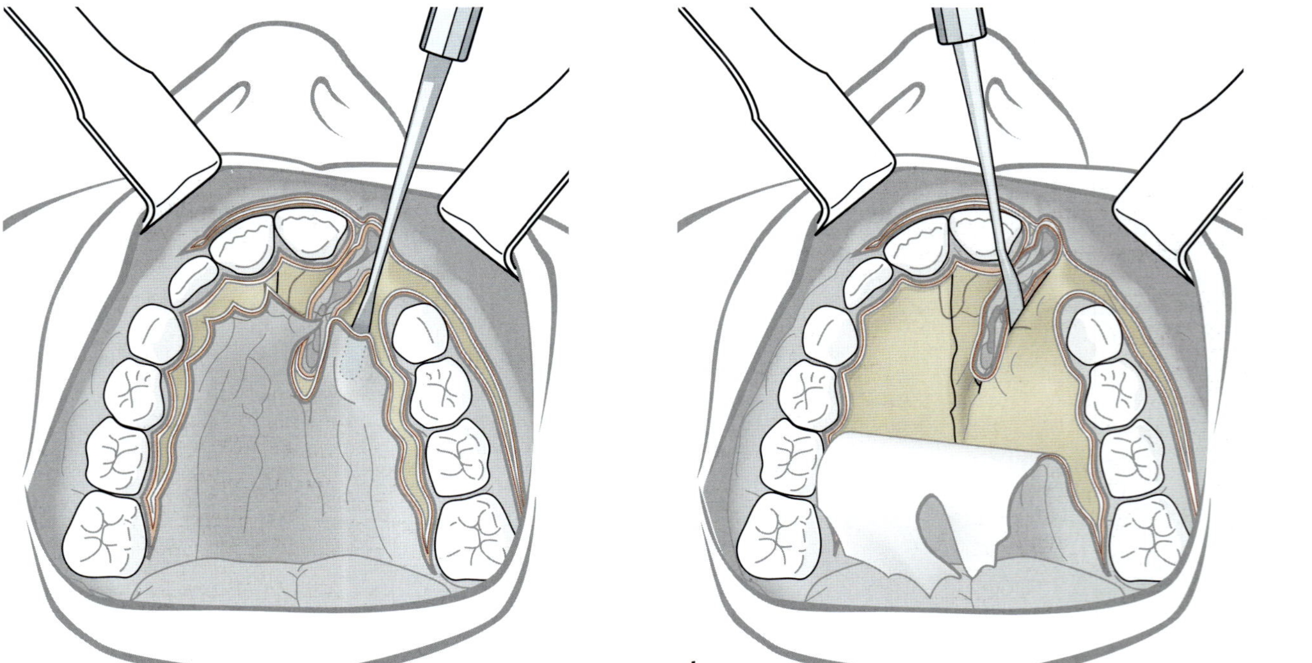

c d

Fig 4.6-1a–g (cont) Techniques for bone grafting and management of residual oronasal fistula in a 9-year-old patient with unilateral cleft lip and palate. The lip and palate were repaired in infancy and early childhood.
c Subperiosteal elevation of palatal flaps.
d With palatal flaps elevated, the nasal mucosa is separated from the floor of the nose on each side for later closure.

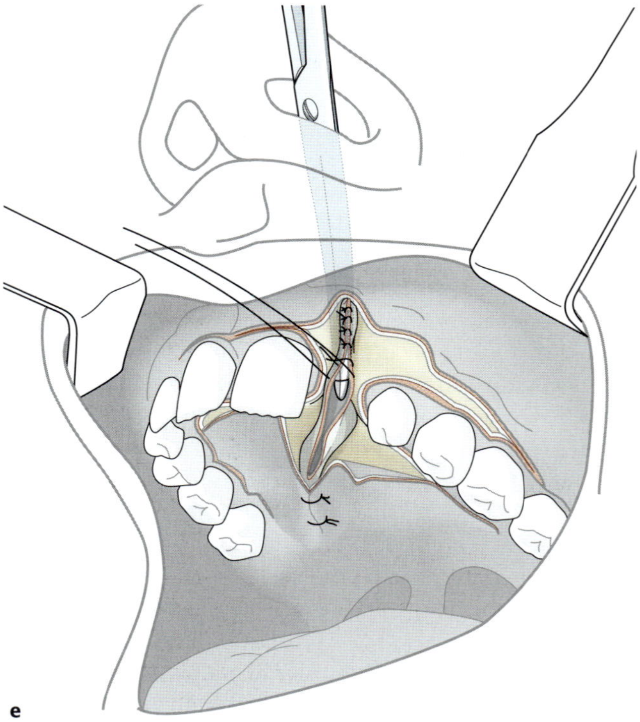

e

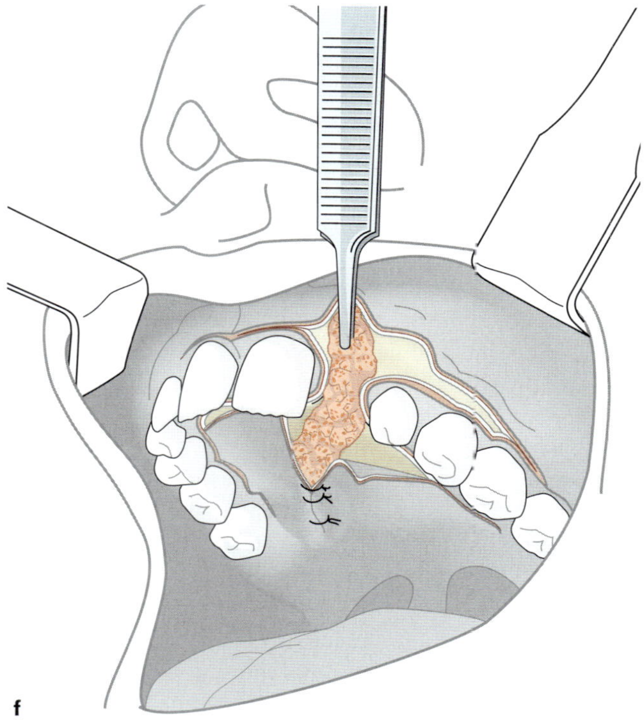

f

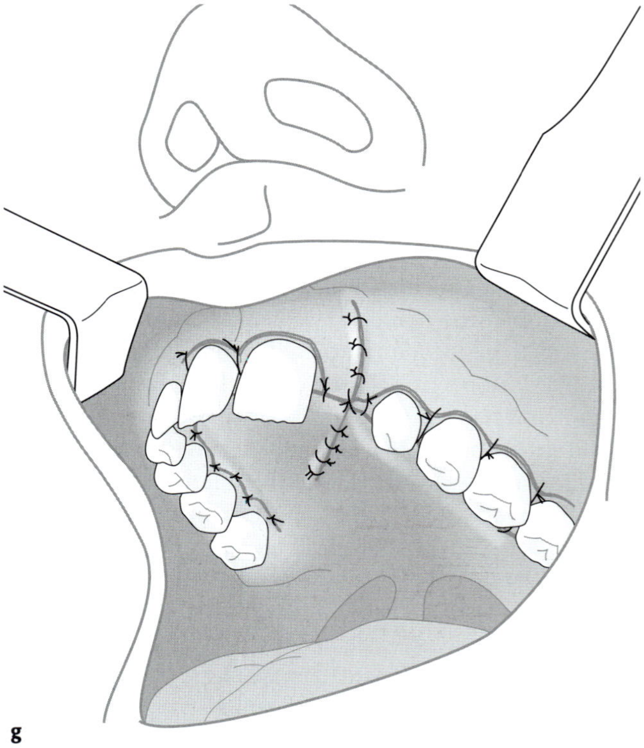

g

Fig 4.6-1a–g (cont) Techniques for bone grafting and management of residual oronasal fistula in a 9-year-old patient with unilateral cleft lip and palate. The lip and palate were repaired in infancy and early childhood.

- **e** Tight suturing of nasal flaps. A hemostat is placed through the left nostril to demonstrate the sutured nasal floor.
- **f** Once the nasal flaps are sutured, iliac cancellous bone graft is packed into palatal, alveolar, and floor-of-the-nose skeletal defects. Left labial flap is incised at periosteum to allow advancement for wound closure over the cleft site.
- **g** Left and right labial flaps and palatal flaps are closed. By advancing the left labial mucogingival flap, keratinized tissue has been placed over the alveolar ridge where the permanent canine tooth will eventually erupt.

4.2.2 For the BCLP patient

Elevation of the labial and palatal flaps is significantly different from that of the UCLP patient. When elevating the labial and palatal flaps for placement of the bone graft and closure of fistulae, the circulation to the premaxillary segment must be carefully maintained through its undisturbed labial mucosa. During flap elevation, it is critical that the labial mucosa overlying the premaxilla not be separated from the underlying periosteum and bone (**Fig 4.6-2a**). Also, on the palatal aspect of the premaxilla an incision is made to fully separate the oral and nasal mucosa. The incision location separates the palatal mucosa (which is keratinized) and the nasal mucosa (which is not) (**Fig 4.6-2b**).

The lateral segment labial flaps are elevated as previously described for the lesser segment flap for the UCLP patient. The posterior palatal flaps are also elevated in a similar way as described for the UCLP patient.

As in the UCLP patient, the inferior turbinates are reduced in size as needed to facilitate nasal side flap closure, to make room for the bone graft, and to improve nasal breathing. The nasal mucosa wound edges are freshened of scar and granulation tissue and then positioned back up into the floor of the nose for suturing to obtain a tight nasal side closure.

The two palatal flaps are sutured to each other in the midline at the previous fistula site for oral side closure of the oronasal communication. The anterior aspects of the palatal flaps are then sutured to the elevated premaxillary palatal mucosa (**Fig 4.6-2c**). If the distance separating these flaps is significant, it will not be possible to achieve a tight oral wound closure in the region of the incisive foramen and bone graft take and complete fistula closure (in the BCLP patient) will be compromised. It is sometimes necessary to gain additional tissue for wound closure by elevating and inserting an anteriorly based dorsal tongue flap.

For the BCLP patient immobilization of the premaxilla during the healing process is critical to achieving a bony union of the premaxillary segment to the lateral maxillary segments. Placement of a custom designed prefabricated acrylic splint directly over the occlusal surfaces of the maxillary teeth to secure the three maxillary segments to each other is a reliable method of immobilization. The splint is wired or bonded to the maxillary orthodontic brackets to achieve immobilization of the maxillary segments. The splint is left in place for 6–8 weeks after surgery (**Fig 4.6-2d**).

5 Alveolar grafting

5.1 Postsurgical care after alveolar grafting

Important postoperative instructions relate to oral hygiene, diet, physical activity level, and medications. Brushing the teeth with a soft-bristled pediatric toothbrush is important. The use of a water pic is not recommended because misdirected water pressure may cause separation of the wounds and bone graft exposure. The patient's diet is advanced to blended foods which should be continued for approximately 4 weeks for the UCLP patient and as long as 6–8 weeks for the BCLP patient. This will allow time for oral mucosa wound healing and initial bone graft consolidation. Concerning the physical activity level, it is important to begin ambulation soon after surgery but to pursue only sedentary activities for 4–6 weeks. This protects both the oral and hip wound regions. Orally administered antibiotics are continued after hospital discharge at the discretion of the surgeon. A prescription for pain relief is given.

5.2 Orthodontic goals after alveolar grafting

Approximately 6 weeks after the bone graft is placed and oronasal fistulae are closed, the patient returns to the orthodontist for evaluation. Reinsertion of the palatal appliance in general is not necessary. Early collapse of the arch width is not seen, as one would expect after procedures such as a surgically assisted rapid palatal expansion (SARPE). The orthodontic alignment of the maxillary anterior teeth will be accomplished overtime as needed. Eruption of the canine tooth through the bone graft is generally orthodontically guided into the location of the congenitally absent lateral incisor (ie, orthodontic closure of the cleft-dental gap without the need for prosthetic management). The orthodontist should do his or her best to limit the amount of time the patient is in active orthodontic treatment. Rather than a continued process of interceptive to final phase of treatment, a "get-in-and-get-out" approach is generally preferred. It is understood that detailing of the arches will proceed during the final phase of orthodontic treatment toward skeletal maturity. This will often be in conjunction with orthognathic surgery planned for the teenage years.

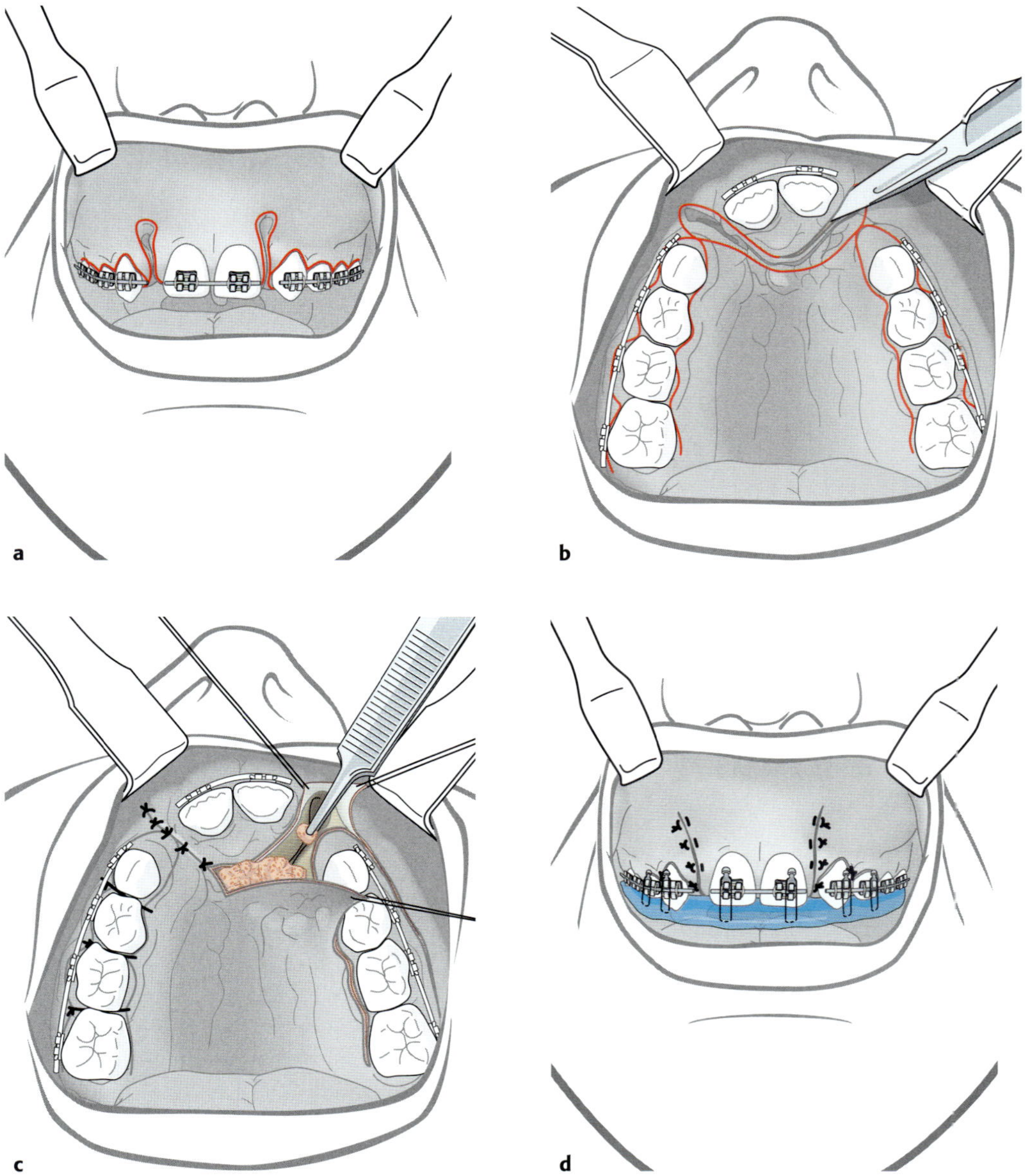

Fig 4.6-2a–d Technique for bone grafting and management of the residual oronasal fistula in a patient with bilateral cleft lip and palate.

a Frontal view indicating location and extent of planned labial incisions. Note the importance of maintaining the integrity of the labial mucosa to the premaxillary bone. Without doing so, the circulation requirements to the premaxilla may be compromised.

b Palatal view indicating location and extent of planned incisions for secondary bone grafting and fistula closure.

c After nasal side closure and bone graft placement on the right side, the oral wounds are closed. View of palate indicating final placement of bone graft on the left side before closure.

d Frontal view after bone grafting procedure and wound closure. Prefabricated acrylic splint is used to secure the three maxillary segments to one another to allow for bone graft healing.

5.3 Controversies

A controversy for the reconstruction of the UCLP/BCLP patient centers around a philosophy of the importance of achieving a "28-Tooth Angle Class I occlusion" with traditional "cuspid-protection" rather than "group function" during lateral excursions. Studies confirm that approximately 93% of the time in UCLP/BCLP, the lateral incisor is either congenitally absent or inadequate at the cleft site. A hypoplastic incisor or supernumerary tooth may be present adjacent to the cleft but with inadequate root development. To achieve a "28-tooth" occlusion would require the maintenance of each cleft-dental gap (ie, lateral incisor region), and no additional extractions (nonextraction therapy) during orthodontics. This would be followed by a single tooth dental implant placement or use of another prosthetic option. Unfortunately, in the maxillary deficient UCLP/BCLP patient dental crowding generally exists. For this reason extractions and/or closure of dental gaps are required just for the purpose of avoiding long-term periodontal sequela.

In a noncleft population, only a few studies compare the results of orthodontic space closure (OSC) to prosthetic replacement (PR) for management of congenitally absent maxillary lateral incisors. The absence of high-quality clinical research to evaluate an implant replacement option (as opposed to a bridge) continues to fuel the discussion of what constitutes optimal treatment of a missing lateral incisor in the cleft patient. It has been documented in several studies that for an individual with an alveolar cleft, OSC results in a healthier periodontium and greater patient satisfaction than classic PR. Orthodontic space closure in cleft patients after successful alveolar bone grafting has the added advantage that the canine can be positioned into the lateral incisor location resulting in an improved alveolar ridge morphology. A single tooth dental implant option for management of the cleft dental gap in the UCLP/BCLP individual is an attractive theoretical alternative but requires the presence of an intact maxilla (ie, stability of premaxilla to each lateral segment in the case of BCLP) with adequate alveolar bone volume, interproximal crestal height, and sufficient attached gingiva at each cleft site for favorable implant placement, dental esthetics, and long-term maintenance. Unfortunately, these physiological/anatomical parameters are not often met in patients with UCLP/BCLP. Furthermore, required dental procedures (eg, gingival grafting, alveolar augmentation, implant placement) are rarely covered by medical insurance which adds to the family's financial burden. This approach would require meticulous coordination of a spectrum of dental specialists (eg, orthodontist, periodontist, prosthodontist, and surgeon) who have expertise and dedication in treating cleft deformities. Even if implant placement and crown restoration is successful it will create a long-term high maintenance dentition for the patient. This combination of factors usually favors OSC when feasible or surgical space (dental gap) closure (via segmental Le Fort I) when appropriate.

Orthodontic space closure is preferably accomplished by successful mixed dentition grafting, canine eruption through the graft, and orthodontic dental gap closure. Oosterkamp et al [2010] completed a retrospective study of adults with BCLP who were missing a permanent lateral incisor at each cleft site. The patients were treated either with orthodontic space closure (n = 17) or by prosthetic replacement (n = 10). The purpose of the study was to compare dental esthetics and function of OSC versus PR of lateral incisors in BCLP. Neither financial nor time commitment burden-of-care issues were taken into account. The predominant mode of prosthetic replacement was resin-bonded bridges. Dental esthetics was evaluated by the patients themselves and by a professional panel. Mandibular function was evaluated by means of the mandibular function impairment questionnaire (standardized survey). The level of mandibular impairment was calculated using the functional impairment rating scale (standardized rating scale). With respect to dental esthetics, no significant differences between patients treated with orthodontic space closure and prosthetic replacement was found. With respect to function, the level of mandibular impairment was significantly higher in patients treated with prosthetic replacement compared with those treated with orthodontic space closure.

6 Summary

This author's preferred method for managing cleft defects of the hard palate, alveolar ridge, and floor of the nose is to place autogenous particulate cancellous iliac bone graft within the defects and simultaneously close all residual oronasal fistulae in the mixed dentition before eruption of the maxillary canine. A short phase of interceptive orthodontic treatment to normalize the maxillary arch form precedes bone graft placement. With subsequent permanent canine eruption through the graft, followed by orthodontic elimination of the dental gap (in the region in the congenitally inadequate lateral incisor), a periodontal sound low maintenance dental rehabilitation is achieved.

When successful, this form of staged reconstruction converts the cleft maxilla into a noncleft maxilla, without adding additional growth inhibition to the upper jaw. If surgical management of maxillary hypoplasia is later required, it is carried out using a standard Le Fort I osteotomy without the need for special considerations related to the previous alveolar cleft.

7 References and suggested reading

Abyholm FE, Bergland O, Semb G. Secondary bone grafting of alveolar clefts. *Scand J Plast Reconstr Surg Hand Surg*. 1981;15(2):127–140.

Adell R. Regeneration of the periodontium. *Scand J Plast Reconstr Surg Suppl*. 1974;11:1–177.

Bergland D, Semb G, Abyholm FE, et al. Elimination of the residual alveolar cleft by secondary bone grafting and subsequent orthodontic treatment. *Cleft Palate J*. 1986 Jul;23(3):175–205.

Berkowitz S. The comparison of treatment results in complete cleft lip/palate using conservative approach vs Millard–Latham PSOT procedure. In: Sadowsky PL, ed. *Cleft Lip and Palate*. Philadelphia: Saunders; 1996:169.

Berkowitz S, Mejia M, Bystrik A. A comparison of the effects of the Latham-Millard procedure with those of a conservative treatment approach for dental occlusion and facial aesthetics in unilateral and bilateral complete cleft lip and palate: part 1. Dental occlusion. *Plast Reconstr Surg*. 2004 Jan;113(1):1–18.

Boyne PJ, Sands NR. Secondary bone grafting in residual alveolar and palatal defects. *J Oral Surg*. 1972 Feb;30(2):87–92.

Capelozza Filho L, Normando AD, da Silva Filho OG. Isolated influences of lip and palate surgery on facial growth: comparison of operated and unoperated male adults with UCLP. *Cleft Palate Craniofac J*. 1996 Jan;33(1):51–56.

Cassolato SF, Ross B, Daskalogiannakis J, et al. Treatment of dental anomalies in children with complete unilateral cleft lip and palate at SickKids Hospital, Toronto. *Cleft Palate Craniofac J*. 2009 Mar;46 (2):166–172.

Daskalogiannakis J, Ross RB. Effect of alveolar bone grafting in the mixed dentition on maxillary growth in complete unilateral cleft lip and palate patients. *Cleft Palate Craniofac J*. 1997 Sep;34(5):455–458.

Daskalogiannakis J, Mehta M. The need for orthognathic surgery in patients with repaired complete unilateral and complete bilateral cleft lip and palate. *Cleft Palate Craniofac J*. 2009 Sep;46(5):498–502.

David DJ, Anderson PJ, Schnitt DE, et al. From birth to maturity: a group of patients who have completed their protocol management. Part II. Isolated cleft palate. *Plast Reconstr Surg*. 2006 Feb;117(2):515–526.

DeLuke DM, Marchand A, Robles EC, et al. Facial growth and the need for orthognathic surgery after cleft palate repair: literature review and report of 28 cases. *J Oral Maxillofac Surg*. 1997 Jul;55(7):694–698.

Felstead AM, Deacon S, Revington P. The outcome for secondary alveolar bone grafting in the South West UK region post-CSAG. *Cleft Palate Craniofac*. 2010 Jul;47(4):359–362.

Friede H, Lilja J. Dentofacial morphology in adolescent or early adult patients with cleft lip and palate after a treatment regime that included vomer flap surgery and pushback palate repair. *Scand J Plast Reconstr Hand Surg*. 1994 Jun;28(2):113–121.

Friede H, Pruzansky S. Long-term effects of premaxillary setback on facial skeletal profile in complete bilateral cleft lip and palate. *Cleft Palate J*. 1985 Apr;22(2):97–105.

Fudalej P, Hortis-Dzierzbicka M, Obloj B, et al. Treatment outcome after one-stage repair in children with complete unilateral cleft lip and palate assessed with the Goslon Yardstick. *Cleft Palate Craniofac J*. 2009 Jul;46(4):374–380.

Good PM, Mulliken JB, Padwa BL. Frequency of Le Fort I osteotomy after repaired cleft lip and palate or cleft palate. *Cleft Palate-Craniofac J*. 2007 Jul;44(4):396–401.

Grayson BH, Cutting CB. Presurgical nasoalveolar orthopedic molding in primary correction of the nose, lip, and alveolus of infants bone with unilateral and bilateral clefts. *Cleft Palate Craniofac J*. 2001 May;38(3):193–198.

Guzel MZ, Altintas F. Repair of large, anterior palatal fistulas using thin tongue flap: long-term follow-up of 10 patients. *Ann Plast Surg*. 2000 Aug;45(2):109–114; discussion 114–117.

Hall HD, Posnick JC. Early results of secondary bone grafts in 106 alveolar clefts. *J Oral Maxillofac Surg*. 1983 May;41(5):289–294.

Harrison JW. Dental implants to rehabilitate a patient with an unrepaired complete cleft. *Cleft Palate Craniofac J*. 1992 Sep;29(5):485–458.

Hathaway RR, Eppley BLE, Hennon DK, et al. Primary alveolar cleft bone grafting in UCLP: arch dimensions at age 8. *J Craniofac Surg*. 1999 Jan;10(1):58–67.

Hathaway R, Daskalogiannakis J, et al. The Americleft Study: an inter-center study of treatment outcomes for patients with unilateral cleft lip and palate. Part 2. Dental arch relationship. *J Cleft Palate Craniofac*. 2011 May;48(3):244–251.

Heidbüchel KL, Kuijpers-Jagtman AM, Freihofer HPM. Facial growth in patients with bilateral cleft lip and palate: a cephalometric study. *Cleft Palate Craniofac J*. 1994 May;31(3):210–216.

Henkel KO, Gundlach KKH. Analysis of primary gingivoperiosteoplasty in alveolar cleft repair. Part I: facial growth. *J Craniomaxillofac Surg*. 1997 Oct;25(5):266–269.

Hsieh CH, Ko EW, Chen PK, et al. The effects of gingivoperiosteoplasty on facial growth in patients with complete unilateral cleft lip and palate. *Cleft Palate Craniofac J*. 2010 Sep;47(5):439–446.

Jorgenson RJ, Shapiro SD, Odinet KL. Studies on facial growth and arch size in cleft lip and plate. *J Craniofac Genet Dev Biol*. 1984;4(1):33–38.

Lund TW, Wade M. Use of osseointegrated implants to support a maxillary denture for a patient with repaired cleft lip and palate. *Cleft Palate Craniofac J*. 1993 Jul;30(4):418–420.

Mars M, Plint DA, Houston WJB, et al. The Goslon Yardstick: a new system of assessing dental arch relationships in children with unilateral clefts of the lip and palate. *Cleft Palate J*. 1987 Oct;24(4):314–322.

Matic DB, Power SM. The effects of gingivoperiosteoplasty following alveolar molding with a pin-retained Latham appliance versus secondary bone grafting on midfacial growth in patients with unilateral clefts. *Plast Reconstr Surg.* 2008 Sep;122(3):863–870.

McIntyre GT, Devlin MF. Secondary alveolar bone grafting (CLEFTSiS) 2000–2004. *Cleft Palate Craniofac J.* 2010 Jan;47(1):66–72.

Millard DR Jr, Latham RA. Improved primary surgical and dental treatment of clefts. *Plast Reconstr Surg.* 1990 Nov;86(5):856–871.

Millard DR, Latham RA, Huifen X, et al. Cleft lip and palate treated by presurgical orthopedics, gingivoperiosteoplasty, and lip adhesion (POPLA) compared with previous lip adhesion method: a preliminary study of serial dental casts. *Plast Reconstr Surg.* 1999 May;103(6):1630–1644.

Normando AD, da Silva Filho OG, Capelozza Filho L. Influence of surgery on maxillary growth in cleft lip and/or palate patients. *J Craniomaxillofac Surg.* 1992 Apr;20(3):111–118.

Nordquist GG, McNeill RW. Orthodontic vs. restorative treatment of the congenitally absent lateral incisor—long-term periodontal and occlusal evaluation. *J Periodontol.* 1975 Mar;46(3):139–143.

Oosterkamp BC, Dijkstra PU, Remmelink HJ, et al. Orthodontic space closure versus prosthetic replacement of missing upper lateral incisors in patients with bilateral cleft lip and palate. *Cleft Palate Craniofac J.* 2010 Nov;47(6):591–596.

Posnick JC. Orthognathic surgery for the cleft lip and palate patient. In: *Seminars in Orthodontics.* Philadelphia: WB Saunders 1996;2(3):205–214.

Posnick JC. Cleft orthognathic surgery: the unilateral cleft lip and palate deformity. In: Posnick JC, ed. Orthognathic Surgery: *Principles and Practice.* St Louis: Elsevier; 2014;33:1297–1370.

Posnick JC. Cleft orthognathic surgery: the unilateral cleft lip and palate deformity. In: Posnick JC, ed. Orthognathic Surgery: *Principles and Practice.* St Louis: Elsevier; 2014;33:1371–1440.

Posnick JC. The staging of cleft lip and palate reconstruction: infancy through adolescence. In: Posnick JC, ed. *Craniofacial and Maxillofacial Surgery in Children and Young Adults.* Philadelphia: WB Saunders; 2000;32:785–826.

Posnick JC, Gray JA. Is it safe to re-harvest the anterior iliac crest to manage Le Fort I interpositional defects in young adults with a repaired cleft? *J Oral Maxillofac Surg* 2015;73:S32–S39.

Posnick JC. Cleft lip and palate: bone grafting and management of residual oro-nasal fistula. In: Posnick JC, ed. *Craniofacial and Maxillofacial Surgery in Children and Young Adults.* Philadelphia: WB Saunders Co; 2000;33:827–885.

Proffitt WR. Orthodontic treatment of clefts: yesterday, today and tomorrow. In: Proceedings of the 48th Annual Meeting, American Cleft Palate–Craniofacial Association; March 1991; Hilton Head, SC.

Robertsson S, Mohlin B. The congenitally missing upper lateral incisor: a retrospective study of orthodontic space closure versus restorative treatment. *Eur J Orthod.* 2000 Dec;22(6):697–710.

Ronchi P, Chiapasco M, Frattini D. Endosseous implants for prosthetic rehabilitation in bone grafted alveolar clefts. *J Craniomaxillofac Surg.* 1995 Dec;23(6):382–386.

Ross RB. Treatment variables affecting facial growth in complete unilateral cleft lip and palate: Part 3. Alveolus repair and bone grafting. *Cleft Palate J.* 1987 Jan;24(1):33.

Ross BR. Treatment variables affecting facial growth in complete unilateral cleft lip and palate. Part 7: an overview of treatment and facial growth. *Cleft Palate J.* 1987 Jan;24(1):71–77.

Skoog T. The use of periosteal flaps in the repair of cleft of the primary palate. *Cleft Palate J.* 1965;2:332–339.

Suzuki A, Takahama Y. Maxillary lateral incisor of subjects with cleft lip and/or palate: Part 1. *Cleft Palate Craniofac J.* 1992 Jul;29(4):376–379.

Takahashi T, Fukuda M, Yamaguchi T, et al. Use of an osseointegrated implant for dental rehabilitation after cleft repair by periosteoplasty: a case report. *Cleft Palate Craniofac J.* 1997;35:268.

Takahashi T, Fukuda M, Yamaguchi T, et al. Use of endosseous implants for dental reconstruction of patients with grafted alveolar clefts. *J Oral Maxillofac Surg.* 1997 Jun;55(6):576–583.

Turvey TA, Vig K, Moriarty J, et al. Delayed bone grafting in the cleft maxilla and palate: a retrospective multidisciplinary analysis. *Am J Orthod.* 1984 Sep;86(3):244–256.

Vargervic K. Orthodontic management of unilateral cleft lip and palate. *Cleft Palate J.* 1981 Oct;18(4):256–270.

Verdi FJ Jr, Slanzi GL, Cohen SR, et al. Use of the Branemark implant in the cleft palate patient. *Cleft Palate Craniofac J.* 1991 Jul;28(3):301–303.

Zachrisson BU, Stenvik A. Single implants—optimal therapy for missing lateral incisors? *Am J Orthod Dentofacial Orthop.* 2004 Dec;126(6):A13–15.

4.7 Orthognathic surgery for unilateral and bilateral total clefts

Jeffrey C Posnick

1 Introduction

The successful reconstruction of cleft lip and palate is inextricably connected with orthodontic care and skeletal surgery. It is now clear that orthognathic surgery is a necessary component of treatment for many individuals born with unilateral cleft lip and palate (UCLP), bilateral cleft lip and palate (BCLP), and isolated cleft palate (ICP) that have undergone lip or palate repair in infancy.

2 Facial growth implications of cleft palate repair in infancy

Good and colleagues [2007] reviewed the prevalence of Le Fort I osteotomy in patients with cleft lip/palate treated at Boston Children's Hospital. They found that 48% of their repaired UCLP and 76.5% of their repaired BCLP patients required orthognathic surgery in the teenage years. Similarly, the Hospital for Sick Children (Toronto, Canada) found that 48.3% of their complete UCLP and 65.1% of their BCLP patients required or underwent orthognathic surgery, while 70% of BCLP patients referred to their team sometime after cleft lip repair were found to require orthognathic surgery.

3 Coordinated team approach

Care of the cleft patient (ie, UCLP, BCLP, and ICP) is best delivered by an integrated group of specialists who evaluate and provide definitive care. It is no longer acceptable for individual practitioners (eg, surgeons, orthodontists, restorative dentists, speech pathologists, or otolaryngologists) to carry out extended treatment without considering all aspects of the patient's care and without discussing options with all members of the team.

3.1 Treatment protocol

Patients presenting with a cleft jaw deformity referred for possible orthognathic surgery are, at a minimum, seen by an orthodontist, orthognathic surgeon, otolaryngologist, and speech pathologist. Additional consultations are held with a prosthodontist, pediatrician/general dentist; periodontist, and other medical specialists (ie, sleep specialist, geneticist), as indicated. For evaluation of the cleft dentofacial deformity, records and tests should include medical-quality photographs with views of the face and occlusion, cephalometric and dental radiographs, dental models and a centric relation bite, direct facial measurements, nasoendoscopic speech and velopharyngeal assessment, and a thorough evaluation of the upper airway.

Discussion between the treating medical and dental consultants and patient/family clarifies the need for and extent of orthognathic and intranasal procedures. The overall plan for speech, jaw, upper airway, dental rehabilitation, and the enhancement of facial esthetics should be accepted by all practitioners and the family representing the patient prior to initiating any treatment.

3.2 Timing of orthognathic surgery

Correction of the cleft jaw deformity is best carried out after skeletal maturity. Maxillofacial growth is generally complete between the ages of 14 and 16 years in girls and 16 and 18 years in boys. However, skeletal growth is variable and best documented by knowledge of the pubertal growth spurt and/or review of sequential cephalometric radiographs taken at intervals. The patient/family's preferences for timing of the reconstruction based on psychosocial needs (ie, self-esteem, body image) and functional disability (ie, speech, swallowing, chewing, and breathing) are also taken into account.

3.3 Residual deformities in the adolescent born with a cleft

Correction of residual skeletal, soft-tissue, and dental deformities in the UCLP and BCLP adolescent will be especially challenging for the orthognathic surgeon and cleft team. The central deformity is maxillary hypoplasia but it is often combined with residual oronasal fistulae, bony defects, intranasal obstruction, soft-tissue scarring, and velopharyngeal dysfunction. In addition, the maxillary lateral incisor at the cleft site is usually congenitally absent or deficient, resulting in cleft dental gap. Secondary deformities of the nose, mandible, and chin region are also common. The prevalence of these residual cleft deformities in mature patients with UCLP and BCLP varies widely depending on the primary cleft surgeon's philosophy, available expertise, the individual's intrinsic biological growth potential, and the family/patient's interest. Published clinical surveys of individuals born with complete UCLP or BCLP and treated at established cleft centers indicate that despite best efforts, a number of children will not be available for mixed dentition (before eruption of the cleft side canine) grafting. Also, some of those that do will fail grafting and require other means of reconstruction and dental rehabilitation. For these reasons, a subgroup of UCLP and BCLP patients will present at or after adolescence with multiple cleft-related problems that may include:

- Maxillary hypoplasia
- Residual oronasal fistulae
- Residual bony defect(s)
- Cleft dental gap(s)
- Chin dysplasia
- Mandibular dysplasia
- Nasal obstruction and sinus blockage
- Velopharyngeal dysfunction

3.4 Orthodontic considerations in a cleft patient with a jaw deformity

The adolescent or adult cleft patient that presents with maxillary hypoplasia and ineffective bone grafting will have two maxillary segments separated by a cleft if born with UCLP or three maxillary segments separated by clefts if born with BCLP. Each segment of the maxilla will have a varied degree of hypoplasia/dysplasia in all three planes in space. From an orthodontic perspective, each segment should be treated individually in anticipation of segmental surgical repositioning.

On the other hand, if the cleft patient underwent effective bone grafting in the mixed dentition followed by canine eruption through the graft, then the maxillary arch form should be evaluated by the orthodontist as an integrated unit.

The decision to extract a fully erupted normally formed tooth (ie, first premolar) depends on the volume and height of available alveolar bone to house the dental roots within arch (or segment of the arch). When indicated, it is preferred to extract a first bicuspid to ensure that there is adequate alveolar bone for leveling and aligning all the retained teeth without irreversibly weakening the periodontal support. Planning for extractions in the maxillary arch depends on alveolar space requirements and on tooth movements needed to position the incisors ideally over basal bone. Mandibular extractions are generally not required.

The potential disadvantage of closure of a cleft dental gap (whether carried out orthodontically or surgically) is that it shifts the preoperative anterior dental gap (lateral incisor region) to a post-treatment posterior dental gap (second molar region). Articulated dental models with the maxilla (or maxillary segments) in the proposed postoperative locations are analyzed prior to treatment. This will confirm that the posterior mandibulomaxillary occlusion will be acceptable. For this reason, the maxillary second molars should be orthodontically included in the arch form. Occasionally, there will be a nonimpacted maxillary third molar tooth that can also be incorporated to oppose the mandibular second molar.

3.5 Immediate presurgical reassessment

Two to 6 weeks before the planned operation, the orthodontist places passive surgical wires and confirms that the preoperative orthodontic objectives have been met. The surgeon takes final records including alginate impressions of the maxillary and mandibular teeth, a centric relation bite registration, a face bow registration for transfer to the semi-adjustable articulator and direct facial measurements. Past medical and dental records (eg, radiographs, consult reports, photographs, dental models, special studies) are reviewed. Computed tomographic scan views of the cleft alveolus can be especially helpful to assess bone volume in the BCLP patient. Decisions are finalized concerning preferred vector changes (repositioning) of the jaw(s) and the precise linear (mm) distances and angles to be accomplished in each jaw for the desired result. Model planning is carried out on the articulated dental casts and splints are fabricated. The splints assist in achieving the precise occlusion and preferred facial esthetics which have been decided preoperatively.

4 Orthognathic surgical approach

4.1 Unilateral cleft lip and palate

Historically, the literature warned of possible complications with maxillary osteotomies in patients with UCLP. As with other aspects of orthognathic surgery, Hugo Obwegeser's milestone contributions to cleft skeletal reconstruction are important. By the late 1960s, he succeeded in advancing the cleft maxilla to the preferred location without the need for a compromised mandibular setback approach. By the mid-1980s, Posnick clarified and routinely utilized Obwegeser's technique of segmental Le Fort I osteotomy for treatment of the ineffectively grafted UCLP jaw deformity. A key aspect is use of the circumvestibular incision which permits direct exposure for dissection, osteotomies, disimpaction, fistula closure, septoplasty, inferior turbinate reduction, pyriform aperture recontouring, bone grafting, and application of plate and screw fixation. This access allows for the routine closure of the cleft dental gap through differential repositioning of each segment.

The modified Le Fort I osteotomy in two segments as carried out in a patient with unilateral cleft lip and palate (UCLP) who has not undergone successful bone grafting in the mixed dentition is shown in **Figs 4.7-1–4.7-4**.

The extent of maxillary advancement carried out by the surgeon is based on the preferred occlusion, airway needs, and facial esthetics determined preoperatively. The ideal vertical dimension is also achieved intraoperatively based on the preoperative plan. The maxillary osteotomized segments are fixed in place with titanium plates and screws at each zygomatic buttress and pyriform aperture according to the principles originally described by Luhr [1968]. An additional microplate is applied to stabilize each interpositional corticocancellous (iliac) graft.

Mandibular and chin osteotomies to correct secondary deformities and facial asymmetries are also frequently required to achieve objectives. The purpose of a mandibular osteotomy is not to set back the lower jaw but rather to fully correct the face.

Improving the nasal airway through septoplasty, reduction of inferior turbinates, and recontouring of the pyriform rims/nasal floor/anterior nasal spine is also simultaneously carried out when indicated.

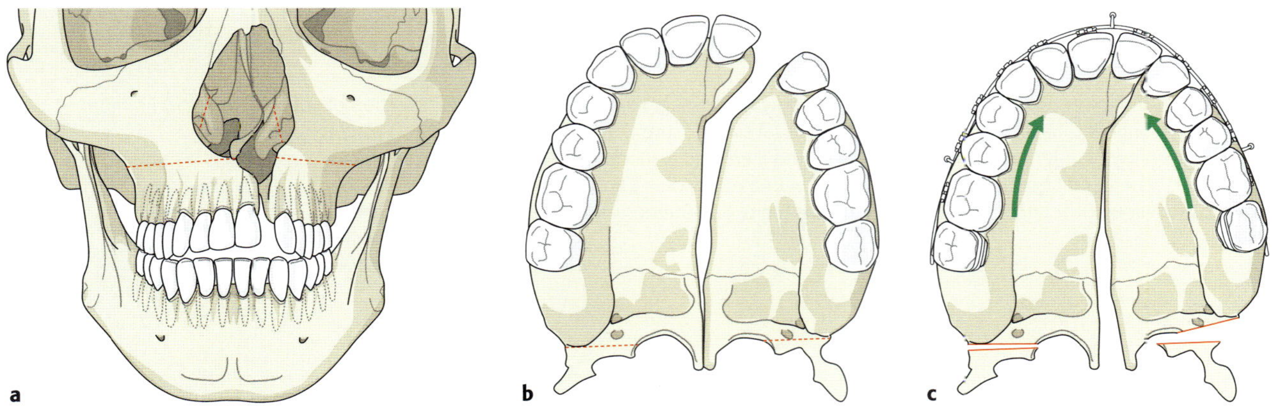

Fig 4.7-1a–c
a Frontal view of maxillofacial skeleton before osteotomy. Le Fort I osteotomy line indicated.
b–c Palatal view of bony segments before (**b**) and after (**c**) repositioning.

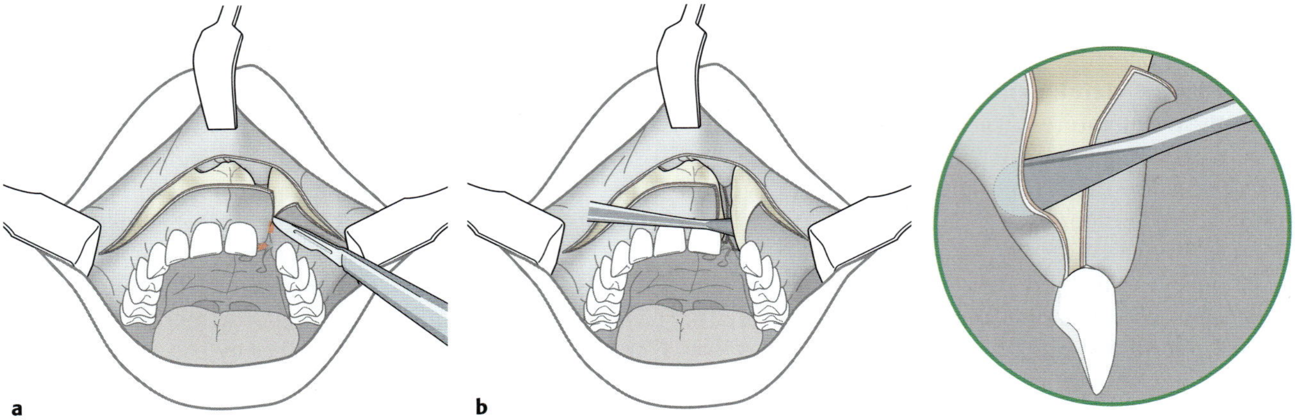

Fig 4.7-2a–b Circumvestibular and perifistula incisions for exposure to complete osteotomies and later fistula closure.

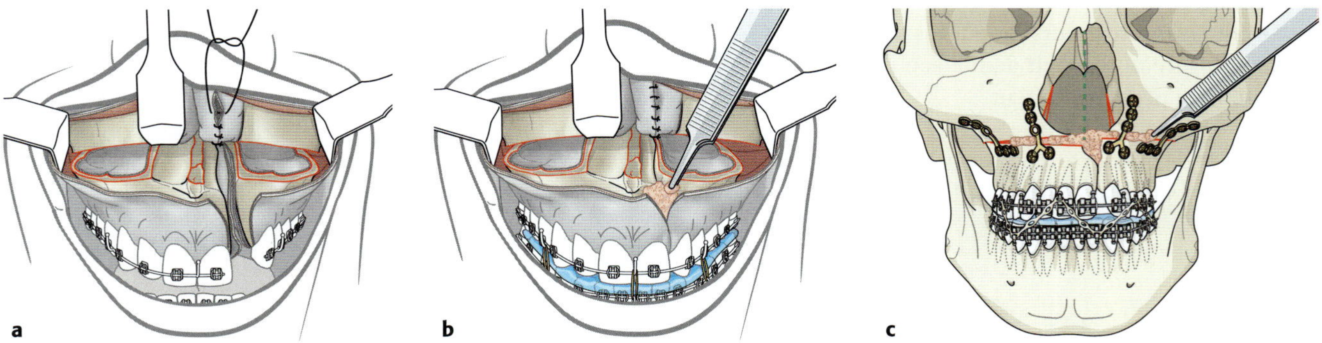

Fig 4.7-3a–c

a–b Down-fractured lower maxilla after Le Fort I osteotomy in two segments after submucous resection of septum, reduction of inferior turbinate through the nasal mucosa opening, and nasal side closure. Cancellous iliac bone graft placed in cleft area.

c After osteotomy the inferior turbinates have been reduced, and a submucous resection of the deviated septum has also been performed. The nasal floor has been recontoured with a rotary drill. Cancellous iliac bone graft has been placed along the nasal floor. Corticocancellous (iliac) graft is also placed in gaps along the anterior maxilla on each side. Correct occlusion is achieved.

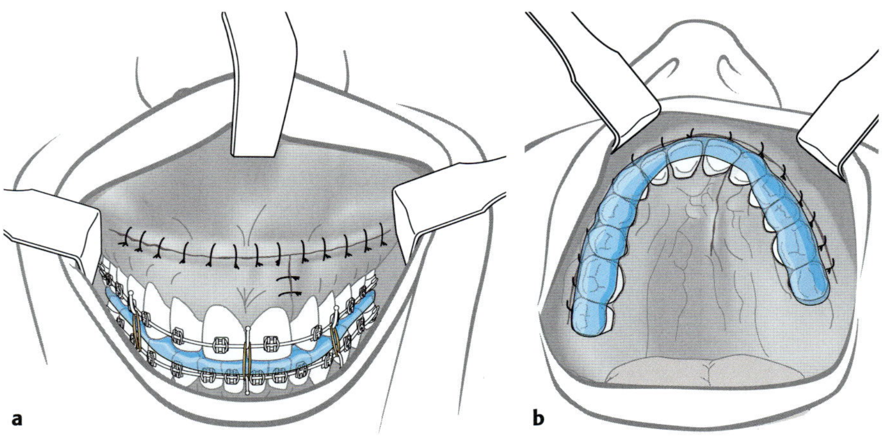

Fig 4.7-4a–b Wound closure. Acrylic splint in place after differential segmental repositioning.

4.2 Bilateral cleft lip and palate

Surgical attempts to correct the jaw disharmony seen in patients with BCLP date back to Steinkamm's descriptions in 1938. Hugo Obwegeser's [1969, 1985] early milestone contributions to cleft skeletal reconstruction are important but unfortunately few clinicians shared his enthusiasm for the management of cleft jaw deformities at the time (**Fig 4.7-5**).

Posnick [1990] clarified the safety of the segmental Le Fort I osteotomy technique in patients with a BCLP jaw deformity in whom effective bone grafting in the mixed dentition was not accomplished. The documented favorable results confirmed the importance of following sound biological principles. In the unsuccessfully grafted BCLP individual, preservation of the labial soft tissue-mucosal pedicle to the premaxilla is essential. The validity of this flap circulation was proven by Bell et al [1971] in rhesus monkeys. For the BCLP patient presenting with a "three-segment" residual clefted maxillary deformity, the modified Le Fort I osteotomy (in three segments) can be used with safety and efficiency (**Fig 4.7-5**).

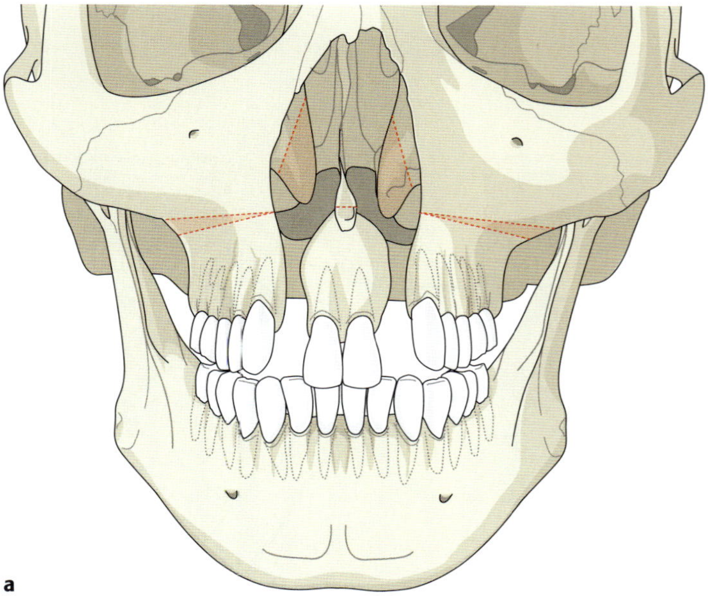

a

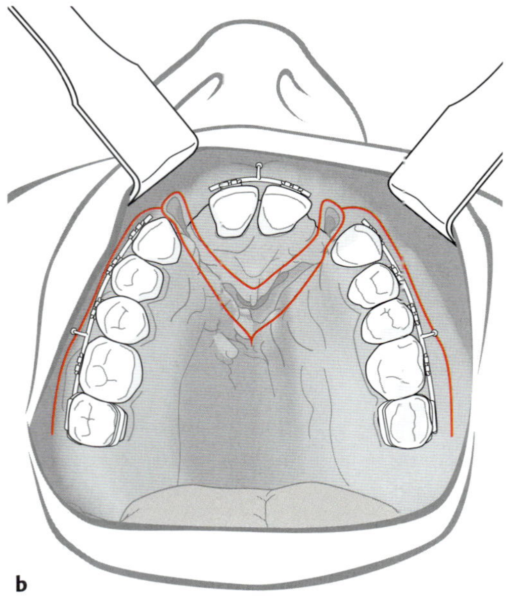

b

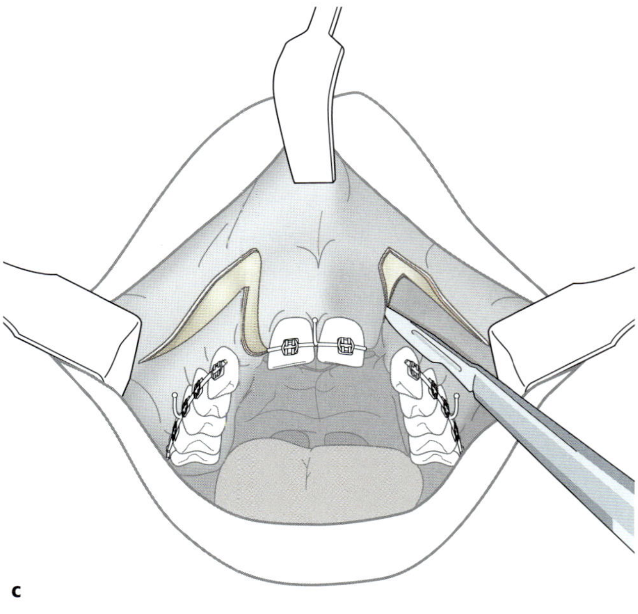

c

Fig 4.7-5a–l Modified Le Fort I osteotomy in three segments as carried out in a patient with bilateral cleft lip and palate (BCLP) who has not undergone successful bone grafting in the mixed dentition.

- **a** Ungrafted malpositioned maxilla in a BCLP patient; osteotomy cuts and inferior turbinate reduction outlined.
- **b** Vestibular and palatinal surgical approaches outlined.
- **c** Vestibular incisions.

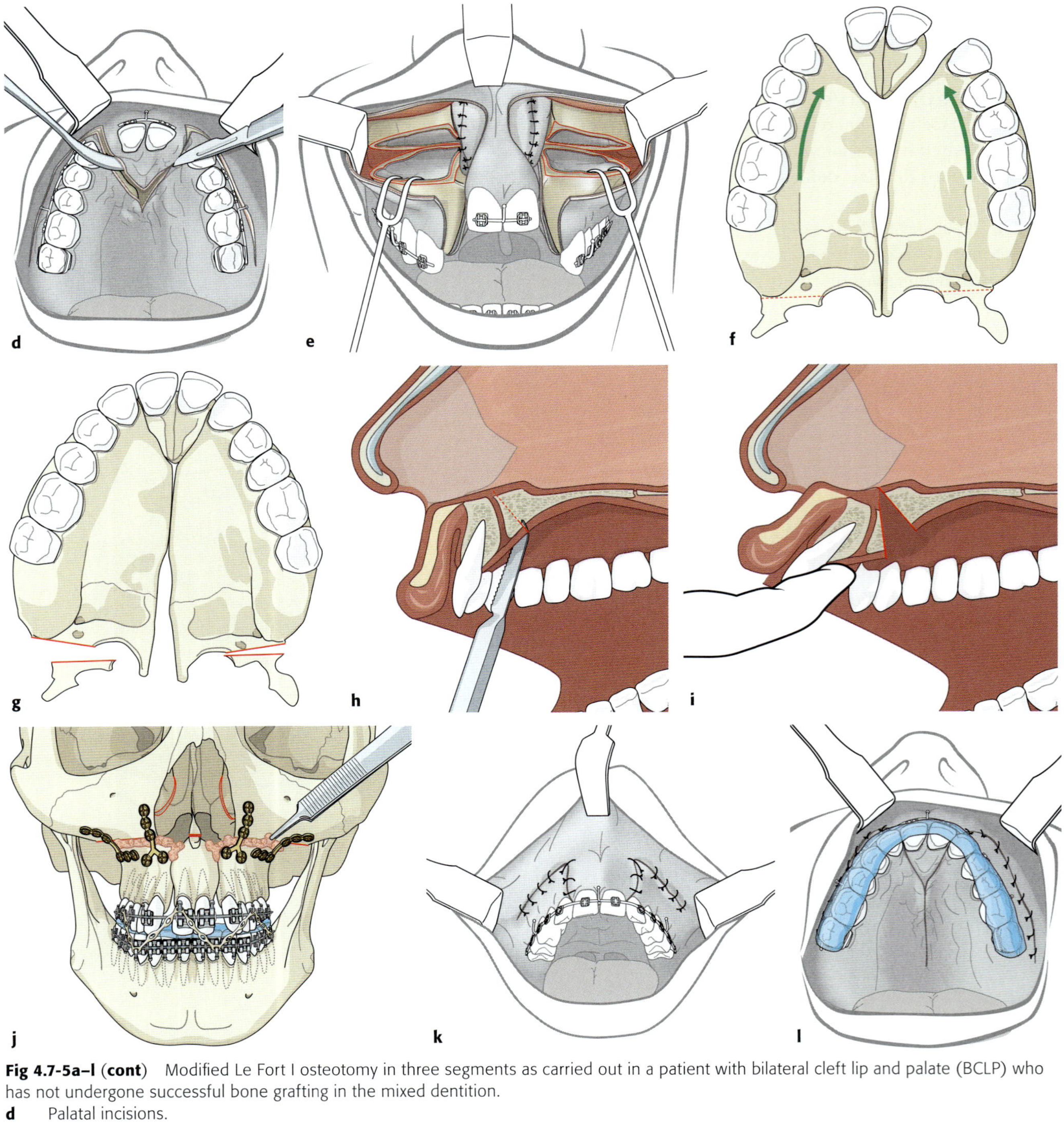

Fig 4.7-5a–l (cont) Modified Le Fort I osteotomy in three segments as carried out in a patient with bilateral cleft lip and palate (BCLP) who has not undergone successful bone grafting in the mixed dentition.

- **d** Palatal incisions.
- **e** Down-fractured lateral segments demonstrating exposure for nasal side closure of oronasal fistula.
- **f–g** Palatal views of bone segments before and after repositioning for closure of cleft dental gaps.
- **h–i** Premaxillary osteotomy carried out on palate side (vomar osteotomy) using a reciprocating saw.
- **j** Le Fort I 3-part maxillary osteotomies with repositioning and fixation of the segments. Septoplasty and inferior turbinate reduction is also shown, as well as bone grafting to the maxilla.
- **k–l** Oral wounds sutured at end of procedure. Note: no sutures are required on palatal side.

The BCLP patient with an intact (successfully grafted) alveolar ridge on one side essentially presents to the surgeon with the same anatomy as a nongrafted UCLP patient. The surgical approach to the maxilla for this patient is the same as described for the nongrafted UCLP patient (see above).

For the BCLP adolescent presenting with an intact (successfully grafted) alveolar ridge on both sides a standard Le Fort I down fracture is carried out.

Mandibular and chin osteotomies to correct secondary deformities and facial asymmetries are also frequently required to achieve objectives. The purpose of mandibular osteotomies is not to set back the lower jaw but rather to fully correct the face. Improving the nasal airway through septoplasty, reduction of inferior turbinates and recontouring of the pyriform rims/nasal floor/anterior nasal spine is also simultaneously carried out when indicated.

4.3 Isolated cleft palate

The primary jaw deformity observed in the ICP adolescent is maxillary hypoplasia/dysplasia resulting from the original cleft deformity and the subsequent surgical interventions. The usual reconstructive procedure to consider is a standard Le Fort I maxillary osteotomy. Early on, Obwegeser clarified that full mobilization of the down-fractured maxilla was essential to achieving an orthognathic correction on the operating room table and to limit skeletal relapse over time.

Any residual palatal oronasal fistula in the ICP patient at the time of orthognathic correction will be difficult to close simultaneously with the Le Fort I procedure. This is because elevation of palatal flaps is generally required to do so and this would compromise the blood supply to the down-fractured maxilla.

4.4 Clinical management after initial surgical healing

Managing details of the in-hospital and at-home convalescence during initial healing after surgery are essential for a successful outcome. The surgeon is responsible for seeing the patient through this phase of treatment. Cephalometric and dental radiographs and facial and occlusal photographs are obtained at standard postoperative intervals to document progress.

Orthodontic maintenance of the surgical result and further detailing of the occlusion is initiated after initial healing (5 weeks after surgery). A seamless transition from the surgeon to the orthodontist for ongoing care is essential.

Speech and velopharyngeal function can be objectively reassessed 6 months after surgery and any remaining issues can be addressed at that time. We prefer to evaluate velopharyngeal function using nasoendoscopic instrumentation when feasible. Further cleft soft-tissue procedures (eg, cleft rhinoplasty, lip scar revision, pharyngeal flap/flap revision) can be carried out as early as 6 months after orthognathic surgery. Once the orthodontic appliances are removed, any planned definitive restorative dental work can also be finalized.

5 Controversies and unresolved issues

5.1 Velopharyngeal function after Le Fort I advancement

Uncertainties about velopharyngeal function and management of an in-place pharyngeal flap should no longer be limiting factors when orthognathic surgery is necessary in a patient with a cleft. A nasoendoscopic–guided examination by a speech pathologist and surgeon familiar with cleft anatomy will document current function and reasonably predict expected velopharyngeal function in a patient scheduled for a Le Fort I advancement. When significant postoperative velopharyngeal deterioration is anticipated, the patient and family are counseled about the sequencing of treatment. Clinical studies have now documented that velopharyngeal function will deteriorate in a similar fashion whether either distraction osteogenesis or standard Le Fort I osteotomy techniques are used. Despite the frequent need for significant Le Fort I advancement to normalize the skeleton, improve the upper airway, and to enhance facial esthetics in patients with a cleft, we have not had to, or seen an advantage to transecting an in-place pharyngeal flap to achieve maxillary mobilization and the desired result. Our research and that of others confirm that a pharyngeal flap in place at the time of Le Fort I does not increase complications nor does it result in a higher incidence of relapse.

Definitive reassessment of velopharyngeal function after cleft Le Fort I advancement can be carried out as early as 3–6 months after surgery. A primary or revision pharyngeal flap, in conjunction with cleft rhinoplasty and/or labial revision if indicated, can safely be carried out 6 months after surgery.

5.2 Mixed dentition Le Fort I osteotomy

By the mid-1980s research clarified that if Le Fort I advancement is undertaken for midface deficiency in a growing cleft palate patient, another procedure will likely be required once skeletal maturity is reached [Posnick, 1990]. More recently, several investigators have tested this theory by preceding with mixed dentition Le Fort I advancement in cleft patients utilizing distraction osteogenesis (DO) techniques. All research to date indicates that Le Fort I advancement carried out in the mixed dentition in the cleft individual, whether by standard or DO technique, results in no significant further horizontal growth. As the mandible continues to grow, an Angle Class III malocclusion will occur with the need for either additional Le Fort I advancement or mandibular setback.

5.3 Skeletal relapse after Le Fort I osteotomy

There are more than 100 published articles reviewing skeletal stability and relapse in cleft patients who have undergone Le Fort I advancement using either standard osteotomies or DO. When reviewed in total, clinical research data does not demonstrate significant differences in relapse patterns between the two techniques (standard vs DO) for Le Fort I advancement. Proponents of DO frequently subjectively state that when more than 10 mm of horizontal advancement is required, the use of standard osteotomies with plate and screw fixation and bone graft may lead to a higher degree of relapse. A broad based review of the literature does not support this theory. In perspective, it should be noted that only 5% of cleft patients undergoing Le Fort I advancement require more than 10 mm of horizontal advancement at the incisors. All clinicians agree that this subgroup of cleft patients (5%) is the most challenging. The reasons for this go beyond the degree of horizontal maxillary deficiency. These individuals are likely to also present with multiple residual end-stage deformities, previously failed cleft procedures, and additional regions of maxillary hypoplasia (ie, vertical and transverse hypoplasia).

Aksu et al [2010] documented a horizontal maxillary (skeletal) relapse of 22% in cleft lip and palate patients after Le Fort I advancement using DO. This was at the 3-year follow-up in a series of adult repaired cleft lip and palate adolescent or adult patients who presented with maxillary hypoplasia.

He et al [2010] reported their results on adolescents with repaired cleft lip and palate and maxillary hypoplasia who then underwent Le Fort I advancement using an external distraction (DO) device. In this study patients (n = 17) were treated at one center between 2000 and 2006 and had more than 1 year of follow-up. Interestingly, the first four patients (two UCLP and two BCLP) treated developed fibrous nonunion. All four required reoperation and rigid fixation to achieve union. The authors then extended the consolidation period to a minimum of 3 months for the remaining patients (n = 13). They were able to achieve bony union (13 [76%] of 17) in this group. The mean horizontal relapse in this group (13/17) was 11.9% with 5 (38%) of 13 patients developing not better than an "end-to-end" occlusion. A second orthognathic procedure was necessary in this subgroup (5 [38%] of the 13). Therefore, 9 (53%) of 17 of the study patients required two orthognathic procedures.

Chen et al [2011] reported a 30.7% incidence of horizontal (skeletal) relapse 1 year after Le Fort I advancement using DO techniques (rigid external distraction device) in cleft patients. This was in a consecutive series of cleft patients that presented to their team with maxillary hypoplasia.

Posnick et al [1990, 1994] documented the long-term results and the degree of horizontal relapse when using a standard Le Fort I osteotomy (in segments) in cleft jaw deformity patients. This was in a complex group of cleft adolescent and adult patients who also presented with multiple end-stage deficits (surgical technique described earlier in this chapter). They measured maxillary horizontal change and stability from the more than 1-year postoperative cephalometric radiographs and clinical examination. The results were reported according to cleft type: UCLP (6.9 mm mean advancement with 5.3 mm maintained); BCLP (94% maintained a positive overjet long term); and ICP (6.1 mm mean advancement with 5.1 mm maintained). Interestingly, the degree of relapse documented by Posnick et al using standard techniques in a consecutive series of end-stage cleft jaw deformity adolescence and adult patients (ie, previous failed bone grafts, residual fistula, dental gaps) was generally less than reported by clinicians using a DO approach as Obwegeser stated in the 1960s and was reconfirmed by Precious [2007], "Relapse in cleft patients after Le Fort I advancement may well be more related to failure to adequately mobilize the maxilla and free it of abnormal soft tissue attachments than anything inherent in the osteotomy or the specific (cleft) diagnosis."

6 Staging of maxillary reconstruction

6.1 Unilateral cleft lip and palate

The described modified Le Fort I (2-segmental) osteotomy as a method of managing end-stage oro-nasal fistulae, alveolar defects, and cleft dental gaps in patients with UCLP who also have maxillary hypoplasia is not intended to replace accepted sequencing of cleft treatment. We always prefer secondary bone grafting in the mixed dentition prior to eruption of the canine followed by orthodontic closure of the cleft dental gap when feasible. However, the method described does offer an option for definitive reconstruction when the opportunity for grafting in the mixed dentition (ie, before the eruption of the permanent canine tooth) is lost and a jaw deformity also exists.

A two-stage approach to the adolescent or adult presenting with maxillary hypoplasia, a residual alveolar cleft, oronasal fistula, cleft dental gap, and nasal obstruction is not cost- or time-effective. In our experience, the potential overall morbidity for the described end-stage cleft patient would be increased if a two stage approach were undertaken. It is in these UCLP individuals that a modified two segment Le Fort I osteotomy offers a safe and reliable opportunity for the resolution of residual end-stage problems (ie, maxillary hypoplasia, alveolar defect, residual fistulae, cleft dental gap, nasal obstruction). The long-term occlusal and periodontal benefits to the patient of the resulting "low maintenance" (nonprosthetic) dental rehabilitation cannot be overstated.

6.2 Bilateral cleft lip and palate

The described modified Le Fort I (3-segmental) osteotomy as a method for managing the maxillary deformity in adolescent or adult BCLP patients who also present with missing teeth, oronasal fistulae, alveolar defects, cleft dental gaps, a mobile premaxilla, and nasal obstruction is not intended to replace accepted sequencing of cleft treatment. This does, however, offer an option for definitive reconstruction once the opportunity for grafting the alveolus in the mixed dentition (ie, before the eruption of the permanent canine) is lost and a jaw deformity coexists. A two-stage approach for the maxillary deficient adolescent with BCLP and residual alveolar clefts, oronasal fistulae, cleft dental gaps, mobile premaxilla, and nasal obstruction is not cost or time efficient, and there may be increased morbidity. It is in these patients with BCLP that a modified Le Fort I osteotomy in three segments with differential repositioning of each segment offers a reasonable opportunity for the resolution of residual problems and also achieving a low maintenance periodontal sound dentition.

6.3 Standard versus DO approach to Le Fort I advancement

The author agrees with Obwegeser when he stated, "Today, many surgeons will resort to the use of distraction devices to gradually advance the cleft maxilla. Although in some circumstances this may be appropriate, it should be remembered that most cleft patients can be treated efficiently, even when requiring significant maxillary advancement, with a classic Le Fort I type procedure."

Standard thinking is for a surgeon to commit to an approach (DO versus standard technique) for a Le Fort I advancement in a cleft patient before arriving in the operating room. The surgeon then "sticks to the plan" no matter what happens intraoperatively. Unfortunately, this line of thinking leads many surgeons to select a DO approach. Based on review of the literature and 30 years personal experience as a cleft jaw surgeon, the author makes the following observations and recommendations.

6.3.1 Observations concerning DO approach for the cleft jaw deformity

- Distraction osteogenesis with gradual maxillary advancement is always a patient's second choice compared with a standard Le Fort I osteotomy with stable rigid internal fixation. The length of convalescence after surgery using DO will also be longer. It will be at least 3 months of a limited diet and physical activity. This generally is followed by several additional months of face mask therapy. The DO device is also physically awkward, socially embarrassing, and typically blocks the patient's visual fields (eg, red, blue or green external DO devices) (see chapter 4.8). Furthermore, there is no overall reduction in the potential for perioperative complications with DO compared with a standard approach.
- If the cleft maxilla is adequately down-fractured, mobilized and then stabilized with interpositional bone grafts and plate and screw fixation, there is a high probability of healing as planned with a predictable result and less extensive convalescence than with DO.
- An experienced cleft jaw surgeon is likely to be more confident with his ability to down-fracture and fully mobilize the cleft maxilla than a less experienced surgeon. Therefore, the less experienced surgeon will more likely chose a DO approach. This is to avoid the uncertainty (ie, personal stress) of the intraoperative maxillary mobilization process.
- Even for the experienced cleft orthognathic surgeon, there will be the rare but occasional patient where the extent of maxillary hypoplasia and associated deformities (ie, missing teeth, lack of alveolar bone) will lead them to choose a DO technique. Despite the DO techniques protracted healing requirements and limited versatility to simultaneously correct all presenting cleft deformities, the device's gradual stretching ability can mobilize even the most recalcitrant maxilla.

6.3.2 Recommendations concerning DO approach for the cleft jaw deformity

For almost all patients with maxillary hypoplasia, standard techniques are preferred to efficiently correct the presenting cleft deformity. Reserving DO as a "bail-out" when the down-fractured maxilla cannot be adequately mobilized is the approach the author recommends in most cases. The occasional patient at risk can be informed in advance of this contingency plan (ie, placement of a DO device) to accomplish full maxillary advancement. This approach allows the surgeon flexibility to make the right decision at the right time for the cleft patient in need in order to achieve the most efficient convalescence and favorable long-term result.

7 Conclusions

There are now convincing clinical studies which document the high prevalence of jaw deformities in mature patients with repaired cleft palate (ie, UCLP, BCLP, and ICP). The methods described to manage the presenting adolescent and adult cleft jaw deformities, malocclusion and any residual oronasal fistulae, bony defects, cleft dental gaps, nasal obstruction, and esthetic needs are generally safe and reliable when performed by a dedicated orthognathic surgeon and team. Successful cleft orthognathic and intranasal procedures provide a stable foundation on which any needed final soft-tissue lip and nose reconstruction may be carried out.

8 References and suggested reading

Abyholm F, Bergland O, Semb G. Secondary bone grafting of alveolar clefts. *Scand J Plast Reconstr Surg.* 1981;15(2):127–140.

Aksu M, Saglam-Aydinatay B, Akcan CA, et al. Skeletal and dental stability after maxillary distraction with a rigid external device in adult cleft lip and palate patients. *J Oral Maxillofac Surg.* 2010;68:254–259.

Bell WH, Levy BM. Revascularization and bone healing after posterior maxillary osteotomy. *J Oral Surg.* 1971 May;29(5):313–320.

Bell WH, You ZH, Finn RA, et al. Wound healing after multisegmental Le Fort I osteotomy and transection of the descending palatine vessels. *J Oral Maxillofac Surg.* 1995 Dec;53(12):1425–1433.

Berkowitz S, Mejia M, Bystrik A. A comparison of the effects of the Latham-Millard procedure with those of a conservative treatment approach for dental occlusion and facial aesthetics in unilateral and bilateral complete cleft lip and palate: part 1. Dental occlusion. *Plast Reconstr Surg.* 2004 Jan;113(1):1–18.

Boyne PJ, Sands NR. Secondary bone grafting of residual alveolar and palatal clefts. *J Oral Surg.* 1972 Feb;30(2):87–92.

Cassolato SF, Ross B, Daskalogiannakis J, et al. Treatment of dental anomalies in children with complete unilateral cleft lip and palate at SickKids Hospital, Toronto. *Cleft Palate Craniofac J.* 2009 Mar;46(2):166–172.

Chanchareonsook N, Samman N, Whitehill TL. The effect of cranio-maxillofacial osteotomies and distraction osteogenesis on speech and velopharyngeal status: a critical review. *Cleft Palate Craniofac J.* 2006 Jul;43(4):477–487.

Chanchareonsook N, Whitehill TL, Samman N. Speech outcome and velopharyngeal function in cleft palate: comparison of Le Fort I maxillary osteotomy and distraction osteogenesis—early results. *Cleft Palate Craniofac J.* 2007 Jan;44(1):23–32.

Chen ZQ, Qian YF, Wang GM, et al. Sagittal maxillary growth in patients with unoperated isolated cleft palate. *Cleft Palate Craniofac J.* 2009 Nov;46(6):664–667.

Chen PK, Por YC, Liou EJ, et al. Maxillary distraction osteogenesis in the adolescent cleft patient: three-dimensional computed tomography analysis of linear and volumetric changes over five years. *Cleft Palate Craniofac J.* 2011 Jul;40(4):445–454.

Cheung LK, Chua HD. A meta-analysis of cleft maxillary osteotomy and distraction osteogenesis. *Int J Oral Maxillofac Surg.* 2006 Jan;35(1):14–24.

Cho BC, Kyung HM. Distraction osteogenesis of the hypoplastic midface using a rigid external distraction system: the results of a one- to six-year follow-up. *Plast Reconstr Surg.* 2006 Oct;118(5):1201–1212.

Daskalogiannakis J, Ross RB. Effect of alveolar bone grafting in the mixed dentition on maxillary growth in complete unilateral cleft lip and palate patients. *Cleft Palate Craniofac J.* 1997 Sep;34(5):455–458.

Daskalogiannakis J, Mehta M. The need for orthognathic surgery in patients with repaired complete unilateral and complete bilateral cleft lip and palate. *Cleft Palate Craniofac J.* 2009 Sep;46(5):498–502.

David DJ, Anderson PJ, Schnitt DE, et al. From birth to maturity: a group of patients who have completed their protocol management. Part II. Isolated cleft palate. *Plast Reconstr Surg.* 2006 Feb;117(2):515–526.

DeLuke DM, Marchand A, Robles EC, et al. Facial growth and the need for orthognathic surgery after cleft palate repair: literature review and report of 28 cases. *J Oral Maxillofac Surg.* 1997 Jul;55(7):694–697; discussion 697–698.

Dodson TB, Bays RA, Neuenschwander MC. Maxillary perfusion during Le Fort I osteotomy after ligation of the descending palatine artery. *J Oral Maxillofac Surg.* 1997 Jan;55(1):51–55.

Drommer R. Selecting angiographic studies prior to Le Fort I osteotomy in patients with cleft lip and palate. *J Maxillofac Surg.* 1979 Nov;7(4):264–270.

Drommer R, Luhr HG. The stabilization of osteotomized maxillary segments with Luhr mini-plates in secondary cleft surgery. *J Maxillofac Surg.* 1981 Aug;9(3):166–169.

Drommer RB. The history of the "Le Fort I osteotomy". *J Maxillofac Surg.* 1986 Jun;14(3):119–122.

Erbe M, Stoelinga PJ, Leenen RJ. Long-term results of segmental repositioning of the maxilla in cleft palate patients without previously grafted alveolo-palatal clefts. *J Craniomaxillofac Surg.* 1996 Apr;24(2):109–117.

Ewing M, Ross. Soft tissue response to orthognathic surgery in persons with unilateral cleft lip and palate. *Cleft Palate Craniofac J.* 1993;30:320–332.

Felstead AM, Deacon S, Revington P. The outcome for secondary alveolar bone grafting in the southwest UK region post-CSAG. *Cleft Palate Craniofacial.* 2010;47:359–362.

Figueroa AA, Polley JW, Friede H, et al. Long-term skeletal stability after maxillary advancement with distraction osteogenesis using a rigid external distraction device in cleft maxillary deformities. *Plast Reconstr Surg.* 2004;114:138.

Freihofer HP Jr. Results of osteotomies of the facial skeleton in adolescence. *J Maxillofac Surg.* 1977 Nov;5(4):267–297.

Friede H, Lilja J. Dentofacial morphology in adolescent or early adult patients with cleft lip and palate after a treatment regimen that included vomer flap surgery and pushback palatal repair. *Scand J Plast Reconstr Hand Surg.* 1994 Jun;28(2):113–121.

Friede H, Pruzansky S. Long-term effects of premaxillary setback on facial skeletal profile in complete bilateral cleft lip and palate. *Cleft Palate J.* 1985 Apr;22(2):97–105.

Fudalej P, Hortis-Dzierzbicka M, Obloj B, et al. Treatment outcome after one-stage repair in children with complete unilateral cleft lip and palate assessed with the Goslon Yardstick. *Cleft Palate Craniofac J.* 2009 Jul;46(4):374–380.

Fudalej P, Hortis-Dzierzbicka M, Dudkiewicz Z, et al. Dental arch relationship in children with complete unilateral cleft lip and palate following Wassaw (one-stage repair) and Oslo protocols. *Cleft Palate Craniofac J.* 2009 Nov;46(6):648–653.

Garrison BT, Lapp TH, Bussard DA. The stability of the Le Fort I maxillary osteotomies in patients with simultaneous alveolar cleft bone grafts. *J Oral Maxillofac Surg.* 1987 Sep;45(9):761–766.

Gillies HD, Rowe NL. L'ostéotomie du maxillaire supérieur enoisagée essentiellement dans le cas de bec-de-lièvre total. *Rev Stomatol.* 1954;55:545–552.

Good PM, Mulliken JB, Padwa BL. Frequency of Le Fort I osteotomy after repaired cleft lip and palate or cleft palate. *Cleft Palate Craniofac J.* 2007;44:396–401.

Guyette TW, Polley JW, Figueroa A, et al. Changes in speech following maxillary distraction osteogenesis. *Cleft Palate Craniofac J.* 2001;38:199–205.

Hall HD, Posnick JC. Early results of secondary bone grafts in 106 alveolar clefts. *J Oral Maxillofac Surg.* 1983 May;41(5):289–294.

Harada K, Baba Y, Ohyama K, et al. Maxillary distraction osteogenesis for cleft lip and palate children using an external, adjustable, rigid distraction device: a report of 2 cases. *J Oral Maxillofac Surg.* 2001 Dec;59(12):1492–1496.

Harada K, Ishii Y, Ishii M, et al. Effect of maxillary distraction osteogenesis on velopharyngeal function: A pilot study. *Oral Surg Oral Med Oral Pathol Oral Radiol Endod.* 2002 May;93(5):538–543.

Harada K, Sato M, Omura K. Long-term maxillomandibular skeletal and dental changes in children with cleft lip and palate after maxillary distraction. *Oral Surg Oral Med Oral Pathol Oral Radiol Endod.* 2006 Sep;102(3):292–299.

Hathaway R, Daskalogiannakis J, Mercado J, et al. The Americleft Study: an intercenter study of treatment outcomes for patients with unilateral cleft lip and palate. Part 2. Dental arch relationship. *Cleft Palate Crainofac J.* 2011 May;48(3):244–251.
He D, Genecov DG, Barcelo R. Nonunion of the external maxillary distraction in cleft lip and palate: analysis of possible reasons. *J Oral Maxillofac Surg.* 2010 Oct;68(10):2402–2411.
Heidbüchel KL, Kuijpers-Jagtman AM, Freihofer HPM. Facial growth in patients with bilateral cleft lip and palate: a cephalometric study. *Cleft Palate Craniofac J.* 1994 May;31(3):210–216.
Heliövaara A, Ranta R, Hukki J, et al. Skeletal stability of Le Fort I osteotomy in patients with unilateral cleft lip and palate. *Scand J Plast Reconstr Surg Hand Surg.* 2001 Mar;35(1):43–49.
Henkel KO, Gundlach KKH. Analysis of primary gingivoperiosteoplasty in alveolar cleft repair. Part I: facial growth. *J Craniomaxillofac Surg.* 1997;25:266–269.
Hochban W, Ganss C, Austermann KH. Long-term results after maxillary advancement in patients with clefts. *Cleft Palate Craniofac J.* 1993 Mar;30(2):237–243.
Houston WJ, James DR, Jones E, et al. Le Fort I maxillary osteotomies in cleft palate cases. Surgical changes and stability. *J CranioMaxillofac Surg.* 1989 Jan;17(1)9–15.
Hsieh CH, Ko EW, Chen PK, et al. The effect of gingivoperiosteoplasty on facial growth in patients with complete unilateral cleft lip and palate. *Cleft Palate Craniofac J.* 2010 Sep;47(5):439–446.
Huang CS, Harikrishnan P, Liao YF, et al. Long-term follow-up after maxillary distraction osteogenesis in growing children with cleft lip and palate. *Cleft Palate Craniofac J.* 2007 May;44(3):274–277.
Kanno T, Mitsugi M, Hosoe M, et al. Long-term skeletal stability after maxillary advancement with distraction osteogenesis in nongrowing patients. *J Oral Maxillofac Surg.* 2008 Sep;66(9):1833–1846.
Kapp-Simon KA. Psychological interventions for the adolescent with cleft lip and palate. *Cleft Palate Craniofac J.* 1995 Mar;32(2):104–108.
Ko EW, Figueroa AA, Guyette TW, et al. Velopharyngeal changes after maxillary advancement in cleft patients with distraction osteogenesis using a rigid external distraction device: 1-year cephalometric follow-up. *J Craniofac Surg.* 1999 Jul;10(4):312–320.
Laspos CP, Kyrkanides S, Tallents RH, et al. Mandibular and maxillary asymmetry in individuals with unilateral cleft lip and palate. *Cleft Palate Craniofac J.* 1997 May;34(3):232–239.
Laspos CP, Kyrkanides S, Tallents RH, et al. Mandibular asymmetry in noncleft and unilateral cleft lip and palate individuals. *Cleft Palate Craniofac J.* 1997 Sep;34(5):410–416.
Luhr HG. [On the stable osteosynthesis in mandibular fractures]. *Dtsch Zahnarztl Z.* 1968 Jul;23(7):754. German.
Lund TW, Wade M. Use of osseointegrated implants to support a maxillary denture for a patient with repaired cleft lip and palate. *Cleft Palate Craniofac J.* 1993 Jul;30(4):418–420.
Mansour S, Burstone C, Legan H. An evaluation of soft-tissue changes resulting from Le Fort I maxillary surgery. *Am J Orthod.* 1983 Jul;84(1):37–47.
Marrinan EM, LaBrie RA, Mulliken JB. Velopharyngeal function in nonsyndromic cleft palate: relevance of surgical technique, age at repair, and cleft type. *Cleft Palate Craniofac J.* 1998 Mar;35(2):95–100.
Mars M, Asher-McDade C, Brattström V, et al. A six-center international study of treatment outcomes in patients with clefts of the lip and palate. Part 3. Dental arch relationships. *Cleft Palate Craniofac J.* 1992 Sep;29(5):405–408.
Matic DB, Power SM. The effects of gingivoperiosteoplasty following alveolar molding with a pin-retained Latham appliance versus secondary bone grafting on midfacial growth in patients with unilateral clefts. *Plast Reconstr Surg.* 2008 Sep;122(3):863–870.
McComb RW, Marrinan EM, Nuss RC, et al. Predictors of velopharyngeal insufficiency after Le Fort I maxillary advancement in patients with cleft palate. *J Oral Maxillofac Surg.* 2011 Aug;69(8):2226–2232.
McIntyre GT, Devlin MF. Secondary alveolar bone grafting (CLEFTSiS) 2000-2004. *Cleft Palate Craniofac J.* 2010;47(1):66–72.
Millard DR, Latham RA, Huifen X, et al. Cleft lip and palate treated by presurgical orthopedics, gingivoperiosteoplasty, and lip adhesion (POPLA) compared with previous lip adhesion method: a preliminary study of serial dental casts. *Plast Reconstr Surg.* 1999 May;103(6):1630–1644.
Mølsted K, Dahl E, Brattström V, et al. A six-center international study of treatment outcome in patients with clefts of the lip and palate: evaluation of maxillary asymmetry. *Cleft Palate Craniofac J.* 1993 Jan;30(1):22–28.
Mølsted K, Brattström V, Prahl-Andersen B, et al. The Eurocleft study: intercenter study of treatment outcomes in patients with complete cleft lip and palate. Part 3: dental arch relationships. *Cleft Palate Craniofac J.* 2005 Jan;42(1):78–82.
Motohashi N, Kuroda T, Capelozza Filho L, et al. P-A cephalometric analysis of nonoperated adult cleft lip and palate. *Cleft Palate Craniofac J.* 1994 May;31(3):193–200.
Nollet PJ, Katsaros C, van't Hof MA, et al. Treatment outcome after two-stage palatal closure in unilateral cleft lip and palate: a comparison with Eurocleft. *Cleft Palate Craniofac J.* 2005 Sep;42(5):512–516.
Normando AD, da Silva Filho OG, Capelozza Filho L. Influence of surgery on maxillary growth in cleft lip and/or palate patients. *J Craniomaxillofac Surg.* 1992 Apr;20(3):111–118.
Obwegeser HL. Correction of the facial appearance of harelip and cleft palate patients by surgery on the jaws. In: *Exerpta Medica International Congress Series No 141. Reconstructive Surgery. Thermal Injury and Other Subjects.* 1966;110–117.
Obwegeser HL. Surgery as an adjunct to orthodontics in normal and cleft palate patients. *Rep Congr Eur Orthod Soc.* 1967 Jul;42:343–353.
Obwegeser HL. Surgical correction of deformities of the jaws in adult cleft cases. Paper presented at: the First International Conference on Cleft Lip and Palate; 1969:14–17; Houston, Texas.
Obwegeser HL. Orthognathic surgery and a tale of how three procedures came to be: a letter to the next generations of surgeons. *Clin Plastic Surg.* 2007 Jul;34(3):331–355.
Phillips JH, Klaiman P, Delorey R, et al. Predictors of velopharyngeal insufficiency in cleft palate orthognathic surgery. *Plast Reconstr Surg.* 2005 Mar;115(3):681–686.
Polley JW, Figueroa AA. Rigid external distraction: its application in cleft maxillary deformities. *Plast Reconstr Surg.* 1998 Oct;102(5):1360–1372.
Posnick JC, Ewing MP. Skeletal stability after Le Fort I maxillary advancement in patients with unilateral cleft lip and palate. *Plast Reconstr Surg.* 1990 May;85(5):706–710.
Posnick JC. Orthognathic surgery in the cleft patient. In: Russel RC, ed. *Instructional Courses, Plastic Surgery Education Foundation.* St Louis: CV Mosby Co; 1991;4:129–157.
Posnick JC, Tompson B. Modification of the maxillary Le Fort I osteotomy in cleft-orthognathic surgery: the unilateral cleft lip and palate deformity. *J Oral Maxillofac Surg.* 1992 Jul;50(7):666–675.
Posnick JC, Tompson B. Modification of the maxillary Le Fort I osteotomy in cleft-orthognathic surgery: the bilateral cleft lip and palate deformity. *J Oral Maxillofac Surg.* 1993 Jan;51(1):2–11.
Posnick JC, Dagys AP. Skeletal stability and relapse patterns after Le Fort I maxillary osteotomy fixed with miniplates: the unilateral cleft lip and palate deformity. *Plast Reconstruct Surg.* 1994 Dec;94(7):924–932.
Posnick JC, Taylor M. Skeletal stability and relapse patterns after Le Fort I osteotomy using miniplate fixation in patients with isolated cleft palate. *Plast Reconstr Surg.* 1994 Jul;94(1):51–58.
Posnick JC, Tompson B. Cleft-orthognathic surgery: complications and long-term results. *Plast Reconstruct Surg.* 1995 Aug;96(2):255–266.

Posnick JC. The treatment of secondary and residual dentofacial deformities in the cleft patient: surgical and orthodontic therapy. *Clin Plast Surg*. 1997 Jul;24(3):583–597.
Posnick JC, Ricalde P. Cleft-orthognathic surgery. *Clin Plastic Surg*. 2004 Apr;31(2):315–330.
Posnick JC, Agnihotri N. Managing chronic nasal airway obstruction at the time of orthognathic surgery: a twofer. *J Oral Maxillofac Surg*. 2011 Mar;69(3):695–701.
Posnick JC, ed. Cleft orthognathic surgery: the unilateral cleft lip and palate deformity. In: *Orthognathic Surgery: Principles and Practice*. St Louis: Elsevier; 2014:1297–1370.
Posnick J. Cleft orthognathic surgery: the bilateral cleft lip and palate deformity. In: *Orthognathic Surgery: Principles and Practice*. St Louis: Elsevier; 2014:1371–1440.
Posnick J. Cleft orthognathic surgery: the isolated cleft palate deformity. In: *Orthognathic Surgery: Principles and Practice*. St Louis: Elsevier; 2014: 1441–1470.
Precious DS. Treatment of retruded maxilla in cleft lip and palate. *J Oral Maxillofac Surg*. 2007 Apr; 65:758–761.
Roberts-Harry D, Semb G, Hathorn I, et al. Facial growth in patients with unilateral clefts of the lip and palate: a two-center study. *Cleft Palate Craniofac J*. 1996;31:372–375.
Robertsson S, Mohlin B. The congenitally missing upper lateral incisor: a retrospective study of orthodontic space closure versus restorative treatment. *Eur J Orthod*. 2000 Dec;22(6):697–710.
Ross RB. Treatment variables affecting facial growth in complete unilateral cleft lip and palate. *Cleft Palate J*. 1987 Jan;24(1):71–77.
Sandham A, Murray JA. Nasal septal deformity in unilateral cleft lip and palate. *Cleft Palate Craniofac J*. 1993 Mar;30(2):222–226.
Schnitt DE, Agir H, David DJ. From birth to maturity: a group of patients who have completed their protocol management. Part I. Unilateral cleft lip and palate. *Plast Reconstr Surg*. 2004 Mar;113(3):805–817.
Shaw WC, Asher-McDade C, Brattström V, et al. A six-center international study of treatment outcomes in patients with clefts of the lip and palate. *Cleft Palate Craniofac J*. 1992 Sep;29(5):393–397.
Sinko K, Caacbay E, Jagsch R, et al. The GOSLON yardstick in patients with unilateral cleft lip and palate: review of a Vienna sample. *Cleft Palate Craniofac J*. 2008 Jan;45(1):87–91.
Steinkamm W. *Die Pseudo-Progenie und ihre Behandlung* [Inaugural dissertation]. Berlin; University of Berlin; 1938. German.
Suzuki A, Takahama Y. Maxillary lateral incisor of subjects with cleft lip and/or palate: Part 1. *Cleft Palate Craniofac J*. 1992 Jul;29(4):376–379.
Suzuki A, Watanabe M, Takahama Y. Maxillary lateral incisors of subjects with cleft lip and/or palate: Part 2. *Cleft Palate Craniofac J*. 1992 Jul;29(4):380–384.
Tessier P, Tulasne JF. Secondary repair of cleft lip deformity. *Clin Plast Surg*. 1984 Oct;11(4):747–760.
Trindale IE, Yamashita RP, Suguimoto RM, et al. Effects of orthognathic surgery on speech and breathing of subjects with cleft lip and palate: Acoustic and aerodynamic assessment. *Cleft Palate Craniofac J*. 2003 Jan;40(1):54–64.
Westbrook MT Jr, West RA, McNeil RW. Simultaneous maxillary advancement and closure of bilateral alveolar clefts and oronasal fistulas. *J Oral Maxillofac Surg*. 1983 Apr;41(4):257–260.
Williams AC, Bearn D, Mildinhall S, et al. Cleft lip and palate care in the United Kingdom—the Clinical Standards Advisory Group (CSAG) study. Part 2: dentofacial outcomes and patient satisfaction. *Cleft Palate Craniofac J*. 2001 Jan;38(1):24–29.
Willmar K. On Le Fort I osteotomy: a follow-up study of 106 operated patients with maxillo-facial deformity. *Scand J Plast Reconstr Surg*. 1974;12(0):suppl 12:1–68.
Wiltfang J, Hirschfelder U, Neukam FW, et al. Long-term results of distraction osteogenesis of the maxilla and midface. *Br J Oral Maxillofac Surg*. 2002 Dec;40(6):473–479.
Witzel MA, Munro IR. Velopharyngeal insufficiency after maxillary advancement. *Cleft Palate J*. 1977 Apr;14(2):176–180.
Wolford LM, Cassano DS, Cottrell DA, et al. Orthognathic surgery in the young cleft patient: preliminary study on subsequent facial growth. *J Oral Maxillofac Surg*. 2008 Dec;66(12):2524–2536.
Zachrisson BU, Stenvik A. Single implants—optimal therapy for missing lateral incisors? *Am J Orthod Dentofacial Orthop*. 2004 Dec;126(6):A13–A15.

4.8 Distraction osteogenesis of the maxilla with external devices

Alexander Hemprich, Thomas Hierl

1 Introduction

Large maxillary forward movements are challenging, especially midface advancements in cleft lip and palate (CLP) patients, which are technically more difficult and more prone to recurrence compared to those in non-cleft patients. This may be due to scars after previous operations, lack of bone and a tight soft-tissue envelope. In some patients, previous velopharyngoplasties may have created a dense connection between the soft palate and posterior pharyngeal wall, which may make a movement of the osteotomized maxillary segment in the forward direction more difficult.

Helfrick [1991], Epker et al [1988] and Luhr et al [1995] have pointed out that the limit for conventional maxillary osteotomies in the cleft patient lies between 5 and 8 mm forward movement. In addition, a negative relation between the amount of maxillary protraction and postoperative long-term stability in conventional Le Fort osteotomies has been discussed. Therefore, midface advancements of more than 8 mm can be truly problematic in cleft patients.

Distraction osteogenesis (DO), however, can be used to treat marked midface retrusions in patients with unfavorable soft-tissue conditions, especially in CLP patients. For those cases, DO seems to be the method of choice since it is the only technique by which large sagittal mandibulomaxillary discrepancies can be corrected by a single maxillary movement. An alternative is a bimaxillary operation combining a maxillary advancement with simultaneous setback of the mandible, but this may lead to an unfavorable profile and even sleep apnea.

The first midface distraction using elastic bands between mandible and maxilla was published by Wassmund in 1935 (**Fig 4.8-1**).

Despite the successful case, it was not before 1978 that Nanda [1978] has carried out animal studies of midface biomechanics and bone regeneration in rhesus monkeys. He demonstrated the protraction of the maxilla by controlled external forces and could undertake a sutural distraction even without osteotomies in adult monkeys.

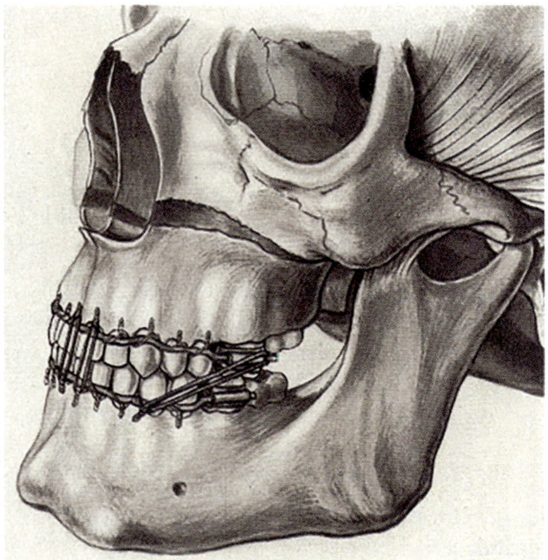

Fig 4.8-1 First maxillary distraction was performed in 1927 by Wassmund in Berlin, Germany (kind permission from JA Barth).

Polley et al [1995] applied the principle of callus distraction to the craniomaxillofacial skeleton and developed a multidirectional distractor for midface advancement, which was anchored to the skull via a halo frame and connected to the maxillary dentition (**Fig 4.8-2**).

In edentulous patients and those with a reduced upper dentition, the original idea of Polley et al [1997] to connect the distraction appliances to the teeth is not possible. For this subgroup, the distraction device needs to be connected directly to the bone.

2 Preoperative diagnostics

Preoperative evaluation starts with a clinical examination of the unanimated and animated face. A dental status is taken, the occlusion and occlusal plane is studied, symmetry is checked and the amount and quality (scars) of the soft-tissue envelope examined.

Radiographic imaging in three planes is mandatory unless a computed tomographic (CT) scan with 3-D reconstruction is taken, the latter being today's gold standard in radiologic imaging for deformity cases.

In conventional radiographic imaging a lateral cephalogram is used to assess the relationships between skull base, midface and mandible. Based on the preoperative analysis, the desired sagittal and vertical maxillary movements are determined. For the second plane, a Water`s view radiograph is taken. The operation should only be undertaken in patients with no major pathology in the paranasal sinuses. A CT scan is superior to plain radiographs for sinus evaluation. An OPT should be taken to screen for hidden dental pathologies.

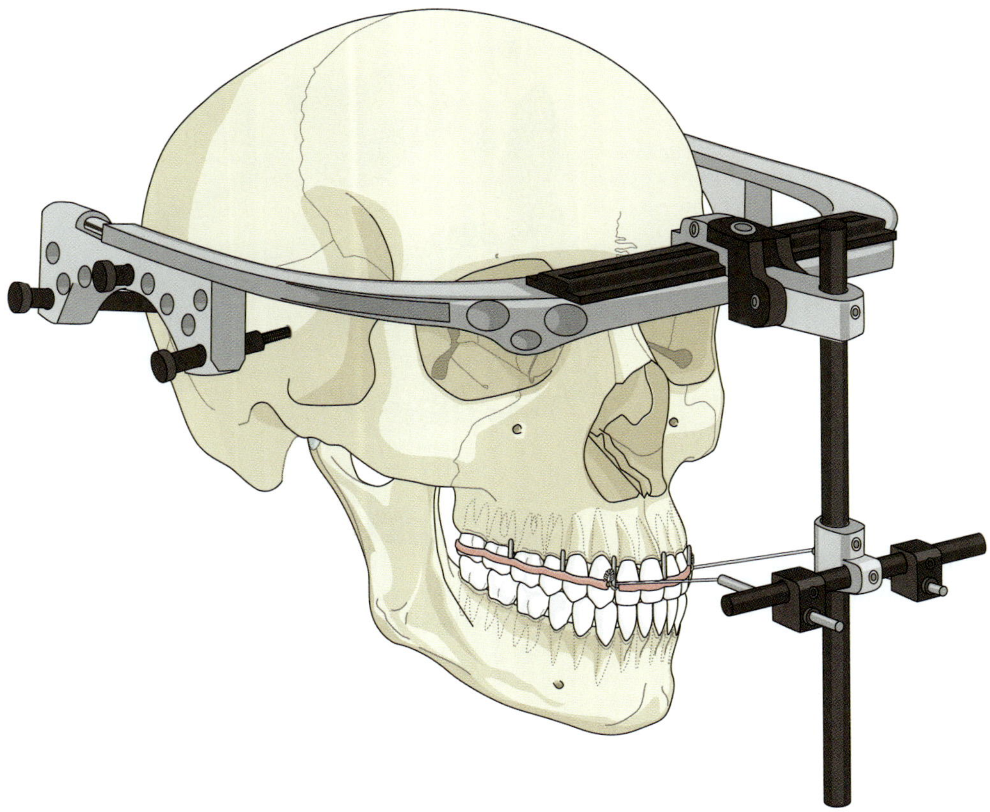

Fig 4.8-2 External midface distractor. The maxilla is connected to the distraction system via a tooth-borne appliance.

Axial and coronal CT scans are the preferred images for preoperative planning in complex orthognathic cases, especially for the evaluation of bone quality and strength of the midfacial pillars. Based on the CT data, stereolithographic models can be manufactured for 3-D analysis. After definition of the desired distraction vectors, haptic mock operations can be performed. Alternatively, this can be done virtually.

A proper preoperative speech assessment should be performed to assess velopharyngeal competence of a patient before and after midface distraction.

Nasal breathing is typically impaired in many cleft patients. This may improve during distraction. It is useful, however, to have objective data taken by rhinomanometry and acoustic rhinometry before and at the end of treatment.

3 Surgical technique

Midface DO can be performed with external or internal devices. External devices are typically anchored to the patient's skull via a halo frame, and directly connected to the patient's maxillary bone (bone anchored) or the patient's upper dentition (tooth anchored). Internal devices are placed transorally. They are fixed both to the mobile osteotomized maxillary segment and the nonmobile superior portion of the midface (see chapter 4.9).

Advantages of external devices:

- Vector of distraction can be altered during the distraction process
- Multivector distraction is possible
- Strict parallel alignment of the distractor arms is not necessary
- Simple procedure

Disadvantages of external devices:

- Discomfort for the patient due to the visible halo frame
- A long retention period is often not possible because of patient discomfort, pin loosening, or pin infection

Advantages of internal devices:

- Good initial patient acceptance due to the invisibility of the device

Disadvantages of internal devices:

- Allows only single vector distraction
- Distraction vectors on both sides need to be almost parallel
- Adjustment of the vector during distraction process is not possible
- Growing patient discomfort during distraction and retention phases because of the intraoral foreign body, which may cause painful mucosa lacerations

Distraction with external devices

To achieve a strict parallel forward movement of the maxillary block and to avoid tilting, distraction forces should be applied along a vector through the center of the osteotomized maxillary segment (**Fig 4.8-3**).

Consequently, this means that wires should ideally be applied directly through the paranasal soft tissues and fixed to the underlying bone. To avoid this, Polley et al [1997] used a long wire attached to a tooth-borne anchorage that was bent around the lips to a line above the nares. However, in edentulous patients this technique cannot be applied.

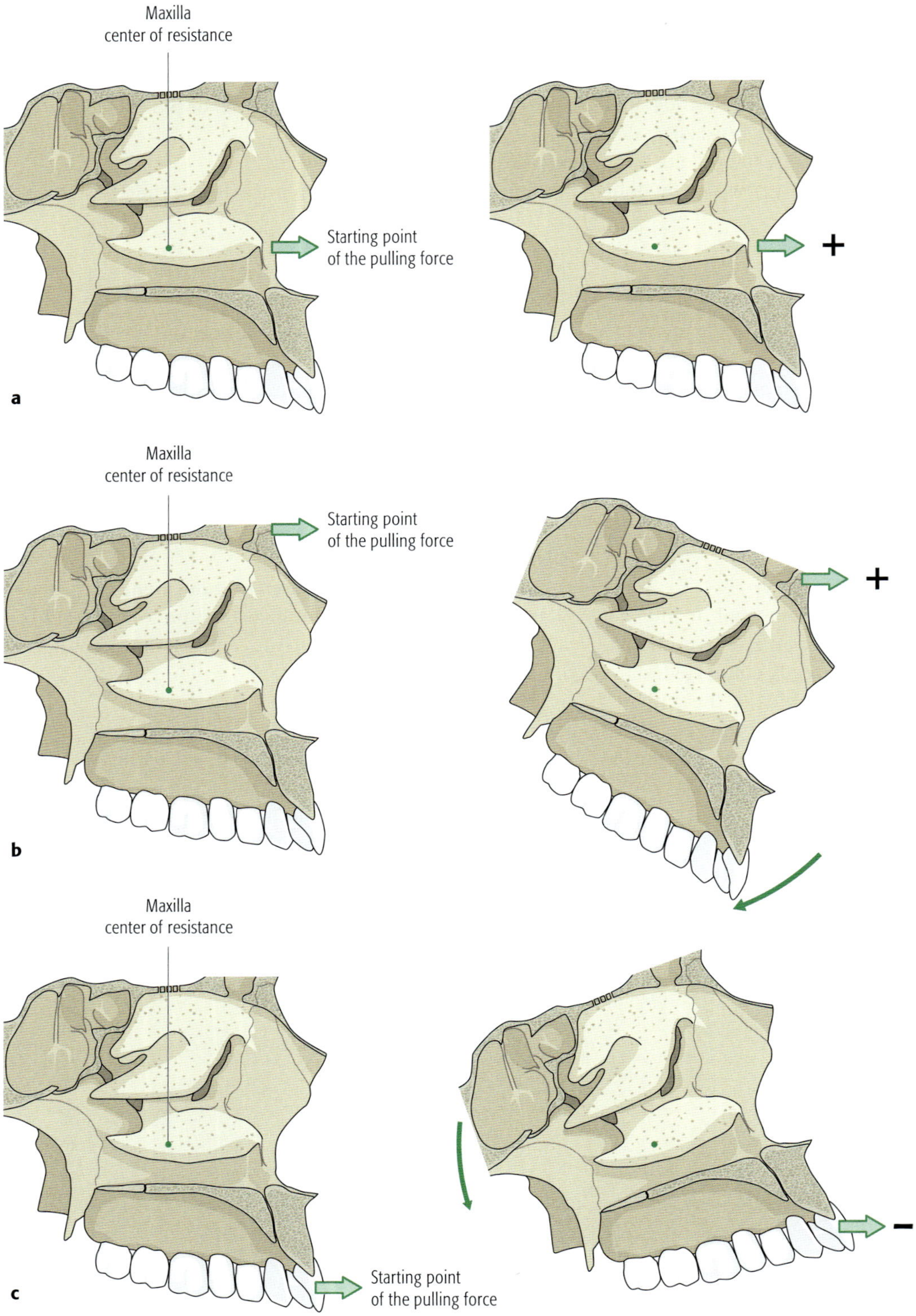

Fig 4.8-3a–c

a Movement of the maxillary block depending on the point of force transmission. A parallel movement results from a pull along a line through the center of the segment (center of resistance).

b Closing of the bite anteriorly (upward movement of the posterior part and downward movement of the anterior part of the maxilla) results from a pull above the center of resistance.

c An anterior open bite (downward movement of the posterior part and upward movement of the anterior part of the maxilla) results from a starting point below the center of resistance, ie, the height of the teeth or the alveolus.

Hierl et al [2000] introduced a special modular retention set that allows maxillary distraction along a defined and stable vector (**Fig 4.8-4**).

A 1.8 mm titanium square rod can be bent individually from the anterior maxillary wall around the lips and up to the desired plane of distraction. It is fixed to the bone via a modified osteosynthesis miniplate with an especially designed rider. It is completely stable even in bone of just about 1 mm thickness. Three screws are placed on the medial aspect and four to five screws on the lateral aspect of the rider.

The system is extremely useful not only in atrophic maxillae of edentulous adults but also for individuals with small teeth and for patients with a reduced number of teeth or chronic periodontitis. Finally, it can be used even in children older than 6 years without causing any harm to the tooth roots of the secondary dentition (**Fig 4.8-5**).

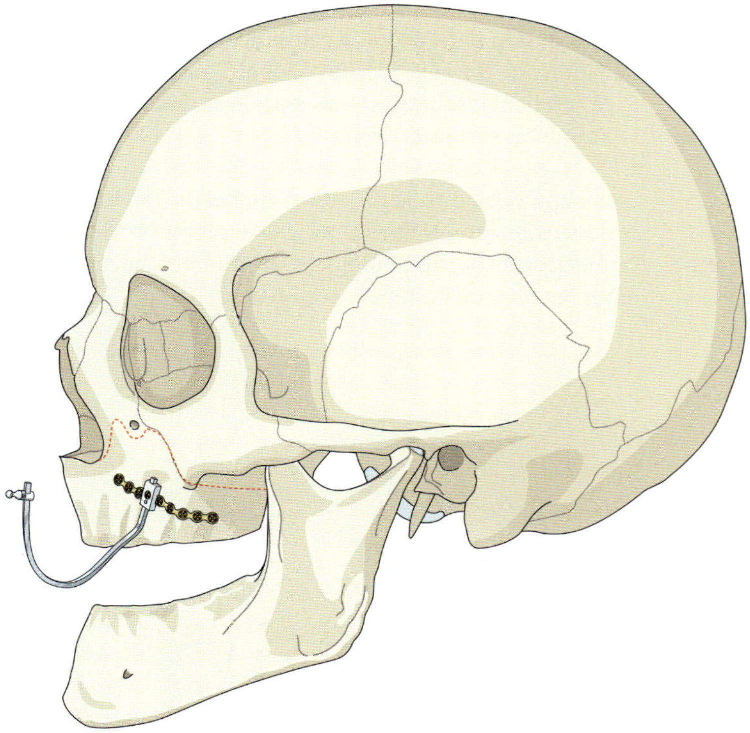

Fig 4.8-4 The complete retention system mounted on the anterior and lateral maxillary wall.

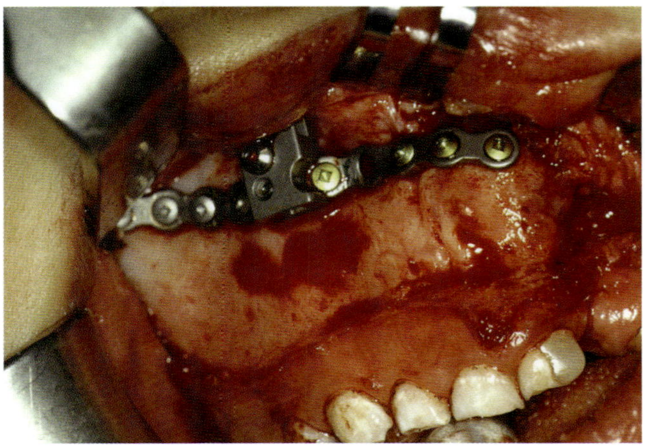

Fig 4.8-5 The retention plate with a rider fixed to the anterior and lateral maxillary walls of a 6-year-old patient.

If necessary the vector can be changed during distraction, not only in the vertical plane but also individually for the right and left maxillary halves in the horizontal plane. Sagittally different distances can be covered on both sides of the maxilla, for instance when the lesser segment of a cleft case should be moved further forward. The external device can also be combined with an additional device for palatal widening, such as a tooth-anchored hyrax device or a bone-anchored palatal distractor.

The treatment protocol for distraction with externally anchored devices is shown in **Fig 4.8-6**:

1. Contouring of the retention plate to the anterior and lateral facial wall and choice of the appropriate position of the rider (**Fig 4.8-5**).
2. Bending of the rods around the lip and fixation to the riders.
3. Fixation of the complete system to the anterior and lateral maxillary walls with at least three monocortical screws to the medial and four to five screws to the lateral aspect.
4. Fixation of the halo frame with 3–4 pins to the skull about 2 cm above the glabella parallel to the Frankfurt horizontal plane.
   - Note: Do not exceed 0.35 Nm during screw placement—use a torque control screwdriver to avoid skull penetration [de Mol et al, 1991].
5. Perform a midface osteotomy according to the treatment protocol.
6. After a 4-day latency period, connection of the rods to the distraction units and start of the distraction process at a rate of twice 0.5 mm = 1 mm per day (**Fig 4.8-6d**).
7. Retention period: 3–4 weeks in children and young adults; 6–8 weeks in older, edentulous patients.
8. Cleft bone grafting (if necessary) on removal of the modular system fixation.

Steps 2–4 can be substituted by alternative techniques to connect the osteotomized maxillary segment to the halo frame (tooth-borne appliances, miniplates, mesh) if the modular fixation system is not used.

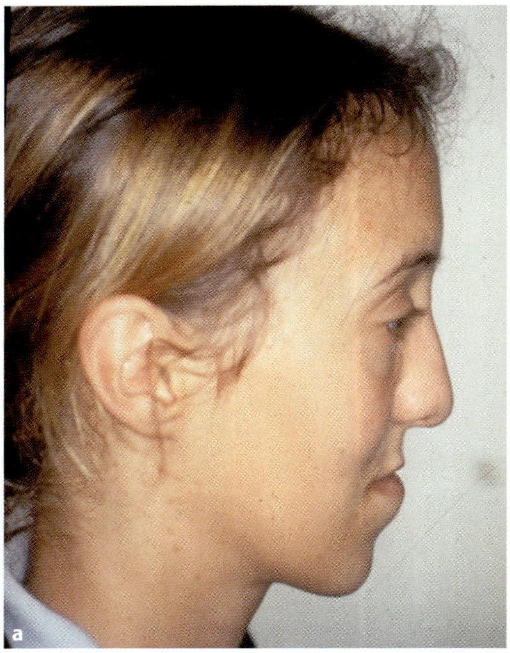

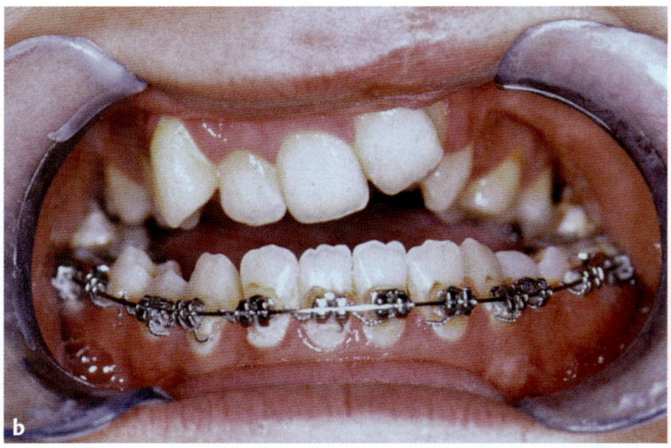

Fig 4.8-6a–h
a Maxillary retrusion in a cleft lip and palate case.
b The dental situation at the beginning of treatment.

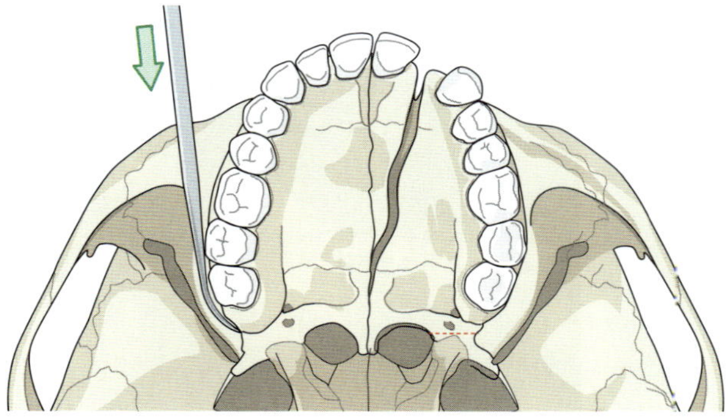

c

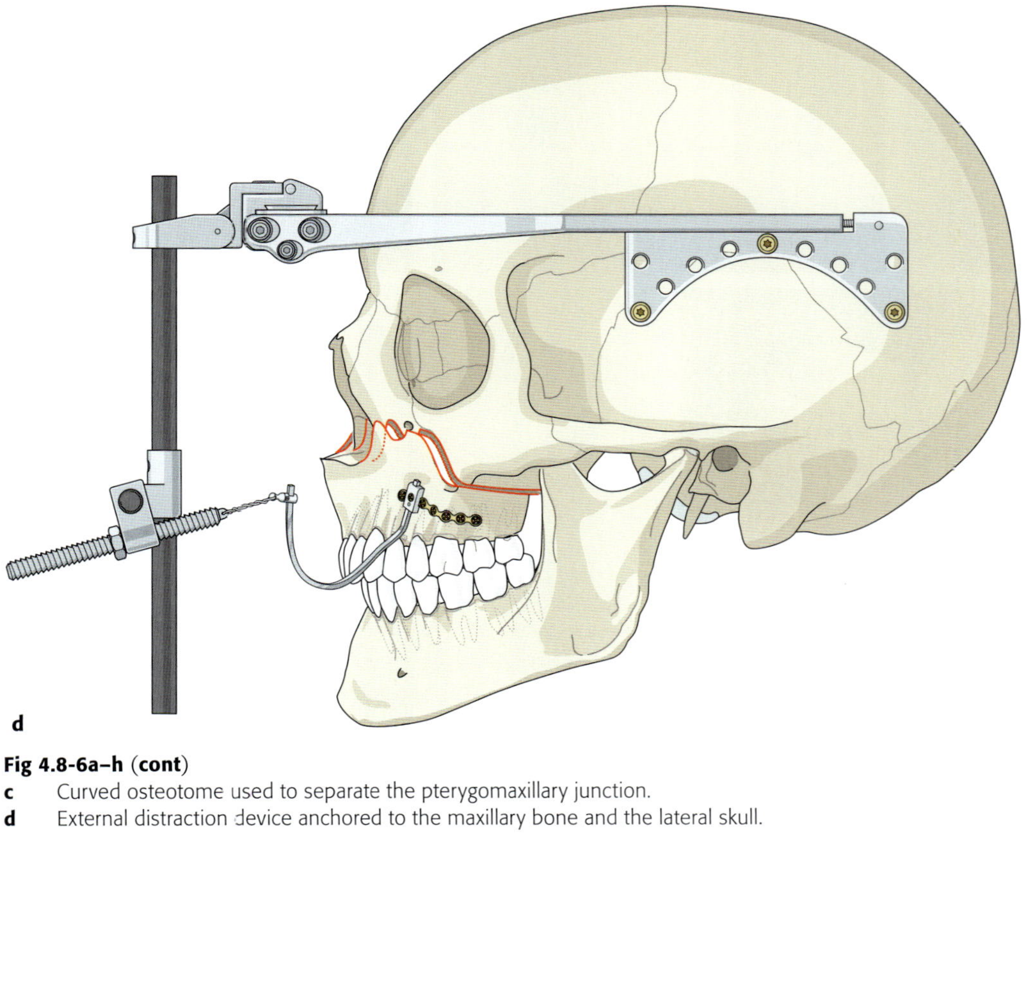

d

Fig 4.8-6a–h (cont)

c Curved osteotome used to separate the pterygomaxillary junction.

d External distraction device anchored to the maxillary bone and the lateral skull.

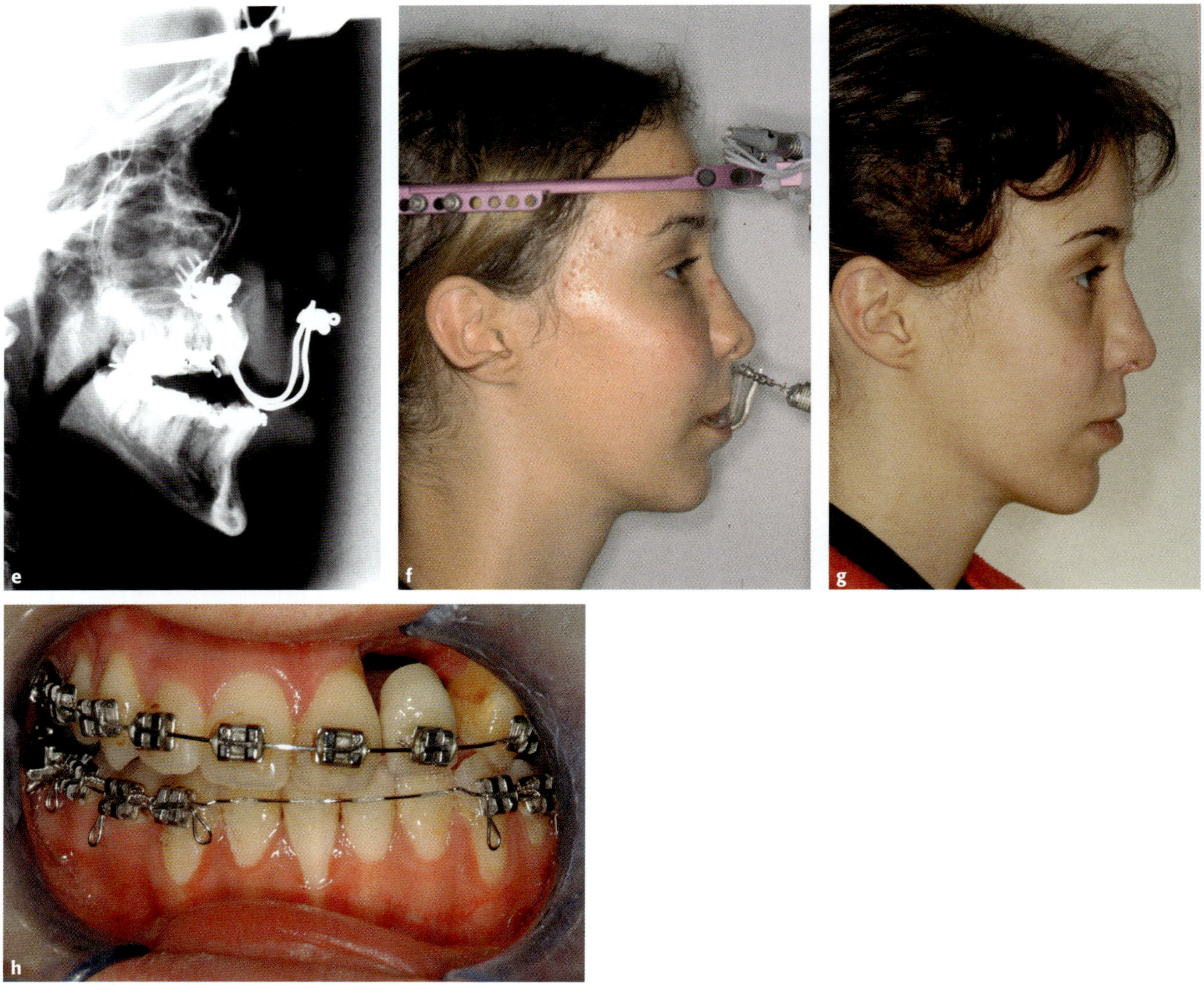

Fig 4.8-6a–h (cont)
Note: the wire connection between the rod and the distractor spindle unit is just above a line through the center of resistance of the maxilla.
e Lateral cephalogram at the beginning of distraction.
f The patient at the end of active distraction phase.
g The patient 2 years after midface distraction.
h Situation at the end of the orthodontic treatment. Dental rehabilitation needs to be performed.

4 Personal experience

Fifty-five patients were treated with DO of the midface with external devices from May 1998 to January 2009, with an age range from 6–65 years. Forty-five patients presented with clefts of the lip, alveolus and palate, among them 36 unilateral CLP; 6 bilateral CLP; and 3 with palatal clefts. Eight patients suffered from congenital midfacial hypoplasia, and two had a Morbus Crouzon.

In 28 of the 45 cleft patients, a velopharyngoplasty was previously performed. Ten patients were almost totally edentulous in the maxilla. One patient had an obstructive sleep apnea syndrome. Except in the first six patients, where wire retention to the maxilla was used, the modular retention system applied was in all patients, edentulous or dentate. It is our preferred method. In eleven patients, a simultaneous transversal expansion of the maxilla with a tooth-borne Hyrax screw was achieved. After removal of the halo and the modular retention system, an alveolar bone graft was performed in 38 cases. In two elderly patients, the distraction gap had to be filled with cancellous bone and the maxillary position secured by four miniplates paranasally and at the zygomatico-alveolar crests. In seven patients, simultaneous onlay bone grafting and sinus augmentation procedures for implant insertion were carried out.

The first seven dentate cases were treated with Delaire masks after removal of the halo frame. Later this method was abandoned because of bad patient compliance and the growing knowledge about sufficient stability after 4 and 8 weeks' retention in young and older patients, respectively. In all patients, the planned maxillary movements could be achieved. Distances from 9–31 mm (average, 17 mm) were measured. A CT scan 8 weeks after distraction suggests bone formation at the midfacial buttresses (**Fig 4.8-7**). Moreover, intraoperative findings during onlay or cleft bone grafting or implant insertion in 20 patients showed complete bony fusion around the piriform aperture in 36 of 40 maxillary halves (**Fig 4.8-8**).

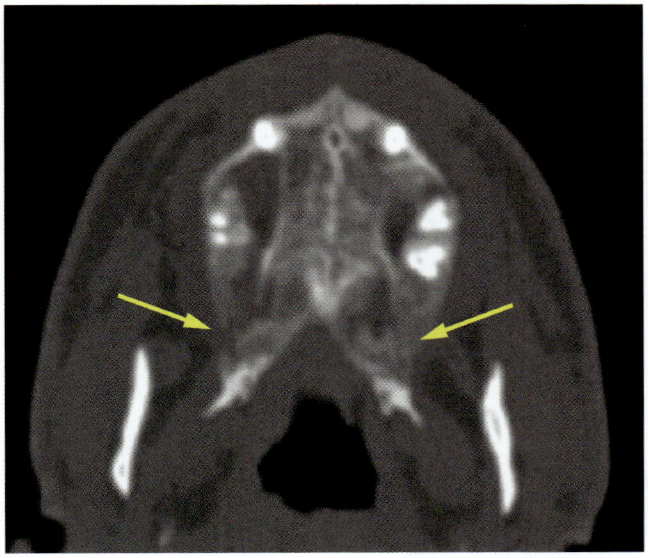

Fig 4.8-7 Axial computed tomographic scan 8 weeks after distraction osteogenesis. The arrows point to the newly formed bone in the retromaxillary region.

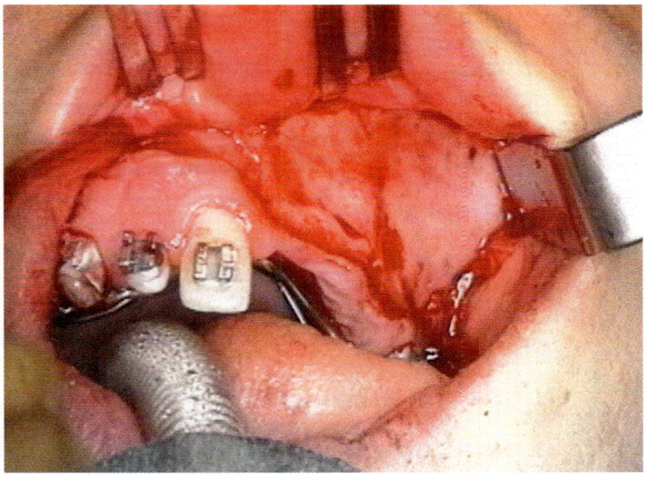

Fig 4.8-8 After removal of the retention system, newly formed bone was present around the piriform aperture and the anterior maxillary wall.

Only in two patients older than 40 years was an additional miniplate fixation in combination with a gap bridging osteoplasty performed at the time of removal of the modular fixation system. The analysis of the lateral cephalogram according to Segner et al [1991] revealed an increase of the S-nasion-point A (SNA) angle of about 12.1° from an average of 71.7° to 83.8°. Six months later a decrease of 19% and 12 months later of 25% was seen (**Table 4.8-1**).

The biggest changes occurred during the first 6 months. After that a further tendency for relapse could hardly be noted (**Fig 4.8-9**). In adult edentulous patients, an overcorrection of about 20% should be planned to overcome the above-described skeletal relapse (SNA angle) of about 20%. In dentate patients, some overcorrection is advisable especially when vertical distraction is carried out. Here skeletal relapse could be observed, although to a lesser extent, whereas a correct overbite was always maintained.

Changes	No., n	SNA	ANB
Initial increase	38	12.1° = (100%)	13.6° = (100%)
Changes after 6 mo	27	-2.3° (19%)	-2.3° (16.8%)
Changes after 12 mo	20	-3.1° (25%)	-3.8° (28.6%)
Changes after 24 mo	6	-3.2° (23%)	-3.2° (23%)

Table 4.8-1 Changes of SNA and ANB during the observation period.*
*SNA indicates Sella-nasion, A point; ANB indicates A point, nasion, B point.

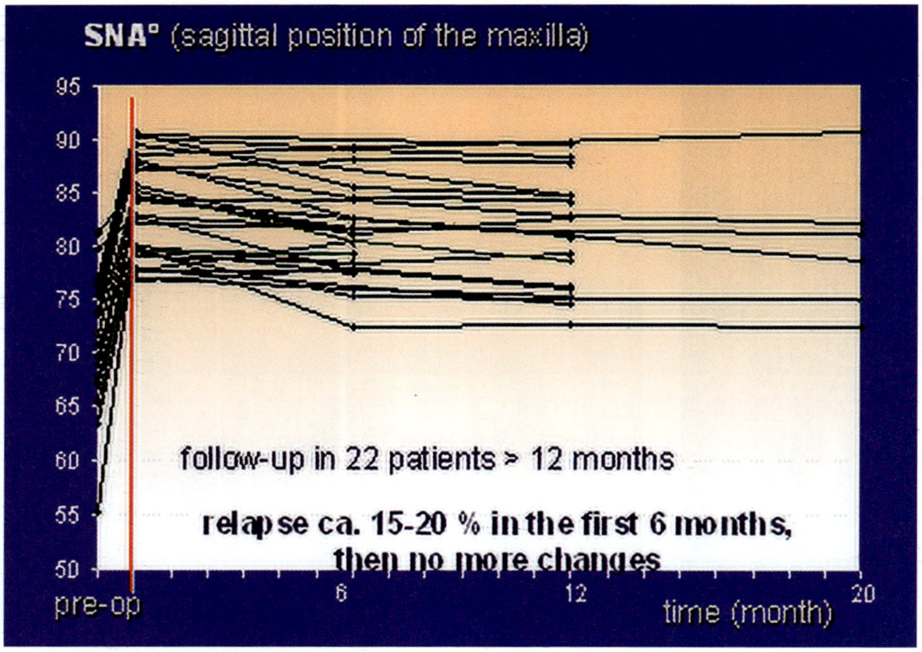

Fig 4.8-9 S-nasion-point A angle changes in 22 cases. If a relapse occurs, it does not exceed 20% in the sagittal plane. Note that only small changes were found after 6 months (courtesy of Thomas Hierl, MD).

It is difficult to discuss the amount of relapse in midfacial DO in comparison with conventional orthognathic surgery. Different authors [Figueroa et al, 2001; Ko et al, 2000] found a relapse after distraction from 12–28%, whereas a relapse in conventional Le Fort I osteotomy is reported between 10% and 29% [Gurstein et al, 1998; Heliövaara et al, 1998]. However, the average forward movement of the maxilla in the studies did not exceed 6 mm.

In our experience midfacial DO has an advantage over conventional orthognathic surgery in the subgroup of cleft patients with large sagittal discrepancies.

To better understand the forces that are necessary to move the maxilla and the complete soft-tissue envelope forward, Knapp et al [2004] developed a measuring device based on strain gauges fixed to the external distractor (**Fig 4.8-10**) using an especially designed data logger which could be carried by the patient for several days. A continuous measurement of force progression during distraction was possible. It was demonstrated that forces between 50 and 114 N are necessary to complete the planned maxillary advancements. The materiel (screws, plates, halo frame) withstood those forces.

Since the above-described forces also exert high loads to the six to eight screws that fix the halo frame to the skull, finite element analysis was done to visualize the skull deformation caused by loading the halo frame. An inward deformation of the lateral skull along the pins was demonstrated. This is probably linked to the fact that the fixation of the frame is usually done at the weakest part of the calvarial bone in the hair-covered area to avoid any visible scar according to Polley et al [1997].

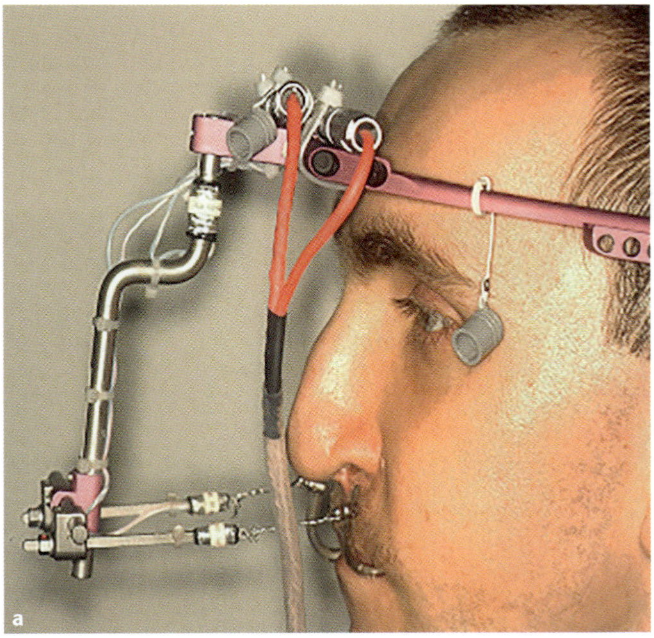

a

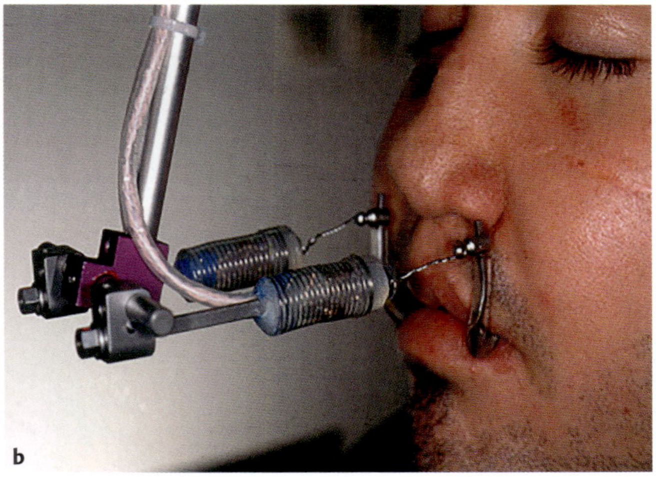

b

Fig 4.8-10a–b Strain gauges mounted at each distractor spindle unit and the central carbon rod for the measurement of force progression during distraction.

Since the preoperative planning of complex orthognathic surgery is usually done with 3-D CT scans, preoperative and postoperative data can easily be compared and analyzed. It is even possible to overlay bony and soft-tissue layers and predict some of the changes that can be expected. In **Fig 4.8-11** the 3-D CT of a 19-year-old woman with a complete cleft lip and palate on the left side is shown preoperatively and postoperatively. The bone changes in such a patient can be better visualized using a viscoelastic model (**Fig 4.8-12**).

It was fascinating to see that the distraction of the maxilla has also notable effects on the nasal region, the orbits and the zygomas in form of a forward-upward movement. Finally, the changes of the midfacial position can be portrayed by vectors to show the direction of movements of all parts of the face (**Fig 4.8-13**).

Nasal breathing improved in almost all patients. No nasal obstruction was ever reported after distraction subjectively by a patient or with rhinomanometry.

The assessment of velopharyngeal competence by means of an aerophonoscope and the analysis of a speech therapist showed no changes in noncleft cases. In five cleft patients, there was a slight deterioration of speech whereas two patients showed an improvement of velopharyngeal competency. In nine more patients, we found some increase in nasal resonance and perflation, all patients in this subgroup showed pathological conditions preoperatively. In two elderly patients, a velopharyngoplasty was finally indicated.

If this is compared with speech results after conventional Le Fort I osteotomies in cleft patients, there is a speech deterioration of about 16% in our group in contrast to 23–81% in conventional Le Fort I cases, although in those series the amount of forward movement was less than 50% of our average of about 17 mm. However, it must be noted that a large subgroup of the distraction cases has had velopharyngoplasties before distraction. In the distraction series, we did not find any correlation between postoperative speech problems and the amount of forward movement. Sugar [Sugar A, MD, personal communication, 2001] found better results with internal DO for patients who required cleft maxillary advancement compared with conventional orthognathic surgery. He also noted that more of the DO patients had previous velopharyngoplasties, which means that the groups were not completely comparable.

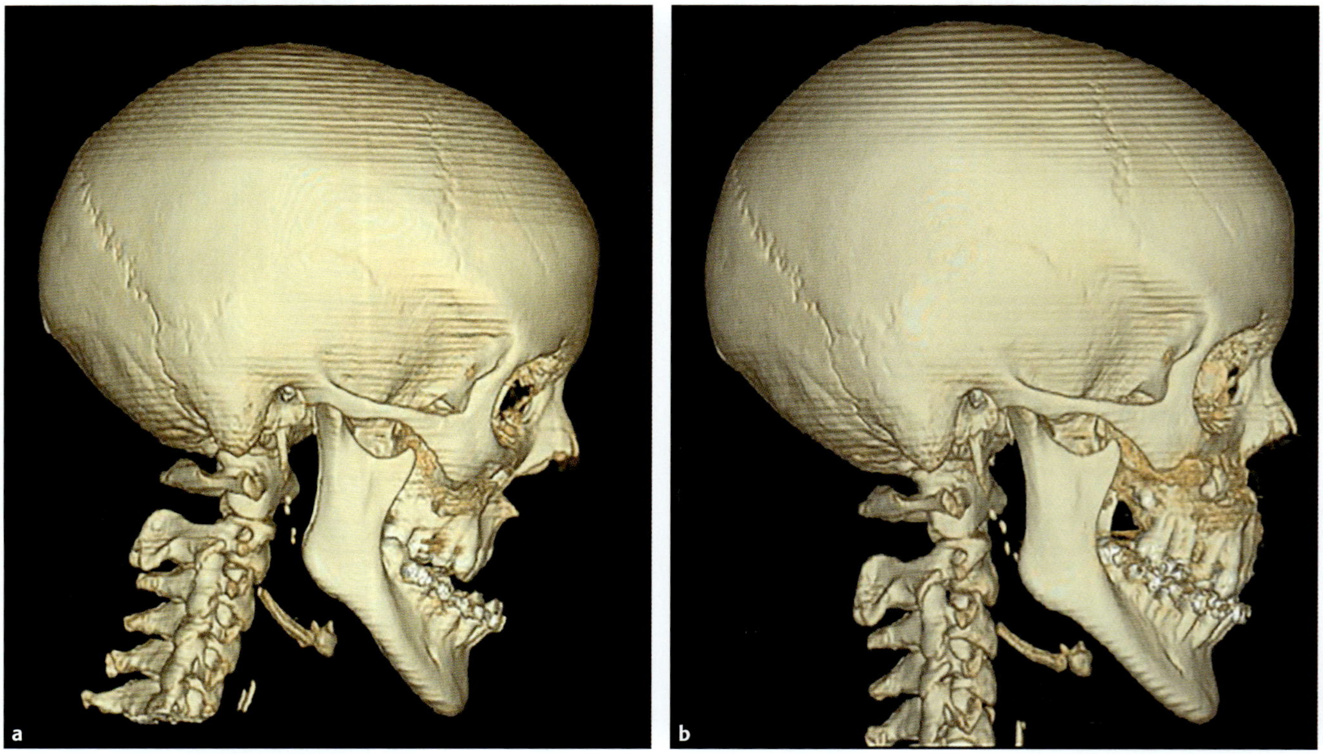

Fig 4.8-11a–b Marked changes in the bony structure of the complete midface are noted in this 18-year-old woman with a unilateral cleft lip and palate before and at the end of treatment.

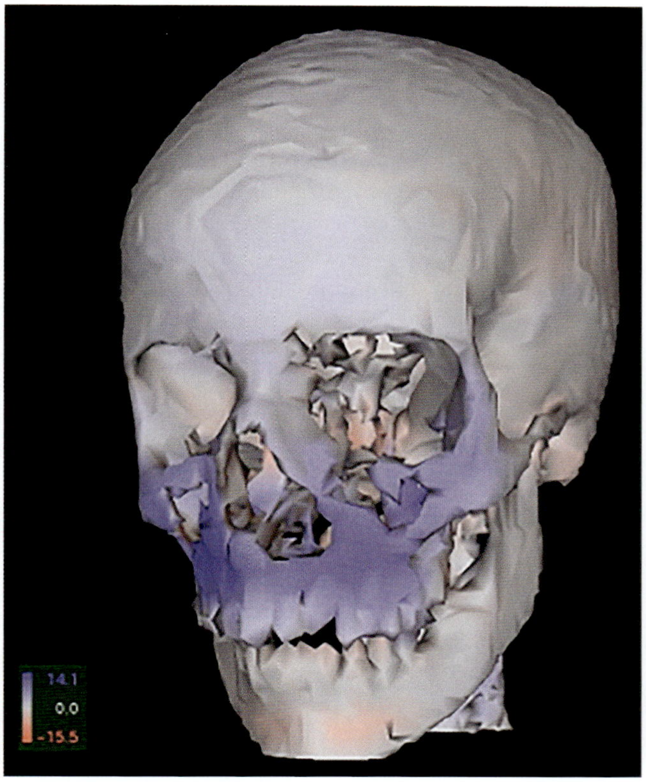

Fig 4.8-12 Viscoelastic model of a patient at the end of distraction. The blue shade indicates forward bone movement/growth.

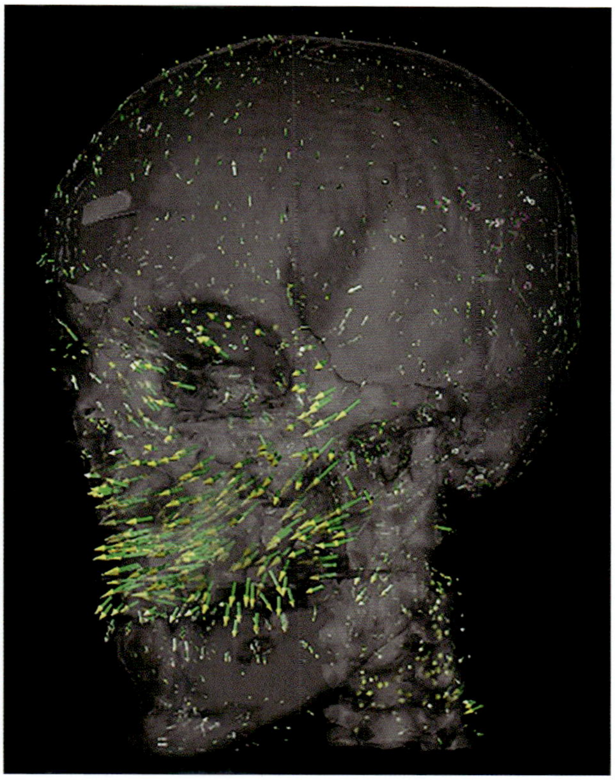

Fig 4.8-13 Changes in the midface during distraction osteogenesis with vectors demonstrating the direction of movements in parts of the facial skeleton.

5 Complications and pitfalls

In our midface distraction series, reoperation was performed in 12.7% of the 55 patients. This is rather high a percentage compared with 6–9%, which are described in the literature for conventional Le Fort I osteotomy [Tung et al, 1995]. It must be noted, however, that almost all these problems occurred within the first 3 years of our practice. This may be because all newly introduced procedures will go along with a learning curve for the performing surgeons.

The following problems were observed:

- Loosening of the halo frame
- Cut into the lip by the rod
- Insufficient maxillary mobilization
- Loosening of a miniplate of the fixation system
- Insufficient protraction (too early ossification)

The following solutions for these problems can be proposed. In our first cases the halo frame was fixed by tightening the six to eight screws to the skull according to the personal feeling/judgement of the surgeon. Because of the skull deformation in the finite element models and the detection of bone deformation and cracks in the outer table of the skull in some CT scans, it is strongly advised not to exceed a maximum torque force of 0.35 Nm for the fixation of the halo screws. Thus, the use of a torque control screwdriver is a matter of choice. The tight fit of the halo frame should be checked weekly.

The rods need to be bent around the lip meticulously during the first operation to avoid cutting into the lip.

It is important to choose the area of the zygomaticoalveolar crest for fixation of the anchoring plates, since here is the strongest bone available.

Pain was not a major problem for the patients during distraction. Some pain/pressure was felt especially in the velopharyngeal pedicle on the onset of distraction but subsided once distraction was finished. Only four patients needed mild analgetics for the whole distraction period. Even tightening of the halo fixation pins in weekly intervals was done without any anesthesia (**Table 4.8-2**).

Reason	No.	Age, y	Therapy
Loosening of the halo frame	1	16	Refixation
Cut into the lip by the situation square rod	1	12	Adjustment
Insufficient mobilization	1	24	Second procedure (mobilization)
Loosening of the miniplate of the fixation system	2	32, 65	Refixation with more screws in better bone
Insufficient protraction (ossified too early)	2	20, 25	Second procedure Le Fort I osteotomy

Table 4.8-2 Complications with subsequent reoperations.

6 Summary

Midfacial DO with external devices is a safe and reliable method that enables the surgeon to perform maxillary movements in the sagittal and vertical plane. It is even possible to achieve a transversal widening of the maxilla simultaneously using an additional palatal distraction device.

It can be stated that midfacial DO can be performed without major complications. Since there is no need for extensive mobilization of the maxilla or midface after osteotomy the risk of extensive bleeding is much less than in conventional Le Fort I/II/III osteotomies.

7 References and suggested reading

Chin M, Toth BA. Le Fort III advancement with gradual distraction using internal devices. *Plast Reconstr Surg.* 1997 Sep;100(4):819–830; discussion 831–832.

Cohen SR. Craniofacial distraction with a modular internal distraction system: evolution of design and surgical techniques. *Plast Reconstr Surg.* 1999 May;103(6):1592–1607.

de Mol van Otterloo JJ, Tuinzing DB, Greebe RB, et al. Intra- and early postoperative complications of the Le Fort I osteotomy. *J Craniomaxillofac Surg.* 1991 Jul;19(5):217–222.

Devani P, Watts R, Markus AF. Speech outcome in children with cleft palate: aerophonoscope assessment of nasal emission. *J Craniomaxillofac Surg.* 1999 Jun;27(3):180–186.

Epker BN, Stella JP, Fish LC. Dentofacial deformities associated with cleft lip and palate. In: Epker BN, Stella JP, Fish LC, eds. *Dentofacial Deformities: Integrated Orthodontic and Surgical Correction.* Mosby: St Louis; 1988;3:1571–1708.

Erbe M, Stoelinga PJW, Leenen RJ. Long term results of segmental repositioning of the maxilla in cleft palate patients without previously grafted alveolo-palatal clefts. *J Craniomaxillofac Surg.* 1996 Apr;24(2):109–117.

Figueroa AA, Polley JW, Ko E. Distraction osteogenesis for treatment of severe cleft maxillary deficiency with RED technique. In: Samchucov ML, Cope JB, Cherkashin AM, eds. *Craniofacial Distraction Osteogenesis.* St Louis: Mosby; 2001:485–493.

Gurstein KW, Sather AH, An KN, et al. Stability after inferior or anterior maxillary repositioning by Le Fort I osteotomy: a biplanar stereocephalometric study. *Int J Adult Orthodon Orthognath Surg.* 1998;13(2):131–143.

Helfrick JF. Treatment of secondary cleft deformities: orthognathic surgery. *Ann R Australas Coll Dent Surg.* 1991 Oct;11:244–258.

Heliövaara A, Ranta R, Hukki J. Le Fort I osteotomy: skeletal stability and soft tissue changes in different cleft types. *J Craniomaxillofac Surg.* 1998;[Suppl 1]:26:71–72.

Hierl T, Hemprich A. Callus distraction of the midface in the severely atrophied maxilla: a case report. *Cleft Palate Craniofac J.* 1999 Sep;36(5):457–461.

Hierl T, Hemprich A. A novel modular retention system for midfacial distraction osteogenesis. *Br J Oral Maxillofac Surg.* 2000 Dec;38(6):623–626.

Hierl T, Klöppel R, Hemprich A. Midfacial distraction osteogenesis without major osteotomies: a report on the first clinical application. *Plast Reconstr Surg.* 2001 Nov;108(6):1667–1672.

Hochban W, Ganss C, Austermann KH. Long-term results after maxillary advancement in patients with clefts. *Cleft Palate Craniofac J.* 1993 Mar;30(2):237–243.

Knapp W, Hierl Th, Günter T, et al. Measurement and analysis of forces during midfacial distraction osteogenesis. *Int J Tech Health Care.* 2004;12:197–198.

Ko EW, Figueroa AA, Guyette TW, et al. Velopharyngeal changes after maxillary advancement in cleft patients with distraction osteogenesis using a rigid external distraction device: a 1-year cephalometric follow-up. *J Craniofac Surg.* 1999 Jul;10(4):312–322; discussion 321–322.

Luhr HG, Jäger A. (Indikation, Technik und Ergebnisse der bimaxillären Chirurgie). *Fortschr Kiefer Gesichtschir.* 1995;40:1–12. German.

Nanda RS. Protraction of maxilla in rhesus monkeys by controlled extraoral forces. *Am J Orthod.* 1978 Aug;74(2):121–141.

Polley JW, Figueroa AA, Charbel FT, et al. Monobloc craniomaxillofacial distraction osteogenesis in a newborn with severe craniofacial synostosis: a preliminary report. *J Craniofac Surg.* 1995 Sep;6(5):421–423.

Polley JW, Figueroa AA. Management of severe maxillary deficiency in childhood and adolescence through distraction osteogenesis with an external, adjustable, rigid distraction device. *J Craniofac Surg.* 1997 May;8(3):181–185; discussion 186.

Schwarz C, Gruner E. Logopaedic findings following advancement of the maxilla. *J Maxillofac Surg.* 1976 Mar;4(1):40–55.

Segner D, Hasund A. *Individualisierte Kephalometrie.* Hamburg: Eigenverlag; 1991. German.

Tung TC, Chen YR, Bendor-Samuel RL. Surgical correction of the Le Fort I osteotomy: a retrospective review of 146 cases. *Changgeng Yi Xue Za Zhi.* 1995 Jun;18(2):102–107.

Van de Perre JP, Stoelinga PJ, Blijdorp PA, et al. Perioperative morbidity in maxillofacial orthopaedic surgery: a retrospective study. *J Craniomaxillofac Surg.* 1996 Oct;24(5):263–270.

Wassmund W. *Lehrbuch der praktischen Chirurgie des Mundes und der Kiefer Bd. 1.* Leipzig: JA Barth; 1935. German.

Watzke I, Turvey TA, Warren DW, et al. Alterations in velopharyngeal function after maxillary advancement in cleft palate patients. *J Oral Maxillofac Surg.* 1990 Jul;48(7):685–689.

4.9 Midface advancement with internal distractors

Jaime Gateno, James J Xia, John F Teichgraeber

1 Introduction

Distractor devices can be classified as internal or external, depending on where they are installed. Internal devices are placed on the bone, under the soft tissues. External devices are placed over the soft tissues outside the skin. In this chapter, we discuss the use of internal distractor devices for maxillary and midface advancement.

Internal distractors have significant advantages over external devices. First, they are hidden from view, so they are better accepted by patients and parents. Second, they impair function less than external devices, eg, halo devices significantly impact speech, chewing, and affective expression. Third, in contrast to external devices, internal devices do not disturb or disrupt activities of daily living, such as dressing and sleeping [Eggermont et al, 2007]. Finally, internal distractors are safer than external devices. Notably, halo devices have caused skull fractures, pin penetration into the intracranial cavity, and injuries from falls [van der Meulen et al, 2005; Aizenbud et al, 2008; Cai et al, 2010].

Notwithstanding, internal devices also have disadvantages. First, they can only move bone in a straight line. Because of their limited range of motion, these devices can only produce good outcomes when the maneuvers required to correct a deformity are simple. Second, internal distractors are nonadjustable; that is, the direction of distraction cannot be changed during treatment. If the devices are not perfectly aligned, the patient will eventually develop an iatrogenic deformity. Third, internal distractors always require a second operation for device removal.

Despite the seemingly insurmountable disadvantages of internal distractors, one can achieve good outcomes consistently by: (1) simplifying the movement required of the distractors; (2) selecting, adapting, and installing the distractors with precision; and (3) devising rescue interventions when outcomes are not in accordance with the plan.

2 Maxillary distraction

2.1 Indications

Upper jaw advancement through distraction is indicated when the upper jaw is retruded, particularly when the movement needed to correct the retrusion is greater than the surrounding soft tissues can flexibly accommodate. This situation occurs in extreme retrusion or when the soft tissues that surround the upper jaw are unyielding due to scarring. Stiff soft tissues are prevalent in patients with cleft lip and palate because scar tissue forms after cleft repair. While normal soft tissues may allow upper jaw advancements of 10–12 mm, scarred lips and palates may only allow for half that measurement (5–6 mm) [Yu et al, 2004].

Internal distraction is contraindicated when there is insufficient bone to anchor the device, or when the patient's behavior is incompatible with intraoral device activation.

Two-step treatment protocol

In this section, planning of upper jaw distraction with an internal distractor is discussed.

A maxillary distractor is typically a modular device with three components: body, footplate, and arm. The body contains the distracting screw; it lies in the vestibule of the mouth, outside the soft tissues. The footplate and arm lie under the soft tissues and anchor the device to the bones. The footplate fixes the device to the midface; the arm attaches the device to the upper jaw (**Fig 4.9-1**).

Successful maxillary advancement with internal distractors demands extensive presurgical planning [Scolozzi et al, 2017]. Because of its complexity, planning internal distraction necessitates the use of 3-D surgical simulation software. With this software, planning begins by building an accurate model of the face. The model is made by segmenting a computed tomographic (CT) scan and incorporating virtual dental models into the facial model [Gateno et al, 2003]. The CT scan is taken with the mandible in centric relationship. The facial model consists of separate 3-D objects—the midface skeleton, upper jaw, and mandible—and should have a correctly defined anatomical frame of reference (ie, sagittal, axial, and coronal planes).

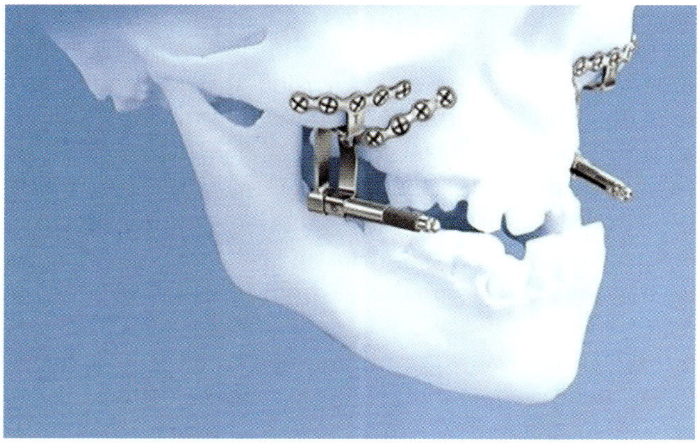

Fig 4.9-1 Maxillary distractor.

2.2 Simplifying the required movements

Moving the maxilla requires two distractors, one on each side of the upper jaw. Right and left devices are installed at the same height, at the same forward position, and at the same pitch. In addition, right and left devices should be parallel with the sagittal plane; however, slight anterior convergence is acceptable.

Two internal rectilinear distractors, installed as described above, may produce different movements, depending how they are activated. When the right and left devices are activated in unison, the maxilla will translate. The direction of the movement is dictated by the direction of the devices. When the right and left devices are activated unequally, the maxilla will rotate; the axis of rotation being perpendicular to the plane that includes the long axes of both distractor bodies. Even though some rotations are possible with these devices, they are not pure. Uneven device activation simultaneously changes the roll, yaw, and position of the upper jaw, rather than pivoting the upper jaw about a single cardinal axis. Simultaneous multi-axis movements are difficult to control clinically. Thus, we have learned that it is best to treat the distractors as if they are only able to produce translation.

Placing a retruded jaw into normal alignment requires complex movements, for two reasons. First, maxillary retrusion is rarely an isolated deformity. Many patients with this condition also have vertical deficiency and malrotation. Second, even in isolated retrusion, the upper jaw must translate and rotate in all directions to land in normal occlusion.

Moving the upper jaw from its initial (malformed) alignment into normal arrangement usually requires six transformations (movements):

1. Anterior translation
2. Vertical translation
3. Transverse translation
4. Yaw rotation
5. Roll rotation
6. Pitch rotation

Unfortunately, rectilinear internal devices only permit two types of transformations:

1. Anterior translation
2. Vertical translation

The obvious question is: How can a retrognathic upper jaw be corrected using devices through which only two of the six required transformations can be effected?

A solution is to correct the deformity in two steps. Initially, the surgeon carries out all movements that the device cannot. These movements are performed intraoperatively, after the osteotomy is completed but before the distractors are installed. In the second step, the distractors complete the movements they are capable of (**Table 4.9-1**); these changes occurring postoperatively during the distraction phase.

In the first step of the two-step protocol, a standard Le Fort I osteotomy is completed. Subsequently, the upper jaw is moved into an intermediate position. This intraoperative movement completes all the transformations the device cannot (ie, transverse translation, yaw rotation, roll rotation, and pitch rotation). To move the upper jaw further into the intermediate position, an occlusal splint is used that has been designed using planning software and manufactured via 3-D printing.

To make the occlusal splint in the software, the upper jaw is first moved to the intermediate position. This position is established using a backward approach. Rather than moving the upper jaw from its original position to the intermediate position, the maxilla is moved backward, from final alignment (**Fig 4.9-2**).

From final alignment, the transformations are removed that the distractors can affect. First, forward-translation is subtracted by sliding the upper jaw straight backward until one of the maxillary tuberosities touches its pterygoid plate (**Fig 4.9-3**).

Intraoperative transformations (impossible with linear distraction)	Postoperative transformations (possible with linear distraction)
Transverse translation	Anteroposterior translation
Yaw rotation	Vertical translation
Roll rotation	
Pitch rotation	

Table 4.9-1 Transformations needed to correct complex maxillary retrusion.

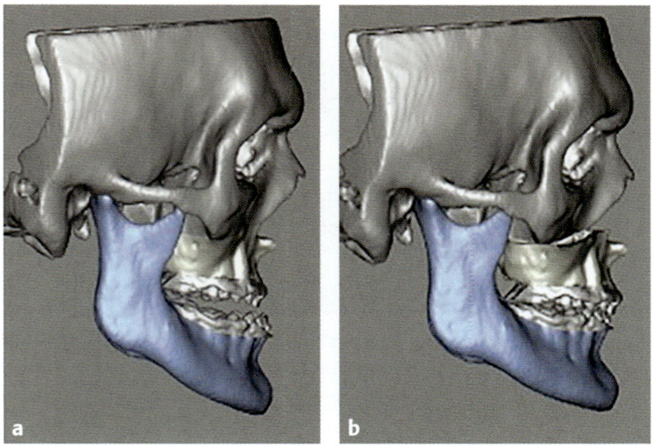

Fig 4.9-2a–b The surgical simulation begins by placing the upper jaw in ideal alignment.
a Original condition.
b Ideal alignment.

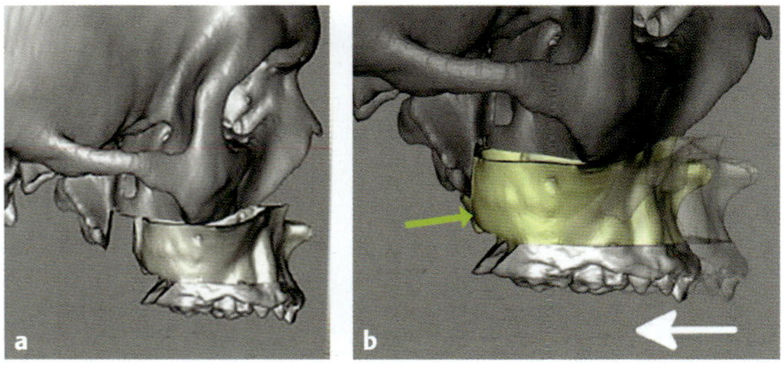

Fig 4.9-3a–b From final alignment, the upper jaw is moved straight back until one of the maxillary tuberosities contacts its pterygoid plate.

Downward-translation is removed by moving the upper jaw up, until it contacts the midface (**Fig 4.9-4**).

At this juncture, the osteotomy gap is assessed. Traditional distraction begins with the upper jaw in the original position, where bone contact between the segments is ample. In our two-step protocol, however, distraction begins from an intermediate position where bone contact may be minimal. For bone to form during distraction, a soft-bone callus must bridge the osteotomy gap. When step-one movements create a substantial gap between the bone segments (**Fig 4.9-4**), a bridging callus may not form, resulting in failure of osteogenesis. To prevent this complication, bone contact is increased by moving the upper jaw further up (**Fig 4.9-5**).

Naturally, this requires bone resection in areas of overlap. Fortunately, bone collisions can be easily mapped using the planning software (**Fig 4.9-6**) and removed at the time of surgery.

Once the osteotomized segment is in the intermediate position, an occlusal splint is designed using the 3-D planning software. The splint must have a certain thickness because as is discussed later its flanks will be used to carry the distractors to their correct position (**Fig 4.9-7**).

An intermediate occlusal splint is not all that is needed to place the osteotomized segment in the intermediate position. When the splint is interposed between the dental arches

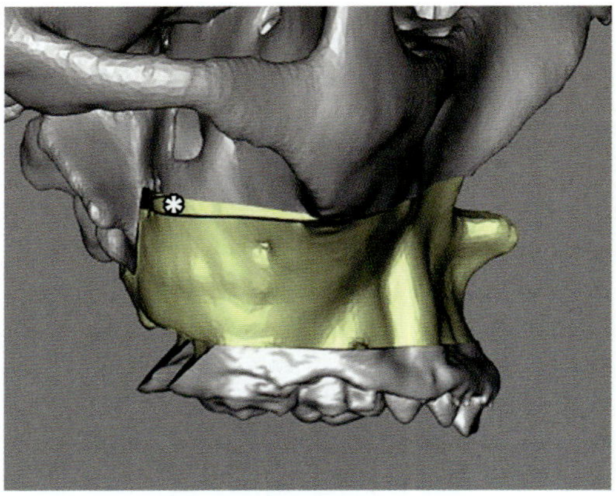

Fig 4.9-4 The upper jaw is moved up until it contacts the midface. Then, the osteotomy gap (asterix) is assessed. A large gap can cause failure of osteogenesis.

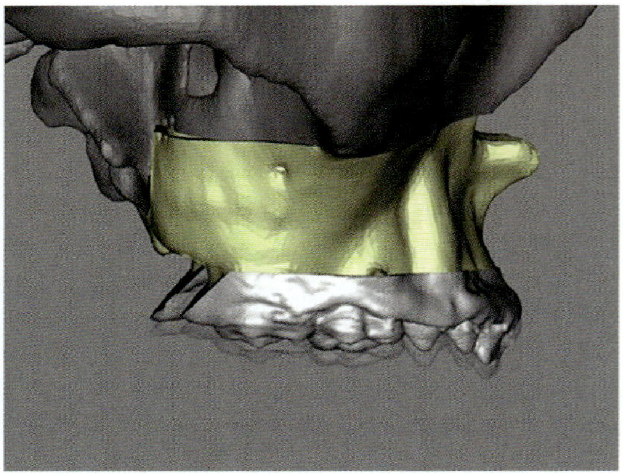

Fig 4.9-5 To increase bone contact, the lower part of the midface is moved further upward. This improves bone contact between the upper and lower midface.

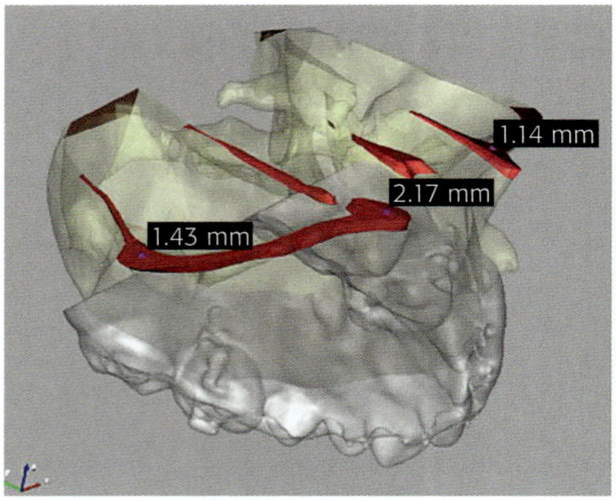

Fig 4.9-6 The areas of bone overlap shown here in red can be mapped in the planning software for future removal.

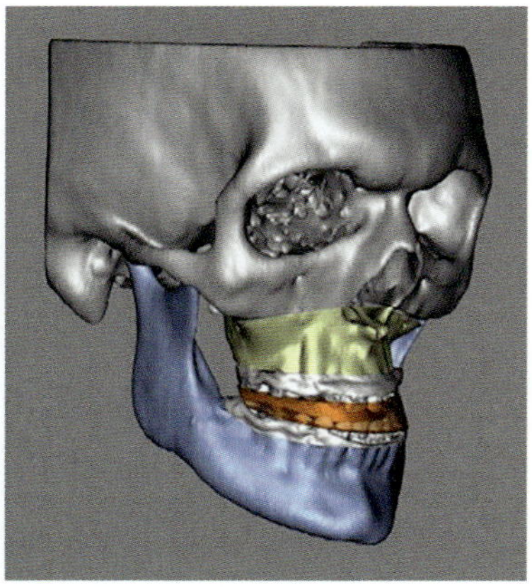

Fig 4.9-7 With the osteotomized segment in the intermediate position, an occlusal splint (clear orange) is fabricated. The splint must be relatively thick.

and the jaws are wired shut, both jaws can still move. Thus, an additional method is needed to fix the mobile segment in the correct alignment. A common technique is to track the vertical position of the maxillary central incisors [Johnson, 1985]. Specifically, the vertical position of U_0 (ie, the point located halfway between the mesioincisal angles of the upper incisors, yellow dot on **Fig 4.9-15g**). Before surgery, in the planning software the vertical displacement of U_0, that is, the change in vertical position that U_0 experienced when the mobile segment is moved from the original to the intermediate position, is calculated. During surgery, this distance is used to determine where the mobile segment should be placed. This method is described in detail in the surgery section.

2.2.1 Selecting, adapting, and installing the distractors

For internal distraction to be successful, the appropriate distractor components need to be selected, the parts well adapted, and the entire device accurately installed. Accomplishing all these goals through improvisation during surgery is virtually impossible.

To fashion the distractor for surgery, first the distraction vector needs to be calculated. The vector is the longest side (hypotenuse) of a right triangle whose sides are the forward translation (run) and the downward movement (rise). The length of the vector is the distance the device should be activated to attain the desired outcome. The direction of the vector (θ) is the angle at which the distractors must be installed. The angle is calculated using the equation θ = cotangent (rise/run). These calculations are illustrated in **Fig 4.9-8**.

In the next step of these preparations, the distractor vectors are rendered in the planning software by constructing two cylinders that have the orientation of vector and the length of distractor bodies. The cylinders are placed at each side of the upper jaw, where the future distractor bodies will be located. The bodies are placed where they can attain parallelism, where they can be activated with ease, and where they will be most comfortable for the patient. With these goals in mind, the cylinders are placed (mock distractor bodies) in the molar area close to the neck of the upper teeth (**Fig 4.9-9**).

After the mock distractor bodies have been set in place, the 3-D virtual model of the skull is printed in plastic. The model shows the upper midface, the Le Fort I segment, and the distractor vectors (as cylinders). The Le Fort I segment is in the intermediate position.

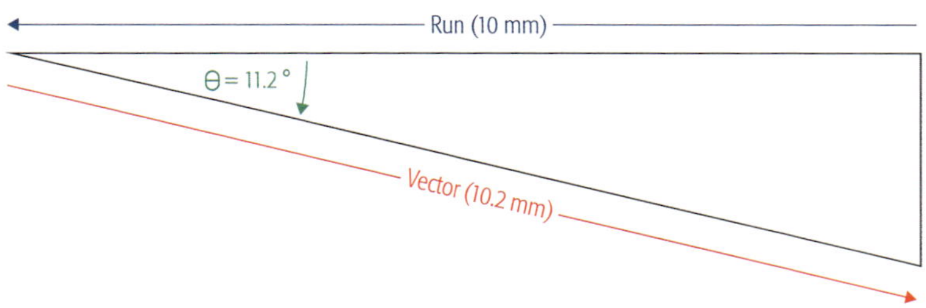

Fig 4.9-8 Distraction vector calculations. The run is the forward translation. The rise is the downward movement. The hypotenuse of the right triangle is the distractor vector.

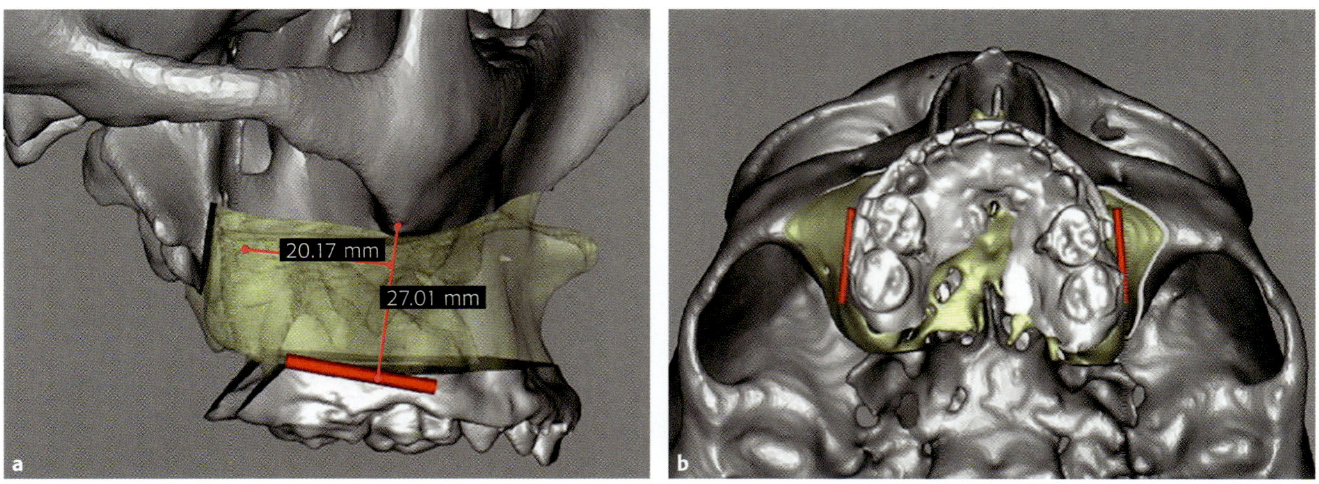

Fig 4.9-9a–b The distractor vector is rendered in computer model using two cylinders. The cylinders have the inclination of the vector and the length of the distractor bodies.

Next, the devices are conformed to the printed model. The process begins by selecting the distractor bodies. The bodies, which contain the distracting mechanisms (screws), are available in 10, 15, 20, and 25 mm lengths. The length of the body should match or surpass the length of distractor vector. However, it should not be unnecessarily long because long bodies encroach the cheeks and are uncomfortable.

After selecting the distractor body, the footplate is selected. The footplate is a T-shaped plate with a back-step (offset) in its vertical limb. The horizontal limb of the T attaches to the malar bone. The bottom of the T holds the distractor body. The footplates are available in three heights (short, medium, and tall), each with two possible posterior offsets (7 and 12 mm). The vertical limb of the T has two segments: an upper segment that runs from the horizontal limb to the offset and a lower segment that runs from the offset to the bottom of the T. For all footplates, the height of the upper segment is 6.8 mm. The height of the lower segment is variable; in short, medium, and long plates, it measures 8.6, 13.6, and 18.6 mm.

To select a footplate with the correct height, the vertical distance is measured between the malar buttress and the mock distractor body (cylinder) (**Fig 4.9-9**). The optimal footplate is the one whose lower vertical segment height approximates this distance. The offset of the footplate moves the distractor body backward to increase patient comfort and to keep the distractors as parallel as possible. To select the appropriate offset for a patient, the horizontal distance is measured between the malar buttress and the maxillary tuberosity (**Fig 4.9-9**). When the distance is equal to or more than 12 mm, the plates are chosen with the large offset; if the distance is less than 12 mm, we opt for the small offset. After the footplate has been selected, it is adapted to the model. The horizontal limb is form-fitted to the malar bone. The bottom end of the footplate is bent so that it holds the distractor body in ideal alignment (mirroring the alignment of the mock distractor body).

Next, the distractor's arm is selected and adapted. This plate, which is shaped like a quarter-turned "L" anchors the device to the upper jaw. The distractor's module has right and left arms of three different heights (6, 10, and 14 mm). To select the appropriate arm, the vertical distance is measured between the distractor body and the horizontal Le Fort I cut. The plate height approximates this distance. After the correct arm has been selected, it is attached to the distractor and adapted to the upper jaw. The arm should form-fit the facial surface of the maxilla below the Le Fort I cut. Its screw-holes should rest over the thickest available bone. Once the right and left distractors are adapted, the devices are fastened to the plastic model and the parallelism of the bodies tested (**Fig 4.9-10**). We begin this task by inserting the footplate screws. The distractor is held in perfect alignment with its mock cylinder, while the malar pilot-holes are drilled. After installing the footplate screws, alignment rods are attached to the distractor bodies to test their parallelism. The rods should parallel one another in the sagittal plane but can slightly converge in the plane that includes the long axes of both distractor bodies (**Fig 4.9-10**). Commonly, one must slightly bend the distractors to ensure parallelism.

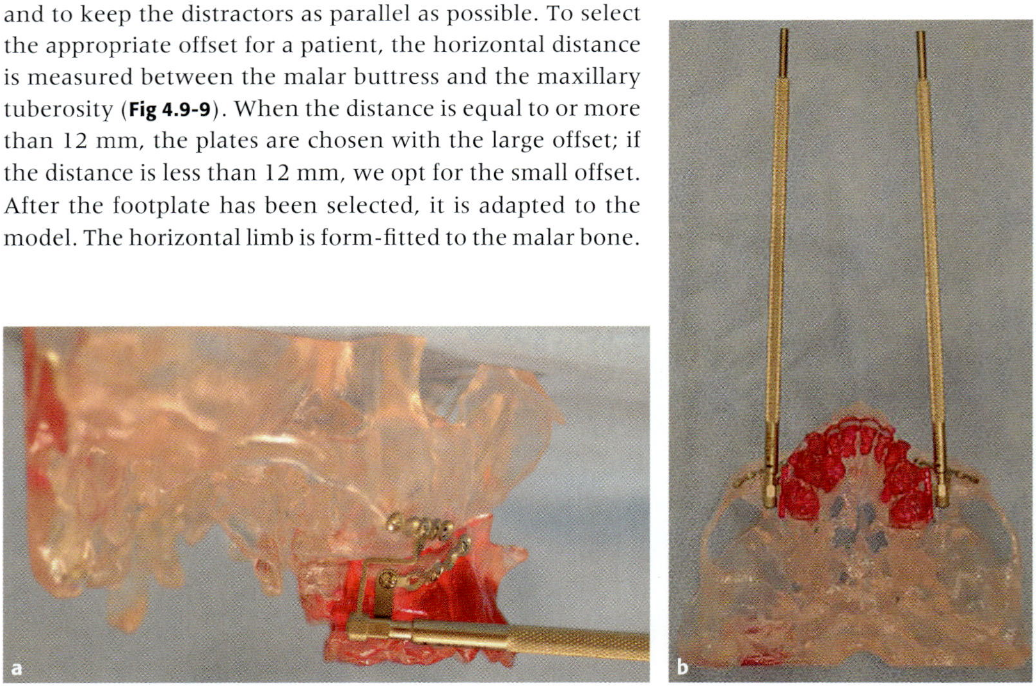

Fig 4.9-10a–b
a Alignment rods are attached to the distractor bodies to test their parallelism.
b The rods should be parallel to each other in the sagittal plane but can converge slightly anterior.

After the desired positions are defined on the model, the same alignments must be achieved during surgery (**Fig 4.9-11**). This can be done by fixing the devices to the intermediate occlusal splint because the splint is removable and can be easily placed in identical positions both on the model and on the patient.

The distractors are attached to the flanks of the occlusal splint. The installation requires new arms, and the contralateral arms work perfectly; when reversed, they extend down rather than up. To select the correct height of the splint-borne arm, the vertical distance is measured between the distractor body and the side of the occlusal wafer. Once the appropriate arms have been selected, the distractors are detached from the model, the bone-borne arms are removed and replaced with the new (splint-borne) arms. Subsequently, the new arms are adapted to the sides of the splint, and the distractors are reinstalled on the model by reinserting the footplate screws. Finally, pilot holes are drilled on the side of the splint where the holes of the splint arm lie (**Fig 4.9-12**).

When using prebent maxillary distractors, the devices may not fit well if the Le Fort I cut made on the patient is different than the one simulated in the computer model. When the osteotomy is either too high or too low, the screw-holes of the anchoring plates may be either on the wrong side of the osteotomy or too close to it. To avoid this complication, the height of the Le Fort I cut is measured in the computer model, specifically the distances from the upper canines and first molars to the cut. These distances are used during surgery to define the height of the bone cut.

2.3 Surgical intervention

The following items are needed for surgery:

1. Prebent right and left distractors, each with two arms: a bone-borne arm and an upside-down splint-borne arm.
2. A sterile, intermediate splint with pilot holes drilled in its flanks.
3. A record of the vertical position of the horizontal Le Fort I cut, in relation to the upper teeth.
4. A record of the vertical displacement of point U_0, from its original to its intermediate position.
5. A map that predicts bone collisions between the upper jaw and the midface.

First step, surgery begins by inserting a K-wire into the nasal bones and measuring the vertical distance between the K-wire and U_0. This distance is recorded as the baseline height. To this measurement, the surgeon adds or subtracts the planned vertical displacement of U_0. The result is the target height.

In the second step, a maxillary vestibular incision is made to expose the upper jaw in the standard fashion. The outline of the Le Fort I cut is marked on the bone. On each side of the jaw, a compass is used to locate the two points that indicate the correct height of the cut. The anterior point is found by tracing an arc whose radius is the predetermined distance between the tip of the canine and the Le Fort I cut. The posterior point is found in the same manner but here the radius is the predetermined distance between the first molar and the bone cut. The highest points of each arc determine the height of the bone cut.

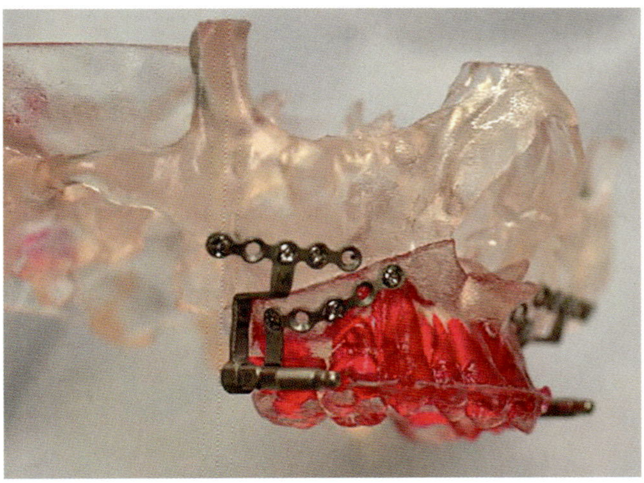

Fig 4.9-11 Right and left distractors are installed on the plastic model. The footplate is anchored to the malar bone; the arm is attached to the lower maxilla.

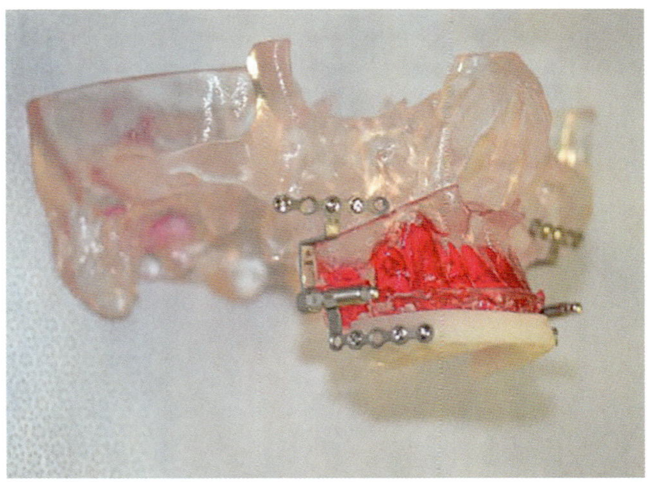

Fig 4.9-12 To carry the distractor from the model to the patient, the distractors are installed on the occlusal splint. The bone-borne arms are replaced with split-borne arms.

In the third step, the Le Fort I osteotomy is completed and the segment is mobilized. Then, guided by a computer map, bone is excised from all areas where bone collisions have been predicted.

In the fourth step, the intermediate occlusal splint is interposed and the upper and lower teeth are wired together. Subsequently, the mandibular condyles are placed in the centric position and the maxillomandibular complex is rotated until U_0 reaches the target height. The purpose of this maneuver is to test whether the upper jaw can be placed in the intermediate position without obstruction.

In the fifth step, the prebent distractors are installed. First, each distractor is assembled by putting its footplate, body, and splint-borne arm together. Then, the distractors are inserted in the wound and the distractor arms are attached to the flanks of the intermediate splint, with screws. Connecting the distractor to the pilot holes of the splint aligns the distractor bodies and fit the footplates to the midface (**Fig 4.9-13a**). Then, the distractors' footplates are fastened to the malar bones. For a second time, the mandibular condyles are placed in centric relationship and the maxillomandibular complex is rotated until U_0 is at the target height. In this position, two or three stay-screws are placed in each footplate (**Fig 4.9-13a**). Subsequently, one of the distractors is uninstalled and the splint-borne arm is replaced with the bone-borne arm. Next, the device is reinstalled on the patient by reintroducing the malar screws. If everything goes according to plan, the new distractor arm should be well adapted to the upper jaw bone. If good adaptation is confirmed, two or three stay-screws are placed in the arm (**Fig 4.9-13b**). The same sequence is repeated on the contralateral side.

In the sixth step, the parallelism of the distractor bodies is tested. Alignment rods are attached to each distractor body, and the orientation of the devices is assessed. As seen from the side, the devices should parallel one another. When seen from the top or bottom, slight anterior convergence is acceptable (**Fig 4.9-14**).

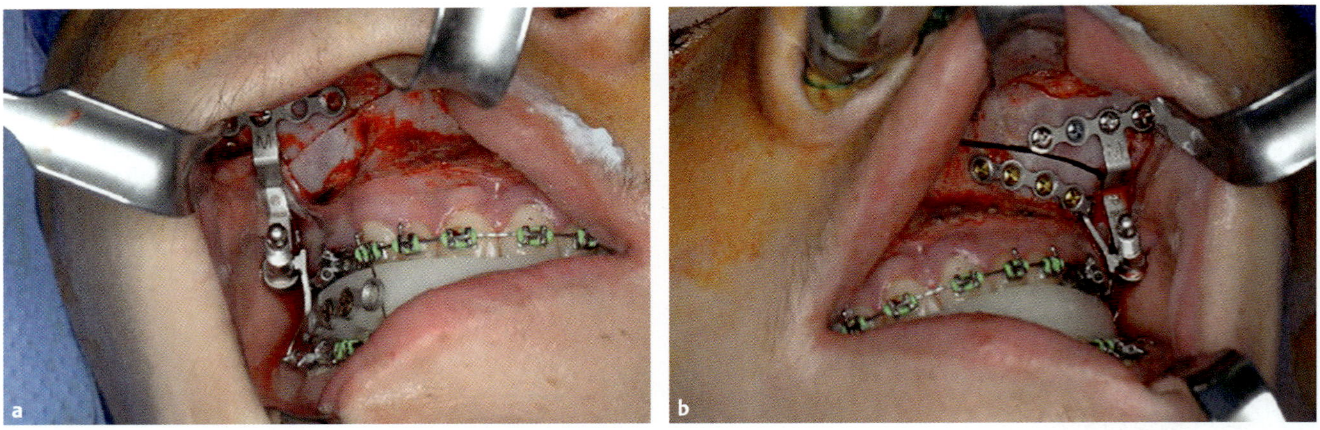

Fig 4.9-13a–b During surgery, after the lower maxilla has been mobilized, the occlusal splint is placed between the teeth and the jaws are wired together.
a The distractor is assembled using its splint-borne arm and the devices are installed in the flanks of the occlusal splint. This maneuver aligns the distractor in the correct position.
b The splint-borne arm has been replaced with the bone-borne arm.

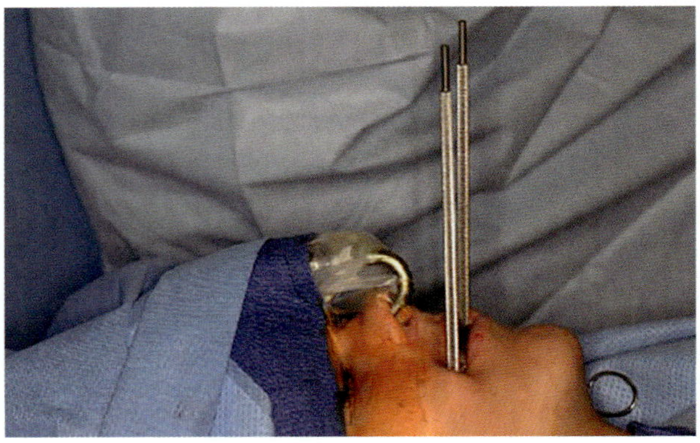

Fig 4.9-14 Alignment rods are used intraoperatively to check the orientation of the distractor bodies.

If the devices are slightly misaligned, small in-situ bends are made by manipulating the alignment rods. These adjustments must be done carefully to avoid fracturing the bone. For larger adjustments, the following steps are recommended: (1) loosen the stay-screws; (2) realign the distractor; (3) place new screws in the open holes; and (4) retighten the loose screws. Once the devices are well aligned, the remaining bone screws are installed.

In the seventh and last step of surgery, the distractors' ability to move the jaw is tested. With alternating adjustments, the right and left distractors are activated by 5 mm. The lower maxilla should move accordingly. After good mobility is confirmed, the advancement is undone and the wound is closed. A patient who requires maxillary distraction may also need mandibular orthognathic surgery. When using internal devices for upper jaw distraction, delaying lower jaw surgery is recommended to the time when the distractors will be removed. If internal distraction results in malocclusion, the bite deformity may be readily corrected by mandibular surgery.

A clinical example of a patient with cleft-palate that had maxillary internal distraction is shown in **Fig 4.9-15**.

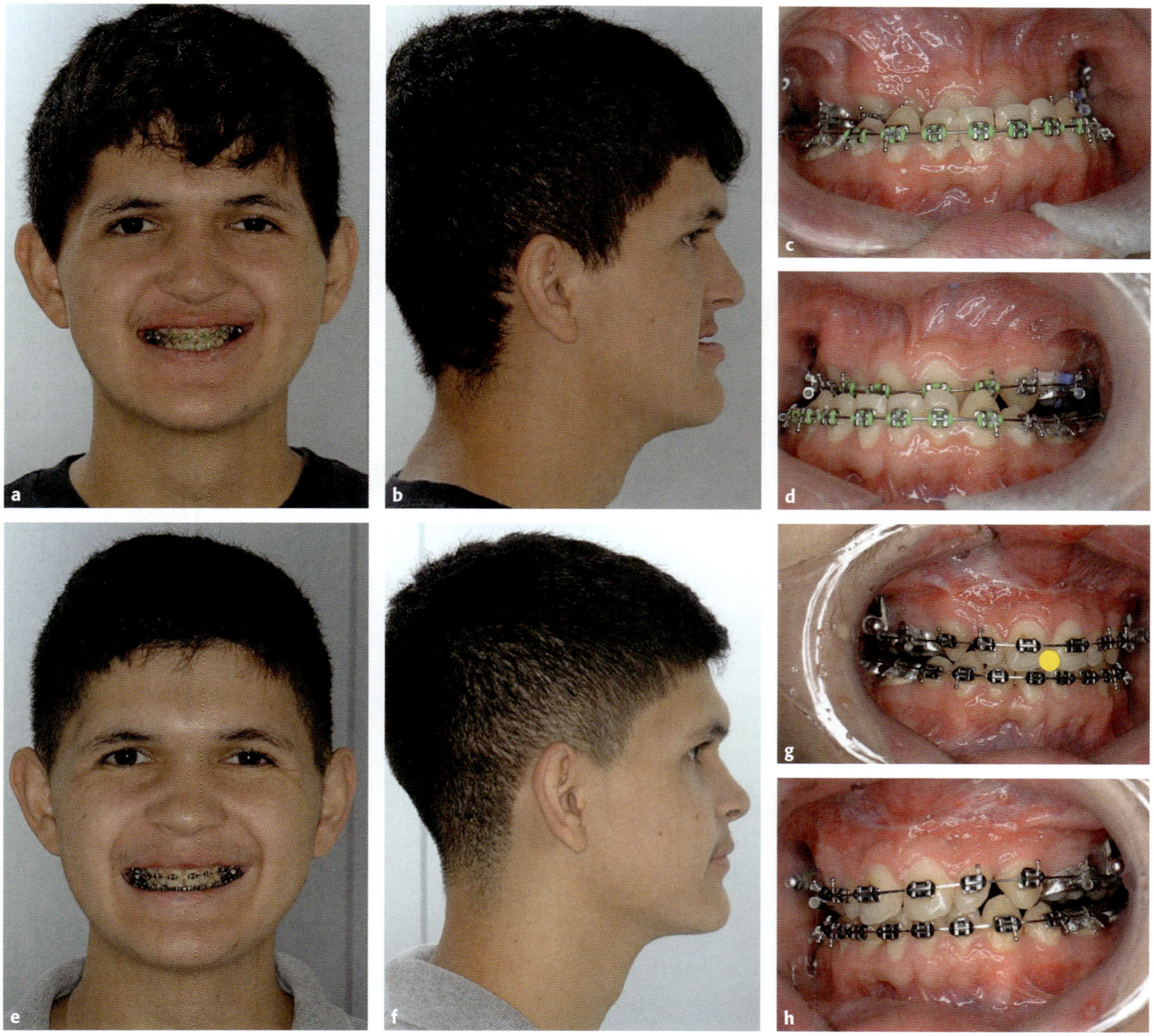

Fig 4.9-15a–h Clinical example of internal maxillary distraction (patient with cleft palate). Preoperat ve condition (**a–d**). Distraction outcome, yellow dot on **Fig 15g** equals U_0 (**e–h**). No elastics were used during distraction.

2.4 Postoperative care

In the first postoperative week, the distractors are not activated. This latency promotes bone-callus formation and soft-tissue healing. Distraction begins on postoperative day 5–7. From that time forward, distraction is performed at a rate of 1 mm/day, at a frequency of four times per day, until the mobile segment is in the desired position [Ilizarov, 1997].

2.4.1 Applying rescue interventions when outcomes are poor

Despite meticulous planning and careful surgery, the maxilla may not reach ideal alignment at the end of distraction. The primary reason for this complication is unforeseen jaw rotation. Initially, it may be assumed that parallel rectilinear distractors activated in unison will produce pure upper jaw translation; however, this is not always the case. Our (unpublished) case series shows that in approximately half of the patients, the pitch of the mobilized segment shifts during distraction. In 33% of our study patients, the rotation was counterclockwise when one looks at the patient's right side: in 22%, it was clockwise. The mechanisms responsible for this improper rotation have not been elucidated. But we hypothesize that the tilting is induced by the resistant forces of the surrounding soft tissues, and that it is enabled by bone deformation, device bending, and the looseness of the distraction mechanism that by design allows a certain movement between the distractor's components.

Unforeseen upper jaw rotations during distraction will cause malocclusion, some of which can be readily corrected; specifically, posterior open bites that occur because of clockwise rotation. Posterior elastics can derotate the maxilla before callus consolidation or can erupt posterior teeth into occlusion.

Conversely, anterior open bites that occur because of counter-clockwise rotation are harder to correct. Anterior elastics can be attempted; however, they are often unsuccessful. If bimaxillary surgery has been planned anyway because of concomitant lower jaw deformity, the anterior open bite can be closed after mandible osteotomy. If bimaxillary surgery has not been planned, the distractor devices can be removed early, at the end of activation and before the callus has ossified. Subsequently, the lower maxilla can be placed into the desired occlusal relationship with the mandible, and be fixated to the upper midface with plates [Baker et al, 2007]. This procedure is called callus molding.

To summarize, in about half of the patients' excellent outcomes can be achieved without rescue interventions. In those patients (roughly 25%) who will develop posterior open bites, the malocclusion can be corrected with posterior (vertical) elastics. In the remaining one-quarter of patients who will develop anterior open bites, the malocclusion can either be corrected with additional orthognathic surgery or callus molding. Mandibular surgery is used when the procedure is indicated to correct a lower jaw deformity; callus molding is used when the lower jaw is normal. Callus molding does not add complexity to the treatment, since all patients who have this rescue intervention would have had a second operation for device removal.

Another strategy that minimizes the number of anterior open bites is adding 1 or 2° clockwise rotation to the intermediate position. Although this may increase the number of patients with posterior open bites, corrective procedures are easier to handle.

2.5 Complications of internal maxillary distraction

Patients who undergo internal maxillary distraction can experience adverse events. Some complications, like infection, are common to most operations; others are specific to technique. Here only the specific complications are described.

One complication of internal maxillary distraction is encountering bone that is too thin for the anchoring screws. This challenging situation rarely occurs in the midface because the footplates lie over the thick malar bone. It sometimes happens in the Le Fort I segment, however, where the distractor arm rests over the facial surface of the maxilla, a wall can be paper thin.

When the bone is too thin for bone-arm screws, the splint-borne arms are used to carry out the distraction via the inserted occlusal splint. For this approach, the splint must be modified. Vertical holes are drilled in the periphery of the wafer, so that it can be wired to the upper teeth. The indentations in the lower surface are ground down to allow the splint to glide. Once these modifications are completed, the bone-borne arms of the distractors are replaced with the splint-borne arms, and the assembled distractors are installed on the patient. The footplates are attached to the upper midface; the arms are anchored to the flanks of the splint.

Another complication of internal maxillary distraction is malocclusion. The causes of malocclusion are many: (1) using rectilinear devices to effectuate complex jaw movements; (2) not adapting or installing the distractors well; (3) unforeseen jaw rotation during device activation; and (4) inadequate activation.

One more complication of internal maxillary distraction is hardware failure (eg, screw loosening). This complication is rare. When it occurs, a remedial strategy is removing the internal distractor and completing distraction with an external device.

Another complication of internal maxillary distraction is malocclusion (the return, following correction, to the original deformity) [Gateno et al, 2005]. Relapse, which occurs during the consolidation phase, is variable. We believe forces that produce the relapse originate from within the soft-tissue envelope. Although relapse cannot be prevented, this problem may be overcome by overcorrecting the deformity.

Additional complications of internal distraction are discomfort [Scolozzi et al, 2016] and soft-tissue ulceration. Internal distractors can be uncomfortable and cause ulcers in the mucosa, specifically when the distractor body is too long, too far forward, or too high. Selecting the shortest possible bodies and installing those bodies in a comfortable region can prevent these complications.

A complication of the two-step technique is bony nonunion between the lower maxilla and the upper midface. Nonunion usually occurs because of an osteotomy gap that is too wide. The large gap is produced by intraoperative movements that are performed to simplify distraction. Fortunately, nonunion is rare. When it occurs, it is usually detected when the distractors are removed. The treatment is straightforward. The upper jaw is stabilized with four bone plates and the area of nonunion is bone grafted.

3 Midface distraction

3.1 Indications

Distraction of the midface is indicated in the treatment of midface retrusion, especially when it causes proptosis, lagophthalmos, sleep apnea, and malocclusion. This presentation is a feature of the craniofacial synostosis syndromes (eg, Crouzon, Apert, Pfeiffer).

Traditional operations for midface retrusion move the midface during the operation. This approach requires extensive mobilization, rigid fixation, and bone grafting. Alternatively, distraction osteogenesis relocates the midface after the operation with gradual movement. The slow movement circumvents the need for immediate extensive soft-tissue stretching and may eliminate the need for bone grafts.

3.1.1 Planning

As in lower maxillary distraction, planning midface distraction is best done using 3-D surgical simulation software. Compared with maxillary distraction, planning midfacial distraction is simple. To correct midface retrusion, the only thing to do is to move the midface straight forward.

Midface retrusion affects the face at different levels. The retroposition of the nose and the orbital rims cause exorbitism; retrusion of the upper jaw causes malocclusion. In some patients, the amounts of nasal, orbital, and maxillary retrusion are similar. In other patients, they are not. When the retrusion is even, at all levels, correcting the deformity at one level corrects the whole deficiency. But when the amount of retrusion varies, at different levels, correcting the malformation at one level leaves deformity in others. An important concept in midface advancement is that the correction of the orbital deformity has precedence over the correction of others [Mulliken et al, 1996; Gateno et al, 2007]. The reason is that residual deformity, at other levels, can be easily corrected with additional procedures while the orbital deformity cannot. In practical terms, when the midface is advanced, one should not aim at correcting the malocclusion, only the exorbitism. Fortunately, in most cases the distocclusion will be corrected when the exorbitism is fixed. Yet, when the upper jaw is still retruded after the exophthalmos has been corrected, one should avoid the temptation to continue the midface advancement, for it will bring about enophthalmos.

The orbit also has precedence when correcting vertical deficits [Gateno et al, 2007]. Many patients with facial synostosis have upper jaws that are too small and superiorly positioned, yet their orbital heights are normal. If one tries to correct the vertical maxillary deficiency by distracting the midface forward and downward, the orbit will be disfigured (**Fig 4.9-16**).

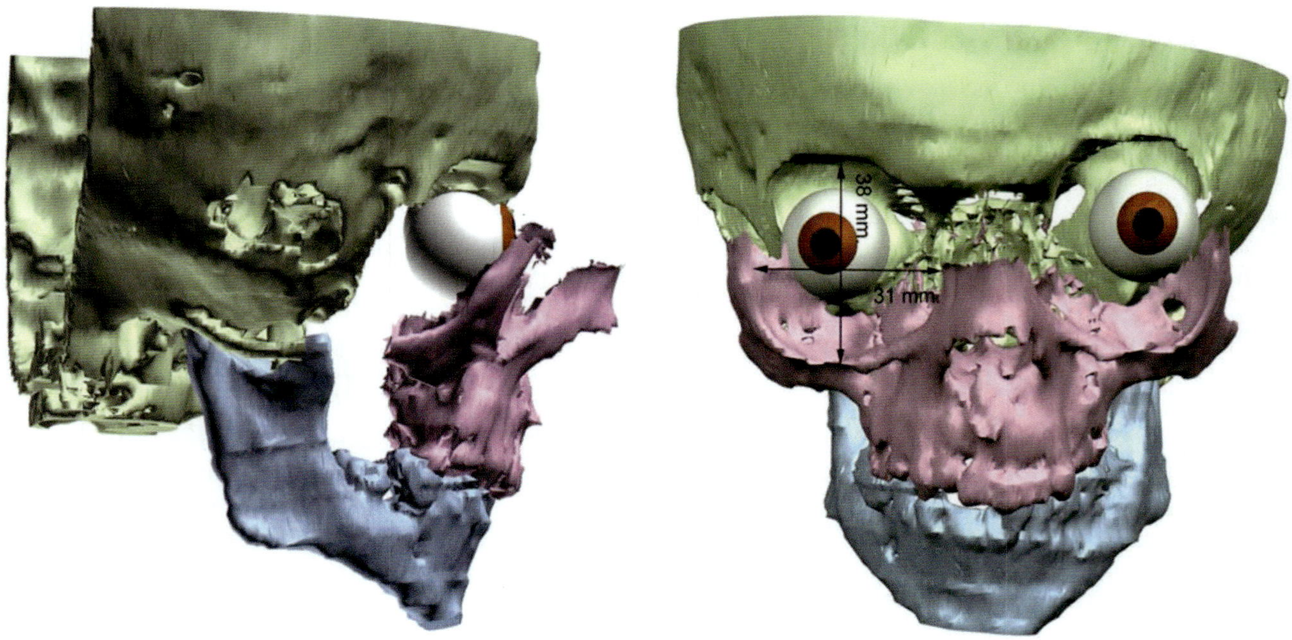

Fig 4.9-16 During midface distraction, the maxilla should not be moved forward and downward. This vector distorts the orbits, as shown here.

To avoid this complication, it is best not to correct the vertical maxillary deficiency during midface distraction. It should be corrected later with a Le Fort I osteotomy (**Fig 4.9-17**).

Planning midface distraction begins by constructing a virtual model of the face. Like the model used to plan lower maxillary distraction, the model shows the bones, the teeth, and the facial soft tissue. To plan midface distraction, however, the eyes are rendered so that orbital retrusion can be measured (**Fig 4.9-18**).

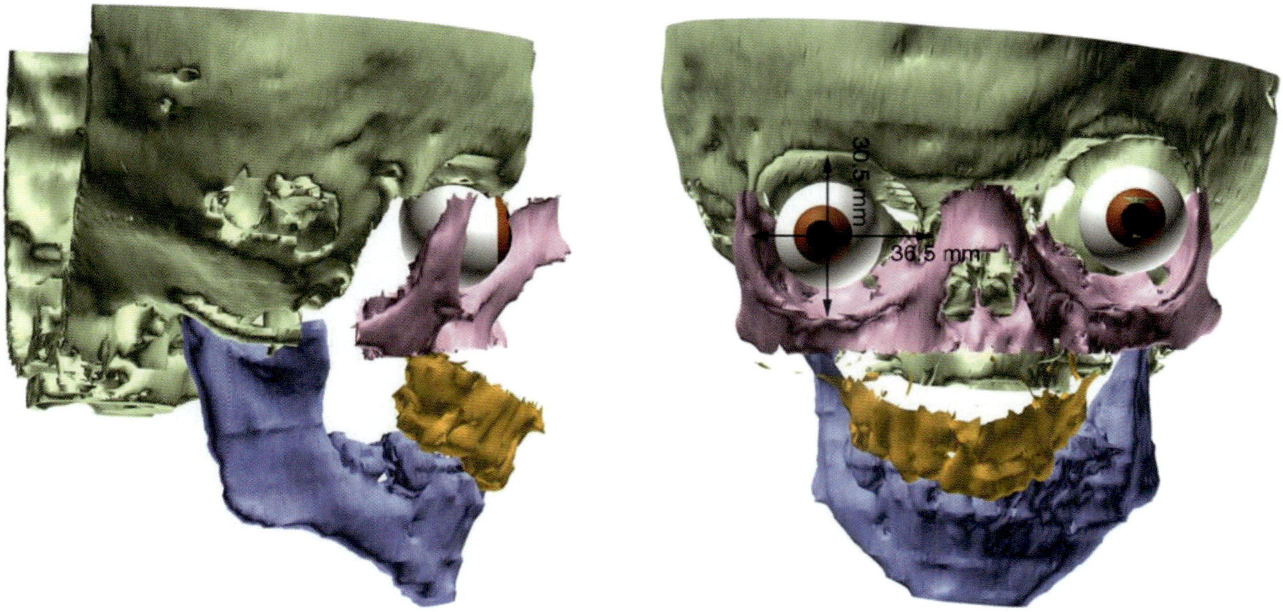

Fig 4.9-17 To correct a residual malocclusion, it is best to perform a Le Fort I osteotomy later.

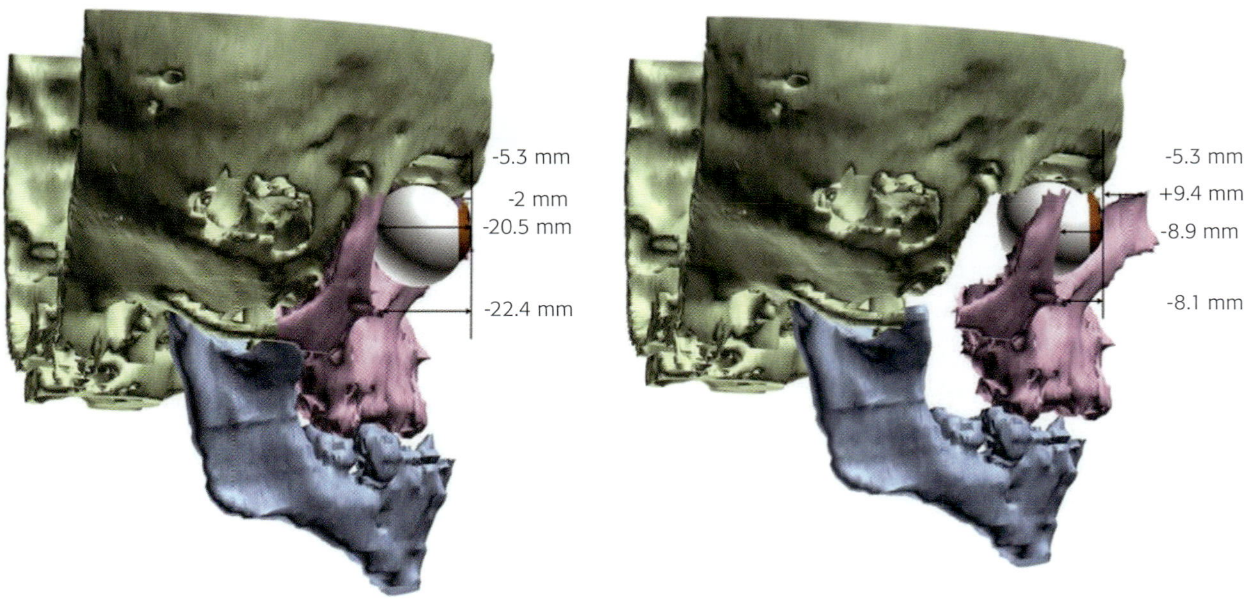

Fig 4.9-18 Orbital rim retrusion can be measured by constructing a paracoronal plane that is tangential to the cornea and then measuring the distances between the plane and the four cardinal points of the orbital rim.

Orbital rim retrusion is measured in the following manner. Initially, four cardinal points are digitized on the orbital rim (superior, medial, inferior, and lateral). These points represent the four orbital rim margins: supraorbital, medial, infraorbital, and lateral. Next, a paracoronal plane is constructed that is tangential to the cornea. Next, the distances are measured between the plane and the four cardinal points (**Fig 4.9-18**). Finally, the measurements are compared with normative values (**Table 4.9-2**) [Mulliken et al, 1996; Gateno et al, 2007; Eckstein et al, 2011].

The location and the size of the retrusion help plan the operation. For example, for a patient with significant retrusion of the whole orbital rim, a monobloc advancement may be recommended (**Fig 4.9-19**) [Kumar et al, 2014; Hariri et al, 2016; Visser et al, 2017]. Yet, for a patient with retrusion that only involves the medial, inferior and lateral rims, a Le Fort III advancement is recommended (**Fig 4.9-18**) [Gateno et al, 2007; Raposo-Amaral et al, 2013].

The distance by which the midface should be advanced depends on the amount of orbital retrusion. Unfortunately, the precise amount of orbital retrusion is difficult to establish because it may be different at each orbital rim margin. For example, the retrusion of the lateral orbital rim may be different than the retrusion of the infraorbital rim. In practice, the surgeon needs to define a distraction length that balances all deficits, taking into consideration that slight residual exophthalmos is preferable to any enophthalmos [Mulliken et al, 1996]. Once the amount of advancement has been established, the distraction is simulated in the planning software. The osteotomies are completed; the midface is moved forward.

In the next step of planning, the distractors are fashioned for surgery. Internal midface distractors have three components: body, posterior footplate, and anterior footplate. The body has the distracting mechanism. The posterior footplate anchors the device to the temporal bone. The anterior footplate anchors the device to the malar bone.

	Distances, mean ± SD, mm	
Cardinal points	**Caucasians**	**Orientals**
Superior	4.6 ± 4.2	5.0 ± 4.5
Nasal	5.9 ± 3.0	6.8 ± 4.1
Inferior	12.6 ± 3.7	11.1 ± 4.3
Lateral	20.6 ± 2.6	17.5 ± 3.3

Table 4.9-2 Average globe to orbital rim distances in adults.

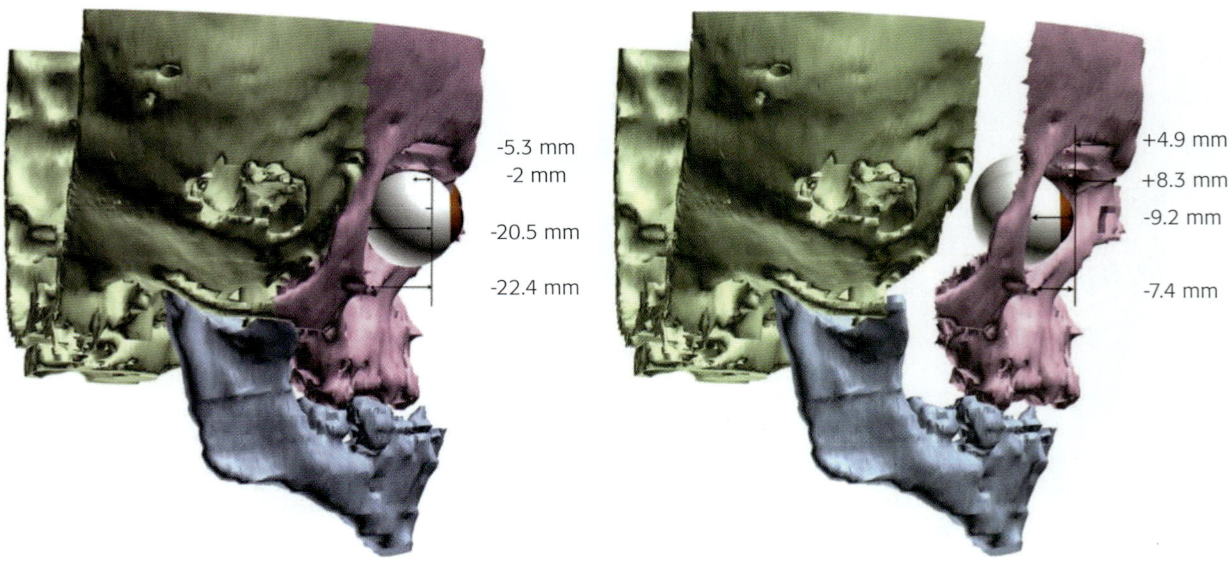

Fig 4.9-19 When the supraorbital rim is normal and the three other margins are retruded, a Le Fort III advancement is indicated. When the whole is retruded, consider a monobloc as shown here.

The distractors are shaped by adapting them to a plastic model of the patient's skull that is created by 3-D printing. On the printed model, both distractors are aligned horizontally and positioned above the zygomatic arch. The anterior footplate is trimmed and adapted to the malar surface of the zygomatic bone, spanning the zygomaticomaxillary suture. Suture straddling prevents separation of the malar bone from the maxillary bone during distraction.

Some anterior footplates have a jutting piece that extends medially behind the temporal border of the malar bone. The purpose of this part is to deliver distraction forces directly to the bone, decreasing the forces that are transmitted to the fixation screws. This load sharing is possible only if the vertical jutting piece has full contact with the slanted malar bone. To achieve adequate contact, the temporal border of the malar bone must be reshaped to create a vertical edge for the jutting piece. The posterior footplate is adapted to the temporal bone behind the temporal line.

3.2 Surgery

Surgery begins by exposing the midface with a coronal incision. Then, the distractors are temporarily installed. In most patients, the distractor bodies are placed over the temporalis muscles. Yet, in patients with bulging temporal fossae, the devices may have to be placed under the muscle. After completing the exposure, the distractors are temporarily installed by putting two to three screws in each footplate. Next, the devices are removed, the osteotomies completed, and the midface mobilized. Finally, the distractors are reinstalled with at least four screws per plate (**Fig 4.9-20**).

In some internal midface distractors, the anterior footplate can be left on the bone during the osteotomy and mobilization because the distractor's body can be detached from the anterior footplate.

Before reinstalling the distractors, the midface needs to be fully mobilized. Otherwise, the distraction will fail. After the devices are installed, the mobility is tested by advancing the midface by 5 mm. Afterward the midface is set back and the incision is closed.

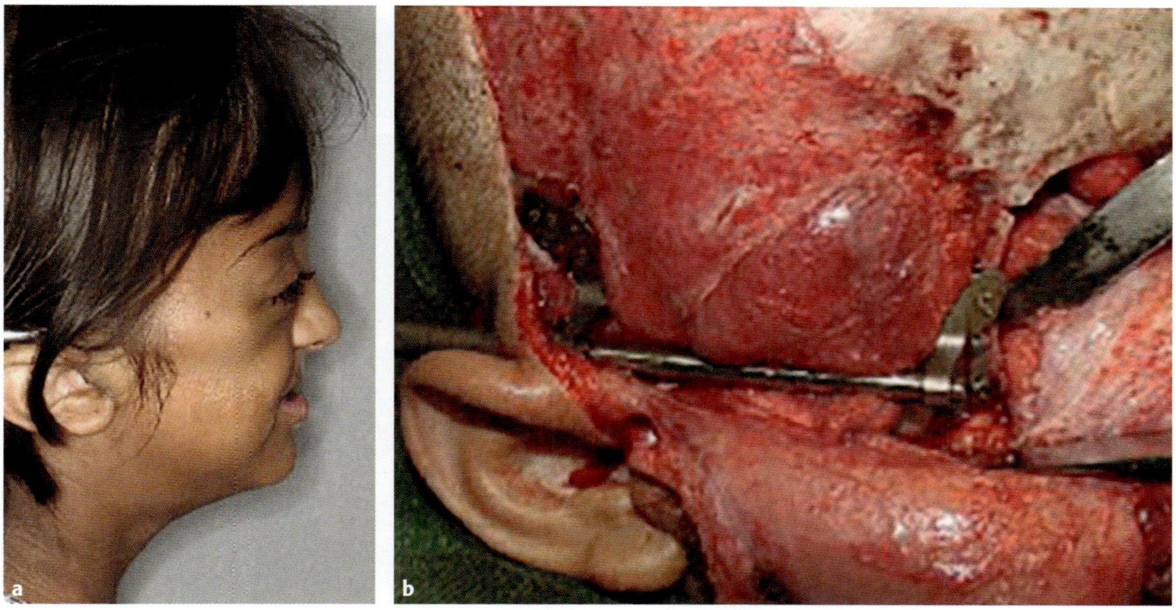

Fig 4.9-20a–b
a The patient with the distractor.
b Intraoperative view. The distractor is aligned horizontally above the zygomatic arch. The posterior footplate is anchored to the temporal bone. The anterior footplate is anchored to the malar bone.

Device activation starts after a latency period of 5–7 days [Kumar et al, 2014]. We recommend activating the devices four times a day to move the midface one, or 1 mm/day [Ilizarov, 1997]. Once the midface is in the correct position, the activating rods are removed and the devices are buried. Three months later, a second operation is performed to remove the devices. A clinical example of a patient with Crouzon syndrome that had internal midface distraction is shown in **Fig 4.9-21**.

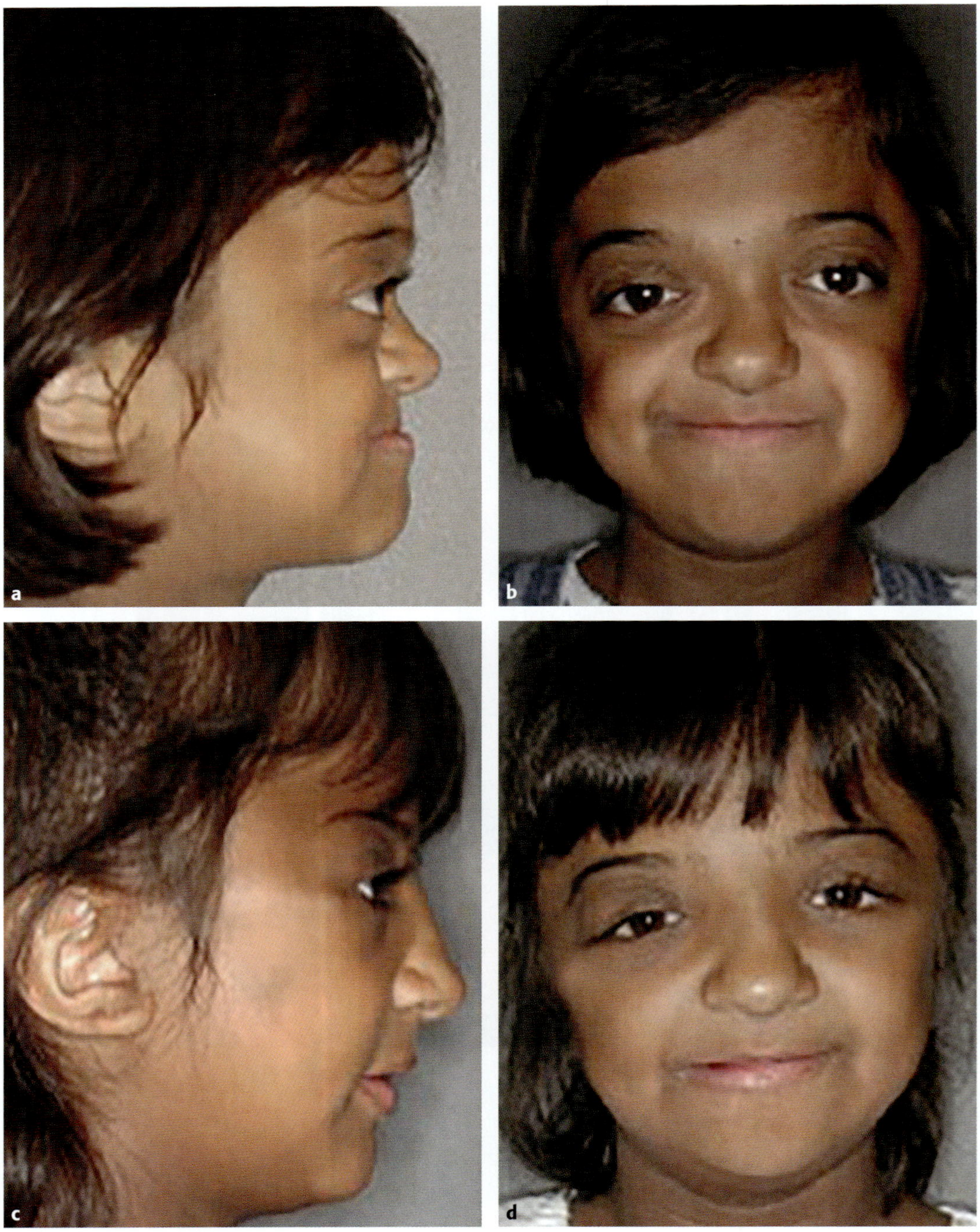

Fig 4.9-21a–d Clinical example of a patient with Crouzon syndrome who had internal midface distraction.
a–b Before surgery.
c–d After surgery.

3.3 Complications

Patients who undergo internal midface distraction can have complications that are common to any surgical procedure or problems that are unique to the operation. One complication that can occur in midface distraction is a malar fracture. It can happen during osteotomy, mobilization, or device activation. To reduce the risk of fracture, the midface should be mobilized gently, but well. If too much force is applied during mobilization, the malar bones can separate from the rest of the midface. If the midface is not well mobilized, the malar bones may fracture during device activation. Surgeons can decrease the risk of malar separation by bridging the zygomaticomaxillary suture with the anterior footplate mesh.

Another complication of internal midface distraction is loosening of the fixation screws. To prevent this complication, at least four screws should be placed in each footplate.

One more complication of internal midface distraction is an unexpected position. This complication occurs when the distractors are not well oriented or when resisting forces tilt the midface. When the treatment outcome is unacceptable, the patient is brought back to surgery before the callous ossifies. During surgery the distractors are removed, the misalignment is corrected, and the midface is stabilized by internal fixation.

4 References and suggested reading

Aizenbud D, Rachmiel A, Emodi O. Minimizing pin complications when using the rigid external distraction (RED) system for midface distraction. *Oral Surg Oral Med Oral Pathol Oral Radiol Endod*. 2008 Feb;105(2):149–154.

Baker SB, Reid RR, Burkey B, et al. Rapid maxillary distraction protocol utilizing the halo distraction system and rigid internal fixation. *Cleft Palate Craniofac J*. 2007 Sep;44(5):476–481.

Cai M, Shen G, Wang X, et al. Intracranial fixation pin migration: a complication of external Le Fort III distraction osteogenesis in Apert syndrome. *J Craniofac Surg*. 2010 Sep;21(5):1557–1559.

Eckstein LA, Shadpour JM, Menghani R, et al. The relationship of the globe to the orbital rim. *Arch Facial Plast Surg*. 2011 Jan-Feb;13(1):51–56.

Eggermont B, Jansma J, Bierman MW, et al. Patient satisfaction related to rigid external distraction osteogenesis. *Int J Oral Maxillofac Surg*. 2007 Oct;36(10):896–899.

Gateno J, Xia J, Teichgraeber JF, et al. A new technique for the creation of a computerized composite skull model. *J Oral Maxillofac Surg*. 2003 Feb;61(2):222–227.

Gateno J, Engel ER, Teichgraeber JF, et al. A new Le Fort I internal distraction device in the treatment of severe maxillary hypoplasia. *J Oral Maxillofac Surg*. 2005 Jan;63(1):148–154.

Gateno JT, Xia J. Surgical planning for distraction osteogenesis. In: Bell WHG, ed. *Distraction Osteogenesis of the Facial Skeleton*. 1st ed. Hamilton, Ontario: BC Decker; 2007:131–139.

Hariri F, Cheung LK, Rahman ZA, et al. Monobloc Le Fort III distraction osteogenesis for correction of severe fronto-orbital and midface hypoplasia in pediatric Crouzon syndrome. *Cleft Palate Craniofac J*. 2016 Jan;53(1):118–125.

Ilizarov GA. The principles of the Ilizarov method. *Bull Hosp Jt Dis*. 1997;56(1):49–53.

Johnson DG. Intraoperative measurement of maxillary repositioning: an ancillary technique. *Oral Surg Oral Med Oral Pathol*. 1985 Sep;60(3):266–268.

Kumar AR, Steinbacher D. Advances in the treatment of syndromic midface hypoplasia using monobloc and facial bipartition distraction osteogenesis. *Semin Plast Surg*. 2014 Nov;28(4):179–183.

Maxillary Distraction System Technique Guide. Available at: DePuy Synthes http://www.depuysynthes.com/hcp/cmf/products/qs/Maxillary_Distractor; DePuy Synthes; 2017.

Mulliken JB, Godwin SL, Pracharktam N, et al. The concept of the sagittal orbital-globe relationship in craniofacial surgery. *Plast Reconstr Surg*. 1996 Apr;97(4):700–706.

Raposo-Amaral CE, Tong A, Denadai R, et al. A subcranial Le Fort III advancement with distraction osteogenesis as a clinical strategy to approach pycnodysostosis with midface retrusion and exorbitism. *J Craniofac Surg*. 2013 Jul;24(4):1327–1330.

Scolozzi P, Herzog G. Computer-assisted virtual planning for surgical guide manufacturing and internal distractor adaptation in the management of midface hypoplasia in cleft patients. *Cleft Palate Craniofac J*. 2017 Jul;54(4):457–464.

van der Meulen J, Wolvius E, van der Wal K, et al. Prevention of halo pin complications in post-cranioplasty patients. *J Craniomaxillofac Surg*. 2005 Jun;33(3):145–149.

Visser R, Ruff CF, Angullia F, et al. Evaluating the efficacy of monobloc distraction in the Crouzon-Pfeiffer craniofacial deformity using geometric morphometrics. *Plast Reconstr Surg*. 2017 Feb;139(2):477e–487e.

Yu JC, Fearon J, Havlik RJ, et al. Distraction osteogenesis of the craniofacial skeleton. *Plast Reconstr Surg*. 2004 Jul;114(1):1E–20E.

4.10 High midface osteotomies

Richard A Hopper, Faisal Al-Mufarrej

1 Introduction

Midface deformities, such as hypoplasias, may be congenital (eg, Crouzon syndrome, Apert disease, Pfeiffer syndrome, Binder syndrome, Hajdu Cheny syndrome) [Satoh et al, 2002] or acquired (radiation therapy or posttraumatic). Subcranial Le Fort III advancement osteotomy was first reported by Gillies and Harrison [1950]. Two decades later, Tessier popularized the technique after refining it to the point of practical clinical application. The Ilizarov principles of distraction osteogenesis to the craniofacial skeleton were successfully applied by McCarthy [1992]. This soon led to reports of successful midface distraction, with Habal [1995] reporting his experience in midface advancement using an external fixator, and Chin and Toth [1997] their experience with Le Fort III distraction using an internal device. Le Fort II advancement may also be used to move only the central portion of the midface leaving the zygomas in place.

2 Le Fort III osteotomy

The Le Fort III advancement is now a standard elective technique to treat syndromic upper midface hypoplasia. The segmental facial movements once only possible with traditional techniques are now becoming also possible using distraction osteogenesis.

2.1 Indications and planning

Le Fort III and II osteotomies are indicated in the setting of severe midface hypoplasia. Timing of surgery in the setting of facial growth is controversial. Ideally, surgery on the maxilla should only be performed once midface growth is complete (about 16–18 years) [Bachmayer et al, 1986; Marchac et al, 1994]. However, since the orbitale grows forward less than 4 mm between the ages of 8.5 and 15.5 years, it is reasonable to advance the midface to adult orbital dimensions in adolescence [Chin et al, 1997].

When midface hypoplasia is associated with obstructive sleep apnea (OSA), earlier surgery (ages 3–7 years) may be indicated to prevent the associated morbidity [Chin et al, 1997]. In children with severe OSA, it is important to consider adjunct measures (continuous positive airway pressure support, adenoidectomy and tonsillectomy, or temporary tracheostomy) to minimize postoperative airway complications and delay surgery until the optimum age [Czerwinski et al, 2010]. Computed tomography (CT) and cephalometric analyses of upper airway space volume in patients undergoing Le Fort III advancement demonstrate a significant increase in volume after surgery [Iannetti et al, 2006 and 2011; Nout et al, 2010; Flores et al, 2009].

Results of prepubertal midface surgery deteriorate with age as the mandible invariably outgrows the poorly developing midface [Reid, 2007; Reitsma et al, 2012]. Surgical overcorrection is therefore required to create an iatrogenic overjet to minimize future maxillary surgery [Meazzini et al, 2005; Swennen et al, 2001; Shetye et al, 2010]. Unlike with Le Fort I osteotomies, speech, nasality and velopharyngeal function are usually not negatively affected by Le Fort III advancement [Pereira et al, 2008].

Proptosis with unmanageable exposure keratopathy can be another indication for early Le Fort III surgery [Buncic, 1991]. Le Fort III advancement increases orbital volume and treats proptosis in the absence of supraorbital rim retrusion [Festa et al, 2012]. If the presentation is complicated by concomitant forehead retrusion, a more appropriate approach is monobloc advancement (if severe OSA present) or a frontoorbital advancement followed by Le Fort III (if no severe OSA).

Although the Le Fort III advancement has a beneficial effect on occlusal relationships and airway, it should be primarily considered an inferior orbital surgery with an end goal of normalizing the globe-malar relationship (**Fig 4.10-1**). Failure to recognize this can result in iatrogenic orbital deformities if the surgeon is focused on normalizing occlusion independent of the effect on the periorbital area. The Le Fort II osteotomy in contrast will not affect the globe-malar relationship, which can provide more flexibility in the movements of this segment compared with the Le Fort III. In a child undergoing high midface osteotomies, it is rarely possible to establish normal occlusion and a Le Fort I osteotomy is usually necessary in later life. In patients requiring a midface advancement after skeletal maturity, a Le Fort I osteotomy may be performed concomitantly as a segmental movement independent of the upper midface to address the occlusion in the same setting.

Preoperatively, patients should undergo vision assessment by an ophthalmologist, a formal sleep study, and a CT scan of the skull and face with 3-D reconstruction. Preoperative computer-assisted virtual surgery is helpful in cases of multilevel/ multisegment midface osteotomies. Syndromic children found to have enlarged ventricles or suspected of a Chiari I malformation will require magnetic resonance imaging of the brain with appropriate treatment (shunt) before midface surgery if they are symptomatic. Cephalometry is important in assessing the direction and magnitude of advancement before and after conventional midface surgery, and in older children, during the activation phase of distraction. The end goal is to normalize the inferior orbital rim position [Chin et al, 1997].

2.2 Technique

2.2.1 Exposure

A bitemporal zig-zag coronal incision starting and ending 1.5 cm cephalad and posterior to the ears is usually the only necessary incision for a Le Fort III surgery. A Le Fort II osteotomy typically requires additional lower eyelid and upper intraoral incisions for the zygomaticomaxillary separation. For conventional Le Fort III advancement with fixation and grafting, the zygomatic arch must be exposed. The dissection is through the superficial layer of the deep temporal fascia at the level of the zygomatico-frontal suture, and then over the temporal fat pad to a subperiosteal plane on the zygomatic arch [Lacey et al, 1994]. For patients undergoing Le Fort III distraction, the same central dissection is performed but the superficial temporal dissection and arch exposure is not required since grafting and fixation will not be needed. The coronal flap is raised in a subperiosteal plane which is continued laterally under the temporalis muscle, separating it from the lateral orbital rim down to the zygomatic body. This limited submuscular dissection is possible since the zygomatic osteotomy is made just behind the body. Compared with conventional dissection, it minimizes the risk of iatrogenic temporalis muscle atrophy and frontal branch of the facial nerve injury.

2.2.2 Osteotomies

Traditional osteotomies

After exposure, the osteotomies proceed from lateral to medial; from least risky to most risky. The zygomatic arches are osteotomized mid-arch with a reciprocating saw, followed by a reverse-C osteotomy from the inferior orbital fissure, parallel to the lateral orbital rim, and out the frontozygo-

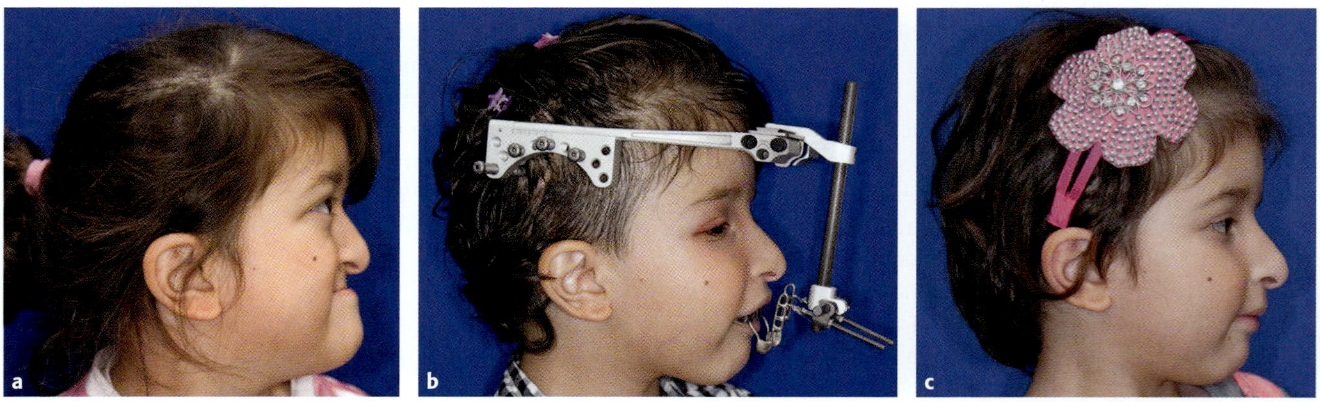

Fig 4.10-1a–c Patient with Crouzon syndrome before (**a**), during (**b**), and after (**c**) Le Fort III osteotomy and advancement with an external device. The patient had documented obstructive sleep apnea and midface retrusion.

matic suture. Using a small osteotome, the orbital floor is cut from the inferior orbital fissure, parallel to the inferior orbital rim, behind the lacrimal fossa. Care must be taken in young syndromic children to ensure the orbital osteotomy is into the maxillary sinus, since the inferior rim often has a sharp projection and is easily broken if the cut is made too anteriorly. From the midline, an osteotome is then used to crack the lamina papyracea vertically to join the inferior floor cut, posterior to the lacrimal fossa. The pterygomaxillary separation is started with an osteotome placed laterally underneath the temporalis muscle, with its tip in the inferior orbital fissure at the point of the floor cut. The osteotomy is continued from the fissure, down the posterior aspect of the maxillary sinus wall, to the level of the pterygomaxillary junction. Bimanual palpation is used, with one finger inside the mouth over the hamulus of the maxilla, to feel the osteotome proceeding down toward the pterygomaxillary fissure from the coronal incision. Be careful to ensure soft tissue is not trapped between the osteotome and the maxilla since the internal maxillary artery is in proximity. To complete the pterygomaxillary separation, a small mucosal incision can be made in the mouth to provide more direct access. The final osteotomy before down-fracture is at the midline. A transverse cut is made just below the level of the frontonasal suture to join the two medial wall fractures. The cribriform can be low-lying in syndromic children, so careful image analysis is critical to ensure the planned cut is subcranial. A thin osteotome is used to separate the septum from the skull base from the frontonasal suture osteotomy back to the posterior nasal spine. Again, this is done with bimanual palpation with one finger in the mouth at the back of the palate (**Fig 4.10-2**). To minimize nasal bleeding, an internal nasal-septal-submucosal dissection can be performed before the osteotomy through an open rhinoplasty approach.

Once all osteotomies are complete, pterygomaxillary disimpaction is achieved with Rowe forceps. Some recommend the placement of the maxillary occlusal splint with palatal coverage before disimpaction to allow for midface mobilization without damaging the teeth or palatal mucosa or cause a sagittal split of the midface segment [Chin et al, 1997]. It is especially important to ensure all osteotomies are complete before down-fracturing the midface. Failure to do so could lead to propagation of a fracture toward the orbital apex.

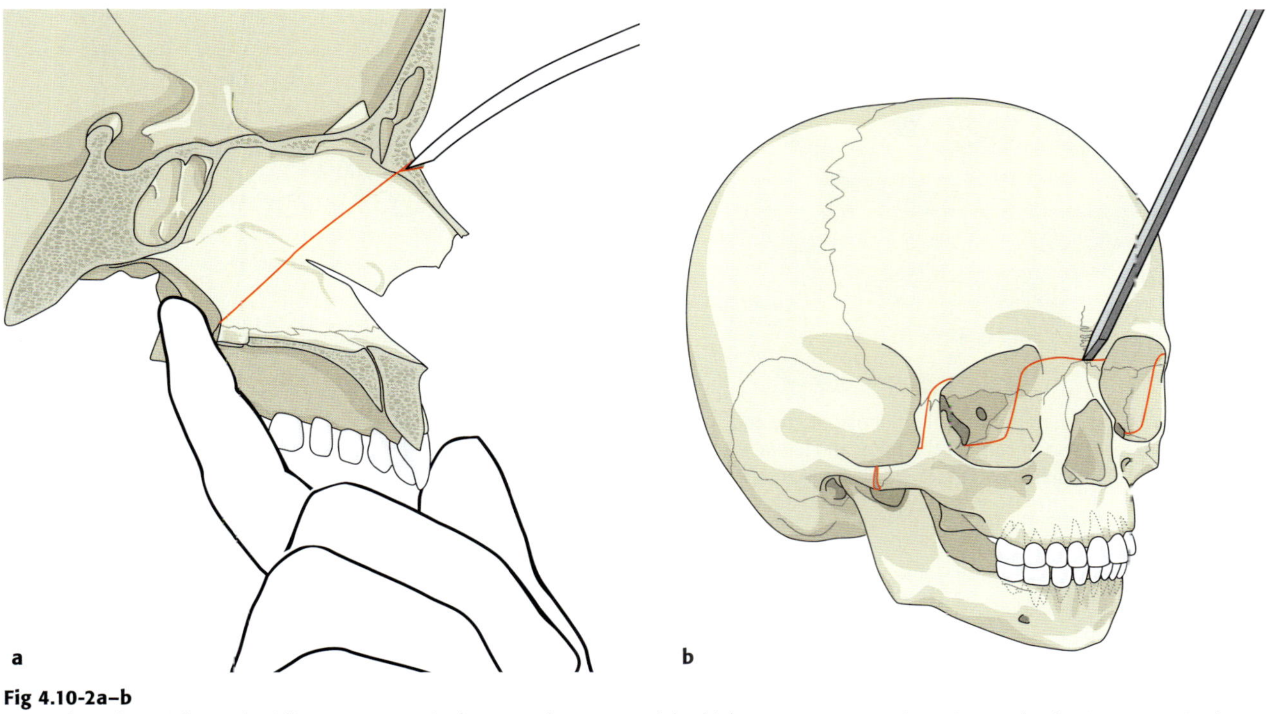

Fig 4.10-2a–b

a The subcranial septal midline osteotomy is the most dangerous of the high Le Fort osteotomies. Bimanual palpation is required to ensure the osteotome is directed toward the posterior nasal spine, and not toward the skull base.

b Same osteotomy as in Fig 2a, half profile projection.

Distraction

With distraction osteogenesis, the subcranial osteotomy is performed similar to the traditional technique but is not fixed. Instead, an internal or external device is applied and used postoperatively to gradually advance the midface into its new position. The benefits of distraction over conventional fixation include [Meazzini et al, 2005; Iannetti et al, 2011; Swennen et al, 2001; Figueroa et al, 2007; Warren et al, 2012]:

- Less soft-tissue dissection
- Less operative time
- Less intraoperative bleeding
- More bone advancement allowing for greater correction
- Possible soft-tissue histogenesis
- No donor site morbidity
- Absence of postsurgical craniofacial defects

The lateral orbital rim osteotomy is made through the temporal extension of the zygoma at the level of the inferior orbital rim (not at the level of the zygomaticofrontal suture), since plate fixation is not required. Anticipating the degree of subcranial advancement, the zygoma and nasal bones below the osteotomies are contoured to avoid a sharp step-off deformity during activation (**Fig 4.10-3**). With use of internal distractors, it is important to make the zygomatic osteotomy vertical and through the body (and not the arch) of the zygoma to allow for adequate bone mass on the proximal and distal segments to engage the distractors [Chin et al, 1997] and to allow for maximum osteogenesis [Jensen et al, 2007]. This also prevents the need for temporal fat pad dissection and the associated morbidity.

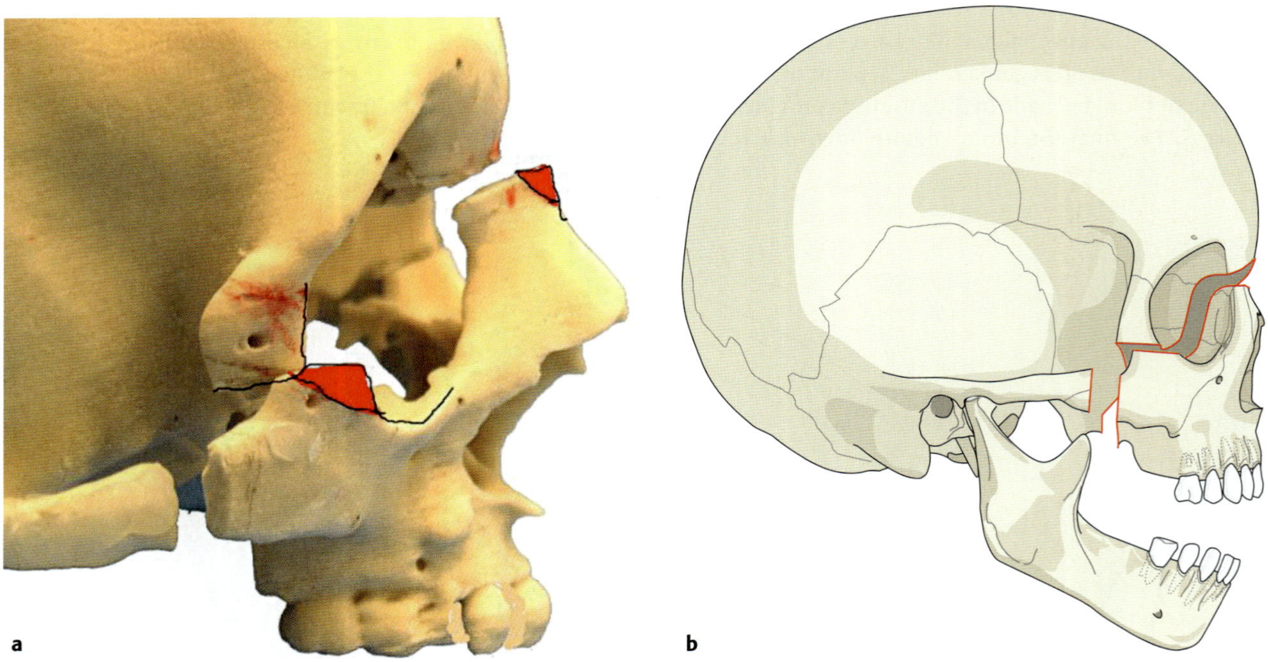

a b

Fig 4.10-3a–b Bone contouring after Le Fort III osteotomy and subcranial separation. It is important to anticipate the desired advancement of the Le Fort III segment and to contour the nasal and lateral orbital osteotomy edges appropriately. If this is not done in cases of Le Fort III distraction, visible and palpable step deformities will result as the segment is advanced during the activation phase.

Internal distractors can be zygoma-zygoma (anterior and posterior plates attached to the osteotomized zygoma) or zygoma-skull (attached to skull and zygoma) [Satoh et al, 2006]. Regardless, engagement of internal distraction device into the osteotomy site is important in maintaining fixation to the skeletal segments [Chin et al, 1997]. A percutaneous cannula is exited though a small preauricular incision and placed in a manner to limit soft-tissue tension. A calibrated torque wrench is used to activate the lead screw and verify the transport vector.

The external halo device is secured to extraoral extensions of a custom-made maxillary splint that has been bonded to the dentition, and wired to the zygomas with subcutaneous suspension wires (**Fig 4.10-4**). If gingivo-buccal access is available, then the splint can also be secured with four circum-maxillary wires through the pyriform aperture and around the zygomaticomaxillary complex bilaterally [Fearon, 2001]. A "Cat's Cradle" or circumferential suspension of the entire midfacial skeleton using wires placed through the soft palate has also been described [Havlik et al, 2004]. Percutaneous bone anchors screwed into the malar prominence [Kobus, 2006] or pyriform aperture wires secured to the buttress utilizing 4-hole miniplates [Satoh et al, 2002] may be used as additional points of traction but are usually unnecessary [Fearon, 2001] and can result in facial scarring. Those options are best reserved for patients with poorly developed maxillary arches or with missing or hypoplastic teeth.

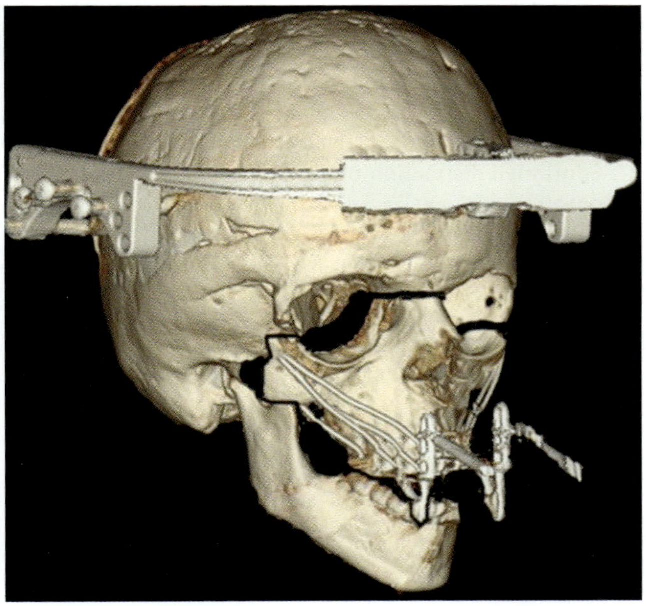

Fig 4.10-4 Le Fort III distraction advancement using an external halo based device (central post not drawn for better visualization). Compared with conventional Le Fort III, the lateral orbital osteotomy is at the level of the inferior orbital rim and the zygomatic arch cut is just behind the zygomatic body. This maximizes the bone interface during distraction, and is possible since plate fixation is not required. The Le Fort III transport segment is attached to the external halo device using a custom-made maxillary splint that is secured using subperiosteal circumzygomatic suspension wires.

Modifications

Various modifications of the classic Le Fort III osteotomies have been described in the literature:

1. Modifications related to nasal projection:
   Midface osteotomy and external distraction without median orbital walls and nasal component [Kobus, 2006]. The orbital floor osteotomies are continued across the frontal process of the maxillae just below the level of lacrimal fossa. The approach is meant to address the excess nasal project that may be seen with some patients undergoing classic Le Fort III but it does not expand their nasopharyngeal airway, has a limited effect on ocular proptosis, and may result in alar flaring.
   Patients with conditions such as Stickler, Apert, or Pfeiffer syndrome can have nasal deficiency that exceeds the degree of midface retrusion. Following a traditional Le Fort III advancement, placement of a cantilever bone graft to the nasal dorsum has been described to correct this differential defect [Allam et al, 2011; Kobus, 2006] but tension in the overlying soft tissue may limit the degree of augmentation following advancement. Patients undergoing midface distraction can receive a simultaneous nasal dorsal graft anchored to the transport segment at the time of osteotomy [Hopper et al, 2012]. Unlike with traditional advancement, the nasal passenger graft moves forward with midface distraction, stretching the overlying skin and improving the nasal profile.
2. Midface distraction with transfacial pins (in children aged 4 months to 10 years with intracranial hypertension and midface retrusion) using only lateral orbit and zygomatic osteotomies at the time of a frontoorbital advancement [Coeugniet, 2012]. The method does not allow for vector control, and while successful advancement has been reported by one group, there is limited published experience at other centers.
3. Endoscopically assisted Le Fort III osteotomy using an ultrasonic scalpel [Taylor et al, 2009]. While it may limit intraoperative bleeding, the approach takes longer and requires eyelid incisions.
4. Seesaw modification of the lateral orbital wall for patients undergoing distraction to prevent a big step-off at the level of the zygomaticofrontal osteotomy. A second lateral orbital wall osteotomy is made 1.5 cm below the frontonasal osteotomy, and the bone fragment is then loosely attached superiorly to the frontal bone with a 4-0 nonabsorbable suture [Mavili et al, 2004].
5. Dual Le Fort III Minus I and Le Fort I distraction [Satoh et al, 2003].
6. Le Fort III osteotomy without the use of a coronal incision. In addition to gingivobuccal and eyelid incisions, medial upper blepharoplasty incisions are used for the nasofrontal osteotomy [Hollier et al, 2002].
7. In rare cases of asymmetric retrusion, differential facial advancement from left to right is required. This can be achieved with a swinging Le Fort III advancement which utilizes a cerclage hinge at one point of the osteotomy to restrict advancement while allowing continued distraction of the opposite side [Hopper et al, 2012].

2.2.3 Fixation

For traditional subcranial Le Fort III advancement, the midface is advanced intraoperatively and fixed using titanium plates with interpositional cortical bone grafts harvested from the calvarium, iliac crest, or rib (**Fig 4.10-5**). Full mobilization often requires periosteal release of the overlying soft tissue and attached muscles. Once the inferior orbits are in their appropriate position, a graft is inserted into the nasion space [Dai et al, 2012]. Interpositional bone grafts are also placed at both zygomatic arches. The reverse-C osteotomies are greenstick fractured back to create a smooth lateral orbital contour and are fixed to the frontal bone using curved 1.5 mm plates. The arches and interpositional grafts are also fixed with straight miniplates.

2.3 Soft-tissue considerations

After osteotomies and fixation or application of distraction device are complete, closure of the dissection planes must include soft-tissue resuspension of the periosteum [Phillips et al, 1991] and lateral canthopexies. In the distraction patient, the canthal resuspension should not be placed on the transport segment but instead secured above the zygomatic osteotomy on the rim attached to the skull base.

2.4 Postoperative care

Patients are intubated for at least 2 days in the intensive care unit and until an air leak is confirmed around the endotracheal tube. Nutrition is supported with enteral feeds until the patient is able to tolerate oral feeds.

2.4.1 Distraction activation

Distraction is started at a rate of 1–1.5 mm/day after a latency phase of 0–5 days [McCarthy et al, 1992; Fearon et al, 2001; Fearon, 2005; Hopper et al, 2010]. The center of resistance of the Le Fort III segment is 55% of the shortest vertical distance from the occlusal plane to the nasion [Shetye et al, 2009]. To prevent rotation of the midface segment, the vector of distraction should be planned at a level parallel to the Frankfurt horizontal, avoiding vertical lengthening of the orbit. Since increases in airway volume do not correlate with the degree of advancement [Nout et al, 2010], the end point of activation is noted when the inferior orbital rim is just anterior to the coronal plane of the corneal surface. When treating OSA, the amount of linear distraction does not appear to correlate with improvement in OSA as much as the increase in the angular measurement from sella to nasion to the midface (SNA or SNO) does [Nout et al, 2010; Ettinger et al, 2011]. Based on radiographic analysis of pterygomaxillary generated bone, a consolidation period of 6 weeks is believed to be adequate [Hopper et al, 2010]. Internal devices require reopening of the surgical incisions to be removed after consolidation, whereas the external devices can typically be removed under light sedation.

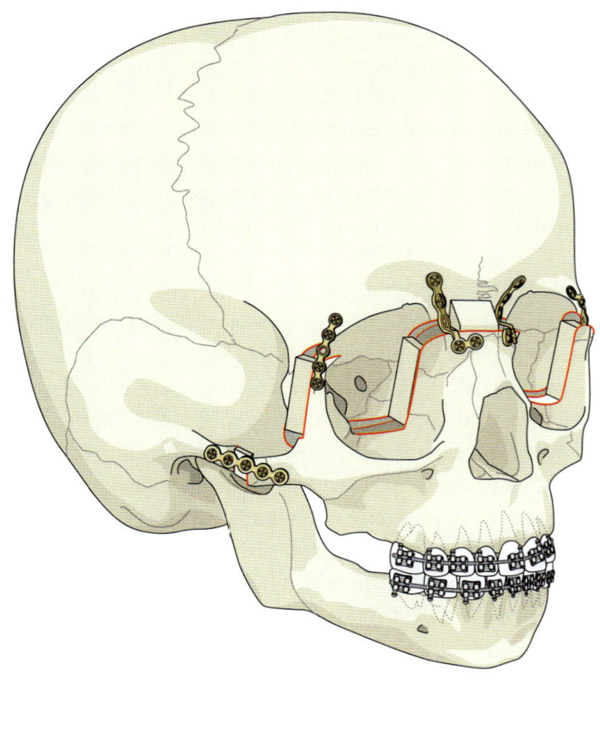

Fig 4.10-5 Conventional Le Fort III advancement, bone grafting and fixation. Rib, cranial, or iliac cortical or corticocancellous autogenous bone graft is placed at the nasofrontal, zygomatic, medial and lateral orbital osteotomies after advancement. The lateral orbital rim cut is done as a C-shaped osteotomy which can then be green-stick fractured back and fixed to achieve a smooth but stable orbital contour. The zygomatic osteotomy is posterior enough to ensure the stabilizing plate is not palpable.

2.5 Complications

2.5.1 Mortality

The incidence of serious morbidity and mortality in subcranial surgery has significantly fallen since first published. A survey of 15 craniofacial centers suggests a 0.1% rate of major morbidity [Czerwinski et al, 2010] and a 0.3% of mortality. Mortality can also occur due to exsanguination, cardiac arrhythmias, hyperthermia, drug interaction, pulmonary thromboembolism, or venous air embolism [Czerwinski et al, 2010; Phillips et al, 1988]. A greater focus on blood salvage and replacement, age-appropriate deep venous thrombosis prophylaxis (sequential compressive devices in children 13 years or older, and in high-risk children 9 years or older) [Sandoval et al, 2008; Victoria et al, 2009], timing of subcranial midfacial advancements, and careful intraoperative and postoperative airway management are important in reducing mortality [Czerwinski et al, 2010].

2.5.2 Intracranial

Cribriform plate fractures and dural tears may occur with subsequent cerebrospinal fluid leak/rhinorrhea, meningitis, meningoencephalocele, encephalocele [Tessier, 1971; Victoria et al, 2009]. Rates of cerebrospinal fluid leak requiring shunting range from 0–2.2% [Chin et al, 1997; Girotto et al, 1998; Watts, 1984; Carr et al, 1986]. The risk of cribriform plate fractures is increased in syndromic patients because craniosynostosis and intracranial hypertension result in inferior displacement of the plate with possible sloping of the anterior cranial base. Ethmoid erosions can also result in a meningoencephalocele [Tessier, 1971; Victoria et al, 2009]. Some authorities recommend an intracranial approach to the nasofrontal osteotomy in cases where the cribriform plate is noted to be low-lying on preoperative imaging [Victoria et al, 2009]. The use of a piezoelectric saw, which uses micrometric ultrasonic vibrations at frequencies that selectively cut mineralized structures, may avoid soft-tissue injury and propagation of fractures. The use of image-guided surgery platforms can help determine the trajectory of frontonasal (and pterygomaxillary) osteotomies, preventing inadvertent injury to the cranial base (and teeth) [Lanigan et al, 1993; Little et al, 1991].

2.5.3 Ocular

Blindness and decreased visual acuity may occur due to direct ocular damage or indirect optic nerve injury during dissection, osteotomy, retraction, or disimpaction. Uncontrolled propagation of pterygoid fractures that can occur with pterygomaxillary disjunction and down-fracture are capable of extending through the lesser wing of sphenoid, optic canal, and sella potentially disrupting the nutrient vessels to the optic nerve [Girotto et al, 1998]. Transient diplopia has also been described with abducens [Watts, 1984] or oculomotor [Carr et al, 1986] nerve neurapraxia.

Transient epiphora may be seen with lacrimal fossa fracture or lacrimal system disruption [Lanigan et al, 1993; Little et al, 1991]. Given the rarity of the complication and the ability of the distal lacrimal system to maintain its patency, the use of lacrimal stents to prevent this is generally unnecessary.

2.5.4 Dental

Dental injury most likely occurs at the pterygomaxillary disjunction but can occur with dentoalveolar traction. Le Fort III surgery in the 4- to 6-year-old can affect first and second molar eruption in up to 21% and 82% patients, respectively [Fearon, 2005]. Osteotomy sites should be placed as distal as possible to the second molar tooth bud to minimize this complication.

2.5.5 Hardware

Internal distractors, even with the use of resorbable plates [Mofid et al, 2001], are associated with the need for second surgery. The use of haloframes is associated with a higher incidence of complications in children than adults [Dai et al, 2012]. Loosening of hardware is noted in 8% cases [Gosain et al, 2002], and pin-tract infections can occur at an overall rate of 5% with 0.9% cases requiring hardware removal [Mofid et al, 2001]. Intracranial movement of halo fixation pins has been reported in children younger than 3 years [Fearon, 2005] and in patients with recent allograft calvarial reconstruction [Breugem, et al, 2008]. Mavili et al [2004] recommended that pins are placed along the cranial equator (3 cm above the ears and 1.5 cm over the supraorbital rim) but there are no "safe zones" for pin placement in the pediatric skull [Wong et al, 1994], and they should only be inserted "finger-tip tight" [Letts et al, 1988]. Should external distraction be necessary in a high-risk patient group, mechanical pin stoppers (which can increase scarring [Mavili et al, 2004; Voor et al, 1998]) may be considered to prevent this complication.

2.5.6 Esthetic/orthognathic

Traditional advancement may be associated with midface under correction, zygomatic effacement, and facial soft-tissue ptosis with deepening of facial folds, collectively giving the appearance of accelerated facial aging [Warren et al, 2012]. With distraction, improper vector in relation to the center of resistance can result in counterclockwise palatal plane rotation, inadequate orbital advancement, clockwise rotation of the mandible, increased facial vertical height, and an increase in the open bite [Shetye et al, 2010; Hopper et al, 2010; Shetye et al, 2007]. Inappropriate vector placement reportedly occurs in 16% of midface distractions, with more than half associated with the use of single vector distractors. While multivector internal distractors may theoretically circumvent this problem, the vector of such devices currently cannot be changed postoperatively [Gosain et al, 2002]. Some surgeons have combined the use of external and internal distractors [Wall et al, 2009], but this approach adds complexity and cost to the distraction process.

2.5.7 Fractures

As the zygomaticomaxillary junction is often dysplastic and the center of resistance is at the midline pterygomaxillary junctions, internal distraction pushing on the zygomas can lead to fractures along the relatively weak zygomaticomaxillary suture, leaving the maxillary bone from the root of the nose behind [Gosain et al, 2002; Mitsukawa et al, 2004].

2.5.8 Relapse

The sagittal movement offered by Le Fort III distraction and advancement are stable at 1-year [Shetye et a., 2010; Hopper et al, 2010; Shetye et al, 2007] and 10-year [Shetye et al, 2010] follow-ups, respectively. No longer is follow-up available for distraction.

3 Le Fort II osteotomy

3.1 Indications and planning

The traditional Le Fort II advancement with bone grafting has been used to advance the central midface while leaving the zygomas behind (**Fig 4.10-6**). Le Fort II halo distraction has also been described as a salvage option for patients who had inadvertent maxillozygomatic fractures from internal distraction [Mitsukawa et al, 2004] or can also be indicated in some patients with cleft lip and palate.

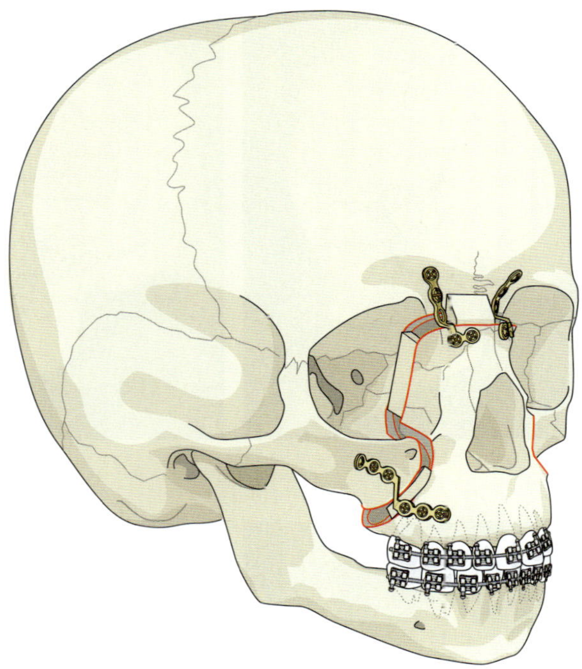

Fig 4.10-6 Conventional Le Fort II advancement, bone grafting and fixation. Rib, cranial, or iliac autogenous bone graft is placed at the nasofrontal and zygomaticomaxillary osteotomies and fixed. Medial orbital wall defects may also need bone grafts or titanium meshes.

For Apert syndrome, Le Fort II distraction with simultaneous zygomatic repositioning is our favored approach as it not only addresses midfacial retrusion but also the vertical maxillary deficiency characteristic of this syndrome [Hopper al, 2012]. The repositioned zygomas hold the globes in the appropriate position while central maxillary repositioning takes place via distraction without the concern of iatrogenic orbital deformities (**Fig 4.10-7** and **Fig 4.10-8**).

3.2 Technique

Bilateral transconjunctival lower eyelid and intraoral incisions are used in addition to the coronal incision. In a standard Le Fort II osteotomy, neither lateral orbital nor zygomatic osteotomies are necessary. The subcranial osteotomy and disimpaction are completed as described previously. The zygomaticomaxillary osteotomy is made through the eyelid and intraoral incisions lateral to the infraorbital foramina. For distraction, the same custom splint used in Le Fort III distraction is used for Le Fort II distraction but the suspension wires are secured to the piriform rim medially, and the lateral maxillary buttress below the osteotomy laterally. Fixation of the traditional Le Fort II advancement is at the nasofrontal junction and the zygomaticomaxillary osteotomies (**Fig 4.10-6**).

3.3 Postoperative care

Postoperative care following Le Fort II surgery is similar to that for Le Fort III surgery. With Le Fort II, the movement vector is chosen to achieve the desired nasal dorsal length, vertical maxillary height, and maxillary occlusal plane. Unlike Le Fort III, an inferior movement of a Le Fort II segment will not cause iatrogenic hypoglobus.

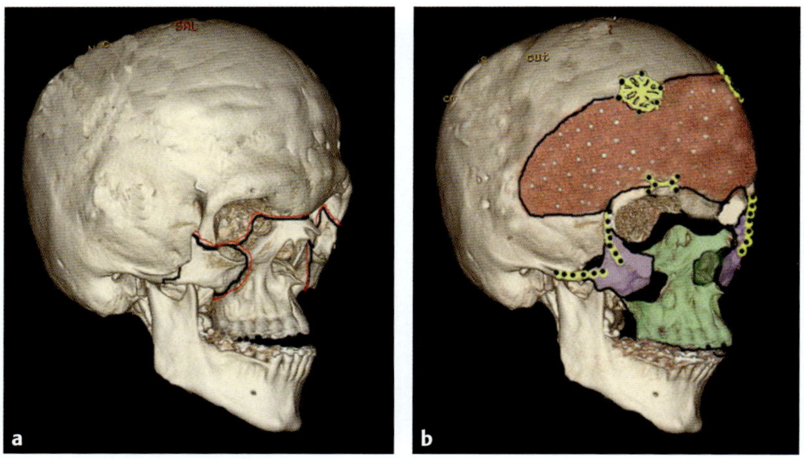

Fig 4.10-7a–b Treatment of the Apert facial deformity using intraoperative lateral orbitozygomatic repositioning and fixation (purple) followed by postoperative distraction advancement and lengthening of Le Fort II segment (green). A central forehead onlay implant is also often placed at the same operation (red). Unlike Le Fort III osteotomy, Le Fort II segment (green) can be moved independent of the lateral orbits to correct the unique central retrusion and rotational deformity of the Apert midface using an external distraction device. A similar advancement of a Le Fort III segment would have resulted in iatrogenic orbital deformities from the inferior vector and rotation.

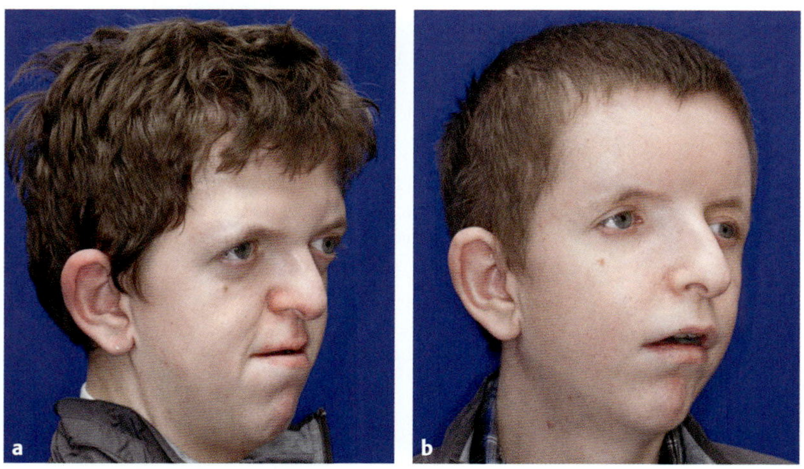

Fig 4.10-8a–b Patient with Apert syndrome before (**a**) and after (**b**) Le Fort II osteotomy and distraction advancement with simultaneous lateral orbitozygomatic repositioning (see text for surgical details). Unlike Crouzon syndrome, the Apert facial deformity requires more central than lateral advancement and vertical lengthening. The Le Fort II osteotomy allows a vertical lengthening of the central midface while the repositioned and fixated lateral orbits maintain globe position.

4 References and suggested reading

Allam KA, Wan DC, Khwanngern K, et al. Treatment of apert syndrome: a long-term follow-up study. *Plast Reconstr Surg.* 2011 Apr;127(4):1601–1611.

Bachmayer DI, Ross RB, Munro IR. Maxillary growth following LeFort III advancement surgery in Crouzon, Apert, and Pfeiffer syndromes. *Am J Orthod Dentofacial Orthop.* 1986 Nov;90(5):420–430.

Breugem CC, Bush K, Fitzpatrick DF. Le Fort III rigid external distraction complicated by intracranial movement of halo fixation pins. *Cleft Palate Craniofac J.* 2008 May;45(3):332–336.

Buncic JR. Ocular aspects of Apert syndrome. *Clin Plast Surg.* 1991 Apr;18(2):315–319.

Carr RJ, Gilbert P. Isolated partial third nerve palsy following Le Fort I maxillary osteotomy in a patient with cleft lip and palate. *Br J Oral Maxillofac Surg.* 1986 Jun;24(3):206–211.

Celik M, Tuncer S. Nasal reconstruction using both cranial bone and ear cartilage. *Plast Reconstr Surg.* 2000 Apr;105(5):1624–1627.

Chin M, Toth BA. Le Fort III advancement with gradual distraction using internal devices. *Plast Reconstruct Surg.* 1997 Sep;100(4):819–830; discussion 831–832.

Coeugniet E, Dhellemmes P, Vinchon M, et al. Midfacial distraction without osteotomy using a transfacial pin and external devices. *J Craniofac Surg.* 2012 Jan;23(1):184–189.

Czerwinski M, Hopper RA, Gruss J, et al. Major morbidity and mortality rates in craniofacial surgery: an analysis of 8101 major procedures. *Plast Reconstr Surg.* 2010 Jul;126(1):181–186.

Dai J, Wang X, Yu H, et al. Simultaneous Le Fort I, II, and III osteotomies for correction of midface deficiency in Apert disease. *J Craniofac Surg.* 2012 Sep;23(5):1391–1395.

Ettinger RE, Hopper RA, Sandercoe G, et al. Quantitative computed tomographic scan and polysomnographic analysis of patients with syndromic midface hypoplasia before and after Le Fort III distraction advancement. *Plast Reconstr Surg.* 2011 Apr;127(4):1612–1619.

Fearon JA. The Le Fort III osteotomy: to distract or not to distract? *Plast Reconstr Surg.* 2001 Apr 15;107(5):1091–1103; discussion 1104–1106.

Fearon JA. Halo distraction of the Le Fort III in syndromic craniosynostosis: a long-term assessment. *Plast Reconstr Surg.* 2005 May;115(6):1524–1536.

Festa F, Pagnoni M, Valerio R, et al. Orbital volume and surface after Le Fort III advancement in syndromic craniosynostosis. *J Craniofac Surg.* 2012 May;23(3):789–792.

Figueroa AA, Polley JW. Management of the severe cleft and syndromic midface hypoplasia. *Orthod Craniofac Res.* 2007 Aug;10(3):167–179.

Flores RL, Shetye PR, Zeitler D, et al. Airway changes following Le Fort III distraction osteogenesis for syndromic craniosynostosis: a clinical and cephalometric study. *Plast Reconstr Surg.* 2009 Aug;124(2):590–601.

Gillies H, Harrison SH. Operative correction by osteotomy of recessed malar maxillary compound in a case of oxycephaly. *Br J Plast Surg.* 1950 Jul;3(2):123–127.

Girotto JA, Davidson J, Wheatly M, et al. Blindness as a complication of Le Fort osteotomies: role of atypical fracture patterns and distortion of the optic canal. *Plast Reconstr Surg.* 1998 Oct;102(5):1409–1421; discussion 1422–1423.

Gosain AK, Santoro TD, Havlik RJ, et al. Midface distraction following Le Fort III and monobloc osteotomies: problems and solutions. *Plast Reconstr Surg.* 2002 May;109(6):1797–1808.

Habal MB. A future domain distractor for the facial skeleton. *J Craniofac Surg.* 1995 Sep;6(5):414–416.

Havlik RJ, Seelinger MJ, Fashemo DV, et al. "Cat's cradle" midfacial fixation in distraction osteogenesis after Le Fort III osteotomy. *J Craniofac Surg.* 2004 Nov;15(6):946–952.

Hollier L, Kelly P, Babigumira E, et al. Minimally invasive Le Fort III distraction. *J Craniofac Surg.* 2002 Jan;13(1):44–48.

Hopper RA, Prucz RB, Lamphongsa S. Achieving differential facial changes with Lefort III distraction osteogenesis: the use of nasal passenger grafts, cerclage hinges, and zygomatic repositioning. *Plast Reconstr Surg.* 2012 Dec;130(6):1281–1288.

Hopper RA, Sandercoe G, Woo A, et al. Computed tomographic analysis of temporal maxillary stability and pterygomaxillary generate formation following pediatric Le Fort III distraction advancement. *Plast Reconstr Surg.* 2010 Nov;126(5):1665–1674.

Iannetti G, Polimeni A, Pagnoni M, et al. Upper airway volume after Le Fort III advancement in subjects with craniofacial malformation. *J Craniofac Surg.* 2011 Jan;22(1):351–355.

Jensen JN, McCarthy JG, Grayson BH, et al. Bone deposition/generation with LeFort III (midface) distraction. *Plast Reconstr Surg.* 2007 Jan;119(1):298–307.

Kobus KF. New osteotomies for midface advancement in patients with Crouzon syndrome. *J Craniofac Surg.* 2006 Sep;17(5):957–961.

Lacey M, Antonyshyn O, MacGregor JH. Temporal contour deformity after coronal flap elevation: an anatomical study. *J Craniofac Surg.* 1994 Sep;5(4):223–227.

Lanigan DT, Romanchuk K, Olson CK. Ophthalmic complications associated with orthognathic surgery *J Oral Maxillofac Surg.* 1993 May;51(5):480–494.

Letts M, Kaylor D, Gouw G. A biomechanical analysis of halo fixation in children. *J Bone Joint Surg Br.* 1988 Mar;70(2):277–279.

Little C, Mintz S, Ettinger AC. The distal lacrimal ductal system and traumatic epiphora. *Int J Oral Maxillofac Surg.* 1991 Feb;20(1):31–35.

Marchac D, Renier D, Broumand S. Timing of treatment for craniosynostosis and facio-craniosynostosis: a 20-year experience. *Br J Plast Surg.* 1994 Jun;47(4):211–222.

Mavili ME, Tuncbilek G. Seesaw modification of the lateral orbital wall in Le Fort III osteotomy. *Cleft Palate Craniofac.* 2004 Nov;41(6):579–583.

Mavili ME, Vargel I, Tuncbilek G. Stoppers in RED II distraction device: is it possible to prevent pin migration? *J Craniofac Surg.* 2004 May;15(3):377–383.

McCarthy JG, Schreiber J, Karp N, et al. Lengthening the human mandible by gradual distraction. *Plast Reconstr Surg.* 1992 Jan;89(1):1–8; discussion 9–10.

Meazzini MC, Mazzoleni F, Caronni E, et al. Le Fort III advancement osteotomy in the growing child affected by Crouzon's and Apert's syndromes: presurgical and postsurgical growth. *J Craniofac Surg.* 2005 May;16(3):369–377.

Mitsukawa N, Satoh K, Hayashi T, et al. Salvaged Le Fort II halo distraction for an unfavorable outcome of midfacial distraction using an internal device in syndromic craniosynostosis. *Plast Reconstr Surg.* 2004 Apr 1;113(4):1219–1224.

Mofid MM, Manson PN, Robertson BC, et al. Craniofacial distraction osteogenesis: a review of 3278 cases. *Plast Reconstrt Surg.* 2001 Oct;108(5):1103–1114; discussion 1115–1117.

Nout E, Bouw FP, Veenland JF, et al. Three-dimensional airway changes after Le Fort III advancement in syndromic craniosynostosis patients. *Plast Reconstr Surg.* 2010 Aug;126(2):564–571.

Pereira V, Sell D, Ponniah A, et al. Midface osteotomy versus distraction: the effect on speech, nasality, and velopharyngeal function in craniofacial dysostosis. *Cleft Palate Craniofac J.* 2008 Jul;45(4):353–363.

Phillips JH, Gruss JS, Wells MD, et al. Periosteal suspension of the lower eyelid and cheek following subciliary exposure of facial fractures. *Plast Reconstr Surg.* 1991 Jul;88(1):145–148.

Phillips RJ, Mulliken JB. Venous air embolism during a craniofacial procedure. *Plast Reconstr Surg.* 1988 Jul;82(1):155–159.
Reid RR. Facial skeletal growth and timing of surgical intervention. *Clin Plast Surg.* 2007 Jul;34(3):357–367.
Reitsma JH, Ongkosuwito EM, Buschang PH, et al. Facial growth in patients with Apert and Crouzon syndromes compared to normal children. *Cleft Palate Craniofac J.* 2012 Mar;49(2):185–193.
Sandoval JA, Sheehan MP, Stonerock CE, et al. Incidence, risk factors, and treatment patterns for deep venous thrombosis in hospitalized children: an increasing population at risk. *J Vasc Surg.* 2008 Apr;47(4):837–843.
Satoh K, Mitsukawa N, Hosaka Y. Dual midfacial distraction osteogenesis: Le Fort III minus I and Le Fort I for syndromic craniosynostosis. *Plast Reconstr Surg.* 2003 Mar;111(3):1019–1028.
Satoh K, Mitsukawa N, Tosa Y, et al. Le Fort III midfacial distraction using an internal distraction device for syndromic craniosynostosis: device selection, problems, indications, and a proposal for use of a parallel bar for device-setting. *J Craniofac Surg.* 2006 Nov;17(6):1050–1058.
Satoh K, Tsutsumi K, Tosa Y, et al. Le Fort III distraction osteogenesis of midface-retrusion in a case of Hajdu Cheny syndrome. *J Craniofac Surg.* 2002 Mar;13(2):298–302.
Shetye PR, Boutros S, Grayson BH, et al. Midterm follow-up of midface distraction for syndromic craniosynostosis: a clinical and cephalometric study. *Plast Reconstr Surg.* 2007 Nov;120(6):1621–1632.
Shetye PR, Davidson EH, Sorkin M, et al. Evaluation of three surgical techniques for advancement of the midface in growing children with syndromic craniosynostosis. *Plast Reconstr Surg.* 2010 Sep;126(3):982–994.
Shetye PR, Giannoutsos E, Grayson BH, et al. Le Fort III distraction: Part I. Controlling position and vectors of the midface segment. *Plast Reconstr Surg.* 2009 Sep;124(3):871–878.
Shetye PR, Kapadia H, Grayson BH, et al. A 10-year study of skeletal stability and growth of the midface following Le Fort III advancement in syndromic craniosynostosis. *Plast Reconstr Surg.* 2010 Sep;126(3):973–981.
Swennen G, Schliephake H, Dempf R, et al. Craniofacial distraction osteogenesis: a review of the literature: Part 1: clinical studies. *Int J Oral Maxillofac Surg.* 2001 Apr;30(2):89–103.
Taylor JA, Maercks RA, Runyan CM, et al. Endoscopically assisted Le Fort III osteotomy using an ultrasonic scalpel: a feasibility study in cadavers. *J Craniofac Surg.* 2009 Nov;20(6):2211–2214.
Tessier P. The definitive plastic surgical treatment of the severe facial deformities of craniofacial dysostosis. Crouzon's and Apert's diseases. *Plast Reconstr Surg.* 1971 Nov;48(5):419–442.
Victoria T, Mong A, Altes T, et al. Evaluation of pulmonary embolism in a pediatric population with high clinical suspicion. *Pediatr Radiol.* 2009 Jan;39(1):35–41.
Voor MJ, Khalily C. Halo pin loosening: a biomechanical comparison of experimental and conventional designs. *J Biomech.* 1998 Apr;31(4):397–400.
Wall SA, Butler L, Byren J, et al. Combined internal and external Le Fort III distraction osteogenesis—the "elusive vector". *J Craniofac Surg.* 2009 Sep;20 Suppl 2:1806–1808.
Warren SM, Shetye PR, Obaid SI, et al. Long-term evaluation of midface position after Le Fort III advancement: a 20-plus-year follow-up. *Plast Reconstr Surg.* 2012 Jan;129(1):234–242.
Watts PG. Unilateral abducent nerve palsy: a rare complication following a Le Fort I maxillary osteotomy. *Br J Oral Maxillofac Surg.* 1984 Jun;22(3):212–215.
Wong WB, Haynes RJ. Osteology of the pediatric skull. Considerations of halo pin placement. *Spine (Phila Pa 1976).* 1994 Jul 1;19(13):1451–1454.

4.11 Craniosynostosis

Ignacio Ismael García Recuero, Gregorio Sánchez Aniceto

1 Indications and planning

Parents and physicians can easily observe and examine the size and shape of the newborn head. If severe skull deformity or asymmetry is diagnosed, all diagnostic and treatment efforts will at first be focused on preserving the patient's life, avoiding possible complications, and giving support and counseling to the parents at every treatment stage.

Pediatric craniofacial surgery has made great advances from the first surgical repair of a sagittal craniosynostosis performed by Lane and Lannelongue in 1890, and the first Gillies Le Fort III osteotomy for a Crouzon disease in the 1930s. Paul Tessier [Tessier, 1967; Tessier, 1971] in 1967 described the correction of isolated and syndromic craniosynostosis using complex craniofacial osteotomies. He and other pioneers, like F Ortiz Monasterio and JG McCarthy, foresaw the necessity of a team approach for the surgical management of congenital craniofacial malformations to improve functional and esthetic results while minimizing morbidity, thus establishing the pillars of contemporary craniofacial surgery.

The term "craniosynostosis" is defined as the premature closure of calvarial sutures, occurring at an estimated frequency of 0.4 per 1000 births. It can happen as an isolated disease in nonsyndromic forms, or as part of syndromic diseases, with associated manifestations either in the face, neck, trunk, or extremities. In some types of craniosynostosis there is a gender predilection, eg, males are more frequently affected by sagittal synostosis (4:1). However, for unilateral coronal synostosis, girls outnumber boys in a 3:2 ratio [Persing, 2008]. There is no clear gender predilection for the remaining types.

The skull base acts as a supporting platform for brain development. It contains multiple growth centers driving both cranial and upper facial growth. The pathophysiology of craniosynostosis was first described in 1851 by Virchow, who established that "bony expansion ceases in a direction perpendicular to a synostosed suture, with compensatory expansion in the opposite direction" [Virchow, 1851]. There are eight main cranial sutures; right and left coronal; right and left lambdoid; right and left squamosal; two in the midline; sagittal and metopic (**Table 4.11-1**). Another one is the nasofrontal suture. The extension of these sutures at the synchondroses in the cranial base and their influence in the origin of craniosynostosis was reported (**Figs 4.11-2–4.11-5**). In the late 1990s some reports suggested that the origin of the synostosis could be associated with mutations of different growth factors and protein receptors like transforming growth factor-B1 (TGF-B1) fibroblast growth factor receptor 2 (FGFR2), FGFR-3 or TWIST within the suture [Cohen, 1991; Gosain et al, 2004]. Retinoid exposure may lead to premature cranial suture fusion by means of enhanced osteogenesis. Also, the interaction between bone morphogenetic proteins (BMPs) and the extracellular BMP antagonist has been investigated but it seems that BMPs only play a role in postoperative bony wound healing and not in the pathogenesis of craniosynostosis [Cray et al, 2011].

Cranial suture	Clinical synostosis
Unilateral coronal	Anterior plagiocephaly
Unilateral lambdoid	Posterior plagiocephaly
Bilateral coronal	Anterior brachycephaly
Bilateral lambdoid	Posterior brachycephaly
Sagittal	Scaphocephaly
Metopic	Trigonocephaly
Multiple synostosis	Oxycephaly, turricephaly, kleeblattschädel anomaly, syndromes (Crouzon, Apert)

Table 4.11-1. Affected suture and clinical synostosis.

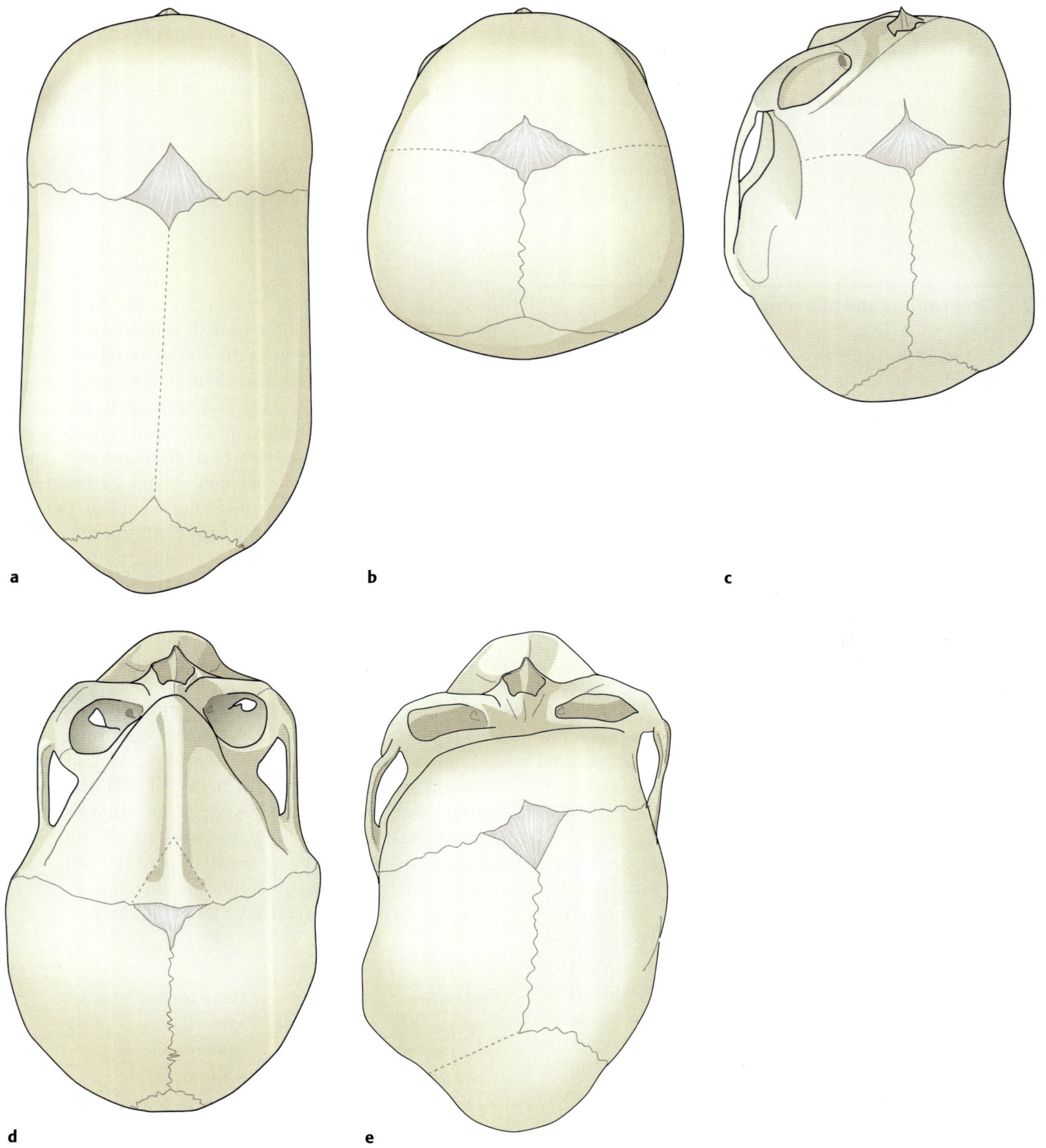

Fig 4.11-1a–g Six abnormal skull shapes due to craniosynostosis. The fused sutures are indicated as dotted lines, as well as the resulting deformity of the skull.
a Sagittal synostosis.
b Coronal synostosis.
c Unilateral coronal synostosis left.
d Metopic synostosis.
e Unilateral lambdoidal synostosis.

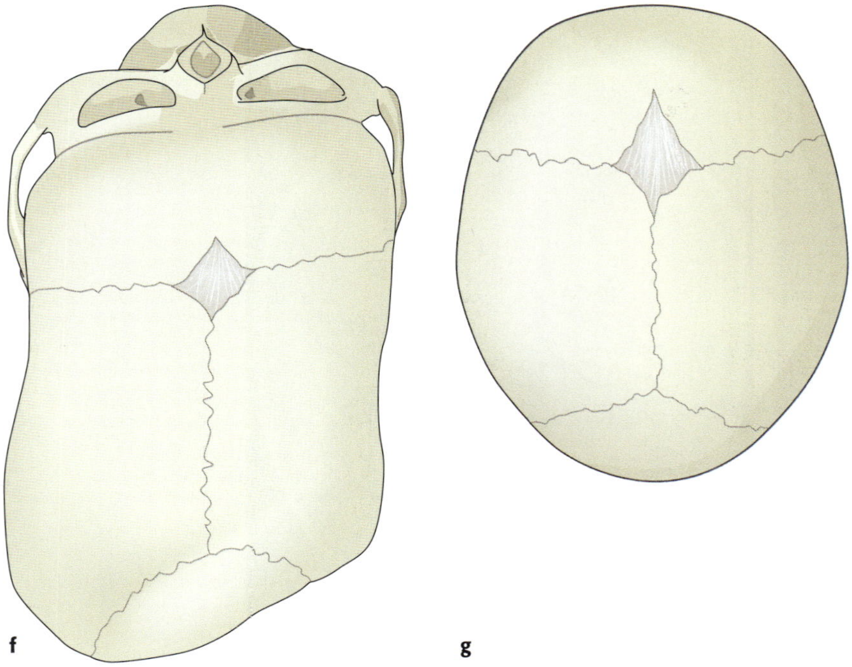

f g

Fig 4.11-1a–g (cont) Six abnormal skull shapes affected with craniosynostosis. The fused sutures are indicated as dotted lines, as well as the resulting deformity of the skull.

f Positional plagiocephaly.

g Normal skull showing all sutures.

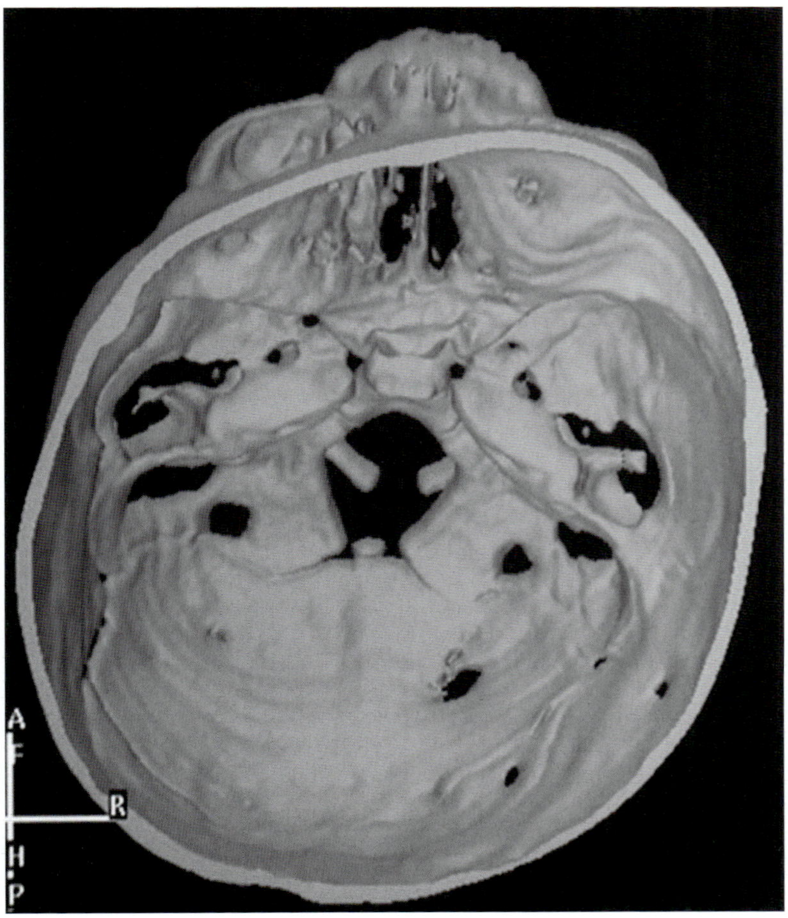

Fig 4.11-2 A 3-D computed tomographic scan of a patient with left unilateral coronal synostosis (left anterior plagiocephaly). Note how the supraorbital rim is depressed, elevated, and displaced laterally at the affected side; nasal root is deviated toward the affected side reflecting the shortened left anterior cranial fossa. At the contralateral side, the forehead is compensatory bossed and the supraorbital rim is rotated anteroinferior.

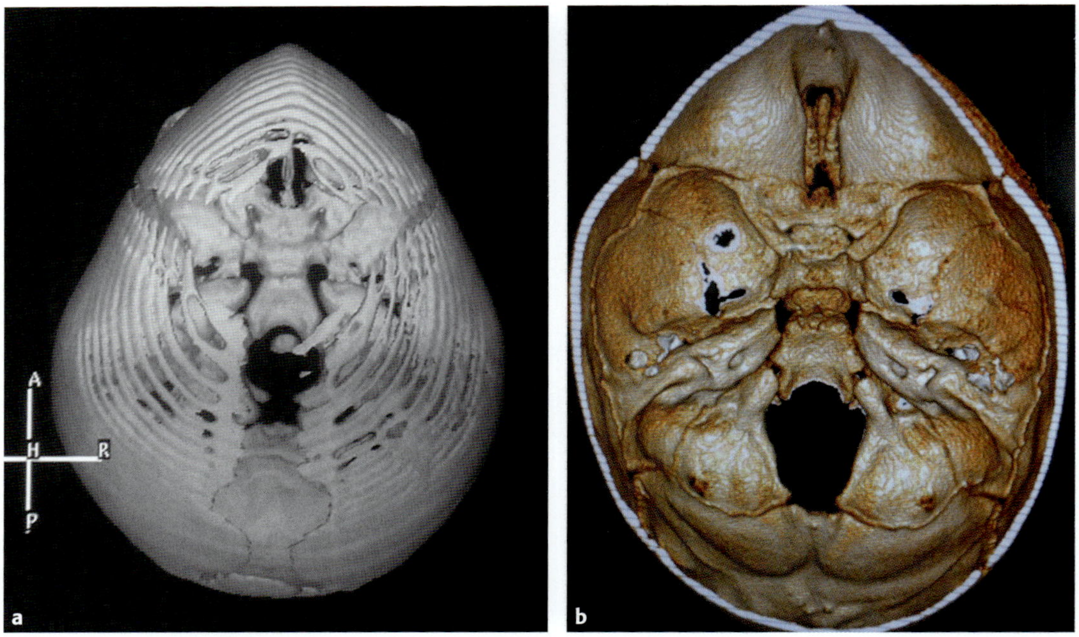

Fig 4.11-3a–b 3-D computed tomographic scans of a patient with metopic synostosis (trigonocephaly). Triangular forehead with a prominent anterior ridge, depressed supraorbital rims and hypoteleorbitism with narrowing of the anterior cranial fossa are diagnostic features.

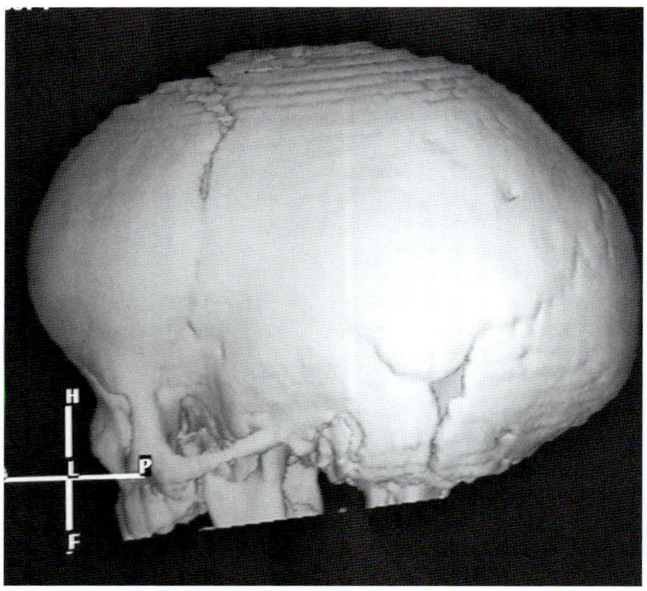

Fig 4.11-4 A 3-D computed tomographic scan of a patient with sagittal synostosis (scaphocephaly or dolichocephaly). The most common synostosis presents an increased anteroposterior length of skull and decreased transversal size of skull laterally.

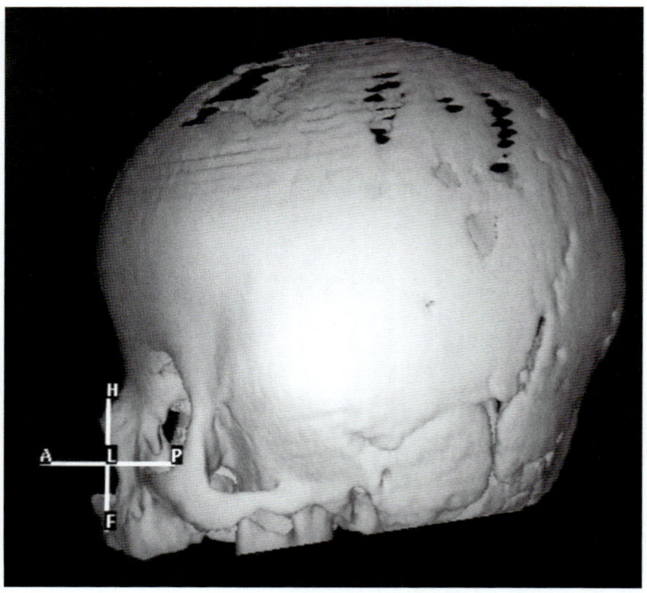

Fig 4.11-5 A 3-D computed tomographic scan of a patient with bilateral coronal synostosis (brachycephaly). Reduced anteroposterior growth produces an increased height of the skull or turricephaly, with associated exorbitism and deep nasofrontal angle.

Brain development is dependent on the normal growth of the skull. Brain weight is around 400 g at birth, doubles by 6 months and triples by 2.5 years of age, getting close to the adult dimensions (1400–1600 g) during the first 3 to 5 years of life. Early diagnosis and surgery during the first 2 years of life for craniosynostosis is aiming to improve morphology, to prevent functional disturbances, and to enhance the psychosocial development of the child [Cohen, 1991].

Preventing, detecting, and treating the possible increased intracranial pressure and airway disturbances are the two main indications for early treatment especially in patients with syndromic craniosynostosis. Although these issues are more common in severe multisynostotic and syndromic cases, single synostosis cases should not be underestimated. They are sometimes extremely difficult to correct at the synostosis site and the near and far compensatory changes in the skull.

Positional deformities must be identified (with their typical ipsilateral flattening with posterior contralateral bulging) because these patients can be managed only with positional techniques during sleep or helmet therapy.

Positional skull deformation is a condition in which the shape of an infant's skull deforms as a result of prolonged external forces. The infant's head is malleable and growing rapidly, hence it is susceptible to deformation, especially when infants develop a positional preference of the head when lying in the supine position. The prevalence of skull deformation increased substantially after it was recommended that infants should be placed in a supine sleep position to prevent sudden infant death syndrome. The preferred treatment is usually nonoperative. In a recently published guideline (2012) the Netherlands Centre of Preventive Child Health Care advised to start counseling parents during baby visits on the handling and repositioning infants with an observed positional preference or skull deformation [Argenta et al, 1996; Meyer-Marcotty et al, 2014].

Systematic general patient evaluation is compulsory to identify the appropriate diagnosis, fully assess any associated medical concerns, and start the appropriate early clinical management. Detailed functional and esthetic assessment are crucial for a successful outcome and are first obtained through a focused and detailed history and physical examination. In patients with craniosynostosis, anatomical features of craniofacial anomalies are often clear but symptoms of increased intracranial pressure (eg, headache, nausea, vomiting, mental retardation, blindness development) need to be identified as soon as possible. Most of the syndromic craniosynostosis have an autosomal dominant inheritance pattern (Apert, Crouzon, Pfeiffer), so it is important to ask about family history as well as the obstetric and pregnancy details. Head perimeter is measured at the first evaluation, as microcephalia could indicate a primary growth abnormality of the brain or an uncompensated growth restriction of the skull secondary to craniosynostosis. An increased head perimeter may indicate hydrocephalus or a compensated growth pattern of the skull secondary to craniosynostosis. Palpation of the fontanel and cranial sutures is mandatory because an enlarged fontanel is commonly seen in certain disorders, such as Apert syndrome, whereas a bulging fontanel could indicate increased intracranial pressure and possible hydrocephalus. A palpable ridge is generally associated with a synostosed suture, as well as a premature closure of the fontanel.

Radiographic analysis is mandatory to confirm the clinical diagnosis. The gold standard is a computed tomographic (CT) scan with 3-D reconstruction images; however, radiation dose, especially to both lenses is a point which is critically discussed. To minimize radiation doses, some surgeons still prefer conventional radiographs, others use magnetic resonance images (MRIs) or ultrasound for diagnosis and planning. Imaging will confirm the clinical features of craniosynostosis by objectively demonstrating fusion of a suture, identifying possible coexisting abnormalities, such as Arnold-Chiari malformation or hydrocephalus, and assessing the number of affected sutures and their extension. In selected cases, MRI is useful to detect associated brain and ventricle alterations differentiating ventriculomegaly from hydrocephalus, and includes a precise study of the posterior fossa and spine to visualize the severity of Arnold-Chiari malformations and the presence of syringomyelia cavities [Gosain et al, 2004]. Clinical photographs (including 3-D photography if available), brain echography and sleep apnea or pulsoximeter studies will add important data to complete the presurgical diagnosis. Careful preanesthesia examination of the patient and correct presurgical immunization against pneumococcus will be completed. DICOM data of the CT scan are better managed with any image processing platform for adequate 3-D surgical planning. Stereolithographic models may also be useful in planning the operative intervention.

Evidence of persistent torticollis could be associated with cervical spine deformities, extraocular muscle problems, or structural foreshortening of the sternocleidomastoid muscle. Recognition, diagnosis, and treatment of these problems are of paramount importance because muscle imbalance can result in significant asymmetry affecting normal growth and development of the face and cranium [Buchman et al, 2002].

Intracranial hypertension may be present in cases of single suture craniosynostosis but it is more frequent in syndromic or multiple suture synostosis cases. Complete ophthalmological evaluation is appropriate in all patients with craniosynostosis, especially in syndromic patients, to determine the presence of strabismus or palpebral alterations. Intraocular assessment of the fundus and visualization of the optic disc should be completed to rule out pallor and papilledema, signs of increased intracranial pressure. Shunt surgery to correct hydrocephalus and intracranial hypertension is preferably done before the craniectomy and cranial vault remodeling (**Fig 4.11-6**).

Genetic consultation is necessary in cases of craniosynostosis to refine, confirm, or help in establishing the diagnosis, screening for associated problems, and for suggesting further evaluation or recommended testing. Genetic counseling can console and inform the patient's family and generate a report as a reference to document the inheritance patterns and subsequent risk to future offspring for the parents and the child. The genetic alterations of FGFRs, TWIST or others will determine the treatment and prognosis of these patients, especially in syndromic cases.

The FGF/FGFR signaling system is implicated in the control of basic processes (eg, proliferation, differentiation, migration, polarity, adhesion, apoptosis) in cells destined to become various tissues including bone and cartilage. Mutations in FGFR1, 2, and 3 can lead to varied impairments of skeletal development as demonstrated by the FGFR-related craniosynostosis syndromes (ie, Apert, Beare-Stevenson, Crouzon, Crouzon with acanthosis nigricans, Jackson-Weiss, Muenke, and Pfeiffer syndromes). These syndromes are characterized by premature fusion of one or several cranial vault sutures associated with skull dysmorphology and potentially presenting with malformations affecting the limbs, upper airway, brain, spine, heart, and/or lungs. Patients with Apert syndrome (craniosynostosis syndrome due to mutations in FGFR2) are most severely affected in terms of intellectual disability, developmental delay, central nervous system anomalies, and limb anomalies. All patients with FGFR-related syndromic craniosynostosis have some degree of hearing loss that requires thorough initial evaluations and subsequent follow-up. Intracranial hypertension is an important consideration in patients with craniosynostosis. Patients with multisuture involvement and patients with FGFR2 mutations have the highest risk of increased intracranial pressure. The occurrence of papilledema, a marker of intracranial hypertension, is most common in patients with FGFR2-related craniosynostoses (Apert, Crouzon, and Pfeiffer syndromes). Papilledema may occur in patients without an identified genetic mutation, but is more common in patients with a known genetic mutation. Syndromic craniosynostosis with FGFR mutations or other genetic-related alterations require more exact diagnosis and aggressive treatment if the vital condition of the patient is compromised [Agochukwu et al, 2012].

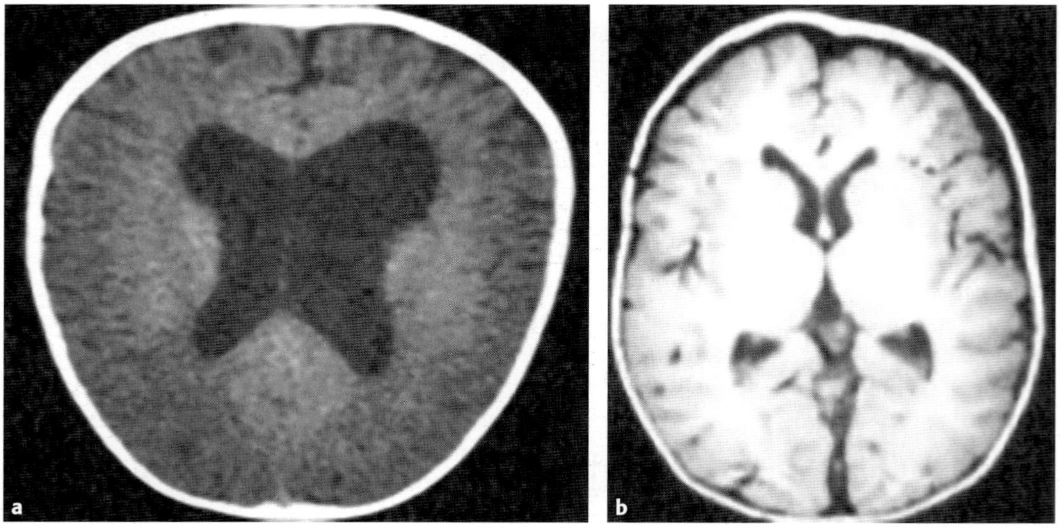

Fig 4.11-6a–b
a A computed tomographic (CT) scan depicting increased intracranial pressure.
b A CT scan of the same patient after shunt surgery.

2 Timetable for surgical corrections

Indications for surgical treatment of nonsyndromic craniosynostosis are the risk of increased intracranial pressure (ICP) and the abnormal skull shape. The risk of increased ICP in scaphocephaly is 12%; trigonocephaly 9%; and plagiocephaly 10%. The estimated risk in bilateral coronal suture synostosis is 37%. Intracranial hypertension is frequently associated with multisuture syndromic craniosynostosis. The prevalence of preoperatively increased ICP in syndromic craniosynostosis is 40–50% in Apert; 50–70% in Crouzon and Pfeiffer; 35–45% in Saethre-Chotzen syndrome; 50–80% in complex craniosynostosis; and 0% in Muenke syndrome. Increased ICP after an earlier cranial vault expansion is estimated at 35–43% in Apert, Crouzon, Pfeiffer, and Saethre-Chotzen syndromes.

Funduscopic examination should routinely be performed in these patients to evaluate papilledema, which warrants urgent surgical intervention. Additional indicators of intracranial hypertension include headache, vomiting, abrupt change in behavior, lethargy, and "copper beaten skull appearance" on skull x-rays. The finding of papilledema should be followed by a CT or MRI scan to assess changes in ventricle size (hydrocephalus).

Intracranial pressure invasive measurements during one night and minimally 12 hours (such as epidural sensor or lumbar puncture) is an effective method to determine the presence of intracranial hypertension. Increased ICP is almost routinely defined as a baseline above 15 mm Hg during slow wave sleep or more than three plateau waves. Radiological findings, such as impressions, ventricle size, or changes therein are unreliable as a screening method for increased ICP. Papilledema found with funduscopy is highly probably a sign of increased ICP, but its absence does not exclude an increased ICP. Invasive ICP measurement remains the gold standard, but naturally has disadvantages such as the need of anesthesia, surgical intervention with risk of complications, and admission to an intensive or high care unit.

Patients with syndromic craniosynostosis should receive long-term postoperative surveillance until approximately 12 years of age, when brain bulk growth is complete. The surveillance program for these patients should include ophthalmoscopic examinations at 6-month intervals in patients with multisuture synostosis (including patients with Crouzon, Apert, Pfeiffer, Saethre-Chotzen, and Muenke syndromes). The MRI examination of the central nervous system malformations associated with syndromic craniosynostosis, including hydrocephalus and Chiari malformations, are performed at 6-month to 12-month intervals [Collman et al, 2011; Mathijssen, 2015].

3 Patient positioning and incisions for craniofacial surgery

Usually the first surgical approach in a craniosynostosis patient is through a coronal incision from ear to ear, with a preauricular/postauricular extension if required [Cray et al, 2011]. The traditional straight-line incision design produces a noticeable scar. The scalloped or pointed zigzag shape by Munro [1987] will diminish the visible scar (**Fig 4.11-7**). Rarely, posterior extensions of this incision in a "T" shape may be used to allow the exposure of the occipital region. Facial incisions in lower eyelids may be added to improve access to the internal orbits and maxilla, in selected cases.

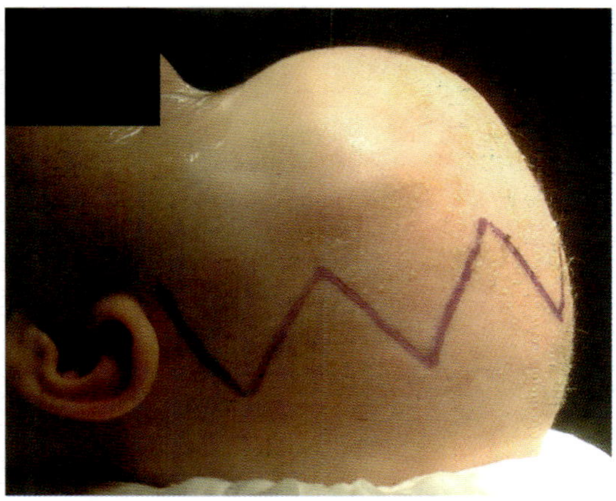

Fig 4.11-7 Coronal incision in a "zigzagged" shape in patient with brachicephaly.

A curved and separate incision in the periosteum is made well above and behind the temporal line. Subperiosteal dissection is made preserving the periosteal-galeal flap, supraorbital nerves and vessels and avoiding aggressive temporalis muscle manipulation, preserving its vascularization and innervation. Minimizing blood loss is mandatory. Covering the exposed bone with wet dressings is useful to avoid drying out of the bone. The eyes are protected as well (eyelid suture, gentle intraorbital retraction) to prevent corneal, conjunctival or globe damage. Reattaching the preserved temporalis muscle with anterior and medial repositioning is recommended in some cases to prevent deformities at the pterional region.

When an anterior reconstruction is planned, positioning of the patient will be in a supine position at the starting point. If a posterior reconstruction or a second procedure of holocranial remodeling is necessary, surgery is started in a prone position ("sphinx" position) (**Fig 4.11-8**). Patient positioning should be changed from supine to prone in cases of holocranial remodeling in a one-stage procedure, with the coordination of an experienced anesthesia team [Gosain et al, 2004], protecting the eyes, decubitus points and preserving normal temperature especially in these long surgical interventions.

4 Surgical technique: anterior cranial expansion

Selection of the proper timing for release of the affected cranial sutures in a patient with craniosynostosis has been controversial, and an individual approach is recommended. The benefits of early release of the cranial sutures are controversial. Our surgical philosophy has now changed to a more comprehensive strategy aiming at releasing the synostotic sutures while concomitantly relocating the bones of the cranial vault into a more anatomically correct position. This will ideally produce a normal growth pattern and is done at 9–12 months of age. Early surgeries are often associated with a high incidence of surgical revision. From our point of view, the number of operations should be minimized not only to avoid patient risks but also because the quality of the bone decreases each time it is subjected to a surgical procedure. Exceptions to the protocol can be made on an individual basis with careful consideration of poor general health conditions, such as high intracranial pressure, which would necessarily indicate early surgical procedures.

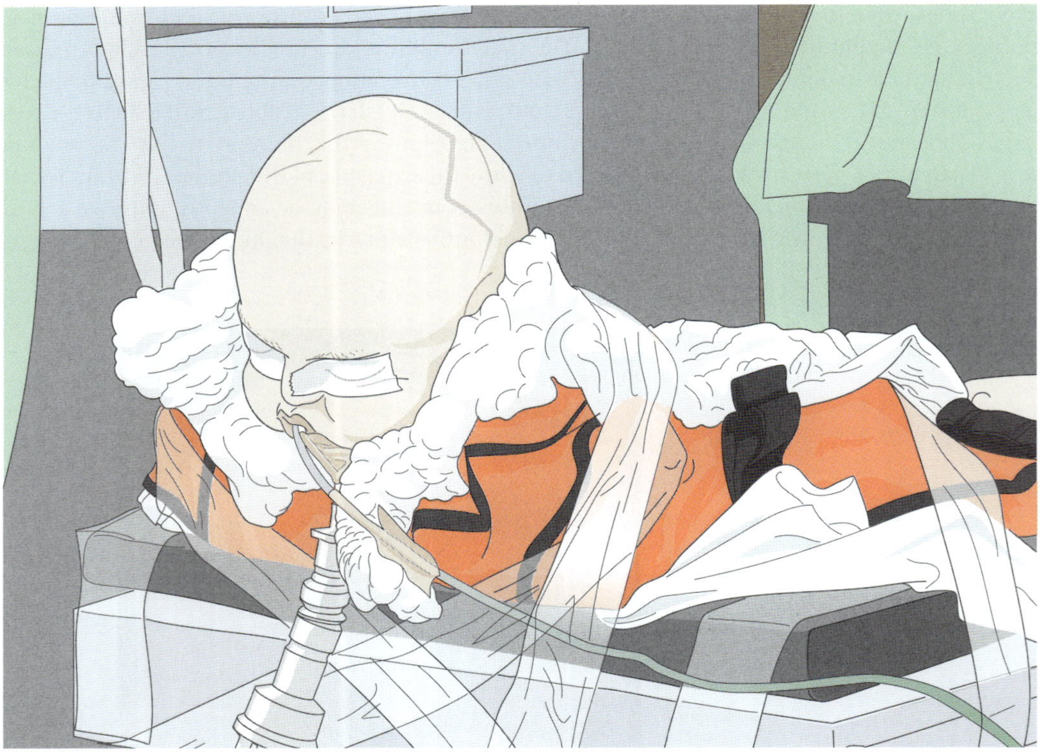

Fig 4.11-8 Positioning of Crouzon patient in sphinx position. It is important to secure the endotracheal tube and the patient while protecting the globes and avoiding decubitus lesions.

Anterior cranial expansion procedures for frontoorbital advancement are indicated in cases of isolated coronal synostosis, bilateral coronal synostosis, and metopic synostosis. Most cases will be treated with bilateral osteotomies and reshaping to achieve symmetry through correction of the involved side and compensatory changes at the uninvolved side and the frontoorbital region. Slight overcorrection of the frontoorbital bandeau will minimize future deformities and residual asymmetries. Unilateral canthal advancement techniques and isolated frontoparietal suturectomies (endoscopically assisted) with or without postoperative helmet therapy could be indicated in selected mild cases (**Fig 4.11-9**). Monoblock or Le Fort III osteotomies with frontoorbital advancement (**Fig 4.11-10**) can be used in syndromic cases, such as Crouzon or Apert, to advance the face and the frontal region at the same time, improving the airway and the depressed frontoorbital region [Molina, 2004].

The patient is placed in a supine position. Using a coronal incision and a subperiostal approach, the scalp is reflected obtaining the exposure of the frontal, pterional and temporal regions, nasion, orbital roofs and lateral orbital rims and walls. Special care should be taken (especially in syndromic cases) when dissecting areas without bone cover to avoid dural injury. Temporalis muscles can be left attached to the subcutaneous tissue or be partially sectioned below the temporalis crest to improve access to the pterional regions in severe cases.

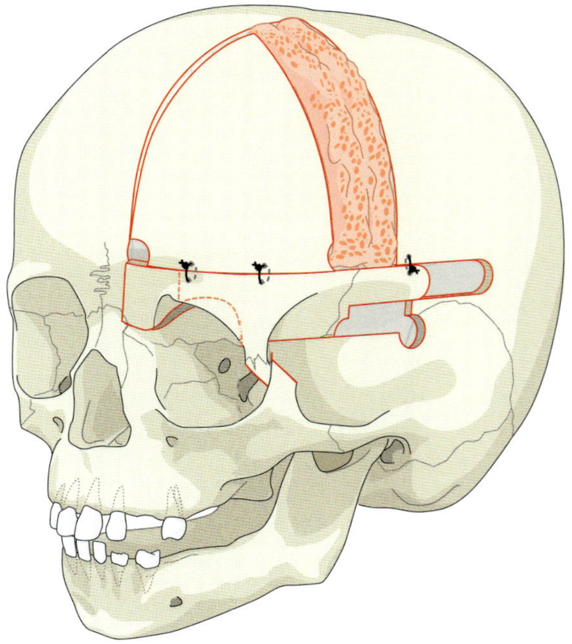

Fig 4.11-9 Unilateral–unicantal frontoorbital advancement as described by Hoffman and Mohr [1976].

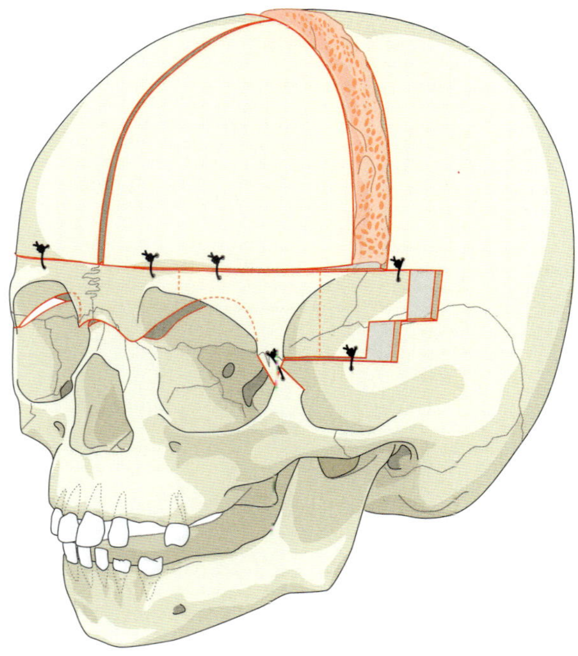

Fig 4.11-10 Bilateral frontoorbital advancement as described by Marchac [1978].

After placing peripheral or central burr holes, dissection and harvest of an anterior frontal bone flap is performed, gaining access to the anterior lateral and central skull base, orbital roofs and cribriform plate without damaging the olfactory nerves. It is recommended to save the bone dust from the osteotomies and burr holes to use as bone graft at the end of the procedures to fill small gaps. The supraorbital osteotomy or "bandeau" is made 1–1.5 cm above the roof of the orbits, extending into the temporal fossa in a "tongue-in-groove," design (by Tessier) to improve retention, unilaterally or usually bilaterally. The supraorbital bar sectioning is completed with osteotomies across the orbital roofs, nasofrontal suture, sphenoid, and frontal processes of the zygoma at the malar eminence on the affected side, and at the frontozygomatic suture on the unaffected side, altering the site of the malar osteotomies depending on the severity of the deformity in the orbital rims [Esparza et al, 1998; Muñoz et al, 2003]. In anterior plagiocephaly cases (**Fig 4.11-11**) nasal straightening with a closing wedge ostectomy in the upper part of the nasal bone on the affected side can be added rotating the nasal pyramid and closing the nasofrontal gap [Marchac, 1978]. Nasal correction achieved in the long-term follow-up with this method is controversial. To avoid possible growth restriction, the nasal or zygoma abnormalities in patients with coronal synostosis are not fully treated in procedures performed early.

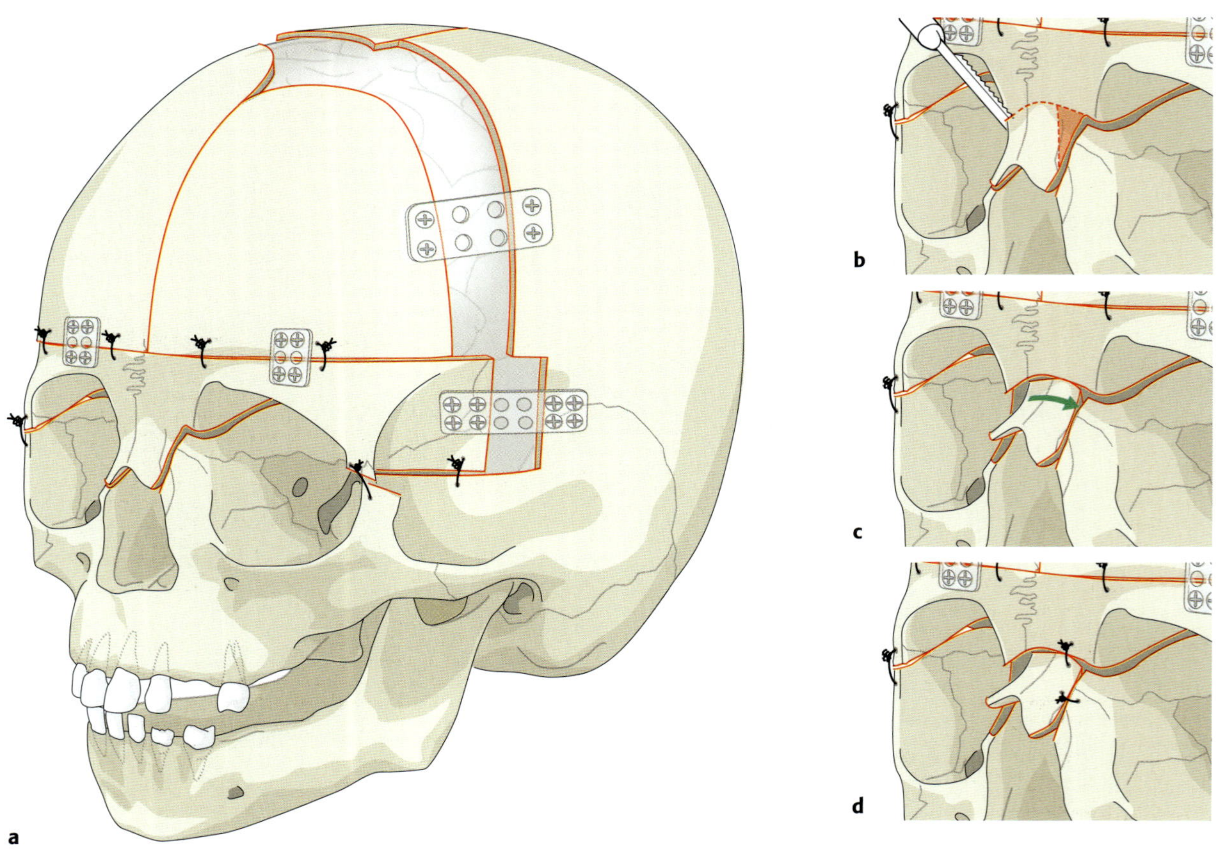

Fig 4.11-11a–d

- **a** Bilateral frontoorbital advancement including the nasal skeleton, fixation with wires and resorbable plates.
- **b** After fixation of the frontoorbital bandeau, an additional osteotomy of the nasal skeleton is performed to be able to position the nasal bones in the facial midline.
- **c** The nasal bone segment is rotated to the affected side. For this movement, a wedge of bone needs to be resected (arrow).
- **d** After positioning, the nasal bone segment is fixed with wires or plates and screws.

Temporal bones are usually depressed, and they can be used in different ways depending on the case and the type of synostosis. They can be used as a donor site for bone graft harvesting or they may be removed, reshaped, and replaced in a more symmetric shape and position. The frontal bone flap and supraorbital bar can be reshaped with peripheral osteotomies or bent in a barrel stave way, or can be replaced using a bone graft harvested from the parietal regions. For this a Marchac template [Cray et al, 2011; Burge et al, 2011] (**Fig 4.11-12a**) is often helpful. After bone harvest the donor site can be filled with the original frontalis bone flap in one or multiple pieces. This new frontal flap is then plated, with resorbable plates or mesh and screws at the inner or outer table, into position with the reshaped frontal bar in a slightly overcorrected position achieving frontal advancements as far as 15–20 mms as planned (**Fig 4.11-12b**). By plating this framework bilaterally at the temporal, parietal, and nasofrontal regions, adequate stabilization of the anterior cranial expansion can be achieved. In selected severe cases of plagiocephaly the supraorbital region can be osteotomized, and a new frontal region including the upper orbital rims with a single parietal bone flap can be constructed [Gosain et al, 2004; Cray et al, 2011]. Scalp closure may be difficult and soft-tissue tension over the plates may increase the risk of an early relapse in cases where large advancements are necessary; to avoid this situation, parallel incisions in the galea should be designed and then anchoring sutures from the galea to monocortical resorbable screws placed at the parietooccipital regions should be used.

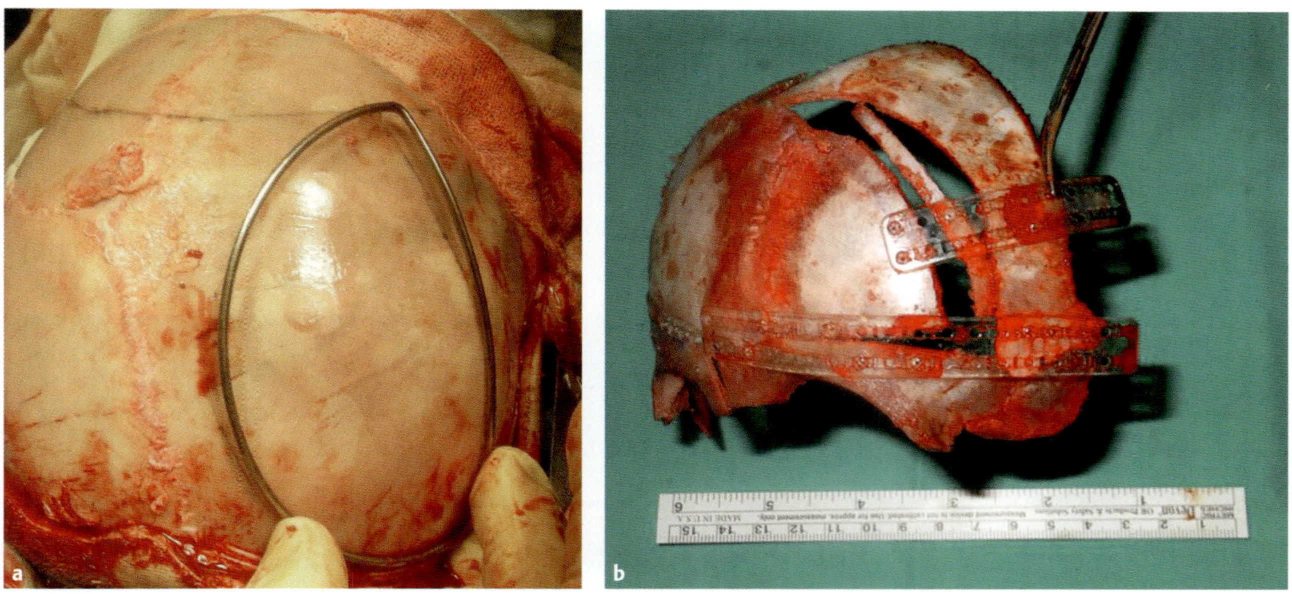

Fig 4.11-12a–b
a Marchac template.
b Resorbable plate fixation at the temporalis region.

Metopic synostosis (trigonocephaly) often shows bilateral retrusion of supraorbital rims (mostly laterally) and hypoteleorbitism (**Fig 4.11-13**). Surgical planning should achieve bilateral canthal advancement, recontoured supraorbital rims, and a reshaped forehead, this being well described by Marchac [1978]. For this a supraorbital bar with a greenstick fracture at the midline (synostosis place) is designed as well as in the lateral parts, if needed. Then the segments are bent and advanced as needed according to the preoperative plan. The forehead is reconstructed with a bone graft usually in one piece from the parietal region or lateral aspect of the frontal bone segment. In severe cases, the supraorbital region can be osteotomized restoring the forehead and supraorbital rims with a single parietal bone graft, filling the donor regions with bone grafts from the previous supraorbital and frontal regions [Cray et al, 2011].

Nowadays surgical guides generated by computer-aided design and computer-aided manufacturing (CAD-CAM) can be used to enhance the efficiency and precision of surgical treatment. This is valid for all anterior craniosynostosis. Computer-assisted modeling and template-based surgery enhances planning, understanding of the preoperative anatomy and potential avoidance of pitfalls, reducing risks related to a longer operation time [Taylor et al, 2012].

5 Posterior calvarial expansion

Conventional posterior calvarial expansion osteotomy is effective in the treatment of nonsyndromic cases where transverse expansion and reshaping are the main goals. Nevertheless, posterior expansion with distraction osteogenesis technique is probably the recommended treatment option for syndromic patients with multisuture synostosis, especially when a Chiari malformation or intracranial hypertension is present [Steinbacher et al, 2011].

With the patient in prone position and using a coronal incision with subperiostal dissection, the occipital bone and lambdoid sutures are exposed to reach the insertion of the posterior neck muscles; osteocutaneus venous channels are cauterized if encountered. In posterior expansion cases, harvest of a "neobandeau" from the vertex is needed. After markings are made to design a new vertex bandeau, it is necessary to remove the deformed bones performing a two-piece parietal-occipital craniotomy in a transverse fashion. Van der Kolk et al [1993] described a posterior osteotomy line starting 5–8 cm above the junction of the left lambdoidal sutures and along the sagittal suture. It then extends in a curvilinear fashion to involve the asterion region. The inferior osteotomy is performed below the transverse sinus.

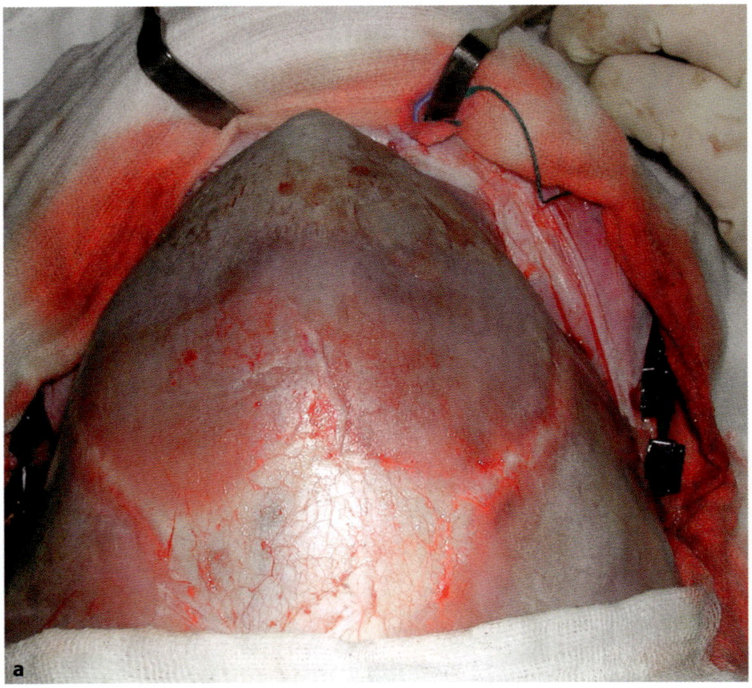

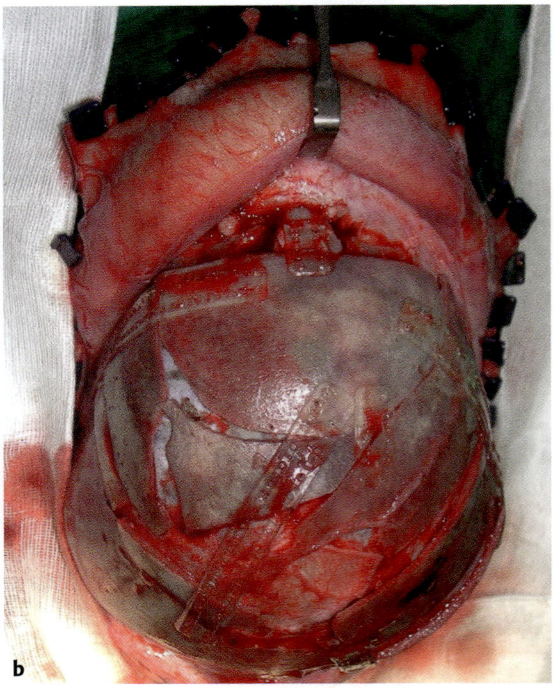

Fig 4.11-13a–b
a Intraoperative view of surgical treatment of a trigonocephaly case before correction.
b Intraoperative view of surgical treatment of a trigonocephaly case after correction.

The bandeau is then harvested and flipped 180°, so that the right side of the bandeau moves to the left side of the skull. When the bandeau is inserted 90° below the vertex, the skull gains more posterior projection at the flattened synostotic side, now corresponding to the higher auricular head height of the unaffected side. The parietooccipital bones are then trimmed to fit the open spaces above and below the new bandeau, and eventually perform barrel stave osteotomies on both sides to get more posterior expansion and contouring. The posterior advance rate is limited by scalp closure and relapse is also possible if osteosynthesis is not stable enough (**Fig 4.11-14**). If a distraction osteogenesis technique is used, after the neurosurgical team has performed parietal-occipital burr holes and limited dural dissection, an occipital craniotomy is designed just above the transverse sinus. The distraction devices are placed in parasagittal orientation with posteroinferior vector of action and the exit of the device will be placed in the anterior scalp flap [Munro, 1997].

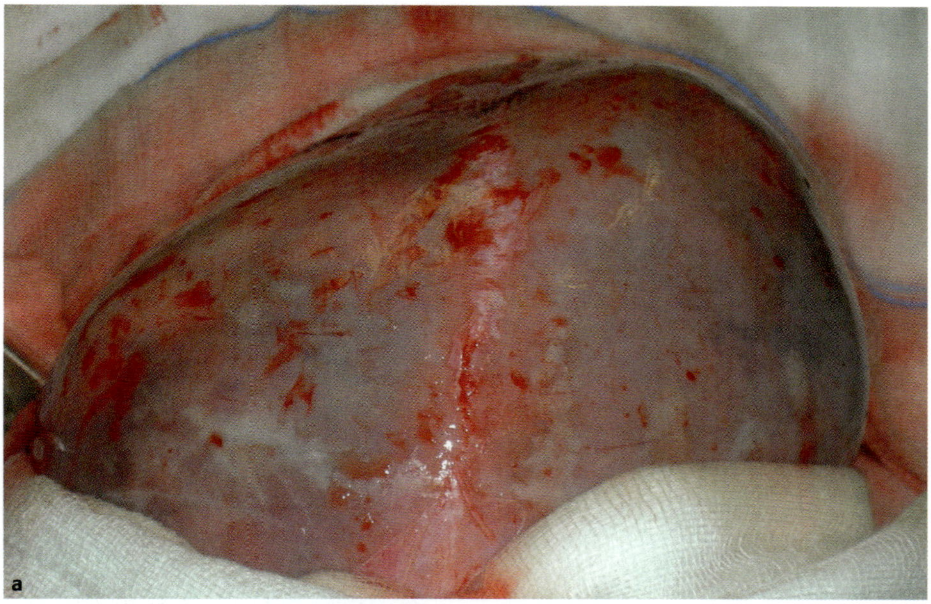

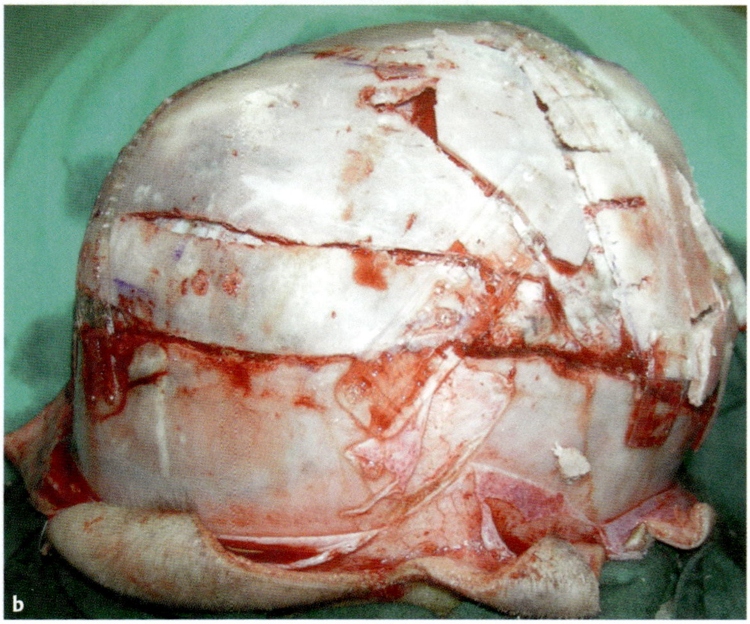

Fig 4.11-14a–b
a Posterior craniosynostosis.
b Posterior craniosynostosis after treatment with resulting expansion and reshaping.

6 Complete or subtotal calvarial expansion

Complete or more commonly near-total cranial expansion is indicated in cases of severe synostosis with brachy-turricephaly deformity, syndromic cases, and recurrences that need total cranial vault remodeling to allow for adequate brain expansion. If younger than 2 years it is a high-risk procedure with potential complications, such as air embolism related to the sphinx position and great vault exposure and the need for a high volume of blood replacement [Muñoz et al, 2003]. The tower-shaped skull abnormality or turricephaly is the most difficult cranial deformity to correct because the excess skull height needs to be changed with multiple and combined osteotomies and calvarial expansions. Nevertheless, this procedure is often indicated for severe turribrachycephaly craniosynostosis or syndromic cases as early as possible (during the first year of life), and better in a "one-step" surgery taking care to avoid possible surgical or medical complications. It is important to not undertreat this type of patient with only partial calvarial expansions, thus ineffectively resolving brain compression. Limited approaches performing frontoorbital advancement alone do not address the occipital flattening or the abnormal height elevation associated with multisuture synostoses (**Fig 4.11-15**).

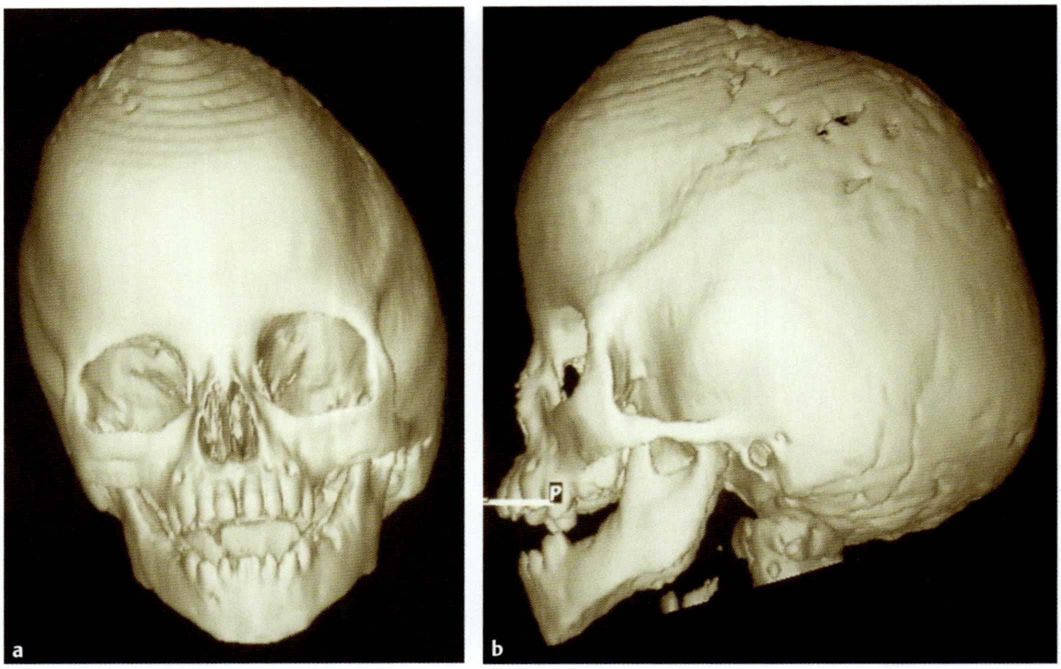

Fig 4.11-15a–b A computed tomographic scan of a patient with multisuture synostosis and brachy-turricephaly deformity.

With the patient in a sphinx position (**Fig 4.11-8**), a subtotal cranial vault remodeling as described by Munro in 1997 [Taylor et al, 2012] starts with a bilateral frontoorbital advancement with removal of the greater wings of the sphenoid bone and lateral aspects of the frontosphenoid suture as described by Tessier; or with a new frontal bone harvested from the parietal regions plated in an advanced position [Muñoz et al, 2003]. Then, radical removal of the cranial bone at the parietalis and temporalis areas is performed, preserving a central strip of bone in one or multiple segments to avoid any damage of the sagittal sinus (**Fig 4.11-16**). Resected bone from the parietal and temporal areas are remodeled, advanced laterally and plated to the basal skull decreasing the vertical height. The dura mater is plicated [Steinbacher et al, 2011] at the frontal and temporal areas to get additional reshaping of the brain also aiding in adaptation of bone flaps. Persing [1990] described parallel vertical osteotomies to perform outward greenstick fractures in a "barrel stave" shape of the basal skull to get additional space and decreasing the resistance to vertical compression, thus allowing safe reduction of the cranial height [Munro, 1997]. As a final step in a total calvarial expansion case, occipital and lambdoid segments are osteotomized near the edge of the foramen magnum in a barrel stave fashion; left like floating bones sutured to the dura, improving AP space for brain elongation; or advanced, rotated, and plated laterally to decrease the AP elongation improving the transverse diameter of the brain. Children typically rest in supine position postoperatively to avoid reshaping relapse. Osteosynthesis technique should be precise avoiding bone gaps, plates will be placed in regions with adequate and stable bone stock.

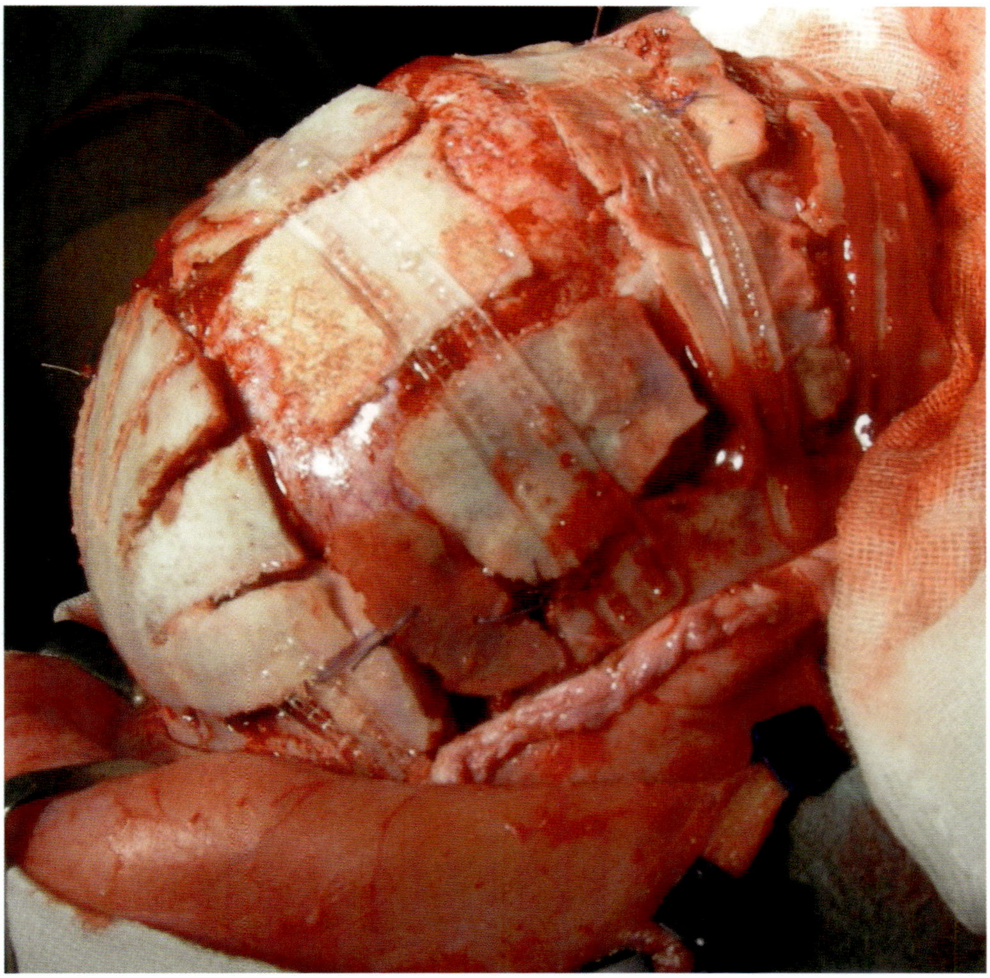

Fig 4.11-16 Subtotal calvarial expansion and holocranial reshaping in the patient from Fig 4.11-15a–b.

7 Helmet therapy

Positional cranial deformities without synostosis of the sutures can be effectively treated by nonsurgical cranial orthotics. Even in ancient cultures, early head modeling was used to conform to prevailing ideals of beauty and revealed lifelong results. Since the introduction of the supine position for babies to prevent sudden infant death syndrome the incidence of postural head deformities has increased in the western civilization. Therefore, recommendations for increased "tummy time" under parents control have been published.

Whereas synostosis of cranial sutures usually has to be corrected surgically; positional head deformities are treated in different ways. Thus differential diagnosis by clinical means, sonography, "blackbone“ MRI or 3-D CT scan becomes crucial in order to determine treatment options.

Cranial deformities are three times more frequent in males than in females, and multiple birth with the risk of asymmetries of the muscles of the neck due to intrauterine shortage of space has a higher risk for later deformations. In most cases cranial deformities develop within the first 6–8 weeks after birth and positional changes will not be successful if shortage of muscles of the neck or cervical spine blockades exist. Spontaneous correction of shape can be expected when the causes for deformation are eliminated. Therefore postural changes, physiotherapy, chirotherapy, and osteopathy are primary treatment options. However, spontaneous correction after elimination of the causes of the deformity usually only occurs until 4–5 months after birth, followed by circumferential growth of the head but with retention of its shape. Later on cranial growth can be directed by an individual cranial orthotic (helmet therapy). According to the cranial growth curve, the success of the treatment is optimal within the first year of life.

Under these aspects, pronounced noticeable brachycephalia persisting 3 months after birth and cranial asymmetries with more than 2 cm slant (diagonal) discrepancy (plagiocephaly), especially when distinct cranial base involvement is obvious, seem to be strong indications for helmet therapy to prevent esthetic stigmatizing or functionally relevant deformities, as eg, cross-bite development.

Registration of the complete head is performed by 3-D photogrammetry within 1.5 ms and the data set edited in a CAD-workstation. The ideal shape of the head is designed under consideration of the cranial growth zones. Precise CAD planning allows evaluation of the volume necessary to correct the deformity. The growth of defined areas of the cranium is blocked by contact with the helmet or released by a non-contact zone where growth can be directed in. For a precise growth guidance the helmet has to be in place for 23 hours per day. The treatment success can be documented by repeated 3-D photogrammetry during the follow up. According to the extent of the deformity, treatment time varies between several weeks and months. A prognosis of the treatment time is based on the knowledge of the volume changes according to age [Blecher et al, 2012].

8 Pitfalls and complications

Pediatric craniofacial surgery presents a similar rate of technical difficulties as trauma and oncological skull base surgery in adults, but the incidence of complications is expected to be low for perioperative or postoperative mortality. Detailed presurgical evaluation of the patient in a coordinated, teamwork approach with the anesthesiologist, pediatrician, and intensive care team is mandatory in all patients who undergo craniofacial surgery.

A thorough evaluation of the airway before surgery and continuous communication between specialists during the perioperative period is imperative for a successful outcome. Furthermore, most pediatric patients with syndromic craniosynostosis present with a narrowed and altered airway, and are better managed with fiberoptic-assisted intubation. In severe and selected cases a perioperative tracheostomy is necessary [Tessier, 1971].

Continuous monitoring and fluid replacement are critical in pediatric patients undergoing craniofacial reconstruction. A significant amount of blood loss can occur during these procedures. Arterial and central venous lines for fluid dynamic cardiovascular monitoring and replacement are mandatory. Erythropoietin administrated weekly for 3 weeks preoperatively can be useful. The use of cell saver systems and aprotinin (e-aminocaproic acid) has also been advocated to reduce the requirements for blood replacement [Persing, 2008; Persing et al, 1990].

Attention to surgical hemostasis and the use of intraoperative autogenous blood transfusion will prevent the necessity of postoperative homologous blood transfusion. In some cases, this is associated with significant risks, such as hemolysis, transfusion-related acute lung injury, post-transfusion hepatitis, allergic reactions, and others. Because the osteotomies create an open communication between the subgaleal and epidural spaces, postoperative hematoma or edema presents low risk to develop intracranial hypertension. Normally, blood administration is not associated with coagulopathy until blood loss equals a circulating blood volume or more.

Venous air embolism is a dangerous situation more prone to occur whenever the patient is in the reverse-Trendelenburg position; Doppler monitoring is supplemented with end-tidal carbon dioxide measurement to check the situation. Hemodynamic responses to large air emboli include ischemic infarcts and cardiac collapse. Adequate patient position, anesthesia management together with meticulous hemostasis and careful coverage of the exposed bone at the subperiosteal dissection with wet sponges usually prevent this situation [Persing, 2008].

Dural lacerations may occur mainly in secondary procedures and the treatment is intraoperative repair, either with direct closure or using a patch of periosteum, temporalis fascia or dural substitutes. Small to moderate bone gaps are not a problem, especially in children during their first year of life, and ossification is expected if there is a good periosteal coverage. Autogenous bone, usually split calvarial grafts, should be used to fill those gaps in older patients. In selected cases cranioplasty implants may be indicated. Skull "growing fractures" are usually associated with intracranial hypertension or inadequate bone fixation or reconstruction.

They are also named "leptomeningeal cysts". They are enlarging skull fractures that occur near posttraumatic encephalomalacia and are usually seen a few months post-trauma (<1% of skull fractures) or craniofacial procedure. In patients with completed craniofacial procedures with dural tears, the leptomeninges and/or cerebral parenchyma is herniated into it. Pulsations from cerebrospinal fluid (CSF) erode the fracture margin, resulting in eventual expansion and nonunion. In CT scan the lesion presents the following features:

- Extracranial brain herniation
- Hydrocephalus
- Unilateral ventricular dilatation and porencephalic cyst [Liu et al, 2012]

The selection of osteosynthesis material is dependent on the age of the patient, presence of bone defects and the maturity of the bone. The use of metallic fixation material appears to be limited to older children, recurrences or complicated cases where extensive bone grafting is needed. Metallic osteosynthesis material is also used in unfavorable situations, such as orbital roof or lateral wall defects, to hold back the pushing brain. It has been documented that metal implants placed on the external aspect of the skull become internalized with natural skull growth by resorption at the internal aspect of the skull and deposition of bone on its external surface. The consequence of internal displacement of plates and/or screws is still unknown, but current reports show that there is no apparent increased incidence of brain injury [Hasan et al, 2004]. Nevertheless, resorbable plates could be internalized in the same way as metallic implants and also the final effect of that fact remains unclear [Jimenez et al, 1995].

Scalp closure is a crucial step for the stability of the osteosynthesis material, especially if resorbable plates and screws have been used. Failure or inadequate fixation technique will result in an immediate postoperative relapse. Precluding excessive tension in scalp flaps at closure, galeal relaxing incisions, bone interdigitation and titanium miniplates used in selected places are useful in major frontoorbital or posterior expansion procedures to prevent immediate relapse (**Fig 4.11-17**).

The incidence of infection is low in craniofacial surgery procedures. Infections are not associated to perforation into the nasopharynx and/or paranasal sinuses, and because of the good vascularization of the scalp and the young age of the patients, the use of perioperative antibiotic prophylaxis is enough as a prevention. The risk of meningitis is also low. It usually occurs with continuing postoperative CSF leaks. Wide spectrum antibiotics, hematoma drainage and repair of CSF leaks are mandatory in patients with this type of infection. Postoperative hyperthermia is also relatively common in patients with craniosynostosis surgery receiving blood derivatives, because of degradation of blood products in contact with dura mater or prolonged use of intravenous central lines.

Bone irregularities and lack of satisfactory results are the most frequent suboptimal outcomes in this type of surgery. The necessity for major surgical revisions depends on the severity and type of craniosynostosis, the age of the patient at the time of surgery, and the technique used. Severe asymmetric deformities involving cranial vault and skull base corrections like anterior plagiocephaly and syndromic craniosynostosis will have a higher rate of reoperations and later corrections, usually delayed to age 3–5 years when the brain and orbital growth are almost complete.

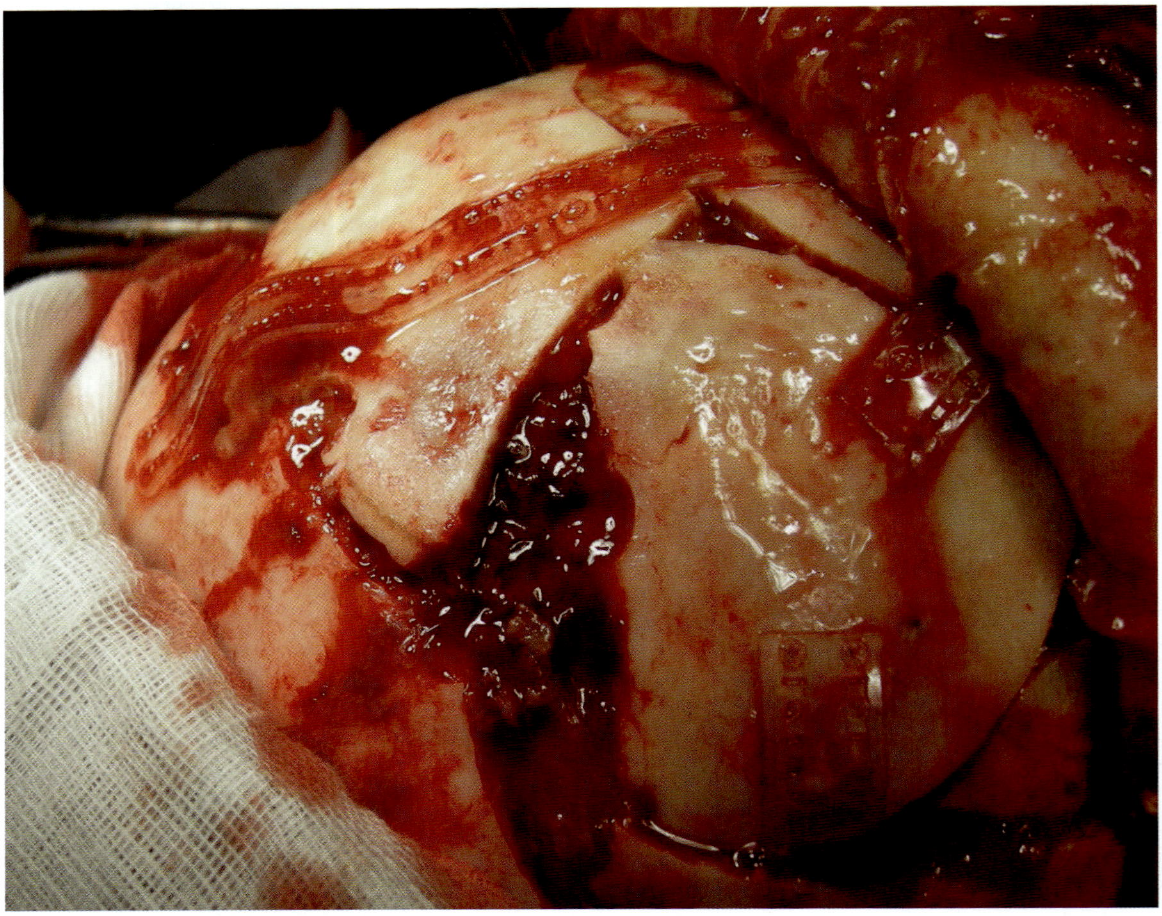

Fig 4.11-17 Immediate relapse of a frontoorbital advance because of excessive tension in the scalp closure and not enough stiffness of the resorbable plate fixation. Note the postoperative hematoma and plate deformation.

9 Acknowledgment

We thank Christoph Kunz, MD, DDS, PhD, University Hospital Basel, Switzerland, for writing the section on "Helmet therapy".

10 References and suggested reading

Agochukwu NB, Solomon BD, Muenke M. Impact of genetics on the diagnosis and clinical management of syndromic craniosynostoses. *Childs Nerv Syst.* 2012 Sep;28(9):1447–1463.

Argenta L, David LR, Wilson JA, Bell WO. An increase in infant cranial deformity with supine sleeping position. *J Craniofac Surg* 1996;7:5–11

Blecher C, Kunz C, Mayr J, et al. Helmtherapie: konservative Kopfmodellierung. Behandlung lagebedingter Kopfdeformitäten. *MKG-Chirurg* 2012(5):289–296. German.

Buchman SR, Muraszko K. Frontoorbital reconstruction. *Atlas Oral Maxillofacial Surg Clin North Am.* 2002 Mar;10(1):43–56.

Burge J, Saber NR, Looi T, et al. Application of CAD/CAM prefabricated age-matched templates in cranio-orbital remodeling in craniosynostosis. *J Craniofac Surg.* 2011 Sep;22(5):1810–1813.

Cray J Jr, Burrows AM, Vecchione L, et al. Blocking bone morphogenetic protein function using in vivo noggin therapy does not rescue premature suture fusion in rabbits with delayed-onset craniosynostosis. *Plast Reconstr Surg.* 2011 Mar;127(3):1163–1172.

Cohen MM Jr. Etiopathogenesis of cranyosinostosis. *Neurosurg Clin North Am.* 1991 Jul;2(3):507–513.

Collman H, Schweitzer T, Bohm H. Imaging studies and neurosurgical treatment. In: Muenke M, Kress W, Collman H, et al, eds. *Monographs in Human Genetics. Craniosynostoses: Molecular Genetics, Principles of Diagnosis and Treatment.* Karger Publishing: Basel; 2011;19:216–231.

Esparza J, Muñoz MJ, Hinojosa J, et al. Operative treatment of the anterior synostotic plagiocephaly: analysis of 45 cases. *Childs Nerv Syst.* 1998 Sep;14(9):448–454.

Gosain AK, Recinos RF, Agresti M, et al. TGF-beta1, FGF-2, and receptor mRNA expression in suture mesenchyme and dura versus underlying brain in fusing and nonfusing mouse cranial sutures. *Plast Reconstr Surg.* 2004 May;113(6):1675–1684.

Hasan RA, Nikolis A, Dutta S, et al. Clinical outcome of perioperative airway and ventilatory management in children undergoing craniofacial surgery. *J Craniofac Surg.* 2004 Jul;15(4):655–661.

Hansen M, Mulliken JB. Frontal plagiocephaly: diagnosis and treatment. *Craniofacial Surg.* 1994 Oct;21(4):543–553.

Hansen M, Padwa BL, Scott M, et al. Synostotic frontal plagiocephaly: anthropometric comparison of three techniques for surgical correction. *Plast Reconstr Surg.* 1997 Nov;100(6):1387–1395.

Hoffman HJ, Mohr G. Lateral canthal advancement of the supraorbital margin. A new corrective technique in the treatment of coronal synostosis. *J Neurosurg.* 1976 Oct;45(4):376–381.

Jimenez DF, Barone CM. Intraoperative autologous blood transfusion in the surgical correction of craniosynostosis. *Neurosurgery.* 1995 Dec;37(6):1075–1079.

Liu XS, You C, Lu M, et al. Growing skull fracture stages and treatment strategy. *Neurosurg Perdiatr.* 2012;9(6)670–675.

Marchac D. Radical forehead remodeling for craniostenosis. *Plast Reconstr Surg.* 1978 Jun;61(6):823–835.

Mathijssen I. Guideline for care of patients with the diagnoses of craniosynostosis: working group on craniosynostosis. *J Craniofac Surg.* 2015;26:1735–1807.

Meara J, Burvin R, Barlett R, et al. Anthropometric study of synostotic frontal plagiocephaly: before and after fronto-orbital advancement with correction of nasal angulation. *Plast Reconstr Surg.* 2003 Sep;112(3):731–738.

Meyer-Marcotty P, Bohm H, Linz C, et al. Spectrum of positional deformities—is there a real difference between plagiocephaly and brachycephaly? *J Craniomaxillofac Surg.* 2014 Sep;42(6);1010–1016.

Molina F. From midface distraction to the "true monoblock". *Clin Plastic Surg.* 2004 Jul;31(3):463–479.

Muñoz MJ, Esparza J, Hinojosa J, et al. Fronto-orbital remodeling without orbito-naso-frontal bandeau. *Childs Nerv Syst.* 2003 Jun;19(5-6):353–358.

Munro IR. Reshaping the cranial vault. In: Converse JM, ed. *Reconstructive Plastic Surgery.* 2nd ed. Philadelphia: WB Saunders Co; 1997.

Persing JA. MOC-PS (SM) CME article: management considerations in the treatment of craniosynostosis. *Plast Reconst Surg.* 2008 Apr;121(4 Suppl):1–11.

Persing JA, Jane JA, Delashaw JB. Treatment of bilateral coronal synostosis in infancy: a holistic approach. *J Neurosurg.* 1990 Feb;72(2):171–175.

Persing JA, Posnick J, Magge S, et al. Cranial plate and screw fixation in infancy: an assessment of risk. *J Craniofac Surg.* 1996 Jul;7(4):267–270.

Prein J, ed. *Manual of Internal Fixation in the Cranio-Facial Skeleton.* Berlin: Springer; 1998.

Steinbacher DM, Skirpan J, Puchala J, et al. Expansion of the posterior cranial vault using distraction osteogenesis. *Plast Reconstr Surg.* 2011 Feb;127(2):792–801.

Taylor JA, Derderian CA, Barlett SP, et al. Perioperative morbidity in posterior cranial vault expansion: distraction osteogenesis versus conventional osteotomy. *Plast Reconstr Surg.* 2012 Apr;129(4):674e–680e.

Tessier P. [Total facial osteotomy. Crouzon's syndrome, Apert's syndrome: oxycephaly, scaphocephaly, turricephaly]. *Ann Chir Plast.* 1967 Dec;12(4):273–286. French.

Tessier P. Total osteotomy of the middle third of the face for faciostenosis or for sequelae of Le Fort 3 fractures. *Plast Reconstr Surg.* 1971 Dec;48(6):533–541.

Tessier P. The definitive plastic surgical treatment of the severe facial deformities of craniofacial dysostosis, Crouzon's and Apert's diseases. *Plast Reconstr Surg.* 1971 Nov;48(5):419–442.

Virchow R. [Über den Cretinismus, namentlich in Franken, und über pathologische Schädelformen.] *Verh Phys Med Gesamle Würzburg.* 1851;2:230–256. German.

Van der Kolk CA, Carson BS, Robertson BC, et al. The occipital bar and internal osteotomies in the treatment of lambdoidal synostosis. *J Craniofac Surg.* 1993;4:112–118.

Wiltfang J, Merten HA, Becker HJ, et al. The resorbable miniplate system Lactosorb in a growing cranio-osteoplasty animal model. *J Craniomaxillofac Surg.* 1999 Aug;27(4):207–210.

4.12 Orbital hypertelorism

Larry A Sargent

1 Introduction

Orbital hypertelorism can be defined as an increased distance between the bony orbits. These are the patients that Greig described [Greig, 1924] as having "a great breadth between the eyes." The term hypertelorism simply describes a "wide-setness" or separation of any bilateral structure. Tessier described orbital hypertelorism as a true lateralization of the entire orbital complex, indicating an increased distance between both the medial and lateral walls [Tessier, 1972]. In the literature hypertelorism has been used interchangeably with the terms orbital hypertelorism, teleorbitism, and hyperteleorbitism. These are complex deformities that can demonstrate a range of interorbital deformities. The deformity of telecanthus, however, represents only an increase in the medial canthi with a normal interorbital distance. Patients who demonstrate increased distance between only the medial orbital walls and not the lateral walls are perhaps more appropriately called interorbital hypertelorism or bony telecanthus. Analyzing the specific anatomy and abnormalities in each of these patients is critical to determining the type and degree of the deformity as well as the best surgical treatment.

2 Classification

A complete clinical and radiographic evaluation is necessary to assess the etiological and anatomical diagnosis [Tan et al, 1997; Yaremchuk et al, 1993]. These findings play a key role in deciding treatment options. Measurements of the medial intercanthal distance and interpupillary distance are made and recorded as well as shape and position of the canthi, the medial orbital walls and the medial orbital rims. Currently, the best method for assessing bony interorbital deformities is computed tomographic (CT) scan with 3-D reconstructions. These images can give precise information about orbital position, rotation, symmetry and interorbital anatomy. Orbital hypertelorism can be measured as the distance between the dacrya (anterior lacrimal crests). Tessier [Tessier, 1974] has used the interorbital distance to rank the severity of the deformity: first degree is 30–34 mm; second degree is 35–40 mm; and third degree is more than 40 mm. These distances apply to adults who have an average interorbital distance of 25 mm in women and 28 mm in men. The interorbital distances in children and infants are obviously smaller and must be scaled down appropriately. Assessing the shape and position of the medial orbital walls as well as the size and configuration of the ethmoid sinuses is also important in planning the correction. The axial CT scan can show the shape and type of enlargement of the ethmoid sinuses. The position and contour of the medial orbital wall is determined by the abnormal enlargement of the ethmoid sinuses. This enlargement can be classified as anterior, central, posterior or uniform, and assessment is essential to formulating a successful treatment plan (**Fig 4.12-1**). A CT scan also shows the level of the cribriform as well as any other intracranial anomalies.

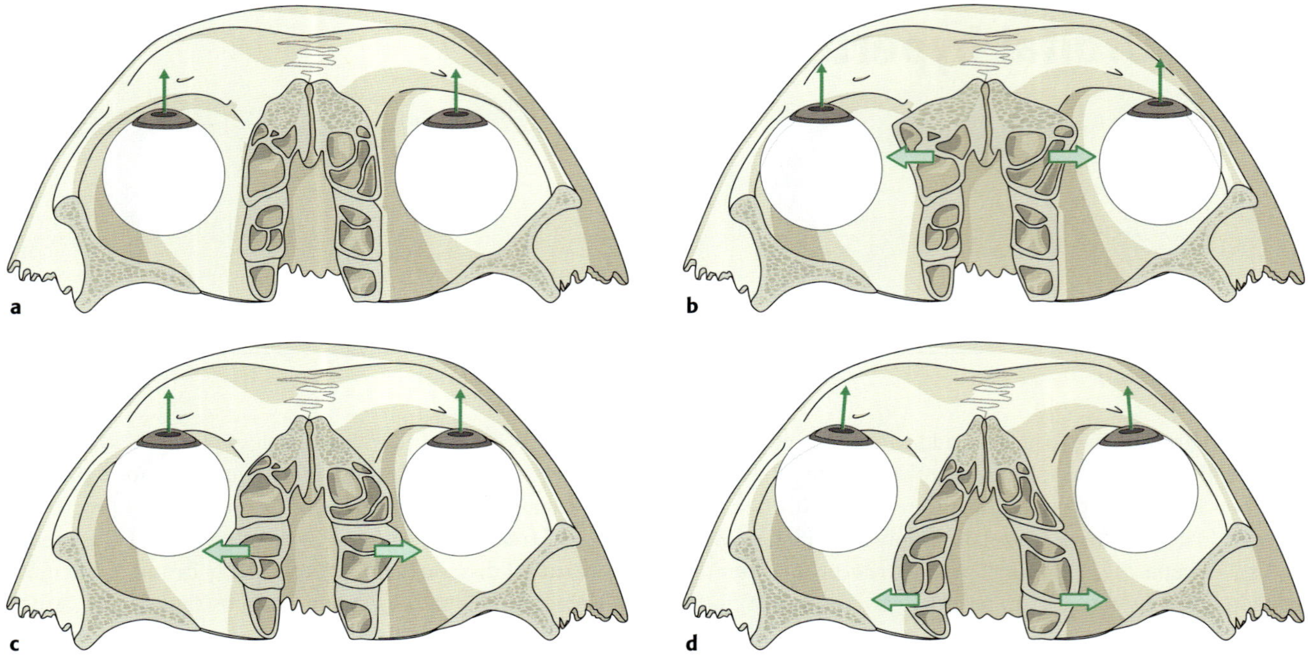

Fig 4.12-1a–d Classification of medial wall deformity and ethmoid sinus by computed tomographic scan.
a Uniform or parallel medial walls.
b Anterior enlargement.
c Central enlargement or oval shaped.
d Posterior enlargement.

It is important to remember that orbital hypertelorism is not a syndrome; it is a symptom or sign of a craniofacial malformation. The symptom is not the malformation itself. Increased interorbital distance can result from several different causes and may be associated with a range of cranial or orbital anomalies. The most common causes of orbital hypertelorism are frontonasal dysplasia, facial clefts, craniofacial dysostosis [Apert, 1906; Crouzon, 1912] and encephaloceles. A complete physical and radiographic evaluation is crucial to identify and assess all other facial anomalies [Tan et al, 1997].

3 Planning

The surgical treatment of orbital hypertelorism is influenced by many factors including severity, etiology, age and associated anomalies [Tessier, 1974; Mulliken et al, 1986; Whitaker et al, 1988]. Treatment before the age of 2 years is difficult with higher risk of problems and relapse and is usually reserved for encephaloceles which require early therapy [McCarthy et al, 1990]. Surgical treatment was pioneered by Paul Tessier [Tessier, 1972, 1974; Tessier et al, 1973] and modified by others [Munro et al, 1979; van der Meulen et al, 1983; Whitaker et al, 1988]. A variety of osteotomies of the orbit have been described in the literature. There are two basic techniques for surgical correction: extracranial and intracranial. Extracranial osteotomies are reserved for mild cases of increased interorbital distance with no prolapse of the cribriform plate between the medial orbital walls. Performing extracranial osteotomies on a patient with an abnormally low positioned cribriform plate increases risk for intracranial injury.

The intracranial/extracranial procedure is the most common technique used for moderate to severe orbital hypertelorism. This procedure is the most difficult but offers the highest degree of safety due to extensive exposure and control of the brain and orbits. The most common type of osteotomies is block osteotomies with movement of the globe in a "boxed" bony unit. The bipartition operation, illustrated later, is less commonly used.

4 Operative technique

4.1 Extracranial approach

The extracranial approach to the correction of orbital hypertelorism is reserved for mild cases of increased interorbital distance. There are two basic approaches: (1) medial orbital wall osteotomies, (**Fig 4.12-2**) and (2) the U-shaped osteotomy (**Fig 4.12-3**). The medial orbital wall osteotomies can also incorporate lateral wall osteotomies with medial movement or simple insertion of bone grafts medial to the lateral wall. These techniques compensate for the enlargement of the orbit by medial movement of the medial orbital walls. The medial orbital wall osteotomy in combination with bone grafts medial to the lateral wall, if needed, is the easier and more versatile procedure compared with the U-shaped osteotomy. The surgical exposure is obtained with a coronal incision, subciliary (or transconjunctival) incisions and upper gingivobuccal sulcus incisions. With these incisions the entire nasoethmoid skeleton, orbit and pyriform area can be exposed. The lacrimal sac and the infraorbital nerve are located to ensure protection during the osteotomy. The osteotomies used are outlined in **Fig 4.12-2a–b** and **Fig 4.12-3a**. Circumferential subperiosteal orbital dissection is performed to allow easier mobilization of soft tissues. Enlarged ethmoid cells are exenterated. The ratio of bone removed to decrease an interorbital distance (mm) is never one to one. An over-resection of bone and over reduction medially of the bony medial orbital walls is always performed. One should strive for a 20 mm bony interorbital distance. The soft-tissue distance is ideally 5 mm per side less than the true soft-tissue distance. Once the medial orbital walls are mobilized medially they are secured to one another in a symmetric manner with transnasal wires through transnasal drill holes posterior and superior to the upper and posterior edge of the lacrimal fossa. The osteotomized segments are then further secured to the supraorbital frontal bone, inferior orbital rim and/or pyriform rim with miniplates. The nose height is reconstructed/augmented with a cantilever calvarial bone graft rigidly fixed in place to the frontal bone with a plate and screws.

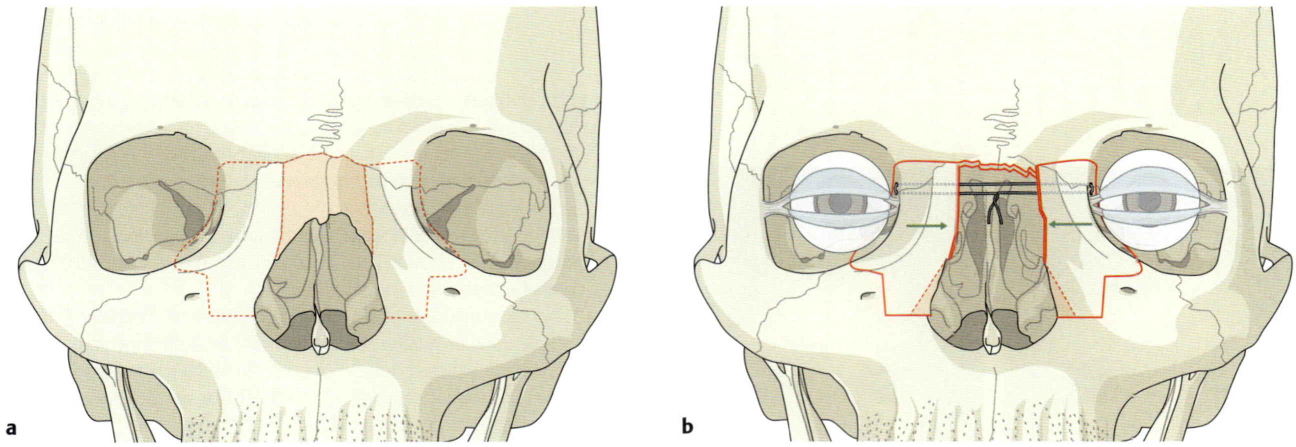

Fig 4.12-2a–h Extracranial correction of orbital hypertelorism by medial orbital wall osteotomies.
a Osteotomies outlined with segment of nasal bone and parts of the ethmoid sinuses to be resected (in red).
b Segments of nasal bone and ethmoids are resected. Medial canthi are reinforced or reattached with a 3-0 transnasal wire suture posterior and superior to the lacrimal fossa.

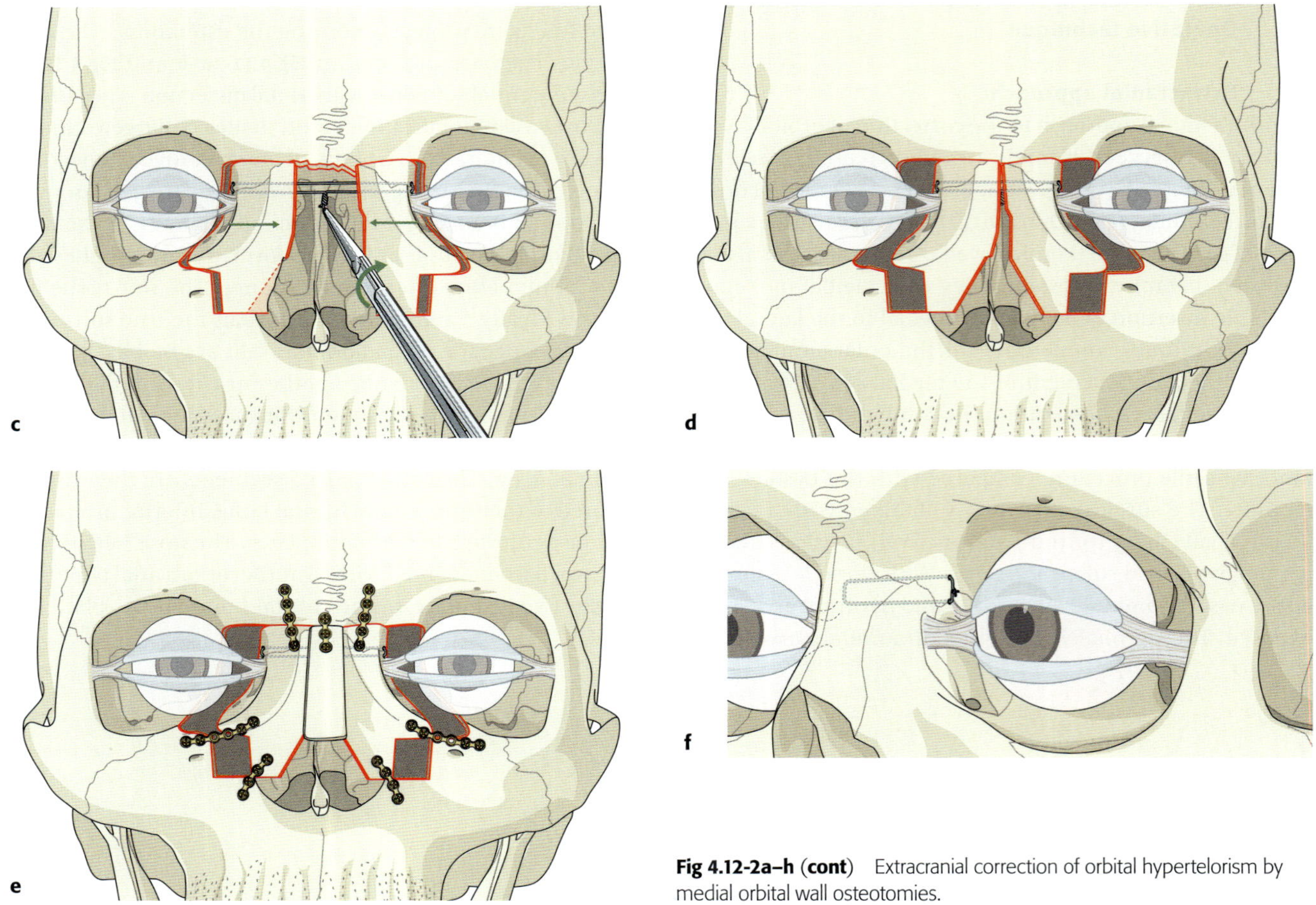

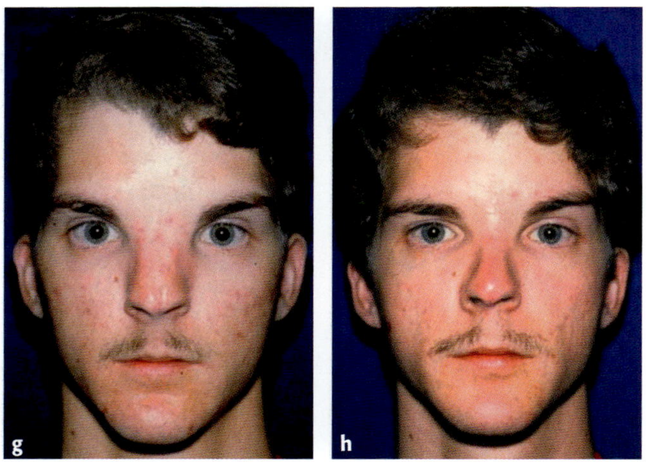

Fig 4.12-2a–h (cont) Extracranial correction of orbital hypertelorism by medial orbital wall osteotomies.

- **c** The bone segments are manually moved medially and positioned with forceps, while the transnasal wire is gently twisted to approximate the bone.
- **d** The movement is completed and the wires are tightened. Note: the transnasal wire position above and behind the posterior limb of the canthal ligament and the lacrimal fossa.
- **e** Stabilization with miniplates at the periphery of the nasoethmoidal complex, and reconstruction of nose with calvarial bone graft. No rigid fixation plates should be placed around the medial canthus or on the side wall of the nose, as their thickness and fibrosis add to the apparent interorbital width. A frontal craniotomy is needed to protect the brain and cribriform if the cribriform plate is abnormally low. Bone gaps may need grafting, if they are over a few millimeters.
- **f** Insertion of left medial canthal ligament from a lateral aspect. The transnasal wire is seen posterior and superior to the lacrimal fossa and posterior limb of the canthus.
- **g** Preoperative, medial orbital osteotomies with extracranial procedure.
- **h** Postoperative, medial orbital osteotomies with extracranial procedure.

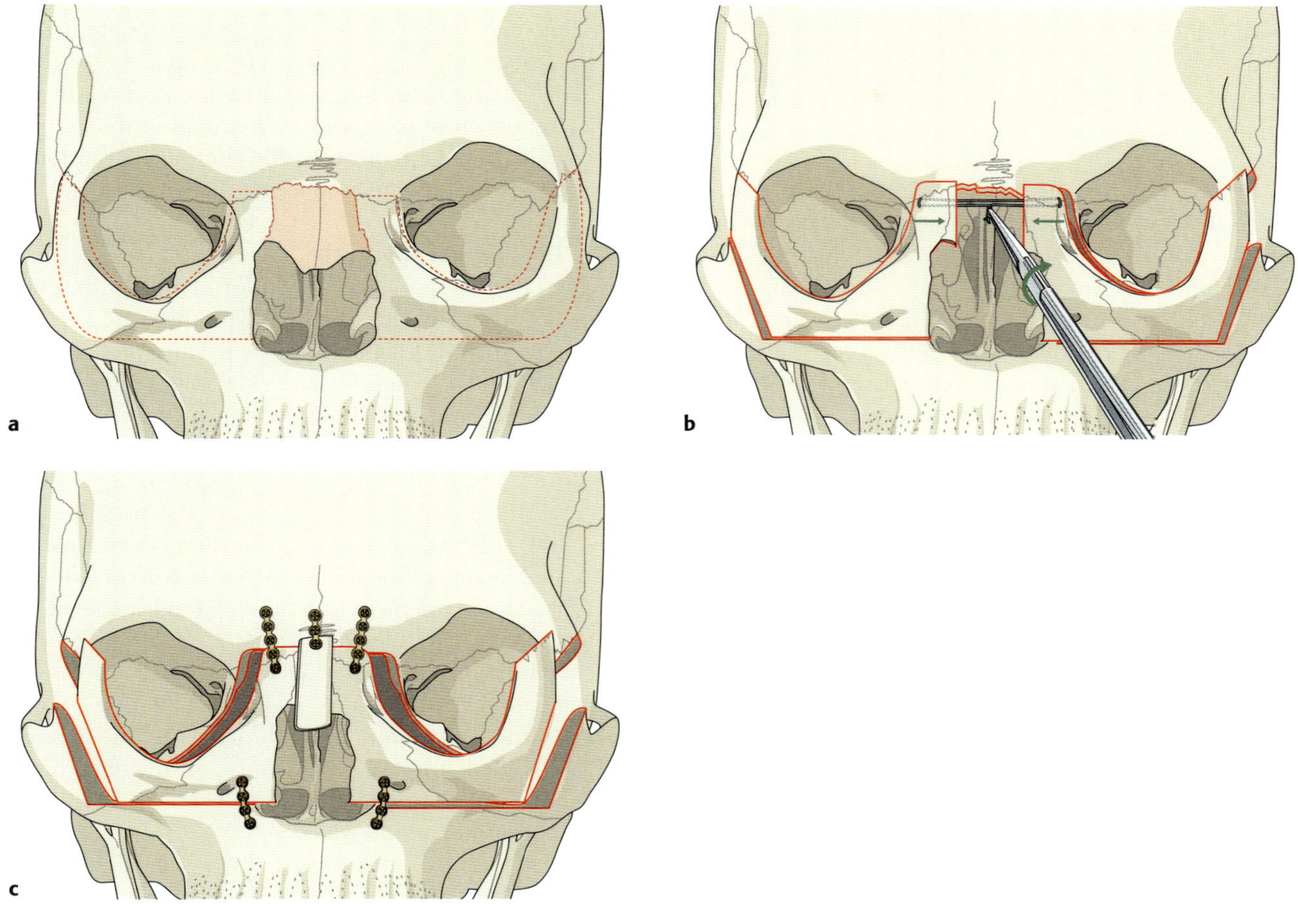

Fig 4.12-3a–c Extracranial correction of orbital hypertelorism by U-shaped osteotomies.
a U-shaped osteotomies of both orbits. Central bone portion in red to be resected.
b The fragments are moved medially and the transverse intercanthal wires tightened after the bone is positioned with forceps.
c Positioning bone segments medially after osteotomies. Stabilization is obtained with miniplates and the transnasal wires tightened (not illustrated in this diagram). The nose height is further augmented with cantilever calvarial bone graft attached to the frontal bone.

Medial orbital wall mobilization and stabilization can be effectively accomplished with predictable results. However, this is only the first step to obtaining a good result in these complex deformities.

The management of soft-tissue deformities in the medial canthal area is of overwhelming importance. It poses a much greater technical difficulty than the actual increased bony distance between the orbits. Management of the medial canthal tendon and the surrounding soft tissue is key to improving results in orbital hypertelorism correction. If the bony contour and medial canthal contour and the thickness of the soft tissue of the medial canthal area appear normal, then the canthal tendon is **not** detached. This is usually **not** the situation. However, even if the tendon is **not** detached, its attachment is always reinforced with a transnasal intercanthal wire. The medial canthal tendon is identified by making a 3–4 mm transverse incision through the skin medial to the medial eyelid commissure anteriorly exactly over the tendon. A 3-0 wire suture on a curved needle is used to secure the tendon with a modified Kessler or figure-of-eight stitch. The tendon insertion is reinforced and/or reattached to the medial orbital wall bone segment behind the posterior and superior edge of the lacrimal fossa by passing the two ends of the 3-0 wire through one or two drill holes behind the posterior aspect of the posterior limb of the medial canthal tendon insertion, superior and posterior to the lacrimal fossa. These wires extend transnasally, come out the contralateral side and can be tightened as a final step before soft-tissue closure, and the two wires are twisted over a screw in the frontal bone. There is one transnasal wire set for each canthus.

This maneuver effectively reinforces the application of the medial canthal tendon to the bone and therefore helps control the position of the medial wall bone segment for reduction and stabilization. Essentially, a single transnasal wire functions as a combination transnasal wire reduction/stabilization and soft-tissue canthopexy. Some surgeons use several sets of two wires each—one set for the stabilization of the bone segment, and one set for the canthal tendon, and one to hold the soft tissue to the bone ("compression bolster/plate"). The opposite side is treated identically, and the several sets of wires are then twisted together reducing and stabilizing the medial orbital wall bone segments (**Fig 4.12-2c–e** and **Fig 4.12-3b**). Over-reduction is **always** needed and can be easily accomplished by continued twisting of the wires, but the bone segments should be held manually in correct position with forceps, while the wires are gradually twisted to approximate the previously reduced bone segment (or the thin bone may fracture if the wires themselves are used to do the reduction). If the contour of the medial orbital rim segment is not normal, a burr is used to correct this by further reshaping or, more commonly, additional intrasegmental osteotomies may be required if the contouring cannot accomplish correction of the shape and thickness.

4.2 Intracranial approach

The intracranial approach is used for moderate to severe degrees of orbital hypertelorism. Essentially there are three surgical options: (1) standard block osteotomies, (2) medial orbital wall osteotomies, and (3) the bipartition operation. Each of these procedures combines a frontal craniotomy for intracranial exposure with the orbital osteotomies. Exposure is obtained with a coronal incision, upper gingivobuccal sulcus and eyelid incisions are also usually needed. A 360° subperiosteal orbital dissection is performed to reach the junction of the middle with the posterior third of the orbit. The entire nasoethmoid skeleton is exposed and the lacrimal sac carefully dissected free, mobilized and left attached inferiorly through the lacrimal canal. The medial canthal tendons are identified and secured with a 3-0 wire suture through a separate 3–4 mm transverse incision medial to the medial eyelid commissure, as described previously. The temporalis muscles are elevated bilaterally to expose the lateral orbital walls.

A standard frontal bone flap is designed and elevated, usually by the neurosurgeon. The supraorbital osteotomy is made 10–15 mm above the supraorbital rims, leaving a 15 mm frontal bar between the superior orbital rim and the supraorbital osteotomy in the frontal bone flap (**Fig 4.12-4** and **Fig 4.12-5**). The intracranial exposure allows safe performance of orbital roof osteotomies. The central frontonasal block is removed preserving the olfactory nerves and cribriform plate. Using the intracranial exposure, the ethmoid sinuses are unroofed and, working from above and below, the sinuses are totally/subtotally exenterated, as necessary. The orbits can now be mobilized as blocks medially. The cribriform plate and the olfactory nerves remain intact centrally and are not part of the mobilization or resection. Stabilization is accomplished with interfragment wires centrally and multiple miniplates peripherally, but miniplates should **only** be placed at the periphery of the osteotomized segments. Bone grafts are used as needed for large defects in the orbital walls and to improve the height and contour of the nose, using full thickness cranial bone in infants and outer table calvarial grafts in adults. Enlargement of the piriform aperture is needed to prevent excessively narrowing the nasal airway.

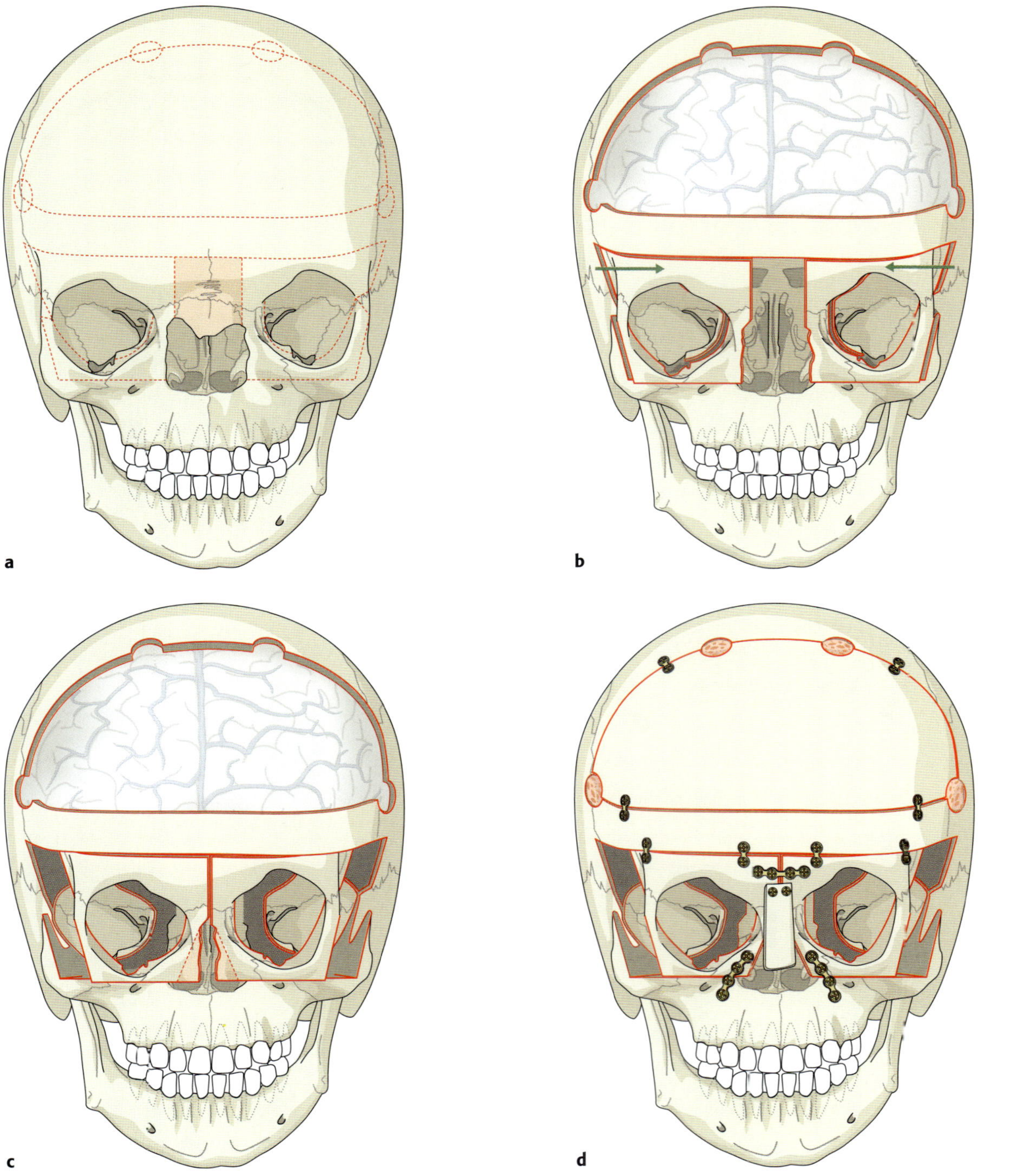

Fig 4.12-4a–d Intracranial/extracranial correction of orbital hypertelorism with block osteotomies.

a Frontal craniotomy and orbital osteotomies outlined. Central bone portion (in red) to be resected with the excess width of the ethmoid sinuses.

b Osteotomies performed and the central section of bone and ethmoid sinuses removed.

c Medial mobilization of both orbital blocks.

d Stabilization with miniplates and reconstruction of nose with cantilever calvarial bone graft. Bone gaps may need grafting (the transnasal reduction wires are omitted).

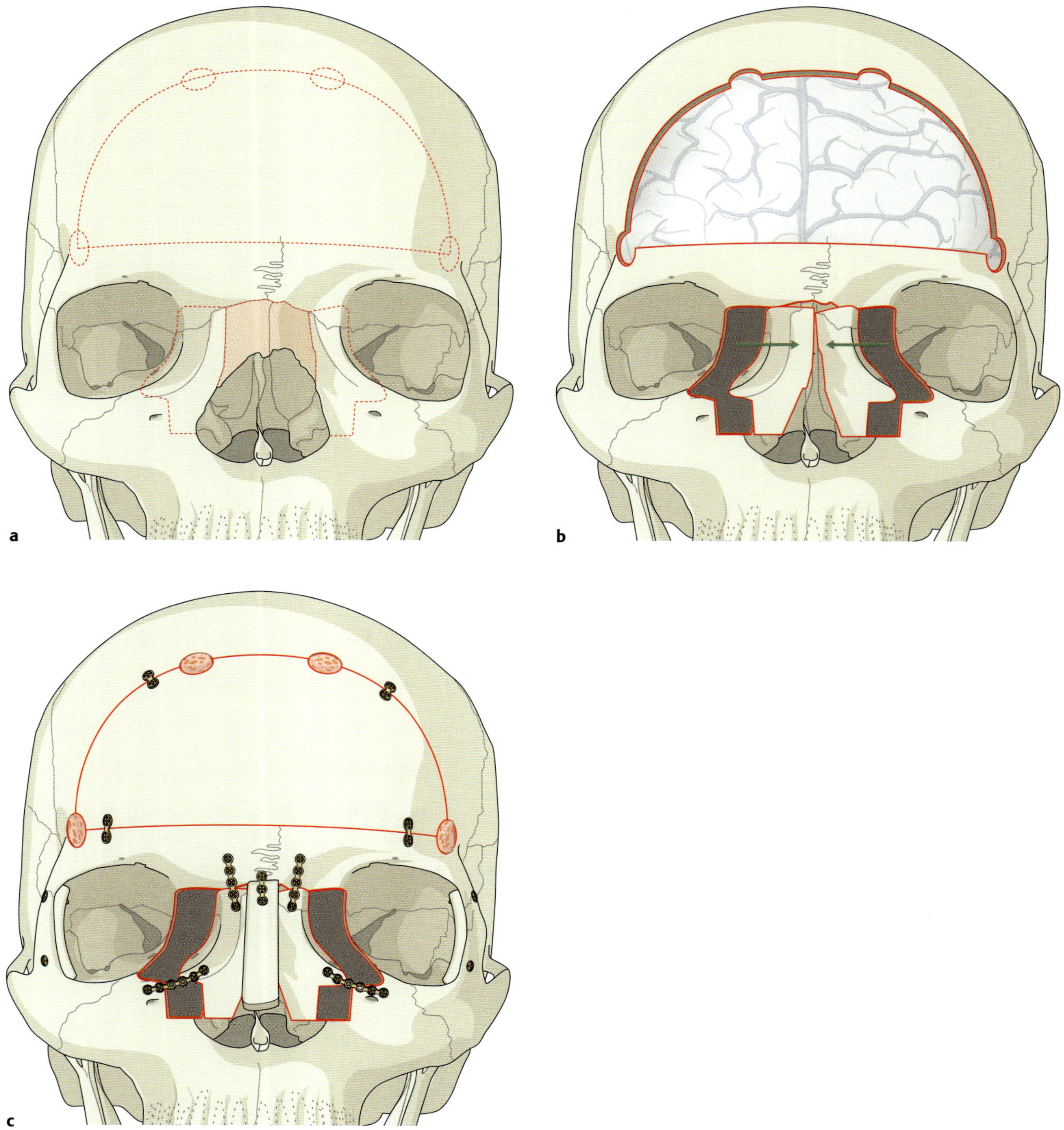

Fig 4.12-5a–c Intracranial/extracranial correction of orbital hypertelorism using medial wall osteotomies.

a Osteotomies outlined with segment of nasal bone. Central bone portion (in red) to be resected. The ethmoid sinuses also require resection.

b Mobilization of bone segments.

c Stabilization with plates and screws. Cantilever bone graft to augment the nasal dorsum. Replacement of the frontal bone segment. Lateral orbital walls are augmented with bone grafts, which are stabilized with screws; burr and drill holes are then filled with bone dust. Residual medial orbital wall defects may need bone grafts. A superior alternative to bone grafts in the lateral orbital wall are osteotomies of the lateral orbital walls with subsequent medial repositioning. In contrast to bone grafts, this will shape the anterior upper facial width, and produce a narrower transverse facial width through the orbits.

The management of the medial canthal tendons is perhaps the most important step in this procedure. The medial canthal tendons have been secured with 3-0 wire sutures through a separate canthal incision, as described previously. If the medial orbital walls are normally developed the tendon can be left attached and just reinforced into bone; this is rarely the case. Normally the medial orbital wall would benefit from additional shape contouring and/or internal osteotomies as well as further mobilization medially. In this situation "custom osteotomies" and shaping are required in the medial orbital walls with further decrease in the interorbital distance, with reshaping and contouring of the medial orbital rim segment (**Fig 4.12-6**). A transnasal canthopexy reduction/stabilization wire set is used as previously described for each canthus. Soft-tissue reduction with compression bolsters with another group of transnasal wires/sutures is performed as described in "the pitfalls and complications" section.

A cantilever calvarial bone graft is used to reconstruct the height of the nose. The frontal bone flap is replaced and secured with miniplates. The temporalis muscles are advanced and secured to the lateral orbital rims. The lateral canthal complex is secured with a 3-0 wire suture on each side and placed in a drill hole inside the orbit at the zygomatic-frontal suture level (higher than the Whitnall tubercle). Burr holes and bone gaps are filled with particulate bone. The scalp flap is closed over suction drains.

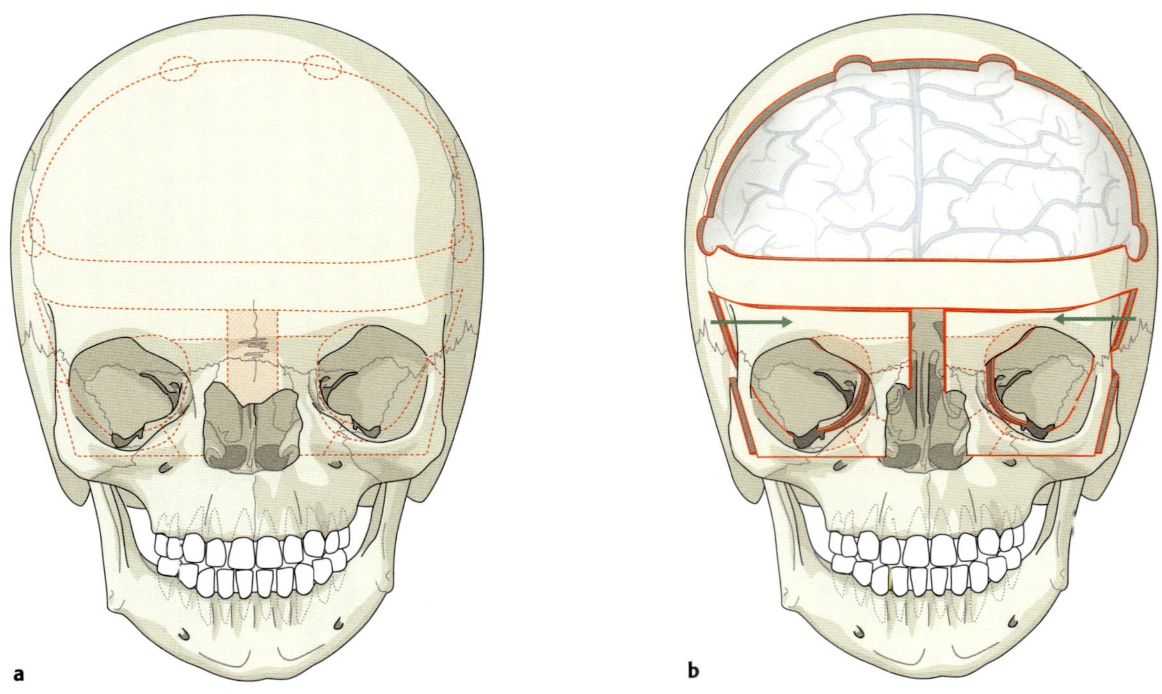

Fig 4.12-6a–i Customization of block osteotomies. The nasoethmoid skeleton may not be normalized because of standard single segment block osteotomies. Additionally, the medial walls may need to be moved more than the lateral walls.

- **a** Osteotomies outlined with segment of nasal bone. Central bone portion (in red) to be resected with the ethmoids.
- **b** Additional medial wall reshaping and custom medial orbital rim osteotomies may be needed to further shape/contour the medial orbital bone in whatever the remaining excess width portion is. One possible set of custom medial wall osteotomies and medial rim reshaping are shown after initial block osteotomies.

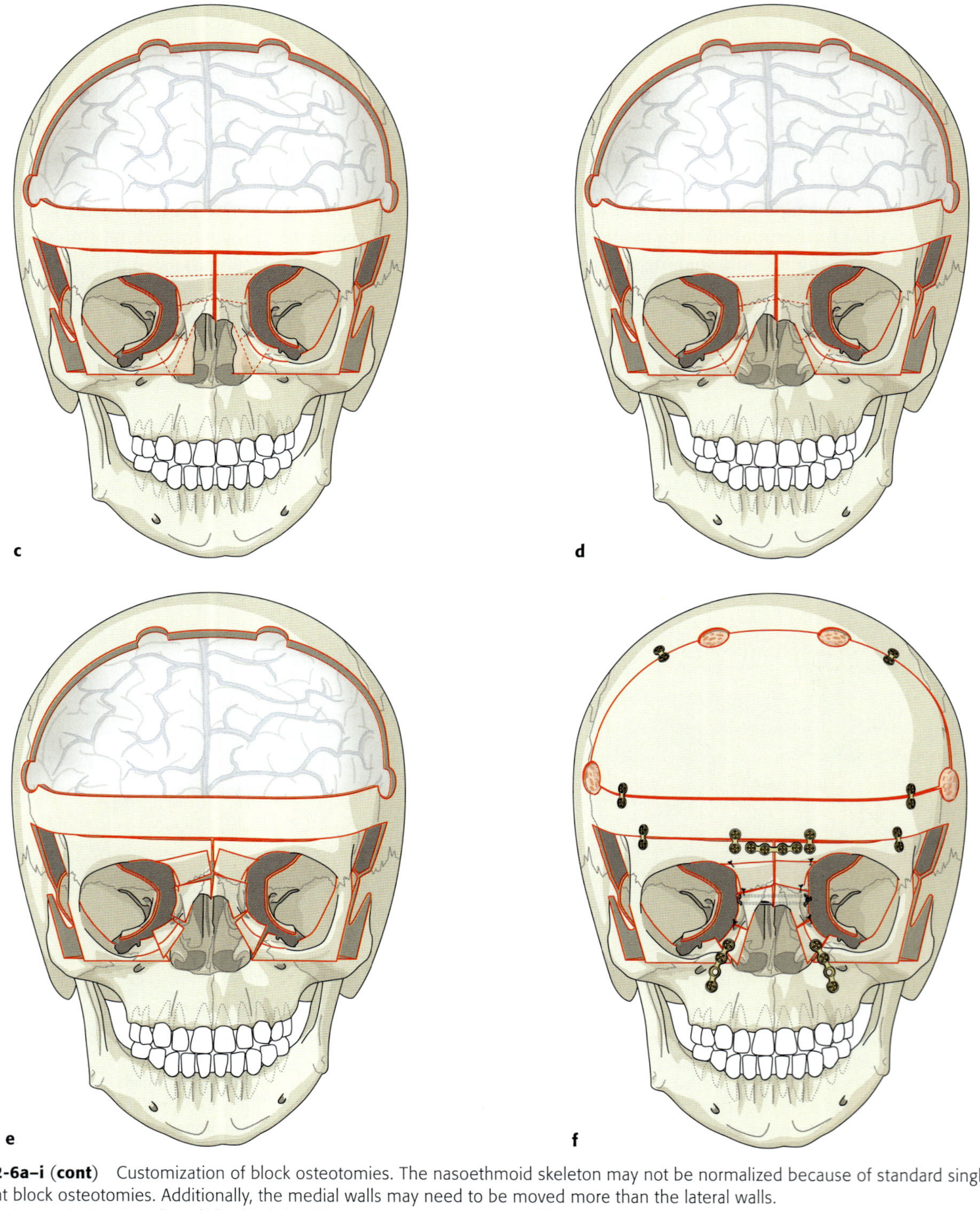

c d e f

Fig 4.12-6a–i (cont) Customization of block osteotomies. The nasoethmoid skeleton may not be normalized because of standard single segment block osteotomies. Additionally, the medial walls may need to be moved more than the lateral walls.

- **c** Custom osteotomies of medial orbital rim. Contouring corrects excess width.
- **d** Excess bone in the nasal aperture is removed.
- **e** The osteotomies are seen in red, including the additional osteotomies in the medial orbital rim.
- **f** The osteotomies are sectioned, and any further contouring of the individual segments completed, and stabilized with interfragment wires.

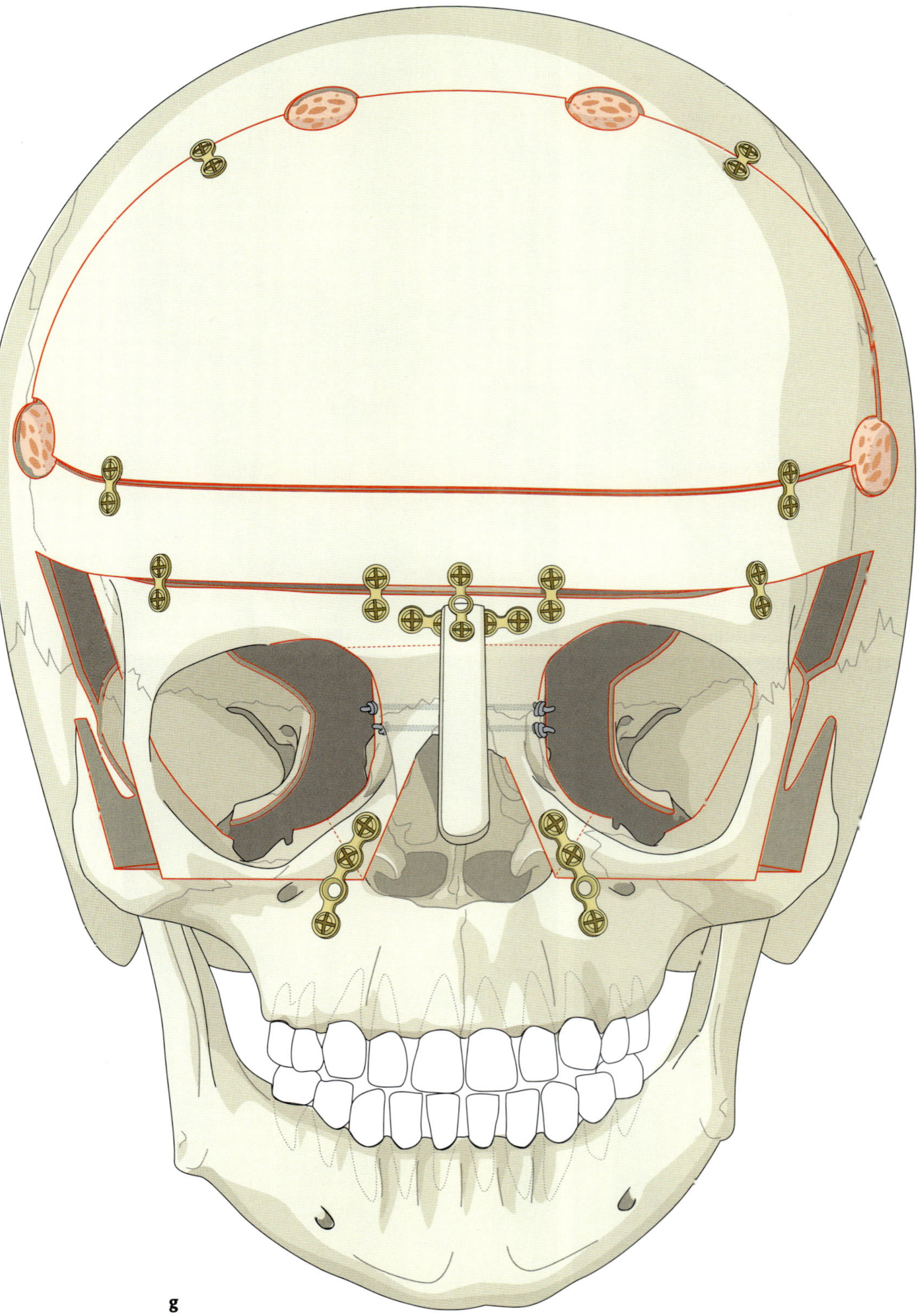

g

Fig 4.12-6a–i (cont) Customization of block osteotomies. The nasoethmoid skeleton may not be normalized because of standard single segment block osteotomies. Additionally, the medial walls may need to be moved more than the lateral walls.

g The nasal dorsum is augmented with a cantilever nasal bone graft stabilized with a miniplate.

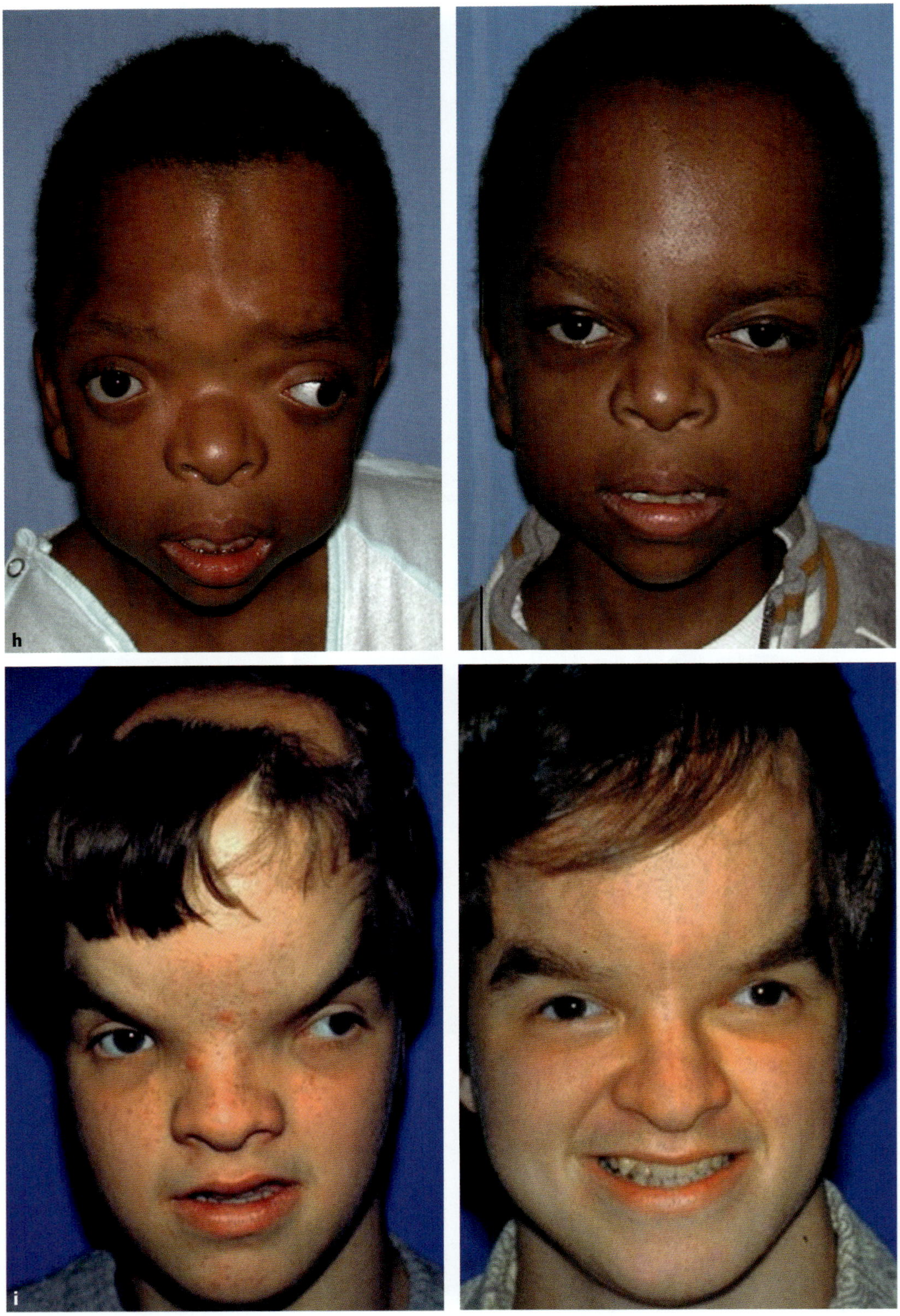

Fig 4.12-6a–i (cont) Customization of block osteotomies. The nasoethmoid skeleton may not be normalized because of standard single segment block osteotomies. Additionally, the medial walls may need to be moved more than the lateral walls.

h A patient with orbital hypertelorism before and after surgery, procedure as in **Fig 6a–i**.

i Patient with intracranial correction with "custom" medial wall osteotomies before and after surgery.

The standard block osteotomy may not always be the best option. In newborns with encephaloceles (**Fig 4.12-8**) or older patients with a mild degree of orbital hypertelorism and a prolapsed or low cribriform plate the intracranial approach with medial orbital osteotomies may be used (**Fig 4.12-5** and **Fig 4.12-7**).

In special circumstances where a monobloc advancement is being performed, a facial bipartition as described by Tessier [1972, 1974] can be used to correct the hypertelorism (**Fig 4.12-7**).

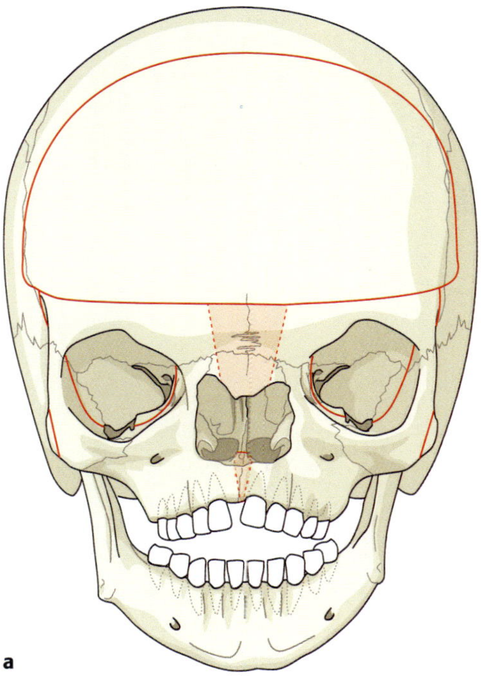

a

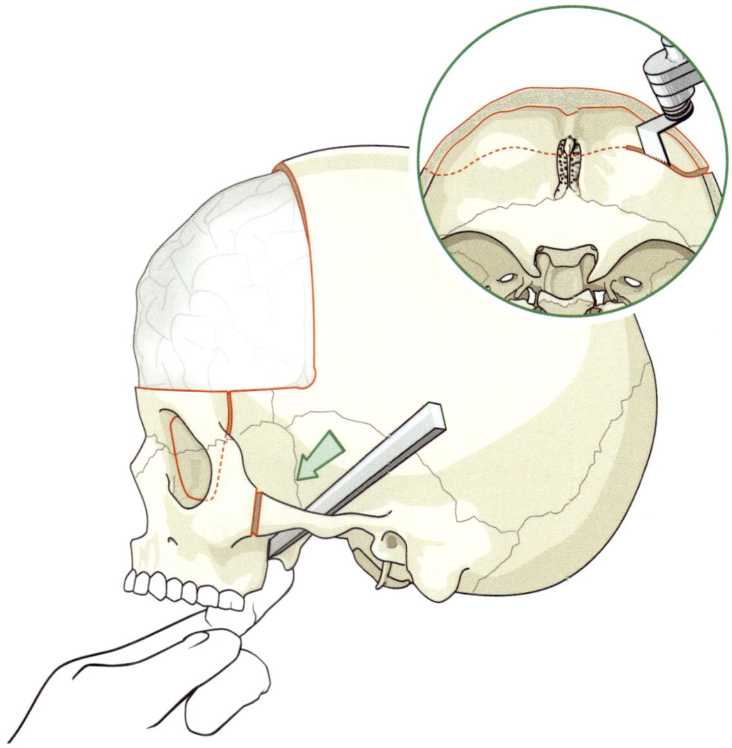

b

Fig 4.12-7a–g

a The design of the facial bipartition operation.

b Facial bipartition—cranial, orbital and maxillary osteotomies (inset). Orbital roof osteotomies.

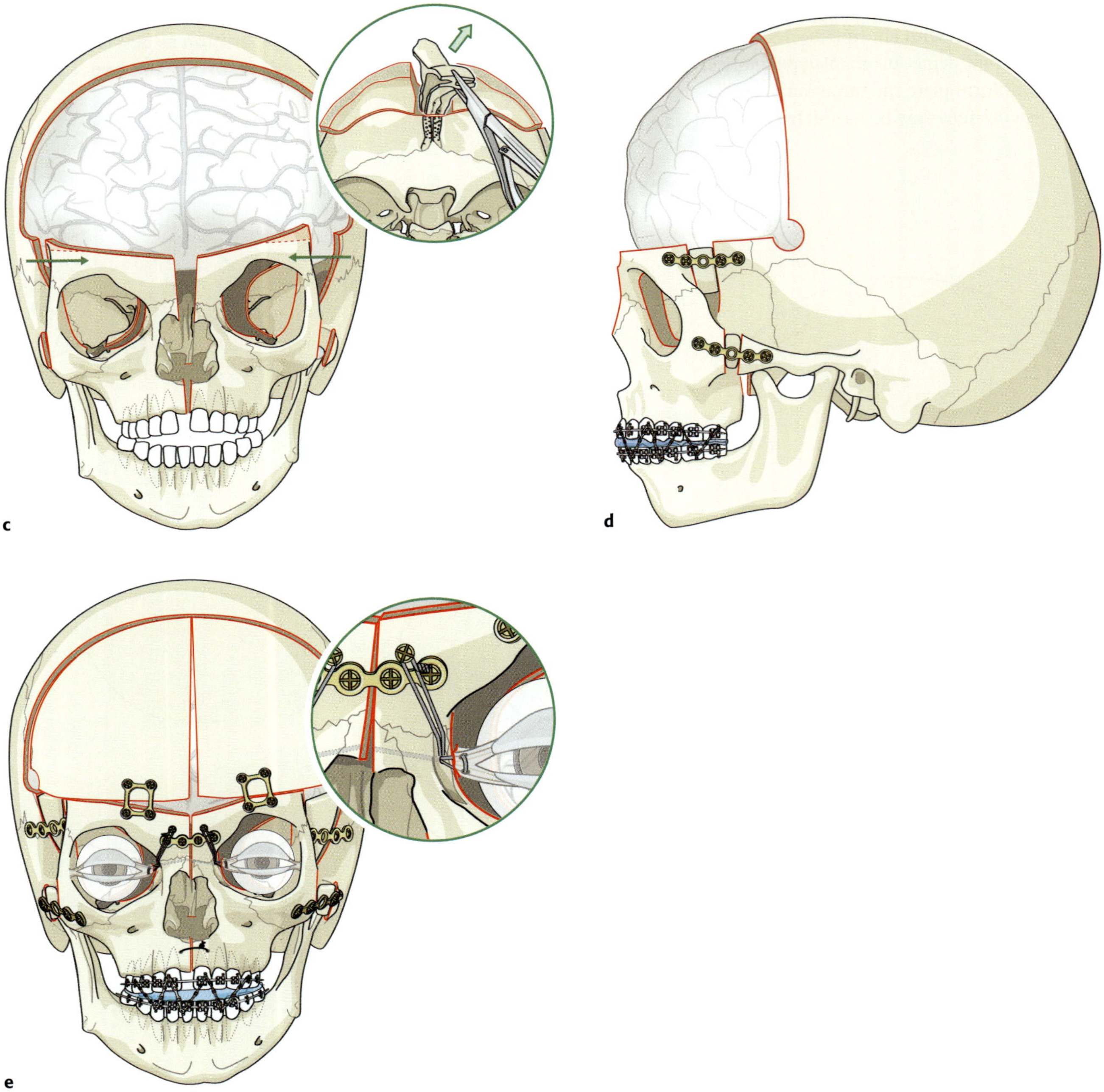

c d e

Fig 4.12-7a–g (cont)

c Facial movement of osteotomized segments. Removal of midline cranial fossa and nose (inset).

d Lateral view of fixation of mobilized segments.

e Frontal view of stabilization, transnasal canthopexies (not shown is nasal bone grafts for correction of the nasal height).

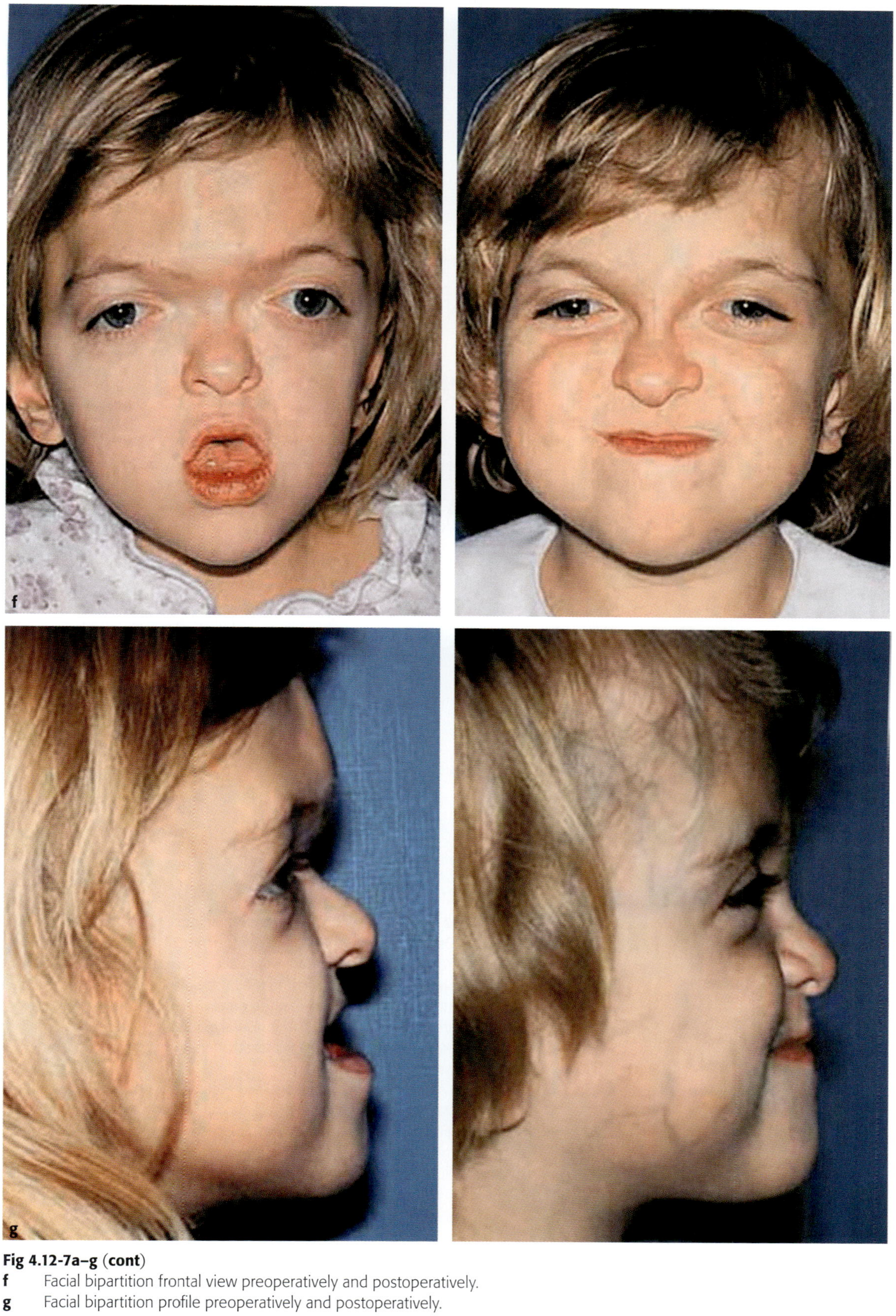

Fig 4.12-7a–g (cont)

f Facial bipartition frontal view preoperatively and postoperatively.

g Facial bipartition profile preoperatively and postoperatively.

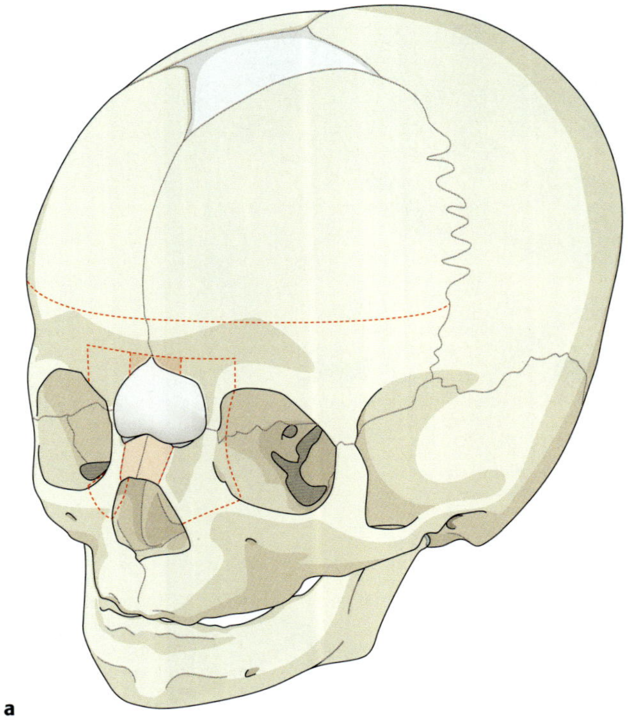

a

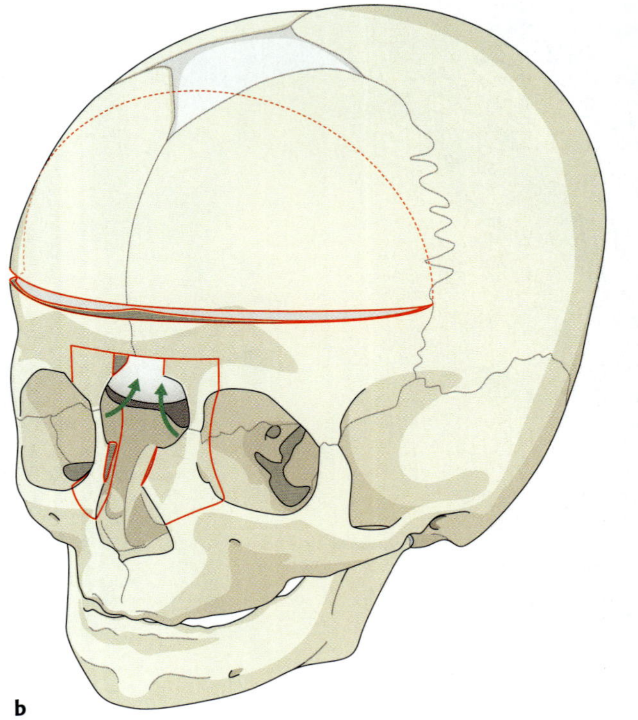

b

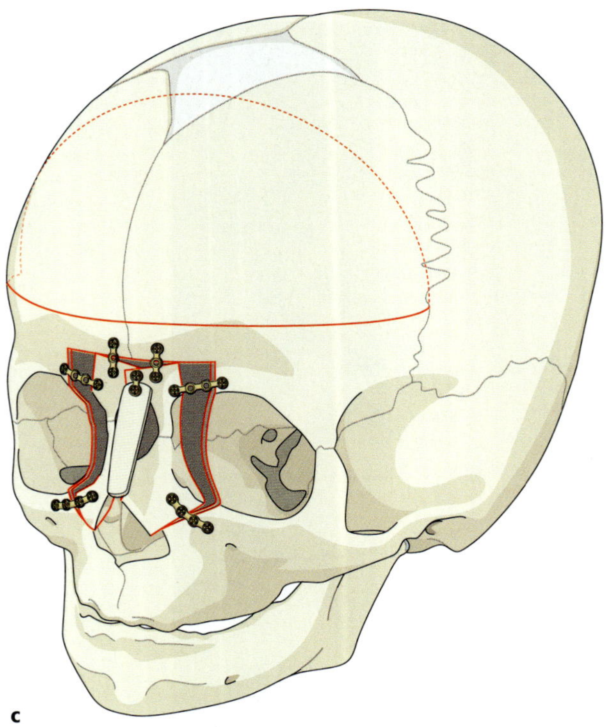

c

Fig 4.12-8a–e Correction of nasoethmoid encephalocele bone defect.

- **a** Osteotomies for mobilization of the medial orbital walls. Horizontal frontal osteotomy line for skull base exposure.
- **b** The encephalocele is corrected by replacing the prolapsed brain intracranially, and securing the dural repair. The orbital walls are centrally mobilized. The frontal osteotomy spread open for access to the skull base, or as standard frontal bone flap (dotted extension) may be performed.
- **c** The encephalocele has been corrected. The orbital walls are stabilized with miniplates and microplates and a cantilever bone graft for the nasal dorsum is in place. The remaining bone defects may need bone grafting. The transnasal canthopexy wires are not illustrated.

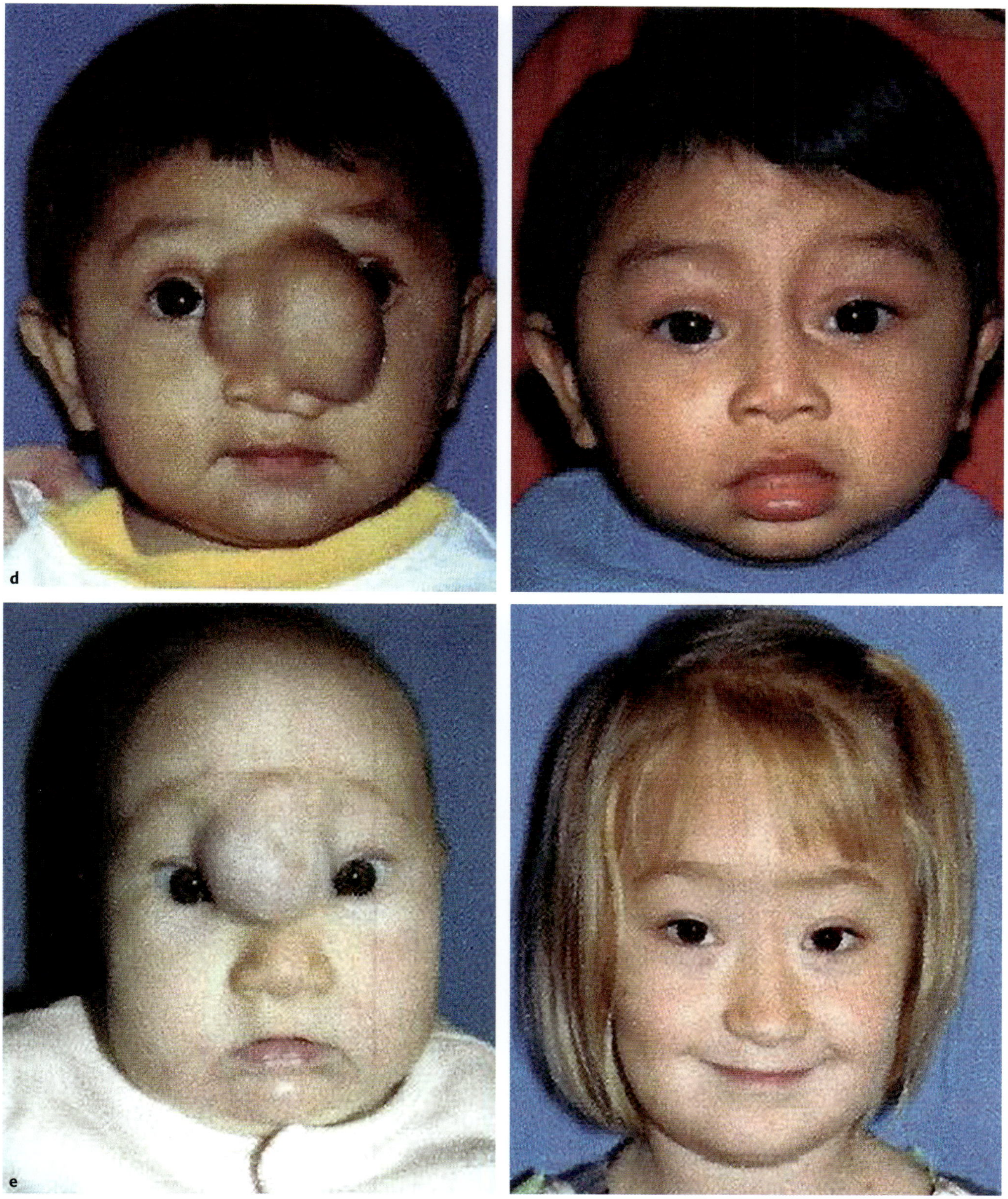

Fig 4.12-8a–e (cont) Correction of nasoethmoid encephalocele bone defect.
d Encephalocele and hypertelorism correction preoperatively and postoperatively.
e Encephalocele and hypertelorism correction.

5 Complications and pitfalls

Of all craniofacial deformities, correction of orbital hypertelorism presents the greatest challenge. There are many pitfalls that can result in poor correction of the problem. Some of these include:

1. Inadequate or under correction of the bony interorbital distance.
2. Lack of normalization of the bony contour of the nasoethmoid skeleton.
3. Medial canthal drift and epicanthal deformities.
4. Inadequate mobilization of soft tissue.
5. Inadequate soft-tissue suspension and redraping.

With rigid plate and screw fixations and custom osteotomies, correction of the bony deformity has become the most predictable part of this procedure. It is attention to the soft-tissue correction and reduction that will improve results in the treatment of orbital hypertelorism. The goal of restoring normal appearance cannot be obtained without taking steps to turn soft-tissue thickness, contour and position in the medial canthal area to normal. Nowhere in the facial skeleton is the interface of soft tissue to bone more important. Attention to this aspect of treatment will significantly improve the results. The restoration of soft-tissue contour in the nasoethmoid orbital skeleton is as important as reduction and stabilization of the bone segments **[Sargent et al, 1988]**. To perform the needed osteotomies, extensive dissection around and below the medial canthal tendon or canthal detachment may be needed. In these cases, hematoma and chronic edema may result in soft-tissue thickening, excessive tension on the medial canthal tendon with thickened scarring, dehiscence and subsequent loss of normal soft tissue to bone adherence in the thin soft tissue of the medial canthal area. This scarring process can mimic the appearance of a wide nasal bridge with telecanthus, despite excellent bony reduction of the orbit and ethmoid skeleton. The goal (and the most difficult aspect of treatment) is to restore the normal delicate appearance and contour of the thin skin in the medial canthal area and "nasoorbital" valley. Internal fixation plates that are placed on the lateral nasal bones area adjacent or anterior to the canthi insertion create a fibrotic reaction and cause a thickened and blunted appearance and should be avoided. The combination of abnormal anatomy and the wide subperiosteal dissection necessary for the osteotomies have made restoring soft-tissue contour the critical step in the hypertelorism operation. If steps are not taken to physically reduce and contour the soft tissue to the bone, then normal contour and appearance cannot be obtained and a wide deformed nasoethmoid complex will persist. This thickness and soft-tissue malposition mimic the appearance of the original deformity (**Fig 4.12-9**).

Principles of surgical technique

1. Simple canthopexy is inadequate—a 1-D repair.
2. Secure canthal tendon with wire suture (3-0 wire suture).
3. Reinforce vs reinsertion of canthal tendon.
4. Dermal canthopexies x3 sites of fixation anterior to the medial canthal tendon insertion and in nasoorbital valley (three sites of fixation) progressive tension technique (**Fig 4.12-9a**), where canthoplasty, soft-tissue canthopexies and compression all work together to achieve proper application of soft tissue to bone.
5. Thinning of soft tissue as needed.
6. Restoration of nasal height necessary to obtain normal contour of the nasoorbital valley (a term used by Converse to describe the area of the junction of the nose, maxilla and orbit lateral to the nose).
7. Soft-tissue compression bolsters to mold soft tissue to the bone of the nasal skeleton, preventing hematoma or fibrosis.
8. Over reduction of bone/soft tissue by 3–5 mms/side is always needed.

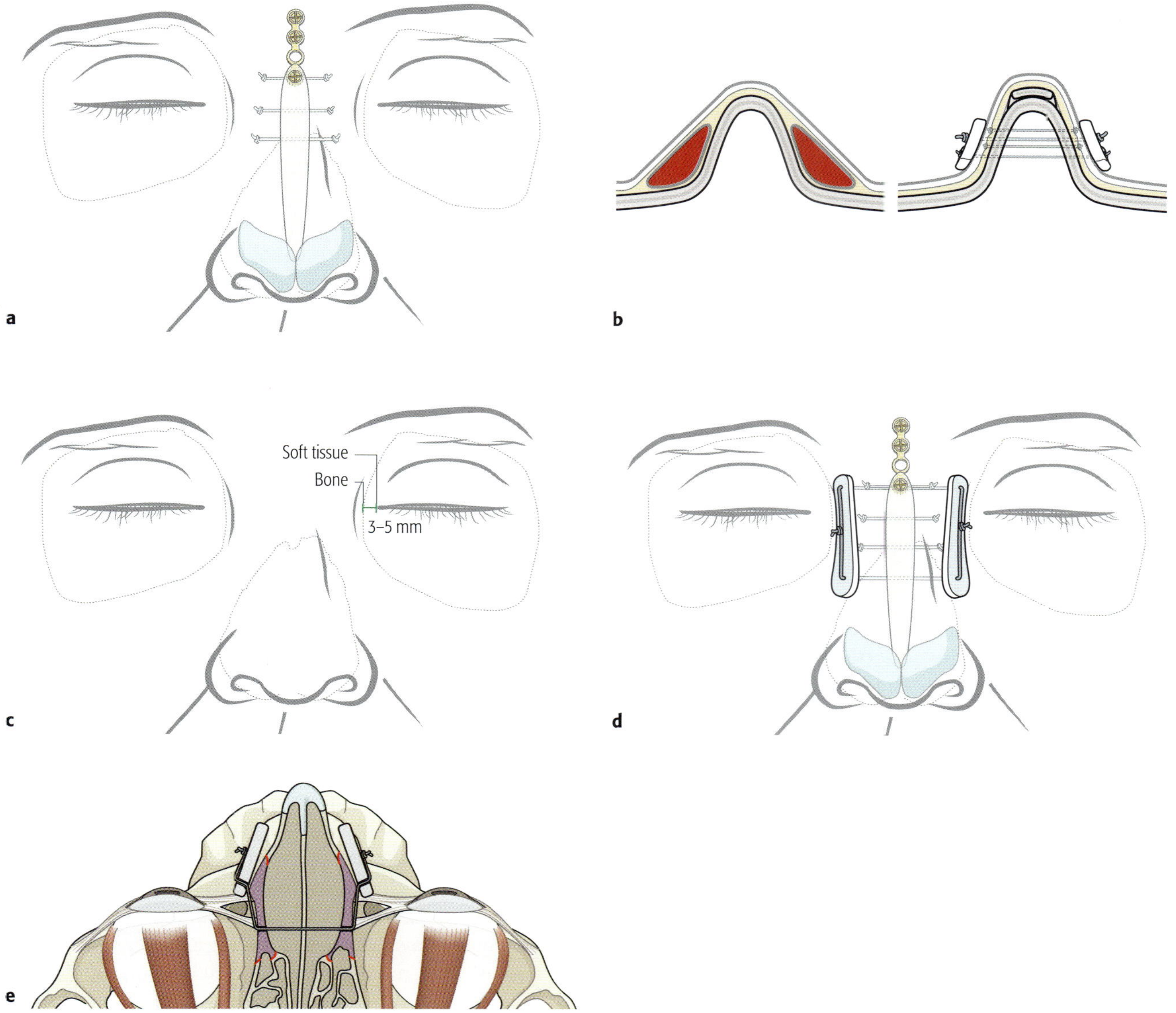

Fig 4.12-9a–e

- **a** Dermal canthopexies assist the contouring and attachment of the lateral nasal skin and soft tissue to the nose. These are led under the nasal bone graft to the other side and go from dermis to dermis. The fixation plate is under the nasal bone graft.
- **b** Lateral nasal compression bolsters limit hematoma (red) and contour the skin to the nasal bone creating a right angle, where the side wall of the nose meets the maxilla (Converse called this area the "nasoorbital valley"). Left: If the potential space between the soft tissue of the nasal sidewall and the bony lateral wall of the nose fills with hematoma followed by scar tissue (illustrated by red area) increasing the base width of the nose, then the intercanthal distance mimics the uncorrected deformity of hypertelorism while the true bony distance may have been corrected. Right: Nasal soft-tissue compression bolsters limit hematoma and contour the skin to the nasal bone. Soft-tissue canthopexies prevent hematoma and ensure that the soft tissue is closely adherent to the bone without dead space. The skin must be redraped to the exact contours of the bone. The skin at the base of the nose forms a right angle between the nose and the maxilla and orbit precisely defining the new normal contours of the nasoorbital valley.
- **c** The ideal distance of the soft tissue to bone in each canthal area is 3–5 mm/side, so the true bony intercanthal distance is 6–10 mm less than the "soft-tissue intercanthal distance".
- **d** Transnasal lead or 2.0 mm Supramid plates are padded by a half thickness of orthopedic felt wrapped in gauze (Xeroform). These soft tissue "bolsters" contour and adapt the skin and soft tissues to the nasal, periorbital and maxillary skeleton, and are secured with two transnasal wires. The bolsters have a protective layer of gauze wrapped half-thickness orthopedic felt.
- **e** Axial view of placement of upper and lower transnasal wire. Placement for soft-tissue external compression bolsters.

There are several techniques that can be used to restore the delicate contour of the medial canthal area (see "Principles of surgical technique"):

1. Dermal pexies (2–3 sutures) are used to secure skin (approximately 10 mm anterior to canthal tendon) in a curved line to underlying nasal bone (**Fig 4.12-10a**). These may go across to the contralateral skin under the nasal bone graft. This helps prevent thickening and separation of soft tissue from underlying bone caused by hematoma, edema and scarring, and recreates the normal soft-tissue contour of this area.
2. Reinforcing the medial canthal tendon attachment may be needed (left orbit, canthal wire) (**Fig 4.12-10a**). With extensive dissection and mobilization of the tendon, the resultant tension can cause stretching or pulling away of the tendon attachment. A 3-0 wire suture is used to secure the tendon to bone with a modified Kessler stitch as described previously. Preferably additional wires (or perhaps the same wire) are twisted and used for transnasal bone segment stabilization (**Fig 4.12-10a–b**).
3. The use of soft-tissue compression bolsters or plates and padding has proven to be a very effective technique to preserve the attachments of the bone to the soft sissue, reestablishing the right angle of the skin at the junction of the maxilla and the nose (**Fig 4.12-10c–d**).
4. It is important to understand the purpose of the compression bolsters. They play no role in bone stabilization or in bone position. These padded plates are to control the position and contour of the soft tissue and prevent hematoma. They are positioned over the medial canthal area and lateral nasal soft tissue to contour the skin exactly to the underlying bone. They prevent hematoma and "dead space", which would ultimately fill with hematoma and remodel to thickened scar. The other purpose of these plates is to serve as a secure nasal splint for the reconstructed nasal bones, molding them to a thin nose and improving nasal height by slight compression medially. The "soft-tissue bolsters" are made of 2 mm lead or 2 mm Supramid polyethylene padded with a half-thickness of "orthopedic felt" which has been wrapped in gauze (Xeroform). Two additional pull-out transnasal wires placed with spinal needles transnasally, inferiorly at the pyriform aperture and superiorly at the canthus, are used to secure the bolsters and provide soft-tissue compression. Correct placement of the transnasal pull-out wires is the key to proper functioning of the compression bolsters to exactly contour the structures to the desired nasal shape and height. The superior 28-gauge wire is placed through the skin of the nose anterior to the medial canthus with a spinal needle anterior to the medial canthal ligament, then through the medial orbital rim posterior and superior to the lacrimal fossa, across the nose, through the septum, then through the medial orbital rim of the other side, then through the skin anterior to the contralateral canthal tendon. The lower wire is placed through the nose, skin and septum just above the pyriform aperture and just inferior to the lateral nasal bone directly above the maxilla. The two wires are placed through the upper and lower aspects of the bolster on each side, then twisted together creating light compression of the soft tissues (**Fig 4.12-10**). Excessive tightening or pressure can cause injury and necrosis of the skin and perhaps excessive narrowing of the nose. The tension of the skin compression (circulation) must be checked daily initially under compression bolsters in the early postoperative period to adjust for swelling and to prevent pressure necrosis of skin by adjustment of wire tension. Thorough cleaning of the skin daily under the compression bolsters must be performed, visualizing the skin and cleaning with peroxide saturated cotton swabs (Q-tips). The two twisted wires on either side are first twisted together adjusting the "fit" of the plate to the skin, applying the skin and soft tissues securely to the bone of the "nasoorbital valley". This maneuver also has the effect of serving as a secure nasal bone "splint". The nasal compression plates stay in place for 7–10 days. Over the years other techniques have not been found to be as effective in restoring soft-tissue contour in this area as the soft-tissue compression bolsters.

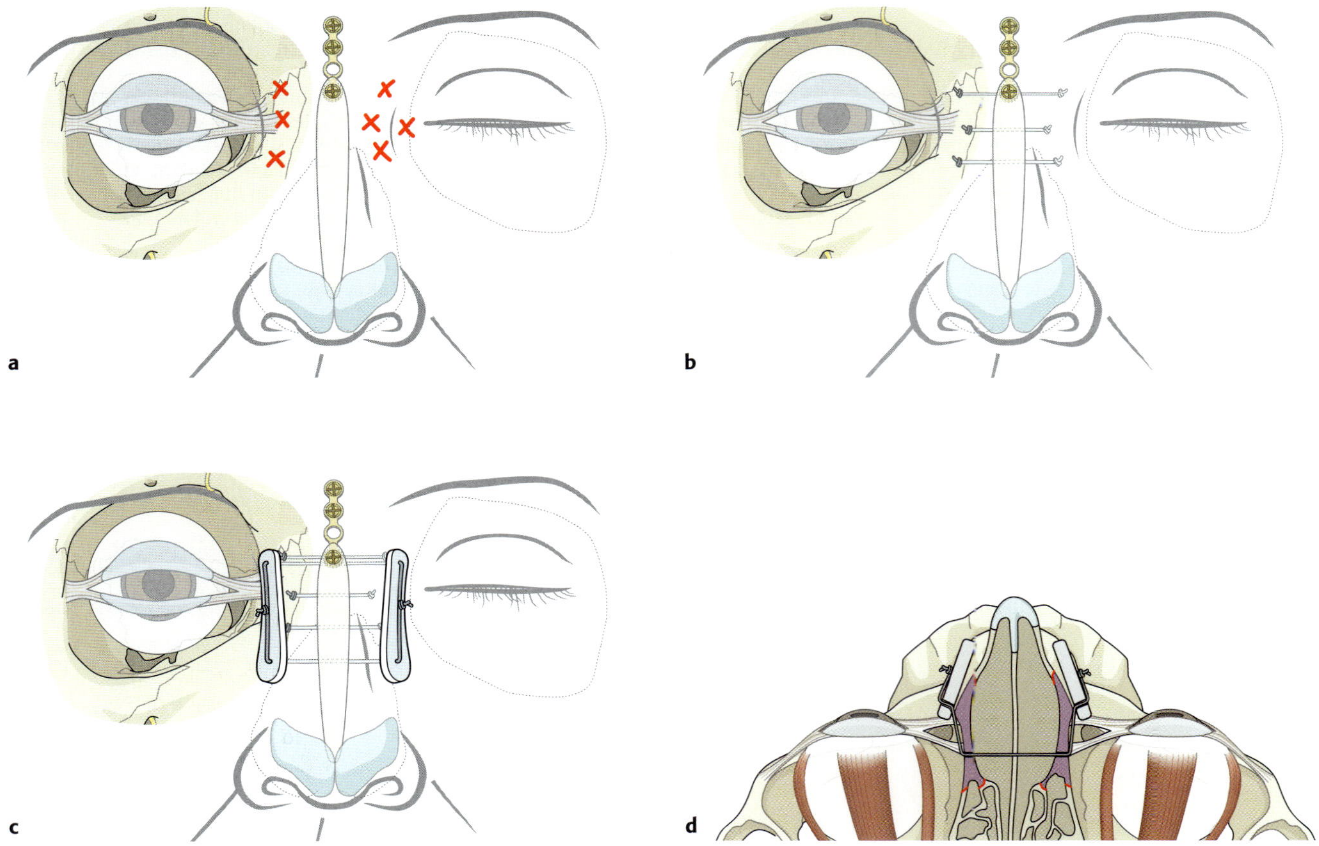

Fig 4.12-10a–d

- **a** Sites of soft-tissue canthopexies anterior 3 "x's". Posterior "x" (left) is medial canthal transnasal wire.
- **b** Soft-tissue canthopexies.
- **c** Transnasal lead or 2.0 mm supramid plates are padded by a half thickness of orthopedic felt wrapped in gauze (Xeroform). These soft tissue "bolsters" contour and adapt the skin and soft tissues to the nasal and periorbital skeleton and are secured with two transnasal wires. The bolsters have a protective layer of gauze wrapped half-thickness orthopedic felt. Dermal canthopexies are seen in addition to the transnasal bolster wires at the upper and lower ends of the compression bolsters.
- **d** Axial view of placement of two upper transnasal wires. Placement for soft-tissue external compression bolsters.

6 References and suggested reading

Apert E. De l'acrocéphalosyndactylie. *Bulletin de la Société de Médecine (Paris)*. 1906 23:1310–1330. French.

Crouzon O. Dysostose cranio-facialae héréditaire. *Bulletin de la Société des Médecins des Hôpitaux de Paris*. 1912. French.

Greig DM. Hypertelorism: a hitherto undifferentiated congenital craniofacial deformity. *Edinburgh Med J*. 1924;31:560.

McCarthy JG, La Trenta GS, Breitbart AS, et al. Hypertelorism correction in the young child. *Plast Reconstr Surg*. 1990 Aug;86(2):214–225.

Mulliken JB, Kaban LB, Evans CA, et al. Facial skeletal changes following hypertelorbitism correction. *Plast Reconstr Surg*. 1986 Jan;77(1):7–16.

Munro IR, Das SK. Improving results in orbital hypertelorism correction. *Ann Plast Surg*. 1979 Jun;2(6):499–507.

Sargent LA, Seyfer AE, Gunby EN. Nasal encephaloceles: definitive one-stage reconstruction. *J Neurosurg*. 1988 Apr;68(4):571–575.

Serafin D, Georgiade NG. Pediatric plastic surgery. In: Jackson IT, ed. *Orbital Hypertelorism*. St Louis: CV Mosby; 1984:457.

Tan ST, Mulliken JB. Hypertelorism: nosologic analysis of 90 patients. *Plast Reconstr Surg*. 1997 Feb;99(2):317–327.

Tessier P. Orbital hypertelorism I. Successive surgical attempts, material and methods, causes and mechanisms. *Scand J Plast Reconstr Surg*. 1972;6(2):135–155.

Tessier P, Guiot G, Derome P. Orbital hypertelorism II. Definite treatment of orbital hypertelorism by craniofacial or by extracranial osteotomies. *Scand J Plast Reconstr Surg*. 1973;7(1):39–58.

Tessier P. Experiences in the treatment of orbital hypertelorism. *Plast Reconstr Surg*. 1974 Jan;53(1):1–18.

van der Meulen JC, Vaandrager JM. Surgery related to the correction of hypertelorism. *Plast Reconstr Surg*. 1983 Jan;71(1):6–19.

Whitaker LA, Vander Kolk C. Orbital reconstruction in hypertelorism. *Otolaryngol Clin North Am*. 1988 Feb;21(1):199–214.

Yaremchuk MJ, Whitaker LA, Grossman R, et al. An objective assessment of treatment for orbital hypertelorism. *Ann Plast Surg*. 1993 Jan;30(1):27–34.

4.13 Encephaloceles

Neal D Futran

1 Introduction

Nasal encephaloceles are herniations of meninges with or without brain tissue through defects in the skull base into the nose. These lesions can be congenital in origin, representing a primary anomaly of the neural tube and its skeletal cover. Most encephaloceles are seen in early childhood. However, these lesions can also manifest in later years of life. Traumatic encephaloceles are categorized as lesions due to head injury or iatrogenic conditions following sinonasal surgery. Anterior skull base encephaloceles usually involve herniation of the frontal lobe tissue through an anterior cranial fossa defect into the ethmoid sinus or nasal cavity. The ethmoid and sphenoid sinuses are the most common sites for encephalocele development [Hughes et al, 1980].

Historically, several mechanisms have been proposed for the pathogenesis of nasal encephaloceles [Sessions, 1982]. The most widely held view is the "encephalocele theory", which suggests that these lesions develop as a protrusion of forebrain secondary to faulty closure of the anterior neuropore. Based on this theory, a nasal encephalocele results from herniation of intracranial tissues into the dural projection through the foramen cecum or fonticulus frontalis (**Fig 4.13-1**).

Furthermore, nasal gliomas represent an encephalocele that becomes sequestrated from the brain and cranial vault early in gestation, and the stalk degenerates early, obliterating a true connection to brain parenchyma. These can also result from severe trauma to the skull base.

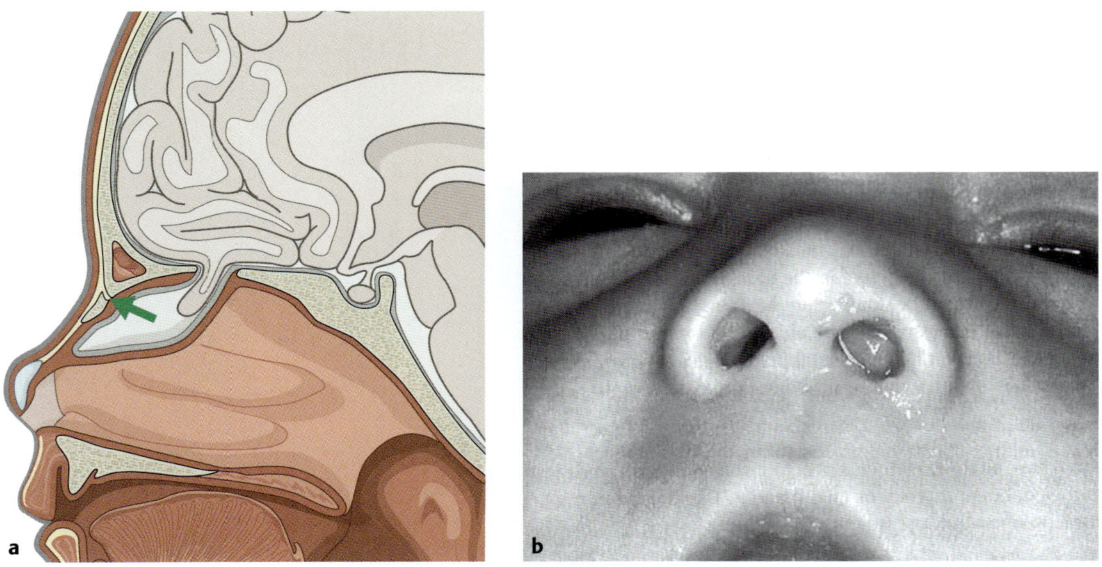

Fig 4.13-1a–b Diagram and clinical picture of an encephalocele.
a Sagittal diagram of the skull base at the midline showing potential pathway of an encephalocele to develop through the foramen cecum. Another pathway is the fonticulus frontalis (arrow).
b A 3-month-old infant with an encephalocele presenting as a left nasal mass.

It is often not possible to distinguish glioma from encephaloceles based on histopathological findings because glial tissue might be the exclusive or predominant component in both types of lesions [Jaffe, 1981]. Although ependymal tissue is not always identified in encephaloceles, when it is present the diagnosis of encephalocele is more likely. When recognizable leptomeninges are absent, encephaloceles can be distinguished from glioma only after clinicopathological correlation. Furthermore, encephaloceles may be classified based on the tissue content of the extracranial herniation: (1) meningoceles only contain meninges, (2) meningoencephalocele (ie, encephalocele) contains neural tissue and meninges, and (3) meningoencephalocystoceles contain meninges, neural tissue, and ventricular system tissue.

2 Indications, planning and correction

The first medical report of an encephalocele may have appeared in the 16th century. This condition occurs in 1 of every 35,000 live births and is equally distributed between male and female patients. Most encephaloceles are seen in early childhood [Muraszko, 1996; Hoving, 2000]. Owing to the intracranial connection, there is pulsation and expansion of the mass with crying, straining, or compression of the jugular vein (Fürstenberg test). Patients may have symptoms of sinusitis (ie, persistent rhinorrhea, nasal airway obstruction) with "nasal polyps" seen on endoscopy.

The proper management of nasal glioma and encephalocele requires a multidisciplinary approach that includes craniomaxillofacial surgery, neurosurgery, and neuroradiology. Patients should undergo a complete examination to exclude any other congenital abnormalities. Nasal endoscopy is performed to determine the location, origin, and extent of the nasal mass and to assess lack of or presence of pulsation, which is of vital importance. Needle aspiration or biopsy should be avoided [Mahapatra et al, 2006].

The evaluation must include cross-sectional imaging studies to assess the location, size, and contents of the lesion [Van Den Abbeele et al,1999]. The integrity of the anterior skull base should be assessed, and herniation of intracranial contents into the nasal region should be documented. Thin-section, high-resolution axial and coronal computed tomographic (CT) images provide useful information about the bony anatomy (**Fig 4.13-2**).

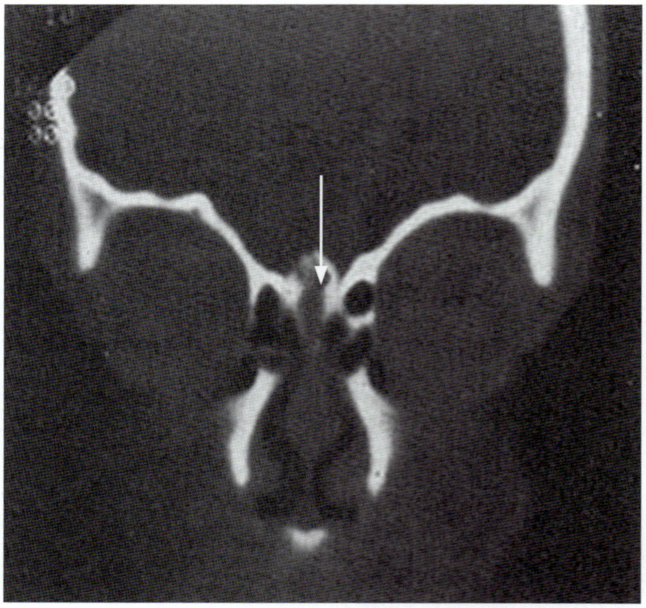

Fig 4.13-2 Coronal computed tomographic scan showing detailed anatomy of the anterior skull base with an encephalocele (arrow).

In young infants, the anterior skull base is only partially ossified or unossified. In this situation, intravenous contrast is used to delineate the cartilaginous skull base. Thin-section, high-resolution multiplanar magnetic resonance imaging provides complementary information to CT regarding the fluid or soft-tissue characteristics of the mass (**Fig 4.13-3**).

Herniation of meninges alone (meningocele) or brain and meninges (encephalocele) is sometimes apparent. Contrast-enhanced images should be obtained to assist in the differential diagnosis of solid masses or when the presence of infection is suspected. The preferred management of encephaloceles is surgical excision [Oucheng et al, 2010]. These lesions have a slow growth rate and are benign, without any potential for malignant transformation. Therefore, it is possible to pursue a comprehensive preoperative evaluation and carefully compose the most appropriate surgical plan. Traditionally, treatment of anterior skull base encephaloceles has included an open approach via a frontal craniotomy (see chapter 4.12). This approach may have substantial morbidity, including permanent anosmia from mobilization of the olfactory bulbs, longer operation and hospitalization time, and late recurrence of up to 50% in some cases. Surgical approaches to encephaloceles in the anterior skull base have changed over time. The nasal passages are natural corridors, providing easy access to the anterior cranial base. The advent of endoscopic sinus surgery has allowed transnasal approaches to the anterior skull base to become routine [Boseley et al, 2004; Van Den Abbeele et al, 1999; Marshall et al, 2001] (**Fig 4.13-4**).

The endoscopic approach, with the rapid advancements in its instrumentation, significantly enhances visualization of the entire sinonasal roof and has become the mainstream approach in the treatment of skull base and sinonasal diseases, including the repair of cerebrospinal fluid (CSF) rhinorrhea. This allows for the removal of the encephalocele and seal of the skull base. This is borne out by studies showing the efficacy of endoscopic repair of CSF leaks. For example, it has been estimated at 90% in 522 cases after a single procedure with the most common complication of meningitis recorded in only 1%. Lanza et al [1996] had the largest number of endoscopically repaired encephaloceles in a 4-year study, which included 11 patients with encephaloceles of the 36 patients who presented with skull base defects. The application of an image guidance system is recommended, which can provide guidance about superior extension toward the skull base as well as complete and safe resection of the mass.

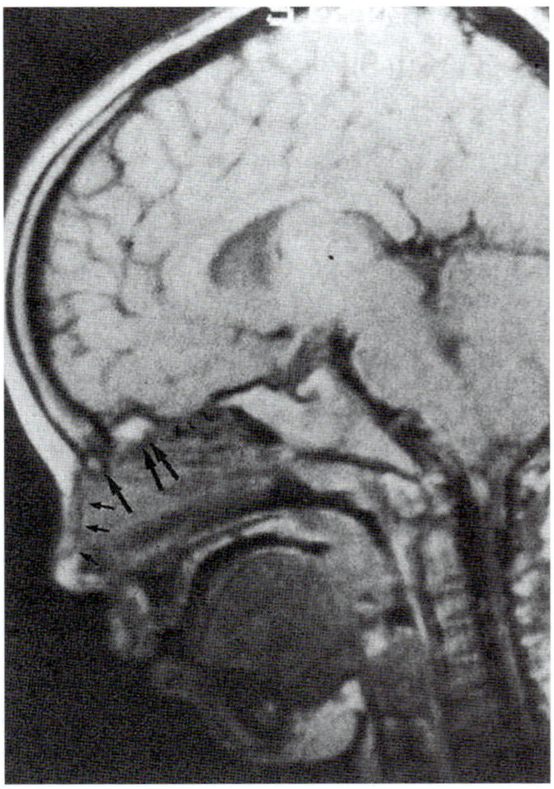

Fig 4.13-3 Sagittal magnetic resonance imaging section through the midline is able to show tissue and fluid characteristics of the mass.

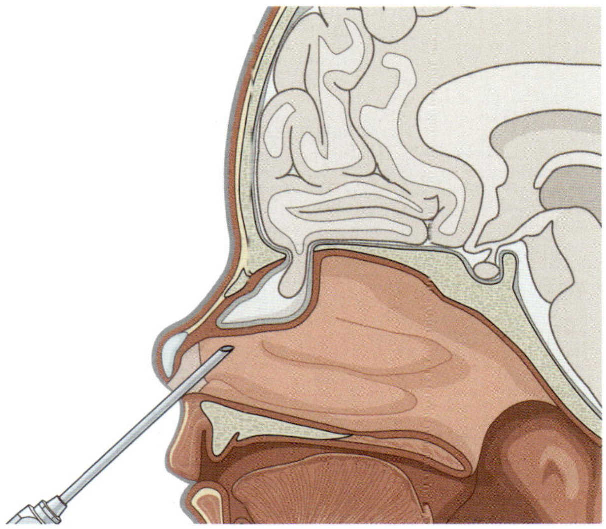

Fig 4.13-4 Sagittal diagram of endoscope placed in the nose to visualize sinus and anterior skull base.

Although there is no one surgical method accepted as the standard of care, various devices, including powered instruments, cautery, and hand instruments, may be used to remove encephaloceles [Boseley et al, 2004]. Most procedures describe the use of some form of cautery to decrease the potential for a blood vessel within the substance of an encephalocele bleeding into the intracranial space during reduction. This involves meticulous monopolar or bipolar cautery to decrease the potential for intracranial bleeding during removal. Excision or amputation of the pouch is necessary because the neural tissue within the encephalocele is redundant, necrotic, and nonfunctioning. Once the encephalocele is removed, the site is prepared and reconstructed with diverse grafting methods that may include bone and fascial grafts. An underlaid composite graft offers a promising closure and efficaciously prevents ascending infection from the nose to the cranium (**Fig 4.13-5**).

Based on the literature [Banks et al, 2009; Woodworth et al, 2006; Woodworth et al, 2008; Lanza et al, 1996; Marton et al, 2005; Nyquist et al, 2010], both overlay and underlay procedures appear to offer similar success rates in the management of CSF rhinorrhea. However, an overlaid graft is inherently easier to displace than an underlay graft, especially on a steep or bumpy surface of the skull base bone. When the skull defect is > 1.0 cm in diameter, a sturdy graft is required to act as a stable barrier between the cranium and nasal cavity to uphold the herniated sac of the encephalocele. A turbinate composite graft placed between the dura and skull bone (underlay procedure) is stable enough and less likely to slip away, and is therefore more favorable than placing the graft beneath the skull bone (overlay procedure). Several intranasal flaps from the inferior turbinate, the middle turbinate, and the nasal septum can also be rotated to repair cranial base defects and/or cover the graft. These matters are particularly important in the management of the anterior skull base defects including the cribriform plate and anterior ethmoid fovea.

For patients with a large intracranial component of the encephalocele, a 2-stage procedure can be considered. The first stage of the procedure should be a frontal craniotomy with resection of the intracranial component and repair of the dural and possible skull base bony defect. The extracranial component may be removed later or preferably at the same setting. The extracranial approach is based on the location and size of the nasal mass. Often the extracranial-extranasal component can be excised through the same coronal incision by extending the coronal flap down to the bony-cartilage junction of the nasal dorsum. This provides excellent exposure for excision of the extracranial component and the best cosmetic result by avoiding other incisions. A transnasal endoscopic approach is advocated for the excision of an extracranial-intranasal component of the encephalocele.

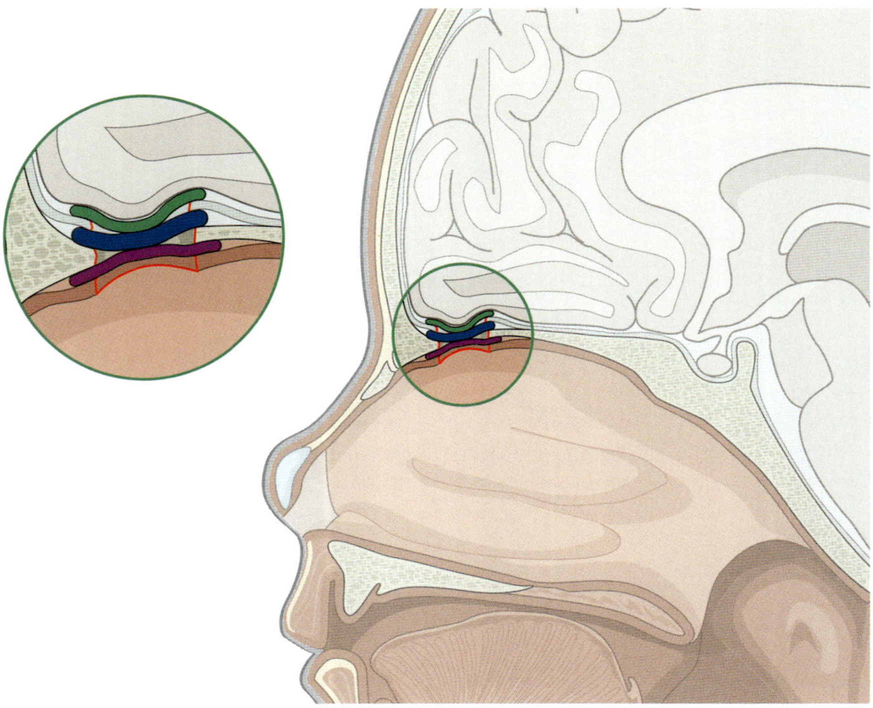

Fig 4.13-5 Sagittal diagram of a layered reconstruction of an anterior skull base defect. Green indicates dura replacement patch; blue, intermediate layer, eg, fascia; and purple, mucosal flap, eg, nasal septal flap.

3 Complications and pitfalls

Detailed methodical history gathering and thorough evaluations of radiographic studies are also imperative for the diagnosis of encephaloceles. Overlooking an encephalocele on endoscopy can lead to a failure of repair and fatal complications, such as delayed meningitis. Meticulous endoscopic controls during the operation are essential to identifying skull lesions. The communication with the nasal cavity in cases of encephalocele carries a significantly higher risk of CSF leakage and neurosurgical complications than that in other types of CSF leaks into the sinuses (**Fig 4.13-6**).

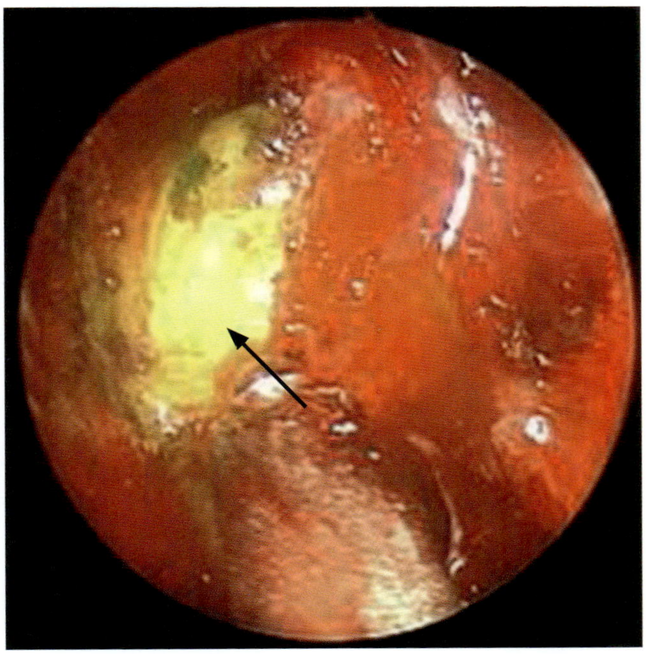

Fig 4.13-6 Intrathecal fluorescein (arrow) allows easy visualization of a cerebrospinal fluid leak through the anterior skull base through nasal endoscopy.

Because CSF leaks provide an intracranial communication for the development of ascending meningitis, it is critical to seal the skull base defect. A successful endoscopic repair includes removal of the encephalocele to expose the defect for placement of grafts or flaps. It is critical to achieve meticulous hemostatis to avoid any bleeding during resection of the encephalocele.

Injury to major vessels or the pituitary-hypothalamus axis is frequent and may have fatal consequences. Appropriate neurosurgical support is, thus, required in such situations. The patient is instructed to avoid nose blowing, strenuous exercise, or valsalva type maneuvers for 2 weeks postoperatively, which reduces stress on the skull base repair.

Cerebrospinal fluid rhinorrhea can occur postoperatively. This should be treated aggressively because of the potential risks of pneumocephalus, ascending meningitis, and fatal brain abscess [Banks et al, 2009; Woodworth et al, 2006; Woodworth et al, 2008; Lanza et al, 1996; Marton et al, 2005; Nyquist et al, 2010]. Most cases of CSF rhinorrhea can be initially managed with the insertion of a lumbar drain. Diverting CSF through a lumbar drain can prevent the formation of a fistula and thus reduce the risk of infection. A lumbar drain can decrease the intracranial pressure as well as minimize CSF pressure fluctuation. Repeated surgical repair is contemplated only if lumbar drainage failed to resolve the leak.

4 References and suggested reading

Banks CA, Palmer JN, Chiu AG, et al. Endoscopic closure of CSF rhinorrhea: 193 cases over 21 years. *Otolaryngol Head Neck Surg.* 2009 Jun;140(6):826–833.

Boseley ME, Tami TA. Endoscopic management of anterior skull base encephaloceles. *Ann Otol Rhinol Laryngol.* 2004 Jan;113(1):30–33.

Hoving EW. Nasal encephaloceles. *Childs Nerv Syst.* 2000 Nov;16(10-11):702–706.

Hughes GB, Sharpino G, Hunt W, et al. Management of the congenital midline nasal masses: a review. *Head Neck Surg.* 1980 Jan-Feb;2(3):222–233.

Jaffe BF. Classification and management of anomalies of the nose. *Otolaryngol Clin North Am.* 1981 Nov;14(4):989–1004.

Lanza DC, O'Brien DA, Kennedy DW. Endoscopic repair of cerebrospinal fluid fistula and encephaloceles. *Laryngoscope.* 1996 Sep;106(9 Pt 1):1119–1125.

Mahapatra AK, Agrawal D. Interior encephaloceles: a series of 103 cases over 32 years. *J Clin Neurosci.* 2006 Jun;13(5):536–539.

Marshall AH, Jones NS, Robertson IJ. Endoscopic management of basal encephaloceles. *J Laryngol Otol.* 2001 Jul;115(7):545–547.

Marton E, Billeci D, Schiesari E, et al. Transnasal endoscopic repair of cerebrospinal fluid fistulas and encephaloceles: surgical indications and complications. *Minim Invasive Neurosurg.* 2005 Jun;48(3):175–181.

Muraszko KM. Encephaloceles. In: Wilkins RH, Rengachary SS, eds. *Neurosurgery.* New York: McGraw-Hill; 1996:3573–3579.

Nyquist GG, Anand VK, Mehra S, et al. Endoscopic endonasal repair of anterior skull base non-traumatic cerebrospinal fluid leaks, meningoceles, and encephaloceles. *J Neurosurg.* 2010 Nov;113(5):961–966.

Nogueira JF Jr, Stamm AC, Vellutini E, et al. Endoscopic management of congenital meningo-encephalocele with nasal flaps. *Int J Pediatr Otorhinolaryngol.* 2009 Jan;73(1):133–137.

Oucheng N, Lauwers F, Gollogly J, et al. Frontoethmoidal meningoencephalocele: appraisal of 200 operated cases. *J Neurosurg Pediatr.* 2010 Dec;6(6):541–549.

Sessions RB. Nasal dermal sinuses: new concepts and explanations. *Laryngoscope.* 1982 Aug;92(8 Pt 2 Suppl 29):1–28.

Van Den Abbeele T, Elmaleh M, Herman P, et al. Transnasal endoscopic repair of congenital defects of the skull base in children. *Arch Otolaryngol Head Neck Surg.* 1999 May;125(5):580–584.

Woodworth BA, Schlosser RJ. Repair of anterior skull base defects and CSF leaks. *Op Tech Otolaryngol.* 2006;18:111–116.

Woodworth BA, Prince A, Chiu AG, et al. Spontaneous CSF leaks: a paradigm for definitive repair and management of intracranial hypertension. *Otolaryngol Head Neck Surg.* 2008 Jun;138(6):715–720.

4.14 Medication-related osteonecrosis of the jaw

Sven Otto, Suad Aljohani

1 Background

1.1 Antiresorptive drugs

Antiresorptive drugs (ARDs), including bisphosphonates and denosumab, are widely used in the treatment of metastatic bone disease, multiple myeloma, osteoporosis, and other metabolic bone diseases, such as Paget disease and osteogenesis imperfecta [Lipton, 2004]. They act by decreasing bone resorption and thereby increasing bone density [Jobke et al, 2014]. Patients with cancer and bone metastasis may complain of pain, skeletal-related events (SREs), such as fractures, and hypercalcemia as a result of increased osteoclast activity [So et al, 2012]. These complications can be managed by ARDs, which have been shown to improve quality of life and decrease mortality and morbidity in cancer patients with bone metastases [So et al, 2012]. In addition, many randomized clinical trials have shown that ARDs can improve bone mineral density and reduce the risk of fractures in patients with osteoporosis [Cosman et al, 2014].

Bisphosphonates are classified according to their structure and contain the more potent nitrogen-containing bisphosphonates including zoledronate, pamidronate, alendronate, risedronate, and ibandronate; and the less potent non-nitrogen–containing bisphosphonates including etidronate, tiludronate, and clodronate [Russell, 2007]. These two classes of bisphosphonates differ also in their mechanism of action. Non-nitrogen–containing bisphosphonates are incorporated into non-hydrolysable analogues of adenosine triphosphate, which induce osteoclast apoptosis [Otto, 2014]. In contrast, nitrogen-containing bisphosphonates act by inhibiting farnesyl pyrophosphate synthase which is essential for the production of isoprenoid lipids necessary for the post-translational prenylation of small GTPases [Rogers et al, 2011]. This results in loss of osteoclast function and apoptosis, and subsequently can suppress bone resorption. Bisphosphonates potency varies also according to their route of administration [Cremers et al, 2011]. Intravenously administered bisphosphonates including zoledronate, ibandronate, and pamidronate are remarkably more potent and are approved mainly for oncological indications. Orally administered bisphosphonates, such as alendronate, risedronate, and ibandronate are less potent and are approved mainly for osteoporosis [Russell et al, 2008]. More recently, yearly single infusions of zoledronate and 3-monthly intravenous ibandronate injections have been approved for osteoporosis treatment [Anastasilakis et al, 2012].

Denosumab is a full human monoclonal antibody that binds to and neutralizes receptor activator of nuclear factor κ B ligand (RANKL), which blocks the formation, function, and survival of osteoclast and suppression of bone turnover [Moen et al, 2011] (**Fig 4.14-1**).

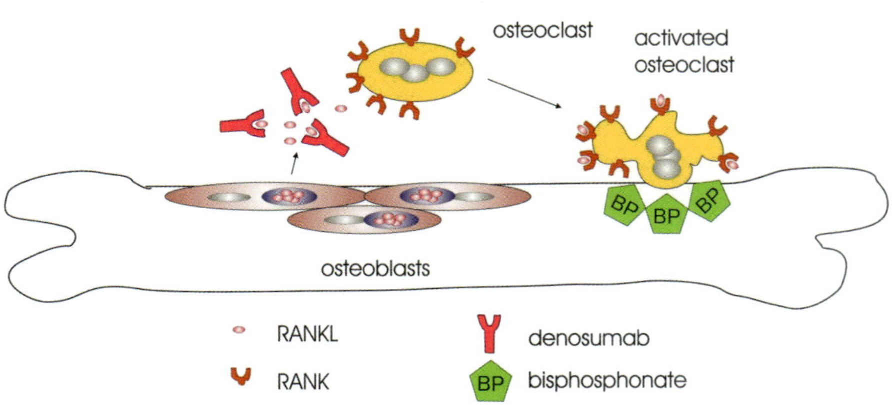

Fig 4.14-1 Mechanisms of action of denosumab and bisphosphonates. RANKL is secreted by osteoblasts and binds to the RANK receptor on osteoclasts, promoting osteoclast differentiation and activation. Denosumab binds RANKL and thereby inhibits the RANKL-RANK pathway. Bisphosphonates bind to the bone and enter, thus inhibiting resorption by activated osteoclasts (modified according to Yee and Raje with kind permission of Dove medical press. Reprinted with kind permission Springer Verlag GmbH) [Otto, 2014].

Although their molecular mechanisms of action are completely distinct, both bisphosphonates and denosumab have antiresorptive effects and are effective in cancer and osteoporosis management. The US Food and Drug Administration has granted approval to Prolia (Amgen Inc), which is denosumab specific for osteoporosis management [Moen et al, 2011]. Prolia is administered in a dose of 60 mg via subcutaneous injection twice yearly. On the other hand, denosumab in monthly larger doses of 120 mg (Xgeva, Amgen Inc) was approved for oncological patients [Lipton et al, 2012]. Unlike bisphosphonates, denosumab is not excreted through the kidneys and can be a safer treatment option in patients with chronic kidney disease [Anastasilakis et al, 2012]. In contrast to bisphosphonates' long biological half-life of 10–12 years that of denosumab is only 26 days. Denosumab does not incorporate into bone minerals. Therefore, the therapeutic effect of denosumab is reversible after treatment cessation while the effect of bisphosphonates can last for many years [Anastasilakis et al, 2012]. Denosumab can be used as a first-line treatment or as an alternative to bisphosphonates.

1.2 Antiangiogenic medications

Antiangiogenic medications are used for several oncological indications; such as gastrointestinal, renal, and non-small cell lung cancer [Shah, 2014]. They slow the growth of a tumor and suppress its further spread through the inhibition of new blood vessels formation [Vokes et al, 2006]. Antiangiogenic medications bind to some signaling molecules necessary for the angiogenesis-signaling cascade, such as vascular endothelial growth factor and subsequently prevent their binding to their receptors on the endothelial cells [Vokes et al, 2006]. Examples of these novel medications are bevacizumab (Avastin), sunitinib (Sutent), sorafenib (Nexavar), pazopanib (Votrient), and everolimus (Afinitor).

2 Medication-related osteonecrosis of the jaw, definition

In 2003, Marx reported a series of cases of jawbone exposure as a new complication associated with intravenous application of nitrogen-containing bisphosphonates, namely pamidronate and zoledronate. This condition was named bisphosphonate-related osteonecrosis of the jaw (BRONJ) [Marx, 2003]. Since then the number of BRONJ cases observed has been increasing [Bagan et al, 2009; Marx et al, 2007]. The first working definition was proposed by an Australian consensus guideline as "an area of exposed bone that persists for 8 weeks" [Sambrook et al, 2006]. The American Association of Oral and Maxillofacial Surgeons (AAOMS) [2007] proposed a working definition for BRONJ and defined the condition if the following three characteristics were prevalent: (1) current or previous treatment with bisphosphonates, (2) exposed and necrotic bone in the maxillofacial region that has lasted for more than 8 weeks, and (3) no history of radiotherapy of the jaw. Thereafter several cases of non-exposed BRONJ were reported and consequently AAOMS added stage 0 or non-exposed variant to its definition in its 2009 position paper [Ruggiero et al, 2009]. Another modification in this paper is the change of "necrotic exposed bone" into "exposed bone."

More recently it became clear that other medications, such as denosumab and antiangiogenic medications, can be associated with osteonecrosis of the jaw [Qi et al, 2014]. Therefore, AAOMS has suggested changing the disease name to medication-related osteonecrosis of the jaw (MRONJ) and has modified MRONJ definition to accommodate the medications other than bisphosphonates that can contribute to osteonecrosis of the jaw. The AAOMS current definition is: the presence of exposed bone, or bone that can be probed through an intraoral or extraoral fistula in the maxillofacial region, present for more than 8 weeks and without a history of radiation therapy to the jaw [Ruggiero et al, 2014].

It is crucial in a clinical setting to exclude all similar pathologies that can present even in patients under the risk of MRONJ or with diagnosed MRONJ. The most relevant differential diagnoses are metastatic disease to the jaw, osteomyelitis, and osteoradionecrosis. Metastatic disease to the jaws can be excluded by histological examination of a biopsy taken from a lesion. Osteomyelitis and osteoradionecrosis can be excluded by proper evaluation of the medical history and through biopsies. Oral ulceration and bone sequestration described previously as "lingual mandibular sequestration and ulceration," can show a similar clinical presentation. Oral ulceration and bone sequestration occurs mainly in the mylohyoid ridge, mandibular tori, palatal tori, and mandibular exostoses [Khan et al, 2015]. A recent systemic review [Palla et al, 2016] has investigated the sparse published literature about oral ulceration and bone sequestration and clarified that it is not a distinct entity but includes multiple ulcerative disorders associated with different local and systemic factors. Other conditions that can be considered in the differential diagnosis are alveolar osteitis, sinusitis, periodontitis, periapical pathology, odontalgia, atypical neuralgias, fibro-osseous lesions, and sarcoma [Ruggiero et al, 2014].

3 Imaging features and techniques

Panoramic radiographs are one of the imaging modalities commonly used by dentists and craniomaxillofacial surgeons to detect jaw lesions, including MRONJ. In fact, panoramic radiographs are sufficient in detection and follow-up of the majority of MRONJ lesions. However, in case of advanced MRONJ lesions, magnetic resonance imaging (MRI), computed tomographic (CT) scans and cone beam imaging may be necessary [Khan et al, 2015]. These radiographic modalities can be important in MRONJ diagnosis and treatment planning. Moreover, panoramic radiographs are only sensitive to large bone lesions, which usually present in advanced stages. However, CT and cone beam imaging help to identify early lesions of MRONJ and the exact borders of extended lesions as well as soft-tissue and maxillary sinus involvement [Guo et al, 2016] (**Fig 4.14-2** and **Fig 4.14-3**).

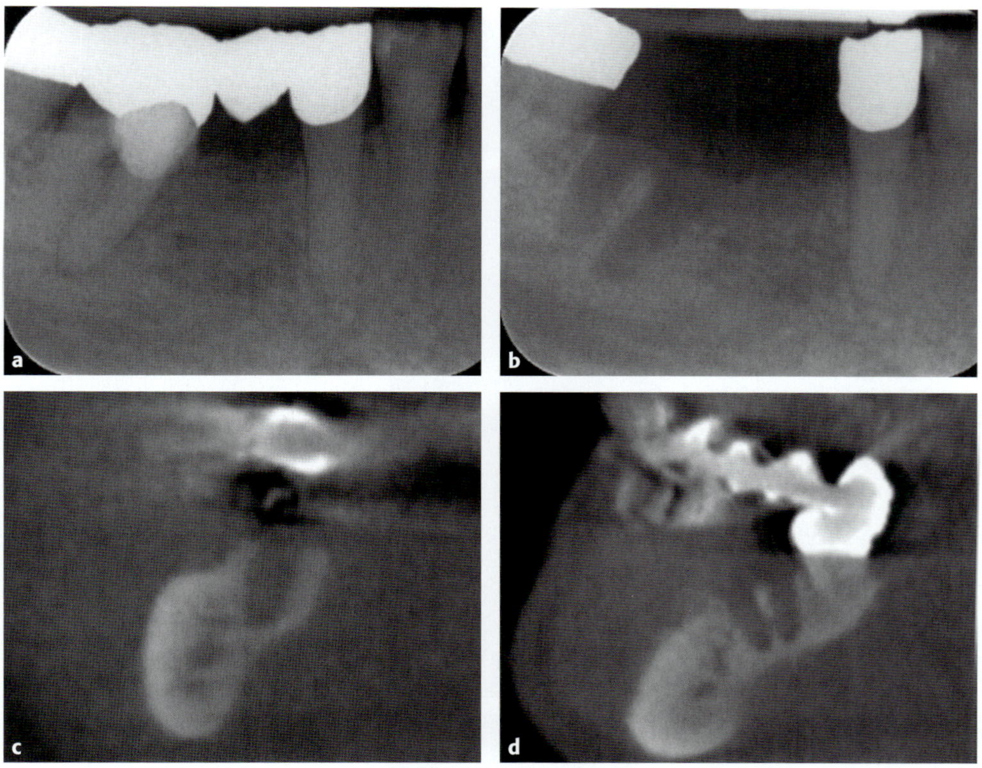

Fig 4.14-2a–d A 70-year-old man presented clinically with a nonhealing extraction wound, exposed bone, and putrid exudate in the mandible in region 45–46. Extraction of tooth 46 had been performed 3 months before. The patient received intravenous bisphosphonate therapy with zoledronate (4 mg/month) for 3.5 years because of osseous metastases from prostate carcinoma.

- **a** Plain film x-ray before extraction.
- **b** Plain film x-ray 3 months after extraction of tooth 46. Lack of bone filling and persisting alveolar sockets are obvious.
- **c–d** Coronal/and sagittal sections derived from cone beam computed tomographic data showing lack of bone filling (reprinted with kind permission of Springer Verlag GmbH) **[Otto, 2014]**.

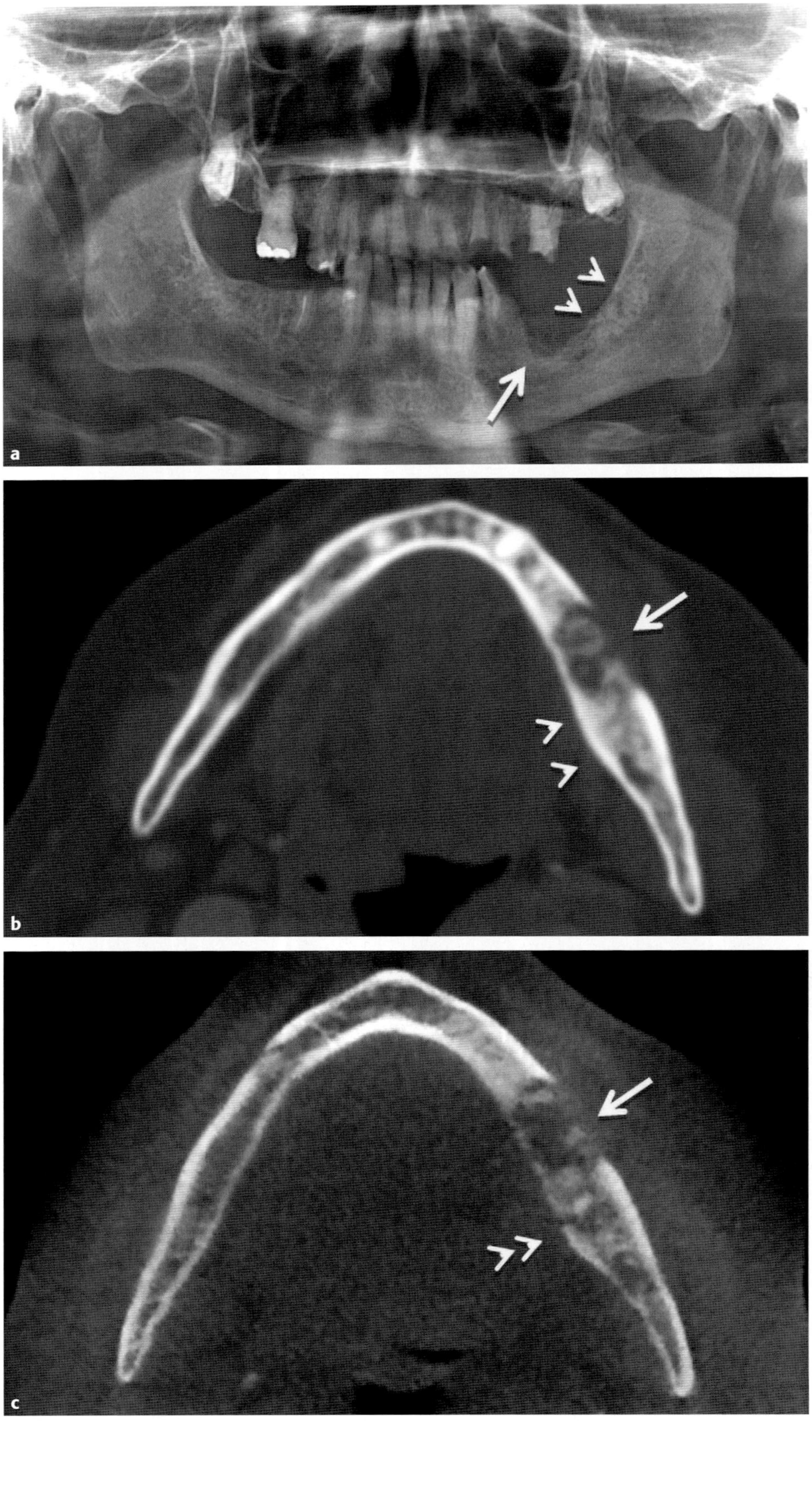

Fig 4.14-3a–c A 69-year-old man received intravenous bisphosphonate therapy with zoledronate (4 mg/month) because of osseous metastases from prostate carcinoma.

- **a** Panoramic radiograph. Large arrow is showing a radiolucent area corresponding to alveolar margin osteolysis. Posterior to the osteolysis, the two arrowheads depict osteosclerosis with disorganized medullary trabeculation and "cotton-wool"-like appearance.
- **b** Multislice computed tomography. The large arrow indicates the osteolytic area; the two arrowheads indicate the osteosclerosis. In contrast to the panoramic radiograph, sequestration is visible as well (within the osteolytic area).
- **c** Cone beam computed tomography. Osteolytic area is indicated (large arrow). Additionally, lingual cortical disruption becomes evident in the layer shown (consecutive arrowheads) (reprinted with kind permission of Springer Verlag GmbH) **[Otto, 2014]**.

Magnetic resonance imaging is an imaging modality with a high sensitivity to osseous edema and inflammation. However, its low specificity limits its use as a diagnostic tool of early MRONJ lesions [Ruggiero, 2015] (**Fig 4.14-4**).

Typically, thickening and prominence of the cortical bone surrounding the inferior alveolar nerve canal can be detected in the early stages of MRONJ [Guo et al, 2016]. Other common radiographic features are osteosclerosis, persisting alveolar sockets after extractions, and bony sequestra and osteolytic areas surrounded by osteosclerotic borders with a cotton-wool-like appearance [Stockmann et al, 2010]. In cases of maxillary involvement, a thickened mucosa of the maxillary sinus can often be detected [Khan et al, 2015]. Periosteal reaction, cortical perforation, and periosteal bone deposition can be better detected using CT and cone beam imaging [Guo et al, 2016]. Both panoramic radiography and CT aid in detection of mandibular fractures. However, MRI is sensitive for the evaluation of soft-tissue inflammation and medullary bone involvement, and hence can better aid in clinical decision making [Guo et al, 2016].

O'Ryan et al [2009] indicated that scintigraphy can be used as an early indicator of MRONJ in patients given intravenous bisphosphonates. Scintigraphy can be sensitive to the associated inflammation or infection that can precede osteonecrosis. Hybrid SPECT/CT can increase the accuracy of conventional bone scintigraphy, as it helps to differentiate between necrotic areas and viable bone and thereby helps surgeons to precisely resect osteonecrotic lesions [Dore et al, 2009].

4 Clinical presentation

Clinically, MRONJ can present as exposed bone or as a bone that can be probed through extraoral or intraoral fistulae with or without pain, suppuration and soft-tissue swelling. However, cases without bone exposure were reported and called non-exposed variants of MRONJ [Fedele et al, 2010]. According to the AAOMS, the diagnosis of such cases can be made by detection of nonspecific symptoms, such as pain and loose teeth not explained by periodontal disease, intraoral or extraoral fistulae not associated with pulpal or periodontal infection, altered neurosensory function, and radiographic findings such as alveolar bone resorption not related to periodontitis [Ruggiero et al, 2014]. The severity and extension of MRONJ can vary significantly. More advanced cases may show maxillary sinus involvement due to superior extension of maxillary lesions, exposed and necrotic bone extending beyond the region of alveolar bone and pathological fractures of the mandible [Otto et al, 2013]. Impairment of inferior alveolar nerve function manifested as hypoesthesia or anesthesia of the lower lip (Vincent symptom) is not an uncommon complication of advanced MRONJ. Interestingly, this complication can also occur in the early disease stages or even as the first symptom of MRONJ [Otto et al, 2009].

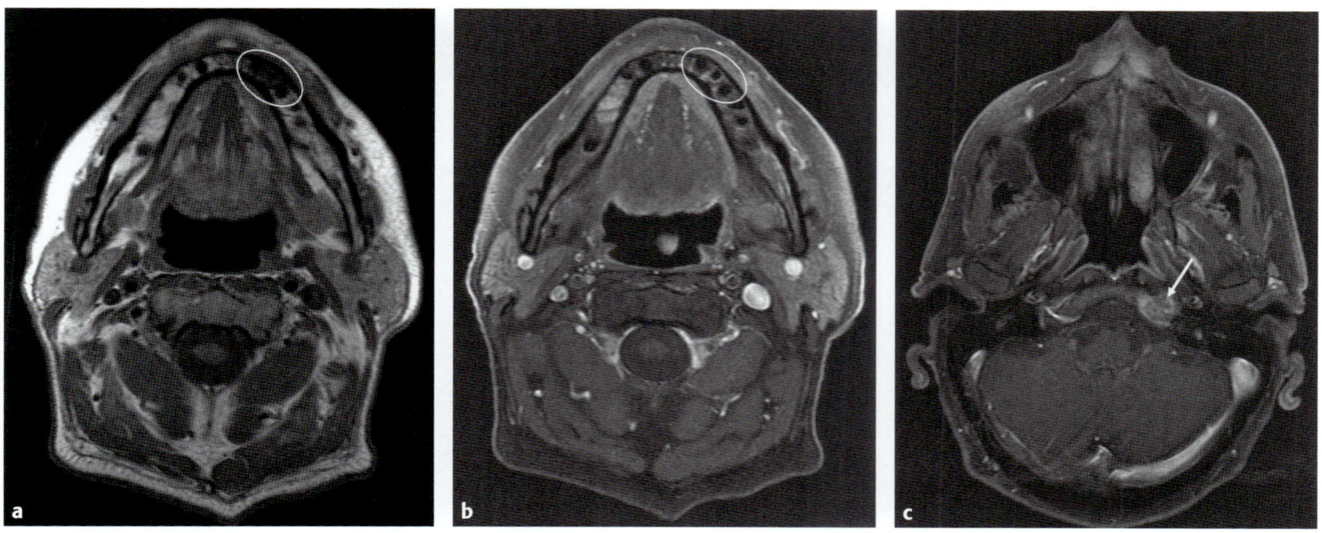

Fig 4.14-4a–c A 61-year-old woman with breast cancer and symptomatic osteonecrosis. Axial T1-weighted image (**a**) shows focal lesion of osteonecrosis in the left side of the mandible as hypointense zone without cortical affection. After gadolinium administration and fat saturation (**b**), the lesion does not demonstrate significant enhancement. Adjacent fat-saturated, post-contrast T1-weighted magnetic resonance image shows enhancing metastatic lesion (arrow) in the left middle skull base (**c**) (reprinted with kind permission of Springer Verlag GmbH) [Otto, 2014].

Different MRONJ staging systems were proposed. According to the AAOMS most recent position paper [Ruggiero et al, 2014], MRONJ can be identified in four stages:

Stage 0
No clinical evidence of necrotic bone but present with non-specific symptoms or clinical and radiographic findings.

Stage 1
Exposed and necrotic bone, localized in the alveolar bone region, or a fistula that probes to bone in asymptomatic patients without evidence of infection. Radiographic findings are localized to the alveolar bone region.

Stage 2
Exposed and necrotic bone or a fistula that probes to bone with infection as evidenced by pain and erythema in the region of exposed bone with or without purulence. Radiographic findings are localized to the alveolar bone region.

Stage 3
Exposed and necrotic bone or fistulae that probe to bone with evidence of infection and at least one of the following: exposed necrotic bone extending beyond the region of alveolar bone, (such as inferior border and ramus in the mandible, maxillary sinus, zygoma, and maxilla), pathological fracture, extraoral fistula, oro-antral or oro-nasal communication, osteolysis extending to the inferior border of the mandible or sinus floor.

The mandible is more often affected than the maxilla by a ratio of 2:1 [Fliefel et al, 2015] (**Fig 4.14-5**). This difference can be attributed to increased vascularity of the maxilla and the compact cortical bone in the mandible. Moreover, MRONJ is more common in premolar and molar regions [Otto et al, 2012; Otto et al, 2011].

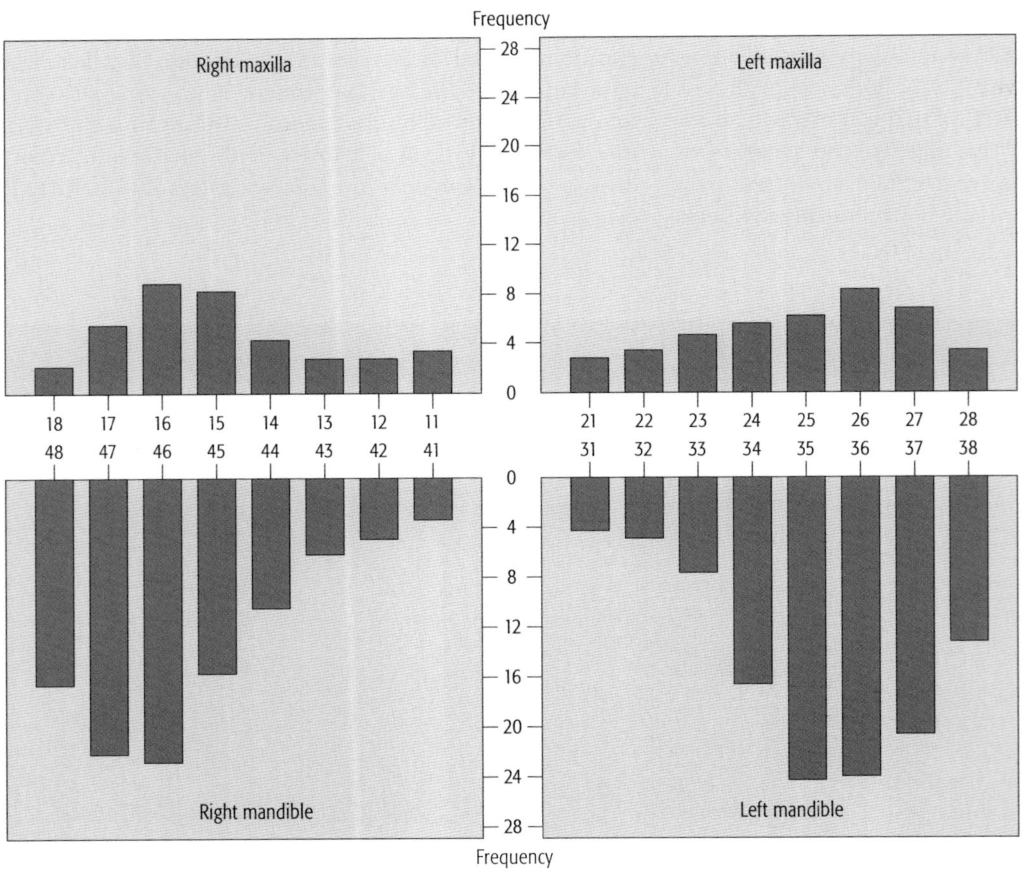

Fig 4.14-5 Distribution of medication-related osteonecrosis of the jaw in the maxilla and mandible (reprinted with kind permission of Elsevier) [Otto et al, 2012].

5 Characteristics and risk factors

Although the first MRONJ case was reported over 15 years ago, there is still no robust evidence regarding its associated risk factors. Many retrospective studies proposed several potential risk factors. To confirm the causative relation of these factors, more prospective and randomized clinical trials are still needed.

5.1 Potential medication-related risk factors

According to the current evidence, the primary risk factor to developing MRONJ is the use of ARDs. The type, duration, dose, potency, and route of administration of ARDs are all risk factors for MRNJ. Many studies [Ruggiero et al, 2014; Otto et al, 2012; Otto et al, 2011] reported the highest risk for patients with long duration of intravenous nitrogen-containing bisphosphonates, particularly zoledronate followed by pamidronate. Therefore, bisphosphonates administered for oncological indication are more associated with MRONJ risk than those administered for osteoporosis. Similarly, patients with cancer exposed to 120 mg subcutaneously monthly denosumab injections have a higher risk for developing MRONJ than patients with osteoporosis half-yearly exposed to 60 mg denosumab injections [Anastasilakis et al, 2012]. In general, the risk of MRONJ in patients with ARDs administered for osteoporosis is approximately 100 times smaller than that for patients with cancer [Ruggiero et al, 2014].

It is known that the incidence of MRONJ increases with increased duration of ARDs exposure [Ruggiero et al, 2014]. A combined analysis of three phase III trials in oncology patients found that the cumulative incidence of MRONJ related to zoledronate and denosumab was, respectively, 0.6% and 0.5% at 1 year; 1.0% and 1.8% at 2 years; and 1.3% and 1.8% at 3 years [Saad et al, 2012]. In patients with osteoporosis and oral bisphosphonates, the incidence increases from 0% at 1 year; 0.05% at 2 and 3 years, and 0.21% at 4 years of drug administration [Lo et al, 2010]. This means that the risk of developing MRONJ positively correlates with the cumulative dose of ARDs.

A randomized, double-blind study of denosumab versus zoledronic acid in the treatment of bone metastases in patients with advanced cancer or multiple myeloma has found comparable prevalence rates of MRONJ in both groups of patients [Henry et al, 2014; Henry et al, 2011]. However, a meta-analysis of seven randomized controlled trials found that the overall incidence of MRONJ in patients with cancer receiving denosumab was 1.7% and there was a numerically increased risk of MRONJ in patients receiving denosumab compared with bisphosphonates [Qi et al, 2014]. Interestingly, MRONJ tends to develop earlier in denosumab therapy compared with bisphosphonates [Otto et al, 2016].

5.2 Systemic factors and comorbidities

Antiresorptive treatment of patients with metastatic bone disease was reported inconsistently as a risk factor for MRONJ [Qi et al, 2014]. The incidence of MRONJ in patients with multiple myeloma is 3.8%; in patients with breast cancer 2.5%; and in patients with prostate cancer 2.9% [Wang et al, 2007]. Multiple myeloma, breast cancer, and prostate cancer are the therapeutic indications for ARDs in 31.2%, 29.5%, and 9.6% of MRONJ patients, respectively [Abu-Id et al, 2008]. Patients with osteoporosis accounted for 5–19.6% of MRONJ patients [Otto et al, 2011; Silverman et al, 2009].

Diabetes mellitus [Khamaisi et al, 2007], osteoporosis [Anastasilakis et al, 2012; Otto et al, 2011; Ruggiero et al, 2004], corticosteroid therapy [Fliefel et al, 2015; Saad et al, 2012; Migliorati et al, 2006; Jadu et al, 2007; Tsao et al, 2013], immunosuppressive therapy [Khan et al, 2015; Otto et al, 2012], chemotherapy [Jadu et al, 2007], and renal dialysis [Jadu et al, 2007] were the most commonly reported risk-increasing comorbidities. Antiangiogenic medications, when combined with ARDs in patients with cancer, seem to be associated with increased MRONJ risk [Ruggiero et al, 2014; Saad et al, 2012]. Smoking as a risk factor for MRONJ was also discussed [Ruggiero et al, 2014]. Most MRONJ patients are elderly, with a mean age of 66.5 ± 4.7 years [Fliefel et al, 2015; Otto et al, 2012; Otto et al, 2011]. Women are affected twice as often as men [Fliefel et al, 2015; Otto et al, 2011]. An explanation is that breast cancer and osteoporosis are far more common in women.

5.3 Potential local risk factors

Medication-related osteonecrosis of the jaw has been frequently reported in relation to tooth extractions, dentoalveolar surgical procedures, local suppuration, and periodontitis. These are considered potential risk factors to MRONJ [Otto et al, 2011; Barasch et al, 2013]. In fact, local chronic infection and its associated inflammatory process is the usual cause of tooth extractions, so it is more probable that the local infection rather than the extraction itself is the real trigger of MRONJ [Otto et al, 2012]. Cases related to local inflammation due to trauma, particularly those caused by ill-fitting dentures or at sites of bony exostoses, were reported [Ruggiero et al, 2014] (**Fig 4.14-6**).

On the other hand, spontaneous MRONJ or MRONJ with an undetectable local preceding event was described [Bagan et al, 2006]. Proper understanding of the role of local factors in MRONJ onset is of great clinical importance as it may aid in prevention of the disease.

6 Pathogenesis

The exact mechanism of MRONJ development is still not fully understood. Over the past decade, considerable progress has been made to better understand MRONJ. However, the definitive pathophysiology of the disease is still elusive, as an essential piece of the puzzle seems to be missing. To date, five hypotheses have been suggested: suppression of bone remodeling because of the direct effect of ARDs on osteoclasts, increased predisposition to oral bacterial infection, antiangiogenic effects, inhibition of oral epithelial cells migration, and suppression of innate or acquired immunity [Allen, 2015]. A combination of these hypotheses and a possible yet unrecognized process is likely to constitute the pathomechanism of MRONJ. Different animal models of MRONJ-like disease induced by ARDs followed by tooth extraction have been developed [de Molon et al, 2015; Aghaloo et al, 2014]. These models are expected to improve our understanding of MRONJ pathophysiology and its treatment.

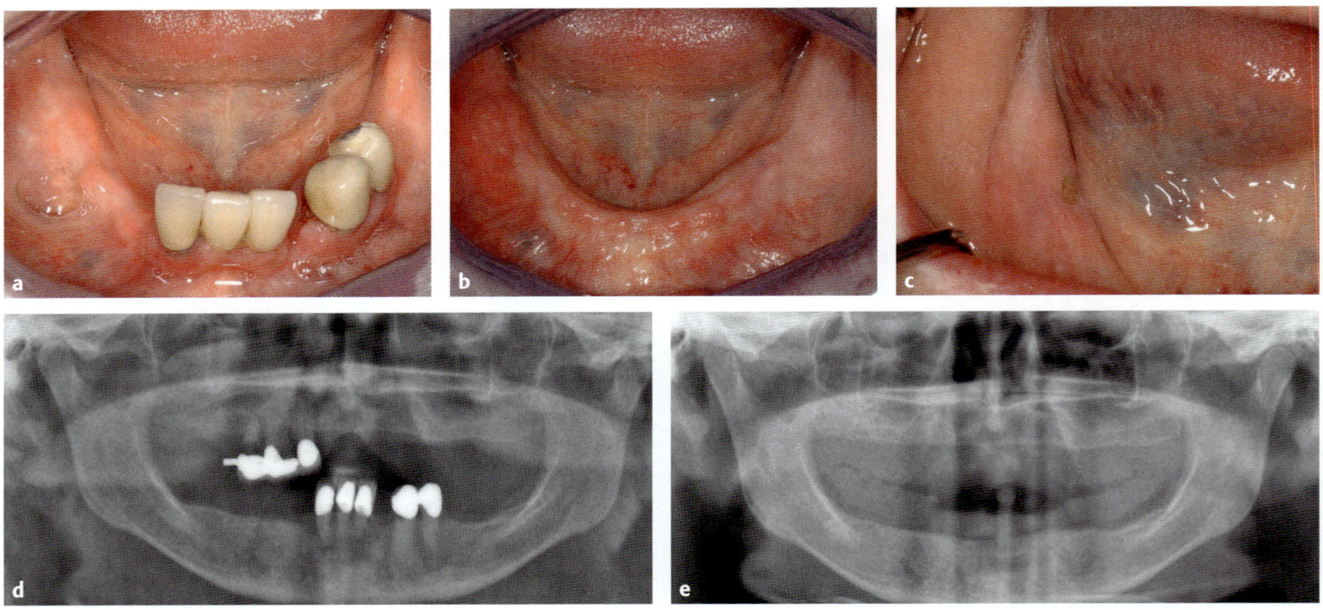

Fig 4.14-6a–e A 60-year-old woman suffering from adenocarcinoma of the lung treated with intravenous administrations of nitrogen-containing bisphosphonates (zoledronate: 4 mg every 4 weeks) was referred for multiple extractions in the upper and lower jaw (**a**). Preoperative intraoral view and corresponding panoramic radiograph (**d**). The extractions were performed including antibiotic prophylaxis, smoothening of sharp bony edges and plastic wound closure. The postoperative course was uneventful and resulted in complete mucosal healing. Intraoral view 18 months after extractions (**b**). Later the patient developed a bisphosphonate-related osteonecrosis of the jaw lesion (according to stage 1 AAOMS 2009 and 2014) that was caused by a pressure sore from her mandibular prosthesis more than 2 years after the extractions (**c**). The corresponding panoramic radiograph is shown (**e**) (reprinted with kind permission of Elsevier) [Otto et al, 2015].

High bone turnover rate in the jawbones and specifically in the dentoalveolar process is needed to repair microdamage of the bone resulting from mechanical loading and exposure to local infections, such as periodontitis, to avoid bone infection and necrosis. However, this repair mechanism is impaired in patients receiving ARDs. It is well known that ARDs have a direct suppressing effect on osteoclasts and subsequently can significantly decrease the bone turnover rate. In general, bone healing is largely based on bone remodeling particularly in jawbones, which have the fastest bone remodeling and are subjected to daily micro-traumas more than any other bones in the skeleton. This hypothesis has been confirmed after appearance of MRONJ cases in relation to other ARDs, such as denosumab [Lipton et al, 2012]. In addition, a study reported improved healing of extraction sockets in animals under zoledronate because of treatment with parathyroid hormone, which basically accelerates osteoclasts function [Dayisoylu et al, 2013]. This hypothesis is the most frequently proposed one to elucidate MRONJ pathogenesis, however it fails to explain that there are no reported cases of osteonecrosis of the jaw in relation to conditions with similar decreased bone remodeling rates, such as hypoparathyrodism [Pazianas, 2011]. Furthermore, bone scintigraphy did not show a significant difference in bone turnover between jawbones and other bones after bisphosphonates and denosumab administration [Ristow et al, 2014].

Increasing evidence shows that local infection and inflammation plays a crucial role in MRONJ onset and progression [Otto et al, 2010]. The environment of the oral cavity is challenging in terms of the presence of oral flora and the frequent exposure to micro-traumas, soft-tissue infections, and surgical interventions. Jawbones are in proximity to the oral cavity and are covered by a thin layer of oral mucosa and periosteum, which may predispose the bone to infection and necrosis in medically vulnerable patients [Sedghizadeh et al, 2009]. Bacteriae, especially *Actinomyces* species, were frequently isolated from MRONJ lesions that may indicate a role of infection in MRONJ pathogenesis [Sedghizadeh et al, 2009; Panya et al, 2017]. Local acidity, which is evident in cases of inflammation and infection, can induce bisphosphonates (especially those containing nitrogen) release from bony hydroxyapatite. Bone necrosis can occur as a direct effect of bisphosphonate cytotoxicity not only to osteoclasts and osteoblasts but also to the cells of the surrounding tissues, such as mesenchymal stem cells, endothelial cells, and epithelial cells [Otto et al, 2010] (**Fig 4.14-7**).

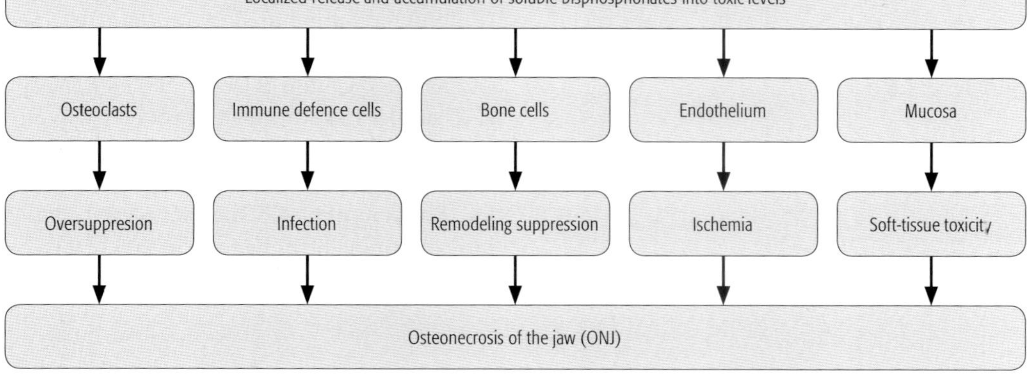

Fig 4.14-7 Potential scheme of the pathogenesis of medication-related osteonecrosis of the jaw (reprinted with kind permission of Elsevier) [Fleisher et al, 2016].

Tumor growth and metastases require the formation of new blood vessels through the process of angiogenesis. Antiangiogenesis is one of the favorable effects of bisphosphonates regarding cancer treatment and aids in prevention of metastasis [Wood et al, 2002; Bezzi et al, 2003]. It is well known that avascular necrosis and lack of blood supply due to decreased angiogenesis is the basic pathomechanism of osteoradionecrosis. Therefore, it is suggested that antiangiogenesis can also play a role in MRONJ development. Indeed, reporting of MRONJ cases in patients with cancer treated by antiangiogenic agents supports these suggestions [Guarneri et al, 2010; Brunello et al, 2009]. However, patients with cancer can have several comorbidities and predisposing factors to osteonecrosis such as radiotherapy and chemotherapy. In addition, denosumab can induce MRONJ although it is not known to have any antiangiogenic effects.

Many studies have shown that MRONJ is more frequent in immunocompromised patients [Ruggiero et al, 2014]. In a recent systematic review, 24.6% of MRONJ patients were being treated with corticosteroids and 39.7% were being treated with chemotherapy [Fliefel et al, 2015]. Both corticosteroids and chemotherapy are known to make the oral mucosa more vulnerable to infection and have a suppressive effect on the immune system. As such, immunosuppression has been described as a factor that may initiate or encourage the progression of MRONJ [Khan et al, 2015].

7 Prevention

Treatment of MRONJ can be challenging and there is yet no consensus regarding the optimal management. Therefore, it is highly recommended to implement strong preventive strategies before and during the treatment with ARDs to decrease the risk for MRONJ. Noteworthy, these recommendations have been mostly based on expert opinion and lack solid supporting evidence.

7.1 Before administration of ARDs

Thorough dental screening should be performed for every patient before ARDs administration. The main aims are to eliminate any oral infections or potential local risk factors that may trigger MRONJ onset and to avoid the necessity of surgical procedures during MRONJ treatment. Optimal oral health should be obtained before ARDs induction. Necessary conservative restorative and prosthodontic procedures as well as root canal treatments should be performed. Teeth with questionable prognosis should be extracted. Ill-fitting dentures should be repaired or replaced to prevent trauma to the underlying oral mucosa. Periodontal treatment, including scaling and root planning should be accomplished. Optimal oral hygiene should be reinforced. The dental team should establish a recall schedule for close periodic clinical and radiological follow-ups (see section 7.2). More important, patients should be informed on the current knowledge about MRONJ, especially its associated risk factors and clinical presentations, and be educated to report any oral pain, inflammation, or bone exposure. Treatment with ARDs should not be started unless a stable oral health is established. In patients scheduled to take oral bisphosphonates, dental implant insertion is permitted in this period but it should be avoided in oncological patients scheduled to have ARDs intravenously.

7.2 During administration of ARDs in patients with cancer

Radiographic and clinical oral screenings should be performed every 6 months. Conservative dental treatments are allowed any time during the ARD treatment. Dental prostheses should be regularly checked and repaired or replaced if necessary. Extractions should be avoided except if they aim to eliminate infection as in cases of dental abscess or severe periodontitis. Before extraction antibiotic coverage is highly recommended. Atraumatic extractions with primary closure of the surgical site are recommended by the German Association of Oral and Maxillofacial Surgery [Groetz et al, 2012]. These strategies proved to be effective in minimizing the risk of MRONJ in a cohort mainly consisting of high-risk patients with malignant underlying disease receiving intravenous bisphosphonates treatment (96.8% success rate and uneventful healing in 209 of 216 extraction sites) [Otto et al, 2015] (**Fig 4.14-8**).

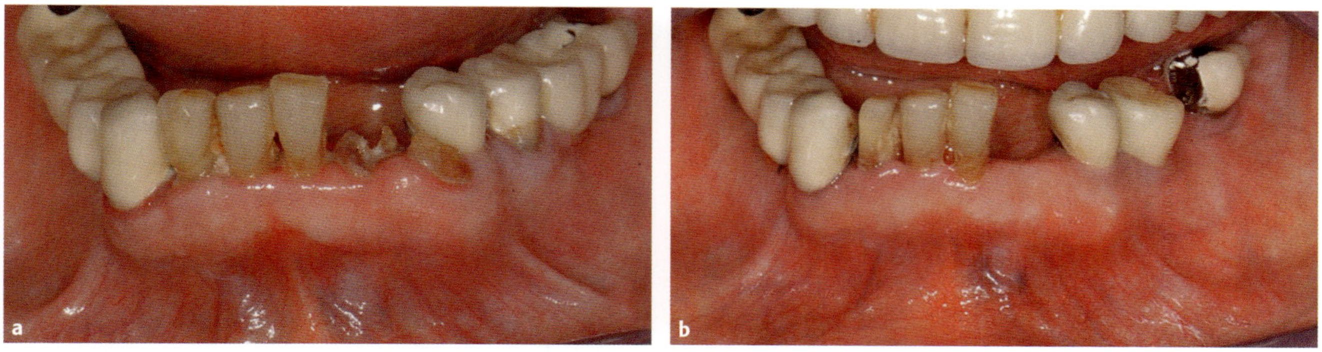

Fig 4.14-8a–b

a Preoperative intraoral view of a 68-year-old woman with breast cancer after intravenous administration of nitrogen-containing bisphosphonates (zoledronate: 4 mg every 4 weeks over 4 years); root remnants of teeth 31 and 32. It is noteworthy that this patient suffered from bisphosphonate-related osteonecrosis in her right upper jaw which was successfully treated previously.

b Postoperative intraoral view showing complete mucosal healing after tooth extraction, smoothening of sharp bony edges, and plastic wound closure (18 months postoperatively) (reprinted with kind permission of Elsevier) [Otto et al, 2015].

A drug holiday of about 3 to 6 months before extraction or other invasive procedures, after consultation with the treating physician, seems to be helpful and indicated in patients taking denosumab, while a drug holiday in bisphosphonate patients seems not to be effective. Implant placement or any elective surgical procedure should be avoided.

7.3 During administration of ARDs in patients with osteoporosis

Regular check-ups twice a year should be scheduled. Optimal oral hygiene and oral health importance should be underlined. Elective dentoalveolar surgeries including implant placement are not contraindicated. However, the patient should be informed that despite the significantly lower risk of MRONJ development in patients with osteoporosis, its consequences can be devastating. Therefore, informed consent of the risk of MRONJ should be obtained. Orthodontic treatment is possible. However, a delay in orthodontic tooth movement is expected [Zahrowski, 2009].

8 Treatment

The treatment of MRONJ is largely based on clinical recommendations and not on robust medical evidence. Many organizations have suggested protocols and management guidelines. Recommendations proposed by the AAOMS, although having some limitations, have won worldwide acceptance [Ruggiero et al, 2014]. In general, MRONJ management should aim at prevention of MRONJ progression, improving quality of life by relieving symptoms, and most important, achieving full mucosal coverage, as it represents the normal physiological status also necessary to prevent recurrence of MRONJ.

The AAOMS treatment protocol varies according to the stage of MRONJ [Ruggiero et al, 2014]. Earlier, nonoperative and limited surgical treatment including antibiotics, removal of bony sequestra, and use of oral antimicrobial rinses were recommended as the main approach to management. More extended surgical treatment concepts, such as resections, were limited only to those cases that failed to respond to the concept. In fact, nonoperative measures can hinder the disease progression and improve the symptoms, but they usually fail to result in complete mucosal healing. Subsequently, most of these patients treated nonoperatively have persisting bone exposure that can significantly affect their quality of life and limit their oncological treatment options, including the use of ARDs [Otto et al, 2015]. Surgical intervention has shown better mucosal integrity and lower recurrence rates compared with nonoperative treatment [Mücke et al, 2011]. To date, surgical management has gained strong agreement as many case series reported good results using surgical therapies [Fliefel et al, 2015; Otto et al, 2016; Otto et al, 2015]. Therapeutic strategies according to AAOMS are summarized in **Table 4.14-1**.

Operative treatment has often been used to manage necrosis, as necrotic tissue cannot heal and should be removed to induce tissue recovery and prevent secondary infection. Conventional surgical techniques vary from superficial debridement to marginal, segmental, subtotal or total resection of the necrotic bone. Superficial debridement is performed as part of a nonoperative approach to reduce but not eliminate the necrotic tissue. On the other hand, surgical resection aims on complete removal of the necrotic bone with or without safety borders. Planning of bone resection can be done using imaging techniques, such as CT or cone beam imaging. In conventional surgical techniques, the subjective parameters such as color or texture of bone are used as signs of vital bone [Otto, 2014]. Moreover, they usually use bleeding of viable bone as a guidance to determine the resection margins [Stockmann et al, 2014]. However, this can be challenging and misleading, as affected bone can show different ranges of vascularity and can be even hypervascularized [Bedogni et al, 2008]. Because of this, the standardization and reproducibility of conventional surgical procedures is impossible, making it unrealistic to compare their outcome results. To identify the real extent of necrotic bone, fluorescence-guided bone surgery was introduced in the treatment of MRONJ [Pautke et al, 2010]. Tetracycline and its derivatives can be incorporated in bone areas with high-remodeling rate due to their calcium affinity [Rauch et al, 2007].

Also, they show fluorescence properties and can be detected in vital bone using a VELscope fluorescence lamp [Pautke et al, 2011]. This technique is reproducible and can be helpful to distinguish between viable and necrotic bone, which may help to standardize surgical treatment of MRONJ [Pautke et al, 2011; Otto et al, 2016] (**Fig 4.14-9**).

MRONJ* stage	Treatment strategies
At risk	No treatment Patient education
Stage 0	Systemic management, including use of pain medication and antibiotics Close monitoring given the potential for progression to a higher stage of disease
Stage1	Antibacterial mouth rinse Clinical follow-up on a quarterly basis No immediate operative treatment is required Patient education Review of indications for continued antiresorptive treatment
Stage 2	Symptomatic treatment with oral antibiotics, oral antibacterial mouth rinse Pain control, debridement to relieve soft-tissue irritation, and infection control
Stage 3	Antibacterial mouth rinse Antibiotic therapy and pain control Surgical debridement or resection for longer-term palliation of infection and pain

Table 4.14-1 Treatment strategies according to the American Association of Oral and Maxillofacial Surgeons [Ruggiero et al, 2014].
*MRONJ indicates medication-related osteonecrosis of the jaw.

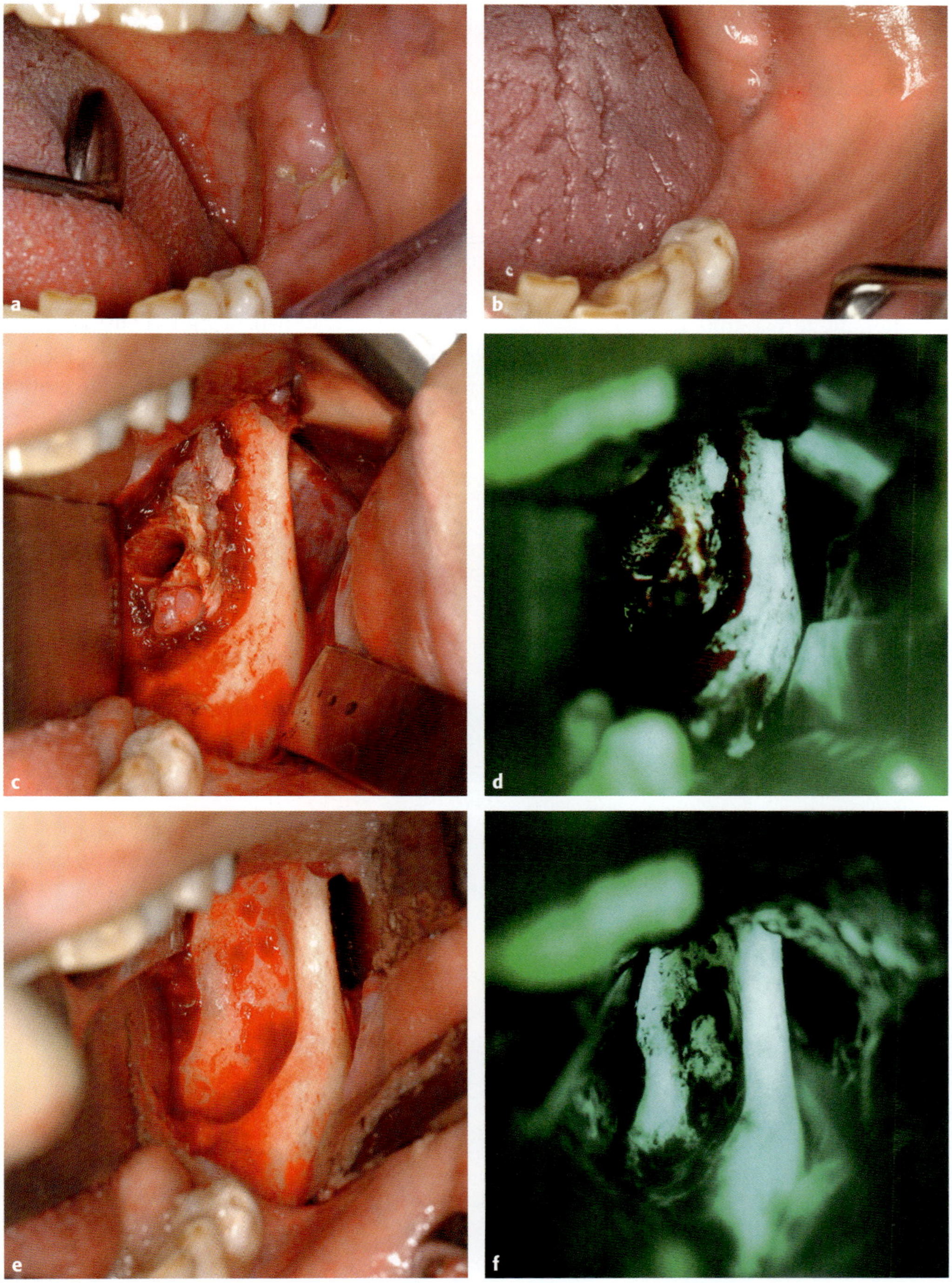

Fig 4.14-9a–f A 58-year-old woman suffering from breast cancer received zoledronate therapy for 56 months and developed a medication-related osteonecrosis of the jaw in the left side of her mandible (region 37/38 mainly lingual aspect). Photographs depicting the clinical intraoral situation before (**a**) and 3 months after surgery (**b**). The intraoperative clinical and fluorescence view before removal of the necrotic bone (**c–d**) and after the removal of necrotic bone and smoothening of sharp bony edges (**e–f**). Note the weak green fluorescence in the lingual aspect region 37/38 corresponding to the necrotic bone area (**d**) as well as the reddish fluorescence in this area corresponding to the bacterial infection of this region before removal of the necrotic and infected bone parts as well as the homogenous greenish fluorescence after the removal and the absence of red fluorescence after the removal of necrotic bone parts (reprinted with kind permission of Elsevier) **[Otto et al, 2012]**.

The use of prophylactic antibiotics preoperatively and postoperatively is important in promoting proper healing of the surgical site. No consensus exists about the duration of administration of antibiotics. Usually it ranges from 2 days before to 5 days after surgery [Eckert et al, 2007]. Penicillin is commonly prescribed [Groetz et al, 2012]. In case of penicillin allergy, quinolones, metronidazole, clindamycin, doxycycline, and erythromycin can be used [Groetz et al, 2012].

Various adjuvant therapies have been reported such as low-intensity laser therapy, ozone therapy, teriparatide treatment, hyperbaric oxygen therapy, and local administration of platelet-derived growth factor [Fliefel et al, 2015]. Some of these techniques showed positive results, however further research is needed to evaluate their efficacy. It is imperative to completely remove the necrotic bone and to cover the bone with local mucoperiosteal flaps to facilitate long-term resolution of infection and pain. In addition, administration of broad-spectrum antibiotics before and after the surgery is highly recommended. In severe cases, maxillary or mandibular resection and reconstruction using an obturator or a reconstruction plate might be needed (**Fig 4.14-10**). Microvascular free flap reconstruction has been reported as an effective reconstructive option in patients with treatment-resistant stage 3 and stage 2 MRONJ [Hanasono et al, 2013].

Extraction of affected teeth in the necrotic bone is recommended, as they may act as potential infection sources [Otto et al, 2015].

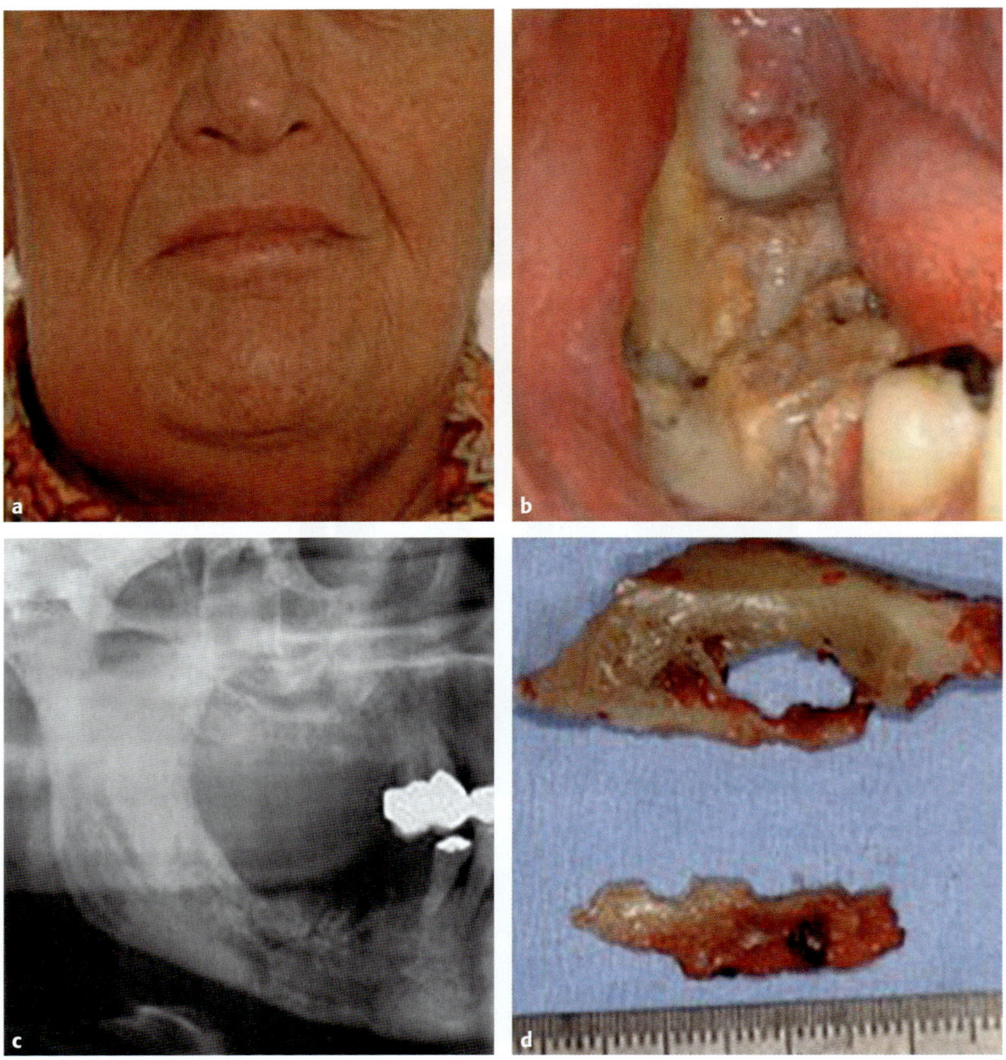

Fig 4.14-10a–g A 65-year-old woman suffering from metastases after breast cancer and receiving intravenous administrations of bisphosphonates (zoledronate) with an extended manifestation of bisphosphonate-related osteonecrosis on the right side of the mandible.

- **a** Extraoral view with a swelling and reddening of the right submandibular area, which was painful on palpation.
- **b** Intraoral view with a large area of exposed necrotic bone, sign of massive superinfection (swelling, pus), and a visible fracture of the mandible with mobile segments.
- **c** Panoramic radiograph of the patient with a mixed radiolucent and radiopaque appearance and a visible fracture line in the right mandibular body.
- **d** Large bone sequestrae were removed including resection of the mandible, followed by rigid internal fixation using a unilock plate 2.4 and complete closure of the wound.

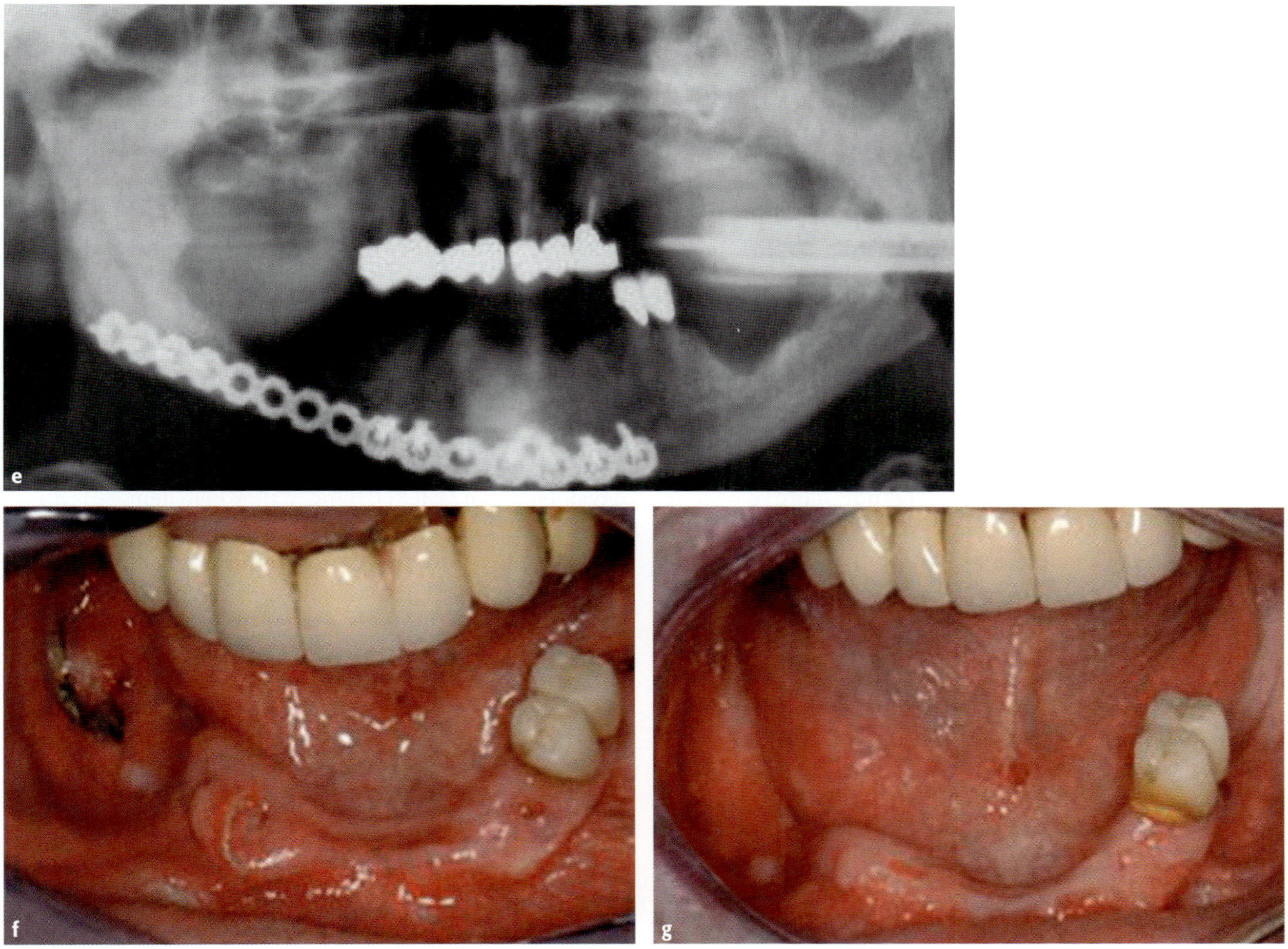

Fig 4.14-10a–g (cont) A 65-year-old woman suffering from metastases after breast cancer and receiving intravenous administrations of bisphosphonates (zoledronate) with an extended manifestation of bisphosphonate-related osteonecrosis on the right side of the mandible.

e Postoperative panoramic radiograph showing the resected area of the right mandible and the rigid internal fixation.

f Intraoral view 3 weeks postoperatively with a late dehiscence and plate exposure in region 47/48.

g Intraoral view 4 months postoperatively with complete mucosal healing after local disinfectant measurements using disinfectant mouth rinses and activated photodynamic therapy (reprinted with kind permission of Thieme Medical Publishers) **[Otto et al, 2013]**.

The effect of discontinuation of bisphosphonates, ie, drug holiday, is a controversial issue. In general, it is not recommended in cancer patients with progressive bone metastases. The skeletal bisphosphonates half-life can extend to several years [Thumbigere-Math et al, 2016]. Therefore, it is unlikely that bisphosphonates discontinuation can result in MRONJ risk reduction [Thumbigere-Math et al, 2016]. However, Hinson et al [2015] reported faster resolution of MRONJ symptoms with discontinuing bisphosphonates before or at treatment initiation compared with continuing the drug throughout treatment. On the other hand, denosumab half-life is much shorter (25–32 days) and the maximum duration of its effect on bone is 6 months. Thus, a drug holiday might be beneficial [Anastasilakis et al, 2012]. However, supporting data are still lacking. A recent study [Hoefert et al, 2017] has shown that denosumab cessation did not improve healing outcomes of both operative and nonoperative patients with an explicit denosumab history.

9 Summary

Medication-related osteonecrosis of the jaw is a potential complication of the use of antiresorptive and antiangiogenetic drugs which mainly occurs in oncological patients (breast cancer, prostate cancer, multiple myeloma, etc), and less frequently also in patients with osteoporosis. This complication is potentially debilitating and can be challenging for clinicians. The exact pathogenesis is still not completely understood. Nonetheless, there is proof supporting the major role of local infection and remodeling suppression in MRONJ onset. Several potential local and systemic risk factors appear to contribute to MRONJ onset.

Effective preventive measures should be used to avoid the development of MRONJ. Hence a thorough dental examination before starting antiresorptive treatment is mandatory. Oral hygiene should be optimized and patients should be included in a recall program. Required dental surgery should, if possible, be performed before the use of bisphosphonates or denosumab. However, dentoalveolar surgery especially tooth extractions are also possible under antiresorptive therapy, when the respective preventive protocols including antibiotic prophylaxis and complete mucosal closure are followed.

Regarding the management of manifest MRONJ lesions, there are both nonoperative and operative treatment options. Nonoperative treatment may lead to symptomatic improvement. Over the past years multiple studies have shown that operative treatment including complete removal of necrotic bone, smoothening of sharp bony edges, and plastic wound closure leads to mucosal healing in most MRONJ patients. In this respect fluorescence-guided removal of necrotic bone is an innovative and helpful tool. However, the general status of the patient may limit the use of surgical techniques and ultimate decision making should be based on the individual situation and should take the quality of life into consideration. Overall, further research is required to provide clarity regarding MRONJ pathophysiology, risk factors, and prophylactic and treatment strategies.

10 References and suggested reading

Abu-Id MH, Warnke PH, Gottschalk J, et al. "Bis-phossy jaws"—high and low risk factors for bisphosphonate-induced osteonecrosis of the jaw. *J Craniomaxillofac Surg*. 2008 Mar;36(2):95–103.

Advisory Task Force on Bisphosphonate-Related Ostenonecrosis of the Jaws AAOO. American Association of Oral and Maxillofacial Surgeons position paper on bisphosphonate-related osteonecrosis of the jaws. *J Oral Maxillofac Surg*. 2007 Mar;65(3):369–376.

Aghaloo TL, Cheong S, Bezouglaia O, et al. RANKL inhibitors induce osteonecrosis of the jaw in mice with periapical disease. *J Bone Miner Res*. 2014 Apr;29(4):843–854.

Allen MR. Medication-related osteonecrosis of the jaw: basic and translational science updates. *Oral Maxillofac Surg Clin North Am*. 2015 Nov;27(4):497–508.

Anastasilakis AD, Toulis KA, Polyzos SA, et al. Long-term treatment of osteoporosis: safety and efficacy appraisal of denosumab. *Ther Clin Risk Manag*. 2012;8:295–306.

Bagan J, Scully C, Sabater V, et al. Osteonecrosis of the jaws in patients treated with intravenous bisphosphonates (BRONJ): a concise update. *Oral Oncol*. 2009;45:551–554.

Bagan JV, Jimenez Y, Murillo J, et al. Jaw osteonecrosis associated with bisphosphonates: multiple exposed areas and its relationship to teeth extractions. Study of 20 cases. *Oral Oncol*. 2006 Mar;42(3):327–329.

Barasch A, Cunha-Cruz J, Curro F, et al. Dental risk factors for osteonecrosis of the jaws: a CONDOR case-control study. *Clinic Oral Investig*. 2013 Nov;17(8):1839–1845.

Bedogni A, Blandamura S, Lokmic Z, et al. Bisphosphonate-associated jawbone osteonecrosis: a correlation between imaging techniques and histopathology. *Oral Surg Oral Med Oral Pathol Oral Radiol Endod*. 2008;105:358–364.

Bezzi M, Hasmim M, Bieler G, et al. Zoledronate sensitizes endothelial cells to tumor necrosis factor-induced programmed cell death: evidence for the suppression of sustained activation of focal adhesion kinase and protein kinase B/Akt. *J Biol Chem*. 2003 Oct 31;278(44):43603–43614.

Brunello A, Saia G, Bedogni A, et al. Worsening of osteonecrosis of the jaw during treatment with sunitinib in a patient with metastatic renal cell carcinoma. *Bone*. 2009 Jan;44(1):173–175.

Cosman F, de Beur SJ, LeBoff MS, et al. Clinician's guide to prevention and treatment of osteoporosis. *Osteoporos Int*. 2014 Oct;25(10):2359–2381.

Cremers S, Papapoulos S. Pharmacology of bisphosphonates. *Bone*. 2011 Jul;49(1):42–49.

Dayisoylu EH, Senel FC, Üngör C, et al. The effects of adjunctive parathyroid hormone injection on bisphosphonate-related osteonecrosis of the jaws: an animal study. *Int J Oral Maxillofac Surg*. 2013 Nov;42(11):1475–1480.

Dore F, Filippi L, Biasotto M, et al. Bone scintigraphy and SPECT/CT of bisphosphonate-induced osteonecrosis of the jaw. *J Nucl Med*. 2009 Jan;50(1):30–35.

de Molon RS, Shimamoto H, Bezouglaia O, et al. OPG-Fc but not zoledronic acid discontinuation reverses osteonecrosis of the jaws (ONJ) in mice. *J Bone Miner Res*. 2015 Sep;30(9):1627–1640.

Eckert AW, Maurer P, Meyer L, et al. Bisphosphonate-related jaw necrosis—severe complication in maxillofacial surgery. *Cancer Treat Rev*. 2007 Feb;33(1):58–63.

Fedele S, Porter SR, D'Aiuto F, et al. Nonexposed variant of bisphosphonate-associated osteonecrosis of the jaw: a case series. *Am J Med*. 2010 Nov;123(11):1060–1064.

Fleisher KE, Kontio R, Otto S, eds. *Antiresorptive Drug-Related Osteonecrosis of the Jaw (ARONJ)—A Guide to Research*. Stuttgart: Thieme; 2016.

Fliefel R, Tröltzsch M, Kühnisch J, et al. Treatment strategies and outcomes of bisphosphonate-related osteonecrosis of the jaw (BRONJ) with characterization of patients: a systematic review. *Int J Oral Maxillofac Surg*. 2015 May;44(5):568–585.

Groetz KA, Piesold JU, Al-Nawas B. [Bisphosphonat-assoziierte Kiefernekrose (BPONJ) und andere Medikamenten-assoziierte Kiefernekrosen]. Available at: www.awmf.org. Access: April 15, 2012. German.

Guo Y, Wang D, Wang Y, et al. Imaging features of medicine-related osteonecrosis of the jaws: comparison between panoramic radiography and computed tomography. *Oral Surg Oral Med Oral Pathol Oral Radiol*. 2016 Aug;122(2):e69–76.

Guarneri V, Miles D, Robert N, et al. Bevacizumab and osteonecrosis of the jaw: incidence and association with bisphosphonate therapy in three large prospective trials in advanced breast cancer. *Breast Cancer Res Treat*. 2010 Jul;122(1):181–188.

Hanasono MM, Militsakh ON, Richmon JD, et al. Mandibulectomy and free flap reconstruction for bisphosphonate-related osteonecrosis of the jaws. *JAMA Otolaryngol Head Neck Surg*. 2013 Nov;139(11):1135–1142.

Henry D, Vadhan-Raj S, Hirsh V, et al. Delaying skeletal-related events in a randomized phase 3 study of denosumab versus zoledronic acid in patients with advanced cancer: an analysis of data from patients with solid tumors. *Support Care Cancer*. 2014 Mar;22(3):679–687.

Henry DH, Costa L, Goldwasser F, et al. Randomized, double-blind study of denosumab versus zoledronic acid in the treatment of bone metastases in patients with advanced cancer (excluding breast and prostate cancer) or multiple myeloma. *J Clin Oncol*. 2011 Mar;29(9):1125–1132.

Hinson AM, Siegel ER, Stack BC Jr. Temporal correlation between bisphosphonate termination and symptom resolution in osteonecrosis of the jaw: a pooled case report analysis. *J Oral Maxillofac Surg*. 2015 Jan;73(1):53–62.

Hoefert S, Yuan A, Munz A, et al. Clinical course and therapeutic outcomes of operatively and non-operatively managed patients with denosumab-related osteonecrosis of the jaw (DRONJ). *J Craniomaxillofac Surg*. 2017 Apr;45(4):570–578.

Jadu F, Lee L, Pharoah M, et al. A retrospective study assessing the incidence, risk factors and comorbidities of pamidronate-related necrosis of the jaws in multiple myeloma patients. *Ann Oncol*. 2007;18:2015–2019.

Jobke B, Milovanovic P, Amling M, et al. Bisphosphonate-osteoclasts: changes in osteoclast morphology and function induced by antiresorptive nitrogen-containing bisphosphonate treatment in osteoporosis patients. *Bone*. 2014 Feb;59:37–43.

Khamaisi M, Regev E, Yarom N, et al. Possible association between diabetes and bisphosphonate-related jaw osteonecrosis. *J Clin Endocrinol Metab*. 2007 Mar;92(3):1172–1175.

Khan AA, Morrison A, Hanley DA, et al. Diagnosis and management of osteonecrosis of the jaw: a systematic review and international consensus. *J Bone Miner Res*. 2015 Jan;30(1):3–23.

Lipton A. Toward new horizons: the future of bisphosphonate therapy. *Oncologist*. 2004;9 Suppl 4:38–47.

Lipton A, Fizazi K, Stopeck AT, et al. Superiority of denosumab to zoledronic acid for prevention of skeletal-related events: a combined analysis of 3 pivotal, randomised, phase 3 trials. *Eur J Cancer*. 2012 Nov;48(16):3082–3092.

Lo JC, O'Ryan FS, Gordon NP, et al. Prevalence of osteonecrosis of the jaw in patients with oral bisphosphonate exposure. *J Oral Maxillofac Surg*. 2010 Feb;68(2):243–253.

Marx RE. Pamidronate (Aredia) and zoledronate (Zometa) induced avascular necrosis of the jaws: a growing epidemic. *J Oral Maxillofac Surg*. 2003 Sep;61(9):1115–1117.

Marx RE, Cillo JE Jr, Ulloa JJ. Oral bisphosphonate-induced osteonecrosis: risk factors, prediction of risk using serum CTX testing, prevention, and treatment. *J Oral Maxillofac Surg*. 2007 Dec;65(12):2397–2410.

Migliorati CA, Siegel MA, Elting LS. Bisphosphonate-associated osteonecrosis: a long-term complication of bisphosphonate treatment. *Lancet Oncol*. 2006 Jun;7(6):508–514.

Moen MD, Keam SJ. Denosumab: a review of its use in the treatment of postmenopausal osteoporosis. *Drugs Aging*. 2011 Jan;28(1):63–82.

Mücke T, Koschinski J, Deppe H, et al. Outcome of treatment and parameters influencing recurrence in patients with bisphosphonate-related osteonecrosis of the jaws. *J Cancer Res Clin Oncol*. 2011 May;137(5):907–913.

O'Ryan FS, Khoury S, Liao W, et al. Intravenous bisphosphonate-related osteonecrosis of the jaw: bone scintigraphy as an early indicator. *J Oral Maxillofac Surg*. 2009 Jul;67:1363–1372.

Otto S. *Medication-Related Osteonecrosis of the Jaws: Bisphosphonates, Denosumab, and New Agents*. Berlin: Springer; 2014.

Otto S, Pautke C, Hafner S, et al. Pathologic fractures in bisphosphonate-related osteonecrosis of the jaw-review of the literature and review of our own cases. *Craniomaxillofac Trauma Reconstr*. 2013 Sep;6:147–154.

Otto S, Hafner S, Grötz KA. The role of inferior alveolar nerve involvement in bisphosphonate-related osteonecrosis of the jaw. *J Oral Maxillofac Surg*. 2009 Mar;67(3):589–592.

Otto S, Schreyer C, Hafner S, et al. Bisphosphonate-related osteonecrosis of the jaws—characteristics, risk factors, clinical features, localization and impact on oncological treatment. *J Craniomaxillofac Surg*. 2012 Jun;40(4):303–309.

Otto S, Abu-Id MH, Fedele S, et al. Osteoporosis and bisphosphonates-related osteonecrosis of the jaw: not just a sporadic coincidence—a multi-centre study. *J Craniomaxillofac Surg*. 2011 Jun;39(4):272–277.

Otto S, Ristow O, Pache C, et al. Fluorescence-guided surgery for the treatment of medication-related osteonecrosis of the jaw: a prospective cohort study. *J Craniomaxillofac Surg*. 2016 Aug;44(8):1073–1080.

Otto S, Tröltzsch M, Jambrovic V, et al. Tooth extraction in patients receiving oral or intravenous bisphosphonate administration: a trigger for BRONJ development? *J Craniomaxillofac Surg*. 2015 Jul;43(6):847–854.

Otto S, Hafner S, Mast G, et al. Bisphosphonate-related osteonecrosis of the jaw: is pH the missing part in the pathogenesis puzzle? *J Oral Maxillofac Surg*. 2010 May;68(5):1158–1161.

Otto S, Marx RE, Troltzsch M, et al. Comments on "diagnosis and management of osteonecrosis of the jaw: a systematic review and international consensus". *J Bone Miner Res*. 2015 Jun;30(6):1113–1115.

Palla B, Burian E, Klecker JR, et al. Systematic review of oral ulceration with bone sequestration. *J Craniomaxillofac Surg*. 2016 Mar;44(3):257–264.

Panya S, Fliefel R, Probst F, et al. Role of microbiological culture and polymerase chain reaction (PCR) of actinomyces in medication-related osteonecrosis of the jaw (MRONJ). *J Craniomaxillofac Surg*. 2017 Mar;45(3):357–363.

Pautke C, Bauer F, Bissinger O, et al. Tetracycline bone fluorescence: a valuable marker for osteonecrosis characterization and therapy. *J Oral Maxillofac Surg*. 2010 Jan;68(1):125–129.

Pautke C, Bauer F, Otto S, et al. Fluorescence-guided bone resection in bisphosphonate-related osteonecrosis of the jaws: first clinical results of a prospective pilot study. *J Oral Maxillofac Surg*. 2011 Jan;69(1):84–91.

Pazianas M. Osteonecrosis of the jaw and the role of macrophages. *J Natl Cancer Inst*. 2011 Feb;103(3):232–240.

Qi WX, Tang LN, He AN, et al. Risk of osteonecrosis of the jaw in cancer patients receiving denosumab: a meta-analysis of seven randomized controlled trials. *Int J Clin Oncol*. 2014 Apr;19(2):403–410.

Rauch F, Travers R, Glorieux FH. Intracortical remodeling during human bone development—a histomorphometric study. *Bone*. 2007 Feb;40(2):274–280.

Ristow O, Gerngross C, Schwaiger M, et al. Effect of antiresorptive drugs on bony turnover in the jaw: denosumab compared with bisphosphonates. *Br J Oral Maxillofac Surg*. 2014 Apr;52(4):308–313.

Rogers MJ, Crockett JC, Coxon FP, et al. Biochemical and molecular mechanisms of action of bisphosphonates. *Bone*. 2011 Jul;49(1):34–41.

Ruggiero SL, Dodson TB, Assael LA, et al. American Association of Oral and Maxillofacial Surgeons position paper on bisphosphonate-related osteonecrosis of the jaw—2009 update. *Aust Endod J*. 2009 Dec;35(3):119–130.

Ruggiero SL. Diagnosis and staging of medication-related osteonecrosis of the jaw. *Oral Maxillofac Surg Clin North Am*. 2015 Nov;27(4):479–487.

Ruggiero SL, Mehrotra B, Rosenberg TJ, et al. Osteonecrosis of the jaws associated with the use of bisphosphonates: a review of 63 cases. *J Oral Maxillofac Surg*. 2004 May;62(5):527–534.

Ruggiero SL, Dodson TB, Fantasia J, et al. American Association of Oral and Maxillofacial Surgeons position paper on medication-related osteonecrosis of the jaw—2014 update. *J Oral Maxillofac Surg*. 2014 Oct;72(10):1938–1956.

Russell RG. Bisphosphonates: mode of action and pharmacology. *Pediatrics*. 2007 Mar;119 Suppl 2:S150–162.

Russell RG, Watts NB, Ebetino FH, et al. Mechanisms of action of bisphosphonates: similarities and differences and their potential influence on clinical efficacy. *Osteoporos Int*. 2008 Jun;19(6):733–759.

Saad F, Brown JE, Van Poznak C, et al. Incidence, risk factors, and outcomes of osteonecrosis of the jaw: integrated analysis from three blinded active-controlled phase III trials in cancer patients with bone metastases. *Ann Oncol*. 2012 May;23(5):1341–1347.

Sambrook P, Olver I, Goss A. Bisphosphonates and osteonecrosis of the jaw. *Aust Fam Phys*. 2006 Oct;35(10):801–803.

Sedghizadeh PP, Kumar SK, Gorur A, et al. Microbial biofilms in osteomyelitis of the jaw and osteonecrosis of the jaw secondary to bisphosphonate therapy. *J Am Dent Assoc*. 2009 Oct;140(10):1259–1265.

Shah MA. The development of bevacizumab in noncolorectal gastrointestinal malignancies: gastroesophageal, pancreatic, and hepatocellular carcinoma. *Clin Adv Hematol Oncol*. 2014 Apr;12(4):239–246.

Silverman SL, Landesberg R. Osteonecrosis of the jaw and the role of bisphosphonates: a critical review. *Am J Med*. 2009 Feb;122(2 Suppl):S33–45.

So A, Chin J, Fleshner N, et al. Management of skeletal-related events in patients with advanced prostate cancer and bone metastases: incorporating new agents into clinical practice. *Can Urol Assoc J*. 2012 Dec;6(6):465–470.

Stockmann P, Hinkmann FM, Lell MM, et al. Panoramic radiograph, computed tomography or magnetic resonance imaging. Which imaging technique should be preferred in bisphosphonate-associated osteonecrosis of the jaw? A prospective clinical study. *Clin Oral Investig*. 2010 Jun;14(3):311–317.

Stockmann P, Burger M, von Wilmowsky C, et al. The outcome after surgical therapy of bisphosphonate-associated osteonecrosis of the jaw—results of a clinical case series with an average follow-up of 20 months. *Clin Oral Investig*. 2014 May;18(4):1299–1304.

Thumbigere-Math V, Michalowicz BS, Hughes PJ, et al. Serum markers of bone turnover and angiogenesis in patients with bisphosphonate-related osteonecrosis of the jaw after discontinuation of long-term intravenous bisphosphonate therapy. *J Oral Maxillofac Surg*. 2016 Apr;74(4):738–746.

Tsao C, Darby I, Ebeling PR, et al. Oral health risk factors for bisphosphonate-associated jaw osteonecrosis. *J Oral Maxillofac Surg*. 2013 Aug;71(8):1360–1366.

Vokes E, Herbst R, Sandler A. Angiogenesis inhibition in the treatment of lung cancer. *Clin Adv Hematol Oncol*. 2006 Nov;4(11 Suppl 23):1–10; quiz 11–12.

Wang EP, Kaban LB, Strewler GJ, et al. Incidence of osteonecrosis of the jaw in patients with multiple myeloma and breast or prostate cancer on intravenous bisphosphonate therapy. *J Oral Maxillofac Surg*. 2007 Jul;65(7):1328–1331.

Wood J, Bonjean K, Ruetz S, et al. Novel antiangiogenic effects of the bisphosphonate compound zoledronic acid. *J Pharmacol Exp Ther*. 2002 Sep;302(3):1055–1061.

Zahrowski JJ. Optimizing orthodontic treatment in patients taking bisphosphonates for osteoporosis. *Am J Orthodon Dentofacial Orthop*. 2009 Mar;135(3):361–374.

5.1 Endoscopy in mandibular condyle and midfacial trauma care

Marcin Czerwinski, Chen Lee, Reid V Mueller, Rainer Schmelzeisen, Robert M Kellman

1 Introduction

Surgical management of craniomaxillofacial trauma has undergone significant evolution over the course of the last 100 years. Nevertheless, several facial areas have remained that could not be approached without obvious surgical stigmata, most notably the mandibular condyle, zygomatic arch, the orbit, and frontal sinus. Those fractures where the benefits of repair outweighed operative risks were treated using open reduction and internal fixation (ORIF). Others, when perceived posttraumatic deformity and dysfunction were less discernable were approached more conservatively, or simply not treated. The decision on how to manage these specific fractures was based on individual surgeon`s experience and patient preferences.

Endoscopy was initiated to the field of craniomaxillofacial surgery by Vasconez et al who performed the first endoscopic brow lift in 1994. This relatively delayed introduction was caused partly by the absence of naturally occurring cavities in the head and neck region. The nasal cavity and paranasal sinuses were too small to allow for the introduction of at least two of the early instruments necessary for the principle of triangulation and unrestricted manipulation. Additional detractors to the popularization of endoscopic craniomaxillofacial surgery were the absence of specialized instrumentation, initially lengthy operative times and significant equipment expenses. Relentlessly, through cadaver studies to first clinical applications, facial endoscopy pioneers introduced novel techniques of exposing and repairing facial injuries through strategically located minute incisions into mechanically dissected optical cavities, avoiding large scars and vital structures. Most notable are the works of Sakai et al [1996] on Le Fort I and III osteotomies, Kobayashi et al [1995] and Lee et al [1997] on zygomatic arch and mandibular condyle, Forrest [1999]. Shumrick [2001], Strong et al [2003], Chen [2003], and Stanley [1989] on frontal sinus and orbit, and Troulis [2004] on mandibular osteotomies. Together with the development of specialized craniomaxillofacial endoscopic instrumentation, these were the pivotal steps in allowing a wider spread application of endoscope-assisted techniques to facial trauma care.

The endoscope is of great benefit to the facial trauma surgeon. It allows for a minimally invasive access to craniomaxillofacial injuries that could previously only be reached using wide open exposures and their associated risks, while still permitting anatomical fracture realignment and rigid fixation. The endoscope has two principal roles in facial trauma management. First, it decreases the morbidity of surgical access in injuries where ORIF is considered the current standard, for example the zygomatic arch. Second, it allows for anatomical repair of injuries that were previously mainly treated nonoperatively or not at all due to perceivably unacceptable operative risks, for example the mandibular condyle.

In this chapter, the rationale, specific indications, surgical techniques and complications of the endoscope-assisted techniques for the repair of mandibular condyle, zygomatic arch, orbital walls, and frontal sinus are presented. The discussion of future directions of craniomaxillofacial endoscopy will follow.

2 Indications

2.1 Mandibular condyle

2.1.1 Rationale

Temporomandibular joint (TMJ) anatomy is highly complex. The condylar head is elliptically shaped in the axial plane, measuring on average 20 mm in width and 10 mm in length. It articulates with the glenoid fossa, which is only slightly larger, measuring 23 mm in width and 15 mm in length. The anterior wall of the fossa is inclined at 30° to the sagittal plane and guides translatory motion. Its medial wall has a slope of 15° in the coronal plane and directs lateral excursive movements. Clearly, only minimal imprecisions can be tolerated at the finely tuned temporomandibular articulation. A malunited condyle alters these precise relationships resulting in significant aberrations in joint dynamics which have a marked potential to produce late internal derangement. Furthermore, the bilateral interdependence of the craniomandibular articulation imposes excessive biomechanical loads on the contralateral condyle, similarly predisposing it to early degenerative changes.

Condylar fractures account for 20–50% of mandibular injuries. For decades these fractures had been treated using mandibulomaxillary fixation (MMF) with seemingly good outcomes. However, careful inspection of the effects of MMF has shown that fracture reduction is rarely achieved and some malunion generally results following displaced fractures. Centric occlusion is thus forced through neuromuscular adaptation at the TMJ. The malunion is not inconsequential, leading to a decreased posterior ramal height due to interfragmentary overlap, abnormal orientation of the condylar head and alteration of TMJ biomechanics, with secondary esthetic and functional disturbances.

In bilateral condyle fractures, with shortened rami, the mandibular plane may rotate clockwise causing an unappealing loss of chin projection through the pogonion. In this position, an anterior open bite of several millimeters may exist. Only seldom and briefly, for instance during chewing, are maximal intercuspidation and chin position forcefully restored. Furthermore, in unilateral condyle fractures, ramus shortening decreases the ipsilateral radius of mandibular rotation resulting in a mechanically disadvantaged jaw deviation during motion.

Next, the anteroposteriorly flexed condylar posture, occurring due to the pull of the lateral pterygoid, and present in more than 80% of adult fractures, results in its premature contact with the anterior wall of the glenoid fossa. Interincisal opening is limited to only the initial 20–25 mm of hinge-type motion. Further, 15–20 mm available through translation along the articular eminence is not fully achieved.

Mandibulomaxillary fixation is not tolerated by certain patient populations, such as those with dementia or psychiatric diagnoses. Inability to freely move the mandible can also be potentially dangerous in those suffering from a seizure disorder or substance abuse, as these patients are at an increased risk for aspiration. Even when tolerated, MMF is frequently uncomfortable and leads to weight loss and difficulties in maintaining proper oral hygiene. The prolonged period of MMF immobilization necessitates a lengthy postoperative regimen of muscular and occlusal rehabilitation to recover muscle function, and condylar range of motion. These issues are far from trivial as they can have negative consequences on patients' general state of health.

Clearly, results of non-surgical treatment of adult condylar injuries with major displacement have not been encouraging. Recent long-term studies comparing ORIF versus MMF confirm the advantage of open techniques, despite the fact that they were used to treat more severe injuries. The reluctance to open repair of the mandibular condyle was also due to the real risk of facial nerve injury, introduction of visible scarring and technical challenge. The risk of permanent facial nerve palsy using transcutaneous surgery averages 1% and transient dysfunction occurs in 0–46% of cases. External incisions almost universally result in perceptible scarring, and in 4% of patients will leave an unsightly mark. As an effect, many surgeons continued to treat condylar injuries in adult patients using MMF.

The introduction of the endoscope to craniomaxillofacial surgery shifted the tides in the traditional doctrine on condylar trauma management. Endoscopic assistance allows the surgeon to achieve the preferable goal of anatomical fracture realignment using a path devoid of cutaneous incisions, which minimizes risk of injury to the facial nerve. The negative sequelae of condylar malunion, a frequent outcome of isolated MMF, can no longer be accepted as the fateful result of treatment.

2.1.2 Treatment indications

Walker [1994] suggested five goals for condylar fracture treatment: pain-free mouth opening with interincisal distance over 40 mm, good movement of the jaw in all excursions, preinjury occlusion of the teeth, stable TMJs, and good facial and jaw symmetry. Mandibulomaxillary fixation may achieve these objectives in some injuries. Fractures in prepubertal patients may not always require accurate reduction due to the immense potential for condylar rehabilitation through growth and restitutional remodeling. For fractures without significant loss of ramus height non-surgical treatment can be expected to produce favorable functional and esthetic results. The last group comprises stable injuries with minimal displacement and no dislocation.

The remaining fracture types benefit from consideration of anatomical reduction and rigid internal fixation to restore preinjury ramus height, upright posture of the condylar head and thus complex anatomical relationships of the temporomandibular articulation. A transcutaneous approach allows the surgeon to effect rigid anatomical repair but entails risk of injury to the facial nerve, whose course and branching pattern are difficult to exactly predict, and of visible scars. An open intraoral approach is intended to minimize these shortcomings but has not gained widespread acceptance because it provides less adequate visualization and makes hardware placement more difficult.

Endoscopic condylar repair thus may replace external techniques in the treatment of some of the fractures which are notorious for poor outcomes when treated with MMF. It is indicated for the treatment of adult condylar neck and subcondylar fractures with displacement or dislocation.

Today, precision, safety, and predictability of endoscopic treatment of condylar fractures also allows for the treatment of children older than 5 years, as in severely dislocated fractures. Remodeling during growth may not always be achieved in this age group and sequelae of the injuries can result in impaired function of the TMJ, associated with an abnormally shaped condylar head, reduced height of the mandibular ramus, and growth anomalies resulting in facial asymmetry. The endoscope may be useful in endoscopically assisted removal of foreign bodies near the condylar process as well as for endoscopic removal of condylar lesions.

3 Preoperative planning

3.1 Fracture anatomy

Careful patient selection is necessary to identify those fractures in which minimally invasive repair is feasible. This assessment includes the anatomical location of the fracture as well as the type and degree of displacement of the fragments, and whether sufficient bony space exists for the placement of fixation hardware.

3.2 Fracture location

The mandibular condyle can be subdivided into three surgically important anatomical zones: head, neck (below the capsule and above the sigmoid notch), and subcondyle. Fractures of the condylar head cannot be treated with endoscopically assisted procedures. Injuries of the neck region are amenable to endoscopic repair if the fracture is low enough to accept the application of at least two holes of a 2.0 mm miniplate into the proximal segment. Subcondylar fractures are most easily approached with the endoscope.

3.3 Fracture displacement

Fracture fragment displacement, defined as the relative position of the proximal to the distal mandible segments, must be considered before endoscopic repair. Fractures demonstrating lateral override, and those where the proximal fragment overlaps the lateral aspect of the ascending mandibular ramus, are easiest to treat. Hardware can be placed on the freely accessible lateral surface of the proximal segment and reduction obtained. Medial override injuries, those where the proximal fragment is overlapped laterally by the ramus, represent a greater challenge. Direct repair is not possible as the ramus obscures visual access to the lateral surface of the condylar fragment and greatly impairs manipulation due to physical obstruction. These injuries must be recognized on preoperative radiography and redisplaced under endoscopic guidance into lateral override. Fortunately, this subgroup accounts for less than 20% of adult condylar injuries. Nondisplaced, nondislocated fractures signify the presence of sufficiently stable periosteal support and do not require open treatment.

3.4 Fracture comminution

Visualization of a congruent fracture line, as well as smooth anterior and posterior borders of the condyle are the most important markers of anatomical reduction. Comminution involving the borders of the fracture significantly impedes, in proportion to its degree, the surgeon's ability to accurately reposition the condylar segments to their preinjury status. A minor amount of comminution is not considered a contraindication. Severely comminuted fractures, however, should not be approached endoscopically. In addition to greatly increasing the difficulty of reduction, comminution does not allow for adequate fixation through the endoscopic approach.

4 Condyle–fossa relationship

Fractures without condylar head dislocation from the glenoid fossa are most favorable for endoscopic repair. When true fracture dislocation is present, repair is significantly more challenging.

4.1 Radiographic imaging

Fracture location, displacement, comminution and condylar head location must be assessed preoperatively to determine the feasibility of the endoscopic approach and to formulate an appropriate operative plan. Accurate radiographic imaging is thus an integral part of patient evaluation. Fine cut axial CT scans with 3-D reformatting provide the most precise illustration of the necessary variables and have been shown more sensitive than traditional panoramic tomography in detecting mandibular fractures. Reformatted images clearly show condylar fracture anatomy, but may underestimate the degree of comminution.

5 Operative technique

5.1 Equipment

Instruments required include a 4 mm diameter 30° angle scope, a 4 mm endoscopic brow lift sheath that maintains the optical cavity, and a video system composed of a camera, light source camera converter and monitor. Two video monitors placed on either side of the head make it easier for the surgeon and assistant to view the procedure. Standard mandible fracture repair instruments are used, in addition to the subcondylar ramus fixation set, which provides many specialized instruments and tools.

5.2 Repair sequence

Additional non-condylar mandibular fractures, if present, are addressed first using standard open reduction and rigid fixation techniques. This restores an intact mandibular arch that may then be used as a lever arm in manipulating fracture fragments to achieve accurate reduction.

5.3 Mandibulomaxillary fixation

The use of tight-wire MMF will often lock the displaced condyle in a malreduced position. Wire MMF must be removed before the commencement of condylar repair. Accurate reduction is judged by the alignment of the fracture fragments. Rubber band anterior MMF is routinely used as it facilitates repair by maintaining occlusion but permitting realignment of fracture fragments.

5.4 Exposure

Initial approach to this fracture is via an intraoral incision along the oblique line of the mandible. The endoscopic cavity is created by elevating the periosteum off the lateral surface of the ascending ramus under direct visualization. Transcutaneous incisions permit screw placement and are made directly over the palpated fracture line at the posterior border of the ramus. To minimize risk of injury to the facial nerve, gentle dissection using a blunt-tipped hemostat is performed through the parotid gland and masseter muscle. The retractor mounted endoscope is then inserted and further subperiosteal dissection of the proximal condylar fragment is carried out up to the joint capsule (**Fig 5.1-1**). Importantly, the degree of overlap and angulation of the proximal condylar segment must be appreciated to avoid mistakenly confusing it with the ascending ramus.

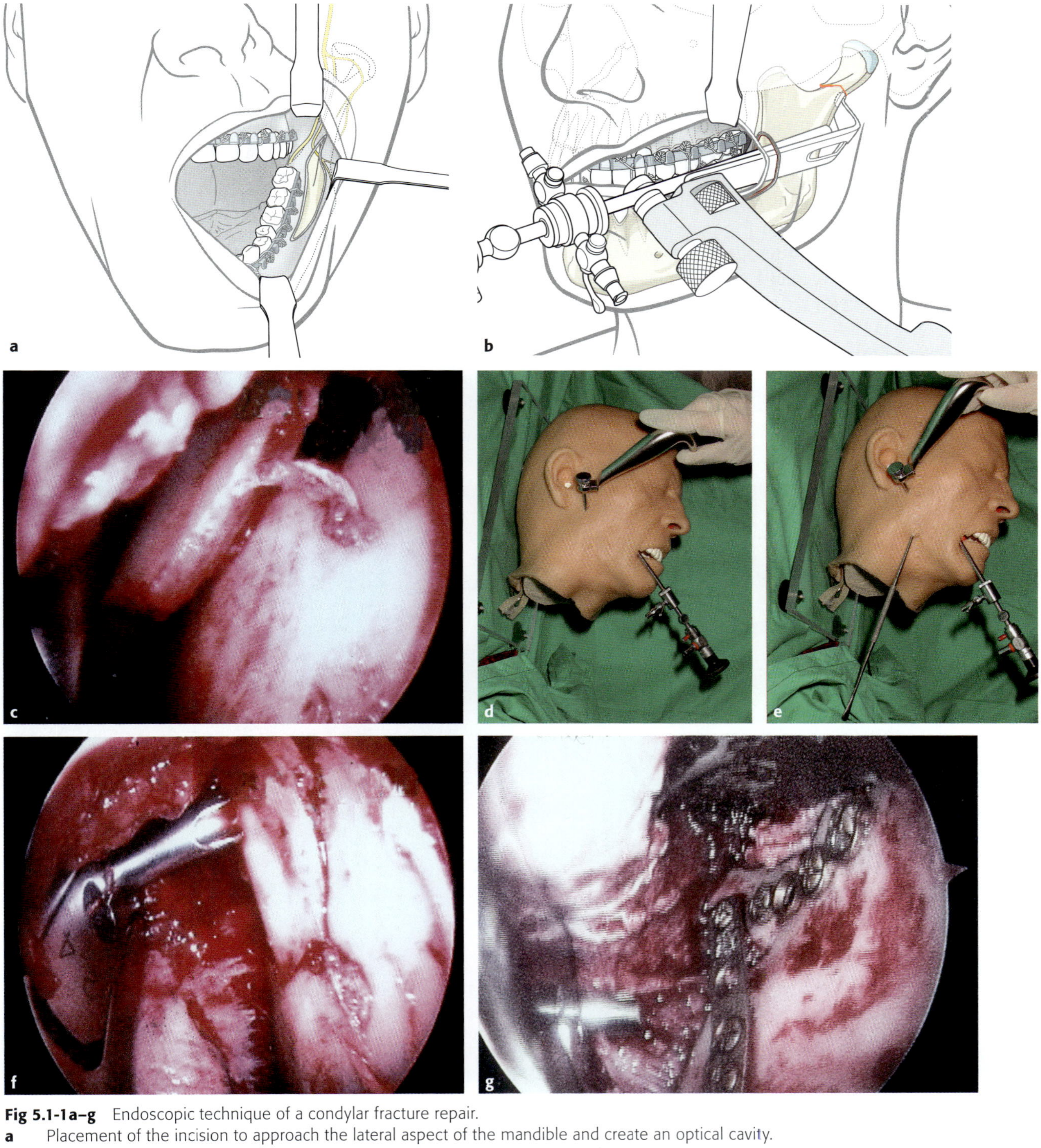

Fig 5.1-1a–g Endoscopic technique of a condylar fracture repair.

- **a** Placement of the incision to approach the lateral aspect of the mandible and create an optical cavity.
- **b** Placement of the endoscope through the optical retractor up to the fracture line.
- **c** Endoscopic visualization of the displaced fracture.
- **d** A second portal is made directly over the fracture site. It is used for the insertion of a trocar, allowing for proximal condylar pole realignment and percutaneous screw fixation.
- **e** An optional third portal may be placed at mandibular angle, allowing for further fracture fragment manipulation. It may also be used to insert the endoscope for superior view of the posterior border of the mandible during fracture reduction.
- **f** Endoscopic view after reduction of the condyle-bearing fragment.
- **g** Situation after fixation with two miniplates.

5.5 Reduction

Medial override injuries are initially reduced into lateral override. This is achieved by placing a curved elevator medial to the proximal fragment, while strongly distracting the fracture so as to allow the proximal fragment to be displaced to the lateral surface of the ascending ramus (**Fig 5.1-2**). For those injuries already in lateral override, interfragmentary realignment is achieved by distracting the distal segment through mechanical traction at the mandibular angle or placement of a posterior occlusal spacer. The proximal segment can be reduced by medially directed pressure using a trocar inserted through the percutaneous incision. Removal of traction or the posterior occlusal wedge will then permit the rubber band MMF to temporarily impact the fracture interfaces.

5.6 Fixation

A transcutaneous trocar serves to introduce the screws. A miniplate (2.0) is initially fixated along the posterior border of the proximal fragment, taking advantage of its thick cortical bone and flat surface. Using the plate as a handle, the condylar fragment is positioned into reduction. Screws are then placed in the distal fragment. A minimum of two screws are placed in each fracture segment to ensure solid fixation. A second plate is then fixated near the anterior portion of the fracture using a similar technique. If possible, placement of two miniplates is advocated to minimize the risk of stress-induced hardware failure (**Fig 5.1-1g**). Following hardware placement, rubber band MMF is released and the mandible moved in all excursions to ensure reproducible complete occlusion with the condyle seated in the fossa and adequate motion.

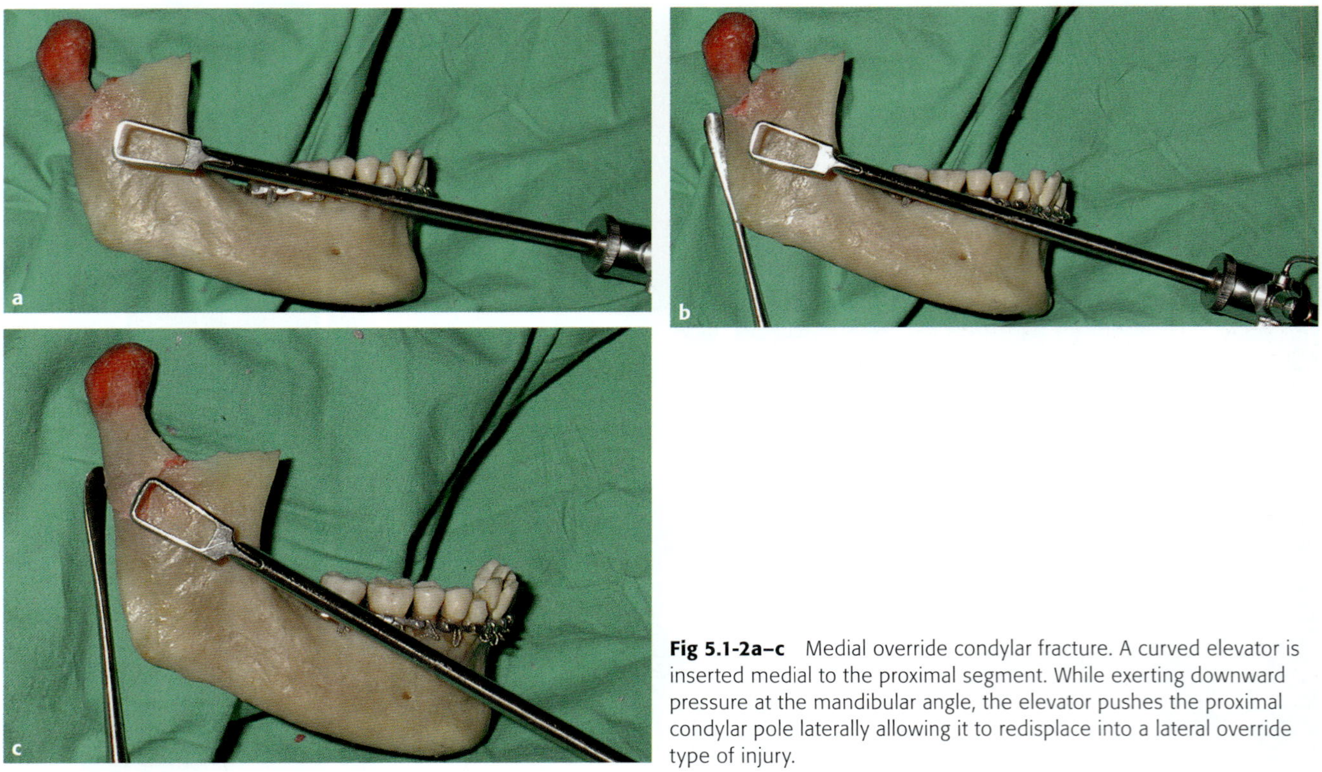

Fig 5.1-2a–c Medial override condylar fracture. A curved elevator is inserted medial to the proximal segment. While exerting downward pressure at the mandibular angle, the elevator pushes the proximal condylar pole laterally allowing it to redisplace into a lateral override type of injury.

5.7 Postoperative regimen

All patients leave the operating room without MMF and are maintained on a puree diet for 6 weeks. Training elastics may help the patient adapt to function postoperatively. Representative case is shown in **Fig 5.1-3**.

5.8 Results of endoscopic treatment of condylar fractures

Multi-year experiences with the transoral, endoscopically assisted treatment of displaced condylar fractures have been reported. In a series [Schön et al, 2005] of 62 fractures, a lateral dislocation of the fracture was observed in 58 patients. Medially displaced condylar heads (n = 17) and bilateral condylar fractures (n = 4) could also be treated with success, however. The use of angulated screwdrivers and drills provided good visibility of the fracture site and precise anatomical reduction in all patients. The average operation time was 1 hour 5 minutes.

In a prospective randomized double-blind study [Schmelzeisen et al, 2009] nonendoscopic ORIF using a transfacial approach was compared with patients with a transoral endoscopic procedure. The primary functional outcome measure was investigated using the asymmetric Helkimo dysfunction score at 8–12 weeks and 1 year after surgery. The nonendoscopic extraoral group (n = 34) and the endoscopically assisted open reduction group (n = 40) showed comparable functional results without any statistical significance. The endoscope-assisted treatment proved to be more time consuming. However, in the nonendoscopic group a greater number of facial nerve injuries were reported showing the reliability and the advantages of endoscope-assisted surgery for selected patients.

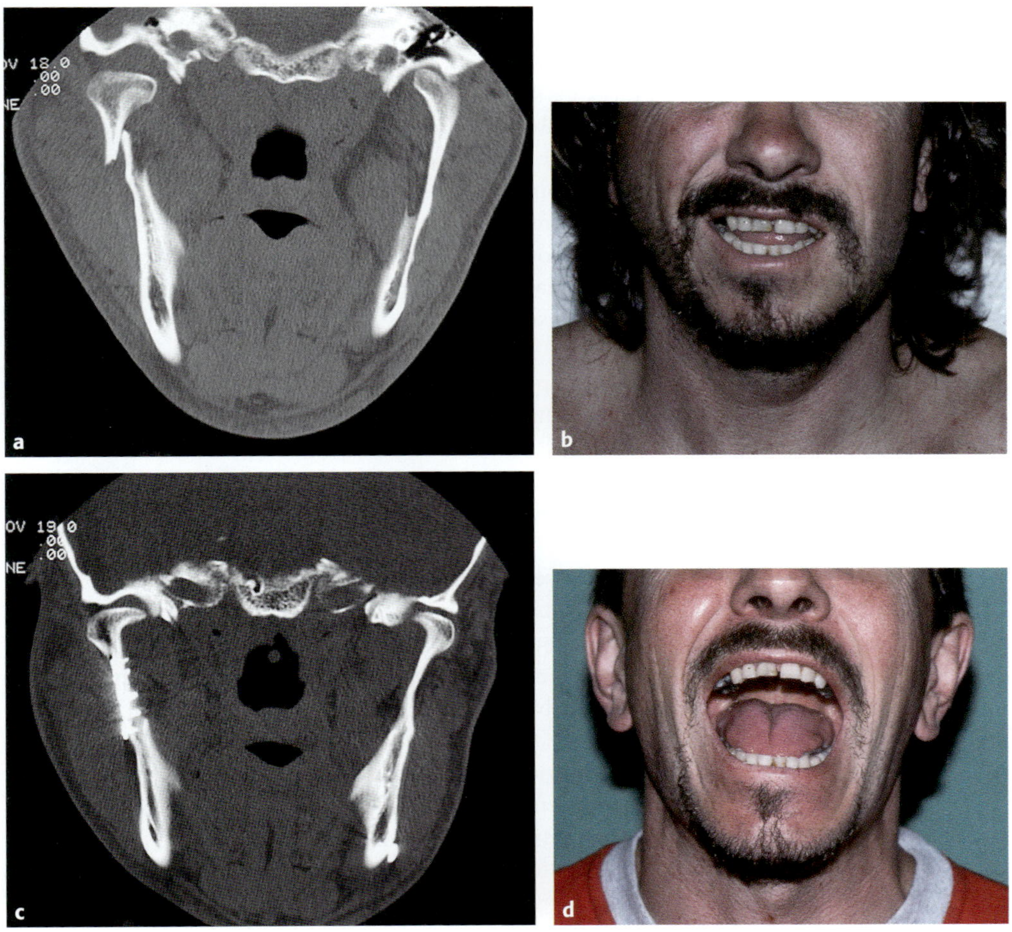

Fig 5.1-3a–d A right subcondylar fracture.
- **a** Preoperative coronal computed tomographic image showing the lateral override of proximal condylar segment.
- **b** Patient presenting with an anterior open bite deformity, decreased interincisal opening and dental midline deviation on jaw opening to the affected side.
- **c** After endoscope-assisted open reduction and internal fixation, restoration of condylar anatomy and mandibular height can be seen.
- **d** Patient after endoscopic repair, premorbid occlusion is restored. Jaw opening is midline and exceeds 40 mm.

6 Contingencies and complications

In a number of cases, endoscopic repair will not be possible. This is most often due to inadequate proximal bone stock or excessive comminution. Careful preoperative CT image evaluation will minimize the number of such cases attempted. When used selectively, endoscope-assisted ORIF can be expected to reliably produce anatomical reduction and adequate stabilization in most cases. If the surgeon is unable to complete the endoscopic procedure, he/she should resort to the method of condylar repair which they would customarily use.

The largest published series [Müller et al, 2006] of endoscopic condylar fracture repair comprises 135 patients. Here the rate of malreduction in primarily endoscopically fixated fractures is 4%. Plate fracture is rare, accounting for less than 2% of cases. Less than 4% of patients do not regain interincisal opening greater than 35 mm. Permanent facial nerve injury has not been reported with this technique and temporary palsy occurs in less than 2% of cases.

In 13 patients [Schön et al, 2008] with endoscope-assisted transoral treatment of displaced bilateral condylar fractures a 6-month follow-up demonstrated a preinjury range of TMJ motion and the possibility of an intake of a normal diet. Limitations of lateral excursion were not noted. There was no clicking of the TMJ and no pain on movement. Twelve months after surgery a stable result regarding TMJ function was noted. In one patient, loosening of one screw was noted at the 12-month follow-up and plate removal was performed without any signs of fracture displacement or resorption.

7 Zygomatic arch

7.1 Rationale

The zygomatic arch forms one of the horizontal facial buttresses, supporting the frequently injured midface from the sturdy temporal bone posteriorly. The arch has a consistent shape. In the axial plane, it is curved in the posterior third of its course and straight in the anterior two thirds. On sagittal section, it is parallel to the Frankfurt horizontal.

Fractures of the zygomatic arch can be isolated or exist with other midfacial injuries. The injury pattern depends on the magnitude and direction of the trauma force vector as well as individual skeletal characteristics. Isolated arch fractures are of three types. First, direct lateral force displaces the arch medially. Second, an anterior force vector focused on the malar prominence will usually cause a posterior telescoping pattern of injury. Third, a posteriorly directed force can also result in an explosive burst with displacement of the arch fragments laterally. Recognition of the latter two injury patterns is important as a nonvisualized reduction attempt, as described by Gillies, will be unsuccessful and exacerbate fracture displacement.

The arch's reliable shape, strategic location and coexistence of arch fractures with high-energy midfacial trauma allow numerous authors to use it as a key landmark support in midface fracture management [Gruss et al, 1990; Stanley, 1989]. The role of the arch in midfacial repair can be viewed as threefold. First, it can be used to guide precise fracture realignment to accurately restore midfacial projection; second, it can serve as an anchor point for the midface due to its sturdy skull base attachment; and third, its anatomical reduction is paramount to esthetic appearance in patients with increased facial width.

Despite the potential role of the zygomatic arch, its repair has been approached with caution, as access to it is challenging. Incisions should not be placed directly over the arch because of a possible facial nerve injury. To avoid facial nerve injuries the coronal approach was used to approach the arch indirectly from above and behind the facial nerve. Disadvantages of the coronal approach include scar alopecia, sensory disturbances posterior to the incision, traction injury to the frontal or zygomatic branches of the facial nerve, temporal hollowing, and excessive blood loss.

Endoscopy gives the surgeon the potential to utilize arch repair while minimizing the negative sequelae of traditional access. In addition, this technique offers other advantages including magnified direct visualization and a potential for rapid, cost-effective treatment.

7.2 Treatment indications

An endoscopic approach to the arch may be considered whenever precise arch repair is deemed an integral part of the treatment plan. Thus, when the zygomatic arch is thought to contribute to proper reduction and/or enhanced stability of other facial fractures or when the arch itself is considered an important esthetic and structural landmark, the surgeon may attempt endoscope-assisted ORIF. Specifically, endoscope-assisted ORIF of the zygomatic arch may be indicated in esthetically evident isolated arch fractures, zygomaticomaxillary complex (ZMC) fractures and Le Fort III level midface injuries.

In isolated arch fractures, repair is particularly important in individuals with prominent premorbid lateral facial contours.

Failure of realignment will lead to unsightly temporal flattening and asymmetry. In addition, miniplate fixation will prevent postoperative arch displacement, an issue which is not addressed by the Gillie's or closed reduction approaches.

In posteriorly displaced ZMC fractures, arch reduction is a valuable tool for anatomical repositioning of the malar prominence and to restore normal facial width and projection. Also, medial repositioning of the ZMC restores adequate orbital volume. This is paramount in complex ZMC fractures where there may be extensive comminution of at least two of the three anterior buttresses. In these injuries, the arch also serves as an additional point of rigid fixation and zygomatic adjustment.

In Le Fort III level injuries, the principal benefit of rigid arch fixation is to stabilize and align the mobile midface to the skull base. This ensures secure midface dimensions and a stable occlusal relationship. The arch is particularly valuable when the other anterior buttresses are comminuted. The remaining role of the arch in Le Fort III fractures is to enhance accurate midfacial realignment.

Endoscope-assisted ORIF is unnecessary when a coronal flap is used for other fracture treatment, such as: nasoorbitoethmoid, posterior table of the frontal sinus or displaced skull fractures.

7.3 Preoperative planning

7.3.1 Radiographic imaging

Fine cut preoperative axial CT scans with coronal and sagittal reformatting is required to visualize arch fragmentation and displacement patterns. The presence of other midfacial injuries is ascertained to create a complete management plan. Aligning the zygoma in the lateral orbit with the greater sphenoid wing proves useful to establish the proper medial position of the zygomatic arch.

7.3.2 Repair sequencing

In nonisolated zygomatic arch injuries, the following sequence of fracture management is generally the most useful. For ZMC and Le Fort III fractures, endoscopic approaches to the arch can assist traditional open techniques.

8 Operative technique

8.1 Equipment

See section on: Mandibular condyle fractures/operative technique/equipment.

8.2 Exposure

A scalp extension of a preauricular incision is carried through the skin and the temporoparietal fascia to expose the deep temporal fascia. A periosteal elevator is then inserted and an optical cavity is created by dissecting superficial to the deep temporal fascia. This nonvisualized part of the dissection is performed only superior to an imaginary line extending from the helical crus to the superior orbital rim. This minimizes the risk of injury to the frontal branch of the facial nerve. Following dissection of the optical cavity, a retractor-mounted endoscope is inserted and directly visualized dissection in the same plane is performed down to the zygomatic arch (**Fig 5.1-4**).

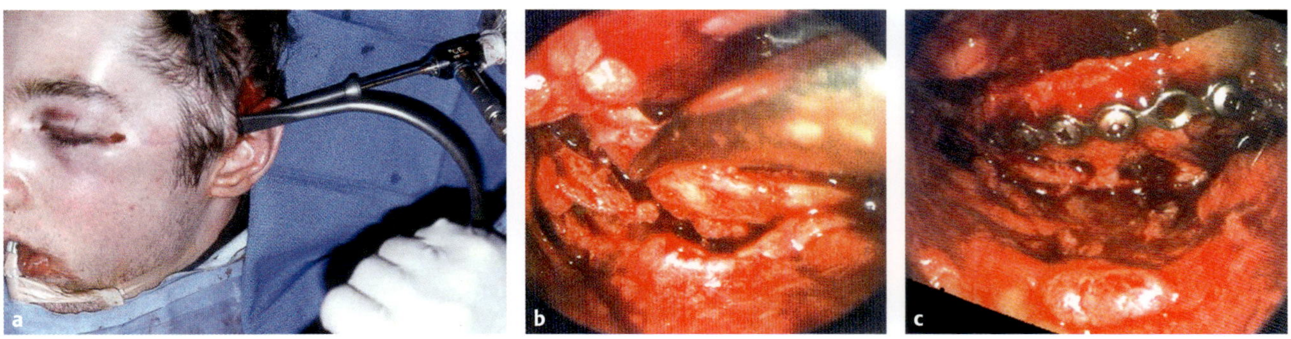

Fig 5.1-4a–c Endoscopic technique for zygomatic arch repair.

a An incision in the temporal hairline is made and dissection is performed superficial to the deep temporal fascia. The endoscope is inserted to minimize the risk of injury to the frontal branch of the facial nerve and exposes zygomatic arch fragments in a subperiosteal plane.

b Fractured zygomatic arch exposed.

c Following in situ reduction, a long mini-adaptation plate is used to fix the arch fragments.

Maintenance of integrity of the deep temporal fascia helps to avoid temporal hollowing. Once the arch is reached, its periosteum is incised and the sites of fracture are exposed in the subperiosteal plane. Chen [2000] modified this approach by performing the dissection beneath the superficial layer of the deep temporal fascia. He incises the deep temporal fascia 1 cm above the zygomatic arch and then proceeds with the subperiosteal dissection to the upper margin of the zygomatic arch.

8.3 Reduction

Following exposure, arch fragments are reduced according to the fragmentation pattern to restore preinjury arch form.

8.4 Fixation

Selection of appropriate fixation hardware depends on the type of fracture. A short miniplate is used in isolated arch injuries whereas a long mini-adaptation plate is preferred in associated midfacial trauma. The long mini-adaptation plate extends onto the lateral orbital rim, restoring and rigidly stabilizing the midface. Following fixation of the plate to an arch segment, accurate reduction is confirmed and the plate is stabilized to other fracture segments using the endoscope (**Fig 5.1-4c**). Representative ZMC and Le Fort III fracture cases are shown in **Fig 5.1-5** and **Fig 5.1-6**, respectively.

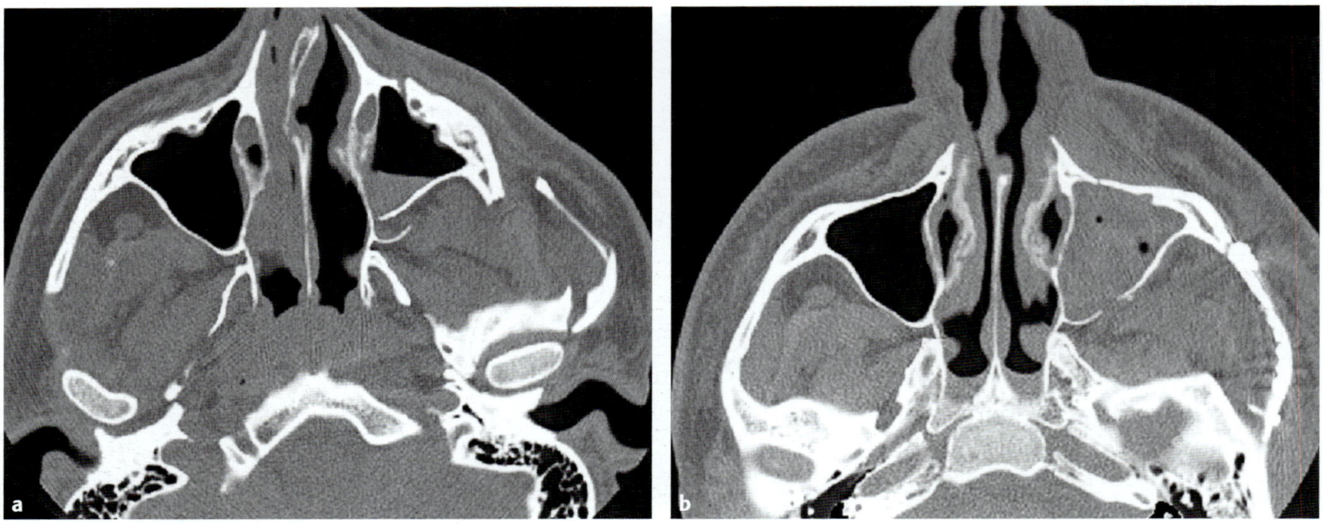

Fig 5.1-5a–b A left ZMC and zygomatic arch fracture.

a Preoperative axial computed tomographic scan demonstrates a left ZMC fracture with posterior displacement of the zygoma body and lateral outburst of arch segments.

b After endoscopic repair, anatomical repositioning of all fracture segments can be seen.

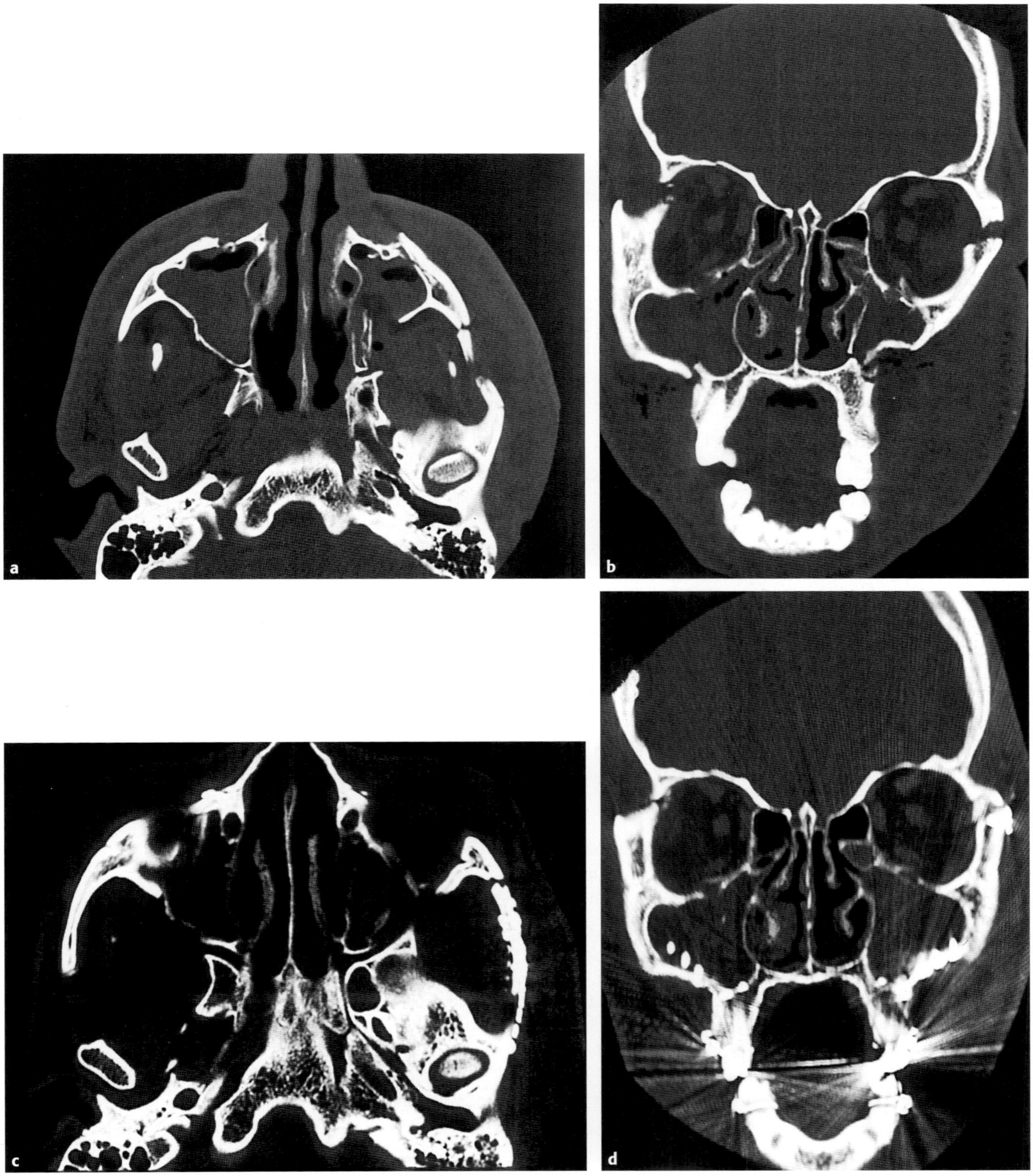

Fig 5.1-6a–d A central midface fracture with zygomatic arch involvement on the left side.
a–b Preoperative axial and coronal computed tomographic scans demonstrate posteromedial left midface displacement.
c–d Postoperative images show accurate midfacial buttress restoration with return of premorbid occlusion.

8.5 Contingencies and complications

Review of the literature identified four eligible patient series (adequate follow-up, outcomes reported) comprising 78 patients. Incidence of temporary facial nerve palsy when dissection was performed beneath the superficial temporal fascia was 3 (5.6%) of 53. Chen [2000] describes no incidences of nerve palsy with his modified approach. He credits this to a greater level of protection from mechanical retraction afforded by a thicker layer of tissue. There have been no cases of permanent palsy. There is lesser risk of temporal hollowing when deep temporal fascia is not violated, thus preserving vascular supply to the fat pad.

If the endoscopic procedure cannot be completed, the surgeon should resort to a coronal or hemicoronal exposure to accomplish arch repair. In our experience this has been infrequent.

9 Orbital floor

9.1 Rationale

Orbital floor fractures may occur in isolation, when trauma applied directly to the globe or inferior orbital rim is transmitted to the floor, or as a necessary component of ZMC fractures. Size of the floor defect and presence of entrapped periorbital tissues determine treatment strategy. Floor fractures greater than 2 cm^2 or 50% of total floor area significantly increase the risk of enophthalmos or hypoophthalmos development through orbital volume augmentation. Entrapped periorbital tissues may cause extraocular muscle imbalance, impeding binocular vision.

Currently, the diagnosis and precise characterization of orbital fractures can be accurately performed using noninvasive fine-cut coronal CT scanning. In cases where adequate preoperative imaging is unavailable or inaccurate, surgical exploration may be considered.

Traditional approaches to the orbital floor involve the use of a transfacial incision, either at the subciliary, transconjunctival, subtarsal or infraorbital level. Several undesirable sequelae are associated with such approaches, including visible scarring, scleral show and ectropion (1–42%). The transconjunctival approach presents significantly lesser morbidity but is however not devoid of complications. For example, ectropion (up to 7%), inferior oblique muscle injury, and entropion have been noted.

The endoscope offers the potential to avoid lower lid incisions in orbital floor fractures. The adjacent maxillary sinus offers a natural optical cavity with great exposure of the entire orbital floor. It may be accessed via an anterior maxillary wall antrostomy or transnasally.

9.2 Treatment indications

Currently, the endoscope is most useful as a diagnostic tool in cases where accurate CT imaging is unavailable or when the information is no longer accurate, for example after reduction of a ZMC fracture. Furthermore, it helps determine which cases require surgical repair.

Whenever floor repair is judged important, endoscopic approach may be considered and used if no contraindications exist. Endoscope-assisted repair of the orbital floor has been performed with success by numerous authors. It does, however, require significant endoscopic experience, specialized equipment and carries a potentially disastrous risk of ocular and optic nerve injury. Injuries which can most easily be repaired with the endoscope include trapdoor and medial orbital floor blowout fractures. Trapdoor fractures are frequently stable after reduction of orbital contents and can be left without fixation. Medial blowout injuries can be treated using a small alloplastic implant. Injuries lateral to the infraorbital nerve (ION), or those involving the medial orbital wall, require more extensive dissection and implant fixation. These are probably best approached through the lower lid.

For some fractures, which need treatment via open approaches, the endoscope may still serve as an adjunct to reducing entrapped periorbital tissue and identifying the posterior floor ledge for implant alignment.

9.3 Operative technique

9.3.1 Equipment

General endoscopic equipment required has been previously described. In addition, a smooth elevator and a 55° forked elevator are useful for mucosal dissection and implant manipulation. Standard orbital fracture instruments are also used.

9.3.2 Exposure

The maxillary sinus is used as the optical cavity in orbital floor injuries. It is entered most commonly through a transoral osteotomy of the anterior maxillary wall using a small osteotome or a piezoelectric device. This antrostomy should be approximately 1 x 2 cm large and situated 1–2 mm below the ION. Be cautious to avoid injuries to the ION or dental roots. Old blood is suctioned from the sinus and the endoscope is inserted and important structures (ION, maxillary sinus ostium) as well as fracture anatomy are visualized (**Fig 5.1-7**).

Alternatively, the sinus may be entered intranasally using a small antrostomy under the uncinate process of the inferior turbinate. The uncinate process may be subluxed medially and removed. The "pulse test" may be used to diagnose clinically significant orbital floor defects. With the endoscope inside the antrum, digital pressure is applied to the globe. Only those fractures that allow intraorbital content herniation with this maneuver require repair.

9.4 Reduction and fixation

Trapdoor injuries are repaired using reduction only. A smooth elevator is used to expose 5 mm of bone at the lateral periphery of the defect. Avoid excessive medial dissection to preserve periosteal integrity. Traction is then placed on the bone flap to allow reduction of orbital contents. The bone flap is then released into position and fracture stability checked. Excessive comminution at the lateral fracture edge will require treatment similarly to medial blowout injuries.

Medial blowout fractures necessitate implant insertion. First, a smooth elevator is used to dissect 5 mm of maxillary sinus mucosa around the circumference of the defect. Similarly, 5 mm of periosteum is dissected circumferentially on the orbital side. All loose bone fragments are removed to permit proper stable ledge identification and prevent their inadvertent displacement into the orbit. This step is essential in minimizing surgical risks. Subsequently, an alloplastic implant is tailored to the defect pattern and inserted onto the orbital face of the fracture. Implant fixation is not required.

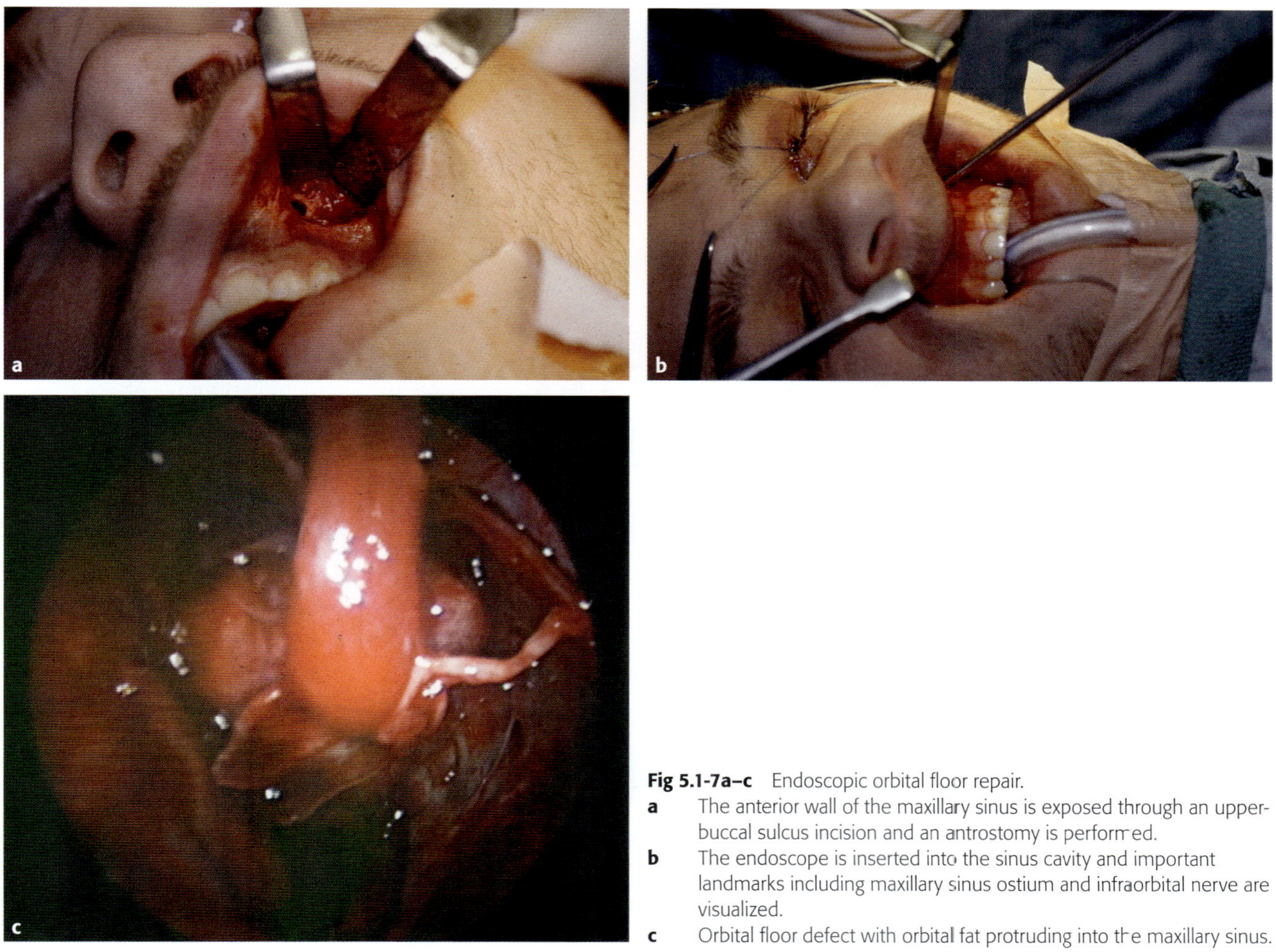

Fig 5.1-7a–c Endoscopic orbital floor repair.
- **a** The anterior wall of the maxillary sinus is exposed through an upper-buccal sulcus incision and an antrostomy is performed.
- **b** The endoscope is inserted into the sinus cavity and important landmarks including maxillary sinus ostium and infraorbital nerve are visualized.
- **c** Orbital floor defect with orbital fat protruding into the maxillary sinus.

Lateral blowout fractures not involving the greater wing of the sphenoid may be repaired similarly to the medial blowout injuries. However, the extent of dissection is significantly greater and extreme care should be taken to prevent injury to the ION during dissection and implant placement. Specialized instrumentation is required for securing the implant. A representative patient example is shown in **Fig 5.1-8**.

"The pulse test" is performed after implant insertion to ensure fracture stability. Routine forced duction test confirms no extraocular muscle entrapment.

9.5 Contingencies and complications

Osteoplastic antrostomy does not leave any contour deformities. Intraorbital misadventures are exceedingly rare but potentially disastrous, including orbital hemorrhage, optic nerve and ocular globe injury and extraocular muscle damage. Risk of nerve and globe injuries can be significantly decreased by ensuring the removal of all intraorbital fracture fragments before implant placement. Avoid excessive posteromedial dissection. In the eight published endoscopic floor fracture repair series, comprising 204 patients, there are no cases of either injury [Strong, 2004; Persons et al, 2002; Saunders et al, 1997; Ikeda et al, 1999; Hinohira et al, 2005; Nishiike et al, 2005; Otori et al, 2003; Chen et al, 2001]. The inferior rectus may be theoretically damaged during intraorbital manipulation; however, this had not been reported. Diplopia was improved in all patients with about 20% having some residual diplopia. Prevalence of long-term nerve disturbances is unknown.

In the endonasal technique, during middle meatal antrostomy, if enlargement of the ostium advances too far anteriorly, the nasolacrimal duct may be injured. There have been no complications with alloplastic implants used for endoscopic floor repair. In difficult cases, endoscopic exposure may be converted to open approaches.

10 Medial orbital wall

10.1 Indications and rationale

Medial orbital wall injuries are frequent. Theoretically their consequences on globe position may in fact be greater than that of orbital floor fractures, as the greater part of the medial wall lies behind the mid-axis of the ocular globe. The sequelae are similar to floor injuries and include extraocular muscle entrapment with secondary horizontal diplopia and enophthalmos due to orbital volume augmentation. The indications for open repair are extraocular muscle entrapment, early enophthalmos or significant wall defect which could result in enophthalmos later.

The transcaruncular approach is most commonly used to expose the medial wall. This technique is simple and without significant morbidities, unlike lower lid transcutaneous approaches. Adequate exposure of the superior and posterior extents of large medial wall fractures and placement of large implants may be more challenging.

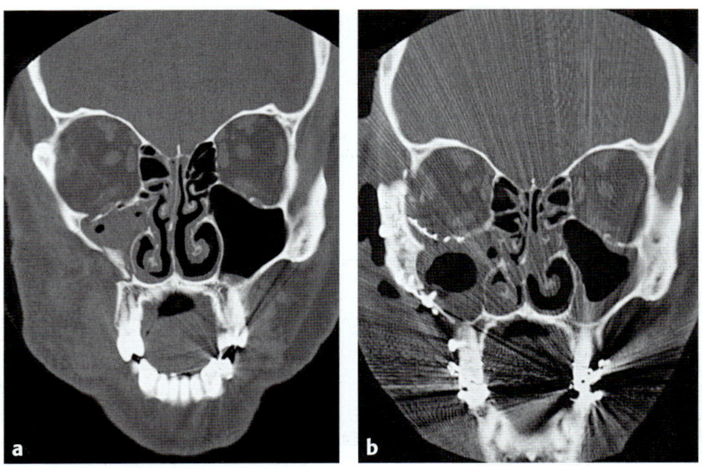

Fig 5.1-8a–b A zygomaticomaxillary fracture on the right side and right orbital floor fractures.

a Preoperative image shows significant floor disruption.

b After endoscopic transantral repair of the floor using a titanium mesh, without lower lid access, the dimensions of the orbital cavity were significantly improved and floor support restored.

Rhee et al [2006] have suggested that endoscopic assistance for surgical medial orbital wall injuries is indicated when the defect is too large for exposure and implant placement using the open transcaruncular method alone. The endoscope allows safer, magnified posterior dissection and identification of fracture extent. The endoscopic technique is unnecessary in concomitant floor injuries as a transconjunctival incision will permit adequate visualization, and in concomitant central facial fractures requiring coronal exposure.

10.2 Operative technique

10.2.1 Equipment

See section on: Orbital Floor Fractures/Operative Technique/Equipment

10.2.2 Exposure and reduction

A 1–2 cm incision through the caruncle is made and blunt dissection is performed behind the posterior lacrimal crest until the medial wall is reached. This decreases the risk of injuries to the nasolacrimal sac and medial canthus. The periorbita is then elevated superoinferiorly and initial dissection is carried posteriorly under direct visualization to create an optical cavity that is then maintained using a malleable retractor. A 0° endoscope is inserted to perform further posterior dissection until the posterior margin of the defect is attained. The superior extent of the dissection is usually marked by the ethmoidal vessels while inferiorly it is dictated by the size of the fracture. Important landmarks during dissection include anterior ethmoidal (24 mm posterior to the anterior lacrimal crest) and posterior ethmoidal arteries (12 mm posterior to the anterior ethmoidal artery). These vessels should be carefully cauterized to facilitate further exposure. The posterior ethmoidal artery marks the safe limit of posterior dissection, as the optic nerve is positioned 6 mm behind it.

10.2.3 Fixation

After the entire medial wall defect is circumferentially delineated, an alloplastic implant is accurately tailored to cover it. The implant is then inserted through the transcaruncular incision and fixated using a screw. As usual, a forced duction test is performed at the end of the procedure.

10.3 Complications

Four series of endoscopic medial orbital wall injuries are reported in the literature totaling 58 patients [Meningaud et al, 2005; Sanno et al, 2003; Lee et al, 2002; Jin et al, 2000]. Potential complications of endoscopic orbital surgery have been presented in the section on orbital floor injuries. In general, injuries to the nasolacrimal sac, medial rectus and optic nerve can be avoided by limiting excessive anterior and posterior dissections, respectively. The risk of intraorbital hemorrhage can be greatly reduced by careful coagulation of the ethmoidal vessels. To our knowledge, none of these injuries have been noted in the literature. A reported incidence of residual postoperative diplopia was 6 (10%) of 58. The transcaruncular incision is well tolerated. There have been no cases of periimplant infection described. Implant migration or extrusion is prevented through stable fixation.

11 Frontal sinus fractures

11.1 Rationale

The anterior table of the frontal sinus shapes the contour of the forehead. Its extent is variable, occupying only the inferior central portion in some individuals, and nearly the entire forehead topographical subunit in others. It is thought to serve as a shock absorber by fracturing and displacing into the frontal sinus cavity thus dissipating traumatic energy and often preventing potentially disastrous injury to the posteriorly located brain parenchyma. This function comes at the price of an esthetically displeasing forehead depression. The severity of this displacement depends on the individual frontal sinus thickness and structure and the magnitude of injury. Lower force injuries may present with isolated anterior table fractures only. In more severe trauma, there may be concomitant injuries to the frontonasal duct and displacement of the sinus posterior table and dural tears resulting in cerebrospinal fluid leakage.

The traditional method of anterior table repair involves direct transverse forehead, vertical corrugator crease or bilateral brow-glabella incisions or extensive exposure through a coronal approach. Direct incisions result in unsightly scars and brow alopecia. A coronal incision, as previously stated, may result in scar alopecia, posterior scalp anesthesia and blood loss. In individuals with short or receding hair, the long scalp scar is frequently more esthetically displeasing than small forehead depressions. In addition, patients with nasofrontal duct injury and voluminous sinuses extending above the lateral supraorbital rims frequently require sinus osteotomies to remove all of sinus mucosa and prevent the formation of a mucocele. This technique may be associated with injury to the supraorbital nerves, bone flap loss, excessive blood loss and significantly increased operative time.

The endoscope may allow approach to the frontal sinus through small incisions hidden behind the hair line. As well, it permits magnified visualization of the frontonasal recess and access to lateral sinus extensions without anterior table osteotomies. The role of the endoscope in frontal sinus fractures continues to be that of an aid, rather than the principal technique.

11.2 Treatment indications

Endoscopic frontal sinus repair may be considered whenever repair of the anterior table fracture is judged important to restore the contour of the forehead but neither sinus obliteration nor cranialization are necessary components of the repair. Thus, the endoscope should be used only in the repair of displaced anterior table fractures. Displaced posterior table fractures and blockage of the frontonasal duct are contraindications to the procedure. Current techniques do not allow sinus cranialization or obliteration using the endoscope. In anterior table fractures the endoscope may also help determine patency of the frontonasal drainage system. In addition, unsuspected cerebrospinal fluid leaks may be diagnosed. Endoscopic repair is contraindicated in comminuted fractures, associated orbital roof fractures and fractures that extend over the orbital rim. Presence of associated depressed frontoparietal fractures is also a contraindication as these can only be repaired through coronal access. The endoscope can serve as an adjunct to the traditional coronal approach in patients with extensive supraorbital sinus recesses requiring removal of sinus mucosa.

11.3 Preoperative planning

A fine-cut axial computed tomography is required to accurately assess the fracture and degrees of displacement of the anterior and posterior frontal sinus walls. Presence of a fracture traversing the frontonasal duct may also be ascertained on preoperative imaging. In equivocal cases the endoscope may be used intraoperatively to assess the status of the drainage system. If required, the endoscopic approach may be converted to traditional coronal exposure.

11.4 Operative technique

The frontal sinus is accessed through three short local incisions placed along the anterior hairline. Dissection, guided by endoscope visualization, is performed in the subperiosteal plane down to the level of the supraorbital rims and frontonasal junction. Identification of supraorbital neurovascular bundles avoids injury. Subsequent placement of retraction sutures directly over the sinus allows for the maintenance of an optimal optical cavity (**Fig 5.1-9a**). The endoscope may then be used to visualize the frontonasal duct. Small local incisions are made directly over the fracture sites in the direction of relaxed skin tension lines. Placement of Steinmann pins into individual bone fragments facilitates reduction. Miniplates and screws are introduced through these incisions to permit percutaneous rigid fragment fixation (**Fig 5.1-9b**). Individual bone fragments may be removed through an enlarged scalp incision, fixated on a side table, and then reintroduced into the defect.

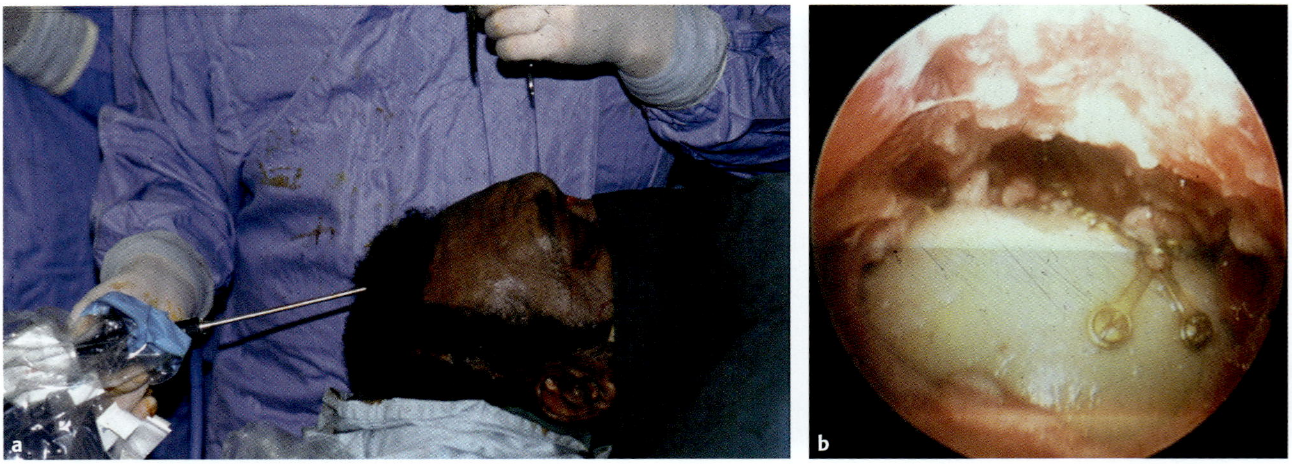

Fig 5.1-9a–b Endoscopic technique for frontal sinus fracture repair.

a The endoscope is inserted through a portal behind the frontal hairline. To increase the size of the optical cavity, a traction suture is placed directly over the fracture region.

b Miniplates and screws are inserted through stab incisions in frontal skin creases, and fracture segments are percutaneously secured.

Alternatively, when anatomical fracture reduction is exceedingly difficult, a camouflage technique may be used. Alloplastic implants may be placed in an onlay fashion to simulate normal forehead contour. This approach can also be used if a cosmetic deformity is identified after a delay has made fracture reduction impossible.

11.5 Contingencies and complications

Local incisions in the glabellar region heal without any esthetic sequelae. The difficulties with this approach include manipulation and percutaneous fixation of small bone fragments, which may significantly prolong operative times. If comminution proves to be too excessive for endoscopic repair, traditional coronal approach or camouflage techniques may then be used. Literature review identified one series of endoscopic frontal sinus fracture repairs, comprising seven patients [Chen et al, 2003]. All outcomes were judged satisfactory. There were no complications and no conversions to traditional techniques were required.

Potential complications include residual forehead depressions, supraorbital nerve lesions, and reactions to alloplastic materials. There have been no incidences of mucocele or mucopyocele reported yet in the case series treated with this approach.

12 Summary

The endoscope has broadened the field of craniomaxillofacial trauma care. It allows for the avoidance of large cutaneous incisions diminishing the risk of visible and dysfunctional scarring, injury to important neurovascular structures and excessive blood loss. It provides a magnified view, potentially permitting more anatomical structural repair and exposure in deep, dangerously located cavities. Endoscopic repair often decreases the extent of surgical trauma, potentially leading to shorter recovery periods. In the long-term, it also has the potential of decreasing operating time.

The future of endoscopic craniomaxillofacial surgery promises more excitement. Specifically designed endoscopic instruments including transcutaneous trocars, reduction screws and plate holders will increase the facility with which reductions are achieved with regular equipment. Binocular endoscopes, already available but at this time limited by their size, will allow greater depth perception decreasing the slope of the learning curve. In addition, voice-activated robotic scope holders will free the field for easier bimanual operation and stabilize the image.

The authors believe the endoscope has already proven its role in craniomaxillofacial trauma care. Work must be done to further improve endoscopic techniques, clarify treatment indications, and objectively assess outcomes.

13 References and suggested reading

Adams W. Basic principles of internal wire fixation and internal suspension of facial fractures. *Surgery*. 1942;12:523.

Appling WD, Patrinely JR, Salzer TA. Transconjunctival approach vs subciliary skin-muscle flap approach for orbital fracture repair. *Arch Otolaryngol Head Neck Surg*. 1993 Sep;119(9):1000–1007.

Bhatti MT, Stankiewicz JA. Ophthalmic complications of endoscopic sinus surgery. *Surv Ophthalmol*. 2003 Jul–Aug;48(4):389–402.

Chen CT, Chen YR. Endoscopically assisted repair of orbital floor fractures. *Plast Reconstr Surg*. 2001 Dec;108(7):2011–2018; discussion 2019.

Chen CT, Chen YR. Endoscopic orbital surgery. *Atlas Oral Maxillofac Surg Clin North Am*. 2003 Sep;11(2):179–208.

Chen CT, Chen YR, Tung TC, et al. Endoscopically assisted reconstruction of orbital medial wall fractures. *Plast Reconstr Surg*. 1999 Feb;103(2):714–720; quiz 721.

Chen CT, Lai JP, Chen YR, et al. Application of endoscope in zygomatic fracture repair. *Br J Plast Surg*. 2000 Mar;53(2):100–105.

Chen DJ, Chen CT, Chen YR, et al. Endoscopically assisted repair of frontal sinus fracture. *J Trauma*. 2003 Aug;55(2):378–382.

Ellis E, Throckmorton GS. Treatment of mandibular condylar process fractures: biological considerations. *J Oral Maxillofac Surg*. 2005 Jan;63(1):115–134.

Ellis E 3rd. Condylar process fractures of the mandible. *Facial Plast Surg*. 2000;16(2):193–205.

Ellis E 3rd, Palmieri C, Throckmorton G. Further displacement of condylar process fractures after closed treatment. *J Oral Maxillofac Surg*. 1999 Nov;57(11):1307–1316; discussion 1316–1317.

Ellis E 3rd, Simon P, Throckmorton GS. Occlusal results after open or closed treatment of fractures of the mandibular condylar process. *J Oral Maxillofac Surg*. 2000 Mar;58(3):260–268.

Ellis E 3rd, Throckmorton G. Facial symmetry after closed and open treatment of fractures of the mandibular condylar process. *J Oral Maxillofac Surg*. 2000 Jul;58(7):719-28; discussion 729–730.

Ellis E 3rd, Throckmorton GS. Bite forces after open or closed treatment of mandibular condylar process fractures. *J Oral Maxillofac Surg*. 2001 Apr;59(4):389–395.

Feifel H, Albert-Deumlich J, Riediger D. Long-term follow-up of subcondylar fractures in children by electronic computer-assisted recording of condylar movements. *Int J Oral Maxillofac Surg*. 1992 Apr;21(2):70–76.

Feifel H, Risse G, Opheys A, et al. [Conservative versus surgical therapy of unilateral fractures of the collum mandibulae—anatomic and functional results with special reference to computer-assisted 3-dimensional axiographic registration of condylar paths]. *Fortschr Kiefer Gesichtschir*. 1996;41:124–127. German.

Forrest CR. Application of endoscope-assisted minimal-access techniques in orbitozygomatic complex, orbital floor, and frontal sinus fractures. *J Craniomaxillofac Trauma*. 1999 Winter;5(4):7–12; discussion 13–14.

Gruss JS, Mackinnon SE. Complex maxillary fractures: role of buttress reconstruction and immediate bone grafts. *Plast Reconstr Surg*. 1986 Jul;78(1):9–22.

Gruss JS, Phillips JH. Complex facial trauma: the evolving role of rigid fixation and immediate bone graft reconstruction. *Clin Plast Surg*. 1989 Jan;16(1):93–104.

Gruss JS, Van Wyck L, Phillips JH, et al. The importance of the zygomatic arch in complex midfacial fracture repair and correction of posttraumatic orbitozygomatic deformities. *Plast Reconstr Surg*. 1990 Jun;85(6):878–890.

Güven O. Fractures of the maxillofacial region in children. *J Craniomaxillofac Surg*. 1992 Aug-Sep;20(6):244–247.

Güven O, Keskin A. Remodelling following condylar fractures in children. *J Craniomaxillofac Surg*. 2001 Aug;29(4):232–237.

Haug RH, Assael LA. Outcomes of open versus closed treatment of mandibular subcondylar fractures. *J Oral Maxillofac Surg*. 2001 Apr;59(4):370–375; discussion 375–376.

Hinohira Y, Yumoto E, Shimamura I. Endoscopic endonasal reduction of blowout fractures of the orbital floor. *Otolaryngol Head Neck Surg*. 2005 Nov;133(5):741–747.

Hovinga J, Boering G, Stegenga B. Long-term results of nonsurgical management of condylar fractures in children. *Int J Oral Maxillofac Surg*. 1999 Dec;28(6):429–440.

Ikeda K, Suzuki H, Oshima T, et al. Endoscopic endonasal repair of orbital floor fracture. *Arch Otolaryngol Head Neck Surg*. 1999 Jan;125(1):59–63.

Jacobovicz J, Lee C, Trabulsy PP. Endoscopic repair of mandibular subcondylar fractures. *Plast Reconstr Surg*. 1998 Feb;101(2):437–441.

Jin HR, Shin SO, Choo MJ, et al. Endonasal endoscopic reduction of blowout fractures of the medial orbital wall. *J Oral Maxillofac Surg*. 2000 Aug;58(8):847–851.

Kellenberger M, von Arx T, Hardt N. [Results of follow-up of temporomandibular joint fractures in 30 children]. *Fortschr Kiefer Gesichtschir*. 1996;41:138–142. German.

Kellenberger M, von Arx T, Hardt N. [Temporomandibular joint fractures in children. A clinical and radiological follow-up in 30 patients]. *Schweiz Monatsschr Zahnmed*. 1994;104(12):1482–1488. German.

Kobayashi S, Sakai Y, Yamada A, et al. Approaching the zygoma with an endoscope. *J Craniofac Surg*. 1995 Nov;6(6):519–524.

Konstantinovic VS, Dimitrijevic B. Surgical versus conservative treatment of unilateral condylar process fractures: clinical and radiographic evaluation of 80 patients. *J Oral Maxillofac Surg*. 1992 Apr;50(4):349–352; discussion 352–353.

Krimmel M, Cornelius CP, Reinert S. Endoscopically assisted zygomatic fracture reduction and osteosynthesis revisited. *Int J Oral Maxillofac Surg*. 2002 Oct;31(5):485–488.

Lauer G, Schmelzeisen R. Endoscope-assisted fixation of mandibular condylar process fractures. *J Oral Maxillofac Surg*. 1999 Jan;57(1):36–39; discussion 39–40.

Lee C, Jacobovicz J, Mueller RV. Endoscopic repair of a complex midfacial fracture. *J Craniofac Surg*. 1997 May;8(3):170–175.

Lee C, Stiebel M, Young DM. Cranial nerve VII region of the traumatized facial skeleton: optimizing fracture repair with the endoscope. *J Trauma*. 2000 Mar;48(3):423–431; discussion 431–432.

Lee CH, Lee C, Trabulsy PP. Endoscopic-assisted repair of a malar fracture. *Ann Plast Surg*. 1996 Aug;37(2):178–183.

Lee CH, Lee C, Trabulsy PP, et al. A cadaveric and clinical evaluation of endoscopically assisted zygomatic fracture repair. *Plast Reconstr Surg*. 1998 Feb;101(2):333–345.

Lee HM, Han SK, Chae SW, et al. Endoscopic endonasal reconstruction of blowout fractures of the medial orbital walls. *Plast Reconstr Surg*. 2002 Mar;109(3):872–876.

Lee SS, Lin SD, Chiu YT, et al. Deep dissection plane for endoscopic-assisted comminuted malar fracture repair. *Ann Plast Surg*. 2002 Nov;49(5):452–459.

Manson PN, Crawley WA, Yaremchuk MJ, et al. Midface fractures: advantages of immediate extended open reduction and bone grafting. *Plast Reconstr Surg*. 1985 Jul;76(1):1–12.

Meningaud JP, Rigolet A, Ernenwein D, et al. [Endoscopically assisted retro-caroncular approach for medial wall fracture of the orbit: preliminary study]. *Rev Stomatol Chir Maxillofac*. 2005 Sep;106(4):205–209. French.

Mohammad JA, Warnke PH, Shenaq SM. Endoscopic exploration of the orbital floor: a technique for transantral grafting of floor blowout fractures. *J Craniomaxillofac Trauma*. 1998 Summer;4(2):16–19; discussion 15.

Mullins JB, Holds JB, Branham GH, et al. Complications of the transconjunctival approach. A review of 400 cases. *Arch Otolaryngol Head Neck Surg*. 1997 Apr;123(4):385–388.

Müller RV, Czerwinski M, Lee C, et al. Condylar fracture repair: use of the endoscope to advance traditional treatment philosophy. *Facial Plast Surg Clin North Am*. 2006 Feb;14(1):1–9.

Nishiike S, Nagai M, Nakagawa A, et al. Endoscopic transantral orbital floor repair with antral bone grafts. *Arch Otolaryngol Head Neck Surg*. 2005 Oct;131(10):911–915.

Otori N, Haruna S, Moriyama H. Endoscopic endonasal or transmaxillary repair of orbital floor fracture: a study of 88 patients treated in our department. *Acta Otolaryngol*. 2003 Aug;123(6):718–723.

Palmieri C, Ellis E 3rd, Throckmorton G. Mandibular motion after closed and open treatment of unilateral mandibular condylar process fractures. *J Oral Maxillofac Surg*. 1999 Jul;57(7):764–775; discussion 775–776.

Persons BL, Wong GB. Transantral endoscopic orbital floor repair using resorbable plate. *J Craniofac Surg*. 2002 May;13(3):483–488; discussion 488–489.

Phillips JH, Gruss JS, Wells MD, et al. Periosteal suspension of the lower eyelid and cheek following subciliary exposure of facial fractures. *Plast Reconstr Surg*. 1991 Jul;88(1):145–148.

Rhee JS, Chen CT. Endoscopic approach to medial orbital wall fractures. *Facial Plast Surg Clin North Am*. 2006 Feb;14(1):17–23.

Rice DH. Management of frontal sinus fractures. *Curr Opin Otolaryngol Head Neck Surg*. 2004 Feb;12(1):46–48.

Rohner D, Tay A, Meng CS, et al. The sphenozygomatic suture as a key site for osteosynthesis of the orbitozygomatic complex in panfacial fractures: a biomechanical study in human cadavers based on clinical practice. *Plast Reconstr Surg*. 2002 Nov;110(6):1463–1471.

Sakai Y, Kobayashi S, Sekiguchi J, et al. New method of endoscopic pterygomaxillary disjunction for a Le Fort Type I osteotomy. *J Craniofac Surg*. 1996 Mar;7(2):111–116.

Sanno T, Tahara S, Nomura T, et al. Endoscopic endonasal reduction for blowout fracture of the medial orbital wall. *Plast Reconstr Surg*. 2003 Oct;112(5):1228–1237; discussion 1238.

Saunders CJ, Whetzel TP, Stokes RB, et al. Transantral endoscopic orbital floor exploration: a cadaver and clinical study. *Plast Reconstr Surg*. 1997 Sep;100(3):575–581.

Schmelzeisen R, Cienfuegos-Monroy R, Schön R, et al. Patient benefit from endoscopically assisted fixation of condylar neck fractures—a randomized controlled trial. *J Oral Maxillofac Surg*. 2009 Jan;67(1):147–158.

Schön R, Fakler O, Gellrich NC, et al. Five-year experience with the transoral endoscopically assisted treatment of displaced condylar mandible fractures. *Plast Reconstr Surg*. 2005 Jul;116(1):44–50.

Schön R, Fakler O, Metzger MC, et al. Preliminary functional results of endoscope-assisted transoral treatment of displaced bilateral condylar mandible fractures. *Int J Oral Maxillofac Surg*. 2008 Feb;37(2):111–116.

Schön R, Gellrich NC, Schmelzeisen R. Minimally invasive open reduction of a displaced condylar fracture in a child. *Br J Oral Maxillofac Surg*. 2005 Jun;43(3):258–260.

Schön R, Herklotz I, Metzger MC, et al. Endoscopic approach to removal of an osteochondroma of the mandibular condyle. *J Oral Maxillofac Surg*. 2011 Jun;69(6):1657–1660.

Shumrick KA. Endoscopic management of frontal sinus fractures. *Facial Plast Surg Clin North Am*. 2006 Feb;14(1):31–35.

Shumrick KA, Ryzenman JM. Endoscopic management of facial fractures. *Facial Plast Surg Clin North Am*. 2001 Aug;9(3):469–474.

Silvennoinen U, Iizuka T, Oikarinen K, et al. Analysis of possible factors leading to problems after nonsurgical treatment of condylar fractures. *J Oral Maxillofac Surg*. 1994 Aug;52(8):793–799.

Silvennoinen U, Raustia AM, Lindqvist C, et al. Occlusal and temporomandibular joint disorders in patients with unilateral condylar fracture. A prospective one-year study. *Int J Oral Maxillofac Surg*. 1998 Aug;27(4):280–285.

Silverman S. A new operation for displaced fractures at the neck of the mandibular condyle. *Dental Cosmos*. 1925;67:876.

Stanley RB Jr. The zygomatic arch as a guide to reconstruction of comminuted malar fractures. *Arch Otolaryngol Head Neck Surg*. 1989 Dec;115(12):1459–1462.

Strong EB. Endoscopic repair of orbital blow-out fractures. *Facial Plast Surg*. 2004 Aug;20(3):223–230.

Strong EB, Buchalter GM, Moulthrop TH. Endoscopic repair of isolated anterior table frontal sinus fractures. *Arch Facial Plast Surg*. 2003 Nov–Dec;5(6):514–521.

Strong EB, Kellman RM. Endoscopic repair of anterior table—frontal sinus fractures. *Facial Plast Surg Clin North Am*. 2006 Feb;14(1):25–29.

Suarez-Cunqueiro MM, Schön R, Gellrich NC, et al. Endoscopic assistance in the removal of a foreign body in the condylar process. *J Craniofac Surg*. 2004 Jan;15(1):98–101.

Throckmorton GS, Ellis E 3rd. Recovery of mandibular motion after closed and open treatment of unilateral mandibular condylar process fractures. *Int J Oral Maxillofac Surg*. 2000 Dec;29(6):421–427.

Throckmorton GS, Ellis E 3rd, Hayasaki H. Masticatory motion after surgical or nonsurgical treatment for unilateral fractures of the mandibular condylar process. *J Oral Maxillofac Surg*. 2004 Feb;62(2):127–138.

Troulis MJ, Kaban LB. Endoscopic vertical ramus osteotomy: early clinical results. *J Oral Maxillofac Surg*. 2004 Jul;62(7):824–828.

Troulis MJ, Nahlieli O, Castano F, et al. Minimally invasive orthognathic surgery: endoscopic vertical ramus osteotomy. *Int J Oral Maxillofac Surg*. 2000 Aug;29(4):239–242.

Troulis MJ, Perrott DH, Kaban LB. Endoscopic mandibular osteotomy, and placement and activation of a semiburied distractor. *J Oral Maxillofac Surg*. 1999 Sep;57(9):1110–1113.

Vasconez LO, Core GB, Gamboa-Bobadilla M, et al. Endoscopic techniques in coronal brow lifting. *Plast Reconstr Surg*. 1994 Nov;94(6):788–793.

Walker RV. Condylar fractures: nonsurgical management. *J Oral Maxillofac Surg*. 1994 Nov;52(11):1185–1188.

Whitehead AN. The organization of thought. *Science*. 1916 Sep 22;44(1134):409–419.

Wilson IF, Lokeh A, Benjamin CI, et al. Prospective comparison of panoramic tomography (zonography) and helical computed tomography in the diagnosis and operative management of mandibular fractures. *Plast Reconstr Surg*. 2001 May;107(6):1369–1375.

Worsaae N, Thorn JJ. [Surgical versus non-surgical treatment of unilateral dislocated fractures of the lower mandibular condyle]. *Ugeskr Laeger*. 1995 Jun 12;157(24):3472–3476.

Worsaae N, Thorn JJ. Surgical versus nonsurgical treatment of unilateral dislocated low subcondylar fractures: a clinical study of 52 cases. *J Oral Maxillofac Surg*. 1994 Apr;52(4):353–360; discussion 360–361.

Zhang QB, Dong YJ, Li ZB, et al. Coronal incision for treating zygomatic complex fractures. *J Craniomaxillofac Surg*. 2006 Apr;34(3):182–185.

Zingg M, Chowdhury K, Lädrach K, et al. Treatment of 813 zygoma-lateral orbital complex fractures. New aspects. *Arch Otolaryngol Head Neck Surg*. 1991 Jun;117(6):611–620; discussion 621–622.

5.2 3-D manufacturing technologies and their applications in craniomaxillofacial surgery

Florian M Thieringer, Jörg Beinemann, Ralf Schumacher, Hans-Florian Zeilhofer

1 Introduction

Diagnosis, planning, and implementation of surgery involving the facial skeleton requires extreme precision. This is especially true in complex patient cases where the functional and esthetic results depend on the specialist's experience and the availability of advanced technology.

The 3-D virtual imaging, surgical planning and navigation techniques have gained widespread use in recent years, particularly in craniomaxillofacial (CMF) surgery and other surgical disciplines. The 3-D fabrication of dimensionally accurate medical models, a process known as rapid prototyping (RP) or manufacturing of anatomical life-size models, is widely accessible, established, and is increasingly used in daily clinical work. Those models make the patient's individual anatomy visually "understandable," provide tactile feedback for the surgeon, help in the planning process, and allow the performance of complex operations on the model as a mock operation before surgery. They are also a valuable tool for patient information [Petzold et al, 1999].

The standard workflow of almost all current rapid manufacturing or rapid prototyping methods in medicine is to create a virtual 3-D model from a patient's radiological data, typically obtained from computed tomography (CT), cone beam CT (CBCT) or magnetic resonance imaging (MRI). An anatomical 3-D model is segmented from the 2-D cross-sectional DICOM image data of the patient on a computer workstation. The resulting virtual model can be manipulated further on the computer screen, imported usually as stereolithography file format (STL) data sets in a slicing and control software application for 3-D printers. It can finally be fabricated at a scale of 1:1 (or scaled to different sizes) in nearly unlimited numbers and from different materials, such as polymers/plastic, ceramics, metal or even bio-degradable materials (**Fig 5.2-1**) [Winder et al, 2005].

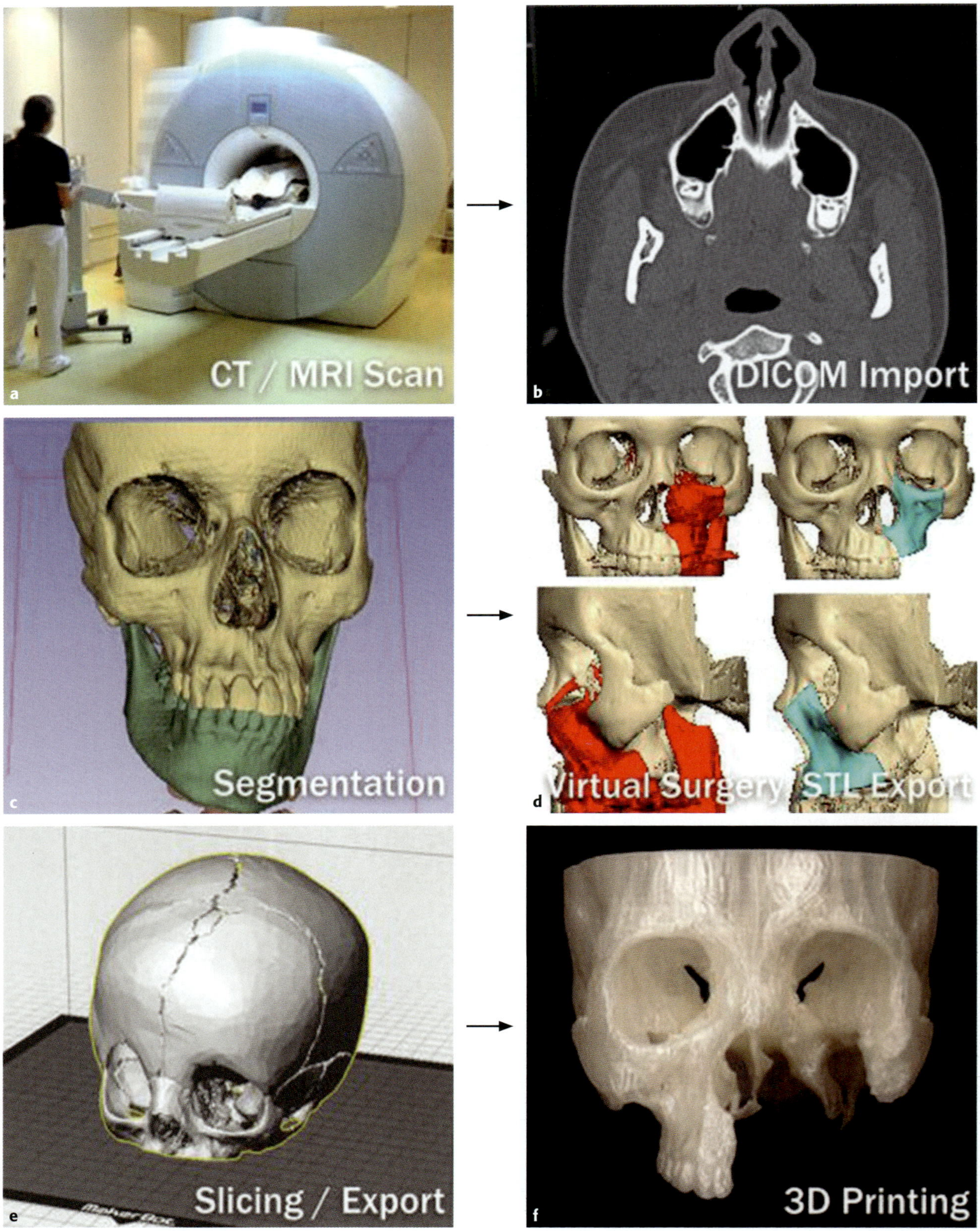

Fig 5.2-1a–f Process workflow from computed tomographic scan to 3-D physical rapid prototyping model.

A medical model accurately corresponds to the image data and print resolution, and represents precisely the anatomical conditions of the patient (**Fig 5.2-2**). Depending on the segmentation process, even combined hard- and soft-tissue models can be produced by using state-of-the-art printing processes with different material characteristics (multiple colors, transparency, different material properties).

2 History of 3-D printing technologies in CMF surgery

Before RP for medicine was introduced in the 1980s, its main field of application was in the aviation and automotive industry [Hull, 1986]. There was a strong need to produce realistic, solid prototypes or pre-series models of almost any shape and geometry. What once was a manual engineering process that consumed significant time and effort can be replaced with RP. Subsequently, RP technology spread quickly into various industrial sectors with great success. The fabrication process of realistic 3-D models in medicine could be established with the knowledge and experiences of professionals from the mechanical engineering field, combined with further development of modern radiological imaging technologies. At the end of the 1980s, the first reports on the production of medical models by using computer numerical control devices appeared (**Fig 5.2-3**) [Brix et al, 1987].

The milling method then used had some major disadvantages and so an additive manufacturing process was introduced that eventually laid the foundation for the success of RP in the medical industry. Leading all 3-D printing processes in healthcare was stereolithography (**Fig 5.2-2**), in which a 3-D model created on a computer is procured layer by layer by a laser beam in a liquid synthetic material bath.

Today a wide variety of 3-D printing technologies and appropriate services are available to fabricate 3-D models using additive or subtractive methods, forming hybrid solutions. Consequently, there is no limitation to one specific printing process.

3 Rapid prototyping technologies

Rapid prototyping is the process of printing realistic, physical 3-D prototypes designed and modified by a computer. These prototypes allow engineers, developers and physicians to visualize their designs and use them as physical models that can be felt and held. The RP models provide a valuable 3-D aid to the planning and design processes, and enable the transfer of a purely visual representation to a visual-tactile interaction called "touch to comprehend" [Petzold et al, 1999].

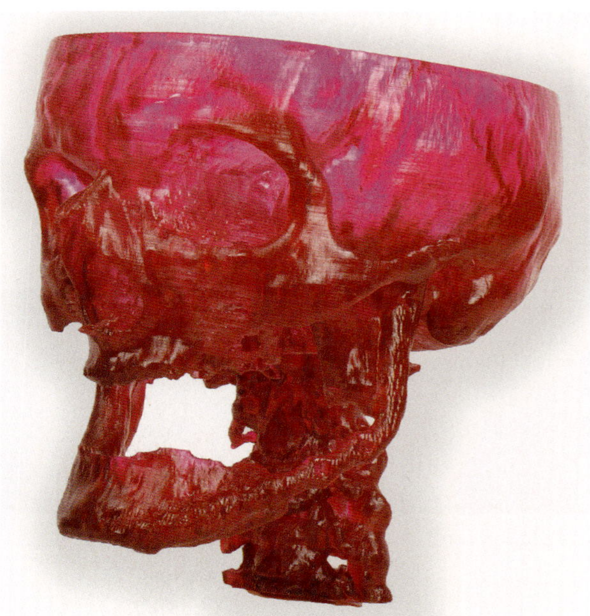

Fig 5.2-2 Stereolithographic model of a patient's skull.

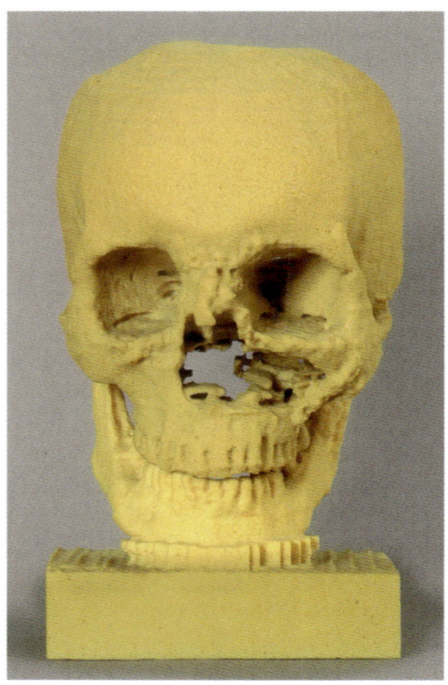

Fig 5.2-3 Computer numerical control milled Styrofoam model of a patient's skull.

In the industrial and healthcare markets, many different RP/rapid manufacturing production units are now available. Additionally, commercial 3-D printing services are offered by numerous service providers. With RP, subtractive manufacturing processes can be differentiated from additive manufacturing processes. As subtractive manufacturing techniques are mainly computer-controlled milling processes, they have gained a greater importance, particularly in the production of bio-models. The resulting model can be produced from a material block (eg, plastic, ceramic or metal) by a multi-axis milling machine. This technology is mainly used in the manufacture of patient-specific implants (eg, polyetheretherketone) or in the dental sector (eg, crowns and bridges). The polyurethane foam blocks (**Fig 5.2-3**) used at the beginning of the RP era to produce skull models did not produce viable applications in CMF surgery, as this technique has significant limitations in the fabrication of closed model geometries, such as sinuses [Brix et al, 1987]. The various additive printing methods nowadays allow creation of an almost free and complex geometry. This results in highly accurate production of 3-D models with almost every conceivable type of material (eg, paper, plastics/polymers, ceramics, or metals) [Barazanchi et al, 2016].

Conventional additive printing processes include stereolithography, selective laser sintering or selective laser melting, fused deposition modeling (FDM) (**Fig 5.2-4**), polyjet or multijet printing and several other 3-D printing technologies. With respect to the accuracy of the fabricated anatomical models, emphasis is rather on the quality of the data source (eg, the image data quality or layer thickness of the underlying CT data set) than the printing process itself.

3.1 Stereolithography

Stereolithography was one of the first RP technologies and additive manufacturing processes introduced in the engineering field in the 1980s. By using a computer-controlled ultraviolet laser beam, a transparent or colored liquid photopolymer resin in a vat is cured successively layer by layer to produce a physical, largely transparent 3-D model from a virtual 3-D data set. Even objects of different colors may be created by modulating the energy of the laser beam. In this way, anatomical models can be produced in numerous colors to label relevant and vulnerable anatomical structures, such as nerves, blood vessels or tooth roots. The 3-D models can be sterilized and used in the operating room.

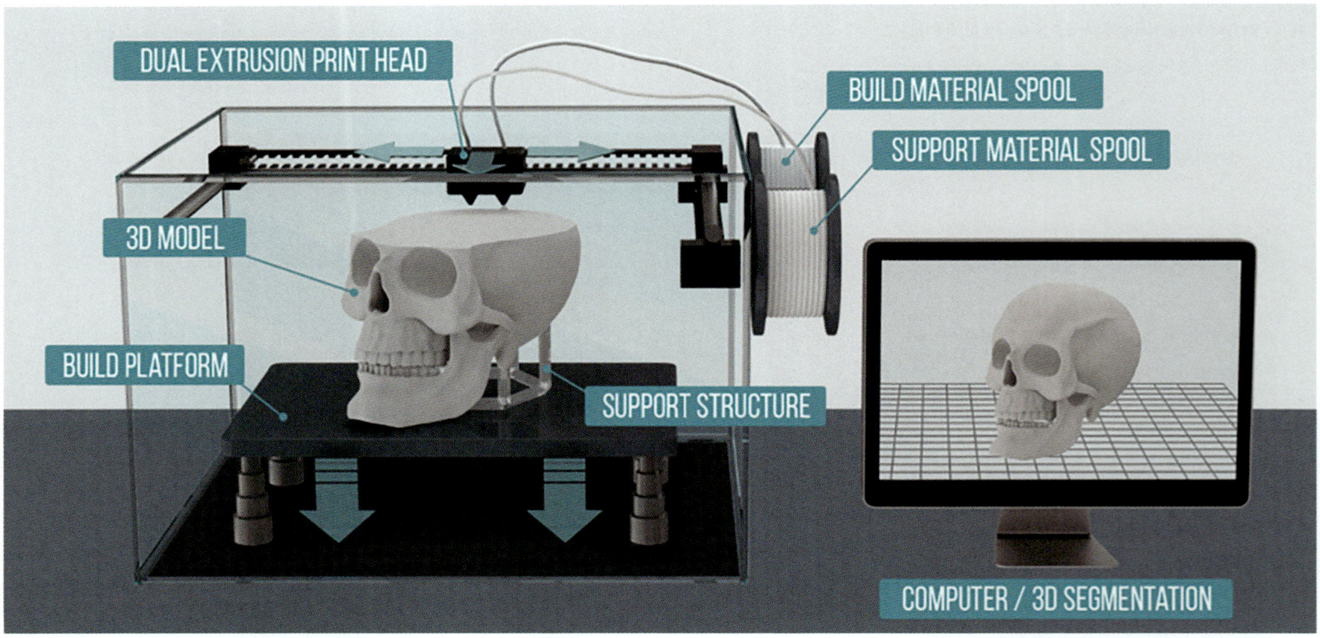

Fig 5.2-4 Principles of the fused deposition modeling printing process (Source: Additively.com).

The high cost of the stereolithography printers and related devices (ie, the photo-curable resins) are a significant drawback. However, more affordable compact consumer stereolithography printers were introduced in recent years, opening new opportunities to fabricate cost-effective anatomical RP models.

3.2 Selective laser sintering, selective laser melting

Selective laser sintering produces 3-D objects by tracing a high-powered laser beam across a bin filled with heat-fusible powder. The powder particles, such as polymers and even ceramics or metal (eg, titanium), fuse in a thin layer. Subsequently, an additional thin layer of powder is applied on top of the solidified layer and fused again by the laser beam, forming the 3-D object. Reinforced structures are unnecessary because support is ensured by the unfused easy-to-remove powdered source material at the boundaries. If the powder is fully melted (not sintered) and solidified completely, this process is called selective laser melting.

3.3 Fused deposition modeling or fused filament fabrication

The FDM/fused filament fabrication process is the most popular printing technique in the RP consumer market (**Fig 5.2-4**), it can also be found in the expensive professional level segment. Moreover, FDM 3-D printers are affordable. The printing process is based on the liquefaction of thermo-softening plastic (thermoplastic) by heat and curing after application and cooling on a build platform. After hardening, the platform is lowered by a fraction of a millimeter in accordance of one print-layer thickness. The next layer of hot plastic is applied on top. This process repeats until the 3-D print task is completed. Some FDM printers have multiple print heads (extruders), so that multicolor models can be printed. Additionally, one extruder produces resolvable support structures that can easily be removed by a special solvent or even by water after the printing process.

3.4 PolyJet or MultiJet printing

Like the inkjet printing technique on a sheet of paper, a polyjet or multijet machine prints using an industrial print head with many small nozzles containing photosensitive liquid polymer on a flat build tray. The printed material layer is usually hardened with ultaviolet light. Afterward, the next layer is applied. With this technology, the production of different colored 3-D objects with different material properties (from soft to hard) is possible.

3.5 Other RP techniques

With respect to all printing techniques, it should be mentioned that the accuracy and production quality of 3-D objects is largely dependent on the image data quality of the 3-D object and not only on the 3-D printer itself.

Moreover, there are other 3-D printing technologies available on the market that are not covered in this chapter [Winder et al, 2005].

4 Production process of RP models

4.1 Image acquisition

The quality and accuracy of a RP model depends primarily on the quality of the underlying image data set. For this reason, the best possible image data should be obtained with only few imaging artifacts. The decisive factor is to choose the correct imaging method (mainly CT, MRI or CBCT, but also ultrasound imaging or scans) and to use a corresponding standardized scanning protocol (**Fig 5.2-5**). For CT images, spatial resolution should be as high and the slice thickness should be as thin as possible (1 mm or less) to minimize partial volume effect and other artifacts in reconstruction, while always considering the radiation dose for the patient. Imaging artifacts in CT scanning from metallic dental fillings and other restorations around the occlusal plane can complicate the segmentation process and hide anatomical structures. To delineate the teeth correctly, the use of radiolucent bite splints during a CT scan is recommended by some authors. Ideally, the image data are stored as DICOM files in the picture archive and communications system (PACS) of the hospital and can be transferred to the segmentation workstation via the internet or intranet. Strict data protection and security protocols for data transmission must be implemented in this workflow [Bibb et al, 2010].

4.2 Segmentation/virtual reconstruction

The segmentation process is a critical and occasionally time-consuming step in generating accurate 3-D objects for further processing. The use of specific segmentation methods for 3-D image reconstruction is essential to obtain a realistic medical model. There are many semiautomated or fully automated software solutions commercially available to enable the image transfer from a 2-D data volume to a 3-D model. The decisive factor is the segmentation of the relevant anatomical structures of the resulting object, which is generally bone or soft tissue. The virtual anatomical model can subsequently be modified with the help of appropriate software applications and can be prepared for the 3-D printing process. At this point, corresponding printer control files are created for each 3-D printer and are exported and imported into this device. The printer control files include information of the 3-D object with specific additional data required for the manufacturing process, such as information about material properties of the print material or the position of supporting structures, if needed (**Fig 5.2-6**).

The decisive factor here is to identify the relevant anatomical structures needed and to differentiate hard tissues from adjacent soft tissues (**Fig 5.2-7**).

One basic approach of image processing algorithms is called thresholding. The CT scans gray scale perimeters are defined and calculated corresponding to the relevant tissue ranges of Hounsfield units. With the resulting image information, a 3-D image can be created by volume rendering and several other current 3-D reconstruction techniques. At the end of the segmentation procedure, the completed 3-D object or several isolated 3-D structures of the underlying DICOM data set can be aligned to predefined reference planes. They are then exported (mostly as STL files), or, depending on the application used, further processed. Since high-resolution 3-D files demand large data storage capacity and processor performance for 3-D visualization and modeling, a data simplification process may be necessary.

Matrix	512 x 512
Slice thickness	Max 1.0 mm
Feed per rotation	Max 1.0 mm
Reconstructed slice increment	Max 1.0 mm
Reconstruction algorithm	Bone or high resolution
Gantry tilt	0°
Export	DICOM
Format	Uncompressed Standard DICOM

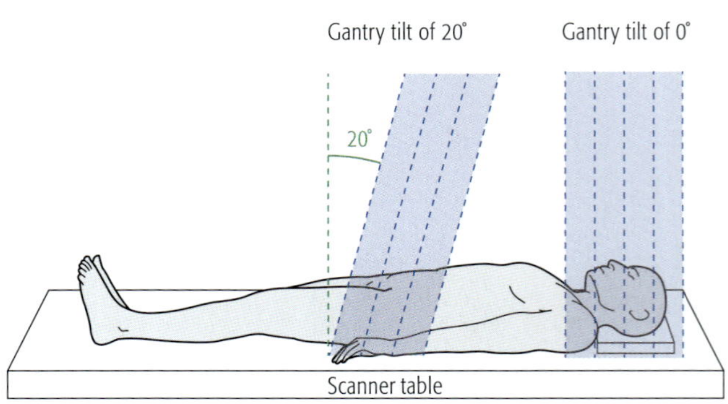

Fig 5.2-5 Computed tomographic scanning protocol/parameters for patient-specific implants (DePuy Synthes PSI).

4.3 Modeling, data modifications, and data export

Once the segmentation process has been completed and a 3-D (STL) data set is present, this can be manipulated and modified further with the appropriate software applications. These steps include, for example, virtual trimming or isolation of relevant anatomical areas, superimposing defect zones with the virtually mirrored, healthy opposite side of the skull, or just modeling and modification of anatomical structures. Additionally, if detailed information on occlusal contacts is needed (eg, in orthognathic surgery), the 3-D files can be merged after the segmentation process with data obtained by an intra-oral (surface) scanning device. Some software solutions provide "wizards" that guide the user through the modeling steps. The resulting 3-D object for printing is optimized, sliced and exported. Defective areas can then be corrected and the data size can be reduced. Finally, a printing control file is exported that contains all necessary information depending on the chosen RP process.

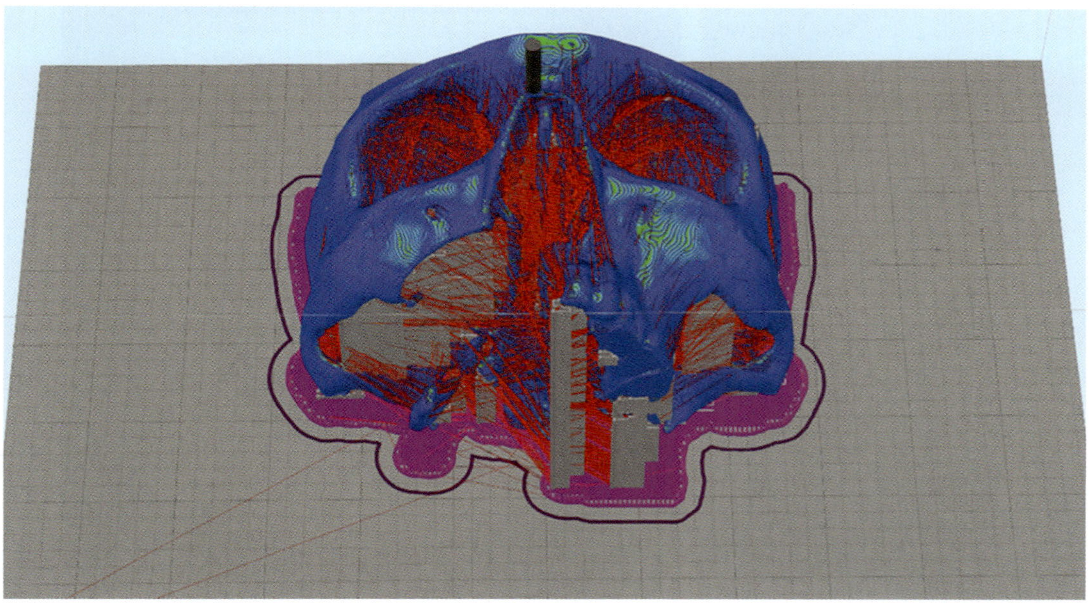

Fig 5.2-6 Visualization of a 3-D printer control file with additional support structures to enable printout of overhanging anatomical geometries.

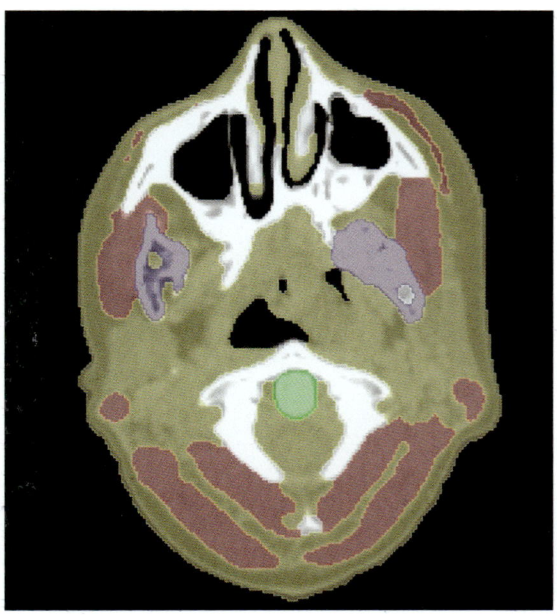

Fig 5.2-7 Cross-sectional view of an axial computed tomographic slide with different anatomical structures labeled during semi-automatic segmentation process.

4.4 Model fabrication and post-processing

The production of 3-D objects is dependent on the specific printing process. Depending on the object size and desired accuracy, the 3-D printing time varies enormously. As a rule, the building materials are applied and/or cured layer by layer. Additional support structures help to manufacture overhanging, complex geometries (**Fig 5.2-8**). Once the 3-D model production process is finished, the print object is removed from the building platform and post-processed. The coarseness of the surface is smoothed and supporting structures are removed. Finally, the 3-D model can be washed and sterilized depending on the print material. Life-size anatomical models may be used as a guide or as a bending template during the operation.

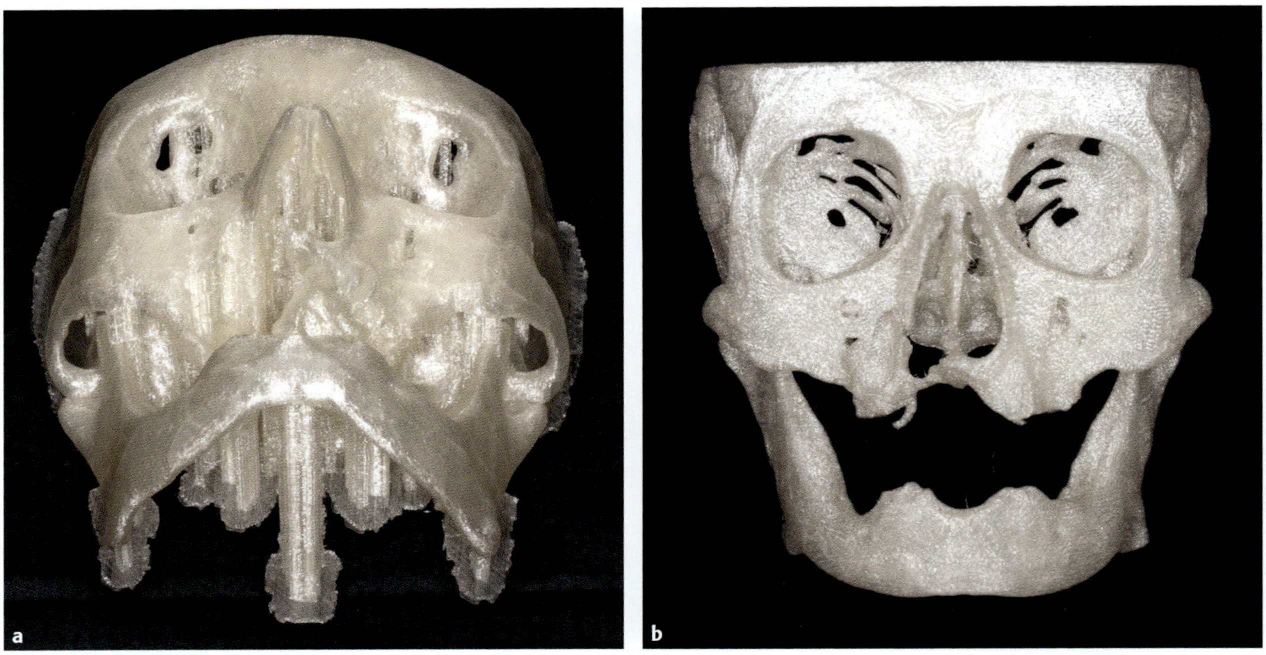

Fig 5.2-8a–b Fused deposition modeling printed skull (polylactic acid plastic) of a patient with maxillary carcinoma for surgery planning before (left) and after removal of the support structures (right).

5 Applications of RP models in CMF surgery

The RP models can be used for preoperative planning and as an aid during surgery. Before the operation, the surgeon can plan the procedure with a realistic anatomical model (**Fig 5.2-9**).

A model operation can be performed, if necessary, the best-fitting implants may be selected before surgery based on the patient's anatomy. Plates can also be accurately prebent on the medical model (**Fig 5.2-10**).

Alternative surgical approaches and minimally invasive surgical techniques may be considered and evaluated. Preoperative planning with medical RP models can shorten operative time. Ultimately treatment and follow-up costs can be saved compared with traditional surgical methods. The likelihood of complications can be reduced using RP models as a planning and guiding aid and they are valuable in the medical informed consent process. The operation can be shown and explained to the patient step-by-step using the anatomical RP model.

The RP models are helpful in student, resident and trainee education [Lambrecht et al, 2010]. Rare diseases, malformations or defects after trauma can be demonstrated based on these models. Surgical procedures can be practiced on RP models, especially if they are produced through cost-effective FDM manufacturing processes.

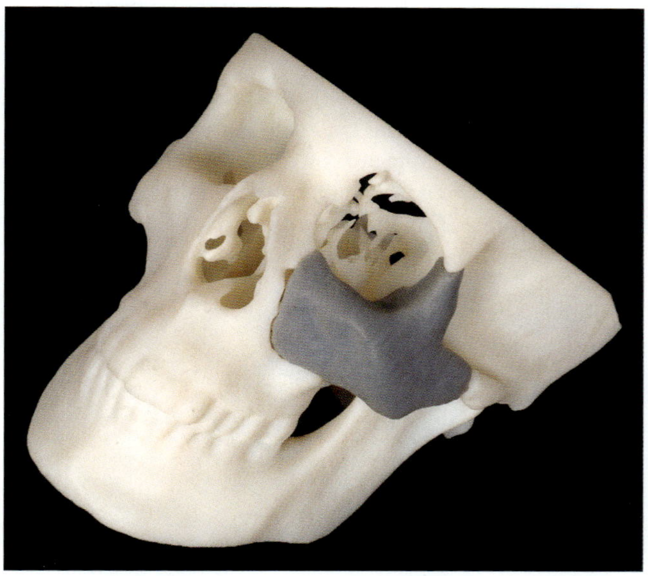

Fig 5.2-9 A 3-D skull/planning model for reconstruction of the left zygomaticomaxillary complex after tumor surgery (healthy side mirrored to the left defect side, reconstruct in grey).

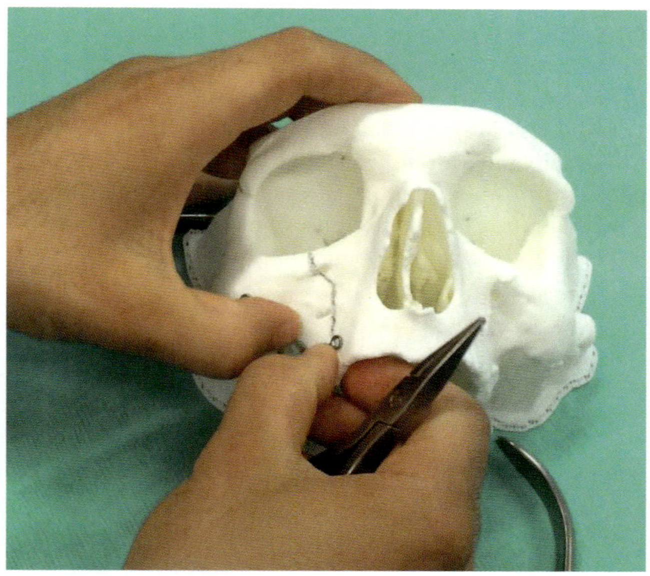

Fig 5.2-10 Residents' training, prebending of osteosynthesis plates before surgical procedure.

5.1 Anatomical models

Realistic, haptic 3-D models of patients' anatomy represent a valuable tool throughout the entire treatment process from diagnosis to treatment planning, the surgical procedure and quality assurance (**Fig 5.2-11**). Anatomical rapid prototyping models have not lost importance in CMF surgery, even in times of computer-based virtual surgical planning, intraoperative navigation and 3-D fabrication of patient-specific implants. Numerous studies have shown that the use of 3-D models in the surgical planning process and implementation not only leads to an improvement of precision in the treatment and prevention of errors but also to a reduction in the operating time. Additionally, 3-D models can help to choose minimally invasive surgical approaches and to practice critical surgical steps in the 3-D model for an optimized treatment outcome.

5.1.1 Surgical planning

Before actual surgery, 3-D printed anatomical models allow to perform all surgical steps realistically on the model itself. In addition, the appropriate surgical approach and the best-fitting implants can be selected preoperatively. These implants can be prebent and used after the sterilization process directly in the operating room when needed, thus guaranteeing precision, saving operation time and costs.

The 3-D printed plastic models can be sawn, drilled, plated, and supplemented by individually manufactured implants. These properties allow to achieve optimal surgical results by planning and practicing the intermediate steps of the procedure especially for complex surgical interventions.

5.1.2 Informed consent

The 3-D printed anatomical models can be used in the process of informed consent as a basis for discussion of the surgical procedure with the patient. They are descriptive, can be handled by the patient during the preoperative consultation and serve as a basis for further discussion (**Fig 5.2-12**).

Especially before tumor operations or extensive reconstructive CMF surgery, 3-D models can be used to explain complex anatomical and procedural details in an understandable way to patients.

5.2 Traumatology

The use of 3-D printed models offers an advantage in the treatment of craniofacial fractures. However, it is crucial that both costs and time are considered in a reasonable way because acute trauma cases typically should be treated in a timely manner. If available, low-cost in-house printing speeds up manufacturing of the models.

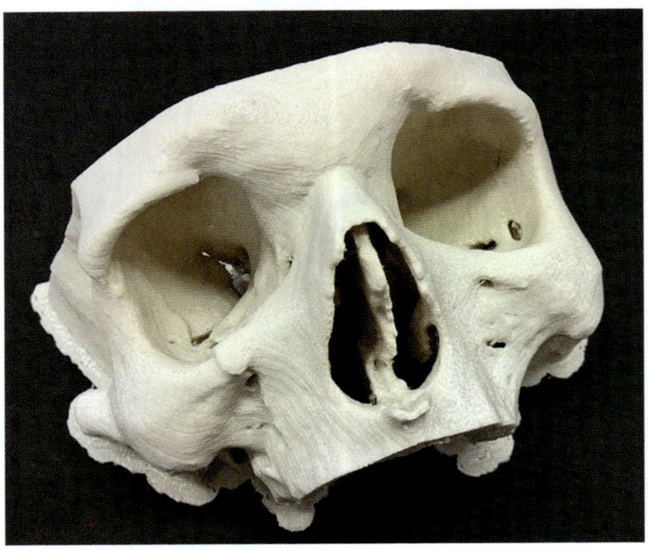

Fig 5.2-11 A 3-D anatomical model (polylactid acid plastic) of a patient with a right zygomaticomaxillary complex fracture.

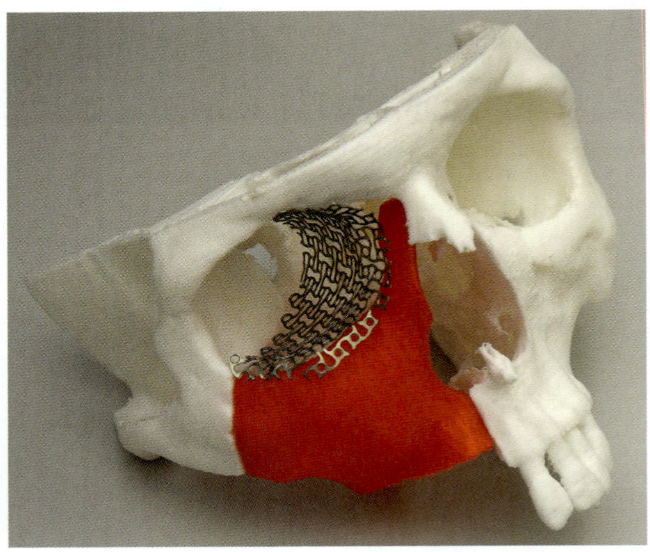

Fig 5.2-12 A 3-D model after tumor resection (defect zone in red) for surgical planning and informed consent. Preformed titanium mesh for orbital wall reconstruction.

The CT scans often are produced just after admission of patients in the emergency department. Subsequently, these radiological cross-sectional images can be used for the segmentation process and as print control files, as the basis to produce anatomical 3-D models. Additionally, it is important that the region of interest be focused as narrowly as possible to shorten the production time of the 3-D models to a few hours. With the use of suitable medically certified materials, 3-D printed models can be used after cleaning and sterilization directly in the operating room.

The appropriate selection and bending of implants, for example in complex mandibular conditions (**Fig 5.2-13**), or adaption of titanium meshes for orbital wall fractures (**Fig 5.2-14**), can save time in the operating room [Dérand et al, 2009]. The use of prebent titanium plates may allow smaller, less invasive surgical approaches and can additionally serve as guides for fracture reduction and fixation. Individually, precontoured titanium plates and titanium meshes represent an accurate, cost-effective alternative to 3-D printed patient-specific implants.

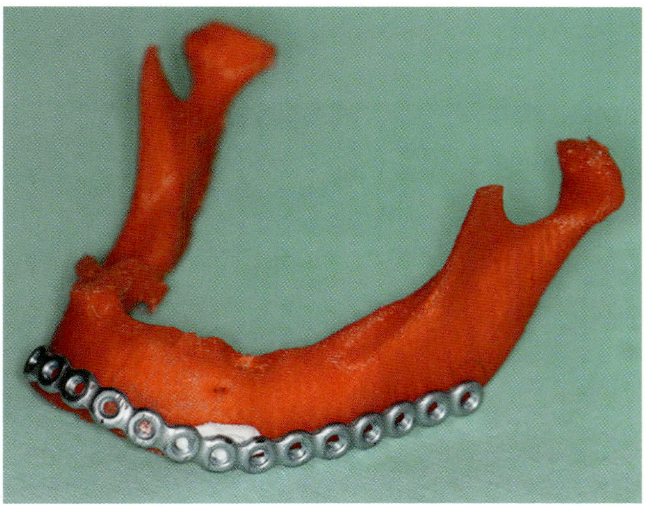

Fig 5.2-13 A 3-D model of a patient's mandible with severe osteomyelitis. Prebending of a titanium reconstruction plate before surgery.

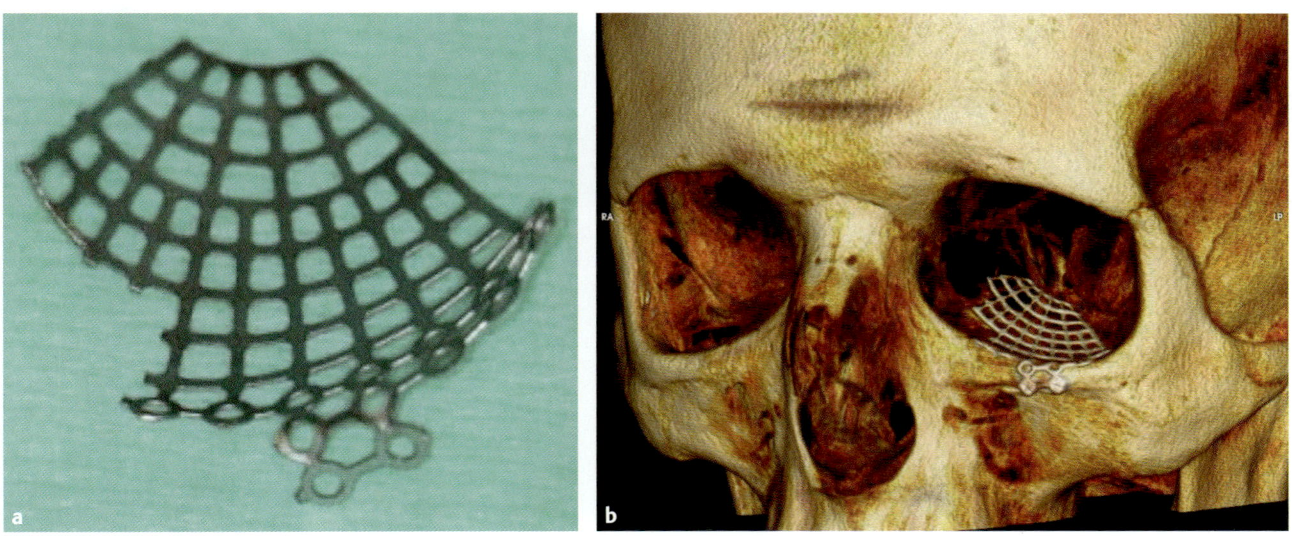

Fig 5.2-14a–b

a Titanium mesh for orbital floor reconstruction prebent and adapted to a 3-D model.

b A 3-D reconstruction of a cone beam computed tomography, postoperative result.

5.3 Orthognathic surgery

Sagittal, vertical or transversal skeletal deformities can be corrected through various types of osteotomies of the maxilla and mandible. These procedures require careful pre-interventional planning to create a stable occlusion, which plays a decisive role for this kind of surgery. With the help of 3-D models that can be combined with plaster models of the dentition, even complex surgery can be planned in a step-by-step fashion. The 3-D models show all relevant anatomical structures and help to prevent intraoperative errors (**Fig 5.2-15**). Accordingly, the appropriate implants can be pre-selected and plates can be prebent before surgery. Prebent plates can serve as surgical guides or templates to facilitate the orientation and positioning of the upper and lower jaw during the operation [Shaheen et al, 2016].

5.4 Craniofacial surgery

The exact anatomical reproduction of congenital or acquired craniofacial deformities in children has made 3-D printed skull models an important tool for the planning of skull correction procedures in many craniofacial centers. The relevant and critical anatomical structures are visualized, and the complex surgical steps can be planned and simulated. With the help of these models, surgical guides can be manufactured, which allow surgery with high degree of precision (**Fig 5.2-16**) [Seruya et al, 2013; Soleman et al, 2015].

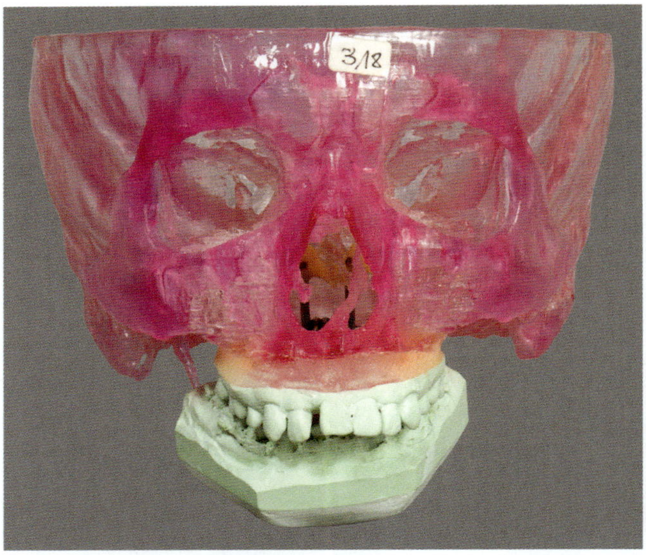

Fig 5.2-15 Hybrid stereolithographic and plaster model of the dentition for the precise planning of orthognathic surgery (Le Fort I osteotomy).

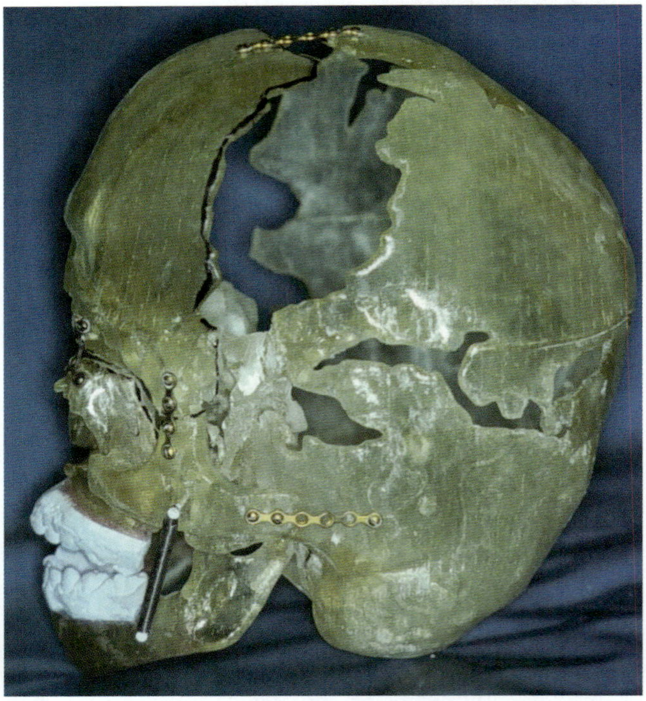

Fig 5.2-16 Planning and simulation of a craniofacial surgical procedure (stereolithography file format/plaster hybrid model) of a patient with Crouzon syndrome.

5.5 Tumor surgery, pathology and adjunctive therapy

The 3-D models are useful in the planning of tumor resection and anatomical reconstructions. Color-coded 3-D models may visualize the extent of tumor infiltration and therefore allow precise planning of ablative surgery (**Fig 5.2-17**). Precise anatomical reconstruction with prebent titanium plates and autogenous grafts or microvascular flaps can be achieved [Chopra et al, 2014]. Furthermore, 3-D anatomical models facilitate orientation and examination of histopathological specimens for pathologists. Resection borders can be marked accurately on the model for their reference (**Fig 5.2-18**). Patient models are also used for radiation therapy as a discussion and planning basis.

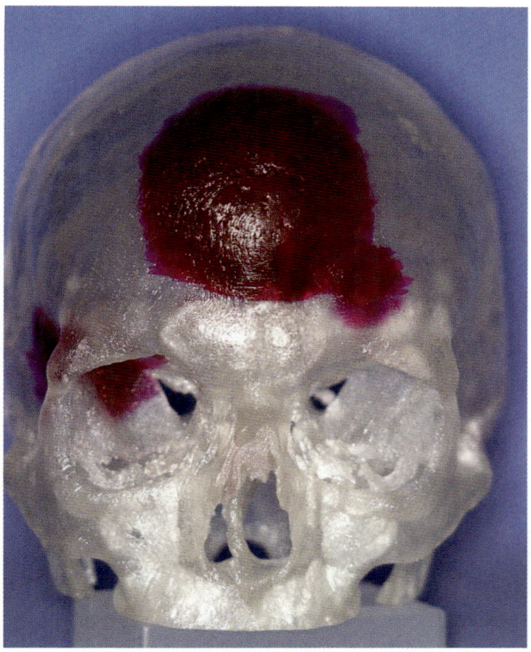

Fig 5.2-17 A color-coded 3-D stereolithographic skull model (red areas indicate tumor (meningeoma) before surgical intervention.

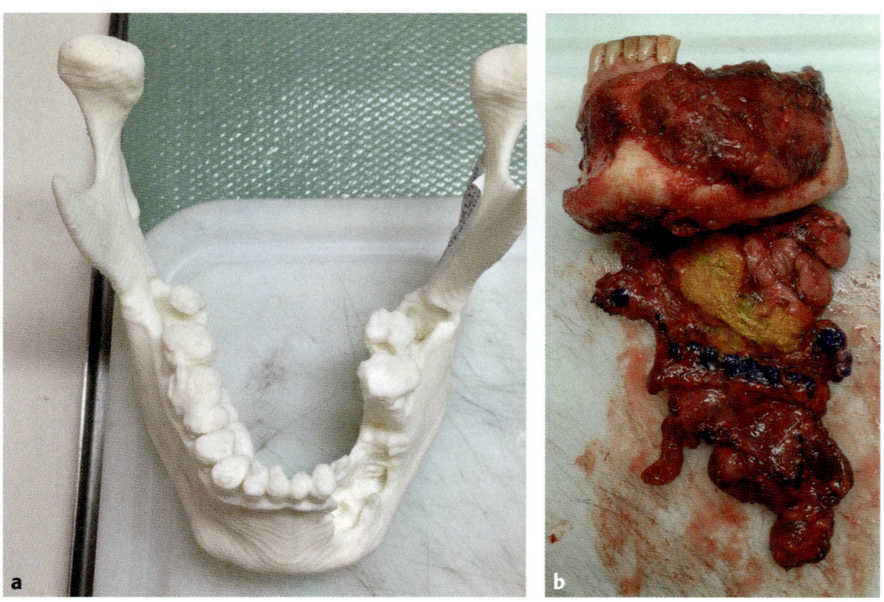

Fig 5.2-18a–b

a Rapid prototype model with squamous cell carcinoma infiltration of the mandible.

b Specimen after tumor resection and neck dissection.

5.6 Reconstructive surgery

For unilateral anomalies or defects in the facial area, the easiest way of reconstruction planning is the virtual mirroring of the healthy anatomical side. This serves as the basis for further planning steps, and for the prebending of titanium plates or the manufacturing of patient-specific implants. Additionally, they can serve as an orientation aid and surgical guide, and prevent misalignment of anatomical structures during the operative procedure (**Fig 5.2-19**).

5.7 Distraction osteogenesis

For the planning of bone distraction, 3-D printed anatomical skull models (**Fig 5.2-20**) are valuable to determine the position of the necessary osteotomies, and ultimately to select the best fitting bone distraction devices. All steps of the surgical procedure and the distraction process itself can be realistically visualized and rehearsed. The distractors can be fitted to the model before surgery.

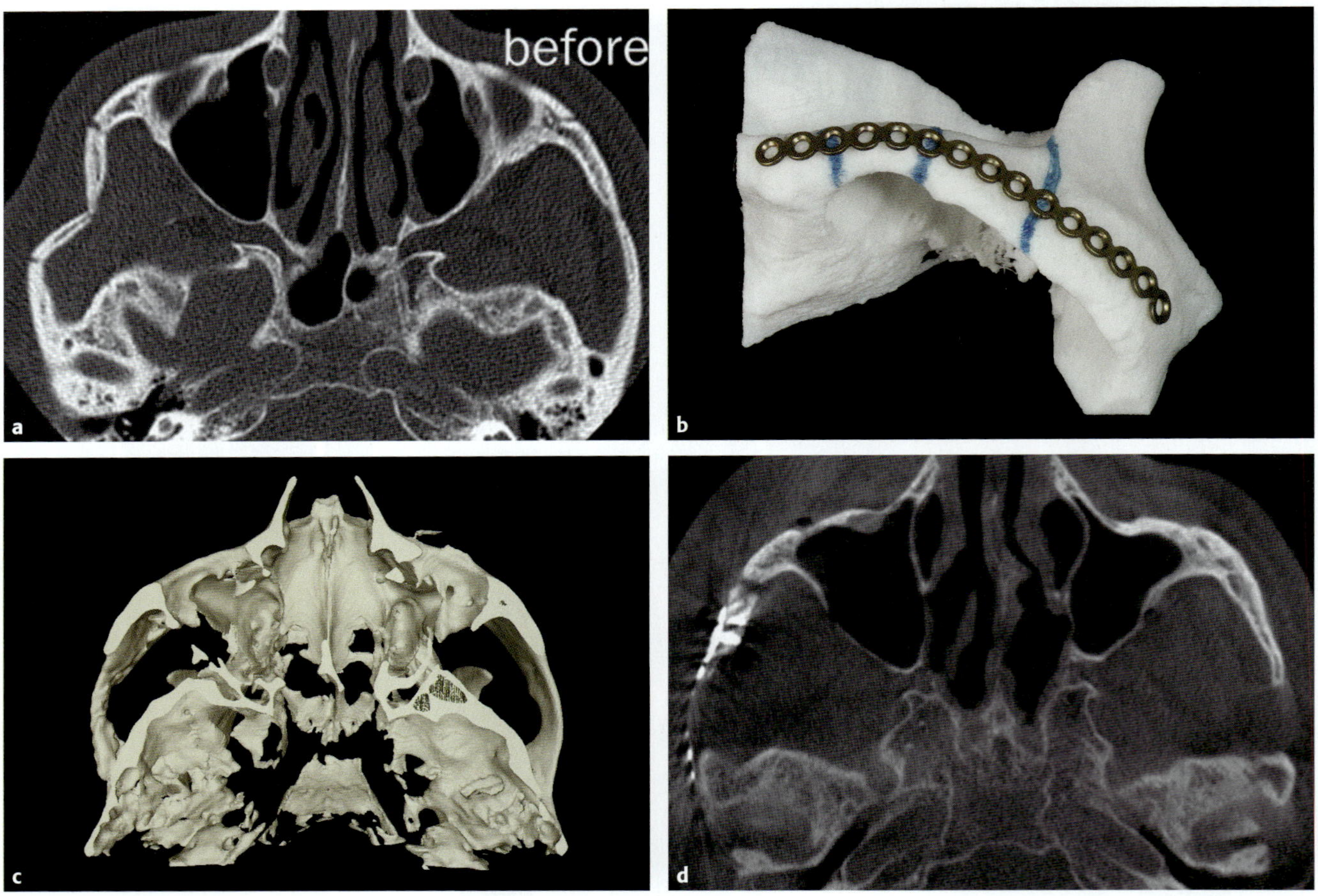

Fig 5.2-19a–d

a Patient with an about 1-year-old (in malposition) consolidated fracture of the zygomatic arch with functional and esthetic impairment.
b Plastic 3-D model mirrored from healthy side and prebent titanium plate.
c–d Situation after osteotomy, reposition of the segments, and osteosynthesis (virtual 3-D reconstruction and cross-sectional cone beam computed tomographic image).

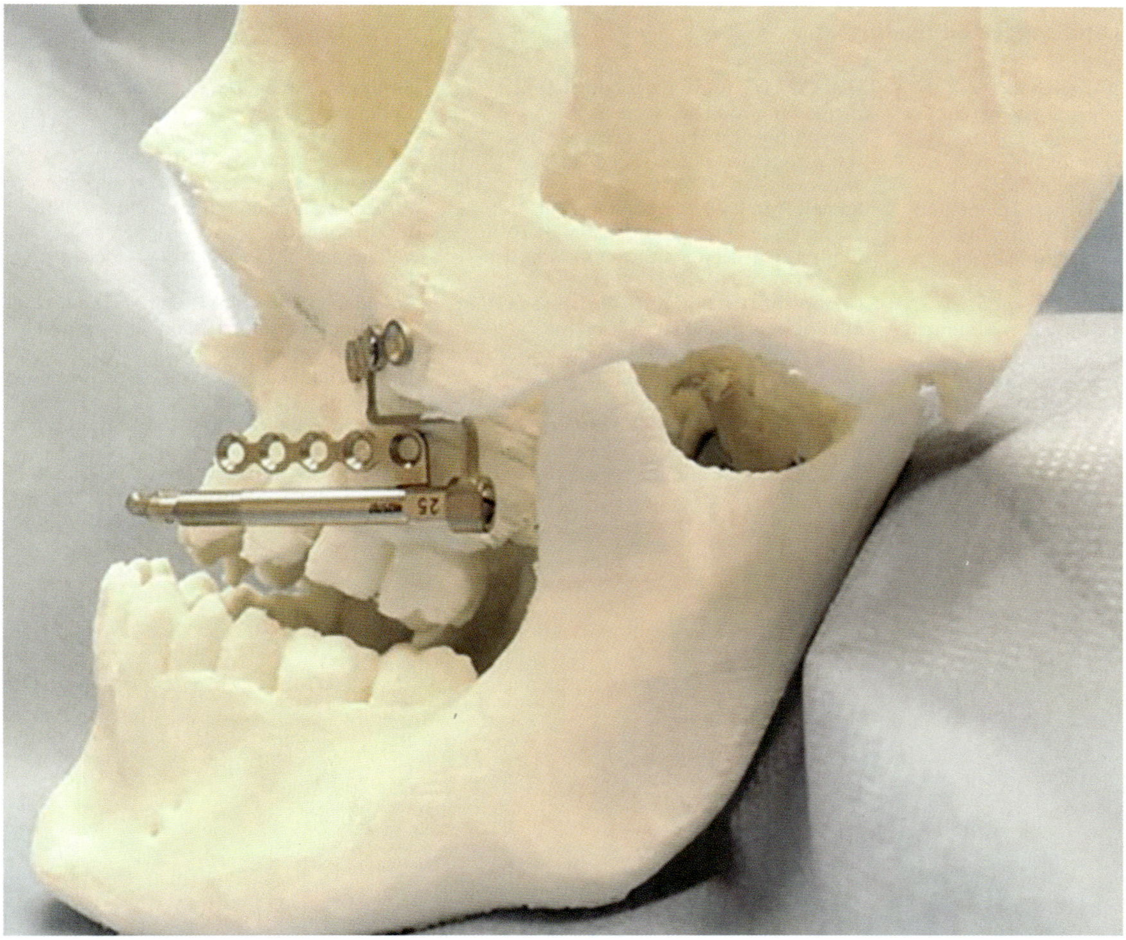

Fig 5.2-20 Example of selection of the best fitting internal distraction device and preadaptation (courtesy of AA Mueller).

6 Summary

Especially for complex problems, patient specific 3-D models are useful for both the planning process and intraoperatively. The use of medical models for planning improves quality and accuracy and reduces operating time and associated costs.

With the introduction of low-priced (consumer) printers in the market, cost-effective 3-D printing to produce planning and demonstration models will play an even bigger role in the field of medicine and surgery [Kamali et al, 2016].

With affordable in-house rapid manufacturing, time-consuming and expensive services provided by external companies can be avoided or limited to special indications. In addition to individual patient care, 3-D models can be used for patient information and surgical training. These models serve as illustrative materials and can be manipulated (sawn, drilled or plated) directly in surgical skill laboratories.

7 References and suggested reading

Barazanchi A, Li KC, Al-Amleh B, et al. Additive technology: update on current materials and applications in dentistry. *J Prosthodontics*. 2016 Sep 23;1–8.

Bibb R, Winder J. A review of the issues surrounding three-dimensional computed tomography for medical modelling using rapid prototyping techniques. *Radiography*. 2010 Feb 1;16(1):78–83.

Brix F, Lambrecht JT. [Preparation of individual skull models based on computed tomographic information.] *Fortschr Kiefer Gesichtschir*. 1987;32:74–77. German.

Chopra K, Folstein MK, Manson PN, et al. Complex craniofacial reconstruction using stereolithographic modeling. *Ann Plast Surg*. 2014 Jan;72(1):59–63.

Dérand P, Hirsch JM. Virtual bending of mandibular reconstruction plates using a computer-aided design. *Am Assoc Oral Maxillofac Surg*. 2009 Aug 1;67(8):1640–1643.

Hull CW. Apparatus for production of three-dimensional objects by stereolithography. Available at: http://www.google.nl/patents/US4575330. Accessed Mar 11, 1986.

Kamali P, Dean D, Skoracki R, et al. The current role of three-dimensional printing in plastic surgery. *Plast Reconstr Surg*. 2016 Mar;137(3):1045–1055.

Lambrecht JTH, Berndt D, Christensen AM, et al. Haptic model fabrication for undergraduate and postgraduate teaching. *Int J Oral Maxillofac Surg*. 2010 Dec 1;39(12):1226–1229.

Petzold R, Zeilhofer HF, Kalender WA. Rapid protyping technology in medicine: basics and applications. *Comput Med Imaging Graph*. 1999;23:277–284.

Seruya M, Borsuk DE, Khalifian S, et al. Computer-aided design and manufacturing in craniosynostosis surgery. *J Craniofac Surg*. 2013 Jul;24(4):1100–1105.

Shaheen E, Sun Y, Jacobs R, et al. Three-dimensional printed final occlusal splint for orthognathic surgery: design and validation. *Int J Oral Maxillofac Surg*. 2016 Nov 1;1–5.

Soleman J, Thieringer F, Beinemann J, et al. Computer-assisted virtual planning and surgical template fabrication for frontoorbital advancement. *Neurosurg Focus*. 2015 May;38(5):E5.

Winder J, Bibb R. Medical rapid prototyping technologies: state of the art and currentlimitations for application in oral and maxillofacial surgery. *J Oral Maxillofac Surg*. 2005 Jul;63(7):1006–1015.

5.3.1 Navigation and computer planning in craniomaxillofacial reconstruction—introduction

Nils-Claudius Gellrich, Majeed Rana

Computer-assisted techniques have given advanced cranio-maxillofacial (CMF) surgery great momentum toward better quality of all steps of the process, including preoperative planning, intraoperative execution, and postoperative quality control. Today even a personal computer has enough calculation power to deal with full-skull Voxel-based data sets (computed tomography [CT], cone beam CT, and magnetic resonance imaging). In the following chapters all aspects of extended use of Voxel-based data sets for the CMF surgeon are described. Analysis of virtual models and biomodels, intraoperative navigation, intraoperative imaging are more technique-related topics and are described in the first part of the following chapters. Process implementation into clinical relevant digital workflow is addressed in the second part.

Besides providing more information for the surgeon, the whole team will benefit from image-analyzing software that allows, independent of the anatomical region, a common trunk data set evaluation and decision making. The impact for teaching, documentation, and interspecialty cross-information is tremendous as visualization allows a language-independent communication.

Computer assistance allows visualization of deformities and defects, creation and visualization of planned reconstructions, and intraoperative visualization of the reconstruction plan. Since all this is accompanied by no further radiation but just the extended use of the required preoperative Voxel-based data set, the following chapters encourage CMF surgeons to take advantage of this breathtaking new development in the field of reconstructive CMF surgery.

5.3.2 Image analysis: data acquisition and processing

R Bryan Bell

1 Introduction

Computer-aided surgical simulation (CASS) nowadays is an important aid in safe and predictable craniomaxillofacial (CMF) surgical reconstruction in a number of clinical applications, including complex maxillofacial trauma [Bell et al, 2009; Bell, 2010; Bell et al, 2010; Bui et al, 2012; Fuller et al, 2007; Gellrich et al, 2002; Markiewicz et al, 2011; Schmelzeisen et al, 2004], head and neck oncological surgery [Bell et al, 2010; Durbin et al, 2005; Gelesko et al, 2012; Gregoire et al, 2011; Hamilton et al, 2012; Hsu et al, 2012; Schramm et al, 2000; Lubbers et al, 2010, To et al, 2002], orthognathic surgery [Bell, 2011; Gateno et al, 2003, 2007, and 2011; Hamilton et al, 2012; Hsu et al, 2012; Xia et al, 2007, 2009, 2011], and temporomandibular joint surgery [Chandran et al, 2011; Schmelzeisen et al, 2002; Yeung et al, 2006; Yu et al, 2009]. Also known as "virtual surgery", CASS can be divided into four phases: (1) data acquisition phase, (2) planning phase, (3) surgical phase, and (4) assessment phase. While there may be some special adjustments based on the specific clinical application, the principles are consistent and are outlined below.

2 Data acquisition phase

A careful clinical examination is an essential part of the data acquisition phase. This is ideally complemented by digital photographic documentation of the facial structures in multiple views, as well as intraoral and occlusal views. High-resolution, thin cut (1 mm) computed tomography (CT) imaging or cone beam CT is obtained for purposes of computer-aided surgical simulation. Low-resolution or wide cut CT scans, which are typically obtained as part of a trauma patient's initial survey, offer a poor representation of the thin-walled orbits and paranasal sinuses and are inadequate for CASS. The high-resolution CT or cone beam CT scan data will be stored in DICOM (digital information and communications in medicine) format. The DICOM data are then imported into a proprietary computer-aided design/computer-aided manufacturing (CAD/CAM) software program.

3 Presurgical planning phase

The presurgical planning phase consists of the analysis of the newly formatted CT data in 3-D, segmenting out the altered portions of the facial skeleton, or using the mirror image of the unaffected side to overlay the deformed portions of the affected facial skeleton. The planning phase differs greatly and depends on the portions of the maxillofacial skeleton that are deformed or missing and the type of reconstruction planned. For instance, in orbital fractures a critical measure of successful reconstruction is the restoration of the orbital volume, whereas in isolated zygomaticomaxillary complex fractures successful reconstruction is largely based on the restoration of the bizygomatic width and facial projection. Restoration of dental occlusion as well as mandibular width, height, and projection are key goals in cases of comminuted mandibular fractures. In general, standardized measurements can be used to segment the fractured portions of the facial skeleton and plan the reconstruction. This part of the surgical planning can either be performed by the surgeon, or alternatively via a web meeting that can be set up with a third-party company in which a computer planning specialist assists the surgeon in manipulating the CT data for the planned reconstruction. Once the surgical plan is finalized, the proprietary software data plan should be back-converted. Back-conversion specifically refers to translating the surgical data plan created by the proprietary software "back" to the standard DICOM format. This DICOM format may then be viewed on workstations not loaded with the proprietary software, and it allows interoperability between the planning software and intraoperative navigation systems.

4 Surgical phase

During the surgical phase, the virtual surgical plan is translated to the patient's situation using a combination of stereolithographic models, cutting guide stents, and/or intraoperative navigation. Stereolithographic models are particularly useful for severely comminuted fractures and panfacial fractures, as they allow for preoperative plate bending and decrease of operating room time. Cutting guide stents in maxillofacial surgery are most useful for reconstruction of head and neck tissues after tumor resection and secondary reconstruction of posttraumatic deformities. They are less useful in the acute setting where the bones can still be mobilized into adequate reduction. Intraoperative navigation is particularly useful for real-time assessment of facial width and projection when repairing zygomaticomaxillary complex fractures and for the evaluation of plate placement during repair of orbital floor and medial orbital wall fractures [Fuller et al, 2007].

5 Assessment phase

The assessment phase has historically consisted of the clinical examination with or without conventional postoperative CT imaging. Modern mobile CT or cone beam CT scanners have more recently facilitated intraoperative quality control by allowing this in the operating room with the patient still under anesthesia. With an intraoperative CT scan the actual surgical result can be compared with the presurgical plan, allowing for immediate surgical correction if indicated. Intraoperative assessment of facial projection, facial width, and orbital volume, as well as correct facial proportions (height, width, projection) or jaw position can be performed, allowing for improved predictability and fewer corrective procedures.

6 References and suggested reading

Bell RB, Markiewicz MR. Computer-assisted planning, stereolithographic modeling, and intraoperative navigation for complex orbital reconstruction: a descriptive study in a preliminary cohort. *J Oral Maxillofac Surg.* 2009 Dec;67(12):2559–2570.

Bell RB. Computer planning and intraoperative navigation in craniomaxillofacial surgery. *Oral Maxillofac Clin North Am.* 2010 Feb;22(1):135–156.

Bell RB, Weimer KA, Dierks EJ, et al. Computer planning and intraoperative navigation for palatomaxillary and mandibular reconstruction with fibular free flaps. *J Oral Maxillofac Surg.* 2010 Mar;69(3):724–732.

Bell RB. Computer planning and intraoperative navigation in orthognathic surgery. *J Oral Maxillofac Surg.* 2011 Mar;69(3):592–605.

Bui RG, Bell RB, Dierks EJ. Technological advances in the treatment of facial trauma. *Atlas Oral Maxillofac Surg Clin North Am.* 2012 Mar;20(1):81–94.

Chandran R, Keeler GD, Christensen AM, et al. Application of virtual surgical planning for total joint reconstruction with a stock alloplast system. *J Oral Maxillofac Surg.* 2011 Jan;69(1):285–294.

Durbin MG, Sonnenburg RE, Melroy CT, et al. Staged endoscopic and combined open/endoscopic approach in the management of inverted papilloma of the frontal sinus. *Am J Rhinol.* 2005 Sep–Oct;19(5):442–445.

Fuller SC, Strong EB. Computer applications in facial plastic and reconstructive surgery. *Curr Opin Otolaryngol Head Neck Surg.* 2007 Aug;15(4):233–237.

Gateno J, Xia JJ, Teichgraeber JF. New 3-dimensional cephalometric analysis for orthognathic surgery. *J Oral Maxillofac Surg.* 2011 Mar;69(3):606–622.

Gateno J, Xia JJ, Teichgraeber JF, et al. Clinical feasibility of computer-aided surgical simulation (CASS) in the treatment of complex cranio-maxillofacial deformities. *J Oral Maxillofac Surg.* 2007 Apr;65(4):728–734.

Gateno J, Xia JJ, Teichgraeber JF. Effect of facial asymmetry on 2-dimensional and 3-dimensional cephalometric measurements. *J Oral Maxillofac Surg.* 2011 Mar;69(3):655–662.

Gateno J, Xia J, Teichgraeber JF, et al. A new technique for the creation of a computerized composite skull model. *J Oral Maxillofac Surg.* 2003 Feb;61(2):222–227.

Gellrich NC, Schramm A, Hammer B, et al. Computer-assisted secondary reconstruction of unilateral posttraumatic orbital deformity. *Plast Reconstr Surg.* 2002 Nov;110(6):1417–1429.

Gelesko S, Markiewicz MR, Weimer K, et al. Computer-aided orthognathic surgery. *Atlas Oral Maxillofac Surg Clin North Am.* 2012 Mar;20(1):107–118.

Gregoire C, Adler D, Madey S, et al. Basosquamous carcinoma involving the anterior skull base: a neglected tumor treated using intraoperative navigation as a guide to achieve safe resection margins. *J Oral Maxillofac Surg.* 2011 Jan;69(1):230–236.

Hamilton T, Markiewicz MR, Jarman J, et al. Dental outcomes in computer-assisted orthognathic surgery. *J Craniofac Surg.* 2012 May;23(3):e223–226.

Hsu SS, Gateno J, Bell RB, et al. Accuracy of a computer-aided surgical simulation protocol for orthognathic surgery: a prospective multicenter study. *J Oral Maxillofac Surg.* 2013 Jan;71(1):128–142.

Lübbers HT, Jacobsen C, Könü D, et al. Surgical navigation in cranio-maxillofacial surgery: an evaluation on a child with a cranio-facio-orbital tumour. *Br J Oral Maxillofac Surg.* 2011 Oct;49(7):532–537.

Markiewicz MR, Dierks EJ, Potter BE, et al. Reliability of intraoperative navigation in restoring normal orbital dimensions. *J Oral Maxillofac Surg.* 2011 Nov;69(11):2833–2840.

Markiewicz MR, Dierks EJ, Bell RB. Does intraoperative navigation restore orbital dimensions in traumatic and post-ablative defects? *J Craniomaxillofac Surg.* 2012 Feb;40(2):142–148.

Markiewicz MR, Bell RB. The use of 3D imaging tools in facial plastic surgery. *Facial Plast Surg Clin North Am.* 2011 Nov;19(4):655–682.

Schmelzeisen R, Gellrich NC, Schramm A, et al. Navigation-guided resection of temporomandibular joint ankylosis promotes safety in skull base surgery. *J Oral Maxillofac Surg.* 2002 Nov;60(11):1275–1283.

Schmelzeisen R, Gellrich NC, Schoen R, et al. Navigation-aided reconstruction of medial orbital wall and floor contour in cranio-maxillofacial reconstruction. *Injury.* 2004 Oct:35(10):955–962.

Schramm A, Gellrich NC, Gutwald R, et al. Indications for computer-assisted treatment of cranio-maxillofacial tumors. *Comput Aided Surg.* 2000;5(5):343–352.

To EW, Yuen EH, Tsang WM, et al. The use of stereotactic navigation guidance in minimally invasive transnasal nasopharyngectomy: a comparison with the conventional open transfacial approach. *Br J Radiol.* 2002;75:345–317.

Xia JJ, Gateno J, Teichgraeber JF. New clinical protocol to evaluate craniomaxillofacial deformity and plan surgical correction. *J Oral Maxillofac Surg.* 2009 Oct;67(10):2093–2106.

Xia JJ, Gateno J, Teichgraeber JF, et al. Accuracy of the computer-aided surgical simulation (CASS) system in the treatment of patients with complex craniomaxillofacial deformity: a pilot study. *J Oral Maxillofac Surg.* 2007 Feb;65(2):248–254.

Xia JJ, McGrory JK, Gateno J, et al. A new method to orient 3-dimensional computed tomography models to the natural head position: a clinical feasibility study. *J Oral Maxillofac Surg.* 2011 Mar;69(3):584–591.

Xia JJ, Shevchenko L, Gateno J, et al. Outcome study of computer-aided surgical simulation in the treatment of patients with craniomaxillofacial deformities. *J Oral Maxillofac Surg.* 2011 Jul;69(7):2014–2024.

Yeung RW, Xia JJ, Samman N. Image-guided minimally invasive surgical access to the temporomandibular joint: a preliminary report. *J Oral Maxillofac Surg.* 2006 Oct;64(10):1546–1552.

Yu HB, Shen GF, Zhang SL, et al. Navigation-guided gap arthroplasty in the treatment of temporomandibular joint ankylosis. *Int J Oral Maxillofac Surg.* 2009 Oct;38(10):1030–1035.

5.3.3 Virtual models and segmentation

Majeed Rana, Nils-Claudius Gellrich

1 Introduction

Virtual models are useful when replacing lost hard-tissue structures of the skull after trauma or ablative tumor surgery. Rapid prototyping procedures like computer-assisted design and manufacturing (CAD/CAM) have dramatically improved surgical strategies in reconstructive surgery of the craniomaxillofacial skeleton [Rana et al, 2012]. Coupling preoperative planning with navigation systems facilitates symmetric bone repositioning and replacement. Before surgery virtual models are segmented out of the DICOM data using appropriate techniques, such as manual segmentation, threshold-based segmentation, or segmentation using the Smartbrush algorithm.

2 Manual segmentation

In manual segmentation, the desired structure is outlined by hand. Based on the gray scale of magnetic resonance imaging scans or Hounsfield units in computed tomographic (CT) scans, the computer automatically recognizes margins of the desired structures. This procedure is time-consuming and can lead to an inadequate segmentation quality if there are areas of poor contrast within the DICOM data. Due to these issues, this segmentation technique is generally not used on a daily clinical routine [Rana et al, 2014] (**Fig 5.3.3-1**).

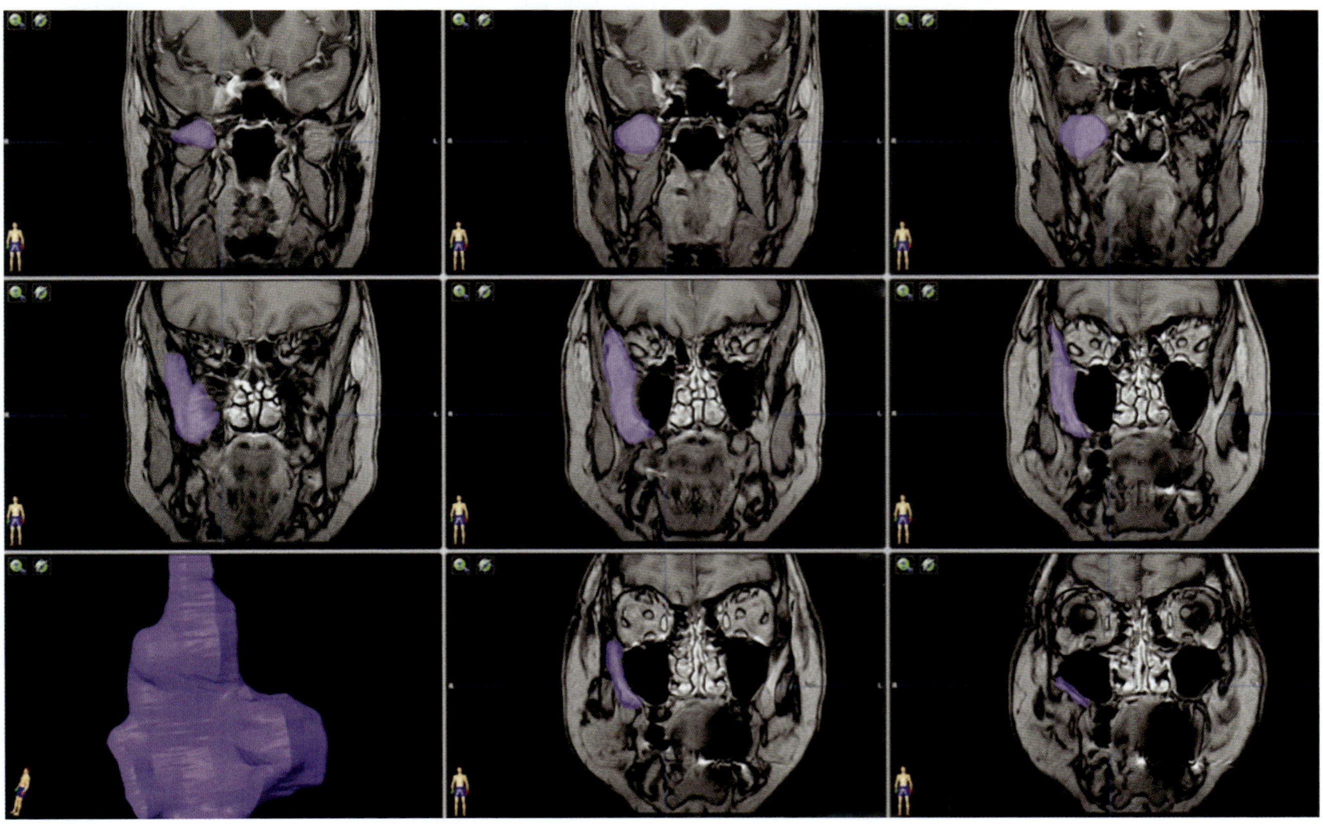

Fig 5.3.3-1 Multiplanar view after manual segmentation of a tumor in the sphenoid fossa (violet) of the right maxilla (3-D and coronal).

3 Threshold segmentation

Segmentation can be achieved using a range of Hounsfield units in a CT or gray scale in other imaging modalities. To limit segmentation to certain areas, a region of interest (ROI) should be defined before the process. Only areas within the predefined range are then automatically selected. The main disadvantage of this method is incorrect segmentation of tissue within the same range of Hounsfield units or gray scale in the vicinity of the desired object [Rana et al, 2014].

4 3-D Smartbrush

Segmentation using the new Smartbrush technique is started by selecting a few points inside the desired area. Around these points, ROI is automatically defined and the final 2-D segmentation is then computed by a region-growing algorithm.

This method of segmentation can then either be conducted for each slice or by the 3-D interpolation of the program itself. The 3-D interpolation algorithm automatically detects the 3-D ROI and segments the designated area with a region-growing algorithm. Smoothing the created object is the last step of the segmentation process. Besides segmenting hard tissue, this method can also segment other anatomical regions like contents of the orbit, which may be available for reconstruction planning. Additionally, segmented structures can be modified by elastic deformation of the selected object using the conventional smart shaper (**Fig 5.3.3-2**).

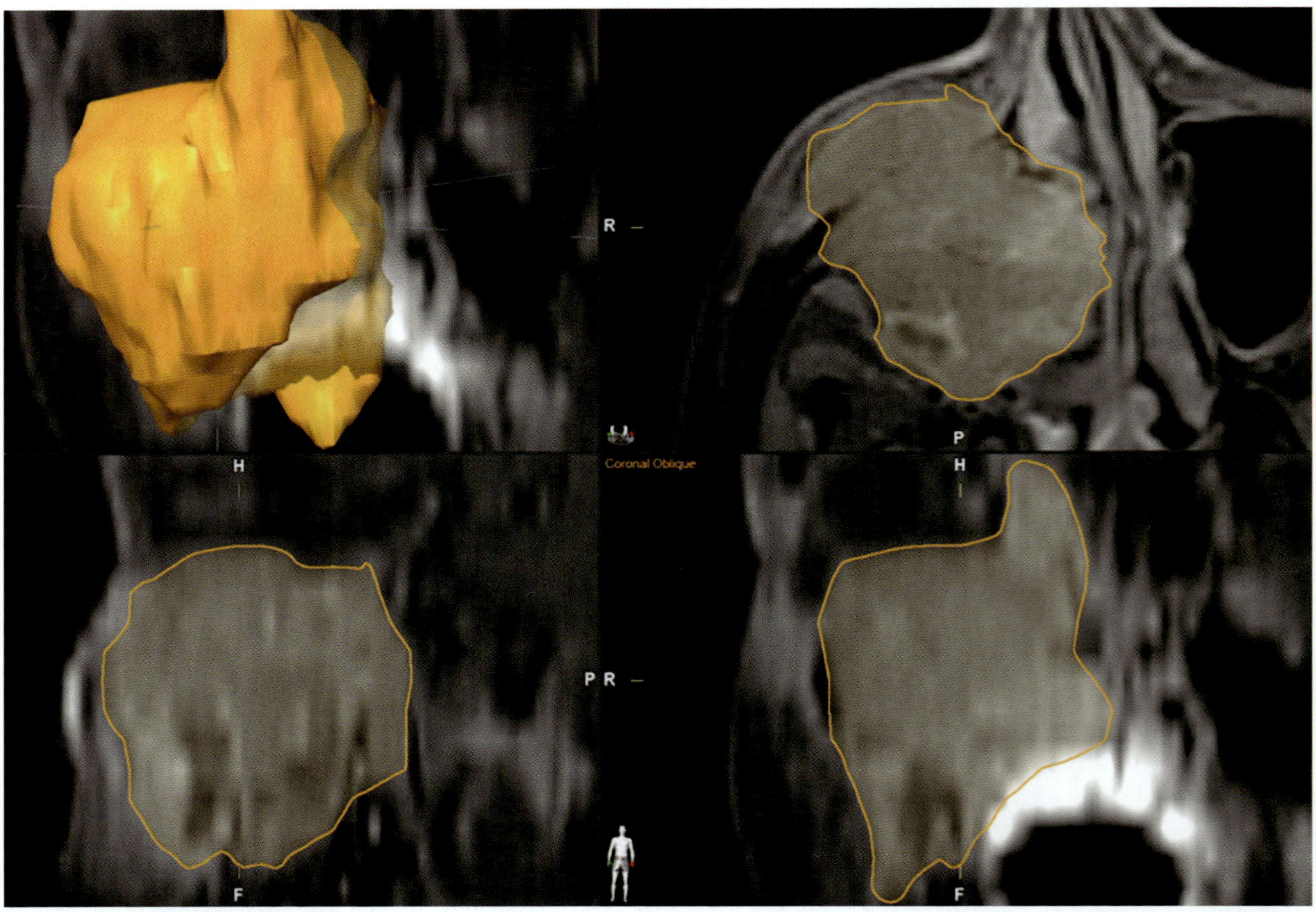

Fig 5.3.3-2 Smartbrush algorithm after completed automatic tumor segmentation (yellow). Multiplanar view (3-D axial, sagittal, and coronal).

5 Clinical use of virtual models

In trauma cases, anatomical structures can easily be segmented using an automatic, atlas-based algorithm (**Fig 5.3.3-3**). The central task of such an algorithm is to find a one-to-one correspondence between the patient's data set and a predefined data set from an atlas containing several anatomical templates. The structures are segmented automatically by elastic deformation of the templates to match the patient's anatomy as precisely as possible. Using the acquired data, cutting and drilling guides for intraoperative use can easily be manufactured within a few days.

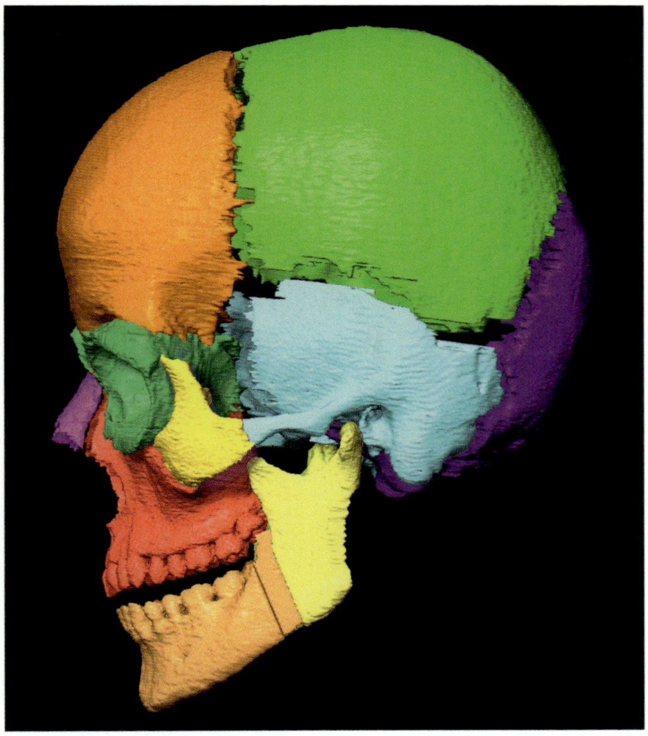

Fig 5.3.3-3 Atlas-based segmentation allows adjustment of the Hounsfield units or gray scale of the target object. A 3-D view of a computed tomographic data set with all possible objects.

In ablative surgery, 3-D (voxel-based) data sets allow to estimate the extension of head and neck tumors. As a tumor is not a normal structure within a patient's anatomy, it cannot be automatically segmented using an atlas. Preoperatively, the tumor margins are therefore most commonly outlined manually using different instruments, such as brushing. After this step of planning, anatomical structures and a target region for tumor resection or taking biopsies are clearly defined. The rendered virtual models can then be transferred into DICOM format to communicate patient-specific tumor information (invasion into vessels, nerves, or skull base) to the oncologist, radiotherapist, and pathologist for further oncological treatment.

6 References and suggested reading

Rana M, Essig H, Eckardt AM, et al. Advances and innovations in computer-assisted head and neck oncologic surgery. *J Craniofac Surg*. 2012;23(1):272–278.

Rana M, Modrow D, Keuchel J, et al. Development and evaluation of an automatic tumor segmentation tool: a comparison between automatic, semi-automatic and manual segmentation of mandibular odontogenic cysts and tumors. *J Craniomaxillofac Surg*. 2014 Apr;43(3):355–359.

5.3.4 Biomodels

Martin Rücker

1 Introduction

Biomodels can be divided into standard ones that are not patient specific (**Fig 5.3.4-1**) and individual ones that are derived mainly from patients' computed tomographic (CT) data. In addition to the visual assessment of a CT scan, the haptic option provided by a patient's specific biomodel can reveal concealed anatomical information. Models created by computer-assisted design and manufacturing (CAD/CAM) not only support medical diagnosis and surgical treatment planning but may also improve communication with the patient [Schramm et al, 2009].

2 Patient-specific biomodels

Rapid prototyping techniques are used to print out patient-specific 3-D biomodels from CT and cone beam-CT data. The most common material used for the rapid prototyping process is polyamide. Variants or hybrids are commercially available with different fillers like glass, carbon-fiber, carbon, and aluminum. Depending on the production process, the models are not necessarily monochrome. Meanwhile anatomical regions of interest like tumors, vessels, or nerves can be highlighted by different colors. For intraoperative use in a sterile environment, it is of crucial importance that the material is autoclavable. This is inevitably necessary for osteotomy guides that enable the accurate transfer of the virtual plan to the operating room.

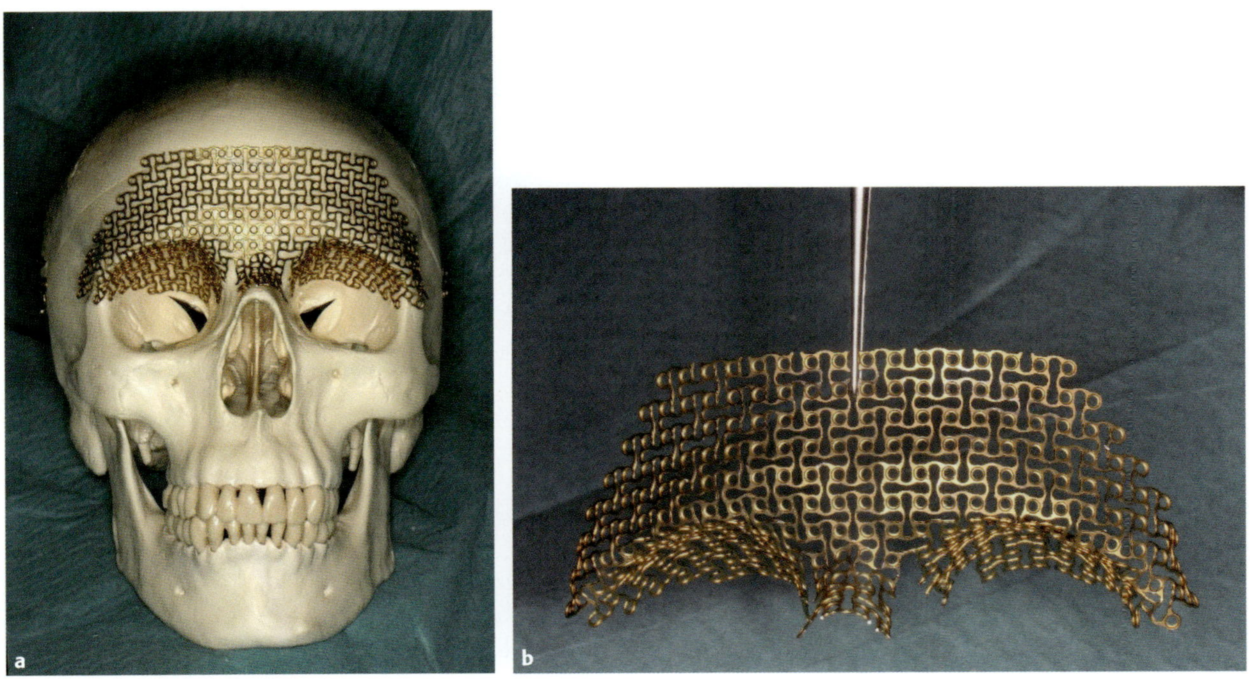

Fig 5.3.4-1a–b Standard nonpatient-specific anatomical biomodel for orienting molding of 3-D titanium structures. Final adjustment of the implant in situ is often necessary.

By using the CT scan data, the actual patient's anatomy can be physically reproduced in a 3-D model. However, more interesting than the reproduction of defects or deformities is the fabrication of a true to original skull model where bone defects and deformities are already individually corrected. The remarkable advance in virtual 3-D planning allows the modification of the CT data by using different algorithms based on mirrored or rigid and elastic deformations. The entire or even partial printout of a reconstructed skull model may serve as a mold at which the osteosynthesis materials can be individually prebent [Kokemüller et al, 2011]. For example, for the reconstruction of the midface or the calvarium 3-D titanium meshes can be used and for bridging mandibular defects titanium plates are suitable. The fit of the prefabricated CAD/CAM implants and osteotomy guides can easily be tested preoperatively on the patient's original nonmodified (osteotomy guides) as well as on the modified biomodels (implants) (**Fig 5.3.4-2**).

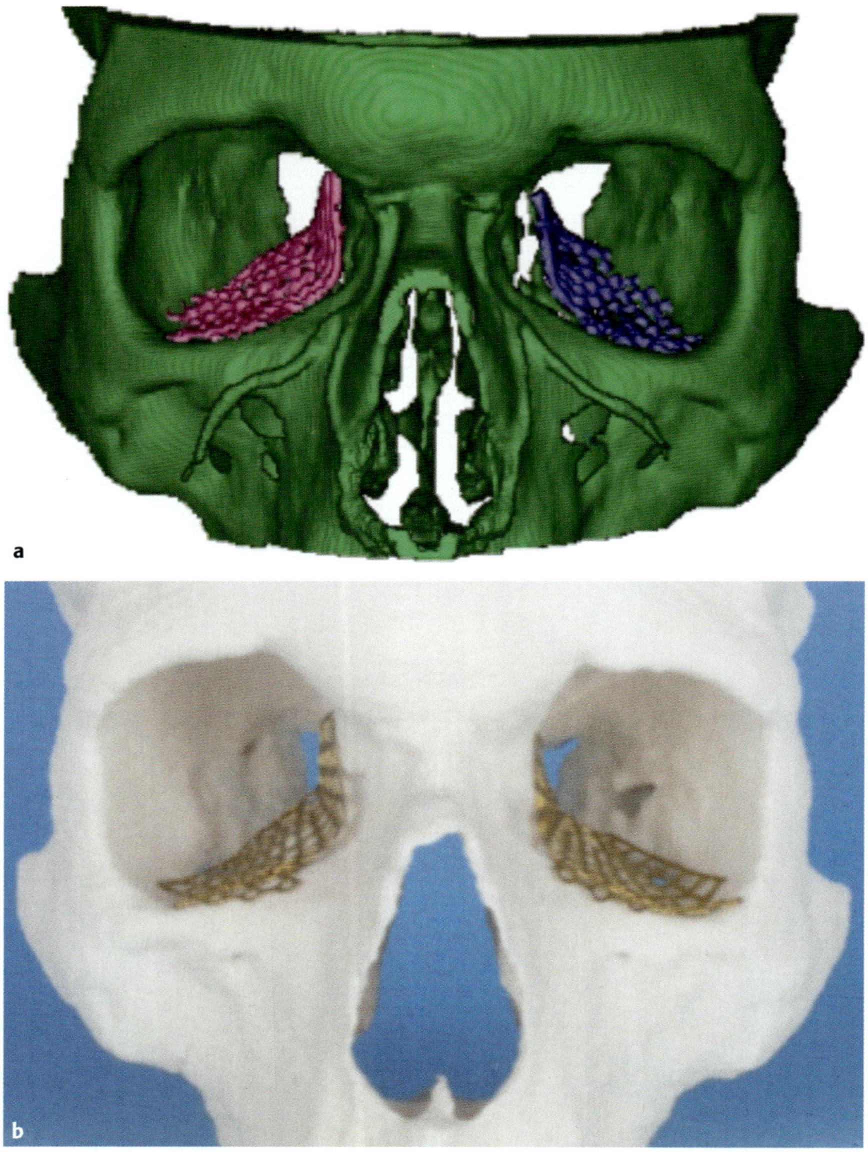

Fig 5.3.4-2a–b Individual patient-specific biomodel for customized implant manufacture.
a Virtual model with virtual implants.
b Printout of the virtual model serving as a mold for controlling the fit of patient-specific implants.

3 Summary and outlook

The appeal of the present workflow is that analysis, planning, and manufacturing of implants to restore the craniofacial skeleton is completely controlled by the surgeon. Meanwhile, several companies offer on-line services to design customized implants derived directly from the patients' CT data. Since in this workflow molding models are no longer required, the surgeon has to collaborate closely with a specially trained clinical engineer throughout the CAD of the implant [Essig et al, 2011]. Actual developments in simulation software pave the way for a model-free automatized design and manufacture of biocompatible patient-specific implants by the surgeon himself.

4 References and suggested reading

Essig H, Rana M, Kokemueller H, et al. Pre-operative planning for mandibular reconstruction: a full digital planning workflow resulting in a patient specific reconstruction. *Head Neck Oncol.* 2011;3:45.

Kokemüller H, von See C, Essig H, et al. [Rekonstruktion komplexer Mittelgesichtsdefekte durch individualisierte Titanimplantate]. *HNO.* 2011;59:319–326. German.

Schramm A, Suarez-Cunqueiro M, Rücker M, et al. Computer-assisted therapy in orbital and midfacial reconstructions. *Int J Med Robot Comput Assist Surg.* 2009;5:111–124.

5.3.5 Intraoperative navigation

Majeed Rana, Nils-Claudius Gellrich

1 Introduction

Navigation technology was incorporated into surgical treatment, initially in neurosurgery, to find specific structures within a volume of tissue, ie, to localize an intracranial tumor [Guijarro-Martinez et al, 2014]. Navigation was introduced into craniomaxillofacial (CMF) surgery when segmentation of data sets became feasible, virtual modeling could occur and digital blueprints resembling the ideal bone reconstruction could be created [Schramm et al, 2008]. The latter means that the breakthrough of navigation for CMF surgeons is because a virtual plan can be visualized intraoperatively by using radiation-free navigation.

2 Navigation systems

Today several navigation systems are available (**Table 5.3.5-1; Fig 5.3.5-1** and **Fig 5.3.5-2**) [Rana et al, 2012]. Navigation systems include a computer that is linked to a detection device. This allows tracking of the position of the patient on the operating table by an infrared camera and instruments that are used for surgery. To achieve intraoperative navigation, the patient on the operating table must be matched with the virtual patient represented by the Voxel-based data set in the navigation system (**Fig 5.3.5-3**) [Rana et al, 2012; Zizelmann et al, 2007; Schmelzeisen et al, 2004].

Technique	Company	Navigational system
Optical	Medtronic	Stealth Station
	IVS Technology	Voxim
	Stryker	eNlite
		NavSuite
	BrainLab	Kolibri, Kick
		Dual Curve
	XIONmedical	Matrix Polar
	Collin	DigiPointeur
	Fiagon	CMF-System
Electromechanical	ISG Technologies	Viewing wand
Electromagnetical	Visualization Technology	Insta Trak
	BrainLab	Kick-EM
	Fiagon	ENT-EM
	Stryker	Scopis-Hybrid
Ultrasound based	Sono Wand	Invite

Table 5.3.5-1 Navigation systems.

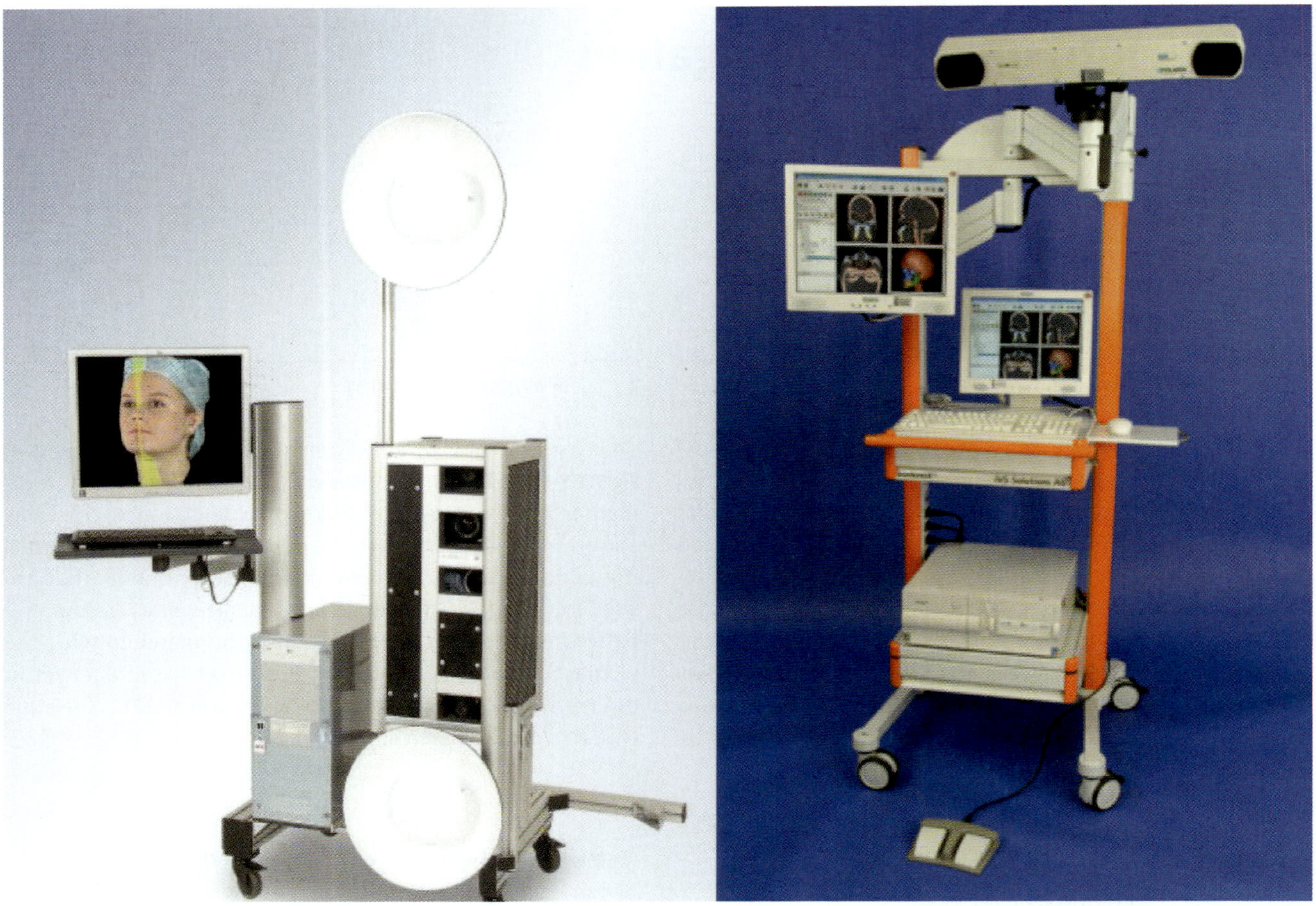

Fig 5.3.5-1 Navigational setup with two monitors where the position of the pointer is at the right monitor (not visible). The optical 3-D surface scanner by 3-D shape and the Voxim navigation system containing an optical camera (Polaris) with two different monitors (Voxim navigation system) are also displayed.

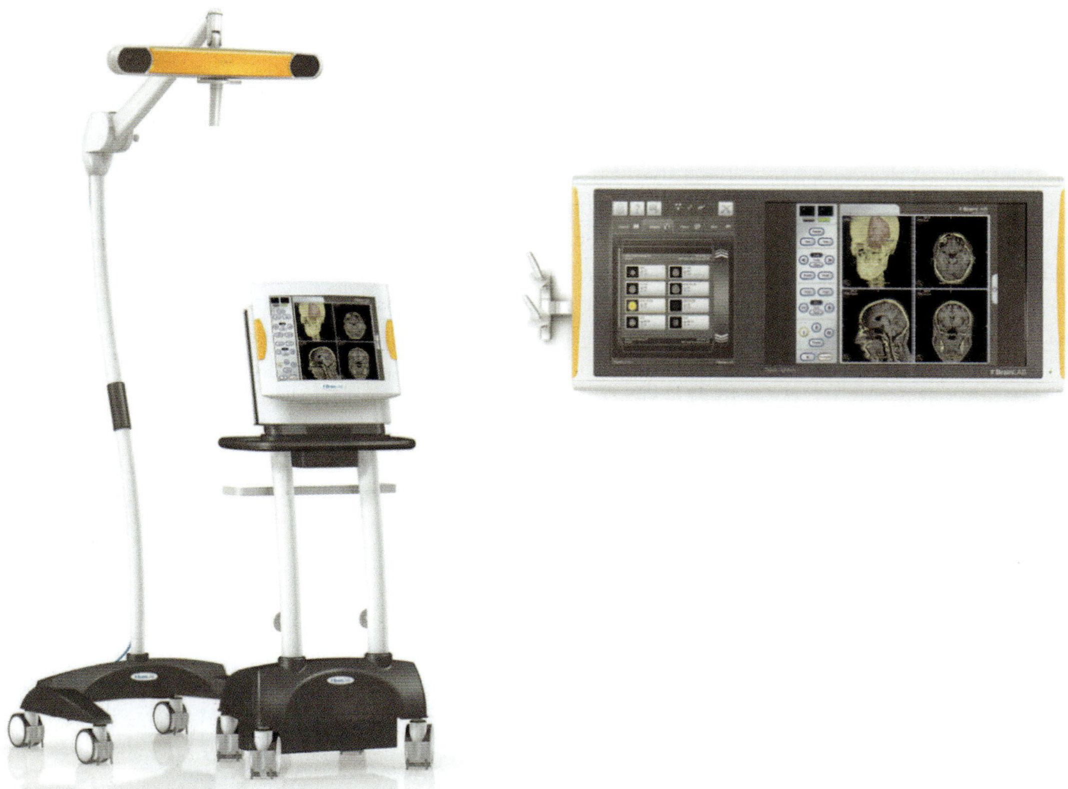

Fig 5.3.5-2 The Brainlab Kolibri System with the TFT monitor using optical cameras and two different monitors.

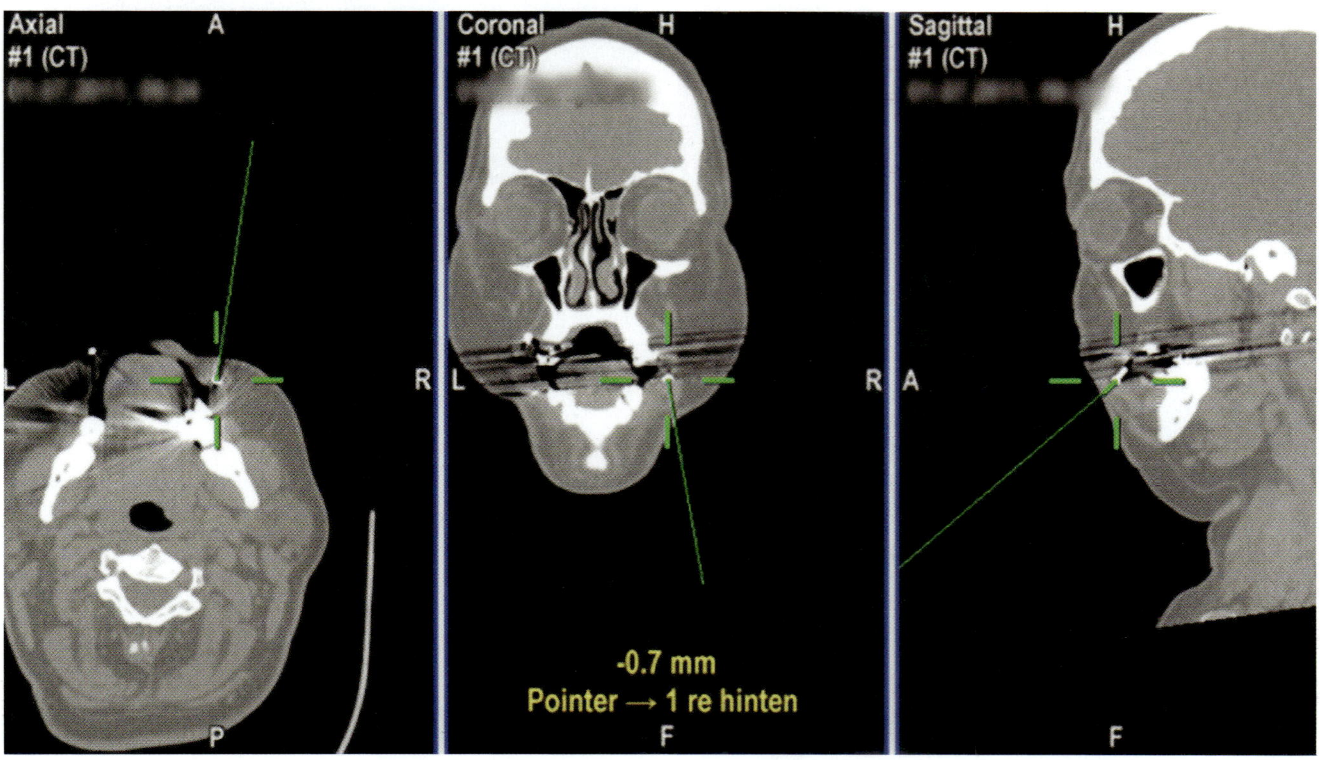

Fig 5.3.5-3 The registration verification is done after the registration procedure, touching the registration landmarks with the pointer (green). The registration accuracy is demonstrated 0.7 mm.

3 Clinical application

To detect the patient's position, the so-called dynamic reference frame or array is fixed to the patient's head, either via an attachment on the Mayfield clamp (**Fig 5.3.5-4**), directly screw-retained on the skull of the patient or a headband attachment (**Fig 5.3.5-5**) [Schmelzeisen et al, 2004]. Registration is based on either preoperative defined landmarks, laser scanning methods or so-called navigation markers that can be either glued to the surface (eg, skin markers, with less accuracy) or hard tissue borne with more accuracy, eg, cruciform bone-anchored screws or cruciform screws mounted on a dental splint (in partially or completely dentated patients) (**Fig 5.3.5-6**) [Gellrich et al, 2002; Essig et al, 2011].

Either of these markers has to be implemented into the scanning protocol of the preoperative Voxel-based data set so that the same structures can be defined on the real patient intraoperatively and on the Voxel-based data set [Essig et al, 2011]. The exception to this is the anatomical landmark-based registration only or the laser surface scanning registration; these latter techniques lack accuracy in long-lasting craniofacial surgeries requiring extensive bone work and especially in cases where re-registration is needed, and coronal flaps have been raised. As a rule of thumb: hard tissue-borne navigation markers are preferred [Rana et al, 2012].

Two different navigation principles can be used, optical systems or electromagnetic systems. For reconstructive CMF surgery, the major experience exists with infrared-based optical navigation systems where a set of cameras is mounted to a mobile stand, which can detect the position of the patient and the instruments in space. Basic components of the setup for intraoperative navigation are the navigation unit, the camera, and the patient on the operating table with a reference device (**Fig 5.3.5-7**) [Rana et al, 2012; Gellrich et al, 2002; Essig et al, 2011].

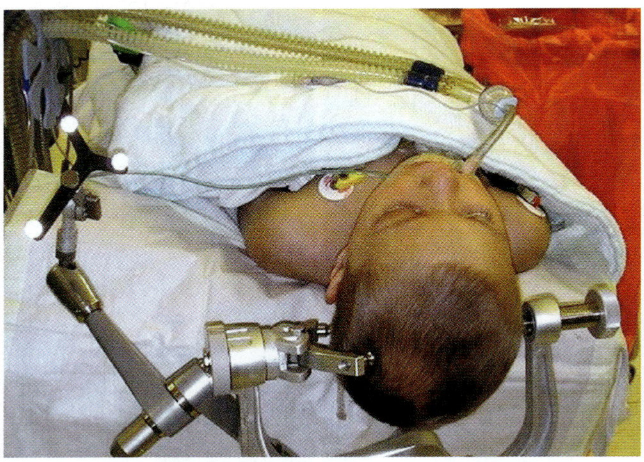

Fig 5.3.5-4 If used with a Mayfield clamp, the dynamic reference array, containing three optical spheres (white dots), is firmly attached.

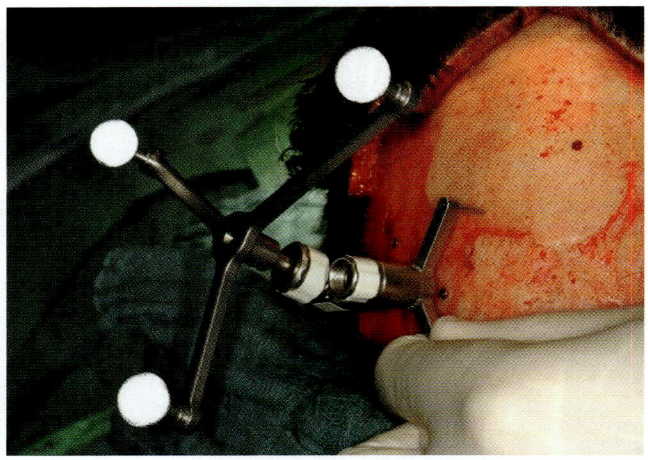

Fig 5.3.5-5 The skull reference array, pre-port system is inserted with an 8 mm screw on the patient's skull. Skull reference arrays contain three optical spheres.

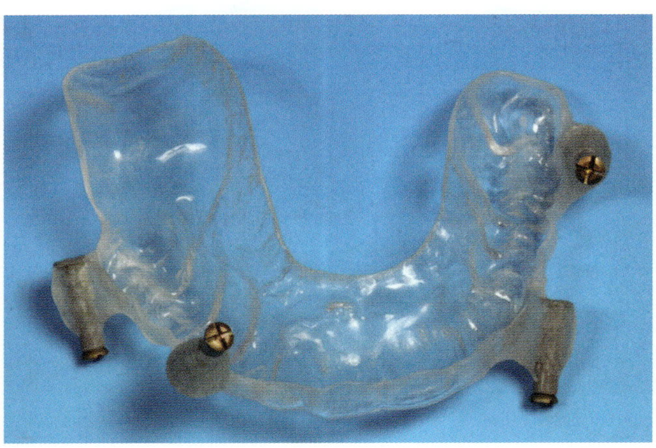

Fig 5.3.5-6 A dental splint containing four screws is used as registration marker. During intraoperative navigation, the screws can be used for (re-)registration purpose.

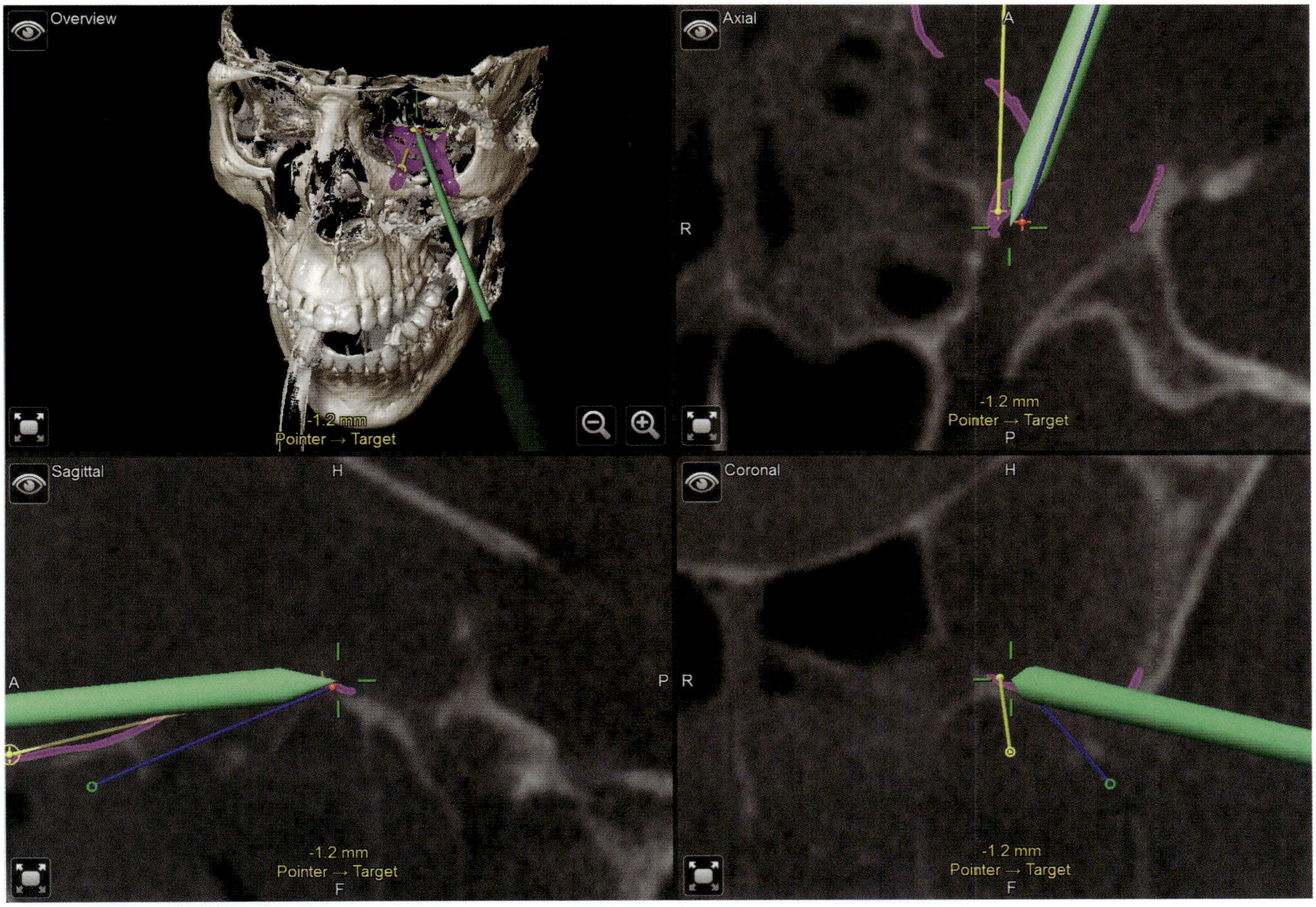

Fig 5.3.5-7 The workflow contains the preoperative planning using the iPlan 3.0.5 Brainlab system and the intraoperative navigation using the Kolibri navigation system Cranial 3.0.

4 Summary

Navigational surgery is implemented into CMF surgery mainly to compose the position of surgical correction with preoperative individual computer-assisted designed digital blueprints of the surgical plan [Guijarro-Martinez et al, 2014; Schramm et al, 2008; Gellrich et al, 2002; Schramm et al, 2000]. This technique is radiation free and can be applied on demand during all surgical steps. Bone-anchored or dental splint-based reference markers should be favored because both allow re-referencing at any time during surgery [Rana et al, 2012; Schmelzeisen et al, 2004; Schramm et al, 2000]. Intraoperative navigation may be used for intraoperative quality control.

5 References and suggested reading

Essig H, Rana M, Meyer A, et al. Virtual 3D tumor marking-exact intraoperative coordinate mapping improve post-operative radiotherapy. *Radiat Oncol.* 2011 Nov 16;6:159.

Gellrich NC, Schramm A, Hammer B, et al. Computer-assisted secondary reconstruction of unilateral posttraumatic orbital deformity. *Plast Reconstr Surg.* 2002 Nov;110(6):1417–1429.

Guijarro-Martinez R, Gellrich NC, Witte J, et al. Optimization of the interface between radiology, surgery, radiotherapy, and pathology in head and neck tumor surgery: a navigation-assisted multidisciplinary network. *Int J Oral Maxillofac Surg.* 2014 Feb;43(2):156–162.

Rana M, Essig H, Eckardt AM, et al. Advances and innovations in computer-assisted head and neck oncologic surgery. *J Craniofac Surg.* 2012 Jan;23(1):272–278.

Schmelzeisen R, Gellrich NC, Schoen R, et al. Navigation-aided reconstruction of medial orbital wall and floor contour in cranio-maxillofacial reconstruction. *Injury.* 2004 Oct;35(10):955–962.

Schramm A, Suare-Cunqueiro MM, Barth EL, et al. Computer-assisted navigation in craniomaxillofacial tumors. *J Craniofac Surg.* 2008 Jul;19(4):1067–1074.

Schramm A, Gellrich NC, Gutwald R, et al. Indications for computer-assisted treatment of cranio-maxillofacial tumors. *Comput Aided Surg.* 2000;5(5):343–352.

Zizelmann C, Gellrich NC, Metzger MC, et al. Computer-assisted reconstruction of orbital floor based on cone beam tomography. *Br J Oral Maxillofac Surg.* 2007 Jan;45(1):79–80.

5.3.6 Intraoperative imaging and quality control

Frank Wilde, Alexander Schramm

1 Introduction

Today, intraoperative 3-D imaging with or without intraoperative navigation is an important element in the workflow of computer-assisted surgery to achieve intraoperative quality control. Clinical and radiological diagnosis by means of computed tomography, (CT), cone beam computed tomography or MRI is followed by preoperative computer-assisted planning to define and simulate the desired outcome of reconstruction. In difficult cases intraoperative navigation helps in the implementation of procedure plans at the site of surgery. Intraoperative 3-D imaging then allows an intraoperative final check to be made and the outcome of the surgery to be validated. Currently, this is preferably done using 3-D C-arm devices based on cone beam computed tomography (CBCT). They help to avoid incorrect positioning of bone fragments and/or implants. This is an outstanding advance to assure the quality of complex operations and reduce the number of secondary interventions.

Functionally important structures are close together in the craniofacial skeleton, especially within the orbit. Detailed knowledge of the anatomy therefore is essential for surgical interventions [Schramm et al, 2010]. This, in turn, places high demands on the imaging procedures used for diagnosis, treatment planning as well as intraoperative and postoperative quality control [Hanken et al, 2013]. Modern craniofacial reconstruction may involve the entire workflow of computer-assisted surgery for reconstruction of the craniomaxillofacial skeleton. This workflow can be subdivided into diagnosis, planning and simulation, surgical execution, as well as validation and quality control (**Fig 5.3.6-1**).

2 Diagnosis

In addition to clinical findings, diagnosis is mainly based on 2-D and 3-D imaging. Multislice CT of the craniofacial skeleton today is the gold standard imaging procedure for diagnosing fractures, defects, and deformities of the craniofacial skeleton. It not only offers excellent resolution concerning bone structures but also allows assessment of concomitant injuries and conditions of soft-tissue structures (eg, eyeball, eye muscles, optic nerve).

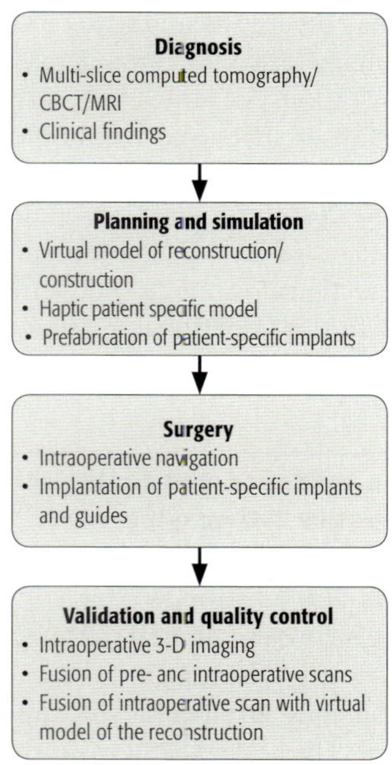

Fig 5.3.6-1 Workflow of computer-assisted surgery for reconstruction of the craniofacial skeleton.

3 Planning and simulation

Computer-assisted planning and surgery simulation is based on the preoperative diagnostic imaging data, CT, CBCT, and/or magnetic resonance imaging (MRI). This should be done with the aid of adequate planning software, which allows various simulations without loss of information. The aim of surgery planning is to create a virtual model that matches the desired outcome of the surgery (see below sections 5.2 and 5.3). The purpose of this is to increase predictability regarding the desired outcome of the surgery as well as the safety of the surgical intervention [Schramm et al, 2010; Schramm et al, 2007]. Aside from basic movements of the virtual models, such as rotation, translation and representations of any type of sectional view, it should help to determine the best route of access to the site of the surgery. When it comes to producing the above-mentioned virtual models, modern planning software allows certain parts of the data set to be automatically segmented and mirrored. Bone-based reconstruction and bone relocation surgery can thus be carried out virtually. The result of the simulation and planning activities can be used as an intraoperative template for an intraoperative navigation system and also for controlling the quality of the outcome of surgery by intraoperative imaging after the preoperative and intraoperative datasets have been fused (see sections 5.2 and 5.3). It should also be possible to freely shift or shape the virtual models generated during planning and to import or export surface tesselation language STL files for purposes of simulating any type of preformed 3-D object (dental implants, titanium mesh structures, etc) (see sections 5.2 and 5.3) or generating patient-specific models and/or implants (see section 5.3) [Schramm et al, 2010].

4 Outcome validation and quality control with intraoperative 3-D imaging

Upon completion of reconstruction (with or without the aid of a navigation system), the surgical outcome should be subjected to 3-D validation for quality control purposes. This should ideally be done intraoperatively, immediately after completion of the surgery. This allows assessment of the bone and/or implant positions, so that corrections can be done immediately if necessary to achieve the desired and planned postoperative result [Schramm et al, 2010; Hanken et al, 2013; Wilde et al, 2013]. This helps to avoid secondary corrections.

The following imaging modalities are fundamentally available today for intraoperative use [Hanken et al, 2013]:

- Ultrasonography
- MRI
- CT
- CBCT

For orbital reconstruction purposes, specific considerations in regard to imaging must be considered:

- Sufficient resolution is needed to visualize in particular the thin bony structures of the orbit and inserted implants.
- The technique must be readily available in the operating room.
- The scan time must be short.
- The surgeon or technical assistant must be able to use it quickly and safely.
- Direct multiplane imaging (axial, coronal, sagittal projection) without complex reconstruction must be possible.
- The direct export of digital imaging and communications in medicine (DICOM) data for fusion with preoperative images and/or preoperative plans is recommended.
- Data storage in the picture archiving and communication system (PACS) of the medical facility must be possible to satisfy the long-term documentation requirements that are mandatory.

Considering the above-mentioned criteria, intraoperative imaging for orbital reconstruction is restricted due to practical considerations almost exclusively to CBCT featuring the use of 3-D C-arms.

4.1 Ultrasonography

Although intraoperative ultrasonography shows the zygomatic arch and the anterior maxillary wall, it does not allow adequate assessments of the complex bony anatomy including the inner orbit [Hanken et al, 2013; Friedrich et al, 2003; Stieve et al, 2012].

4.2 Magnetic resonance imaging

The disadvantage of using MRI for orbital reconstruction is the difficulty to assess bony structures and inserted implants. The long scan time and the complex intraoperative handling, particularly in a non-metallic environment and in view of the need for a radiologist to be present, are arguments against an intraoperative use of MRI in orbital reconstruction surgery.

4.3 Computed tomography

As already mentioned, CT has become the standard imaging technique for diagnosing fractures of the craniofacial skeleton and especially orbital wall fractures. However, the integration of standard CT scanners into an operating room, that is a so-called "hybrid operating room", requires complex structural conditions to be met for reasons of size, even though this equipment meanwhile comes in smaller sizes. A clear advantage of intraoperative CT for orbital reconstruction compared with all other imaging modalities mentioned is its high resolution. This technique is superior to all other modalities in particular in the display of the orbit's thin bony structures and the inserted implant material. Its disadvantages are the relatively high doses of radiation emitted, the high procurement costs and, as with magnetic resonance tomography, the imperative need for a highly competent radiologist [Hanken et al, 2013]. This final disadvantage may always result in unpredictable intraoperative delays.

4.4 Cone beam computed tomography

Intraoperative imaging by means of CBCT mainly refers to intraoperative imaging by means of so-called 3-D C-arms (**Fig 5.3.6-2**). Intraoperative use of C-arms or image intensifiers started in the 1960s [Gebhard et al, 2012]. Initially, only 2-D displays could be obtained so their use was restricted almost entirely to the field of trauma surgery and orthopedics [Gebhard et al, 2012]. The 2-D devices were and still are not suitable for displaying the complex anatomy of the craniofacial skeleton, especially the orbit because superimposition effects limit the practical value. Intraoperative imaging was revolutionized by the introduction of motorized cone beam systems that produce 3-D CT-like image datasets. These systems that are also referred as angiographic image intensifiers were initially used in cardiac and vascular surgery. Since the end of the 1990s, they have increasingly been used in orthopedic and trauma surgery [Gebhard et al, 2012; Rock et al, 2001]. Technical progress has allowed use of such 3-D C-arms to display the craniofacial skeleton intraoperatively, so that over the last 10 years this technology has increasingly been used in CMF surgery [Schramm et al, 2010; Wilde et al, 2013; Heiland et al, 2005; Klatt et al, 2011; Badjate et al, 2005; Heiland et al, 2004; Pohlenz et al, 2009]. The devices normally consist of isocentric C-arms that are motorized and achieve a 190° rotation around the patient. By producing series of images for multiplane representation in axial, coronal, and sagittal projections, they allow hard tissues to be sufficiently represented intraoperatively within approximately 10 minutes (time between the adjustment of the devices and the evaluation of the scans). It is not possible, however, to evaluate soft tissues. The dose of radiation emitted depends on the device used, in particular on its tube power, image repetition frequency, and image intensification time. Although no comparative studies have been conducted, the applied radiation dose per C-arm rotation can be assumed to be less than for a comparable conventional CT scan of the craniofacial skeleton [Hanken et al, 2013]. The CBCT technology is known for emitting a radiation dose in comparable craniofacial skeleton scans that is below that of CT scans [Ludlow et al, 2008; Loubele et al, 2009; Chau et al, 2009; Schulze et al, 2004].

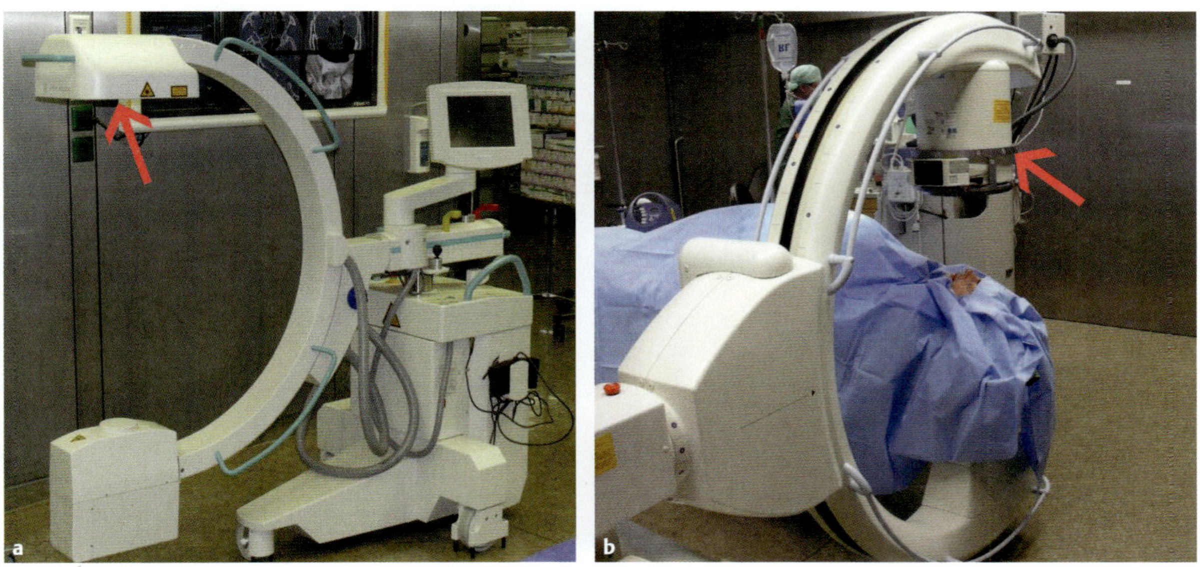

Fig 5.3.6-2a–b Mobile 3-D C-arm devices.
a Vario (FD) 3-D with a flat-panel detector (arrow) (Ziehm, Germany).
b Arcadis Orbic 3-D with a 9-inch x-ray amplifier tube and tracking array for navigational surgery registration (arrow) (Siemens, BrainLAB, Germany).

Both mobile and fixed systems are available with 3-D C-arms [Gebhard et al, 2012]. Fixed systems can be mounted either on the ceiling or the ground, with advantages and disadvantages in terms of hygiene, sterility, and intraoperative handling [Gebhard et al, 2012]. Mobile systems have the great advantage of not being restricted to a given operating room. Other advantages include interdisciplinary use of the imaging unit. Their fundamental disadvantages in comparison with fixed systems are the low tube power (2–25 kW vs recommended power of 80–100 kW), the low image repetition frequency (25 f/s 50 Hz vs recommended rate of 30 f/s 50 Hz) [Gebhard et al, 2012] and a mostly smaller "field of view." This is reflected in a lower resolution and a smaller volume that can be displayed by mobile systems compared with fixed systems. A higher resolution is mainly required for cardiac surgery and angiological interventions [Gebhard et al, 2012; Bonatti et al, 2007], but inevitably results in the application of higher doses of radiation. A level of image resolution comparable with CT would, however, certainly not be disadvantageous in orbital reconstruction. Another limitation of mobile systems is that they overheat due to their lower cooling capacity compared with fixed systems [Gebhard et al, 2012]. This disadvantage is of minor importance in CMF surgery since the units are not permanently used during surgery.

The third and latest type of fixed system is one in which the 3-D C-arm is mounted on a robotic arm that is automatically moved from its resting position to the operating table to avoid collisions (**Fig 5.3.6-3**). Although mounted on the ground, this C-arm is as flexible as those in ceiling-mounted systems. The improvement in range is achieved by attaching the arm to an industrial robot. Another essential advantage is that it can be operated by the surgeon [Gebhard et al, 2012].

Nowadays, flat-panel detectors should preferably be used as image intensifier units (**Fig 5.3.6-2a**) because they allow for a better image quality with lower radiation exposure than intensifier tubes (**Fig 5.3.6-2b**). Moreover, flat-panel detectors generally provide an extended field of view [Gebhard et al, 2012].

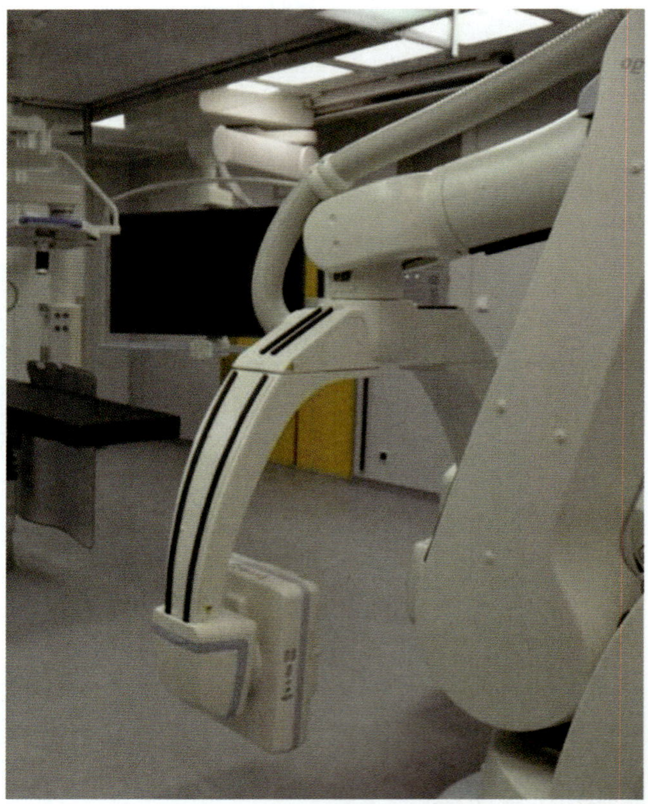

Fig 5.3.6-3 Hybrid operation room with a navigation system and a 3-D C-arm device mounted on a robotic arm (Artis Zeego, Siemens, Germany).

Mobile 3-D C-arms currently provide a maximum field of view that does not allow the complete craniofacial skeleton to be visualized in one rotation. Different manufacturers have specified different visible 3-D volumes. Siemens specifies a visible volume of 12 cm x 12 cm x 12 cm for its Arcadis Orbic 3-D (**Fig 5.3.6-2b**) and the use of a 9-inch x-ray amplifier tube. Ziehm, in contrast, specifies a visible volume of 512^3 voxels for its Vario (FD) 3-D (**Fig 5.3.6-2a**) and the use of a flat-panel detector. It does not, however, provide any further definition of the voxel size in the product specification. In the product specification for its Pulsera 3-D unit, Philips only mentions that the unit can be purchased with either a 9-inch or a 12-inch image intensifier. The authors have so far used the first two devices. In clinical practice, both devices provide more or less similar image volumes so that today mobile 3-D C-arms can be assumed to achieve 3-D image volumes of approximately ± 12 cm x 12 cm x 12 cm, which means that it is normally hardly possible to cover the complete craniofacial skeleton in one rotation.

Some authors have regarded this limited image volume as a disadvantage in the reconstruction of the craniofacial skeleton [Hanken et al, 2013; Heiland et al, 2005; Pohlenz et al, 2009], as it hinders or prevents comparisons between the affected and unaffected sides. This is only partially true because suitable software allows the data set generated intraoperatively by the 3-D C-arm to be easily merged with the preoperative diagnostic CT data set. Accordingly, the affected and unaffected sides can be compared fully [Wilde et al, 2013]. The outcome of surgery can at the same time be compared with preoperative imaging.

Furthermore, intraoperative image quality is normally sufficient, thus further postoperative CT scans are no longer necessary. The DICOM export functionality of the 3-D C-arms, which is required and normally available, enables data to be stored fully and the requirements regarding long-term documentation to be met, for example, in the PACS of the medical center. We can therefore assume that the use of a mobile 3-D C-arm may become the standard procedure for intraoperative imaging in craniofacial skeleton reconstruction.

In tumor resections of the skull base followed by primary reconstruction, the most desirable option for intraoperative 3-D imaging of the craniofacial skeleton including the orbit is a hybrid operating room with a fixed 3-D C-arm (eg, mounted on a robotic arm). Therefore, the authors use these devices in all surgeries that benefit from the combination of soft-tissue display and bony windowing, which cannot be achieved with intraoperative MRI alone. Strictly soft-tissue imaging in tumor resections still indicates the use of intraoperative MRI (**Fig 5.3.6-4**).

We therefore recommend for specialized centers the combination of mobile 3-D C-arms, floor or roof mounted intraoperative CBCT and intraoperative MRI to achieve best intraoperative imaging modalities to cover the full scope of CMF surgery.

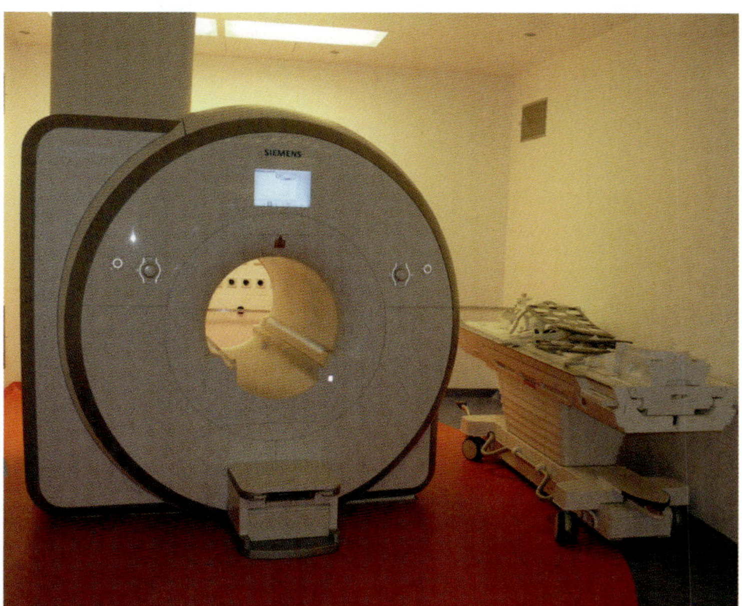

Fig 5.3.6-4 Hybrid operation room (Brainsuite, BrainLAB) with an intraoperative MRI (3 Tesla).

5 Case examples

5.1 Fracture of the zygomaticomaxillary complex

Fractures of the zygomaticomaxillary complex are often accompanied by displaced fractures of the orbital walls (**Fig 5.3.6-5a–b**). In such cases the question is what level of dislocation of the orbital walls needs surgical revision and reconstruction in addition to a repositioning of the zygomaticomaxillary fracture. Such a revision may mean an additional surgical access in the area of the lower eyelid and consequently an increase in morbidity. Following the repositioning of the zygoma, particularly when a closed reduction or purely transoral reduction technique is used, the question is whether the repositioning of the zygoma has also resulted in sufficient reduction of the orbital floor or whether additional orbital reconstruction is required. The answer can be found quickly and easily by means of intraoperative 3-D imaging (**Fig 5.3.6-5c–d**). It helps to avoid unnecessary exploration and reconstruction of the orbit.

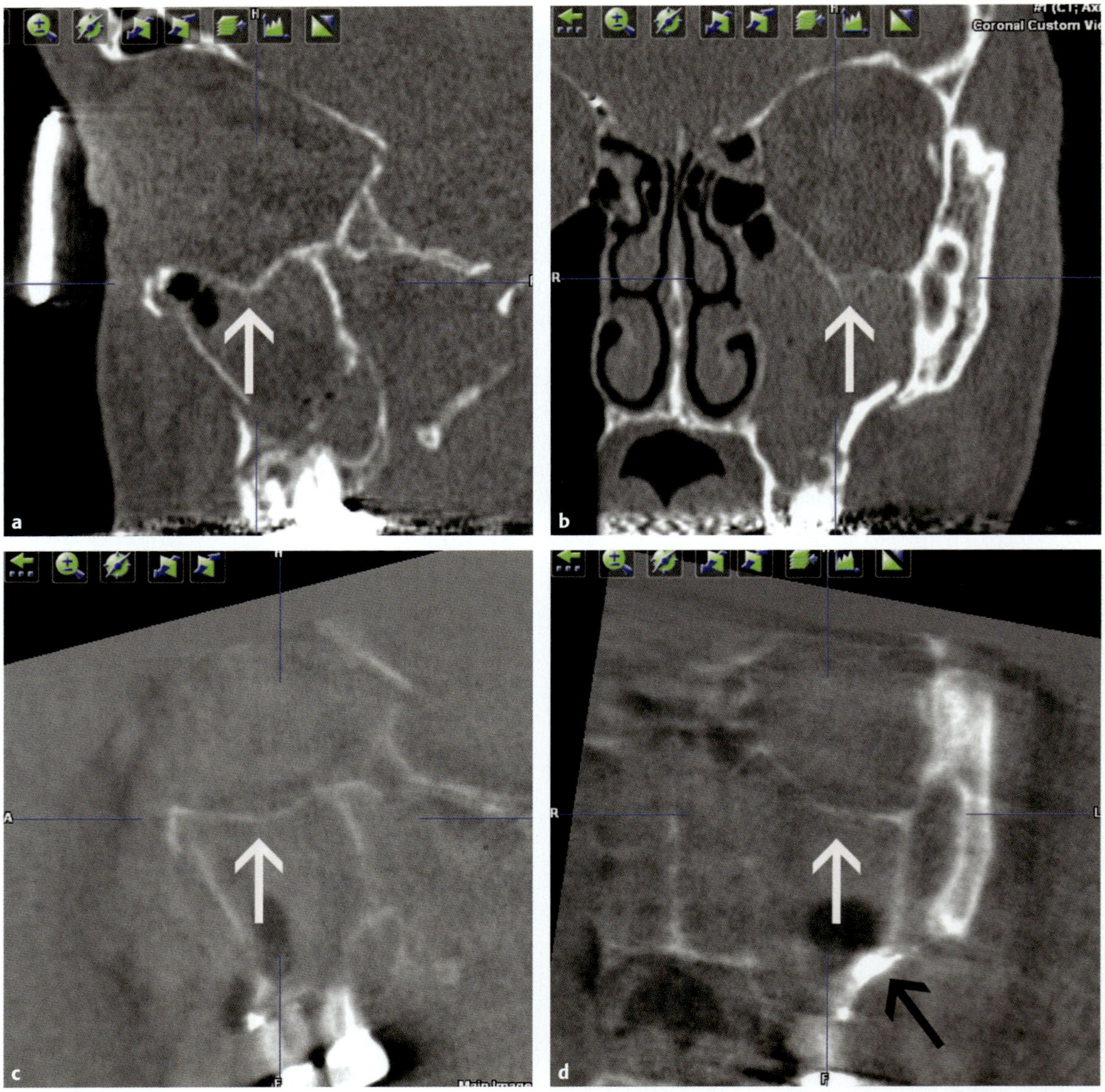

Fig 5.3.6-5a–d Fusion of preoperative computed tomography with intraoperative scan by a mobile 3-D C-arm device after the reduction of the zygoma. Left: Sagittal (**a**) und coronal (**b**) views of preoperative computed tomography with a dislocated fracture of the orbital floor (white arrows). Right: Sagittal (**c**) and coronal (**d**) views of intraoperative imaging following zygoma reduction and osteosynthesis on the zygomatic buttress (black arrow), with the orbital floor now in the anatomically correct position (white arrows), indicating closed reduction of the orbital floor fracture and therefore no need for orbital reconstruction.

5.2 Isolated fractures of orbital walls

Patients with isolated fractures of the orbital walls (medial wall and/or orbital floor) should receive primary care within the first 2 weeks after swelling has gone down [Schramm et al, 2010; Burnstine, 2003]. Limited intraoperative visibility is particularly a frequent reason for incorrect positioning of reconstruction materials in the treatment of orbital wall fractures, especially when the transition zone between the orbital floor and medial wall is involved or in case of an avulsion fracture of the orbital floor. The transition zone between the orbital floor and medial wall is often reconstructed at an excessively acute angle or the posterior part of the orbital floor is reconstructed too deeply. Both mistakes result in an insufficient correction of the bony orbit and may lead to persistent eyeball malposition. Due to concomitant soft-tissue changes and central adjustments, anatomically correct primary reconstruction has clear advantages over secondary correction. Intraoperative visualization is helpful to avoid incorrect positioning and to reduce the number of secondary reconstructions. Alloplastic materials, such as titanium mesh, are today preferred over autogenous bone grafts due to the increased predictability of the result which they offer through anatomically correct shaping. In addition, the need for bone harvest and its associated morbidity as well as the incalculable resorption of bone grafts are avoided.

The first step of virtual reconstruction planning is done by automatically segmenting the CT data set into anatomical and surgical units for complex orbital wall fractures in particular (**Fig 5.3.6-6a**). A virtual model for orbital reconstruction can subsequently be created either by free-forming

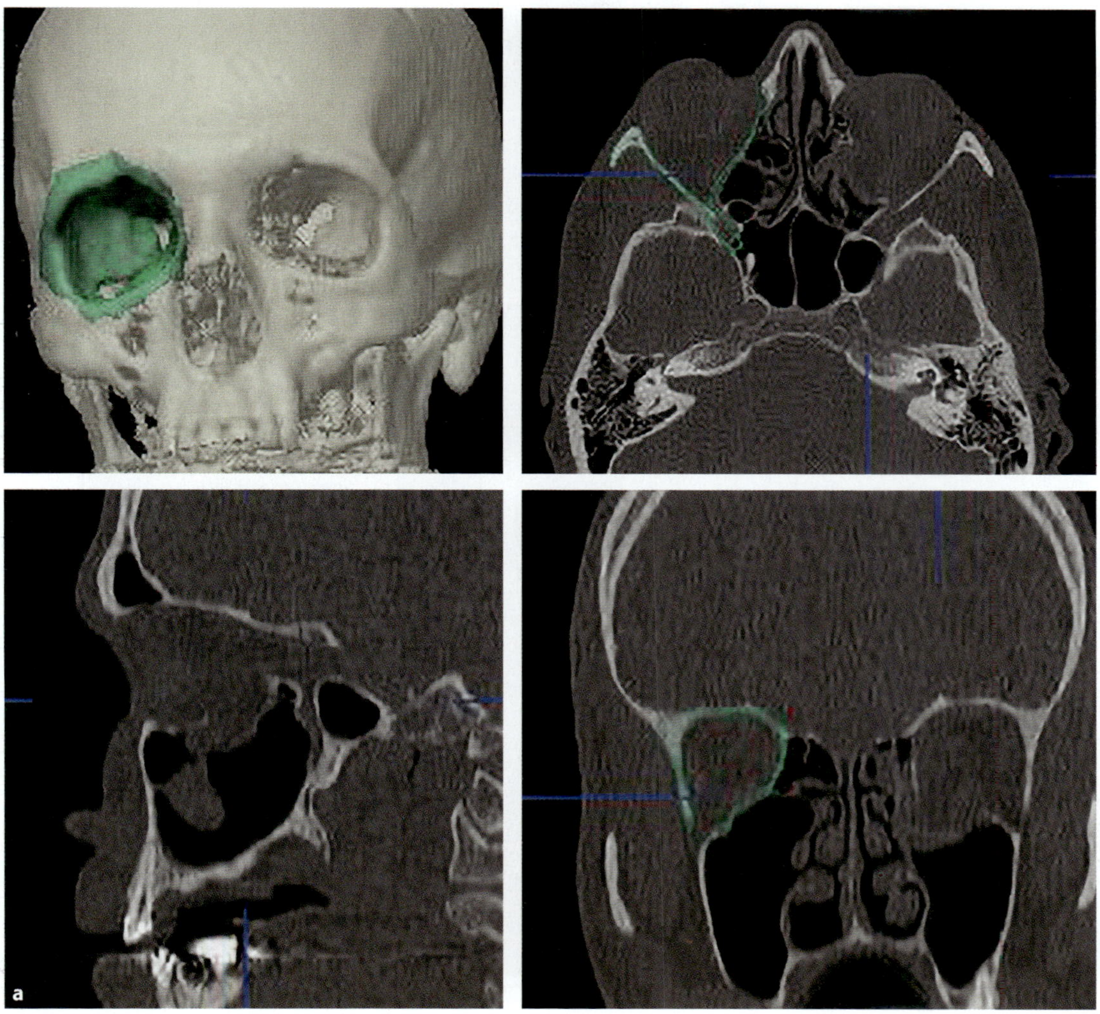

Fig 5.3.6-6a–d
Computer-assisted primary reconstruction of the left orbit using an anatomically preformed implant.
a Multiplanar view of the virtual planning and preparation of a template for orbital wall reconstruction by means of automatic segmentation of the unaffected right orbit (green contour lines).

segments (bilateral fractures) or mirroring the unaffected opposite side (unilateral fractures), the segmentation subsequently being aligned (**Fig 5.3.6-6b**). Anatomical preformed titanium implants can be inserted virtually before surgery to choose size and position (**Fig 5.3.6-6b**). The positions of bony fragments following repositioning as well as inserted titanium mesh and/or bone grafts in the orbit can then be controlled by means of intraoperative navigation (see above).

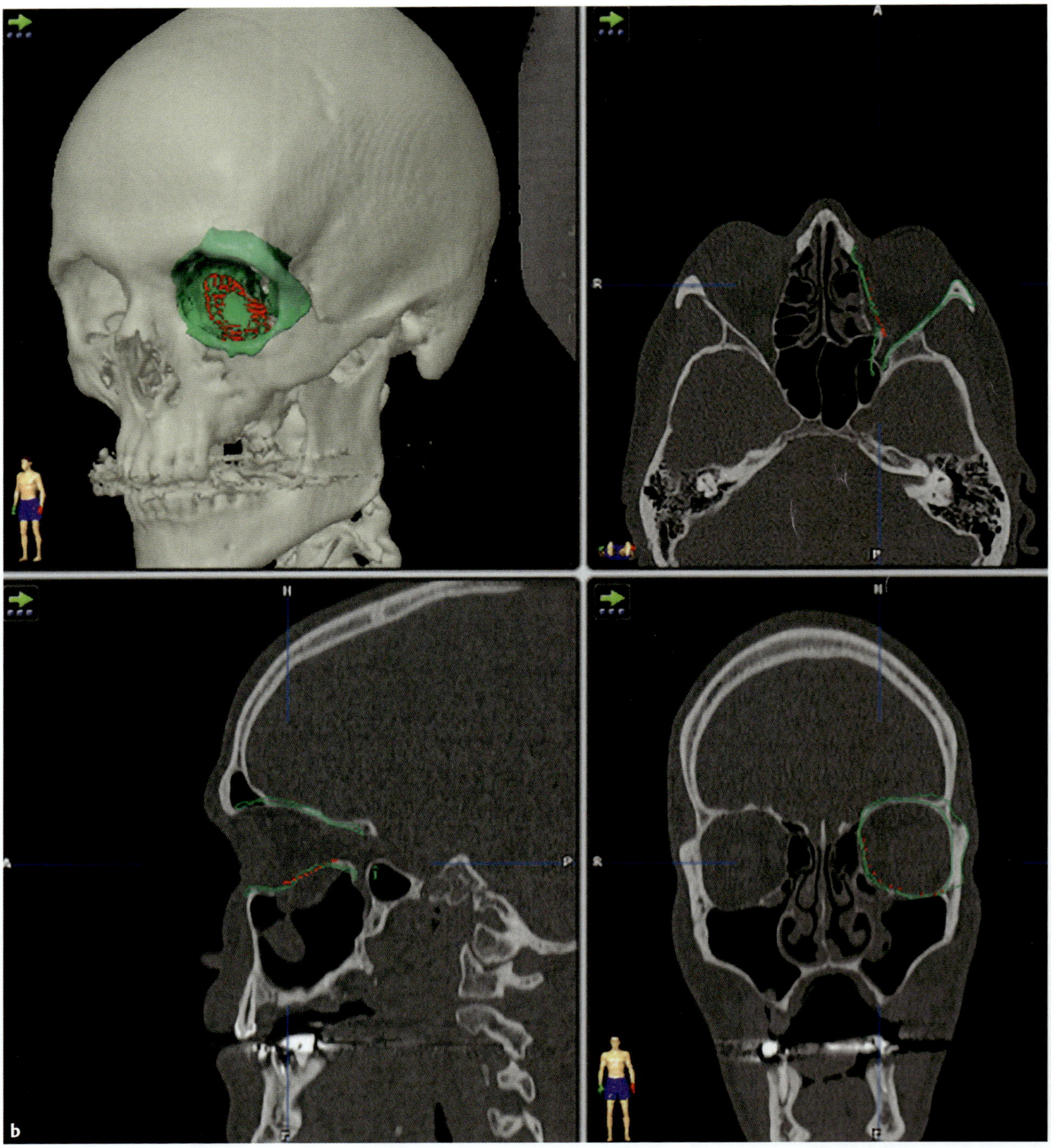

Fig 5.3.6-6a–d (cont) Computer-assisted primary reconstruction of the left orbit using an anatomically preformed implant.

b Multiplanar view of the virtual reconstruction of the left orbit by means of mirroring the segmentation of the intact contralateral side (green contour lines) and virtual insertion of an anatomically preformed orbital implant (red contour lines). The virtual insertion of the anatomically preformed titanium implant allows the fit to be validated and size of the orbital implant to be selected.

The navigation pointer tip is placed on the inserted titanium mesh or the repositioned bone. The position of the pointer tip in relation to the virtual reconstruction template indicates the current position of the navigated structure (**Fig 5.3.6-6c**). This allows control of the repositioned bones as well as position and fit of the inserted implants and may lead to necessary modifications. If anatomical preformed or conventional implants are used, the implants can be tracked intraoperatively by fixing a dynamic reference array to them. The procedure is rounded off by intraoperative 3-D imaging being carried out for final validation purposes. The outcome of the reconstruction can be validated exactly even with a small intraoperative field of views by fusing the preoperative data and preoperative simulation (**Fig 5.3.6-6d**). Because of this, even extensive reconstruction of an orbital floor and medial orbital wall that previously required coronal incision can be performed by means of an exclusively transconjunctival approach, with no visible scars being left due to the combined use of preformed implants, intraoperative navigation, and intraoperative imaging.

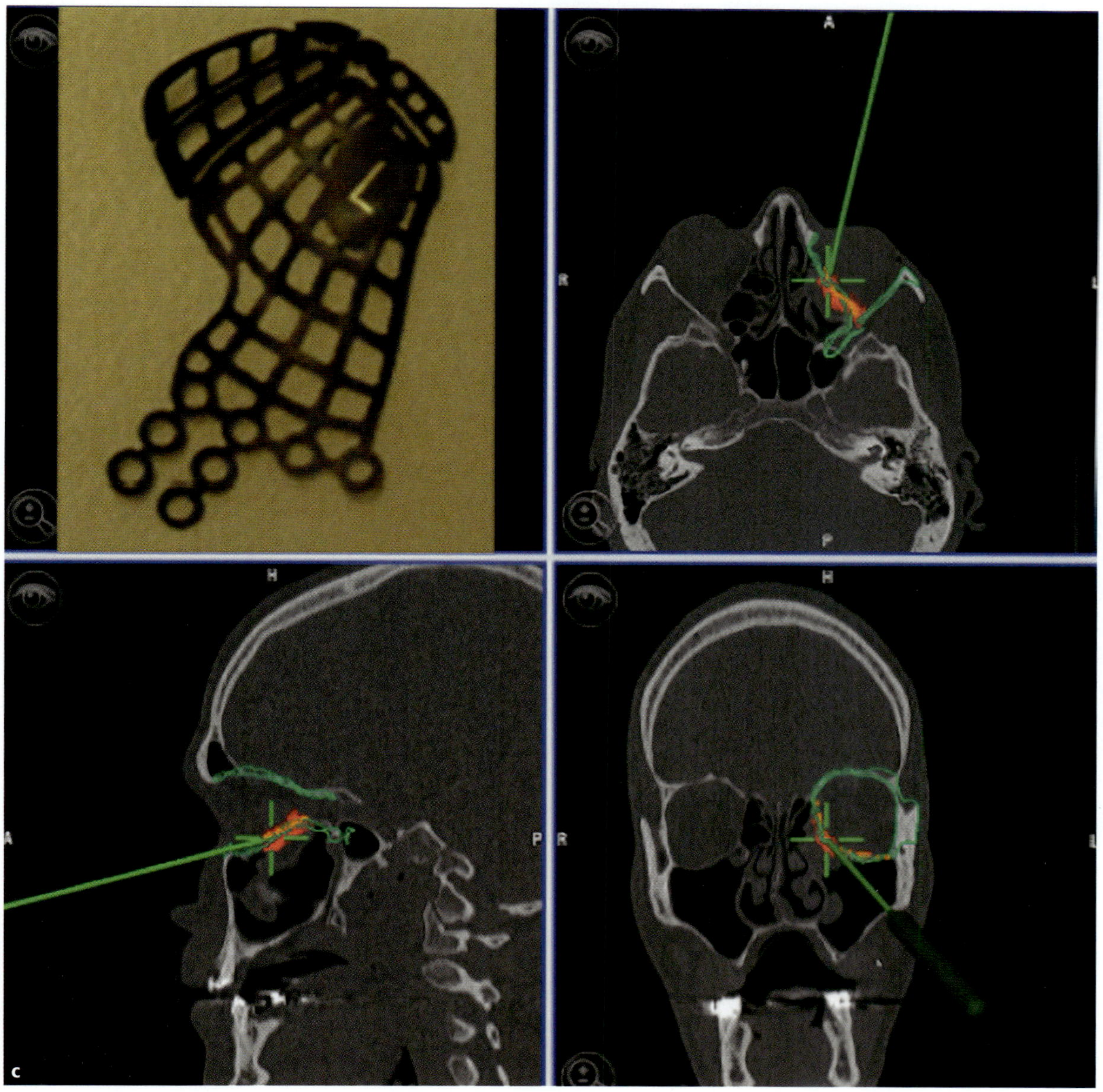

Fig 5.3.6-6a–d (cont) Computer-assisted primary reconstruction of the left orbit using an anatomically preformed implant.

c Multiplanar view of the navigation-assisted positioning of an anatomically preformed orbital implant (**c**: top left). The green contour line shows the virtual template of the planned reconstruction (analogous to the green contour line in **b**). The red contour line represents the surface of the orbital implant inserted on the basis of the navigation pointer tracking the implant surface. The orange contour line intraoperatively shows the virtually planned position of the orbital implant on the screen of the navigation system (analogous to the red contour line in **b**).

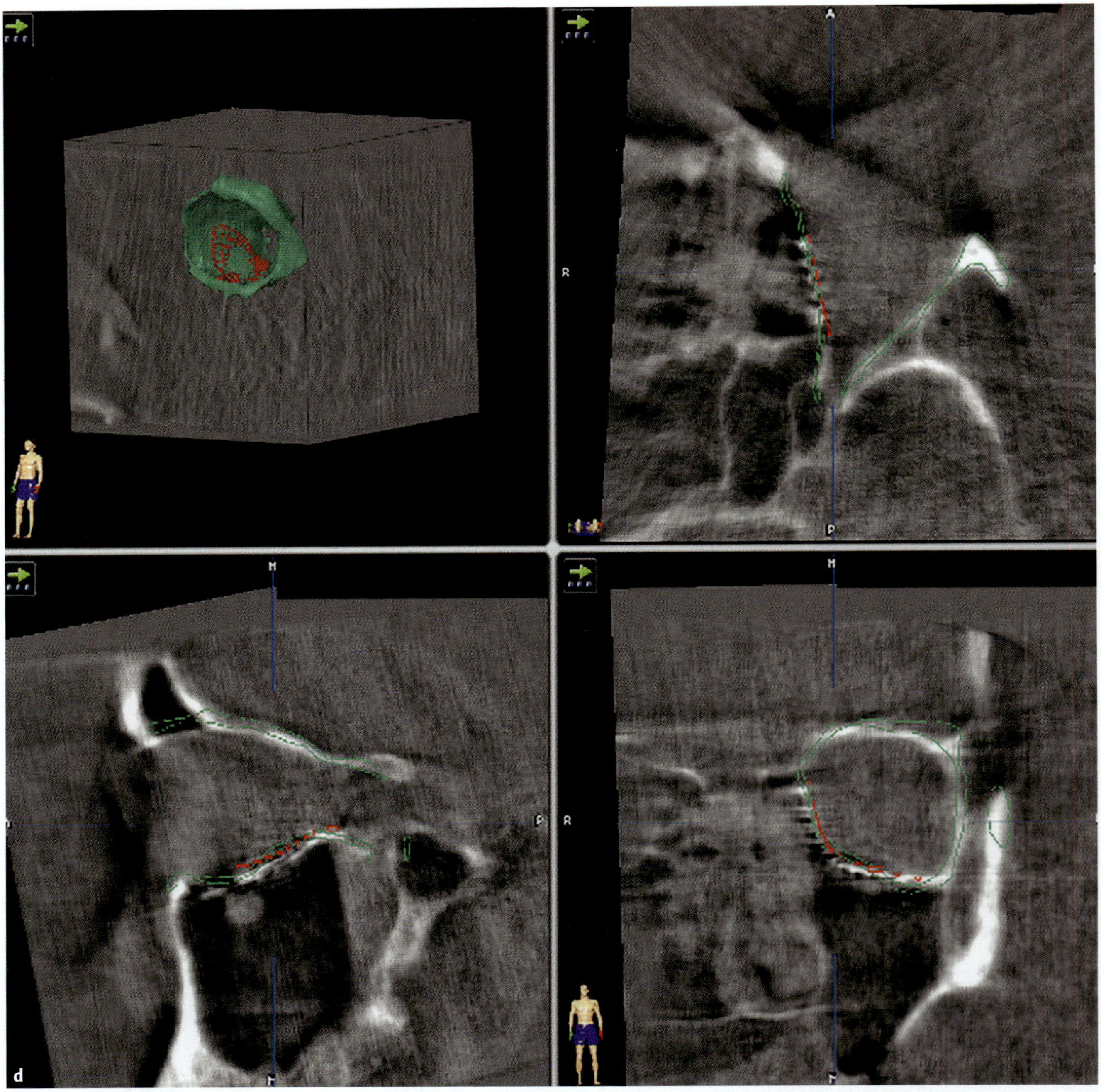

Fig 5.3.6-6a–d (cont) Computer-assisted primary reconstruction of the left orbit using an anatomically preformed implant.

d Multiplanar view of the intraoperative 3-D imaging and superimposition of the virtual planning. The green contour line represents the virtual template (analogous to **b** and **c**) and the red contour line the virtual inserted orbital implant (analogous to **b**). The inserted implant shows a good alignment to the virtual planning.

5.3 Secondary reconstruction of the orbit and midface

Secondary reconstruction is difficult due to soft-tissue atrophy and scarring. The complex anatomical conditions in the orbital and periorbital regions make functional and esthetic reconstruction with autogenous bone grafts a challenging task [Schramm et al, 2010; Gellrich et al, 1999]. Reconstruction using alloplastic material tends to be much easier. Those materials can be combined with autogenous bone grafts (calvaria) as well as soft- and hard-tissue flaps with microvascular anastomosis, if necessary. Computer-assisted simulation and planning (**Fig 5.3.6-7a–c**) allows osseous reconstruction to be planned virtually in detail, the result can

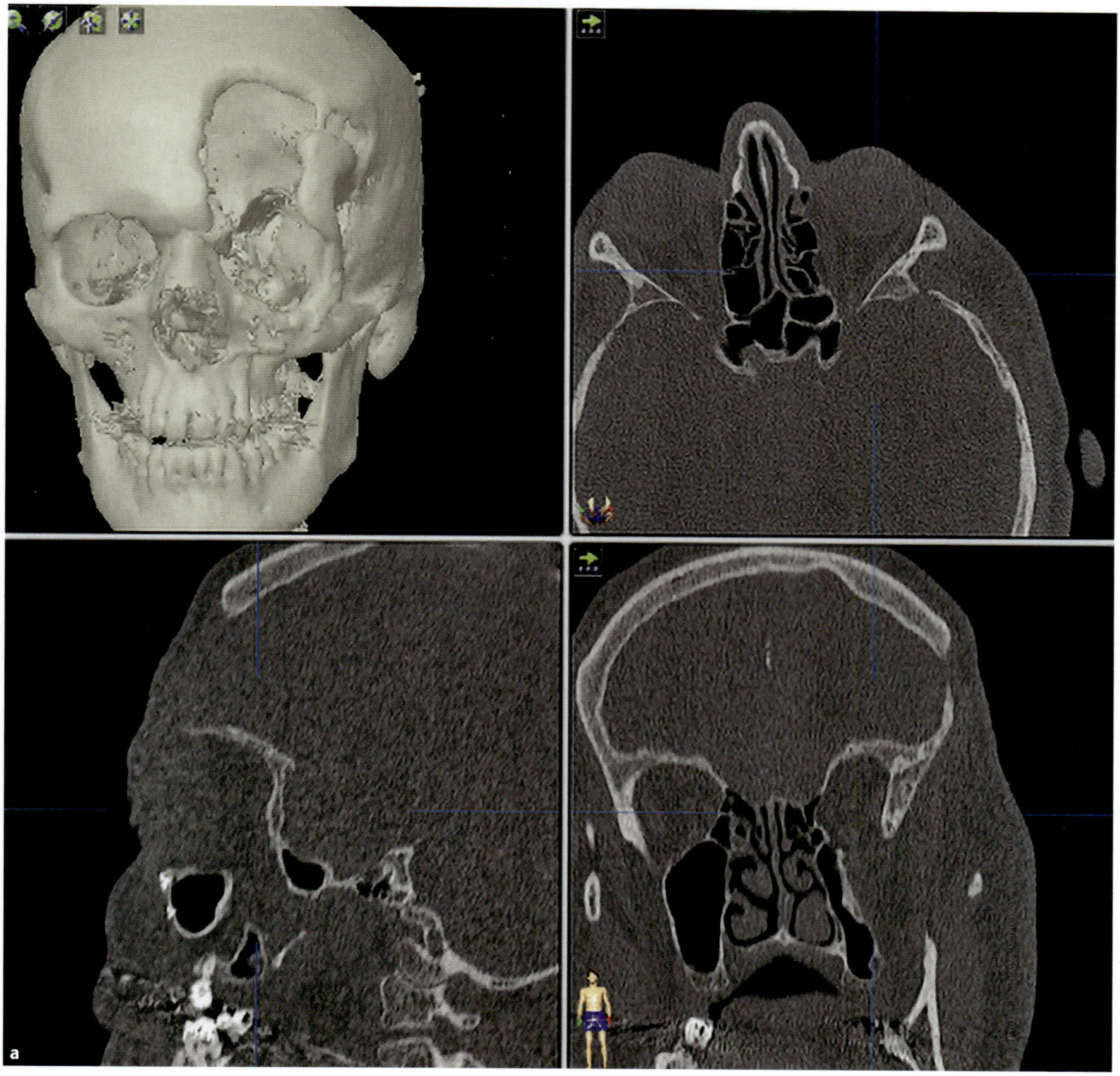

Fig 5.3.6-7a–i Computer-assisted secondary reconstruction of the midface and frontal bone.

a Multiplanar view of an insufficiently treated left-side comminuted midface fracture and secondary trepanation of the skull following a brain abscess.

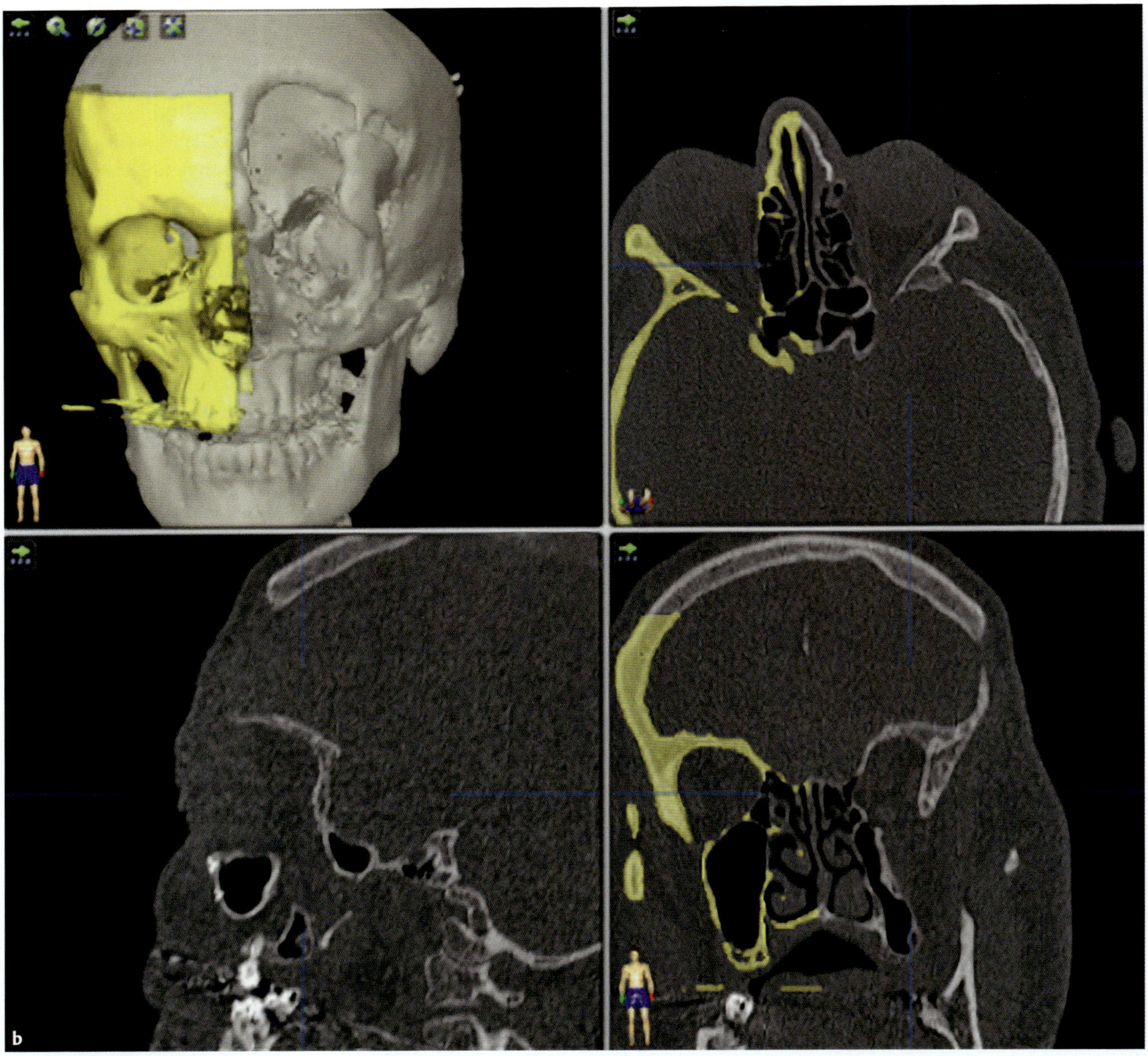

Fig 5.3.6-7a–i (cont) Computer-assisted secondary reconstruction of the midface and frontal bone.
b Multiplanar view of the virtual planning and preparation of the template for midface reconstruction by means of a segmentation of the unaffected right side (yellow contour lines).

be exported in the form of so-called STL files. Through rapid prototyping it is possible to quickly generate accurate and cost-effective patient-specific 3-D models from STL files (**Fig 5.3.6-7d**) [Cohen et al, 2009]. These models allow patient-specific titanium plates and mesh structures to be preformed preoperatively (**Fig 5.3.6-7d**). Alternatively or additionally (like in the presented case), these patient-specific implants can be manufactured industrially (eg, polyetheretherketone or titanium) (**Fig 5.3.6-7e**). Preoperatively preformed implants can be positioned intraoperatively using pointer-assisted navigation (**Fig 5.3.6-7f–g**) and subsequently validated using intraoperative 3-D imaging (**Fig 5.3.6-7h–i**).

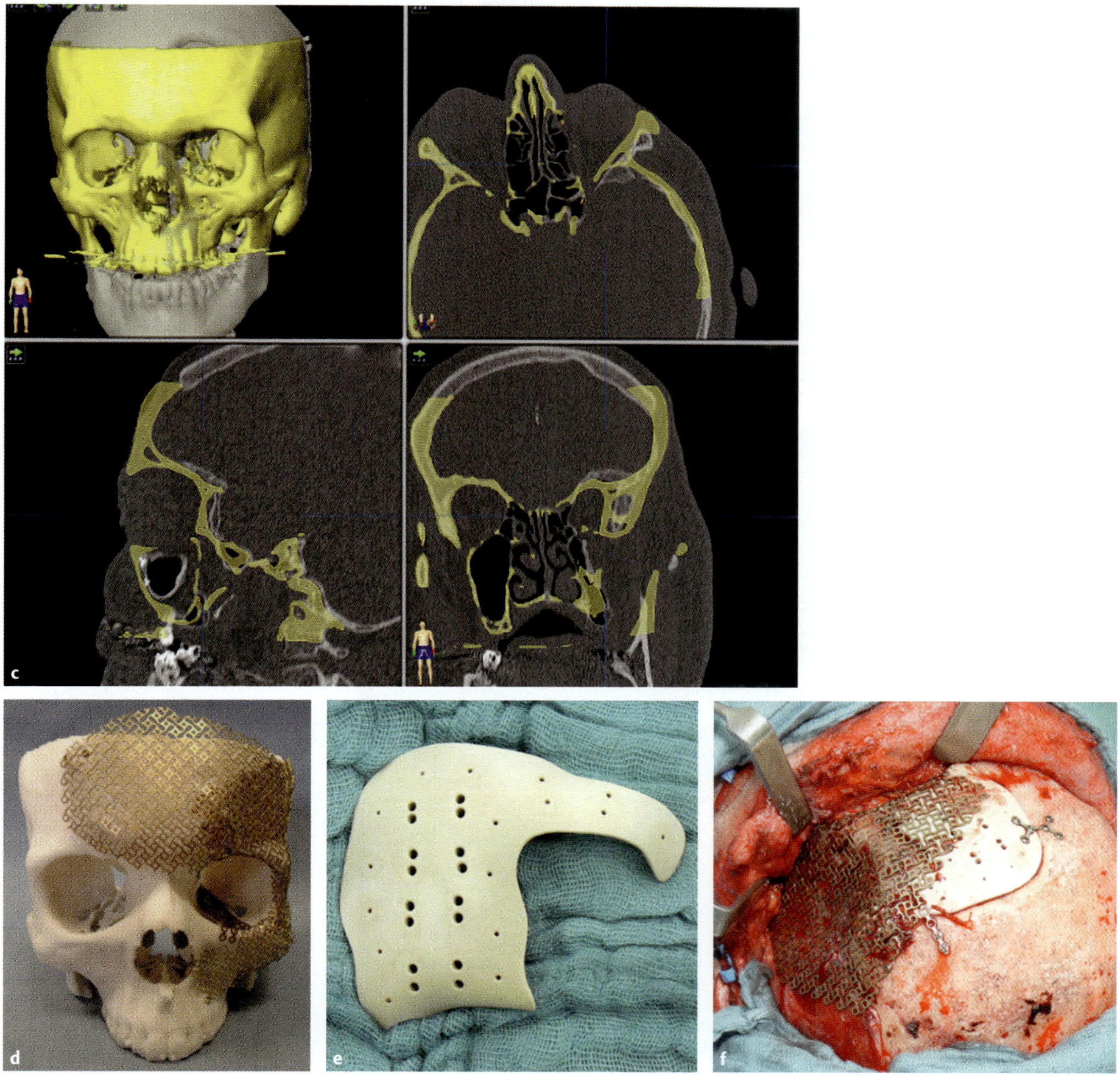

Fig 5.3.6-7a–i (cont) Computer-assisted secondary reconstruction of the midface and frontal bone.

- **c** Multiplanar view of a virtual reconstruction by means of the mirroring of the segmentation of the intact contralateral side (yellow contour lines).
- **d** Conversion of the virtual reconstruction into a STL file that can be printed by a 3-D printer. The 3-D model serves as a template for preforming patient-specific implants.
- **e** Industrially manufactured patient-specific polyetheretherketone implant for reconstructing the calvarial defect.
- **f** Intraoperative view after insertion and fixation of the patient-specific implant following a re-osteotomy of the left zygomatic complex.

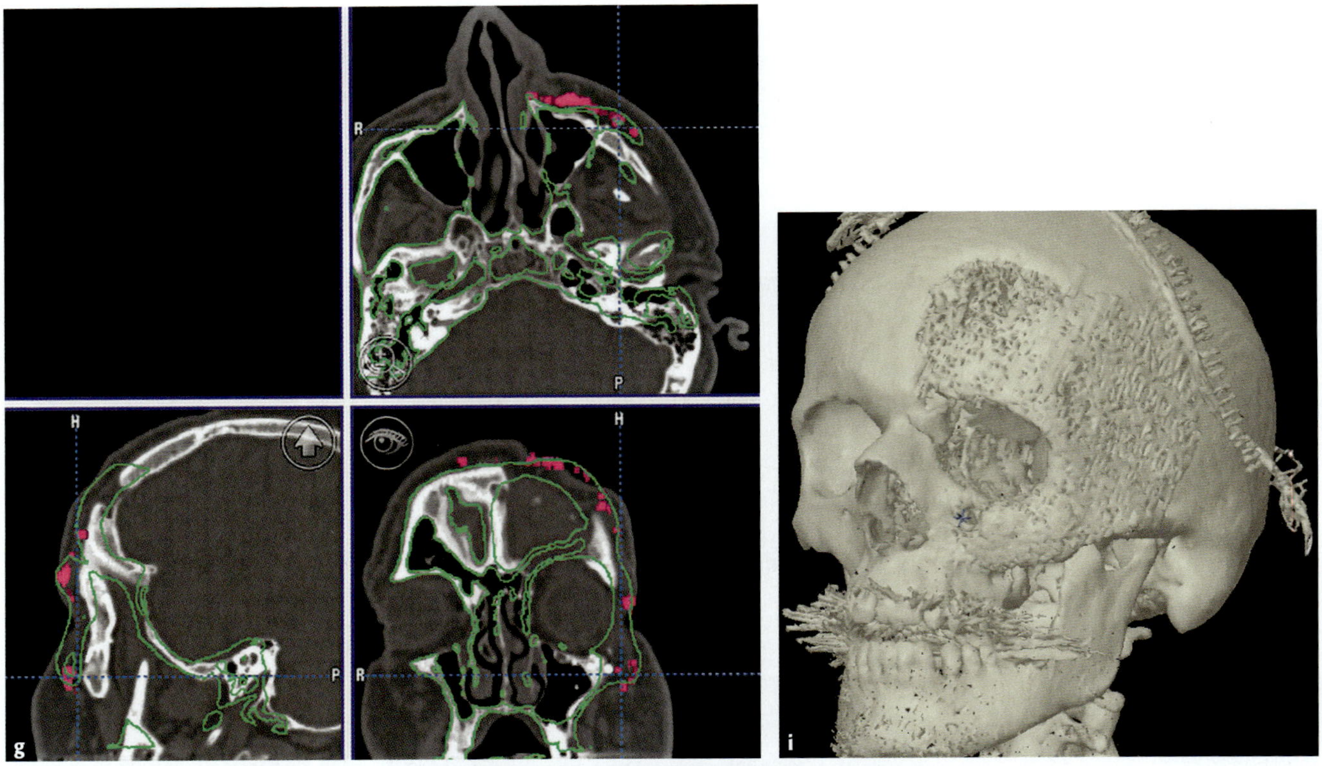

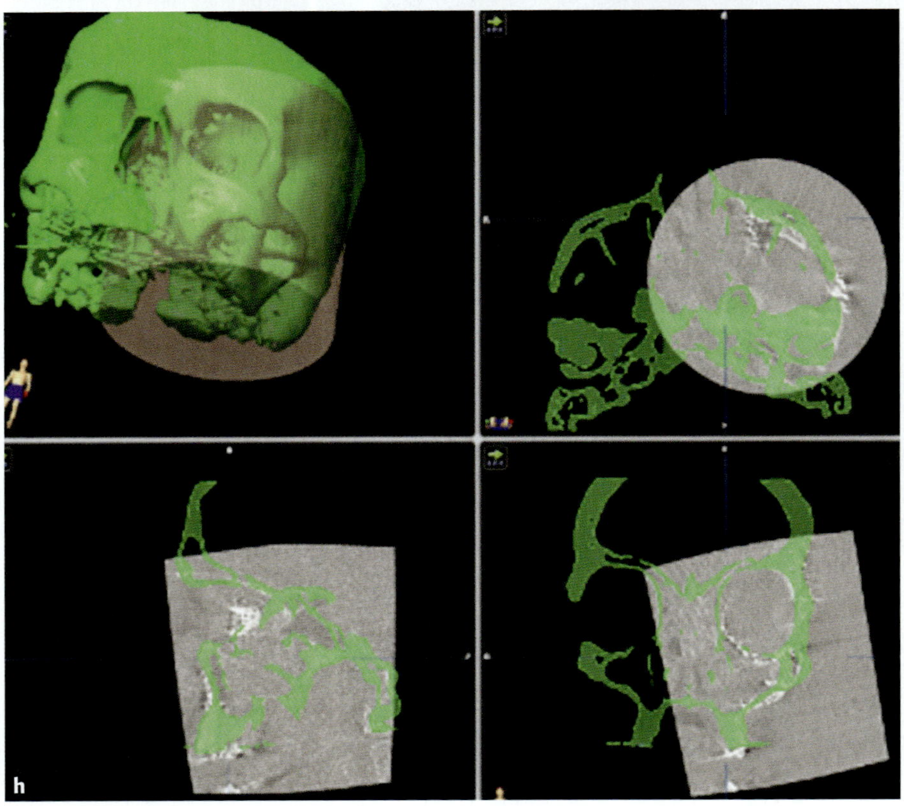

Fig 5.3.6-7a–i (cont) Computer-assisted secondary reconstruction of the midface and frontal bone.

- **g** Multiplanar view of the intraoperative navigation to control the reduction and position of the inserted titanium implants. The pink contour lines represent the surface of the inserted implants. The green contour line shows the preoperatively planned virtual template for the envisaged reconstruction.
- **h** Multiplanar view of intraoperative 3-D imaging and superimposition of virtual planning (green contour). The reconstruction shows alignment to the virtual template.
- **i** A 3-D reconstruction view of postoperative computed tomography.

6 Summary

Today, intraoperative 3-D imaging using 3-D C-arm devices is an important element in the workflow of computer-assisted surgery of the craniofacial skeleton. It helps to avoid malpositioning of bone fragments and/or inserted implants. This is an outstanding advance in the assurance of the quality of such complex operations. If performed correctly, it reduces the number of secondary interventions, reduces morbidity as well as operation time by avoiding unnecessary orbital reconstructions in midface fracture repair.

7 References and suggested reading

Badjate SJ, Cariappa KM. C-arm for accurate reduction of zygomatic arch fracture—a case report. *Br Dent J.* 2005;199:275–277.

Bonatti J, Vassiliades T, Nifong W, et al. How to build a cath-lab operating room. *Heart Surg Forum.* 2007;10(4):E344–E348.

Burnstine MA. Clinical recommendations for repair of orbital facial fractures. *Curr Opin Ophthalmol.* 2003 Oct;14(5):236–240.

Chau AC, Fung K. Comparison of radiation dose for implant imaging using conventional spiral tomography, computed tomography, and cone beam computed tomography. *Oral Surg Oral Med Oral Pathol Oral Radiol Endod.* 2009 Apr;107(4):559–565.

Cohen A, Laviv A, Berman P, et al. Mandibular reconstruction using stereolithographic 3-dimensional printing modeling technology. *Oral Surg Oral Med Oral Pathol Oral Radiol Endod.* 2009 Nov;108(5):661–666.

Friedrich RE, Heiland M, Bartel-Friedrich S. Potentials of ultrasound in the diagnosis of midfacial fractures. *Clin Oral Investig.* 2003 Dec;7(4):226–229.

Gebhard F, Riepl C, Richter P, et al. [The hybrid operating room. Home of high-end intraoperative imaging]. *Unfallchirurg.* 2012 Feb;115(2):107–120. German.

Gellrich NC, Schramm A, Hammer B, et al. The value of computer aided planning and intraoperative navigation in orbital reconstruction. *Int J Oral Maxillofac Surg.* 1999;28:52–53.

Hanken H, Christian L, Assaf A T, et al. Intraoperative Bildgebung in der Mund-, Kiefer- und Gesichtschirurgie. Intraoperative Imaging of the Facial Skeleton. OP-JOURNAL 2013;29:130–135. Available at: https://www.thieme-connect.com/products/ejournals/html/10.1055/s-0033-1350665. Accessed May 15, 2014. German.

Heiland M, Schulze D, Blake F, et al. Intraoperative imaging of zygomaticomaxillary complex fractures using a 3D C-arm system. *Int J Oral Maxillofac Surg.* 2005 Jun:34(4):369–375.

Heiland M, Schmelzle R, Hebecker A, et al. Intraoperative 3D imaging of the facial skeleton using the SIREMOBIL Iso-C3D. *Dentomaxillofac Radiol.* 2004 Mar;33(2):130–132.

Klatt JC, Heiland M, Blessmann M, et al. Clinical indication for intraoperative 3D imaging during open reduction of fractures of the neck and head of the mandibular condyle. *J Craniomaxillofac Surg.* 2011;39(4):244–248.

Loubele M, Bogaerts R, Van Dijck E, et al. Comparison between effective radiation dose of CBCT and MSCT scanners for dentomaxillofacial applications. *Eur J Radiol.* 2009 Sep;71(3):461–468.

Ludlow JB, Ivanovic M. Comparative dosimetry of dental CBCT devices and 64-slice CT for oral and maxillofacial radiology. *Oral Surg Oral Med Oral Pathol Oral Radiol Endod.* 2008 Jul;106(1):106–114.

Metzger MC, Schön R, Weyer N, et al. Anatomical 3-dimensional pre-bent titanium implant for orbital floor fractures. *Ophthalmology.* 2006 Oct;113(10):1863–1868.

Pohlenz, P, Blake F, Blessmann M, et al. Intraoperative cone beam computed tomography in oral and maxillofacial surgery using a C-arm prototype: first clinical experiences after treatment of zygomaticomaxillary complex fractures. *J Oral Maxillofac Surg.* 2009 Mar;67(3):515–521.

Rock C, Linsenmaier U, Brandl R, et al. [Introduction of a new mobile C-arm/CT combination equipment (ISO-C-3D). Initial results of 3-D sectional imaging]. *Unfallchirurg.* 2001 Sep;104(9):827–833. German.

Schramm A, Gellrich NC. Intraoperative Navigation und computerassistierte Chirurgie. In: Schwenzer N, Ehrenfeld M, eds. *Zahn-Mund-Kieferheilkunde, Mund-Kiefer-Gesichtschirurgie.* Stuttgart: Thieme; 2010:479–499. German.

Schramm A, Gellrich NC, Schmelzeisen R. *Navigational Surgery of the Facial Skeleton.* Berlin Heidelberg New York: Springer; 2007.

Schulze D, Heiland M, Thurmann H, et al. Radiation exposure during midfacial imaging using 4- and 16-slice computed tomography, cone beam computed tomography systems and conventional radiography. *Dentomaxillofac Radiol.* 2004 Mar;33(2):83–86.

Stieve M, Issing PR, Mack KF, et al. [Indications of intraoperative ultrasound in head and neck surgery]. *Laryngorhinootologie.* 2012 Jul;91(7):422–426. German.

Wilde F, Lorenz K, Ebner AK, et al. Intraoperative imaging with a 3D C-arm system after zygomatico-orbital complex fracture reduction. *J Oral Maxillofac Surg.* 2013 May;71(5):894–910.

5.3.7 Surgically preformed implants: nonpatient specific

Nils-Claudius Gellrich, Majeed Rana

1 Introduction

Several biomaterials for implants used in reconstruction of the craniofacial skeleton exist. Manson et al [1987], Hammer et al [1999], and Gruss [1986] reported the necessity to use moldable, contourable, and stable material and they initially favored autogenous bone. However, advanced technical skills are necessary to use bone grafts in such a way that contours can be reestablished, according to the functional and esthetic needs (**Fig 5.3.7-1**).

A biological problem associated with the use of bone grafts is secondary loss of volume because of resorption. Alloplastic materials have been developed to overcome these issues but have more late complications of infection and metal reactions (orbital adherence syndromes).

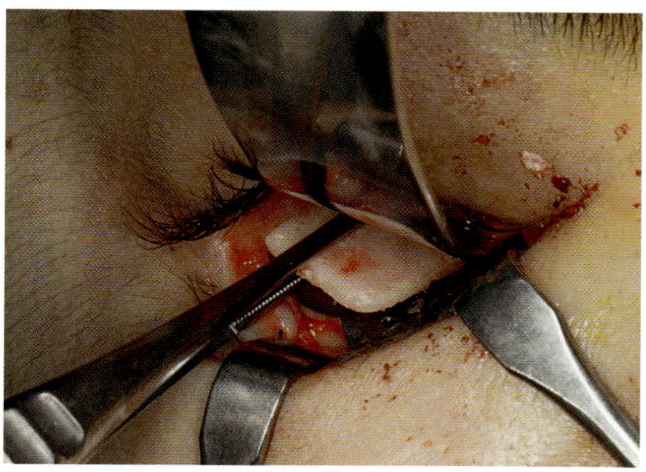

Fig 5.3.7-1 A calvarial split graft is positioned over a 3-D titanium mesh for augmentation and to reduce intraorbital volume.

The orbit and the occlusion are anatomical regions/entities which are challenging when inaccurate reconstruction has been performed. In the orbit. radiopaque reconstruction biomaterials are visible in a postoperative computed tomographic (CT) scan wich is helpful to assess the reason for inadequate operative results.

Today preformed alloplastic implants can be efficiently created if digital modeling and/or manufacturing is used. Manual preformation can be applied easily if appropriate individual patient models have been manufactured before reconstruction. They allow preoperative or intraoperative implant preformation, utilizing adaptable or moldable biomaterials.

2 Technical notes

Early reports [Sugar et al, 1992; Schubert et al, 2002] on the use of titanium mesh (**Fig 5.3.7-2**) have encouraged the authors to use it widely for craniofacial reconstruction. The advent of biomodels has allowed to contour those 2-D meshes to the 3-D anatomy of the patient (**Fig 5.3.7-3**).

The extent and shape of an orbital deformity are assessed by a preoperative high-resolution CT or cone beam scans. The volumetric information of a defect can be evaluated on a biomodel that in addition allows the surgeon to contour a titanium mesh appropriate for the intended reconstruction. Standard nonpreformed fan-plate orbital mesh-style plates serve as a basis to create a one-wall or two-wall individualized orbital implant (**Fig 5.3.7-2** and **Fig 5.3.7-4**).

These implants are available in different thicknesses, so that the appropriate implant can be selected according to the specific patient´s needs [Rana et al, 2015].

With this prebending process a patient-specific implant can be created. However, in combination with intraoperative navigation and/or imaging, the correct position of the implant should be validated. Even a perfectly preshaped implant can cause an adverse effect if the position is not correct. It may even endanger vital structures, such as the optic nerve. Especially for thinner and pliable implants, the surgeon must take into account that contour changes during the insertion or stabilization process are possible.

The implant should be secured with one or two screws in its final position. As a rule, a more complex anatomical reconstruction requires more screw fixation.

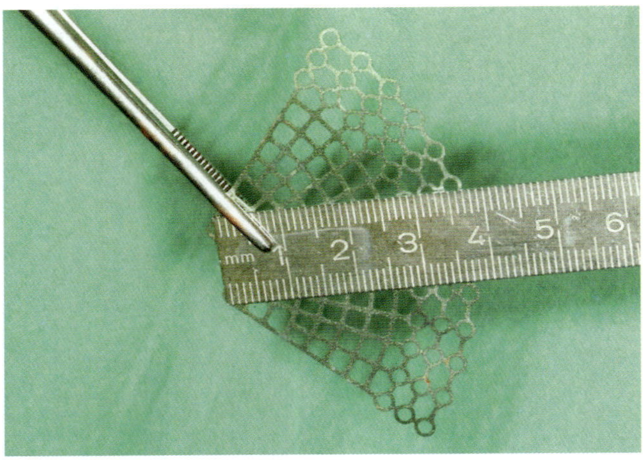

Fig 5.3.7-2 Nonpreformed orbital mesh, length 37 mm.

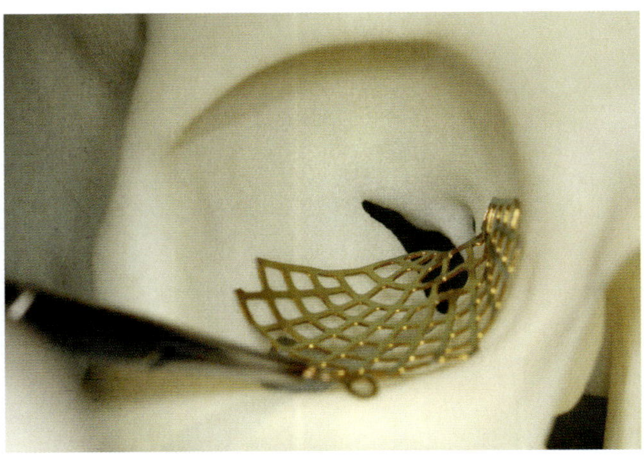

Fig 5.3.7-3 A nonpreformed mesh is molded on a skull model for reconstruction of the orbital floor and the medial orbital wall.

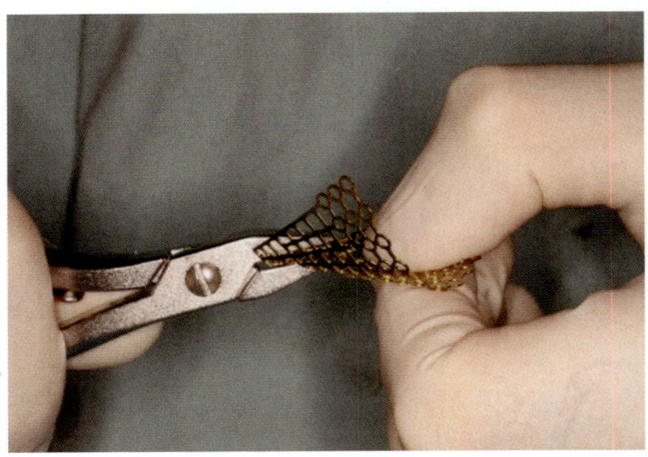

Fig 5.3.7-4 The procedure of bending a nonpreformed 3-D mesh.

3 References and suggested reading

Gruss JS. Complex nasoethmoid-orbital and midfacial fractures: role of craniofacial surgical techniques and immediate bone grafting. *Ann Plast Surg*. 1986 Nov;17(5):377–390.

Hammer B, Kunz C, Schramm A, et al. Repair of complex orbital fractures: technical problems, state-of-the-art solutions and future perspectives. *Ann Acad Med Singapore*. 1999 Sep;28(5):687–691.

Manson PN, Ruas EJ, Iliff NT. Deep orbital reconstruction for correction of post-traumatic enophthalmos. *Clin Plast Surg*. 1987 Jan;14(1):113–121.

Rana M, Gellrich MM, Gellrich NC. Customised reconstruction of the orbital wall and engineering of selective laser melting (SLM) core implants. *Br J Oral Maxillofac Surg*. 2015 Feb;53(2):208–209.

Schubert W, Gear AJ, Lee C, et al. Incorporation of titanium mesh in orbital and midface reconstruction. *Plast Reconstr Surg*. 2002 Sep 15;110(4):1022–1030; discussion 1031–1022.

Sugar AW, Kuriakose M, Walshaw ND. Titanium mesh in orbital wall reconstruction. *Int J Oral Maxillofac Surg*. 1992 Jun;21(3):140–144.

5.3.8 Industrially preformed orbital meshes

E Bradley Strong, Marc C Metzger

1 Introduction

Orbital fractures are common sequelae of facial trauma and result in disruption of the normal orbital architecture. The complex orbital geometry makes posttraumatic reconstruction extremely challenging, particularly in fractures that involve more than one wall [Steidler et al, 1980; Ellis et al, 1985]. Historically, bone grafts were often used for orbital reconstruction. In an effort to obtain a more accurate reconstruction and eliminate donor site morbidity, alloplastic materials, such as titanium, bioabsorbable polymers, and porous polyethylene, were subsequently introduced [Potter et al, 2004]. Implant preferences vary greatly among surgeons and there is still no "ideal" implant for orbital reconstruction. Such an ideal implant would be: (1) readily available; (2) biocompatible; (3) cheap; (4) malleable but strong enough to support the orbital contents and maintain its shape over time; (5) radiopaque so it can be visualized on radiographs; and (6) not resorb. Bioabsorbable implants appear to provide adequate support for smaller defects [Al-Sukhun et al, 2006]; however, they are not visible on computed tomography (CT) and there has been some concern about inflammatory reactions to the polymer [Uygur et al, 2009]. Porous polyethylene sheeting provides adequate support but is difficult to shape and is also radiolucent. Titanium mesh sheets fulfill most of the above-mentioned criteria. However, accurate free-hand bending of any implant can be challenging [Ellis et al, 2003]. One technique to optimize plate contour is the use of a sterilized skull model for intraoperative plate/mesh bending. These models may be generated from generic CT data sets or patient specific models using mirrored CT data from the uninjured contralateral eye [Gellrich et al, 2002; Holck et al, 1999; Perry et al, 1998]. While these techniques are promising, they are costly and time consuming.

2 Industrially preformed meshes

Attempts at free-hand reconstruction of complex orbital fractures are less accurate than preformed mesh [Strong et al, 2013]. Metzger et al [2006] described the use of preformed orbital mesh implants based on an amalgamation of 278 normal adult CT data sets. The data were ultimately used to fabricate preformed orbital mesh implants (**Fig 5.3.8-1**).

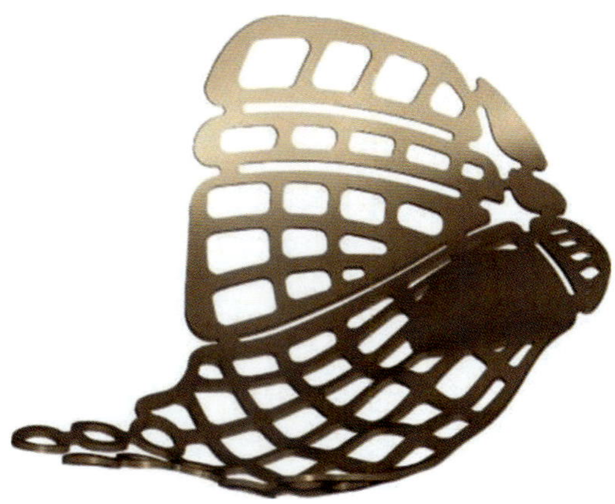

Fig 5.3.8-1 A preformed mesh implant for the left eye.

These preformed mesh implants are available in two sizes (small and large) for the left and right eye. The edges, particularly the posterior edge and medial edge of the implant, may be trimmed to optimize the implant to the fracture size. Unlike traditional mesh implants, the margins of the implant are smooth even after trimming (**Fig 5.3.8-2**).

Because these implants are preformed, shape modifications are not recommended. If this implant is used for small orbital floor defects, the implant must be trimmed so significantly that the added cost of using the preformed implant has to be questioned. In the authors' experience, these implants are most useful for two-wall defects that result in a large disruption of the posterior orbital floor and extend onto the lamina papyracea. These fractures can occasionally extend up to the skull base (**Fig 5.3.8-3**).

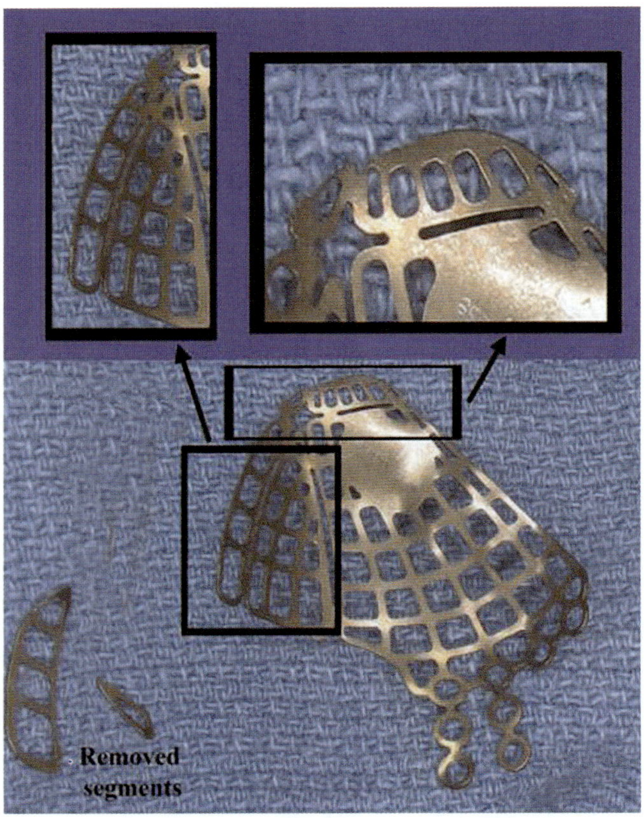

Fig 5.3.8-2 A preformed mesh implant after trimming of the distal flanges. The trimmed flanges are shown in the left inferior corner. Note the smooth border of the implant even after trimming.

3 Surgical technique

Preformed orbital mesh implants are commonly inserted through a transconjunctival incision for floor defects or a combined transconjunctival and transcaruncular approach for two-wall defects. A subciliary incision can also be used based on surgeon preference. The entire bony defect should be exposed and the bony margins visualized. Particular attention should be paid to visualization of the posterior shelf of the orbital floor and the superior margin of the lamina papyracea. The orbital contents are then reduced back within the orbital cavity as the implant is inserted. The implant can be grasped with a pair of forceps applied to the anterior edge. Normally the edge of the implant is inserted first. As the implant is inserted, lateral rotation allows the implant to slide beneath the orbital contents and up along the medial wall (**Fig 5.3.8-4**).

Once the implant is in the ideal position, the margins and orientation of the implant to the existing walls of the orbit are reevaluated. Pitfalls of implant placement may include: (1) the implant is not resting on the bony posterior ledge of the orbital floor and deviates into the maxillary sinus, or (2) the superomedial edge of the implant is placed laterally (not resting on the lamina papyracea) so that the orbital contents prolapse over the superior edge of the implant and become trapped between the lamina papyracea and the mesh.

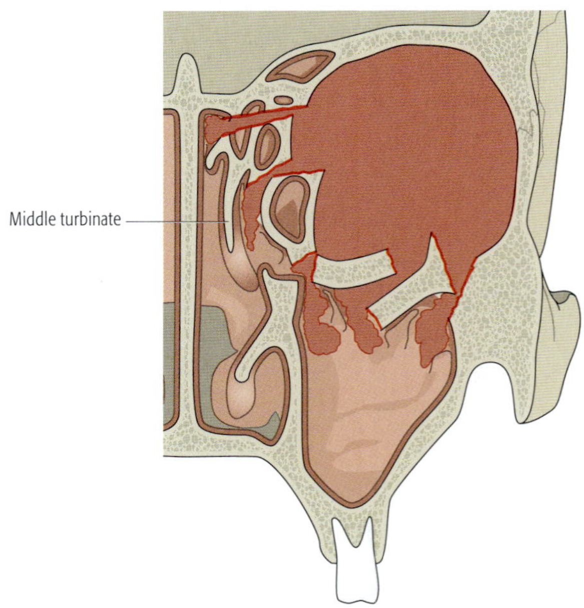

Fig 5.3.8-3 A complex, two-wall orbital fracture that is amenable to repair with a preformed mesh implant.

Once the implant is adequately positioned, it is fixed with a miniscrew at the orbital rim. Caution should be exercised that the screw tightening (lag screw) does not torque the implant and alter its position.

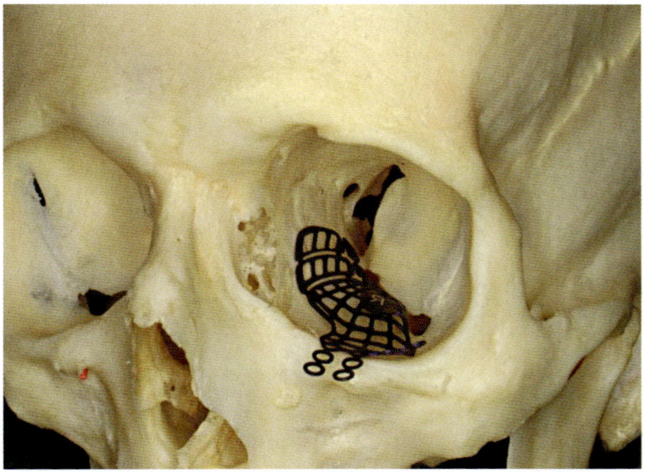

Fig 5.3.8-4 A small, left orbital preformed mesh implant placed into the left orbit. Note how the preformed shape mimics the normal orbital architecture.

4 Results

Several recent studies have evaluated the preformed mesh implant and found it to be safe and effective for complex orbital reconstructions [Metzger et al, 2006; Scolozzi et al, 2009]. Schoen et al [2006] concluded that the use of preformed implants is less time consuming and more precise compared to free-hand bending. Momjian et al [2011] showed equal volume reconstruction and clinical results with the use of traditional vs preformed mesh. Strong et al [2013] noted similar volume results for traditional vs preformed mesh but also found that the contour of the preformed mesh was superior to traditional implants.

Multiple questions remain to be answered about the ideal techniques and materials used for orbital reconstruction. The use of preformed orbital mesh appears to be a safe and effective technique. While improved volume reconstruction has not been proven when using preformed meshes, its use seems to provide a more anatomical surgical repair; mimicking the premorbid orbital architecture more precisely than implants that are not prebent. Late problems from metallic implants include chronic infection, often from failure of mucosalization, orbital adherence syndrome to include diplopia. Meshes are more difficult to remove than nonperforated materials.

5 References and suggested reading

Al-Sukhun J, Lindqvist C. A comparative study of 2 implants used to repair inferior orbital wall bony defects: autogenous bone graft versus bioresorbable poly-L/DL-Lactide [P(L/DL)LA 70/30] plate. *J Oral Maxillofac Surg*. 2006 Jul;64(7):1038–1048.

Ellis E 3rd, el-Attar A, Moos KF. An analysis of 2,067 cases of zygomatico-orbital fracture. *J Oral Maxillofac Surg*. 1985 Jun;43(6):417–428.

Ellis E 3rd, Tan Y. Assessment of internal orbital reconstructions for pure blowout fractures: cranial bone grafts versus titanium mesh. *J Oral Maxillofac Surg*. 2003 Apr;61(4):442–453.

Gellrich NC, Schramm A, Hammer B, et al. Computer-assisted secondary reconstruction of unilateral posttraumatic orbital deformity. *Plast Reconstr Surg*. 2002 Nov;110(6):1417–1429.

Holck DE, Boyd EM Jr, Ng J, et al. Benefits of stereolithography in orbital reconstruction. *Ophthalmology*. 1999 Jun;106(6):1214–1218.

Metzger MC, Schön R, Weyer N, et al. Anatomical 3-dimensional pre-bent titanium implant for orbital floor fractures. *Ophthalmology*. 2006 Oct;113(10):1863–1868.

Metzger MC, Schön R, Schulze D, et al. Individual preformed titanium meshes for orbital fractures. *Oral Surg Oral Med Oral Pathol Oral Radiol Endod*. 2006 Oct;102(4):442–447.

Momjian A, Heuberger J, Scolozzi P. [Post-traumatic orbital reconstruction comparing preformed versus non preformed titanium mesh plates]. *Rev Stomatol Chir Maxillo-Fac*. 2011;112:145–150. French.

Perry M, Banks P, Richards R, et al. The use of computer-generated three-dimensional models in orbital reconstruction. *Br J Oral Maxillofac Surg*. 1998 Aug;36(4):275–284.

Potter JK, Ellis E. Biomaterials for reconstruction of the internal orbit. *J Oral Maxillofac Surg*. 2004 Oct;62(10):1280–1297.

Schön R, Metzger MC, Zizelmann C, et al. Individually preformed titanium mesh implants for a true-to-original repair of orbital fractures. *Int J Oral Maxillofacial Surg*. 2006 Nov;35(11):990–995.

Scolozzi P, Momjian A, Heuberger J, et al. Accuracy and predictability in use of AO three-dimensionally preformed titanium mesh plates for posttraumatic orbital reconstruction: a pilot study. *J Craniofac Surg*. 2009 Jul;20(4):1108–1113.

Steidler NE, Cook RM, Reade PC. Incidence and management of major middle third facial fractures at the Royal Melbourne Hospital. A retrospective study. *Int J Oral Surg*. 1980 Apr;9(2):92–98.

Strong EB, Fuller SC, Wiley DF, et al. Preformed vs intraoperative bending of titanium mesh for orbital reconstruction. *Otolaryngol Head Neck Surg*. 2013 Jul;149(1):60–66.

Uygur S, Cukurluoglu O, Ozmen S, et al. Resorbable mesh plate in the treatment of blow-out fracture might cause gaze restriction. *J Craniofac Surg*. 2009 Jan;20(1):71–72.

5.3.9 Preformed mandible plates

Marc C Metzger, Florian A Probst, Rainer Schmelzeisen, E Bradley Strong

1 Introduction

Surgical reconstruction of the mandible, after trauma or surgical resection, can be time-consuming and extremely challenging. Complications, such as plate exposure, loosening of the hardware, and plate fracture, can occur, particularly in segmental defects without bony reconstruction [Wei et al, 2003; Klotch et al, 1999; Knoll et al, 2004; Schoning et al, 1998; Klotch et al, 1987; Shibahara et al, 2002] (**Fig 5.3.9-1**).

Current reconstruction plates have several drawbacks: bending is time-consuming, placement via a transoral approach is difficult, and plate fractures may happen, particularly when no bony reconstruction is performed or after excessive bending [Shibahara et al, 2002]. A "preformed" reconstruction plate was developed to improve ease of handling and increase stability of mandibular reconstruction plates.

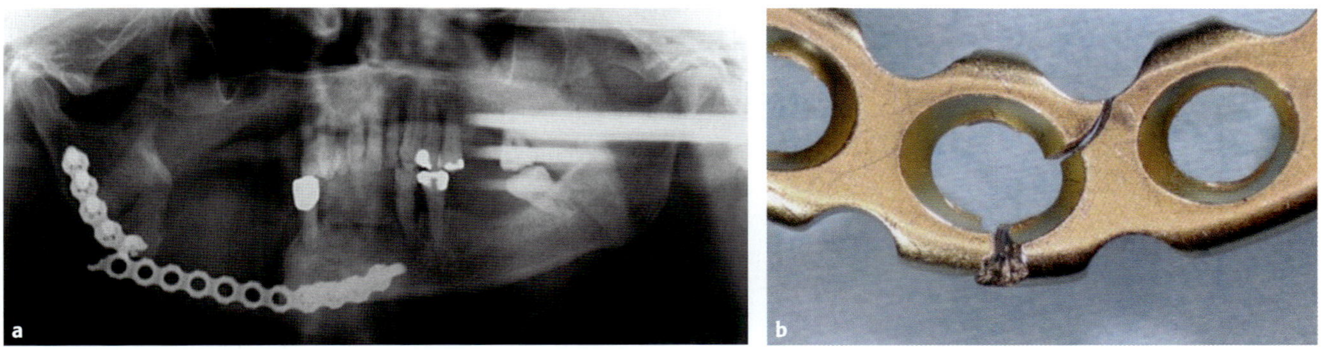

Fig 5.3.9-1a–b
- **a** Panoramic x-ray of a patient after tumor resection including segmental resection of the right mandible body and alloplastic reconstruction, presenting with a plate fracture.
- **b** Plate after removal showing a fatigue fracture.

2 Plate design

A biometric analysis was performed evaluating the shapes of mandibles using the data obtained from more than 7,000 computed tomographic (CT) scans from various ethnic adult populations **[Metzger et al, 2011]**. Anatomical stress zones secondary to mastication were also considered. Based on those data, prebent plates were designed in small, medium, and large sizes. Each plate has four distinct regions (**Fig 5.3.9-2**). The central preshaped region requires no cutting or bending. This eliminates any reduction in strength secondary to deformation and metal fatigue. The symphyseal and ramus regions are also prebent but can be molded intraoperatively to optimize the individual fit. The most distal portion of the plate is straight and can be cut or modified as necessary. The plate holes have threads and can be used with locking or conventional nonlocking screws.

Minimizing the need for intraoperative bending preserves the optimal hole and thread shapes that reduces the risk of metal fatigue and fracture compared with conventional reconstruction plates (**Fig 5.3.9-3**). In addition, the preformed shape allows easier transoral application, in combination with transbuccal instrumentation and/or 90° screwdrivers. Finally, the preshaped form can reduce surgical time by minimizing bending and handling time.

3 Indications

The primary indication for use of an anatomically preformed reconstruction plate is the bridging of mandibular defects. Vascularized or nonvascularized bony reconstruction can then be performed using the preformed plate for contour and graft/flap fixation. Other potential indications include treatment of comminuted, edentulous/atrophic, and/or infected mandibular fractures.

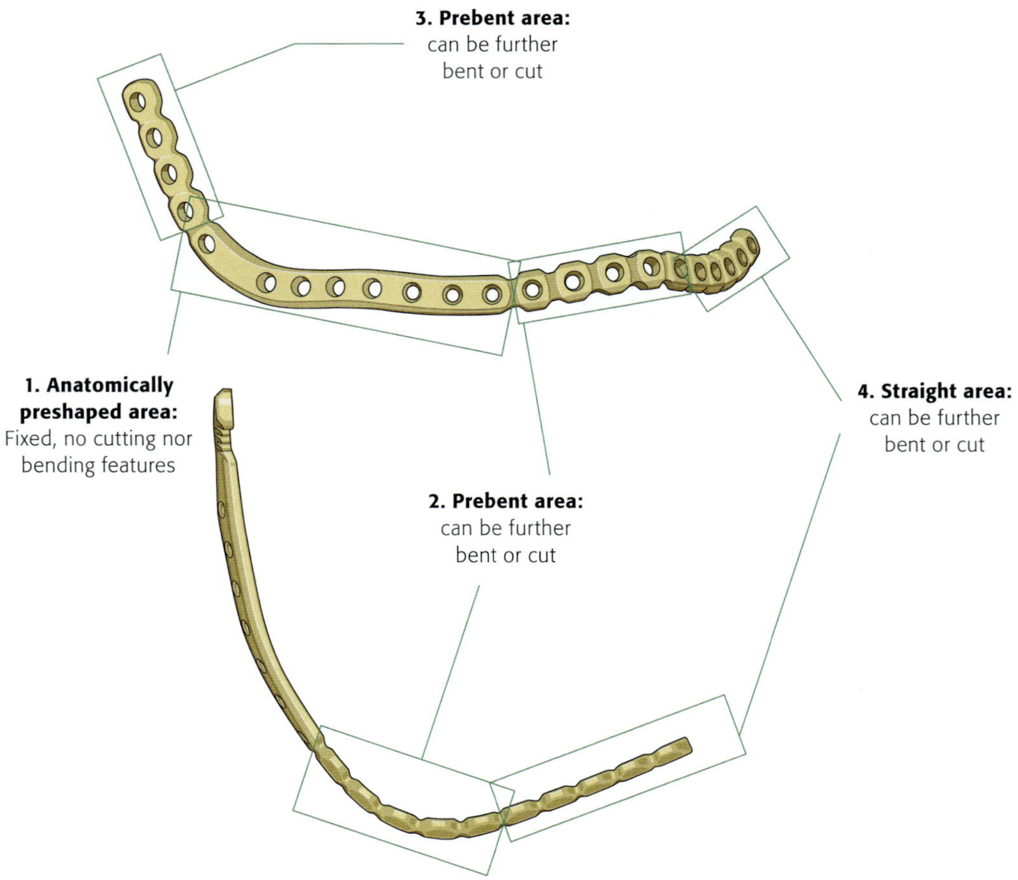

Fig 5.3.9-2 Bending and nonbending zones of the preformed mandibular plate.

4 Surgical technique

After exposing the defect area or fracture, templates can be placed to determine the adequate shape of the plate. The "medium" template should initially be selected and placed along the inferior body of the mandible (**Fig 5.3.9-4**).

The position of the template along the mandibular ramus is first assessed. If the posterior border of the ramus and the template are correctly aligned, the medium plate can be used. If the template lies behind the posterior ramus, a small plate is considered for reconstruction. If the template position is in front of the posterior ramus, the large plate should be considered. Small and large templates are also available for contour assessment before the final plate is selected (**Fig 5.3.9-5**).

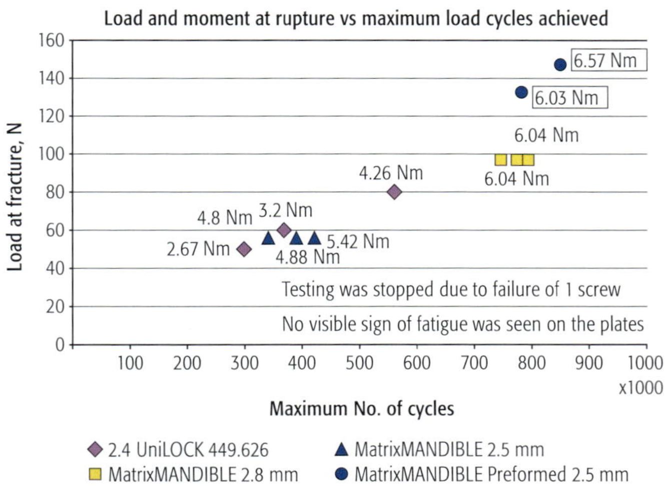

Fig 5.3.9-3 Mechanical stress test of different reconstruction plates including the preformed mandible plates. Blue dots indicating that there was no fatigue failure of these plates.

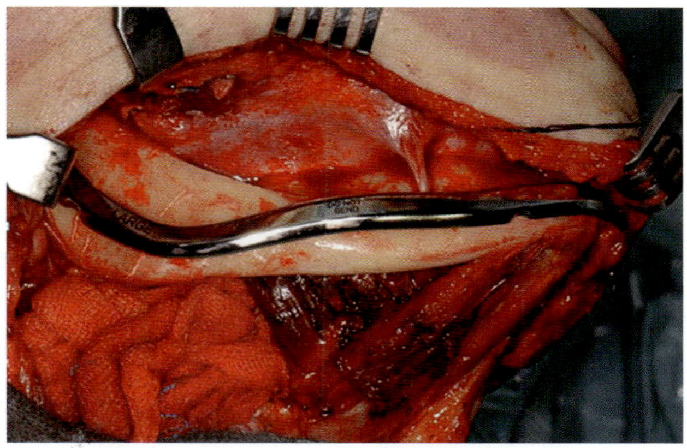

Fig 5.3.9-4 Template to determine size, length, and contour of the preformed plate.

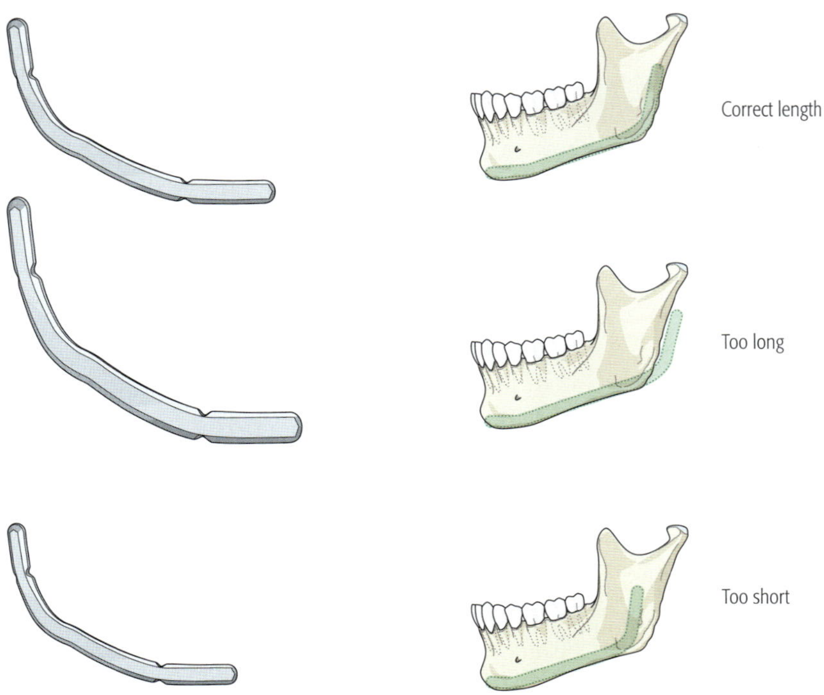

Fig 5.3.9-5 Three different templates allow the determination of the best fitting preformed plate.

Once the appropriate size has been selected, the corresponding template can be adapted and molded onto the contour of the mandible, and used as a template to modify the malleable anterior and/or posterior portions of the plate. The first 2–4 holes anterior to the nonadaptable central section of the plate allow the surgeon to adjust the length with minimal bending. Bending pliers are used to perform out-of-plane bending. "In-plane" bending is generally not required (particularly in the symphyseal region) because of the preformed nature of the anterior and posterior extensions (**Fig 5.3.9-6**). "Bending inserts" that prevent distortion of the screw holes are rarely necessary. They are available for plates which might require extensive bending that exceed 20° in torsional and in-plane bending, and 45° for out-of-plane bending.

Stable fixation usually requires a minimum of three to four screws at both ends, in the proximal (ramus) and distal (symphyseal) segments. While a certain amount of screw angulation in the plate hole can be tolerated, perpendicular placement of all screws with respect to the plate and bony surface will provide optimal plate stability. A drill guide is available to assure placement of the screw centrally within the plate hole. When using preformed reconstruction plates as a temporary bridging device, 2.4 or 2.9 mm locking screws should be inserted. If limited bone length or poor bone quality exists, a minimum of three 2.9 mm locking screws are used. If a condylar head add-on system is used, the last three holes in the region of the ramus should not be bent to avoid deformation.

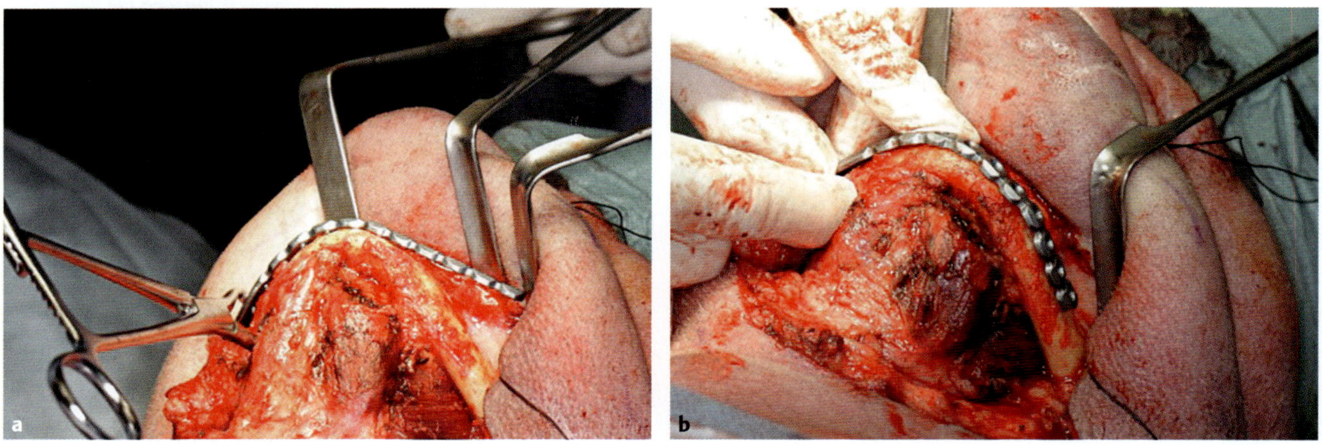

Fig 5.3.9-6a–b Preformed reconstruction plate showing the chin area before (**a**) and after (**b**) out-of-plane bending. The vertical dimension will automatically fit to the right position; in-plane bending is usually not necessary.

5 References and suggested reading

Klotch DW, Gal TJ, Gal RL. Assessment of plate use for mandibular reconstruction: has changing technology made a difference? *Otolaryngol Head Neck Surg.* 1999 Oct;121(4):388–392.

Klotch DW, Prein J. Mandibular reconstruction using AO plates. *Am J Surg.* 1987 Oct;154(4):384–388.

Knoll WD, Gaida A, Maurer P. [Stress tests of reconstruction plates for bridging mandibular angle defects]. *Mund Kiefer Gesichtschir.* 2004 Jul;8(4):237–243. German.

Metzger MC, Vogel M, Hohlweg-Majert B, et al. Anatomical shape analysis of the mandible in Caucasian and Chinese for the production of preformed mandible reconstruction plates. *J Craniomaxillofac Surg.* 2011 Sep;39(6):393–400.

Probst FA, Mast G, Ermer M, et al. MatrixMANDIBLE preformed reconstruction plates—a two-year two-institution experience in 71 patients. *J Oral Maxillofac Surg.* 2012 Nov;70(11):e657–666.

Schoning H, Emshoff R. Primary temporary AO plate reconstruction of the mandible. *Oral Surg Oral Med Oral Pathol Oral Radiol Endod.* 1998 Dec;86(6):667–672.

Shibahara T, Noma H, Furuya Y, et al. Fracture of mandibular reconstruction plates used after tumor resection. *J Oral Maxillofac Surg.* 2002 Feb;60(2):182–185.

Wei FC, Celik N, Yang WG, et al. Complications after reconstruction by plate and soft-tissue free flap in composite mandibular defects and secondary salvage reconstruction with osteocutaneous flap. *Plast Reconstr Surg.* 2003 Jul;112(1):37–42.

5.3.10 Patient-specific mandible implants

Max Heiland, Maximillian Schöllchen, Henning Hanken

1 Introduction

Patient-specific mandible implants are available as individually milled or sintered plates. Milled and sintered plates offer various design options because they are made to correspond to the individual reconstructive problem. The difference between milled and sintered plates is in the production technique. Milled plates are produced by cutting the desired implant out of a metallic block in a subtractive process. Additionally manufactured implants are made by fusing metallic powders, for instance with laser beams. The subtractive process of milling is subject to some geometrical restrictions, eg, shapes that include an undercutting design are not possible. Furthermore, the size is limited to the workpiece and dimensions of the milling cutter. There are numerous metals that can be milled and used for facial reconstruction.

In contrast, sintered metals do not have this geometric restriction, but they show a certain degree of porosity because the starting materials never fuse completely, but just compact to a dense material. This porosity can lead to difficulties in the process of preoperative sterilization. A special way of sintering is the electron beam melting (EBM) process. The technique uses an electronic beam to additively manufacture a CAD piece by a melting process of layers of metal powder. With EBM, it is possible to create trabecular-like implant surfaces, which allow for bony ingrowth [Biemond et al, 2013; Wong et al, 2010].

In terms of mechanical properties, milled and sintered materials are equally stable. For both not only the shape of the implant is customizable but also positioning and angulation of the screw holes can be individually planned. This is a significant advantage compared with prebent plates as it allows a better consideration of structures, such as nerves, tooth roots, osteotomies or existing implants, and the avoidance of interferences with those structures. Virtual planning allows a prediction about possible screw collisions, screw angulation, and allows a prediction of length of the planned screws.

Another advantage is the potentially increased stability of patient-specific milled or sintered plates compared with conventional reconstruction plates. Additional bending that may decrease plate stability is not needed, plate dimensions may be designed individually to increase stability in certain areas, for instance in bridged defect areas.

2 Planning

The planning process requires close cooperation between the surgeon and a planning platform provided by the plate-producing industry. Virtual planning can easily be done in a web-meeting session between the surgeon and design engineer.

For virtual planning, a 3-D data set with a maximum of 1 mm slice thickness is needed. A customized implant should be used within 3 months after data acquisition. If possible, the scan should be done with a gantry tilt of 0° and afterward be reconstructed with a high-resolution bone algorithm. A DICOM data set of axial slices, generated by a computed tomographic (CT) scan or cone beam CT scan, meeting the above-mentioned criteria, is sufficient for the preoperative planning.

Planning software is used to construct a 3-D volume, perform segmentation, simulate the ablative surgery, and finally implant placement, with or without the use of autogenous grafts/flaps.

3 Indication for patient-specific mandible implants

Indications for computer-assisted design and manufacturing (CAD/CAM) reconstruction plates include segmental bone defects as well as fractures in extremely atrophic and comminuted mandibles, when the bone is no longer capable of resisting applied muscular and mechanical forces. Situations where tumor spread or a deformity limits the use of conventional plates, which are usually contoured or adapted to the bone surface, are an indication for patient-specific implants. Long-term data comparing outcomes of patient-specific implants to conventional implants are not yet available.

4 Clinical application

Segmental mandibular defects may result from various pathologies with different dignities and dimensions. Some pathologies, for example, cystic lesions, ameloblastomas or other tumors, usually result in locally circumscribed defects. Other pathologies, like medication-related osteonecrosis, osteomyelitis, or osteoradionecrosis, can involve the complete mandible, including the region of the temporomandibular joint. The loss of bone substance leads, depending on extent and location of the defect, to various functional problems such as impaired speech, masticatory and even deglutition disorders. In addition, a possible disfigurement may severely affect the patients' quality of life [Buchbinder et al, 1989].

To restore a fully functional mandibular unit, a number of surgical procedures using different grafts/flaps have been described to accommodate both biomechanical and functional needs [Wong et al, 2010]. In these situations, reconstruction plates are commonly used to support or even take over the biomechanical functions of the bone.

Preoperative computer-assisted planning of the surgery can help to accurately determine the anatomical situation and anticipate the extent and shape of osteosynthesis material needed. This includes scenarios with bone grafts/flaps as well as reconstructions with a plate alone to bridge defects (**Fig 5.3.10-1**). Especially in long spanning and geometrically challenging defect situations, individual planning is advantageous concerning precision and operation time.

The integration of preoperative individual plate production into the process of CAD/CAM-guided bone transplantation for segmental defects is also possible. It may prevent postoperative deformities or misplacement of bone grafts/flaps. The shape of a plate can also be designed according to a backward planning dental implant placement process in order to place a graft into the ideal position for prosthodontic rehabilitation [Essig et al, 2011].

It is also possible to integrate the screw positions within patient-specific implants into cutting guides which are part of the CAD/CAM-assisted bone flap transplantation procedure. The plate's position and angulation are predefined corresponding to the bone graft, the mandible, and the bridged defect [Hidalgo et al, 1989; Wolff et al, 2005; Taylor, 1982; Silverberg et al, 1985; Swartz et al, 1986].

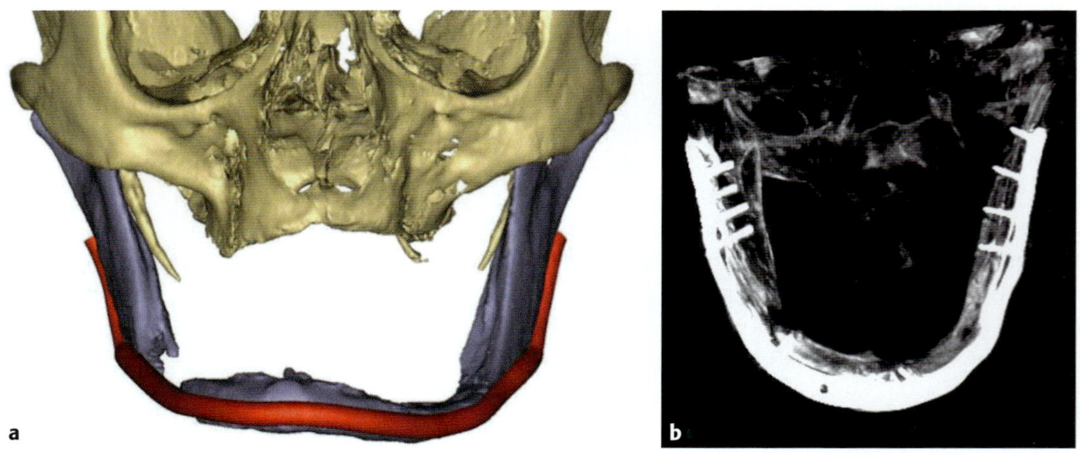

Fig 5.3.10-1a–b Fracture of an atrophic mandible, treatment with a patient-specific milled plate.
a Virtual planning of the plate design.
b Postoperative result (3-D reconstruction based on a postoperative cone beam computed tomographic scan).

The additional option to narrow the distance of the screw holes allows an increase in the number of screws in a graft/flap segment or areas with difficult access, such as the region of the condyle (see chapter 5.3.12).

5 Summary

Two types of patient-specific plates can be produced. Production of these plates can either be via a milling or a sintering process. In terms of stability, both types of plates are equally stable. They are considered to be potentially more stable than conventional plates because individual bending is not necessary.

For virtual planning a 3-D data set with a maximum of 1 mm slice thickness is needed. A considerable advantage of CAD/CAM reconstruction plates compared with conventional plates is the possibility to produce them for situations where tumor spread or deformities do not permit contouring or adaption to the surface of the local bone.

6 References and suggested reading

Biemond JE, Hannink G, Verdonschjot N, et al. Bone ingrowth potential of electron beam and selective laser melting produced trabecular-like implant surfaces with and without a biomimetic coating. *J Mater Sci Mater Med*. 2013 Mar;24(3):745–753.

Buchbinder D, Urken ML, Vickery C, et al. Functional mandibular reconstruction of patients with oral cancer. *Oral Surg Oral Med Oral Pathol*. 1989 Oct;68(4 Pt 2): 499–503; discussion 503–504.

Essig H, Rana M, Kokemueller H, et al. Pre-operative planning for mandibular reconstruction: a full digital planning workflow resulting in a patient specific reconstruction. *Head Neck Oncol*. 2011 Oct;3:45.

Hidalgo DA. Fibula free flap: a new method of mandible reconstruction. *Plast Reconstr Surg*. 1989 Jul;84(1):71–79.

Silverberg B, Banis JC, Jr, Acland RD. Mandibular reconstruction with microvascular bone transfer: series of 10 patients. *Am J Surg*. 1985 Oct;150(4): 440–446.

Swartz WM, Banis JC, Newton ED, et al. The osteocutaneous scapular flap for mandibular and maxillary reconstruction. *Plast Reconstr Surg*. 1986 Apr;77(4):530–545.

Taylor GI. Reconstruction of the mandible with free composite iliac bone grafts. *Ann Plast Surg*. 1982 Nov;9(5):361–376.

Wolff KD, Hölzle F. *Raising of Microvascular Flaps*. Berlin: Springer; 2005.

Wong RC, Tideman H, Merkx MA. Biomechanics of mandibular reconstruction: a review. *Int J Oral Maxillofac Surg*. 2010 Apr;39(4):313–319.

5.3.11 Patient-specific implants for craniofacial reconstruction

Dominik Horn, Jürgen Hoffmann

1 Introduction

Large-bone defects remain a challenge in craniofacial surgery. Such deformities may occur as a result of various etiologies including trauma, neoplasms, infection, systemic immunological diseases, or osteonecrosis due to radiation [Futran et al, 2006].

In some cases, the reconstructive choices based on autogenous materials such as microvascular free flaps with bony components are limited. The reasons can be the absence of suitable recipient site vessels, patient comorbidities, or the size of the defect that is beyond the feasibility of autogenous tissue supply. In addition, donor site morbidity after harvest of extended free flaps needs to be considered.

The major goals in reconstructive craniofacial surgery are rehabilitation of function and appearance [Cordeiro et al, 1998; Santamaria et al, 2006].

Alloplastic materials may be utilized instead of or in combination with autogenous flaps. In general, alloplastic implants must present biological attributes similar to bone in terms of biocompatibility, biomechanics, resistance to heat and radiation. Metallic cranial implants from gold and silver were first used in the 16th century [Sanan et al, 1997]. Individual computer-designed implants with preformed materials for restoration of craniofacial defects were described in the late 1980s [Toth et al, 1988; Epker et al, 1989; Schmitz et al, 1989; Lambrecht et al, 1990].

Currently, 3-D computer designed preformed implants are in widespread use for complex craniofacial reconstruction; they simplify the surgical procedure and reduce the operative time [D'Urso et al, 2000; Eppley et al, 2002; Chim et al, 2005]. Different materials, such as polyetheretherketone (PEEK), titanium, ceramics, porous polyethylene, or polymethylmethacrylate (PMMA), have emerged as materials for complex alloplastic reconstruction of the face with or without parts of the skull.

2 Materials

2.1 Titanium (titanium mesh, solid titanium)

Titanium is characterized by an outstanding biocompatibility and it is highly corrosion-resistant [Rae, 1986; Alpert et al, 1996]. In the view of the modulus of elasticity, it is the metal with the highest similarity to human bone [Haug, 1996; Katou et al, 1996]. Due to its low mass compared with its mechanical strength, titanium is a suitable alloplastic for the lightweight reconstruction of the craniofacial skeleton. Titanium allows a direct osseointegration without surrounding fibrous tissue, which has been demonstrated with dental implants, joint prostheses, and bone screws [Branemark et al, 1977; Albrektsson et al, 1987; Allison et al, 1990].

Therefore, individualized titanium implants offer an excellent option to reconstruct complex and large craniomaxillofacial areas with or without autogenous soft-tissue flaps to fulfill functional and esthetic needs [Triana et al, 2000; Nakayama et al, 2004] (**Figs 5.3.11-1–5.3.11-3**). Titanium can be manufactured as solid, meshed, or mixed implants. Meshed titanium may be modified during surgery for an individual design. Due to its larger surface, it allows tissue ingrowth, whereas solid implants are characterized by higher stability. In contrast to titanium mesh, solid titanium implants have the disadvantage of being heavy and impossible to bend or contour during surgery. Additionally, titanium implants may cause complications, such as infection, extrusion and ocular complaints, such as orbital adherence [Weintraub et al, 1981; Mauriello et al, 1987; Jordan et al, 1992; Spetzger et al, 2010]. The rate of infection has been reported to be low (2.6%) [Matsuno et al, 2006]. The thermal conductivity can also be perceived as disturbing by patients who have received a titanium implant [Spetzger et al, 2010].

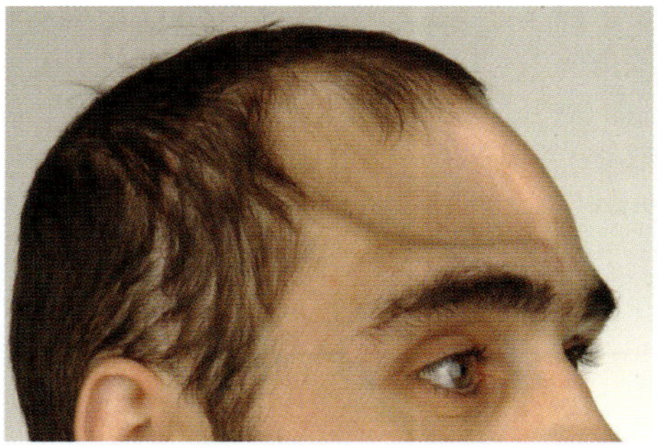

Fig 5.3.11-1 Posttraumatic cranial defect, preoperative.

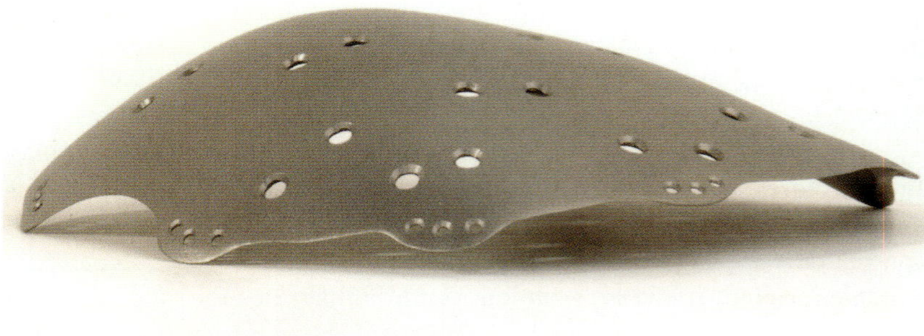

Fig 5.3.11-2 Patient-specific titanium implant.

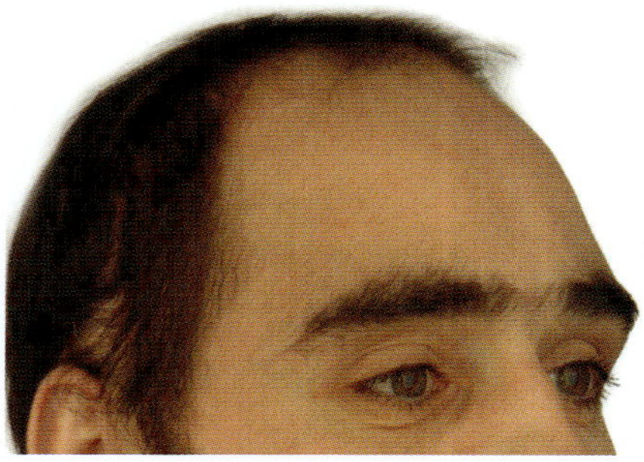

Fig 5.3.11-3 Postoperative result.

2.2 Polyetheretherketone

Polyetheretherketone was introduced for potential medical use at the end of the 1980s [Williams et al, 1987]. It is a 3-D solid synthetic material and a submember of polyacryletherketones. Due to its chemical structure, it combines properties such as resistance to chemical and radiation damage and stability even when exposed to high temperatures [Rigby, 1985; May, 1988]. Despite its strength, PEEK offers a considerable ductility that is similar to bone [Hamdan et al, 1996; Rae et al, 2007]. Low weight, thermal nonconductivity, chemical inertness combined with clinical features such as few artifacts in x-ray diagnostics, applicability in magnetic resonance imaging, and radiation resistance make PEEK an ideal material for alloplastic reconstruction of craniofacial bones [Hanasono et al, 2009]. Computer tomographic-based design and preformed shape are excellent options for skeletal reconstruction because of complex midfacial and craniofacial defects. Unlike titanium, PEEK has no bioactive potential and there is little data available concerning the long-term success in craniofacial reconstruction. Another disadvantage is that unlike meshed titanium, PEEK cannot be molded to unexpected anatomical situations during surgery, though it can be trimmed.

2.3 Ceramics

Ceramic implants can be divided into inert ceramics (eg, aluminia and zirconia) and bioactive ceramics (eg, glass-ceramic or hydroxyapatite). Patient-specific implants (PSIs) are currently commercially available for glass ceramics but potentially can be realized for all other ceramic bone substitutes.

2.3.1 Glass ceramics

Bioactive glass-ceramic consists, among other things, of silicon oxide, sodium oxide, calcium oxide, and phosphate oxide in varying proportions. Although the E-modulus of glass ceramics is similar to bone, its fragility prevents the clinical application in anatomical areas that are mechanically highly loaded. Biological and physical properties can be varied by changing the calcium oxide/phosphate ratio. When applied in a liquid environment, a gelatinous layer of silicic acid results out of the cleavage of silicon oxide. On the gelatinous surface, crystallized calcium phosphate creates an apatite layer, which leads to a reaction with collagen, mucopolysaccharide and glycoproteins and hence to a bony fixation. The fibrous encapsulation is described to be moderate [Hench et al, 1972]. In contrast to hydroxyapatite, the bioactive surface of glass ceramics allows a more effective neoformation of bone [Peltola et al, 2003; Cancian et al, 2004]. It can be used for the reconstruction of frontoorbital tissues [Aitasalo et al, 2007] or cranial vault defects [Gosain, 2004]. High rates of extrusion in case of facial contour filling, however, remains a major drawback [Duskova et al, 2002].

2.3.2 Hydroxyapatite

The main inorganic component of teeth and bone is hydroxyapatite, which is a hydroxylated calcium phosphate salt with a high hardness degree that can be manufactured synthetically or out of allogenic material. Hydroxyapatite is characterized by a high-pressure resistance, low modulus of rupture, and low torsional rigidity. Therefore, it is not suited to reconstruct highly loaded areas. Hydroxyapatite is osseointegrative, presents a low resorption, and can be shaped during surgery [Gosain et al, 2002; Bittermann et al, 2014]. These qualities make it suitable for augmentation or shape corrections. Due to previous reports of high complication rates, it seems unsuitable for reconstruction in the presence of full-thickness defects [Zins et al, 2007]. Recent studies, however, show only minor complications, even in large craniofacial reconstructions of the cranial vault [Staffa et al, 2012; Brie et al, 2013].

2.3.3 Alumina/zirconia ceramics

Ceramics containing aluminum oxide (Al_2O_3) and zirconium oxide (ZrO_2) are inert. In contrast to glass ceramic implants, aluminia and zirconia implants are neither osteoconductive nor osteoproductive. They are characterized by a high elastic modulus, compressive strength, biocompatibility, and corrosion resistance [Mantripragada et al, 2013]. Like titanium implants, ceramic implants can be manufactured by using CAD/CAM techniques [Staffa et al, 2012; Brier et al, 2013].

2.4 Porous polyethylene

Porous polyethylene is a highly sintered hydrocarbon which is an inert material with high biocompatibility. Due to its porous surface, it enables some fibrous tissue and bony ingrowth [Eppley et al, 1990]. Foreign body reactions have not been described [Klawitter et al, 1976; Spector et al, 1979]. It can be used for facial augmentation or bone reconstruction for large craniofacial defects [Wellisz, 1993; Abuzayed et al, 2009]. Porous polyethylene allows individual shaping and intraoperative cutting of an implant to appropriate size. The CT-based preforming of porous polyethylene implants is possible and the clinical application of porous polyethylene shows a low complication rate and acceptable long-term compatibility in the follow-up for more than 30 years [Rubin, 1983; Yaremchuk, 2003]. The infection rate is described from 0% up to 6% [Yaremchuk, 2003; Menderes et al, 2004; Cenzi et al, 2005; Lin et al, 2012].

2.5 Polymethylmethacrylate

Polymethylmethacrylate is a stable, inert, radiolucent, and nonconductive material [Firtell et al, 1981]. It is characterized by a high compression resistance, a density similar to bone and a hydrophilic surface. Its porosity enables the ingrowth of fibrous tissue and blood vessels and hence a potentially more stable fixation. There is no resorption described for PMMA [Manson et al, 1986]. Complication rates were initially published up to 12% [White et al, 1970; Cabanela et al, 1972] but could not be confirmed in one long-term study [Eppley, 2002]. A recent study with a low patient number showed no complications in PMMA implants that were designed with computer support [Turgut et al, 2012].

3 Workflow

Digital radiological image data (DICOM data) are essential to manufacture patient-specific preformed implants.

Virtual segmentation of the data set enables a 3-D image. Based on this data, the PSI can be virtually designed by using a database of empirical anatomical information. For virtual reconstruction, the symmetry of face and skull can be applied to reflect the unaffected anatomical region. Freehand design can also be used.

The digital transfer of 3-D data to the manufacturer is followed by the production of the PSI via CAD/CAM techniques. Depending on the stability, the PSI is manufactured by laser-sintering, subtractive milling, deep-drawing, or metal casting.

For a safe intraoperative application, cleaning and sterilization are required. Depending on the material, unexpected anatomical difficulties related to the fitting of PSI can be solved by individual curving or milling. The PSI is fixed using titanium or resorbable plates and/or screws.

4 References and suggested reading

Abuzayed B, Tuzgen S, Canbaz B, et al. Reconstruction of growing skull fracture with in situ galeal graft duraplasty and porous polyethylene sheet. *J Craniofac Surg.* 2009 Jul;20(4):1245–1249.

Aitasalo KM, Peltola MJ. Bioactive glass hydroxyapatite in fronto-orbital defect reconstruction. *Plast Reconstr Surg.* 2007 Dec;120(7):1963–1972; discussion 1973–1974.

Albrektsson T, Branemark PI, Jacobsson M, et al. Present clinical applications of osseointegrated percutaneous implants. *Plast Reconstr Surg.* 1987 May;79(5):721–731.

Allison RT, Sugar AW. Production of high quality ground sections of bone containing metal implants to demonstrate osseo-integration: a simplified method. *Med Lab Sci.* 1990 Jul;47(3):168–171.

Alpert B, Seligson D. Removal of asymptomatic bone plates used for orthognathic surgery and facial fractures. *J Oral Maxillofac Surg.* 1996;54(5):618–621.

Bittermann GK, Janssen NG, van Leeuwen M, et al. One-year volume stability of human facial defects filled with a β-tricalcium phosphate-hydroxyl apatite mixture (Atlantik). *J Craniofac Surg.* 2014 Mar;25(2):372–374.

Branemark PI, Hansson BO, Adell R, et al. Osseointegrated implants in the treatment of the edentulous jaw. Experience from a 10-year period. *Scand J Plast Reconstr Surg.* 1977;16:1–132.

Brie J, Chartier T, Chaput C, et al. A new custom made bioceramic implant for the repair of large and complex craniofacial bone defects. *J Craniomaxillofac Surg.* 2013 Jul;41(5):403–407.

Cabanela ME, Coventry MB, MacCarty CS, et al. The fate of patients with methyl methacrylate cranioplasty. *J Bone Joint Surg Am.* 1972 Mar;54(2):278–281.

Cancian DC, Hochuli-Vieira E, Marcantonio RA, et al. Utilization of autogenous bone, bioactive glasses, and calcium phosphate cement in surgical mandibular bone defects in Cebus apella monkeys. *Int J Oral Maxillofac Implants.* 2004 Jan–Feb;19(1):73–79.

Cenzi RA, Farina A, Zuccarino L, et al. Clinical outcome of 285 Medpor grafts used for craniofacial reconstruction. *J Craniofac Surg.* 2005 Jul;16(4):526–530.

Chim H, Schantz JT. New frontiers in calvarial reconstruction: integrating computer-assisted design and tissue engineering in cranioplasty. *Plast Reconstr Surg.* 2005 Nov;116(6):1726–1741.

Cordeiro PG, Santamaria E, Kraus DH, et al. Reconstruction of total maxillectomy defects with preservation of the orbital contents. *Plast Reconstr Surg.* 1998 Nov;102(6):1874–1884; discussion 1885–1887.

Costantino PD, Friedman CD, Lane A. Synthetic biomaterials in facial plastic and reconstructive surgery. *Facial Plast Surg.* 1993 Jan;9(1):1–15.

D'Urso PS, Earwaker WJ, Barker TM, et al. Custom cranioplasty using stereolithography and acrylic. *Br J Plast Surg.* 2000 Apr;53(3):200–204.

Duskova M, Smahel Z, Vohradnik M, et al. Bioactive glass-ceramics in facial skeleton contouring. *Aesthetic Plast Surg.* 2002 Jul–Aug;26(4):274–283.

Epker BN, Stella JP. Reconstruction of frontal and frontal-nasal deformities with prefabricated custom implants. *J Oral Maxillofac Surg.* 1989 Dec;47(12):1272–1276.

Eppley BL. Craniofacial reconstruction with computer-generated HTR patient-matched implants: use in primary bony tumor excision. *J Craniofac Surg.* 2002 Sep;13(5):650–657.

Eppley BL, Kilgo M, Coleman JJ 3rd. Cranial reconstruction with computer-generated hard-tissue replacement patient-matched implants: indications, surgical technique, and long-term follow-up. *Plast Reconstr Surg*. 2002;109(3):864–871.
Eppley BL, Sadove AM. Effects of material porosity on implant bonding strength in a craniofacial model. *J Craniofac Surg*. 1990 Oct;1(4):191–195.
Firtell DN, Grisius RJ. Cranioplasty of the difficult frontal region. *J Prosthet Dent*. 1981;46(4):425–429.
Futran ND, Mendez E. Developments in reconstruction of midface and maxilla. *Lancet Oncol*. 2006 Mar;7(3):249–258.
Gosain AK. Bioactive glass for bone replacement in craniomaxillofacial reconstruction. *Plast Reconstr Surg*. 2004 Aug;114(2):590–593.
Gosain AK, Song L, Riordan P, et al. A 1-year study of osteoinduction in hydroxyapatite-derived biomaterials in an adult sheep model: part I. *Plast Reconstr Surg*. 2002 Feb;109(2):619–630.
Hamdan S, Swallowe G. Strain-rate and temperature dependence of the mechanical properties of polyetherketone and polyetheretherketone. *J Mat Sci*. 1996;31:1415–1423.
Hanasono MM, Goel N, DeMonte F. Calvarial reconstruction with polyetheretherketone implants. *Ann Plast Surg*. 2009 Jun;62(6):653–655.
Haug RH. Retention of asymptomatic bone plates used for orthognathic surgery and facial fractures. *J Oral Maxillofac Surg*. 1996 May;54(5):611–617.
Hench L, Splinter R, Allen WC, et al. Bonding mechanisms at the interface of ceramic prosthetic materials. *J Biomed Mater Res*. 1972;2:117–141.
Jordan DR, St Onge P, Anderson RL, et al. Complications associated with alloplastic implants used in orbital fracture repair. *Ophthalmology*. 1992 Oct;99(10):1600–1608.
Katou F, Andoh N, Motegi K, et al. Immuno-inflammatory responses in the tissue adjacent to titanium miniplates used in the treatment of mandibular fractures. *J Craniomaxillofac Surg*. 1996 Jun;24(3):155–162.
Klawitter JJ, Bagwell JG, Weinstein AM, et al. An evaluation of bone growth into porous high density polyethylene. *J Biomed Mater Res*. 1976 Mar;10(2):311–323.
Lambrecht, JT, Brix F. Individual skull model fabrication for craniofacial surgery. *Cleft Palate J*. 1990 Oct;27(4):382–385; discussion 386–387.
Lin AY, Kinsella CR Jr, Rottgers SA, et al. Custom porous polyethylene implants for large-scale pediatric skull reconstruction: early outcomes. *J Craniofac Surg*. 2012 Jan;23(1):67–70.
Manson PN, Crawley WA, Hoopes JE. Frontal cranioplasty: risk factors and choice of cranial vault reconstructive material. *Plast Reconstr Surg*. 1986 Jun;77(6):888–904.
Mantripragada VP, Lecka-Czernik B, Ebraheim NA, et al. An overview of recent advances in designing orthopedic and craniofacial implants. *J Biomed Mater Res A*. 2013 Nov;101(11):3349–3364.
Matsuno A, Tanaka H, Iwamuro H, et al. Analyses of the factors influencing bone graft infection after delayed cranioplasty. *Acta Neurochir (Wien)*. 2006 May;148(5):535–540; discussion 540.
Mauriello JA Jr, Fiore PM, Kotch M. Dacryocystitis. Late complication of orbital floor fracture repair with implant. *Ophthalmology*. 1987 Mar;94(3):248–250.
May R. Polyetheretherketones. In: Mark HF, Bikales NM, Overberger CG, et al, eds. *Encyclopedia of Polymer Science and Engineering*. New York: 1988:313–320.
Menderes A, Baytekin C, Topcu A, et al. Craniofacial reconstruction with high-density porous polyethylene implants. *J Craniofac Surg*. 2004 Sep;15(5):719–724.
Nakayama B, Hasegawa Y, Hyodo I, et al. Reconstruction using a three-dimensional orbitozygomatic skeletal model of titanium mesh plate and soft-tissue free flap transfer following total maxillectomy. *Plast Reconstr Surg*. 2004 Sep 1;114(3):631–639.
Peltola MJ, Aitasalo KM, Suonpää JT, et al. Frontal sinus and skull bone defect obliteration with three synthetic bioactive materials. A comparative study. *J Biomed Mater Res B Appl Biomater*. 2003 Jul;66(1):364–372.
Rae PJ, Brown EN, Orler EB. The mechanical properties of poly(ether-ether-ketone) (PEEK) with emphasis on the large compressive strain response. *Polymer*. 2007;48:598–615.
Rae T. The biological response to titanium and titanium-aluminium-vanadium alloy particles. I. Tissue culture studies. *Biomaterials*. 1986 Jan;7(1):30–36.
Rigby R. Polyetheretherketone. In: Margolis JM, ed. *Engineering Thermoplastics: Properties and Applications*. New York: Marcel Dekker; 1985:299–314.
Rubin L. Polyethylene as a bone and catilage substitute: a 32-year retrospective. In: Rubin L, ed. *Biomaterials in Plastic Surgery*. St Louis, Mo: CV Mosby; 1983:474–492.
Sanan A, Haines SJ. Repairing holes in the head: a history of cranioplasty. *Neurosurgery*. 1997 Mar;40(3):588–603.
Santamaria E, Cordeiro PG. Reconstruction of maxillectomy and midfacial defects with free tissue transfer. *J Surg Oncol*. 2006 Nov;94(6):522–531.
Schmitz HJ, Tolxdorff T, Honsbrok J, et al. 3D-based computer assisted manufacturing of individual alloplastic implants for cranial and maxillofacial osteoplasties. In: Lemke HU, Rhodes ML, Jaffe CC, et al, eds. *Computer-assisted Radiology CAR '89*. Berlin: Springer; 1989:390.
Spector M, Harmon SL, Kreutner A. Characteristics of tissue growth into Proplast and porous polyethylene implants in bone. *J Biomed Mater Res*. 1979 Sep;13(5):677–692.
Spetzger U, Vougioukas V, Schipper J. Materials and techniques for osseous skull reconstruction. *Minim Invasive Ther Allied Technol*. 2010 Apr;19(2):110–121.
Staffa G, Barbanera A, Faiola A, et al. Custom made bioceramic implants in complex and large cranial reconstruction: a two-year follow-up. *J Craniomaxillofac Surg*. 2012 Apr;40(3):e65–70.
Stelnicki EJ, Ousterhout DK. Prevention of thermal tissue injury induced by the application of polymethylmethacrylate to the calvarium. *J Craniofac Surg*. 1996 May;7(3):192–195.
Toth BA, Ellis DS, Stewart WB. Computer-designed prostheses for orbitocranial reconstruction. *Plast Reconstr Surg*. 1988 Mar;81(3):315–324.
Triana RJ Jr, Uglesic V, Virag M, et al. Microvascular free flap reconstructive options in patients with partial and total maxillectomy defects. *Arch Facial Plast Surg*. 2000 Apr–Jun;2(2):91–101.
Turgut G, Ozkaya O, Kayal MU. Computer-aided design and manufacture and rapid prototyped polymethylmethacrylate reconstruction. *J Craniofac Surg*. 2012;23(3):770–773.
Weintraub B, Cucin RL, Jacobs M. Extrusion of an infected orbital-floor prosthesis after 15 years. *Plast Reconstr Surg*. 1981;68(4):586–587.
Wellisz T. Clinical experience with the Medpor porous polyethylene implant. *Aesthetic Plast Surg*. 1993 Fall;17(4):339–344.
White RJ, Yashon D, Albin MS, et al. Delayed acrylic reconstruction of the skull in craniocerebral trauma. *J Trauma*. 1970 Sep;10(9):780–786.
Williams DF, McNamara A. Potential of polyetheretherketone (PEEK) and carbon-fibre-reinforced PEEK in medical applications. *J Mat Sci Lett*. 1987;6:199–190.
Yaremchuk MJ. Facial skeletal reconstruction using porous polyethylene implants. *Plast Reconstr Surg*. 2003 May;111(6):1818–1827.
Zins JE, Moreira-Gonzalez A, Papay FA. Use of calcium-based bone cements in the repair of large, full-thickness cranial defects: a caution. *Plast Reconstr Surg*. 2007 Oct;120(5):1332–1342.

5.3.12 Computer-assisted surgical planning and execution: models, cutting and drill guides, positioning aids, and patient-specific implants

Carl-Peter Cornelius, Gerson Mast, Michael Ehrenfeld

1 General aspects

Comprehensive diagnostic analysis and preoperative planning of surgical procedures in the craniofacial skeleton have moved from mechanical simulation by use of haptic dental casts and stereolithographic models into a complete virtual environment based on high-resolution computed tomography (CT) or cone beam CT datasets as well as surface scans of the dental occlusion and/or the facial contours. Repair or reconstruction can be reliably evaluated and optimized in a digital test phase on a computer workstation using appropriate software programs before implementation in actual surgery [Hirsch et al, 2009; Bell, 2010; Edwards, 2010; Bell et al, 2011; Sharaf et al, 2010; Patel et al, 2012; Dérand et al, 2012; Saad et al, 2013; Rodby et al, 2014; Steinbacher et al, 2015; Pfaff et al, 2016].

2 Protocols

Two basic protocols determine the planning sequence and depend on multiple factors such as the condition of the craniofacial skeleton, the dentoalveolar and the dental status, tumor involvement, a defect after resection, a posttraumatic or congenital deformity or defect, edentulousness and atrophy or osteonecrosis.

2.1 Forward planning

Surface scans, CT and magnetic resonance imaging (MRI) data of the situation before surgery provide information about soft tissues and the craniofacial skeleton that is used to plan osteotomies or resections followed by reconstruction with autogenous bone grafts, bone containing flaps or allogenic material. Forward or prospective planning is targeted to restore the preablative skeletal framework in pathological states with internal destruction, tumor infiltration or bulky outgrowth, where resection in predictable boundaries can be realized [Smolka et al, 2015] (see chapter 5.3.10) (**Fig 5.3.12-1**). Hence, forward planning is applied either in primary reconstruction or in preparation for a second stage reconstruction. For secondary reconstruction, ideally the position of the pretreatment skeletal elements should be maintained, ie, by bridging a mandibular continuity defect with a reconstruction plate, or by an external mandible fixator.

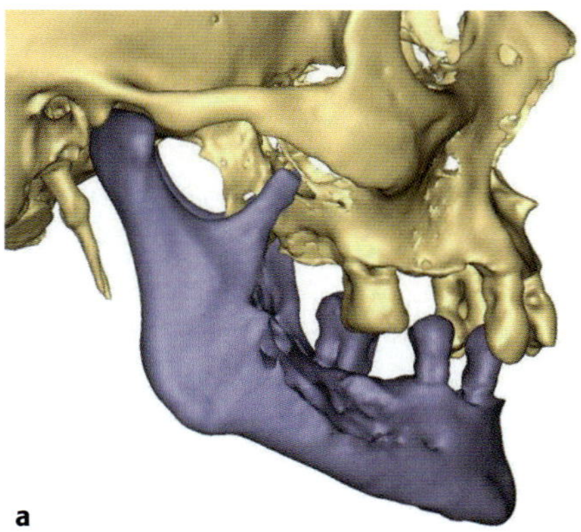

a

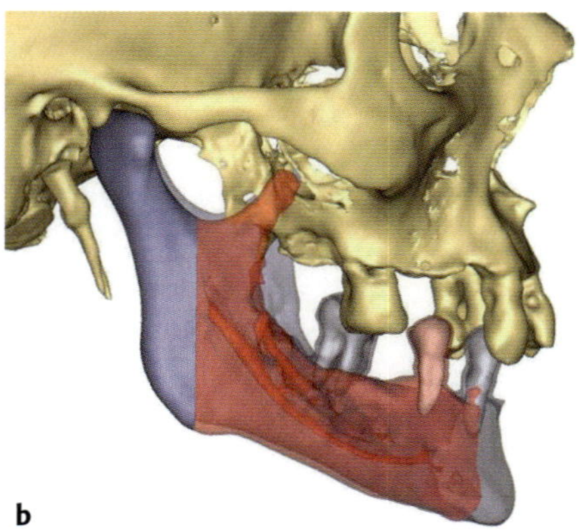

b

Fig 5.3.12-1a–m Forward planning of a mandible resection and reconstruction.
a Original contours and vertical bone height are easily recognized, although there is tooth loss, tumor infiltration and osteolysis in the right mandible.
b Translucent visualization of the proximity between mandibular canal and osteolysis to determine resection margins.

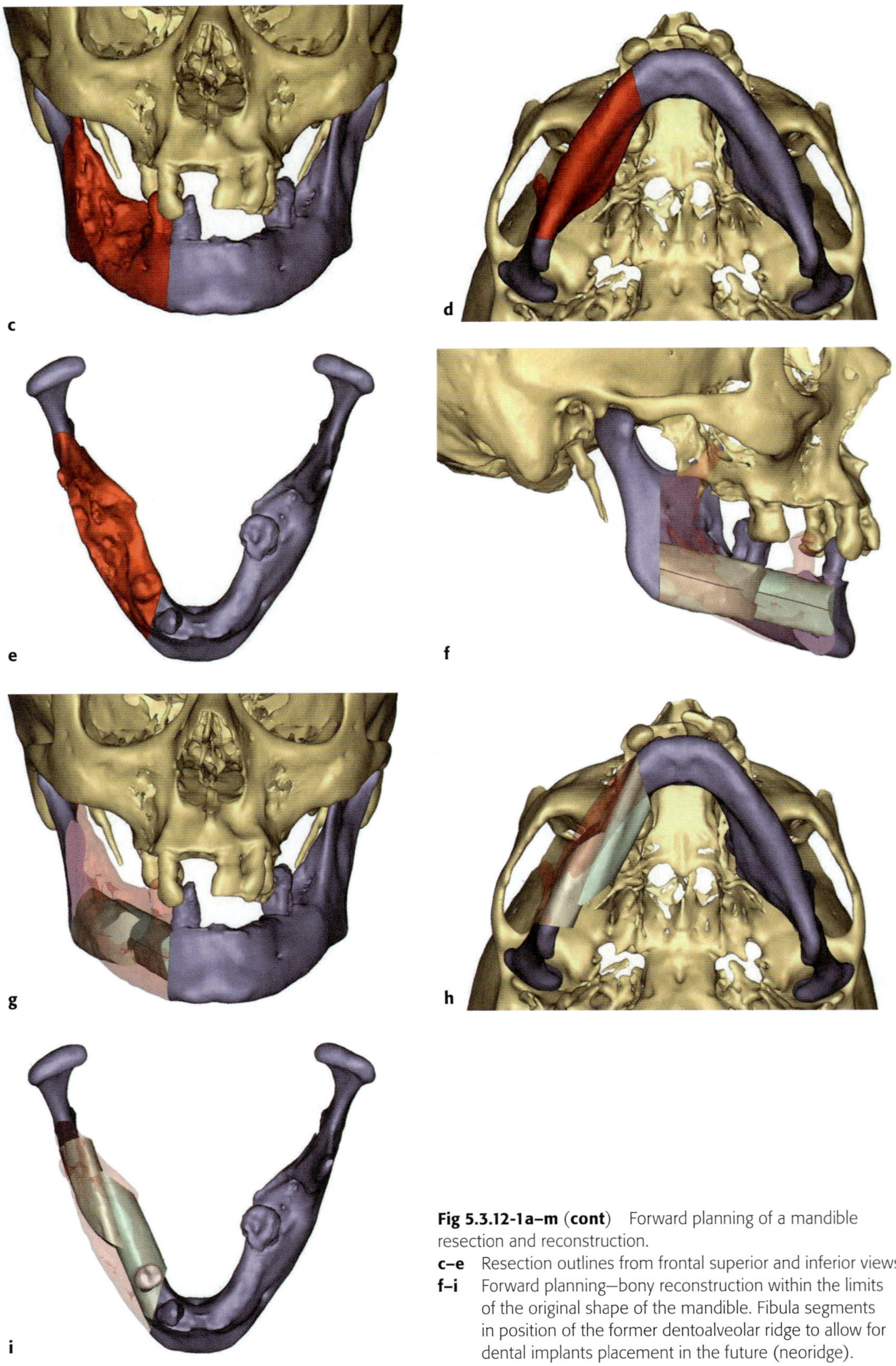

Fig 5.3.12-1a–m (cont) Forward planning of a mandible resection and reconstruction.
c–e Resection outlines from frontal superior and inferior views.
f–i Forward planning—bony reconstruction within the limits of the original shape of the mandible. Fibula segments in position of the former dentoalveolar ridge to allow for dental implants placement in the future (neoridge).

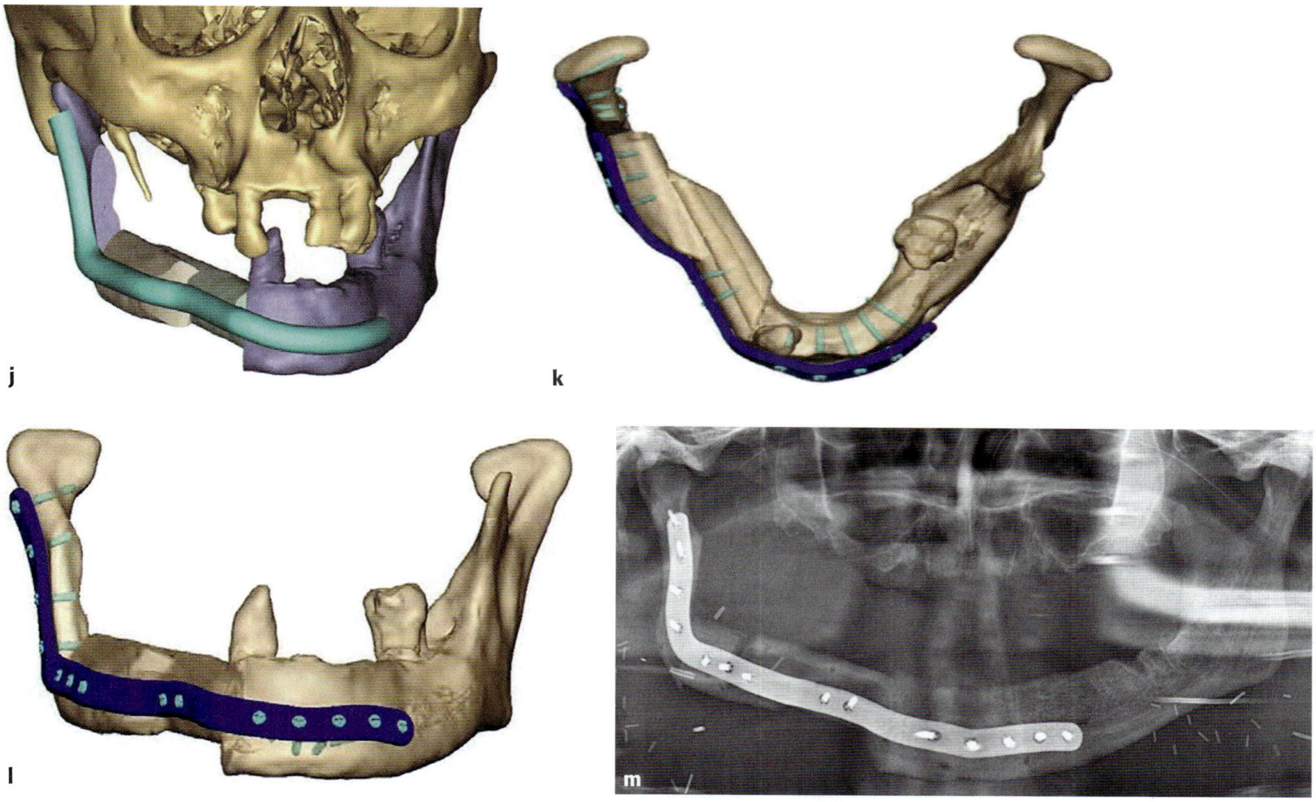

Fig 5.3.12-1a–m (cont) Forward planning of a mandible resection and reconstruction.

j Provisional virtual design of an inward bent reconstruction plate that will stabilize the segments with special emphasis on the lingual shift of the neomandibular segments.

k–l Final design of patient-specific mandibular plate.

m Panoramic x-ray view after surgical realization.

2.2 Backward or reverse planning

The necessity to virtually recreate the original or normal preexisting skeletal architecture (dimension and spatial arrangement) as a retrospective blueprint for subsequent repair and/or reconstruction in kind may arise from bone loss (eg, post-traumatic or resectional defects) [Tepper et al, 2011; Ciocca et al, 2012] and displacement (eg, collapsed defects, shifting of nonconsolidated fragments), dislocation of the mandibular condylar head, deformity, distortion or deficiency (eg, atrophy of the dentoalveolar process). The domain of backward planning will be secondary repair or reconstruction of the skeleton due to loss of initial morphological information.

Under favorable circumstances, imaging of the intact or preablative condition is available, so that the fusion with the current defect/deficiency provides the most reliable foundation for planning. Thus, guesswork and arbitrary repositioning is obviated.

A common "reverse approach" is the adjusted positioning of bone flaps or grafts to augment an atrophic alveolar process in the sense of a preimplantological vertical ridge augmentation [Okay et al, 2013, 2016].

Occasionally the term "backward planning" exclusively refers to a mandibular or maxillary reconstruction sequence with a head start from the optimal position of an implant supported dental restoration (dentures, bridge and crowns). The priority is on functional occlusion and its matching implant bed after bone placement in an ideal mandibulomaxillary relationship as a downstream step in the entire virtual workflow [Essig et al, 2011; Levine et al, 2013]. In such an implant or prosthodontic-driven bony reconstruction of the mandible or maxilla, the following references [Rohner et al, 2000, 2013; Schepers et al, 2016] in the order of increasing accuracy can be used to locate the optimal 3-D position of the neomandibular or neomaxillary bone segments:

- Variant 1: Symmetrical mirror image of the contralateral mandibular or maxillary alveolar ridge and/or the curve of the intact arch with dentition, if present (**Fig 5.3.12-2**).

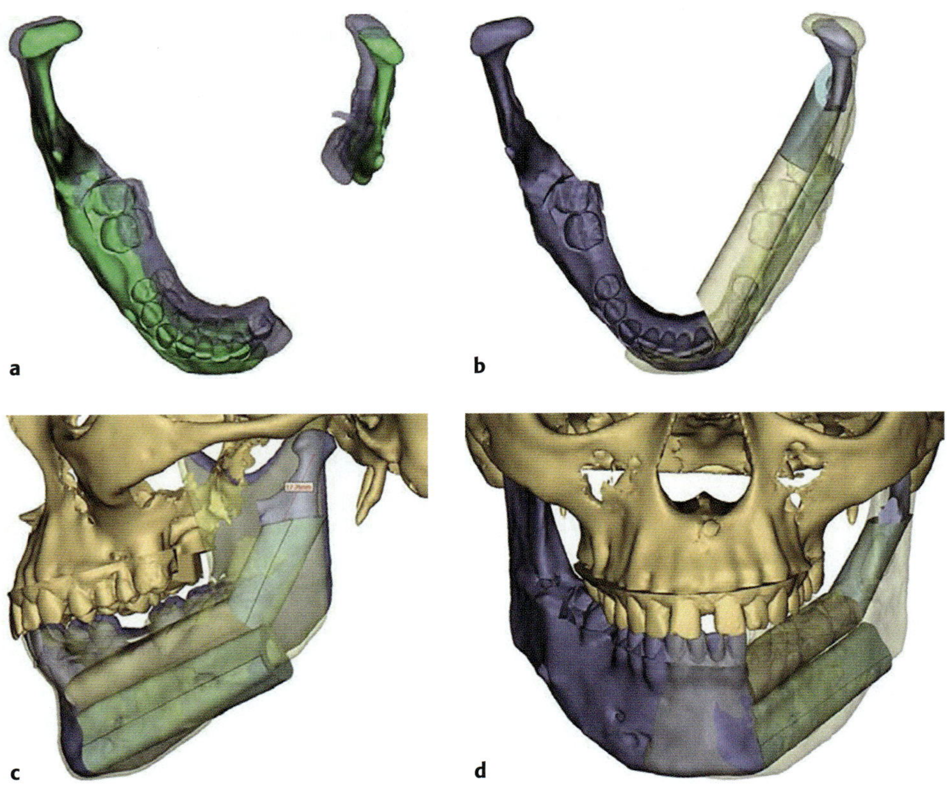

Fig 5.3.12-2a–d References for bony reconstruction in implant/prosthodontic driven backward planning. Variant 1: Mirror imaging of the contralateral mandibular body (including teeth) angle and ramus.

a Mandibular defect left body and angle. The bony remnants are brought into the supposed former position (green).

b–d Transparent mirrored contours and "over and under" barrel fibula flap segments, positioning of the segments is directed by mirrored tooth row in the mandibular body, which will define a dentoalveolar ridge position suitable for dental implant insertion in an optimal position.

- Variant 2: Teeth or dental arch of the opposite jaw in worms eye or birds eye transparency (**Fig 5.3.12-3**) or superimposition.
- Variant 3: Implant dummies in multiplanar transparent views (**Fig 5.3.12-4**).
- Variant 4: Virtual tooth-set-up to indicate tooth axes in multiplanar views (**Fig 5.3.12-5**).

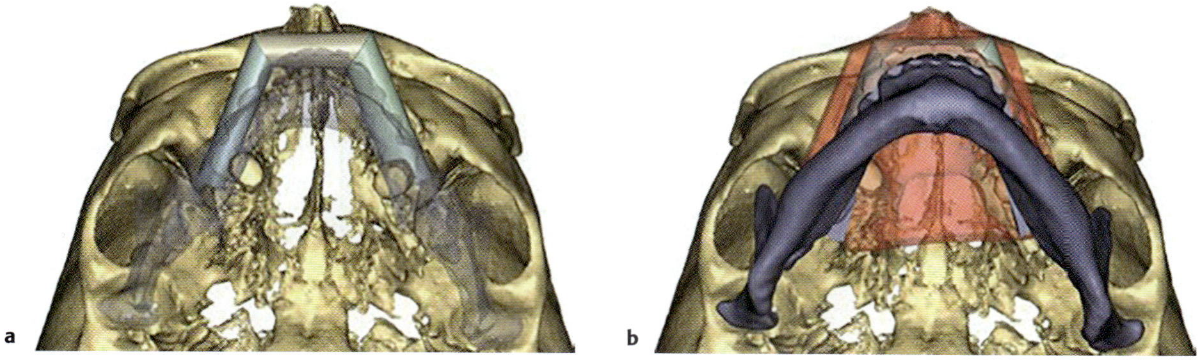

Fig 5.3.12-3a–b
References for bony reconstruction in implant/prosthodontic-driven backward planning. Variant 2: Teeth and dental arch of the opposite jaw in worms eye transparency.

a U-shaped fibular flap neoridges in upper jaw and superimposed mandible with teeth.
b Superimposed (red) surface scan of the planned denture in occlusion with mandibular teeth to confirm proper position of the neomaxillary construct.

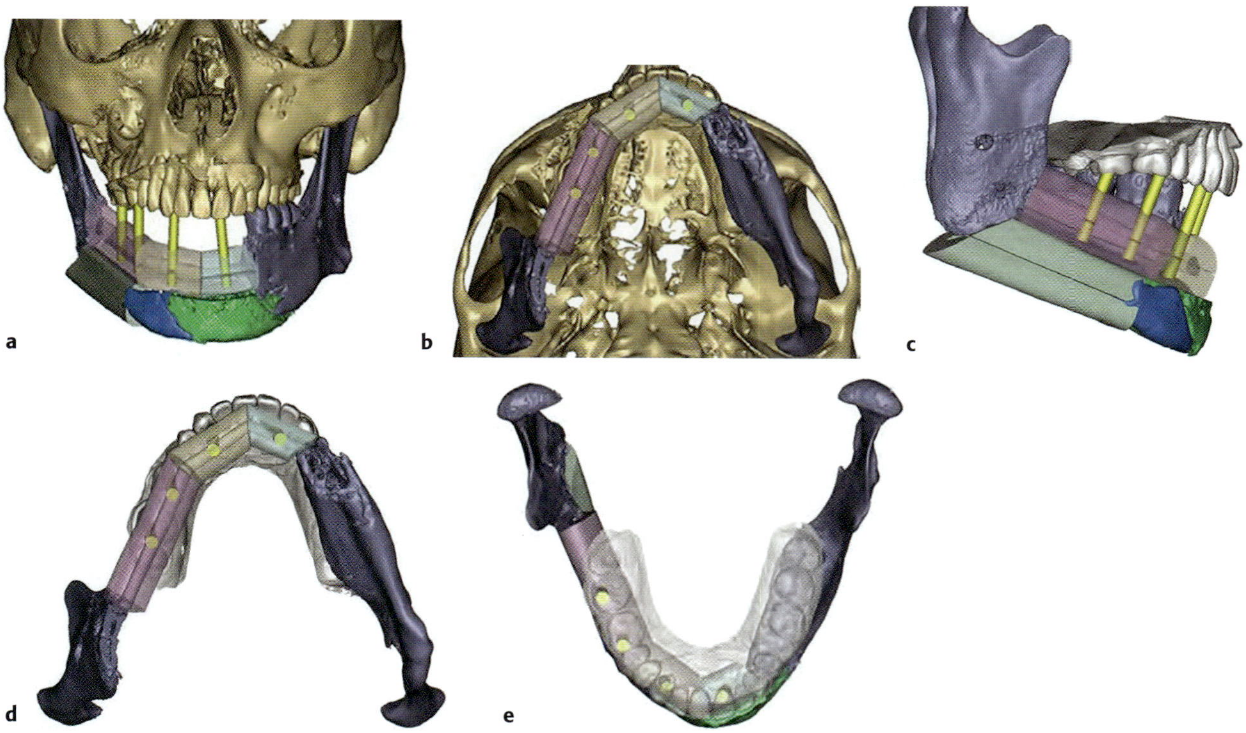

Fig 5.3.12-4a–e
References for bony reconstruction in implant/prosthodontic-driven backward planning. Variant 3: Placement of dental implant dummies in multiplanar views. Mandible with right anterolateral defect combined with multifragmentation in symphysis/chin area rebuilt with over and under barrel fibular segments.

a–b Planned mandibular reconstruction in full skeletal interrelation-neoridge segments aligned to a virtual tooth set up in the maxilla, four yellow implant dummies indicate an accurate bone replacement.
c–e Transviews of mandibulomaxillary block after erasure of midfacial suprastructures (lateral, basal, superior) to double-check for fitting of implant dummy positions.

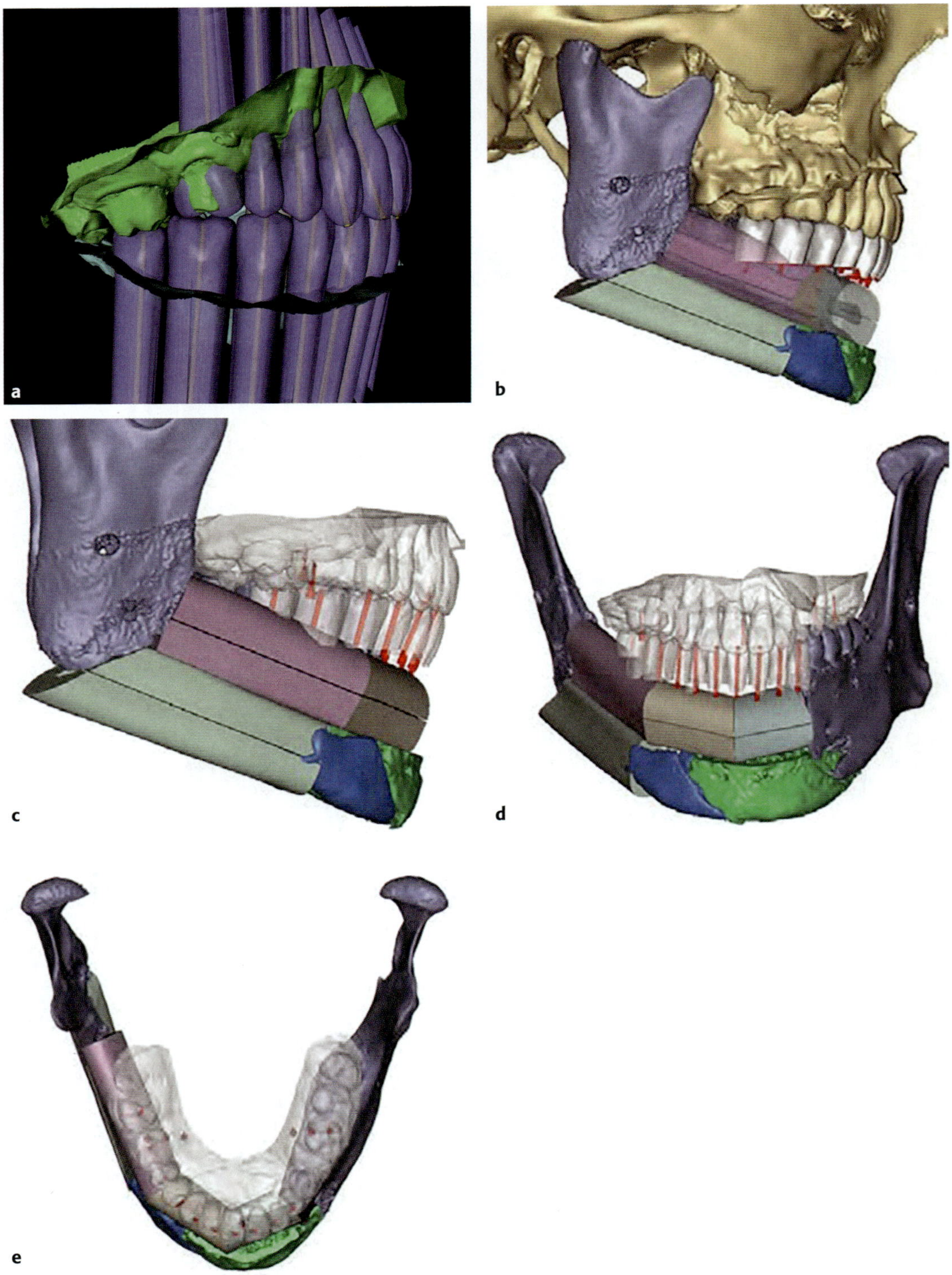

Fig 5.3.12-5a–e
References for bony reconstruction in implant/prosthodontic-driven backward planning. Variant 4: Virtual tooth set up and indication of tooth root axes in multiplanar views. Mandible with right anterolateral defect combined with multifragmentation in symphysis/chin area rebuilt with over and under barrel fibular segments.

a Virtual tooth set up in opposing edentulous maxillary and mandibular areas.
b Alignment of virtual dental arches—tooth crowns only—over bony surface.
c–d Transparent crowns with central axes pointing to neoridge fibular segments.
e Mandibular tooth axes from above through transparent upper dentition.

3 Template-assisted surgery

3.1 Purpose of template toolkits

A restored or reassembled skeletal framework is fundamental for the subsequent modeling of surgical templates, regardless of whether a forward or backward concept has been applied in virtual surgical planning (VSP). The goal of the modeling process is to design, generate and manufacture a supplementary toolkit whose components can be collectively referred to as templates to transfer VSP into real surgery. These toolkits consist of stereolithography (STL) models, duplicates of contoured flaps/grafts, positioning aids, interocclusal wafers, segmentation and resection guides, drill guides and transplant cutting guides (for harvesting and contouring). They are designed to ensure the transfer of planning to surgery with high accuracy and with minimal time expenditure.

Patient-specific implants (PSIs) may be designed and manufactured to facilitate the alignment and insetting of bone segments into a defect efficiently, and therefore contribute to the accuracy and precision of the operation (see chapter 5.3.11).

The alternative approach to computer-assisted and/or template/toolkit-based surgery is image-guided or navigational surgery. The virtual treatment plan is exported to the navigation system without the need for other specific tools to translate and control the intended design during the individualized operation (see subchapter 5.3.5).

4 Digital workflow, virtual planning

The overall digital workflow begins with data acquisition in the craniofacial skeleton and the potential donor site for flaps or grafts using at least one, or ideally, several sources. Volume CT or CBCT data may be supplemented with MRI datasets, digitized conventional dental casts, or dental impressions taken with intraoral 3-D digital scanners (computer-aided impressioning [CAI]), bite registrations, a virtual or scanned tooth set-up for prosthetic rehabilitation, facial surface scans and/or 3-D photographs as needed for the planning process. Physical dental models, such as plaster of Paris casts from conventional dental impressions, or digital impression fabricated rapid prototyping models, may be anatomically mounted into a real articulator and used along with digital images in a virtual articulator for comparison/quality control. The digital datasets are uploaded into a treatment planning platform, where they are further processed by cleaning artifacts, and image segmentation and fusion. Image segmentation is used to refine anatomical structures and pertinent details (eg, location of tumor borders) in the stacks of image slices by various techniques (eg, grey scale threshold selection, edge detection) or manually to enhance the representation in the 3-D visualization, which serves as the initial state for any consecutive data manipulation (**Fig 5.3.12-6a**). In the VSP 'prototype' mandibular reconstruction with fibula flaps, a generic ('standard') fibular bone may be selected and imported from a virtual library conforming to the patient's physical height and body mass index instead of an individual CT-derived fibula, without seriously compromising the accuracy.

Due to the complexity of the programs, it is useful to perform the next steps with simulation of osteotomies, bone movements, resections, mandibular or maxillary reconstruction using grafts, flaps and/or alloplasts and the prediction of soft-tissue changes into an interactive online web session with a professional engineering team.

For the restoration of jaw bone sections, the planning sequence is started with the placement of a virtual prosthetic tooth set-up and/or dental implant dummies to align the underlying bony reconstruction in a backward sequence (**Fig 5.3.12-4** and **Fig 5.3.12-5**). An automation of CAS/VSP procedures is within reach by the introduction of statistical shape models [Semper-Hogg et al, 2017].

The result of the planning phase is a hybrid virtual model that integrates repositioning, resection, repair and reconstruction sites in the desired dimensions, shape and location within the initial anatomical framework (**Fig 5.3.12-6a–c**).

Using this indicator model as the definitive base for treatment, the components of the toolkit are chosen and designed. Models, templates, and PSIs are generated by additive manufacturing (selective laser sintering, erroneously known as 3-D printing) (**Fig 5.3.12-6d–q**).

To manually prebend and adapt osteosynthesis plates or construct PSIs, the virtual hybrid model can be transferred into a tactile STL model. In mandibular defects, the inner side of load-bearing plates prebent in this manner are often used as an indirect guide for osteotomies and alignment of the flap or graft segments according to the former mandibular curvature. The possibility to bend reconstruction plates virtually and create templates for contouring using the actual titanium plates has been reported [Dérand et al, 2009; Rahimov et al, 2011].

Indeed, the digital workflow in craniomaxillofacial repair and reconstruction has come to full circle with the direct production of patient-specific osteosynthesis plates and implants using subtractive computerized numerical control (CNC) milling (**Fig 5.3.12-6j–o**) and/or additive layered fabrication techniques (selective laser sintering [SLS], selective electron beam melting [SEBM], fused deposition modeling [FDM]) by computer-steered machines.

The design options for templates for osteotomies and repositioning of bone elements as well as the conceivable design variants of PSIs are limited not by manufacturing techniques but only by the creativity of the treatment team and the medical engineers [Edwards, 2010].

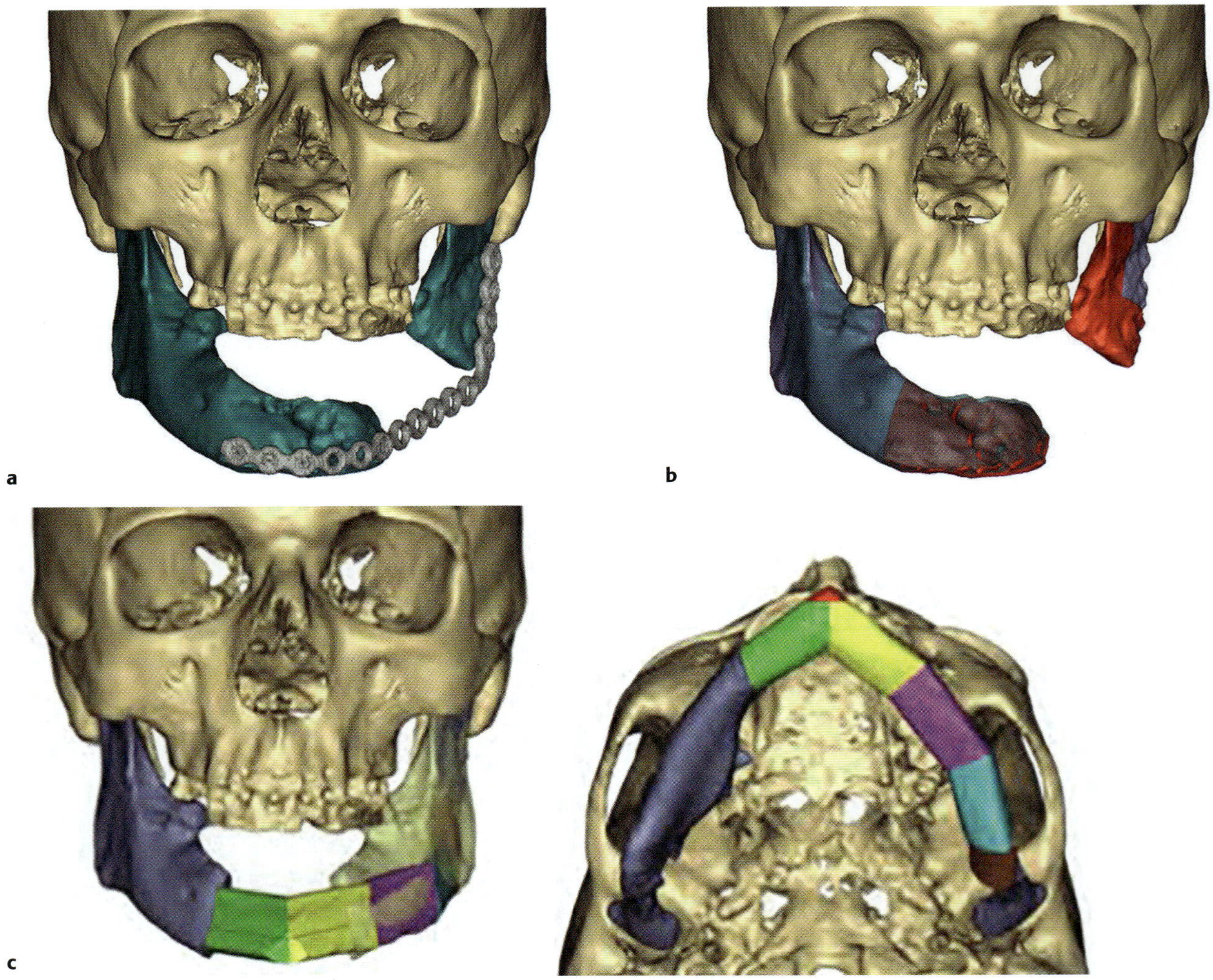

Fig 5.3.12-6a–x
Secondary mandibular reconstruction in progressing osteoradionecrosis (ORN): Virtual planning, toolkit/templates, computerized numerical control-milled patient-specific mandibular reconstruction plate (PSMRP).
Intraoperative application:

- **a** Initial model displaying a clinically exposed and loose reconstruction plate bridging a segmental defect in left mandibular body.
- **b** Virtual plate removal, repositioning of bone segments and additional resection of ORN affected bone portions.
- **c** Five fibula segments virtually placed into the mandibular continuity defect.

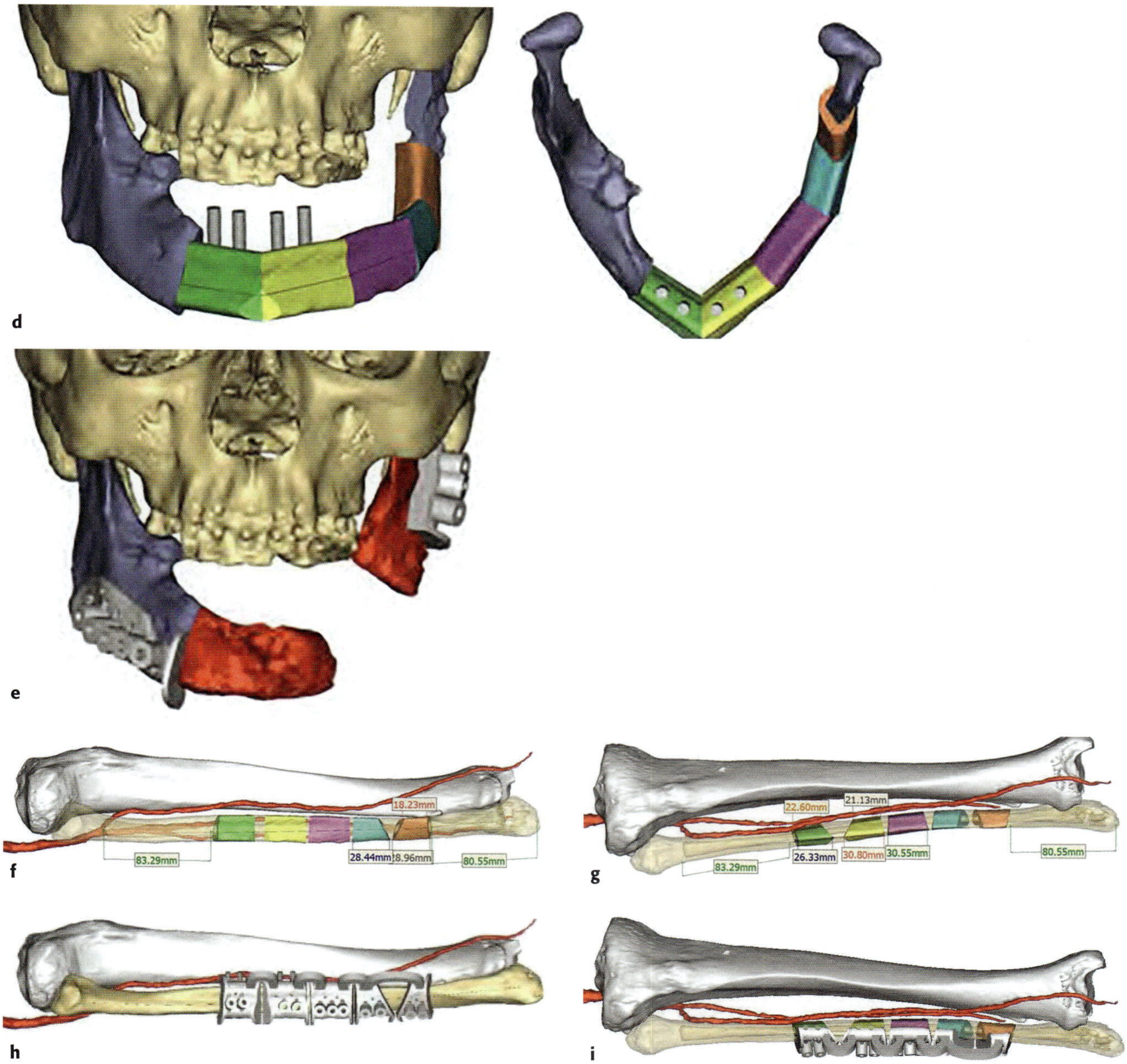

Fig 5.3.12-6a–x (cont)
Secondary mandibular reconstruction in progressing osteoradionecrosis (ORN): Virtual planning, toolkit/templates, computerized numerical control-milled patient-specific mandibular reconstruction plate (PSMRP).
Intraoperative application:

d Future dental implant insertability—dummies to evaluate adequate jaw interrelation.
e Resection guides equipped with hollow cylinders to define the screw hole positions for later fixation of the PSMRP.
f–g Bones of right lower extremity, lateral and anterior aspect, peroneal vessels and color-coded fibular segments for transfer.
h–i Design of cutting guides with flanges for harvesting the transplant with angulated ends and wedge osteotomies for subdivision.

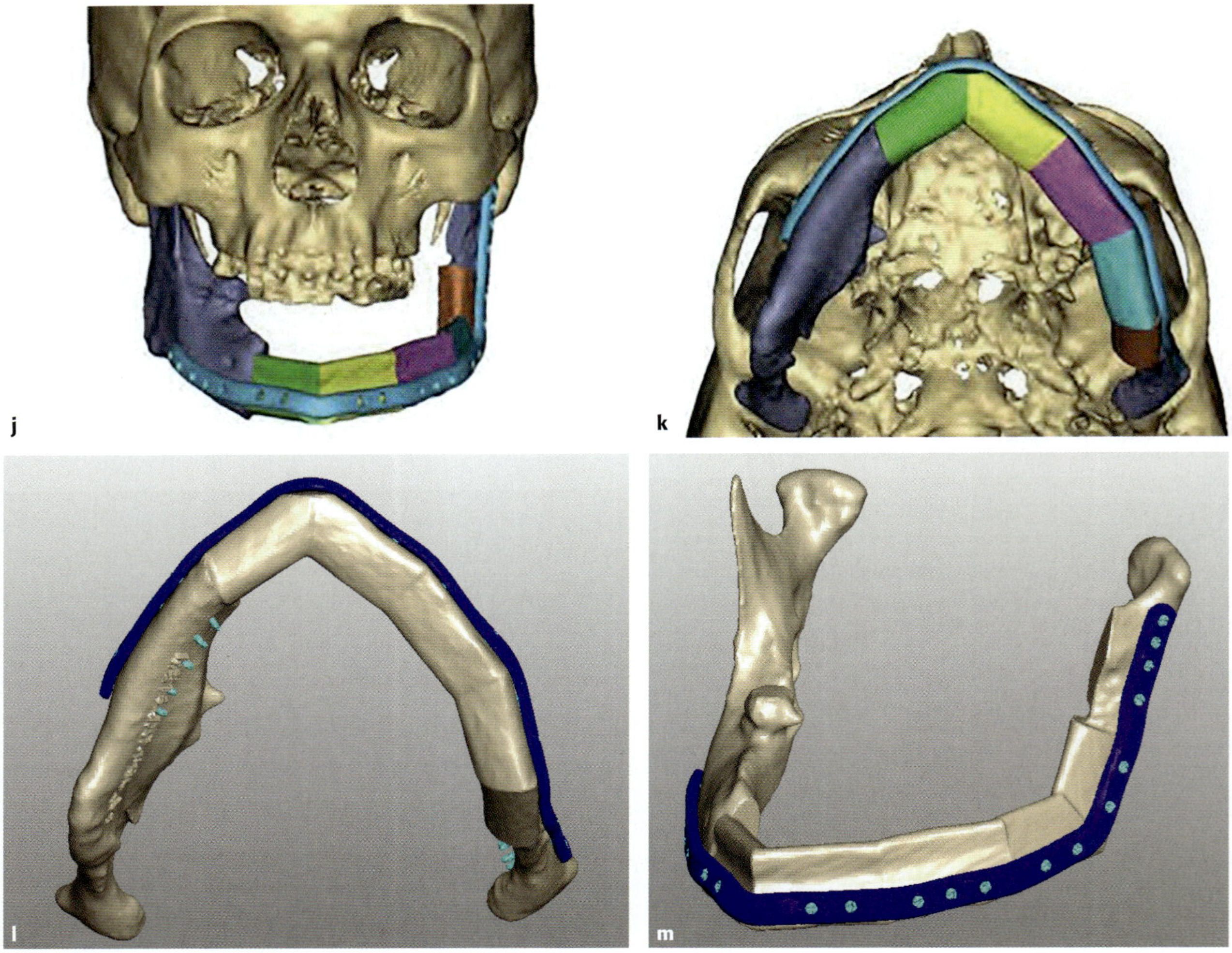

Fig 5.3.12-6a–x (cont)
Secondary mandibular reconstruction in progressing osteoradionecrosis (ORN): Virtual planning, toolkit/templates, computerized numerical control-milled patient-specific mandibular reconstruction plate (PSMRP).
Intraoperative application:
j–k PSMRP adapted to the mandible and the flap.
l–m PSMRP design and screw position.

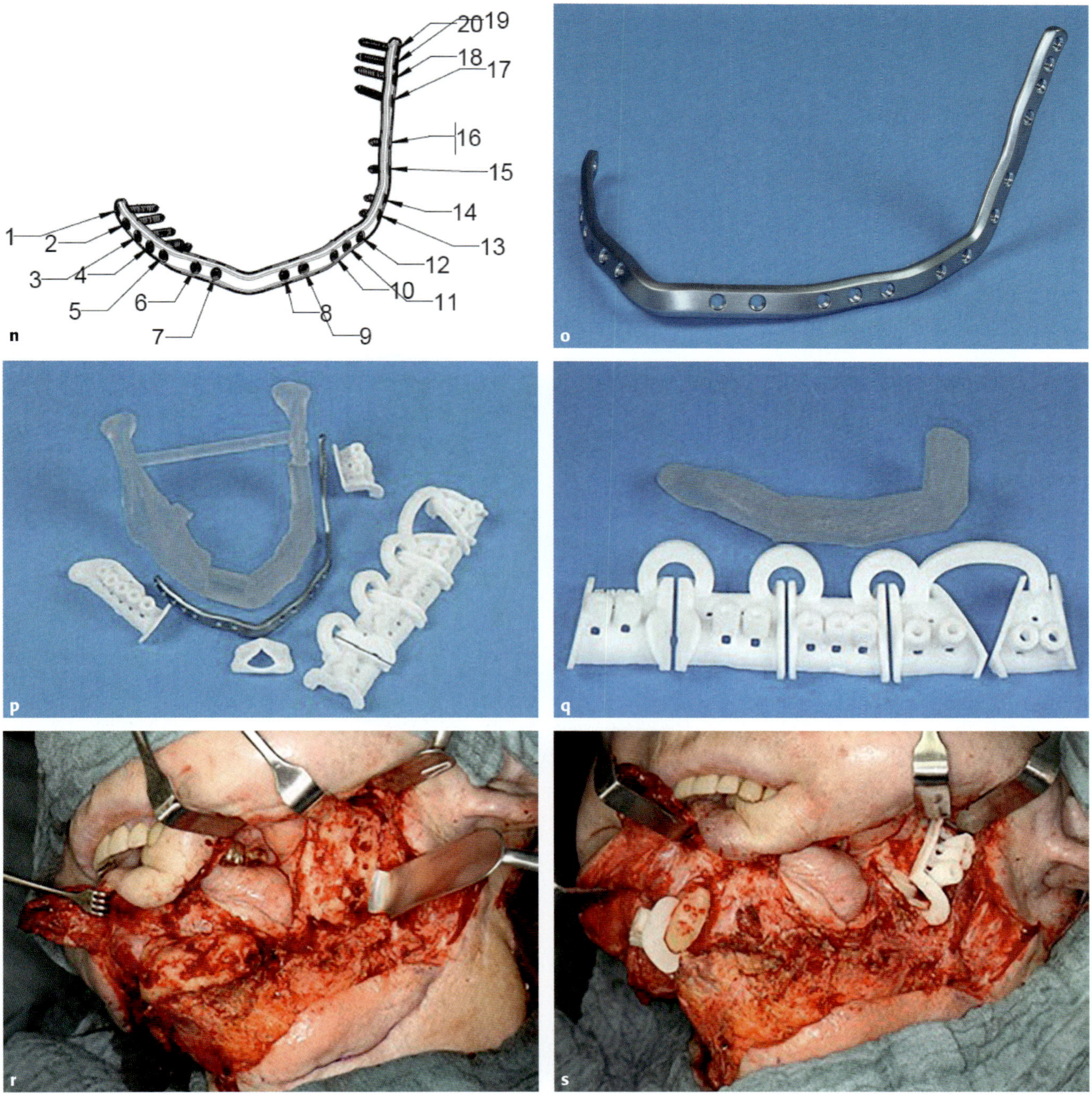

Fig 5.3.12-6a–x (cont)
Secondary mandibular reconstruction in progressing osteoradionecrosis (ORN): Virtual planning, toolkit/templates, computerized numerical control-milled patient-specific mandibular reconstruction plate (PSMRP).
Intraoperative application:

- **n** Blueprint of PSMRP and preplanned screw lengths and angulations.
- **o** PSMRP.
- **p** Guides, STL-model of the planned reconstruction and PSMRP.
- **q** STL- model of the coupled fibula segments as a separate contiguous item and corresponding fibula cutting guide in detail.
- **r** Exposed mandibular bone after plate removal.
- **s** Guided resection of ORN affected bone regions.

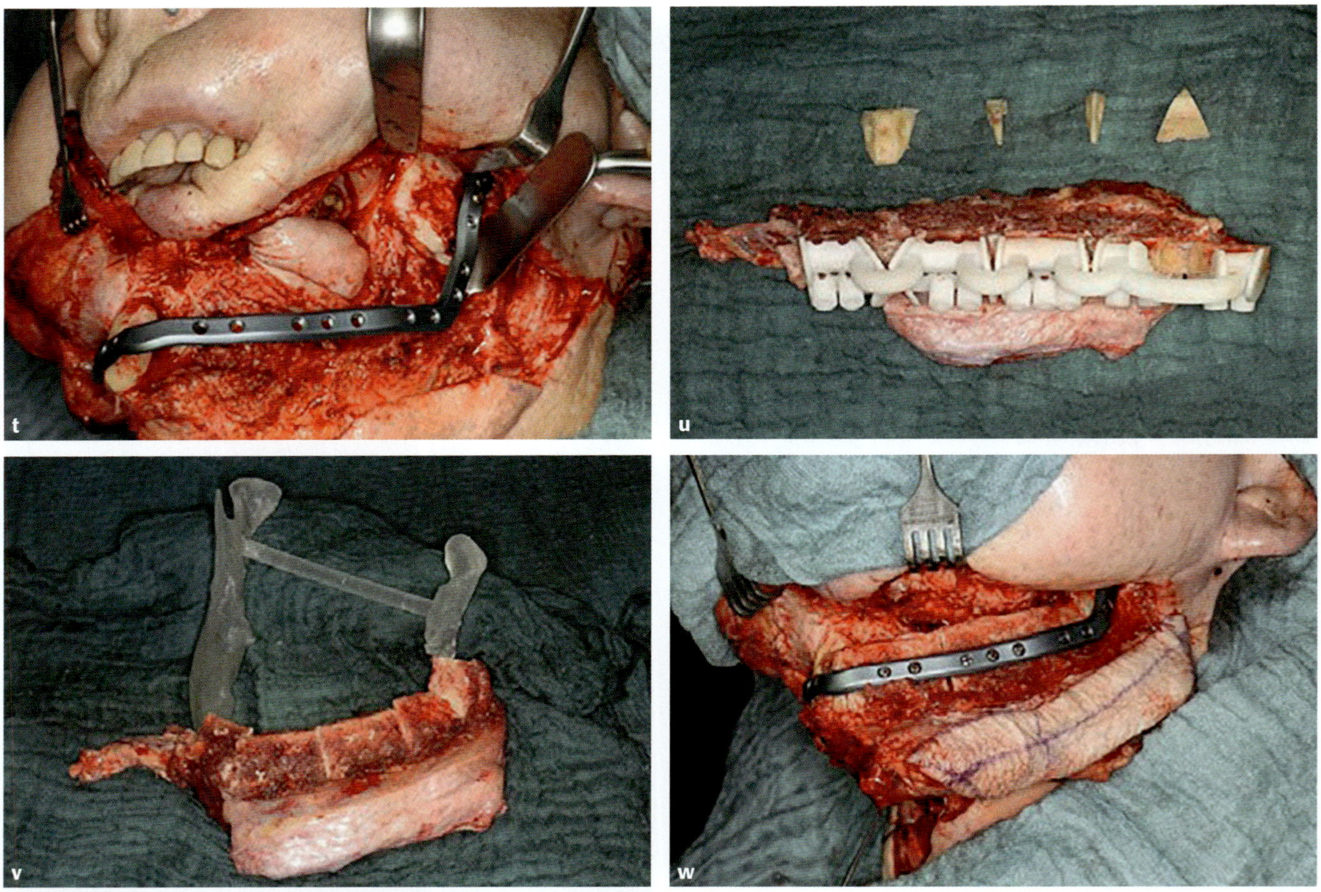

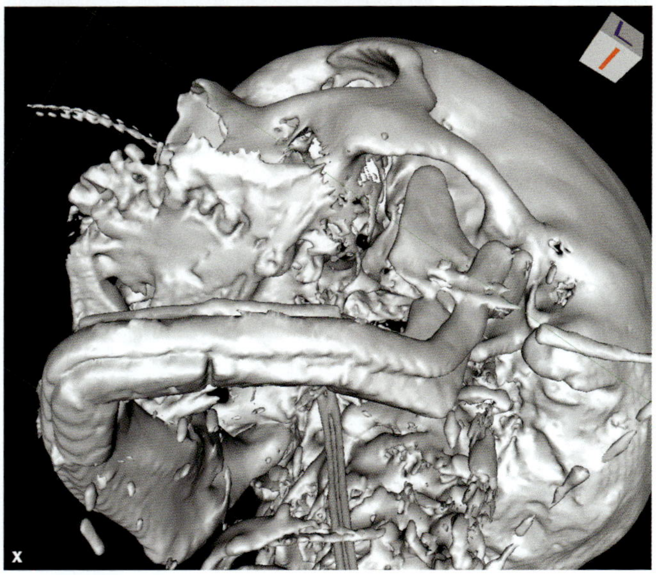

Fig 5.3.12-6a–x (cont)
Secondary mandibular reconstruction in progressing osteoradionecrosis (ORN): Virtual planning, toolkit/templates, computerized numerical control-milled patient-specific mandibular reconstruction plate (PSMRP).
Intraoperative application:

- **t** PSMRP bridging segmental mandibular defect.
- **u** Cutting guide mounted on fibula flap, wedge ostectomies completed.
- **v** Fibula segments fitted into defect of STL–mandible model for double checking.
- **w** Bone flap inset with PSMRP, intermuscular septum and skin island positioned to repair submandibular cutaneous deficit.
- **x** Postoperative CT, 3-D reconstruction.

4.1 Soft-tissue models, soft-tissues paddle/vascular pedicle position linkage

The progress in virtual analysis and surgical planning technology of bone-associated soft-tissue reconstructions has been stagnant, compared with the progress seen in bone reconstruction. The main reason for this is the difficulty to reliably determine existing soft-tissue volume and deficiencies, or the challenge of anticipating the size and configuration of defects. This is due to the lack of parameters pertinent to the deformable soft-tissue components, both at the recipient and donor site.

The factual assessment of the dynamic soft-tissue behavior (consistency, pliability, resilience, visco-elasticity and stretching capacity without compromising vascularity) is currently not amenable to practical physico-mathematical evaluation methods compared to rigid bone structures. At present, it is a matter of clinical experience and judgement.

The prediction and correlation of soft-tissue responses to skeletal movements in orthognathic surgery is an ongoing scientific endeavor where a deeper understanding of the morphological interplay is emerging through vast data processing (see chapter 5.3.13). The problem of anticipating the soft-tissue requirements in primary reconstruction (ie, configuration of skin islands and/or mucosal inner lining; dead space obliteration/volume filling with prevention of too much bulkiness) before tumor ablation in a VSP setting, however, has not been brought to a general solution.

Unlike secondary reconstruction relating to a defined defect, an immediate reconstruction demands a high level of flexibility in soft-tissue tailoring since the eventual defect dimensions may vary due to resections exceeding the planned margins because of more widespread tumor involvement. In the future, intraoperative surface scans may provide a holographic outline of the defect that can be immediately projected to the donor site.

Currently, soft-tissue models or templates in combined complex resection and primary reconstruction are still handmade in the traditional fashion based on the arbitrary delineation of the defect and consist of a plastic foam or a silastic sheet. Quantifying the congenital bone and soft-tissue volume deficits, for example in hemifacial microsomia, were often done by use of standard facial impressions, plaster of Paris casts and a diagnostic wax up. Today the same tasks are rapidly resolved by VSP technology (**Fig 5.3.12-7**). The well-established procedure of mirroring the non-affected side to the deficient side balanced by subtraction of the two superimposed face halves provides the digital basis for the fabrication of STL models.

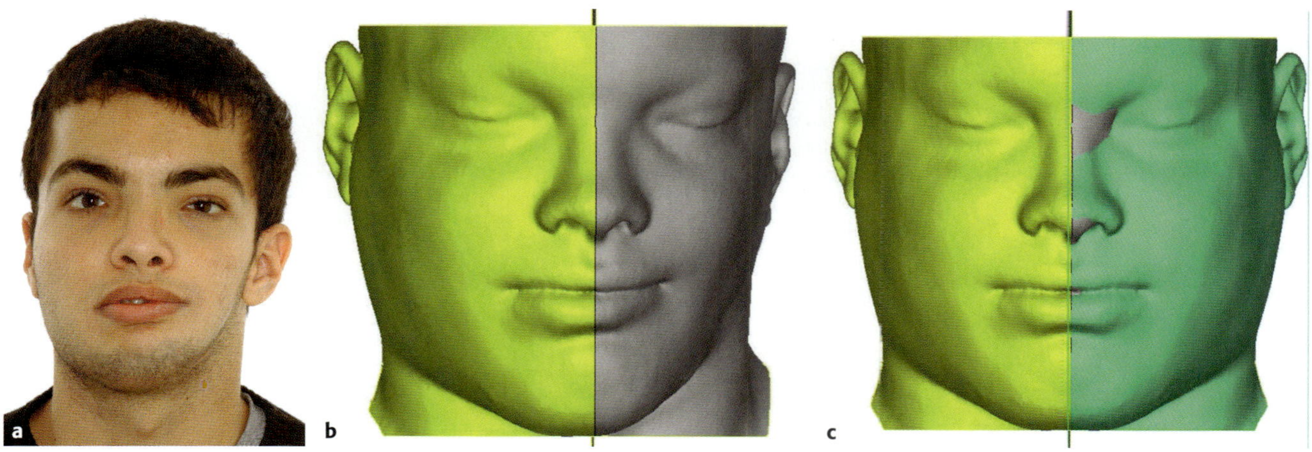

Fig 5.3.12-7a–i
Soft-tissue augmentation in hemifacial microsomia, trial VSP and STL-outcome models.
a Preoperative situation.
b Unaffected right side (yellow) and affected left side (grey) of the face.
c Mirroring along a vertical midline axis.

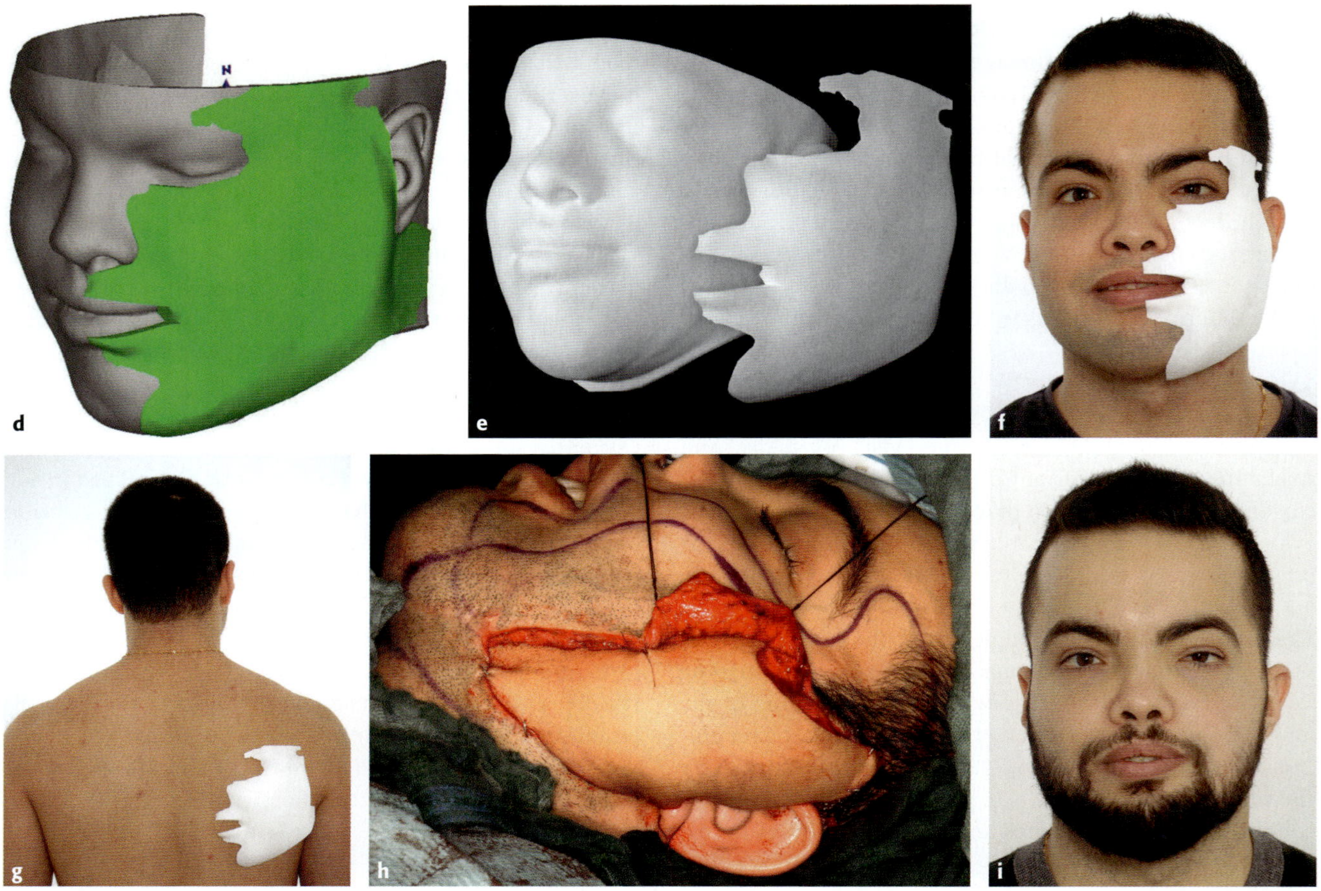

Fig 5.3.12-7a–i (cont)
Soft-tissue augmentation in hemifacial microsomia, trial VSP and STL-outcome models.

d Net volumetric difference between left and right hemiface.
e Sterilizable STL models of the asymmetric face and a mask-like 'template' representing the amount and topographic distribution of volume deficiency.
f STL model of the tissue deficit attached to patient's face.
g STL model attached to the parascapular region for design of a parascapular soft-tissue flap.
h Parascapular flap inserted before deepithelization.
i Postoperative result.

Any virtual planning of an osteoseptomusculocutaneous fibula flap transfer into a mandible or maxillary/midface defect must be oriented to the location of available recipient vessels in the neck. The donor site from the lower extremity is selected according to the following aspects [Yagi et al, 2016]:

- Position of flexor hallucis longus and tibialis posterior muscle cuff and nutrient vessels at the lingual or palatal side of the bone segments
- Orientation of the posterior intermuscular septum with the perforators to the skin paddle alongside the intraoral mucosa or external skin defect
- Length of the peroneal vascular pedicle
- Anterior or posterior exit of the peroneal vessels
- Anterior and/or lateral bone surface for application of osteosynthesis plates

Provided that the vascular trees of each leg permit fibula flap harvesting, there are four possible settings to reconstruct anterolateral mandible segments with fibula osteomusculocutaneous flaps, SB/SHB or BS/BSH–defect pattern according to Urken Classification [Urken et al, 1991].

- A fibula from the contralateral donor leg placed with the vascular pedicle exiting posteriorly below the mandibular angle brings the intermuscular septum carrying the skin paddle up to the top of the bony framework, an arrangement that comes in handy for intraoral mucosal lining.
- A fibula from the contralateral donor leg placed with the vascular pedicle into the anterior/midline direction allocates the intermuscular septum and skin paddle along the bottom of the bony framework, and is particularly suitable for coverage of cutaneous defects in the cheek or submandibular area.
- Posterior positioning of the vascular pedicle of a fibula from the ipsilateral donor leg results in a downward orientation of the intermuscular septum and skin paddle ready for closure of skin defects.
- Anterior positioning of the vascular pedicle of an ipsilateral fibula leads to an upward orientation of the skin paddle for mucosa replacement inside the oral cavity.

"Double barrel" [He et al, 2011] or "over and under barrel" arrangements in mandibular reconstructions with multisegmented osteoseptocutaneous fibula flaps raises the complexity of the procedure. Consequently, the linkage between vascular pedicle placement, the implicit flip over bone segments, the skin paddle orientation and laterality of the donor leg should be evaluated in a sketch or a provisional VSP that indicates the course of the vessels on the medial bone surface (**Fig 5.3.12-8**).

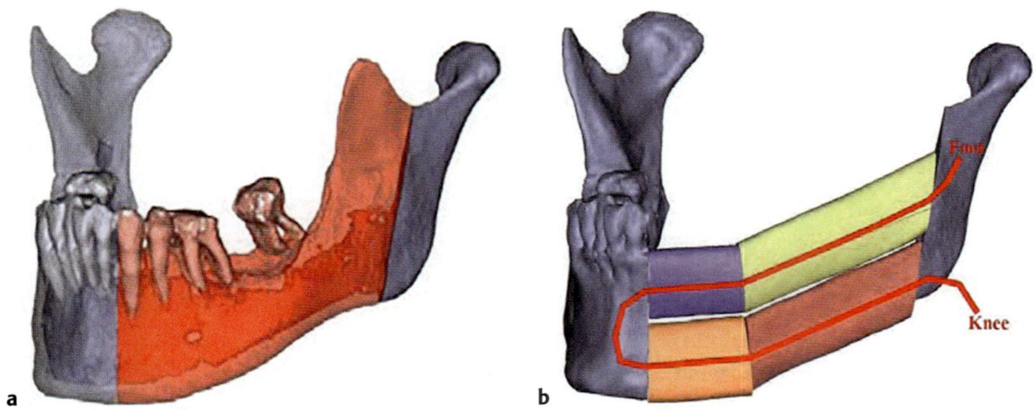

Fig 5.3.12-8a–b Virtual surgical planning of a mandible reconstruction with an osteoseptocutaneous, "over and under barrel" fibula flap.

a Vertical osteotomies for resection of the anterolateral mandibular body and anterior ramus including the coronoid process (SHBR-defect).

b "Over and under barrel" reconstruction in four (sub)segments—vascular pedicle loops along the medial/lingual bone margin emerging at the mandibular angle (knee). Consequently, the septum and skin paddle are put on the top side of the bone construct.

Amazing innovations are heralded by a report on a so-called haptics-assisted surgery planning (HASP) system that, besides the design of bone resection and transplant sub-segmentation, incorporates selection of recipient neck vessels, vascular pedicle and perforator location and skin-tissue paddle positioning in reconstructions with osteoseptocutaneous fibula flaps using stereographic and CT angiography datasets [Olsson et al, 2015]. As the name implies, the system does not only yield the information on the configuration and contouring of bone and soft tissues but also a haptic feedback on advances and stretching in the skin paddles, attached flexor hallucis longus or soleus musculature and vascular pedicles in the digital planning environment. It is not yet disclosed how patient-specific soft-tissue behavior is defined, but it will be interesting to see how this concept improves performance in special circumstances, such as preplanned augmentation.

5 Templates, treatment toolkit components

Templates are made of thin solid plastic or metal, they have a wide range of applications during surgery. They are used to control bone position in space, cut out, form and shape bone segments, as well as guide and position osteotomy lines (**Fig 5.3.12-6r–s**).

5.1 Bone models

Either STL, plaster bound, or methyl methacrylate models are suitable tools to provide a presurgical and intraoperative reference for bone-grafting procedures, both at the recipient and the donor site [Lambrecht et al, 1997; Bell et al, 2009; Hallermann et al, 2006; Lethaus et al, 2012; Antony et al, 2011]. Before actual surgery, the sequence of a surgical intervention can be rehearsed by hands-on simulation. The surgeon can use life-sized 3-D bone models to perform cuts or resections, move segments, and to prebend appropriate plates for osteosynthesis or adapt meshes and implants. Hybrid outcome models, consisting of remnants of the subunits of the native facial skeleton (mandible, midface, orbits, craniofacial transition) conjoined with the planned bony replacement parts are well-suited to customize hardware. Sterilizable models can be taken into surgery to make comparisons, and shape a graft/flap accordingly (**Fig 5.3.12-9**) and perform intraoperative measurements for a graft, flap or alloplasts, such as titanium meshes. Replicas of a bone defect are useful to correct the segmentation, orientation and fitting of a graft/flap before transfer into the real defect. They can also be used to verify if a PSI fits to the clinical situation. A unique application is to bring a copy of the defect into direct proximity of a remote donor site, and arrange the segments of a bone flap into a full-fitting replacement module while it is still connected and perfused by its vascular pedicle. Conversely, the facsimile of a contoured graft or transplant may be used as a spacer to ensure matching with the spatial dimensions of an actual defect (**Fig 5.3.12-6** and **Fig 5.3.12-9**).

5.2 Locating guides—positioning aids

Presumably, the most frequently used aid to position bone segments in craniomaxillofacial surgery are interocclusal wafers to transfer movements of tooth-bearing skeletal blocks in orthognathic or reconstructive procedures. In this context (re) positioning means to arrange skeletal parts into a defined location in space and in relation to one another (**Fig 5.3.12-10**) or to a remote or external orientation (**Fig 5.3.12-11a–c**). Once an object is fully adjusted into a position it is immobilized and secured to maintain its position. On the other hand, positioning aids come into play to guide and gauge the 3-D drilling for burr holes, eg, corresponding to plate holes (**Fig 5.3.12-12a–b**) or osseointergrated dental implants indicating the right track and position to place such objects.

An example of positioning aid applications are spacers to reposition the collapsed mandibular bone stumps and open the true defect extent in secondary reconstruction. Positioning aids help to align bone segments in the intended 3-D arrangement. They are pointers for reference to anatomical landmarks.

5.2.1 Cutting guides

The essential purpose of cutting guides is to allow for the precise 3-D location of osteotomy cuts. Such guides may not solely delineate the osteotomy line on the bone surface but can indicate the angulation and beveling of the osteotomy plane with tilted slots or flanges. Moreover, the guides can be fitted with depth stops or removable outrigger arms for soft tissue, nerve or vessel protection. The design of the guides must comply with the cutting action and the blade or drill bit characteristics (length, width, thickness, rigidity) of the power tool (reciprocating or oscillating saw, piezoelectric-powered osseous scalpel tips, drilling machine, craniotome) used by the surgeon. The cutting guide should permit copious irrigation during the osteotomy process. The cutting guides must have a sufficient contact surface, and at best are complemented with collars which embrace bone rims, angles, curvatures or notches to guarantee proper positioning. In addition, a clamp or screw fixation is needed.

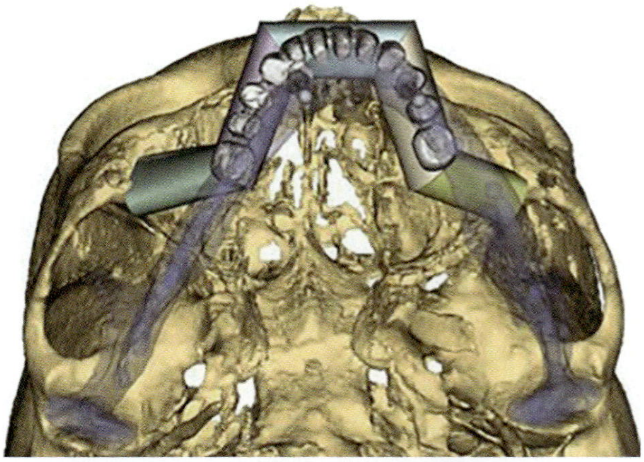

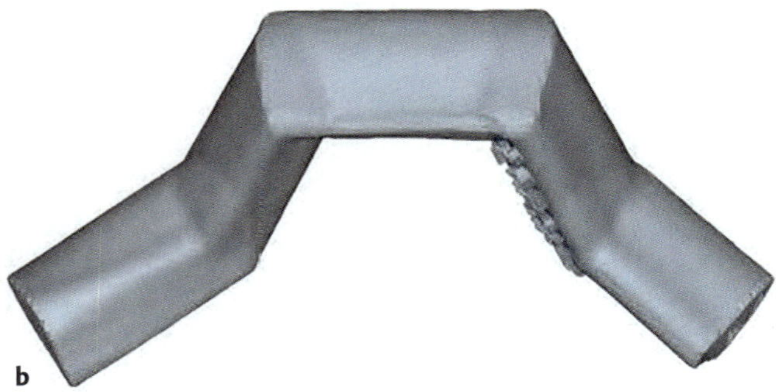

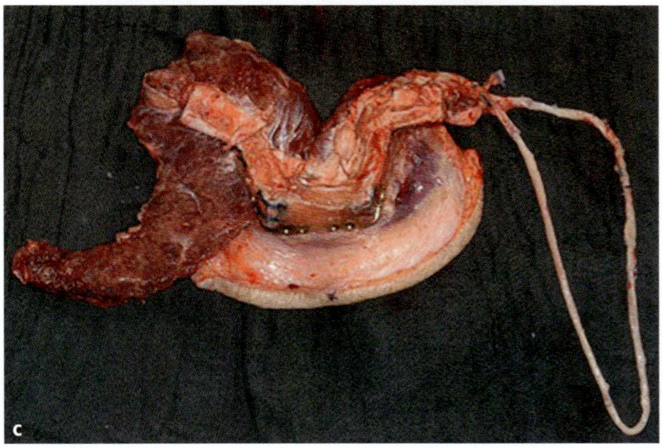

Fig 5.3.12-9a–c Total upper jaw reconstruction including the zygomaticomaxillary buttresses (Brown Class IId) using an omega-shaped fibular segment design.

- **a** Virtual planning of five fibular segments restoring the complete upper alveolar process.
- **b** STL model of the segments to double check the accuracy of fit and prebending of miniplates.
- **c** Osteofasciocutaneous fibula flap and its components before insertion into the defect: skin island for palatal resurfacing, bony segments mounted in omega assembly, peroneus brevis muscle to fill the void in the right maxillary antrum and great saphenous vein loop connected to the peroneal vessels.

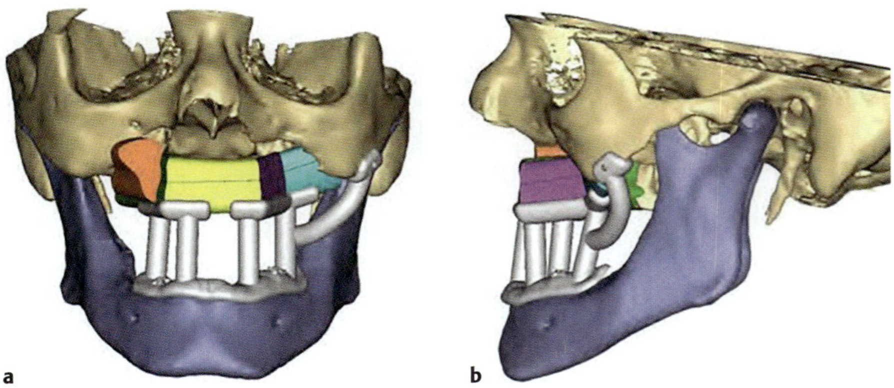

Fig 5.3.12-10a–b
Bilateral lower maxillectomy defect, edentulous mandible, bone reconstruction with fibula segments.

- **a** Design of a positioning aid with broad support in the edentulous mandible by four pillars, resembling a gunning splint, to support and position the fibula segments, frontal view [Zheng et al, 2016].
- **b** The positioning aid is equipped with an outrigger to stop the autorotation of the new mandibulomaxillary block at the zygomaticomaxillary crest and prevent telescoping into the maxillary sinus and nasal passage, lateral left view.

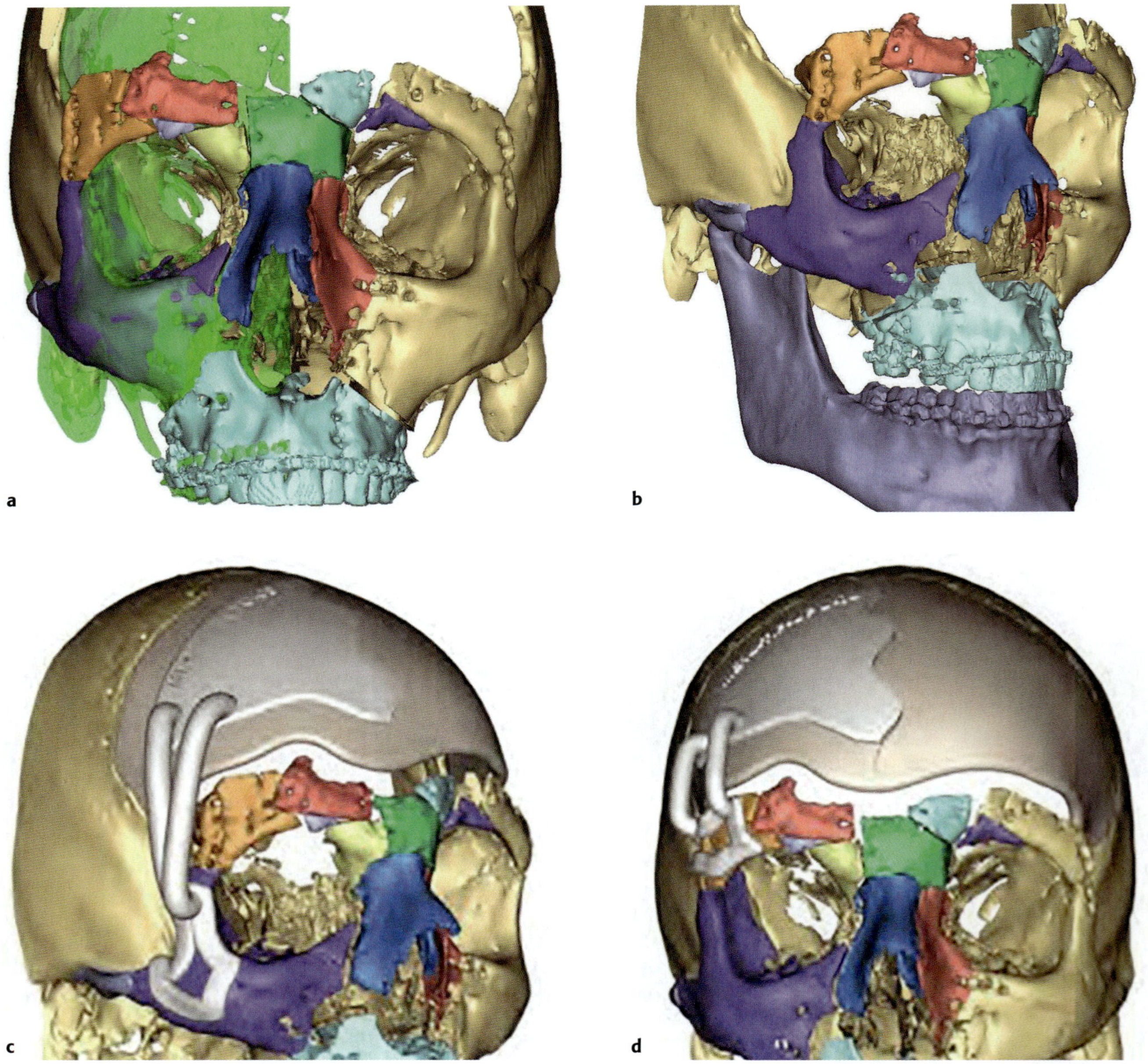

Fig 5.3.12-11a–d Secondary reconstruction of posttraumatic craniofacial deformity (midface and anterior cranial vault), replacement of the forehead with a two-piece PEEK implant and reosteotomies of the centro-lateral (right) midface. Virtual planning:

- **a** Intact portions of left midface flipped to right side (green) along vertical mirroring axis, fragments repositioned into this outline.
- **b** Forehead defect and color-coded reostomized midface segments reassembled.
- **c** Positioning aid for right zygoma—two holding arms supported on the right PEEK forehead implant in relation to its undulating midline boundary.
- **d** Equivalent device to position right superolateral orbital rim segment.

Typical areas of cutting guide applications include:

- Bone segmentation, eg, in orthognathic procedures—Le Fort I osteotomy (see chapter 5.3.13)
- Osteotomies in craniosynostosis or reosteotomies in posttraumatic deformities
- Bone resection (segmental or marginal) in tumors [Tarsitano et al, 2016] or other bone pathology [Smolka et al, 2015] (eg, osteoradionecrosis or medication-related osteonecrosis of the jaws)
- Harvesting and contouring of bone flaps or bone grafts

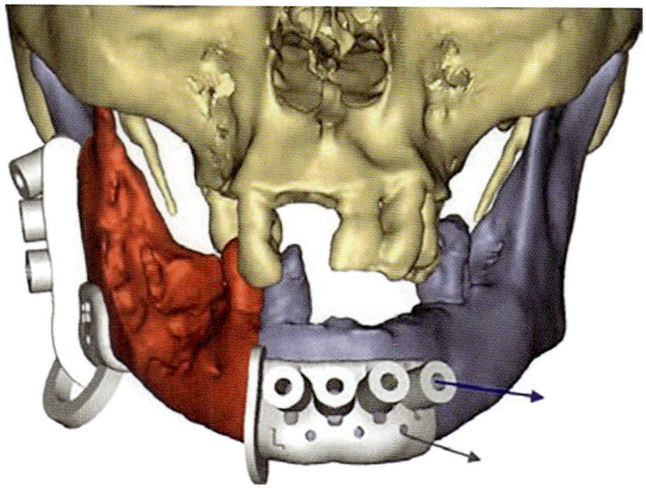

a

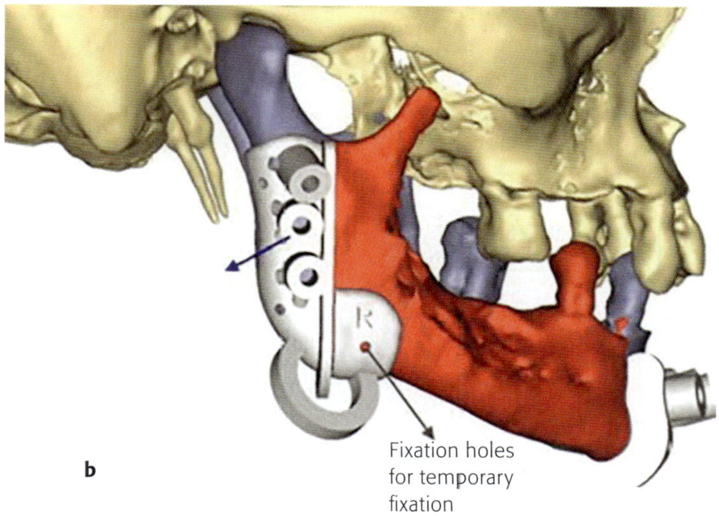

b

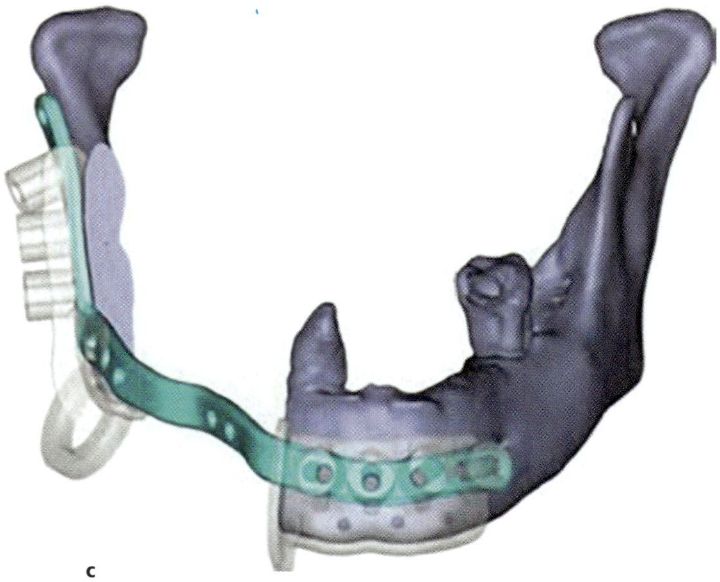

c

Fig 5.3.12-12a–c Resection guide design for removal of a right mandible segment:

- **a** Outlined resection borders with two separate resection guides. Both guides carry hollow trocar guide cylinders to place the screw holes for the PSMRP—anterior view.
- **b** The flange of the posterior resection guide conveys into a slot toward the inferior mandibular border. This results in a larger contact area yielding more reliable congruency between guide and bony surface—lateral view.
- **c** Transparent superimposition reveals interrelationship of the resection guides, the PSMRP and the bony remnants via the hollow cylinders as well as the plate and screw holes.

5.2.2 Resection guides

Segmental or marginal bone resections require osteotomies. Resection guides may come in isolated parts, in a contiguous layout as a single piece that encompasses the resection area or in multiple components interlinked with connecting bars, dovetail joints or detachable couplings (**Fig 5.3.12-13**). The removal and remodeling of hyperostotic bone formations (eg, in fibrous dysplasia, osteomas, etc) may require tangential bone resections over extended areas at a predetermined depth level. Templates in a grid square design with unpunched bar edges or additionally containing drill jig holes with depth stops at each corner point can be extended over the thickened territory to indicate the resection plane with the burr holes going to a controlled depth [Juergens et al, 2011].

Mandible

Continuity resections in the mandible are usually performed through two straight line osteotomies. To obtain free bone margins in tumor ablation, several successive slots with intermediate spacing can be incorporated into a resection guide. If necessary, the resection can be incrementally widened until the bone margins appear free of the tumor invasion. Ideally, a primary reconstruction must consist of an exact 3-D counterpart that exactly fits into the mandibular defect. The incremental approximation of the resection outline should pattern an adaptable length of bone flap, respectively, subsegments to be set into the defect. The solution is to integrate additional cutting slots at intervals into the bone graft or flap contouring templates [Cornelius et al, 2015].

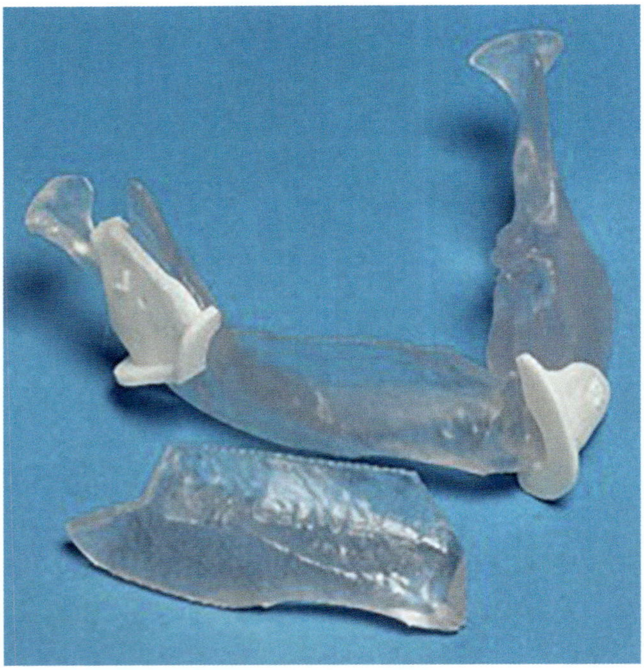

Fig 5.3.12-13 Secondary reconstruction of the mandible (SHB-Defect) with lateral scapular border:
"Toolkit components"—two separate resection guides are attached to a hybrid STL mandibular model consisting of the native bone remnants and a neomandibular division, in between. The neomandible (scapular flap) is also produced as a separate item for intraoperative use and control.

Bulky, space-occupying anterolateral tumors causing expansion of the transverse width of the mandible impose backward planning to eliminate a potential flap malposition which may result in a cross-bite situation.

The angulation of the resection osteotomies at either end of the resection can be designed to increase the bony interface with a bone graft or flap. While a conventional resection is perpendicular to the lateral mandibular surface, decreasing the angle to 60°, 45°, 30° or even less will yield increased contact areas between the graft/flap and the native mandible, creating a contact surface up to triple that of a simple right-angle joint [Haddock et al, 2012; Longo et al, 2013]. A divergent or convergent angulation of the anterior and posterior resection ends is also preferable to a parallel placement, since a rhomboid form allows for some gliding and drifting of the neomandibular segments instead of providing a restraint box with minimal tolerances. An alternative way to increase the bone-to-bone contact between the resection ends and the graft/flap is the "tongue in groove" technique. A horizontal osteotomy above the mandibular angle on one side is combined with a reciprocal step osteotomy underneath the alveolar process anteriorly [Aleid et al, 2012].

Another goal associated with mandible resection may be to avoid injury to the inferior alveolar, mental or lingual nerves. The topographic relationship of these neural structures within or adjacent to the mandible must be appreciated by the resection design. Almost any configuration of a marginal mandibulectomy [Barttelbort et al, 1991] is transferable into a cutting guide. A finite element analysis may be performed to predict if the remaining bone is robust enough to resist fractures [Narra et al, 2014]. When in doubt, protection plating with conventional, preformed or patient-specific reconstruction plates is recommended especially when adjuvant irradiation will follow.

An important prerequisite for patient-specific reconstruction plates bridging a mandibular defect is the use of conforming resection guides, which contain hollow cylinders to determine exactly the position of the plate/screw holes in the bony segments. Targeted predrilling of the screw holes through defined vectors obviates the necessity to position and mount the patient-specific mandibular reconstruction plate (PSMRP) [Wilde et al, 2014, 2015; Cornelius et al, 2015; Schepers et al, 2013, 2015]. This was formerly common in preplating techniques [Marchetti et al, 2006] and makes it possible to take the sterile plate to the donor site from the outset of the procedure. Thus, a complete module for the reconstruction can be built up independently from the ongoing tumor resection (**Fig 5.3.12-6p–s** and **Fig 5.3.12-12**). The hollow cylinders provide a mounting tube for the insertion of metal drill guide trocars.

Maxilla/midface/paranasal sinuses/naso-orbito cranial transition/cranial vault

Due to the pneumatized cavities of the paranasal sinus system and the inner nose, resections in the maxilla, midface and the internal orbit are governed by unique rules. If solid osseous structures, such as the vertical and horizontal buttresses of the maxilla, the orbital frame, the nasal skeleton, the forehead and cranial vault are mainly involved, en bloc tumor resections may be possible. Resection of tumors in the aerated cavities and cell systems including the boundary sites to the intracranial fossae and the orbits is commonly performed stepwise [Cordeiro et al, part I and part II, 2012]. Resection within the solid structures may be guided by prefabricated templates while resection within the sinus system might profit from intraoperative support by navigation systems that track the position of the surgical instruments or probes on preoperatively acquired multiplanar CT scans [Stelter et al, 2006].

Cutting guides for reconstructive procedures, harvesting and contouring of vascularized and nonvascularized flaps/grafts

The conditions of a given defect in terms of bone quantity and configuration, soft-tissue volume and coverage with external and/or internal (eg, intraoral, intranasal, etc) linings determines the selection of bone or bone containing vascularized flaps as well as nonvascularized grafts. The donor site availability and morbidity, the status of the recipient vessels, the caliber and length of the vascular pedicle and the ease of harvesting, contouring and inset must be considered for the selection of a specific bone containing flap or bone graft. Common donor site choices are fibula [Rohner et al, 2000, 2013], ilium (deep circumflex iliac artery [DCIA] flap) [Modabber et al, 2012, 2014, 2015; Thomas, 2013], scapula [Cornelius et al, 2016] and radius [Thomas et al, 2013]. The medial femoral condyle area, distal radius, ribs and the humeral shaft are also eligible but less used. Once harvested, the basic bone element of a flap or graft is contoured and may be folded using opening or closing osteotomies to conform to the resected segment pattern. Cortical osteotomies and greenstick fractures may open intersegmental gaps that should be packed using bone chips [Buchbinder et al, 1991]. The portfolio of cutting-guide designs and toolkits is being broadened continuously to cover the entire spectrum of all potential bone flaps.

Fibula

The fibula provides a linear bone rod approximately 30 cm in length with a teardrop cross-section and an outer cortical shell of substantial thickness and rigidity. Because of its periosteal blood supply, the fibula can be multiply osteotomized which allows for extensive bony reconstructions and excellent positioning. The insertability of osseointegrated dental implants into the fibular bone stock has been shown repeatedly. The fibula can be raised as a composite osteosepto- or osteomusculocutaneous flap incorporating one or several thin and pliable skin flaps based on the perforators of the peroneal artery [Fan et al, 2015]. These distinctive features make the fibula flap the workhorse in vascularized reconstruction of mandibular [Chang et al, 2014] and maxillary [Chang et al, 2004] defects. Application of the fibula for reconstruction of the supraorbital bar or the frontal sinus and forehead region are a powerful addition to its reconstructive scope [Rodriguez et al, 2008; Bluebond-Langner et al, 2009; Shipchandler et al, 2012; Lundgren et al, 2016]. Geometric simplification with a low number of osteotomies has ruled the design concept of fibular flap insets to make free-hand sculpting practicable and safe. In bilateral anterolateral mandibular defects, for instance, a two-site wedge osteotomy layout creates a three-segment reconstruction as the accepted solution. A trapezoid shape is not ideal however, since a horizontal anterior bar undoubtedly causes a "boxy" chin appearance with a loss of projection.

Three wedge osteotomies and a quadruple segmentation of the fibula permit a more parabolic mandibular design and represent a better choice replicating the anatomy of the symphysis and the anterior contours of the mandible. This is done using preformed channel type profile titanium osteotomy guides with angulated slots with average [Xu et al, 2012] or tailored SLS-cutting guides [Leiggener et al, 2009, 2015]. Determination of the exact location and angulation trigonometry of wedge osteotomies and intermediate bone pieces to be discarded is fundamental for the design of custom-made cutting templates. The fibula, analogous to a reconstruction plate, can be bent in plane or out of plane with slight additional rotational movements (pitch, roll, yaw) [Hidalgo, 1989; Hidalgo et al, 1995].

Whenever feasible the tips of the wedges are oriented toward the muscle cuff of the vascular pedicle to reduce the subperiosteal dissection adjacent to the flap vessels. To achieve enough mobility between the fibula segments, an intervening bone segment of adequate size and shape should be removed while the flexible periosteal cuff is preserved. The longitudinal orientation of such a square-shaped bone piece needs to account for the diameter of the fibula plus sufficient additional leeway to preclude kinking of the vessels. Removal of intervening bone pieces is more often required in maxillary than in mandibular reconstructions because of the more complex 3-D architecture of the midface. However, the length of a single fibular flap bone segment should not be shorter than 1.5 cm to capture a musculoperiosteal perforator and not to jeopardize the vascularization.

Fibula bone flap for mandible reconstruction

As noted above, the fibula can be folded on itself to build up a 'double barrel' mandible [He et al, 2011] with basal bone an alveolar ridge division [Lee et al, 2004] corresponding to the two arches concept of the mandible [Chen et al, 2012; Ch'ng et al, 2013]. Unlike the parabolic basal arch where the width has a direct bearing on the lower face profile and the esthetic jaw line, the upper arch forms a narrower "U shape." Thus, the posterior upper arch is shifted inward, making up for balconies overhanging to the lingual side. These balconies house the lower premolars and molars. Their 3-D position is key to dental implant-supported prosthodontic restorations. The double-barreled reconstruction, or more correctly described as an 'over and under barrel design' to restore the vertical height of the neomandible is assembled by a 180° positioning of the distal (foot) fibular segments atop the segment series along the lower border [Chang et al, 2014] (**Fig 5.3.12-8a–b**).

With the use of an osteoseptocutaneous fibula flap the eventual orientation of the skin island, for internal lining or external skin replacement, and the exit of the peroneal vascular pedicle, anteriorly or posteriorly, depend on the selection of the donor leg regarding the type of defect [Cummins et al, 2017] as well as the fact that plates and screws are applied to the lateral portion during the inset. To bridge a unilateral segmental defect with a single barrel the ipsilateral leg is chosen for flap harvest to place the skin paddle externally into the submental/submandibular region and the proximal bone end including the vascular pedicle posteriorly. Raising the flap from the contralateral leg will bring the skin island into the oral cavity and the vascular pedicle posteriorly. Turning the long axis of a fibula flap either from the ipsilateral or the contralateral leg 180° around like a propeller will produce just opposite associations.

The fibula for a single barrel reconstruction in symphyseal or anterolateral defects can be raised from either leg and rotated subsequently for the internal or external placement of skin paddle, on the condition that recipient vessels are available on both sides of the neck. Otherwise the final selection of the donor leg is according to the criteria outlined in section 4.1.

In hemimandibular defects the distal fibula segment is commonly used to replace the ascending ramus and condyle, and directs the vascular pedicle along with the horizontal segments anteriorly, precluding the need for additional length of a pedicle looping back down into the neck. Corresponding to this spatial layout, the fibula is procured from the contralateral lower extremity to place the soft-tissue island intraorally and from the ipsilateral limb to accommodate the skin island into the upper neck or lower face [Stirling et al, 2015]. The fibula provides appropriate length to reconstruct an anatomical hemimandible with over and under barrels of the body and parasymphysis to include a single barrel condylar process after exarticulation. This is significantly facilitated by virtual planning and bone-cutting guides [Wang et al, 2013; Deek et al, 2016] (**Fig 5.3.12-8a–b**).

With an increasing number of fibula segments mimicking the 3-D curvatures in the mandible, the complexity of the design of the osteotomies becomes exponentially difficult if done freehand [Hanasono et al, 2013]. Each deviation triggers a chain reaction of incongruencies and malalignment. Cutting guides bring accuracy into this process and eliminate any intraoperative guesswork [Quaisi et al, 2016].

The accuracy of fibula flap mandible reconstruction has been confirmed by superimposition of the virtual planning and computer models of the final reconstruction [Roser et al, 2010; Zheng et al, 2012; Modabber et al, 2012; Foley et al, 2013; Seruya et al, 2013; Metzler et al, 2014; Ciocca et al, 2015; Mascha et al, 2015; Hanken et al, 2015; Wang et al, 2016; Weitz et al, 2016; Yu et al, 2016] as well as overall functional assessment by axiographic test series [Ritschl et al, 2017]. Patient-specific mandible plates in a basal or lingual position [Probst et al, 2016] expands possibilities for flap insetting.

Fibula bone flap, cutting guides for maxillary/midface reconstruction

With increasing amounts of horizontal and vertical bone loss the restoration of the maxillary alveolar ridges, the midfacial buttresses and orbital rim framework becomes increasingly demanding [Cordeiro et al, 2000; Brown et al, 2010; Hanasono et al, 2010, 2013]. In accordance with the pattern of a horizontal palatomaxillary defect, the alveolar arch is replaced unilaterally (Brown Class Ib), anteriorly (Brown Class Ic) or circumferentially (Brown Class Ic) (see chapter 3.2; Fig 3.2-2) with a U-shaped fibular construct or appropriate subunits. The absence of the pterygoid plates can impede the untilted 3-D seating of a full arch reconstruction, in this case the reconstruction may benefit from positioning guides (**Fig 5.3.12-10a–b**). A bilateral palatomaxillary defect extending along the naso- and the zygomatico-maxillary buttresses (Brown Class IId) requires an omega-assembly of the neomaxillary segments to reestablish a mechanical connection by means of the transverse cantilever arms reaching up into the zygomatic bodies [Hanasono et al, 2010; Shen et al, 2012; Wang et al, 2016] (**Fig 5.3.12-9**).

A simple reconstructive option for a limited unilateral defect (Brown Class IIa) may consist of two-level or over and under arrangement of fibular segments. This configuration obliterates the maxillary sinus and rebuilds both the anterior and lateral vertical pillar system. With the omega assembly, the anterior vertical buttress and the nasal sidewall is either reconstructed with an additional free bone strut or filled with soft-tissue components.

The bony buttresses in vertical palatomaxillary defects involving the orbit with or without retention of the orbital contents (Brown Class III or IV), the zygoma and the superolateral orbital rims (Cordeiro Class IV) can be built up with the fibular segments layered, stacked upon each other or put into a semicircular or curved shape. Mirror image planning based on the unaffected side displays a skeletal boundary line model within which a secondary fibula reconstruction can be patterned. The intermediate segments of such a supporting beam and bar construct may need radically flipping of the segments into deviating axes to create 3-D frameworks providing an infraorbital and/or lateral orbital rim, a cheek prominence and an alveolar arch suitable for dental rehabilitation. Still, the vascular pedicle needs to run a continuous uninterrupted course as the indispensable lifeline of the construct. Multisegmentation extending over the whole length of the fibula reduces the reach of the peroneal vascular pedicle to the recipient vessels. A saphenous vein loop (**Fig 5.3.12-9c**) or a flow through radial forearm free flap will provide the required length to approach the temporal or the neck vessels for microvascular anastomoses of the fibula flap. Use of a radial forearm flap might be advantageous in complex 3-D defects with specific soft-tissue requirements. Deepithelialized, it can supply inner nasal or sinus lining and without deepithelialization external soft-tissue lining. The orbital walls, in the inferomedial circumference, are reconstructed with titanium meshes (preformed or PSI) or bone grafts (calvarial outer table, split rib or split fibula segments).

After removal of the orbital roof, fontal sinuses and frontal cranial vault with exposure of the cranial base, dura and brain, an autogenous reconstruction using a vascularized tissue transfer to fill the dead space to effectively seal the cranial cavity from the paranasal sinuses and skin is usually needed.

Vascularized anterior iliac crest, flap, deep circumflex iliac artery (DCIA) flap

The unique shape and natural curvature of the anterior ilium resembles the native hemimandible [Taylor, 2016]. The large amount of available robust cortical and cancellous bone is also suitable to restore maxillectomy (central or lateral) and midface defects [Brown, 1996; Shaw et al, 2009]. All variants of composite flaps based on the DCIA and its commitant veins are called DCIA flaps. The flaps of interest here are bone containing, although DCIA flaps without iliac crest have been described. An iliac crest bone flap is harvested with a small muscular cuff on the inside of the bone curvature containing portions of iliacus and optionally the three layers of abdominal muscles (external oblique, internal oblique and transversus abdominis muscle), which are traversed by the nutrient DCIA vessel system [Ting et al, 2011] (see chapter 1.1). In the common variant, the DCIA extends from the external iliac artery toward the anterior superior iliac spine (ASIS) to continue its course within the groove between the surface of the iliacus muscle and the medial margin of the iliac crest just underneath the transverse fascia [Thein et al, 1997; Ghassemi et al, 2013]. Along its way to the posterior ileum, an array of osteomusculocutaneous perforators arise from it [Bergeron et al, 2007]. The skin flap overlying the iliac crest that has been conventionally used is relatively fixed to the bone, often bulky and considered poorly reliable because it is nourished by minute terminal twigs of the same perforators responsible for the osseous supply [Zheng et al, 2013]. A large ascending arterial branch bifurcates near the ASIS and pierces the transverse muscle to travel a cephalad course on the undersurface of the internal oblique muscle. The transfer of the thin and pliable internal oblique muscle as a pedicle island or apron flap tied to the inner table of the iliac crest has been proposed for intraoral lining [Urken et al, 1989].

Along the crestal bow, the bone has a thickness of at least 2 cm. The ilium bone stock can be approached and sectioned from the lateral aspect after the upper origin of the medial and minimal gluteal muscles have been detached from the outer bone table. In contrast to the cross-cuts for segmentation of the fibula, intricate curved or even irregular cuts are made to create a primary form in the best possible approximation to the dimensions and shape of the defect in the mandible, maxilla or midface [Modabber et al, 2014]. Once this overall bone segment is isolated (leaving a notch in the iliac crest) it will be further sectioned, carved and shaped for a precise fit into the defect.

DCIA flap for mandibular reconstruction

Common algorithms and virtual planning to select the proper side on which to raise a DCIA flap to restore the mandible and related structures [Yu et al, 2016; Zhang et al, 2016] take into consideration:

- The tissue composition—musculo-osseous, musculo-osseous including internal oblique muscle, or osteo-musculo-cutaneous—to meet with the surgical requirements.
- DCIA vessel anatomy and architecture and presence of ramifications.
- The relative short vascular pedicle with the need to orient it in direct proximity to the recipient vessels.
- Use of a bicortical or a split inner table bone component.
- Inclusion of anterior superior iliac spine (ASIS) and/or anterior inferior iliac spine (AIIS) or window-type bone harvest.
- The decision whether to use the natural crest of the anterior ileum or the osteotomized inferior surface of the flap to reconstruct the alveolus. This has direct influence on the decision from which side to harvest.
- The anterior or posterior exit of the donor vessels from the flap into the neck.
- Exclusive use of the lateral iliac bone surface for application of osteosynthesis plates.
- Need for additional contouring through supplemental vertical osteotomies. This applies particularly to anterior and anterolateral mandibular subregions.
- The attachment and maneuverability of the skin paddle and internal oblique muscle.
- Interarch and occlusal relationships.

In ablative procedures with primary reconstruction, the extent of mandibular resection is predetermined. The bone segment which is planned for resection is projected and moved along the usable bone zone of the lateral surface of the ilium until the position with the most congruent match of the curvatures is detected [Ayoub et al, 2014; Ghassemi et al, 2016]. The eventual flap-cutting guide design is made based on all information listed above.

In secondary reconstructions based on backward planning, defects are replenished with mirror inverted intact counterparts and/or a size-matching replica from a virtual library to render visualization of the size, shape and angulation of the missing mandibular area, as reference for the DCIA flap bone design. The most frequently used technique to contour and angulate iliac bone flaps are opening osteotomies. The outer cortex and the adjacent cancellous layer of a longitudinal bone portion running along the crest are split vertically at a single site or in a series of osteotomies to bend the ilium by cracking or bending the inner cortex, thus opening the angulation. With this technique, the medially located vascular pedicle is efficiently protected. The V-shaped gaps are then filled with cancellous bone chips also harvested from the iliac donor site. A defect size up to half of the mandible can be reconstructed with iliac crest segments from one side. To reconstruct a hemimandible, the ASIS and AIIS may be incorporated to replace the ramus and condylar process. While the natural curvature of the iliac bone yields substantial congruity with the mandibular angle and body region, it will usually require several opening osteotomies to be bent into the parabolic arch form of the anterior symphyseal area. In terms of vertical dimension, the usable iliac bone stock is suitable to rebuild a full height of an adult dentate mandibular arch, offering enough width for the insertion of endosseous dental implants. Concomitantly, the extent of vertical bone height and width provides ample contact between the bone flap and the native mandible.

The use of a toolkit of resection guides, transplant cutting guides, and STL models of the mandible (displaying the defect and the sculpted transplant) offer an ideal back up for rapid performance of a mandibular reconstruction with the highest accuracy. After exposure of the bone surfaces at the donor site and the vascular pedicle, the cutting guide is applied to the bare lateral surface of the ilium and fixed with miniscrews [Modabber et al, 2012, 2015]. The bony portion of the flap is finally cut out taking care to preserve the vascular pedicle. The posterior as well as the anterior osteotomies in the pelvis correspond to the height of the neomandible, the inferior osteotomy to the longitudinal extent. Both the plan and the compatible vertical slots in the cutting guide allow the bone portion to be subsegmented further along its length, fit into the defect model and supplied with osteosynthesis hardware to assemble a module for easy inset into the mandibular defect, being still connected via its vascular pedicle (**Fig 5.3.12-14**).

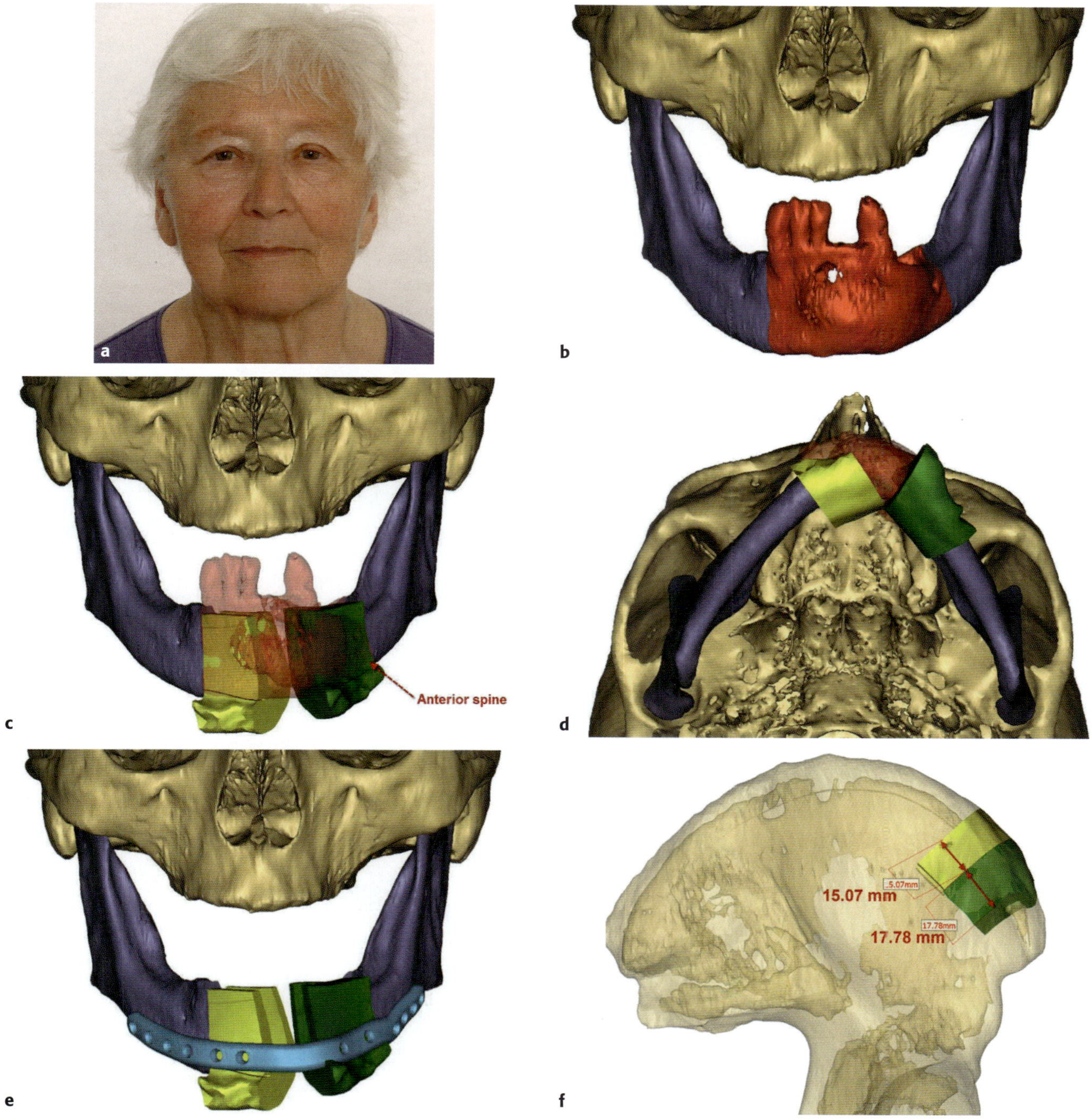

Fig 5.3.12-14a–q Chin resection and reconstruction in a patient with an ameloblastoma.

a Preoperative.
b Outlined resection in a 3-D reformatted computed tomography.
c Virtual reconstruction planning with an osteomuscular iliac bone flap with anterior opening osteotomy.
d Virtual opening osteotomy and bone flap fit seen from below.
e Virtual design of a patient specific reconstruction plate.
f Required bone segment from the anterior ileum with osteotomy line for an opening osteotomy.

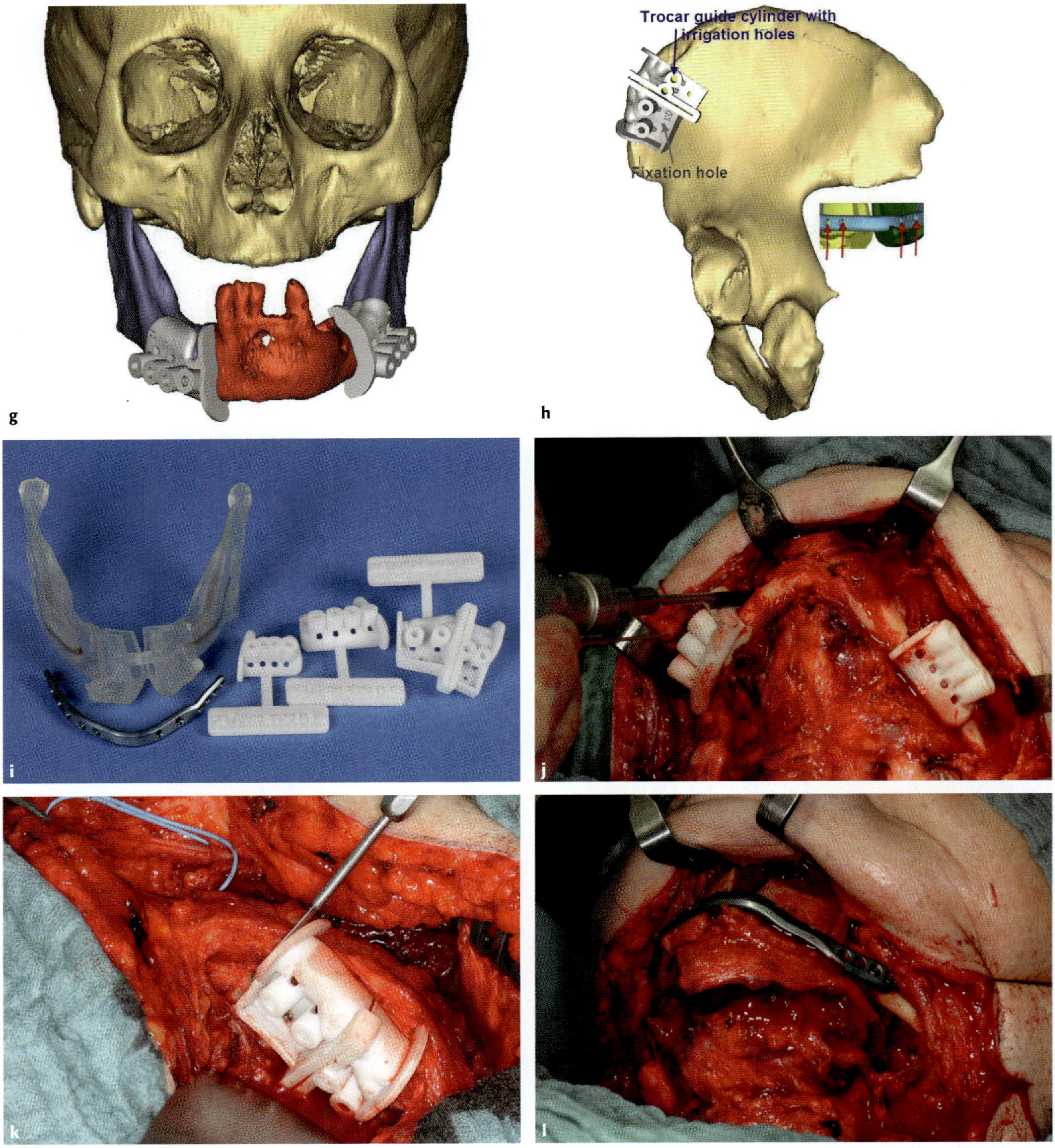

Fig 5.3.12-14a–q (cont) Chin resection and reconstruction in a patient with an ameloblastoma.

- **g** Virtual resection guides with predetermined protruding holes for trochar placement to define the screw holes for the reconstruction plate.
- **h** Bone flap harvesting guide with protruding holes for later trochar placement and fixation holes that are used to fix the guide to the ileum during the harvesting process.
- **i** Hardware toolkit produced for the planned operation. Resection guides, flap harvesting guide, patient specific reconstruction plate, and STL model with chin reconstruct.
- **j** Resection guides fixed to the mandible after neurolysis of the left mental nerve, chin resection in progress.
- **k** Flap harvesting guide fixed to the anterior ileum. The relatively short flap allows for preservation of the anterior iliac spine.
- **l** Iliac bone flap inserted and attached to a PSMRP.

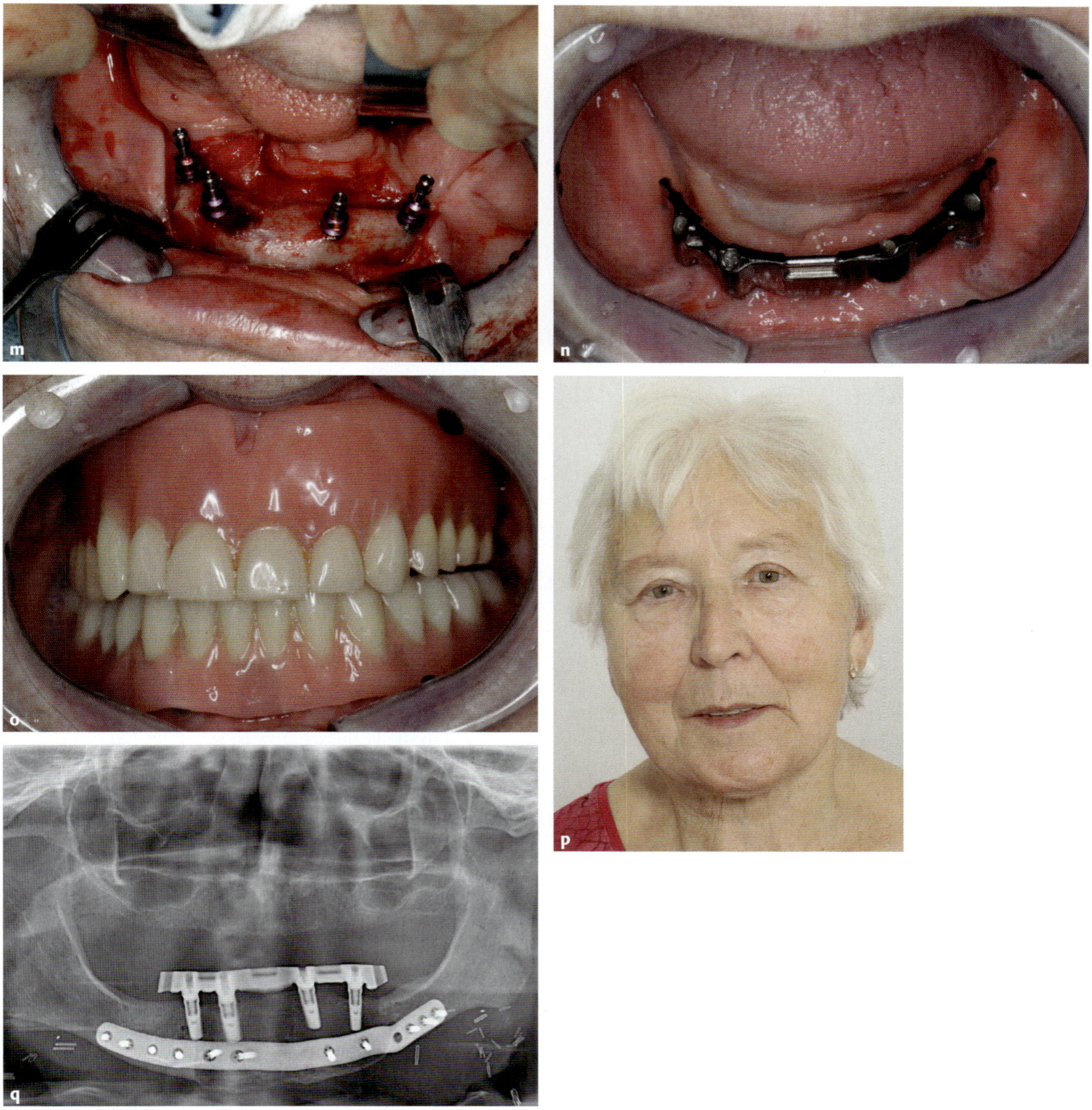

Fig 5.3.12-14a–q (cont) Chin resection and reconstruction in a patient with an ameloblastoma.
m Second stage placement of dental implants into the flap.
n Bar to support the denture.
o Dentures in place.
p Patient after mandible reconstruction and prosthodontic rehabilitation.
q Postoperative orthopantomogram.

DCIA flap for maxillary reconstruction

Modifications of the DCIA flap are suitable for reconstruction within the entire range of horizontal and vertical maxillectomy defects (Brown Class I–V). Put into an upside down frontal position the natural curvature of the outer table of the ipsilateral iliac crest compares with the anterior surface of the maxilla and midface [Brown, 1996; Grinsell et al, 2015]. The ASIS of the DCIA flap or a cut angle posterior to it will become the new maxillary tuberosity and the vascular pedicle will point posteriorly to be connected to the facial or temporal vessels. Loss of suprastructures (zygomatic body, infrorbital rim and orbital floor) can be compensated by the vast proportions and quantity of the iliac bone. Various amounts of the iliacus muscle and the internal oblique island may be used to fill the orbit, the maxillary sinus medial to the restored alveolar process and/or to cover a palatal defect.

Application of the cutting guide design for DCIA flaps for maxillary defects does not differ from the variation for mandibular reconstruction. Additional opening osteotomies are usually not necessary; however, the iliac bone transplant once fixed in the maxilla and midface may need in situ trimming and sculpting to create an adequate shape.

Scapula, flaps containing bone from the lateral border and tip

The volume of vascularized bone from the lateral scapular border and/or inferior angle or tip is limited, but the simultaneous availability of extended soft-tissue components on the subscapular vascular axis provides valuable reconstructive options for composite head and neck defects [Swartz et al, 1986; Holle et al, 1996; Nkenke et al, 2009; L'Heureux-Lebeau et al, 2013; Mitsimponas et al, 2014]. The osseous flap component can be raised as a single flap entity from the infraglenoid lateral scapular border supplied by the circumflex scapular vessels, or from the scapular tip region with the vascular feed via an angular branch coming from the thoracodorsal vessels [Seneviratne et al, 1999]. A bipedicled bone flap formation based on each of the two vascular branches requires the surgeon to enclose the subscapular trunk ahead of its bifurcation [Coleman et al, 1991]. The muscle cuff consisting of the infraspinatus, teres minor/major and subscapularis portions around the lateral scapular border must be preserved to maintain the periosteal blood supply.

The fundamental need for this muscular cover layer interferes with the direct application of cutting guides to the posterior bone surface. If transverse osteotomies of the bone for sub-segmentation are required, the muscular cover layers must be elevated from the medial side to access the bone sandwiched between them. This osteotomy usually will be confined to the region above the transitional vascularization zone that lies between the territories of the circumflex scapular and angular vessels. The bone stock along the lateral scapula is not uniform, with the thickest portion in a short section below the infraglenoid tubercle, then tapering off and partially twisting toward the tip region where it narrows substantially. Preservation of the muscular envelope even in the transitional zone is necessary for a singular vascular pedicle transfer of the border and tip subsegments. These specific conditions led to the development of sophisticated biplanar cutting guides that consist of a frame and a vertical rod rider used in a plug on mode (**Fig 5.3.12-15d**) [Cornelius et al, 2016].

This type of SLS cutting guide provides access to the lateral scapular border and tip from two perpendicular planes. In the first step, the infraspinatus muscle is incised to open either a through shaped or right-angled corridor space along the blank bony surface over the posterior side of the scapula. This space consists of a longitudinal pathway about 2–3 cm parallel to the lateral scapular border with a lateral cross-connection below the infraglenoid tubercle and another lateral transverse or posterior linear extension above or medial to the scapular tip for the placement of the framework part of the cutting guide. The framework makes up a template that rests on two footplates at the cranial and caudal ends held to the bone by screw fixation. Each of these footplates contains a connector socket to accommodate a removable vertical rod rider spanning the entire vertical length of the bone flap. The initial cut out of the bone segment encompasses the footplates. The final cut out proceeds inside the caudal and cranial footplates only after the wedge ostectomies for subsegmentation have been accomplished. For this next step, the rod rider component of the cutting guide equipped with one or two hovering pairs of slots and/or flanges is plugged on. It is convenient to continue the subsegmentation on a side table, after ligation of the vascular pedicle and total mobilization of the entire flap. The transition zone between the lower lateral border and the tip of the scapula can be approached from the posterior aspect and divided by means of the rider extensions, eg, flanges into bipedicled subsegments following the transsection of the muscle cuff. Finally, the vertical rod rider component is lifted off the framework and the twofold subsegmentation is completed with transverse cuts along the inside of the upper and lower footplates. The scapula subsegment assembly is then ready to be folded for a counter-check inside the maxillary defect of the STL model.

Scapular tip for maxillary reconstruction

The bone from the tip of the scapula and the hard palate including the upper alveolar arch bear a strong resemblance in shape and dimensions. The palatal shelf can be reconstructed from half size to the total palate with a segment from the scapular tip molded in a single segment "tray-like" manner if the maxillary suprastructure and the pterygoid process structures are preserved and can provide a stable autogenous linkage. There are two options to reestablish a sustainable connection to the suprastructure. One way is stabilization by additional subsegments which run like roof rafters and beams to contact the adjoining midface pillars superiorly or with the pterygoid process posteriorly (**Fig 5.3.12-15b** and **Fig 5.3.12-15i**). The second solution is manufacturing a specific metal supporting platform (**Fig 5.3.12-15e** and **Fig 5.3.12-15j–m**). Virtual planning, design and production of the template toolkit and PSI follows the principles and tracks outlined above.

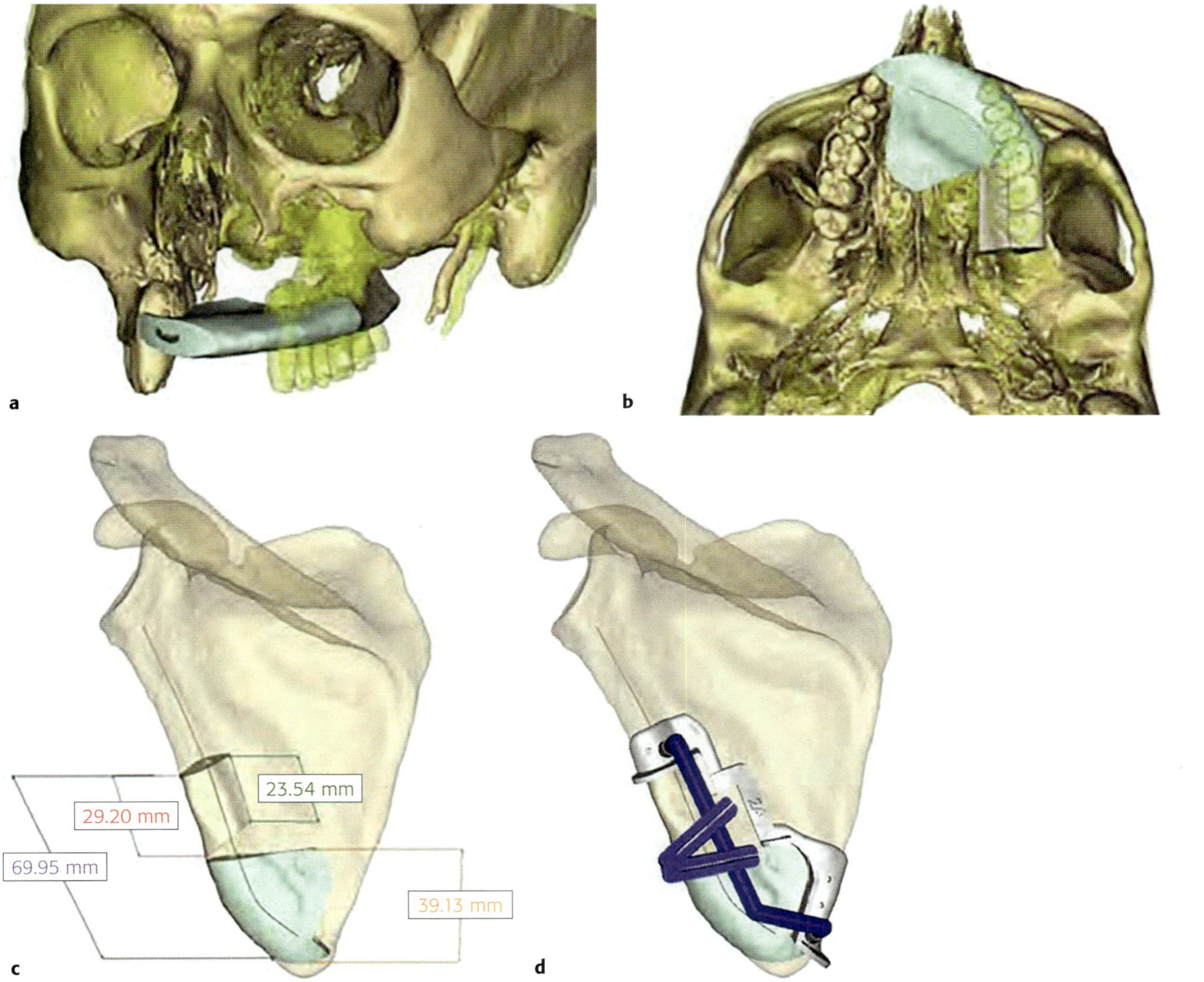

Fig 5.3.12-15a–x Hemimaxillary reconstruction with a scapular bone flap.

- **a** Maxillary reconstruction planning (Brown Class IId defect) with a bone flap from the lateral scapular border and tip
- **b** Virtual plan after mirroring intact contralateral side. Scapular tip as anterior palatal shelf and lower lateral border for posterior support toward pterygoid process, no direct link to remaining suprastructure.
- **c** Posterior view of left scapula, two-color coded subsegments projected on the infraglenoid margin and tip.
- **d** Two-part cutting guide design, posterior view, outer framework (grey-whitish) housing the margins of the complete scapula segment and plug-on rod rider with a slot extension (dark blue).

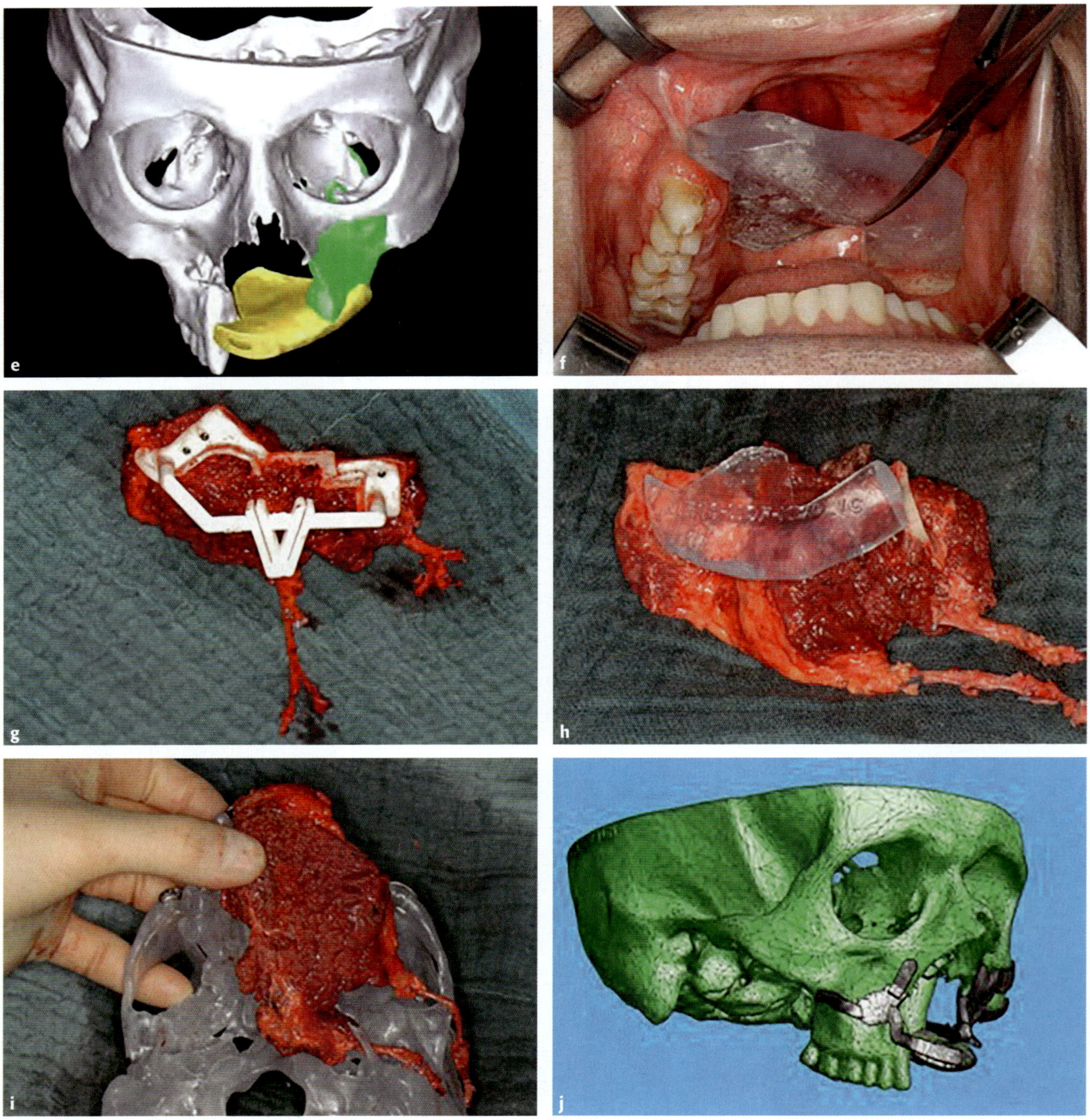

Fig 5.3.12-15a–x (cont) Hemimaxillary reconstruction with a scapular bone flap.

- **e** Lacking connection to suprastructure (green) to be replaced by patient-specific implant (PSI).
- **f** Intraoral fit check with STL model of scapular subsegments at start of surgical procedure.
- **g** Harvested scapular segment with mounted cutting guide components. Note, two separate vascular pedicles due to lack of subscapular artery and vessel bifurcation: short pedicle = circumflex scapular artery; long pedicle = thoracodorsal artery and angular branch.
- **h** Vessel variant suggested use of a singular (long) pedicle with preservation of muscle cuff between lateral border and tip subsegments, STL model of the segments on top of muscle cuff, model ends correspond with bone ends, intersegmental cuts covered by muscle.
- **i** Contoured transplant put into maxillary defect of STL, midface model defect for size check.
- **j** Maxillary reconstruction with a bone flap from the lateral scapular border and tip, PSI design.

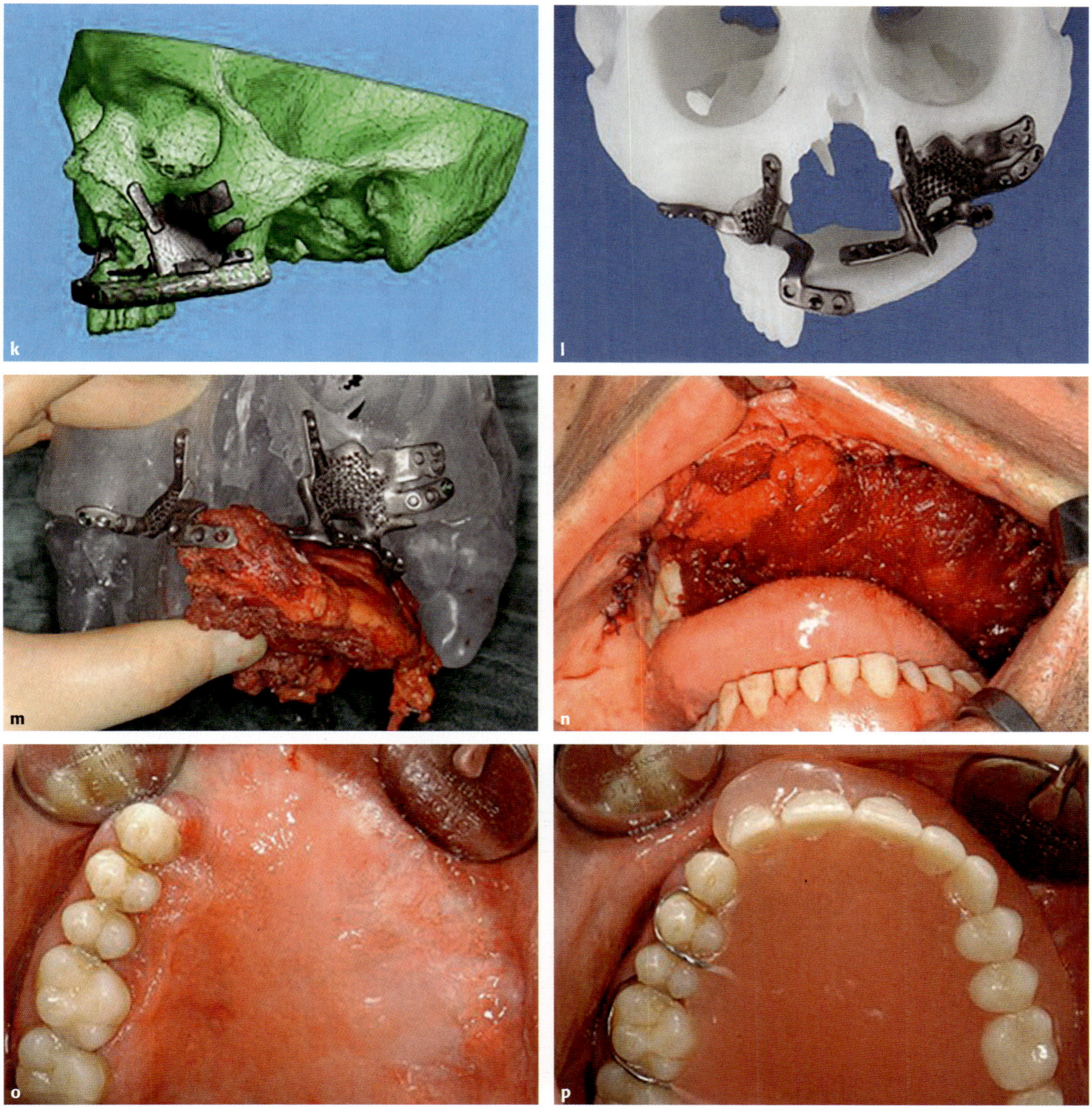

Fig 5.3.12-15a–x (cont)

k Scapular flap and PSI design, lateral view.

l Selected electron beam melted PSIs on STL model.

m Preliminary intraoperative assembly of scapular segments and PSIs in defect of STL midface model.

n Sufficient perfusion after reanastomosis of the long pedicle, no additional reanastomoses of sho-t pedicle required.

o Mucosalized surface.

p Provisional denture in place before implant-borne prosthodontic rehabilitation has started.

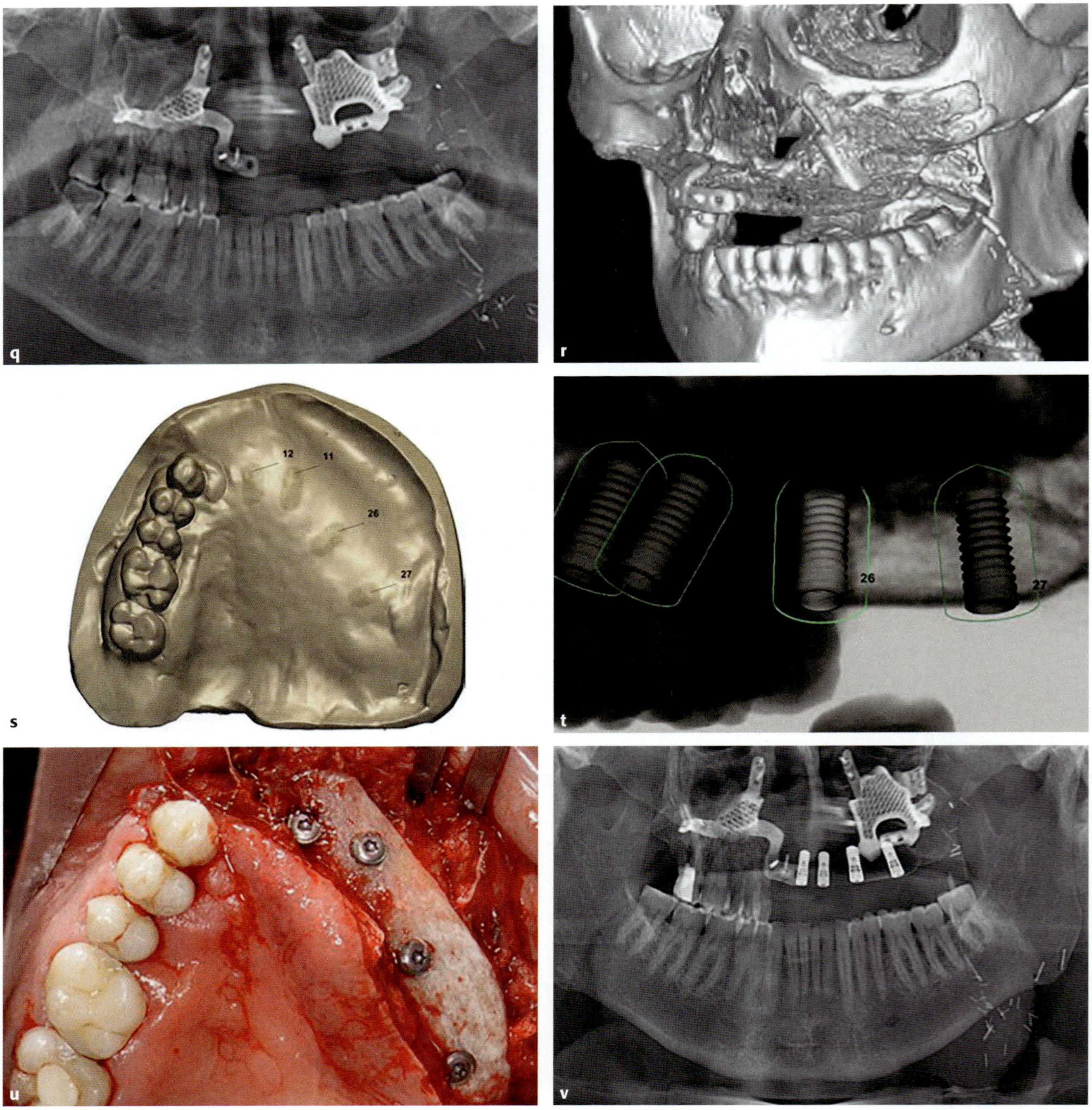

Fig 5.3.12-15a–x (cont)

q Panoramic x-ray view.

r A 3-D CT scan after transfer of scapular free flap.

s–t Virtual implant planning on digitalized plaster cast model and CT scan.

u Intraoperative view after open insertion of endosseous dental implants.

v Panoramic x-ray following dental implant insertion.

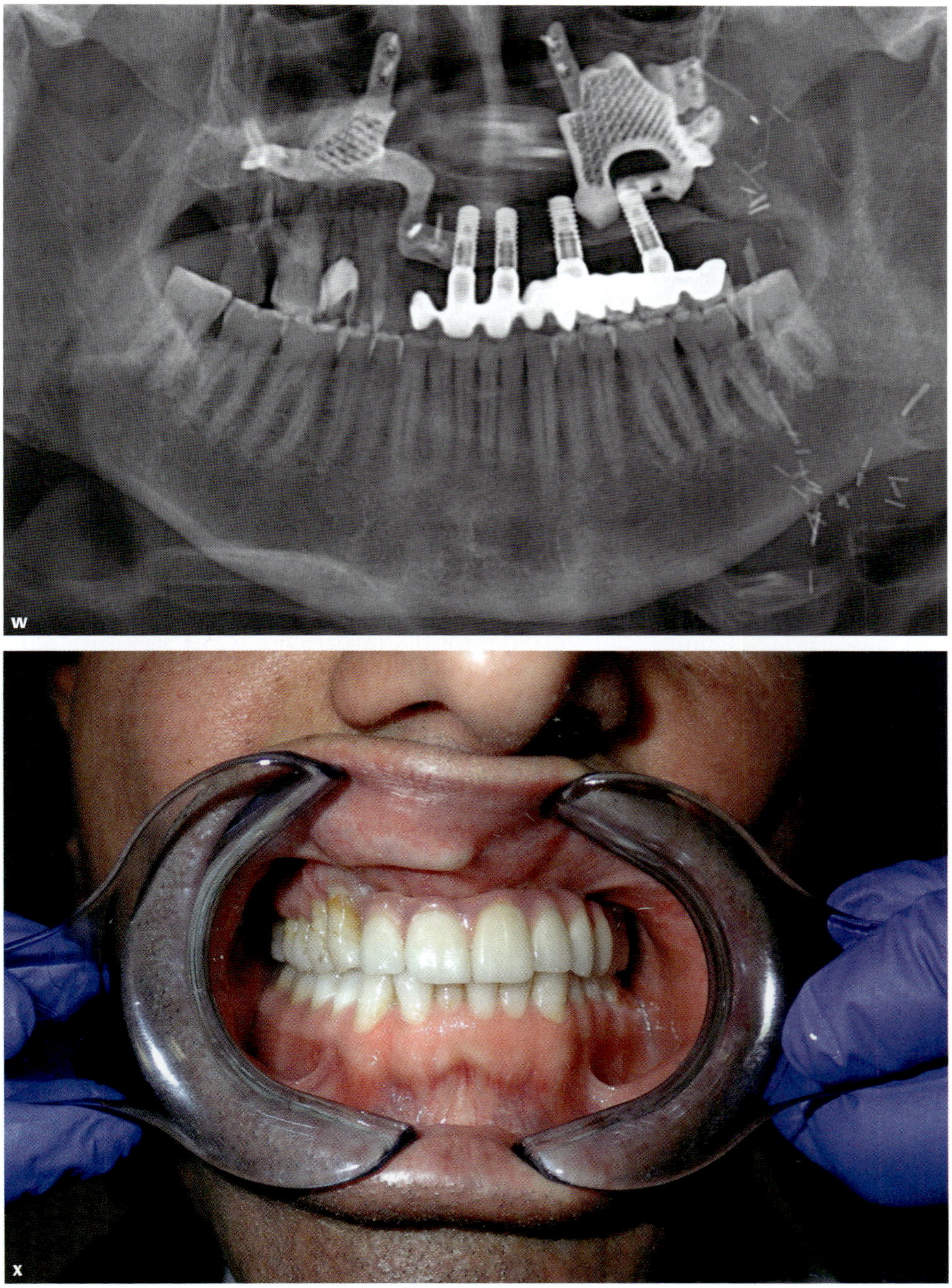

Fig 5.3.12-15a–x (cont)

w Panoramic x-ray after prosthodontic rehabilitation with a fixed bridge.

x Occlusion of the patient.

Lateral scapular border and tip for mandibular reconstruction

All types of mandibular defects below a total length of 14–16 cm can be bridged with osseous segments from the lateral scapular border and tip. The virtual planning must consider the diminishing and twisting bone stock along the way from the scapular top to the tip to place the maximum quantity into a position intended for the insertion of dental implants. Since mandibular reconstruction using scapular bone segments is associated with high rates of pseudarthrosis following subsegmentation [Mitsimponas et al, 2014] it is strongly recommended to use closing osteotomies to improve osseous positioning and consolidation. A three-part subsegmentation that is needed to fold the transplant into a bilateral segmental defect of the anterior curvature of the mandible is accomplished using a wedge osteotomy in the vascular transition zone (see previous paragraph) and a second osteotomy in the infraglenoid bone portion [Cornelius et al, 2016].

To preserve the continuity of the muscular layers during the osteotomy, the only access is from the medial aspect. This corresponds to the longitudinal bone edge of the in toto scapular segment. A gateway arch, hooked to the connecting bridge of the outer framework component of the cutting guide, provides a pass-through for the additional pair of flange extensions put forward by the rod component at 90° to top over the bone edge. The tandem ensemble of the bone flap mounted with both cutting guide components is turned onto its lateral side. The muscle envelope over the intended osteotomy location is subperiosteally peeled off either side. The wedge osteotomies within the created muscular tunnel are then attained under the guidance of the flanges crossing the medial osteotomy line of the in toto segment. Finally, the rod rider component is removed and the three subsegments, interconnected either by the muscle cuff or a bipedicled source vessel, are cut out of the framework component for the inset into the mandibular defect. The varying bone stock of the flap may be insufficient for the primary placement of endosseous dental implants and may require secondary augmentation procedures.

6 Patient-specific implants

Patient-specific (alloplastic) implants, also known as personal or custom-made implants, are unique implants produced for an individual patient [Eufinger et al, 1995, 1997; Eufinger et al, 1998]. Attributes such as personalized, customized, or individualized rather refer to ready-made, off the shelf products that have been modified, eg, molded, shaped or bent, and cut to size to meet with distinctive anatomical conditions [Lethaus et al, 2010; Probst et al, 2012]. The PSIs in conjunction with patient-specific instruments and toolkits pursue the objective of translating from approximation to the utmost level of accuracy and anatomical fit in fixation and/or reconstruction [Westermark et al, 2011; Mertens et al, 2013; Wilde et al, 2014; Ciocca et al, 2015]. The PSIs potentially offer a reduced number of steps in the surgical workflow, saving surgical time. Whereas the fundamental principles and concepts of potential PSI applications have been pointed out and discussed in the literature, a straightforward and consented taxonomy has not been created so far. Currently, PSIs are categorized in a plethora of terms, such as material properties, type of manufacturing process (eg, additive versus substractive), configuration (plate, grid, mesh) and shape, anatomical location, biomechanics (eg, static, kinematic, load bearing) and functionality (dead space—bony void filling, spatial reduction/realignment of segments or fragments, surface restoration, joint replacement, etc), without any attempt to embed these criteria into an interrelating organized overall scheme.

The examples of this chapter show a small fraction of the vast scope of various PSI types and applications in the mandible and in the maxillary/midface area. The PSI technology has rapidly come into widespread use for mandibular reconstruction, particularly in the form of solid, robust reconstruction plates together with free flaps [Ciocca et al, 2012] (**Fig 5.3.12-6j–p** and **Fig 5.3.12-12**). In the maxillae and midface, PSIs have developed from relatively massive fixation elements [Mertens et al, 2013; Tarsitano et al, 2016] with increased risk of exposure to the paranasal sinuses (**Fig 5.3.12-15j–p**) into more delicate support structures with fine filigree arms (**Fig 5.3.12-16a–c**).

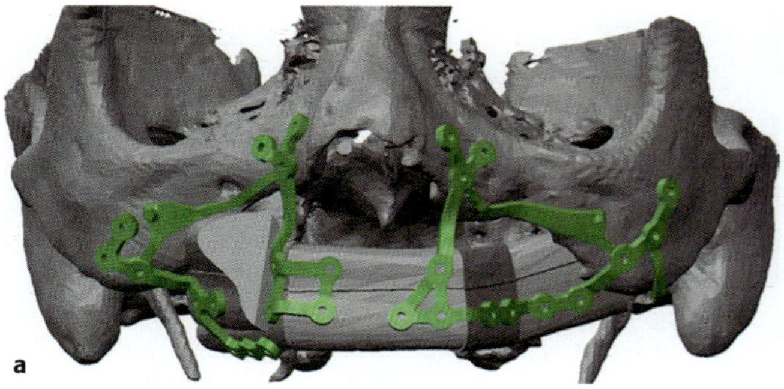

a

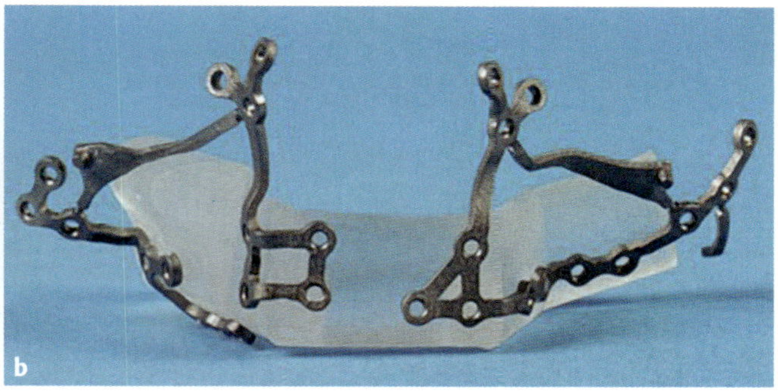

b

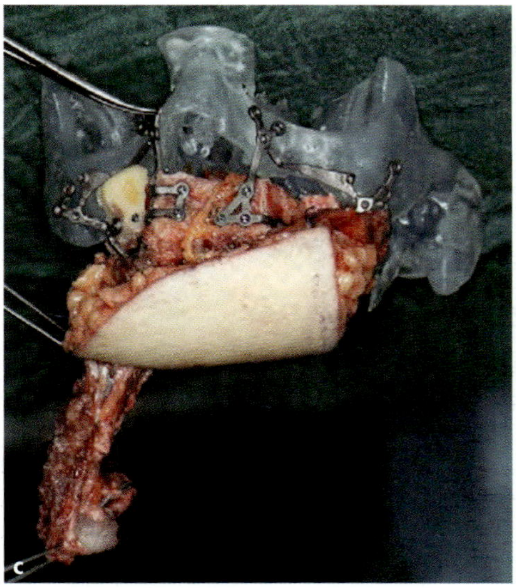

c

Fig 5.3.12-16a–e Patient-specific implant (PSI) design: for placement and fixation of fibula segments in a bilateral horizontal maxillectomy defect (Brown Class IId plus, total palate and alveolar arch).

- **a** PSI design: additional free, nonvascularized fibular segment to build up the zygomaticomaxillary crest as a connection to the maxillary suprastructure.
- **b** CAM: electron beam melted PSIs attached to the STL model of the fibular segments; intermediate removable bars, defined breaking points enable their efficient removal.
- **c** Composite fibula flap mounted to the STL model for position control of bone, soft tissues, and PSI implants. The vascular pedicle goes to the upper right neck area.

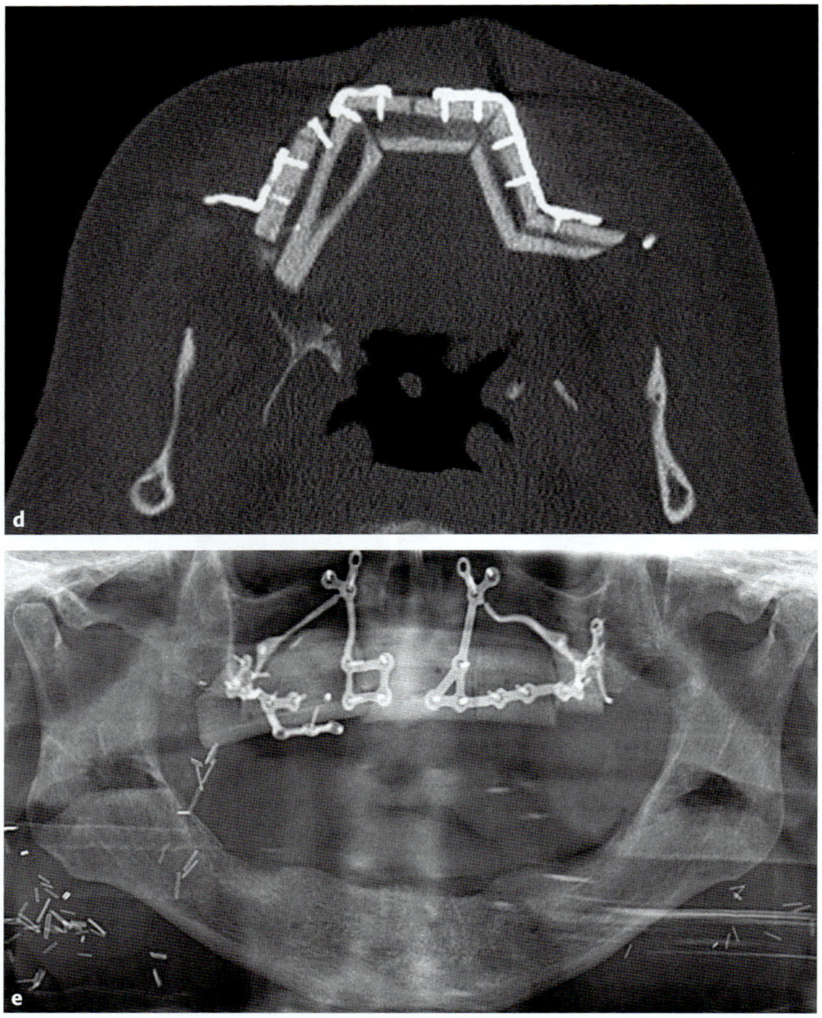

Fig 5.3.12-16a–e (cont) Patient-specific implant (PSI) design: for placement and fixation of fibula segments in a bilateral horizontal maxillectomy defect (Brown Class IId plus, total palate and alveolar arch).
d Axial CT cut showing the alignment of bone and PSI implants used for fixation.
e Postoperative orthopantomogram.

7 Preoperative, intraoperative, and postoperative control

Computer-assisted surgery must be accompanied with systematic monitoring of designs, processes and manufactured products as well as control of their efficacy and outcome in all its stages. The conceptualization and planning of individual surgical solutions will adopt traditional principles and standards, for instance regarding implant dimensions and shapes. Creative techniques heading toward unprecedented CAD/CAM-based template and PSI (**Fig 5.3.12-16**) configurations and procedural innovations should represent cautious extrapolation of existing know-how.

It is essential to avoid misconceptions and anticipate errors at the beginning of virtual planning and simulate outcomes to prevent mishaps during the subsequent surgery. This initial control and prediction cannot be purely confined to the mechanics of bony structures and their replacement or relocation based on CT datasets, but still needs thorough appreciation of the individual soft-tissue conditions by meticulous clinical evaluation. In contrast to forward planning, the normal soft-tissue anatomy does not exist in backward planning situations, ie, secondary reconstruction, with the occurrence of collapse, soft-tissue shrinkage, distortion, fistulae, defects, and sensory or motor nerve deficits. The need for a comprehensive analysis and understanding of mutual relationships between tissue components, flaps, and alloplastic materials is the reason why virtual planning and simulation is not to be delegated by the operating surgeon. A peer-reviewed and intensive dialogue before the definitive approval of a virtual plan is recommended as routine. Cautions in drafting PSIs include refraining from oversizing and overambitious complexity with respect to biomechanics and appropriate stability. The primary plan is to simplify PSIs that might work best according to the complexity of a given situation.

An intraoperative change of plan may be required because of multiple situations, eg, unsuitability of the CAD/CAM toolkit and/or PSI, tumor infiltration exceeding the margins predicted from preoperative imaging, unavailability, minor size or insufficient flow of cervical recipient vessels, variations of transplant vessels (**Fig 5.3.12-15g–h**), short vascular pedicles, and so on. In the worst case, all the prepared material is discarded in exchange for an improvised freehand approach.

Intraoperative process control is facilitated by consistent use of toolkits. As measuring devices and during repeated counter checks, they increase the reliability and safety of the ongoing intervention in a stepwise fashion. A clear awareness of domino effects and chain reactions due to every imprecision starting with defect size, plate hole locations, PSIs, and transplants is crucial. A reliable means for achieving final intraoperative quality assurance must focus on the process output and selective measurements used in direct comparison with the model situation.

Navigation and/or intraoperative multiplanar or 3-D imaging in principle provide numerous options to conduct a check at the completion of a reconstructive procedure regarding virtual planning. In a multi-part reconstructive sequence with relocated bone fragments or segments after tumor ablation, folded transplants in an assigned position, and after fixation using one or multiple PSIs, it appears advantageous to use intraoperative imaging at strategic points for intraoperative assessment. This allows incremental evaluation of the accuracy stage by stage in the assembly, instead of trying to just control the product, which is difficult to alter. Intraoperative and postoperative imaging are critical to confirm consistency with the initial plan The accuracy of the postoperative result is compared with the virtual preoperative plan by fusion of the appropriate datasets. It is self-evident that a final intraoperative imaging ideally replaces an early postoperative control.

8 Summary and outlook

Virtual planning and template-assisted surgery have gone from proof of concept to extensive use. New technologies will become reality, eg, robotic osteotomies are far more precise than man-made bone cuts [Chao et al, 2016]. Thus, template-assisted bone surgery is nothing more than a development step in an ever-changing surgical world.

9 References and suggested reading

Aleid W, Jones K, Laugharne D. The horizontal and stepped osteotomy technique for mandibular reconstruction using fibular free flap. *Craniomaxillofac Trauma Reconstr.* 2011;4(3):157–160.

Antony AK, Chen WF, Kolokythas A, et al. Use of virtual surgery and stereolithography-guided osteotomy for mandibular reconstruction with the free fibula. *Plast Reconstr Surg.* 2011;128(5):1080–1084.

Ayoub N, Ghassemi A, Rana M, et al. Evaluation of computer-assisted mandibular reconstruction with vascularized iliac crest bone graft compared to conventional surgery: a randomized prospective clinical trial. *Trials.* 2014;15:114.

Barttelbort SW, Ariyan S. Mandible preservation with oral cavity carcinoma: rim mandibulectomy versus sagittal mandibulectomy. *Am J Surg.* 1993;166(4):411–415.

Bell RB, Weimer KA, Dierks EJ, et al. Computer planning and intraoperative navigation for palatomaxillary and mandibular reconstruction with fibular free flaps. *J Oral Maxillofac Surg.* 2011Mar;69(3):724–732.

Bell RB. Computer planning and intraoperative navigation in cranio-maxillofacial surgery. *Oral Maxillofac Surg Clin North Am.* 2010 Feb;22(1):135–156.

Bell RB, Markiewicz MR. Computer-assisted planning, stereolithographic modeling, and intraoperative navigation for complex orbital reconstruction: a descriptive study in a preliminary cohort. *J Oral Maxillofac Surg.* 2009;67(12):2559–2570.

Bergeron L, Tang M, Morris SF. The anatomical basis of the deep circumflex iliac artery perforator flap with iliac crest. *Plast Reconstr Surg.* 2007;120(1):252–258.

Bluebond-Langner R, Zamani A, Rodriguez ED. Frontal bandeau reconstruction with a fibula flap in a patient with Freeman-Sheldon syndrome. *J Craniofac Surg.* 2009 Jan;20(1):256–258.

Brown JS, Shaw RJ. Reconstruction of the maxilla and midface: introducing a new classification. *Lancet Oncol.* 2010 Oct;11(10):1001–1008.

Brown JS. Deep circumflex iliac artery free flap with internal oblique muscle as a new method of immediate reconstruction of maxillectomy defect. *Head Neck.* 1996 Sep-Oct;18(5):412–421.

Buchbinder D, Urken ML, Vickery C, et al. Bone contouring and fixation in functional, primary microvascular mandibular reconstruction. *Head Neck.* 1991 May-Jun;13(3):191–199.

Ch'ng S, Ashford BG, Clark JR. Alignment of the double-barrel fibula free flap for better cosmesis and bone height for osseointegrated dental implants. *Plast Reconstr Surg.* 2013 Oct;132(4):688e–689e.

Chang EI, Jenkins MP, Patel SA, et al. Long-term operative outcomes of preoperative computed tomography-guided virtual surgical planning for osteocutaneous free flap mandible reconstruction. *Plast Reconstr Surg.* 2016 Feb;137(2):619–623.

Chang YM, Wallace CG, Hsu YM, et al. Outcome of osseointegrated dental implants in double-barrel and vertically distracted fibula osteoseptocutaneous free flaps for segmental mandibular defect reconstruction. *Plast Reconstr Surg.* 2014 Nov;134(5):1033–1043.

Chang YM, Coskunfirat OK, Wei FC, et al. Maxillary reconstruction with a fibula osteoseptocutaneous free flap and simultaneous insertion of osseointegrated dental implants. *Plast Reconstr Surg.* 2004 Apr;113(4):1140–1145.

Chao AH, Weimer K, Raczkowsky J, et al. Pre-programmed robotic osteotomies for fibula free flap mandible reconstruction: a preclinical investigation. *Microsurgery.* 2016 Mar;36(3):246–249.

Chen YS, Hu KY, Lin TW. The concept of "two arches" in mandibular reconstruction. *Ann Plast Surg.* 2012 Dec;69(6):616–621.

Ciocca L, Mazzoni S, Fantini M, et al. CAD/CAM guided secondary mandibular reconstruction of a discontinuity defect after ablative cancer surgery. *J Craniomaxillofac Surg.* 2012 Dec;40(8):e511–e515.

Ciocca L, Marchetti C, Mazzoni S, et al. Accuracy of fibular sectioning and insertion into a rapid-prototyped bone plate, for mandibular reconstruction using CAD-CAM technology. *J Craniomaxillofac Surg.* 2015;43(1):28–33.

Ciocca L, Mazzoni S, Fantini M, et al. The design and rapid prototyping of surgical guides and bone plates to support iliac free flaps for mandible reconstruction. *Plast Reconstr Surg.* 2012 May;129(5):859e–861e.

Ciocca L, Mazzoni S, Fantini M, et al. A CAD/CAM- prototyped anatomical condylar prosthesis connected to a custom-made bone plate to support a fibula free flap. *Med Biologic Engineer Comput.* 2012 Jul;50(7):743–749.

Coleman JJ 3rd, Sultan MR. The bipedicled osteocutaneous scapula flap: a new subscapular system free flap. *Plast Reconstr Surg.* 1991 Apr;87(4):682–692.

Cordeiro PG, Santamaria E. A classification system and algorithm for reconstruction of maxillectomy and midfacial defects. *Plast Reconstr Surg.* 2000 Jun;105(7):2331–2346; discussion 47–48.

Cordeiro PG, Chen CM. A 15-year review of midface reconstruction after total and subtotal maxillectomy: part I. Algorithm and outcomes. *Plast Reconstr Surg.* 2012;129(1):124–136.

Cordeiro PG, Chen CM. A 15-year review of midface reconstruction after total and subtotal maxillectomy: part II. Technical modifications to maximize aesthetic and functional outcomes. *Plast Reconstr Surg.* 2012;129(1):139–147.

Cornelius CP, Giessler GA, Wilde F, et al. Iterations of computer- and template-assisted mandibular or maxillary reconstruction with free flaps containing the lateral scapular border—evolution of a biplanar plug-on cutting guide. *J Craniomaxillofac Surg.* 2016 Mar;44(3):229–241.

Cornelius CP, Smolka W, Giessler GA, et al. Patient-specific reconstruction plates are the missing link in computer-assisted mandibular reconstruction: a showcase for technical description. *J Craniomaxillofac Surg.* 2015;43(5):624–629.

Cummins DM, Kim B, Kaleem A, et al. Pedicle orientation in free-flap microvascular maxillofacial reconstruction. *J Oral Maxillofac Surg.* 2017 Apr;75(4):875.e1–875.e4.

Deek NF, Wei FC. Computer-assisted surgery for segmental mandibular reconstruction with the osteoseptocutaneous fibula flap: can we instigate ideological and technological reforms? *Plast Reconstr Surg.* 2016;137(3):963–970.

Dérand P, Hirsch JM. Virtual bending of mandibular reconstruction plates using a computer-aided design. *J Oral Maxillofac Surg.* 2009 Aug;67(8):1640–1643.

Dérand P, Rännar LE, Hirsch JM. Imaging, virtual planning, design, and production of patient-specific implants and clinical validation in craniomaxillofacial surgery. *Craniomaxillofac Trauma Reconstr.* 2012;5(3):137–144.

Edwards SP. Computer-assisted craniomaxillofacial surgery. *Oral Maxillofac Surg Clin North Am.* 2010 Feb;22(1):117–134.

Essig H, Rana M, Kokemueller H, et al. Pre-operative planning for mandibular reconstruction: a full digital planning workflow resulting in a patient specific reconstruction. *Head Neck Oncol.* 2011 Oct;3:45.

Eufinger H, Wehmöller M. Individual prefabricated titanium implants in reconstructive craniofacial surgery: clinical and technical aspects of the first 22 cases. *Plast Reconstr Surg.* 1998 Aug;102(2):300–308.

Eufinger H, Wehmoller M, Machtens E. Individual prostheses and resection templates for mandibular resection and reconstruction. *Br J Oral Maxillofac Surg.* 1997 Dec;35(6):413–418.

Eufinger H, Wehmoller M, Machtens E, et al. Reconstruction of craniofacial bone defects with individual alloplastic implants based on CAD/CAM-manipulated CT-data. *J Craniomaxillofac Surg.* 1995 Jun;23(3):175–181.

Fan S, Wang YY, Wu DH, et al. Intraoral lining with the fibular osteomyofascial flap without a skin paddle during maxillary and mandibular reconstruction. *Head Neck.* 2016 Apr;38(S1):E832–E836.

Foley BD, Thayer WP, Honeybrook A, et al. Mandibular reconstruction using computer-aided design and computer-aided manufacturing: an analysis of surgical results. *J Oral Maxillofac Surg.* 2013;71(2):e111–119.

Ghassemi A, Schreiber L, Prescher A, et al. Clinically usable bone region of ilium versus fibula considering mandible reconstruction: "A different view of bone comparison". *Clin Anat.* 2016 Sep;29(6):773–778.

Ghassemi A, Ghassemi M, Modabber A, et al. Functional long-term results after the harvest of vascularised iliac bone grafts bicortically with the anterior superior iliac spine included. *Br J Oral Maxillofac Surg.* 2013 Jun;51(4):e47–50.

Grinsell D, Catto-Smith HE. Modifications of the deep circumflex iliac artery free flap for reconstruction of the maxilla. *J Plast Reconstr Aesthet Surg.* 2015;68(8):1044–1053.

Haddock NT, Monaco C, Weimer KA, et al. Increasing bony contact and overlap with computer-designed offset cuts in free fibula mandible reconstruction. *J Craniofac Surg.* 2012;23(6):1592–1595.

Hallermann W, Olsen S, Bardyn T, et al. A new method for computer-aided operation planning for extensive mandibular reconstruction. *Plast Reconstruct Surg.* 2006;117(7):2431–2437.

Hanasono MM, Silva AK, Yu P, et al. A comprehensive algorithm for oncologic maxillary reconstruction. *Plast Reconstr Surg.* 2013;131(1):47–60.

Hanasono MM, Skoracki RJ. Computer-assisted design and rapid prototype modeling in microvascular mandible reconstruction. *Laryngoscope.* 2013 Mar;123(3):597–604.

Hanasono MM, Jacob RF, Bidaut L, et al. Midfacial reconstruction using virtual planning, rapid prototype modeling, and stereotactic navigation. *Plast Reconstr Surg.* 2010;126(6):2002–2006.

Hanasono MM, Skoracki RJ. The omega-shaped fibula osteocutaneous free flap for reconstruction of extensive midfacial defects. *Plast Reconstr Surg.* 2010 Apr;125(4):160e–162e.

Hanken H, Schablowsky C, Smeets R, et al. Virtual planning of complex head and neck reconstruction results in satisfactory match between real outcomes and virtual models. *Clin Oral Investigations.* 2015 Apr;19(3):647–656.

He Y, Zhang ZY, Zhu HG, et al. Double-barrel fibula vascularized free flap with dental rehabilitation for mandibular reconstruction. *J Oral Maxillofac Surg.* 2011;69(10):2663–2669.

Hidalgo DA, Rekow A. A review of 60 consecutive fibula free flap mandible reconstructions. *Plast Reconstr Surg.* 1995 Sep;96(3):585–596; discussion 97–602.

Hidalgo DA. Fibula free flap: a new method of mandible reconstruction. *Plast Reconstr Surg.* 1989 Jul;84(1):71–79.

Hirsch DL, Garfein ES, Christensen AM, et al. Use of computer-aided design and computer-aided manufacturing to produce orthognathically ideal surgical outcomes: a paradigm shift in head and neck reconstruction. *J Oral Maxillofac Surg.* 2009 Oct;67(10):2115–2122.

Holle J, Vinzenz K, Würinger E, et al. The prefabricated combined scapula flap for bony and soft-tissue reconstruction in maxillofacial defects: a new method. *Plast Reconstr Surg.* 1996 Sep;98(3):542–552.

Juergens P, Ratia J, Beinemann J, et al. Enabling an unimpeded surgical approach to the skull base in patients with cranial hyperostosis, exemplarily demonstrated for craniometaphyseal dysplasia. *J Neurosurg.* 2011 Sep;115(3):528–535.

Kamali P, Dean D, Skoracki R, et al. The current role of three-dimensional printing in plastic surgery. *Plast Reconstr Surg.* 2016 Mar;137(3):1045–1055.

L'Heureux-Lebeau B, Odobescu A, Harris PG, et al. Chimaeric subscapular system free flap for complex oro-facial defects. *J Plast Reconstr Aesthet Surg.* 2013;66(7):900–905.

Lambrecht JT, Schiel H, Kreusch T, et al. New trends in the 3D management of CT data in plastic and reconstructive surgery. *Int Surg.* 1997 Oct-Dec;82(4):332–338.

Lee JH, Kim MJ, Choi WS, et al. Concomitant reconstruction of mandibular basal and alveolar bone with a free fibular flap. *Int J Oral Maxillofac Surg.* 2004 Mar;33(2):150–156.

Leiggener CS, Krol Z, Gawelin P, et al. A computer-based comparative quantitative analysis of surgical outcome of mandibular reconstructions with free fibula microvascular flaps. *J Plast Surg Hand Surg.* 2015 Apr;49(2):95–101.

Leiggener C, Messo E, Thor A, et al. A selective laser sintering guide for transferring a virtual plan to real time surgery in composite mandibular reconstruction with free fibula osseous flaps. *Int J Oral Maxillofac Surg.* 2009 Feb;38(2):187–192.

Lethaus B, Poort L, Bockmann R, et al. Additive manufacturing for microvascular reconstruction of the mandible in 20 patients. *J Craniomaxillofac Surg.* 2012 Jan;40(1):43–46.

Lethaus B, Kessler P, Boeckman R, et al. Reconstruction of a maxillary defect with a fibula graft and titanium mesh using CAD/CAM techniques. *Head Face Med.* 2010;6:16.

Levine JP, Bae JS, Soares M, et al. Jaw in a day: total maxillofacial reconstruction using digital technology. *Plast Reconstr Surg.* 2013 Jun;131(6):1386–1391.

Longo B, Nicolotti M, Ferri G, et al. Sagittal split osteotomy of the fibula for modeling the new mandibular angle. *J Craniofac Surg.* 2013 Jan;24(1):71–74.

Lundgren TK, Pignatti M, Halle M, et al. Composite orbital reconstruction using the vascularized segmentalized osteo-fascio-cutaneous fibula flap. *J Plast Reconstr Aesth Surg.* 2016 Feb;69(2):255–261.

Marchetti C, Bianchi A, Mazzoni S, et al. Oromandibular reconstruction using a fibula osteocutaneous free flap: four different "preplating" techniques. *Plast Reconstr Surg.* 2006 Sep;118(3):643–651.

Mascha F, Winter K, Pietzka S, et al. Accuracy of mandibular reconstruction with CAD/CAM fabricated patient specific reconstruction-plates in combination with CAD/CAM drill guides. *Int J CARS.* 2015;10(Suppl):S139–S140.

Mertens C, Löwenheim H, Hoffmann J. Image data based reconstruction of the midface using a patient-specific implant in combination with a vascularized osteomyocutaneous scapular flap. *J Craniomaxillofac Surg.* 2013 Apr;41(3):219–225.

Metzler P, Geiger EJ, Alcon A, et al. Three-dimensional virtual surgery accuracy for free fibula mandibular reconstruction: planned versus actual results. *J Oral Maxillofac Surg.* 2014 Dec;72(12):2601–2612.

Mitsimponas KT, Iliopoulos C, Stockmann P, et al. The free scapular/parascapular flap as a reliable method of reconstruction in the head and neck region: a retrospective analysis of 130 reconstructions performed over a period of 5 years in a single department. *J Craniomaxillofac Surg.* 2014 Jul;42(5):536–543.

Modabber A, Mohlhenrich SC, Ayoub N, et al. Computer-aided mandibular reconstruction with vascularized iliac crest bone flap and simultaneous implant surgery. *J Oral Implant.* 2015;41(5):e189–194

Modabber A, Ayoub N, Mohlhenrich SC, et al. The accuracy of computer-assisted primary mandibular reconstruction with vascularized bone flaps: iliac crest bone flap versus osteomyocutaneous fibula flap. *Med Devices.* 2014 Jun;7:211–217.

Modabber A, Gerressen M, Stiller MB, et al. Computer-assisted mandibular reconstruction with vascularized iliac crest bone graft. *Aesthet Plast Surg.* 2012 Jun;36(3):653–659.

Monaco C, Stranix JT, Lee ZH, et al. A modified approach to extensive oromandibular reconstruction using free fibula flaps. *J Craniofac Surg.* 2017 Jan;28(1):93–96.

Narra N, Valasek J, Hannula M, et al. Finite element analysis of customized reconstruction plates for mandibular continuity defect therapy. *J Biomech.* 2014 Jan;47(1):264–268.

Nkenke E, Vairaktaris E, Stelzle F, et al. Osteocutaneous free flap including medial and lateral scapular crests: technical aspects, viability, and donor site morbidity. *J Reconstr Microsurg.* 2009;25(9):545–553.

Okay D, Al Shetawi AH, Moubayed SP, et al. Worldwide 10-year systematic review of treatment trends in fibula free flap for mandibular reconstruction. *J Oral Maxillofac Surg.* 2016 Dec;74(12):2526–2531.

Okay DJ, Buchbinder D, Urken M, et al. Computer-assisted implant rehabilitation of maxillomandibular defects reconstructed with vascularized bone free flaps. *JAMA Otolaryngol Head Neck Surg.* 2013;139(4):371–381.

Olsson P, Nysjo F, Rodriguez-Lorenzo A, et al. Haptics-assisted virtual planning of bone, soft tissue, and vessels in fibula osteocutaneous free flaps. *Plast Reconstr Surg Glob Open.* 2015 Aug 10;3(8):e479.

Patel A, Levine J, Brecht L, et al. Digital technologies in mandibular pathology and reconstruction. *Atlas Oral Maxillofac Surg Clin North Am.* 2012 Mar;20(1):95–106.

Pfaff MJ, Steinbacher DM. Plastic surgery applications using three-dimensional planning and computer-assisted design and manufacturing. *Plast Reconstr Surg.* 2016 Mar;137(3):603e–616e.

Probst FA, Metzger M, Ehrenfeld M, et al. Computer-assisted designed and manufactured procedures facilitate the lingual application of mandible reconstruction plates. *J Oral Maxillofac Surg.* 2016 Sep;74(9):1879–1895.

Probst FA, Mast G, Ermer M, et al. MatrixMANDIBLE preformed reconstruction plates—a two-year two-institution experience in 71 patients. *J Oral Maxillofac Surg.* 2012;70(11):e657–666.

Qaisi M, Kolodney H, Swedenburg G, et al. Fibula jaw in a day: state of the art in maxillofacial reconstruction. *J Oral Maxillofac Surg.* 2016 Jun;74(6):1284.e1–1284.e15.

Rahimov C, Farzaliyev I. Virtual bending of titanium reconstructive plates for mandibular defect bridging: review of three clinical cases. *Craniomaxillofac Trauma Reconstr.* 2011;4(4):223–234.

Ritschl LM, Mücke T, Fichter AM, et al. Axiographic results of CAD/CAM-assisted microvascular fibular free flap reconstruction of the mandible: a prospective study of 21 consecutive cases. *J CranioMaxillofac Surg.* 2017 Jan;45(1):113–119.

Rodby KA, Turin S, Jacobs RJ, et al. Advances in oncologic head and neck reconstruction: systematic review and future considerations of virtual surgical planning and computer aided design/computer aided modeling. *J Plast Reconstr Aesthet Surg.* 2014 Sep;67(9):1171–1185.

Rodriguez ED, Bluebond-Langner R, Park JE, et al. Preservation of contour in periorbital and midfacial craniofacial microsurgery: reconstruction of the soft-tissue elements and skeletal buttresses. *Plast Reconstr Surg.* 2008;121(5):1738–1747; discussion 48–49.

Rohner D, Bucher P, Hammer B. Prefabricated fibular flaps for reconstruction of defects of the maxillofacial skeleton: planning, technique, and long-term experience. *Int J Oral Maxillofac Implant.* 2013 Sep-Oct;28(5):e221–229.

Rohner D, Kunz C, Bucher P, et al. [New possibilities for reconstructing extensive jaw defects with prefabricated microvascular fibula transplants and ITI implants]. *Mund Kiefer Gesichtschir.* 2000 Nov;4(6):365–372. German.

Roser SM, Ramachandra S, Blair H, et al. The accuracy of virtual surgical planning in free fibula mandibular reconstruction: comparison of planned and final results. *J Oral Maxillofac Surg.* 2010 Nov;68(11):2824–2832.

Saad A, Winters R, Wise MW, et al. Virtual surgical planning in complex composite maxillofacial reconstruction. *Plast Reconstr Surg.* 2013 Sep;132(3):626–633.

Schepers RH, Raghoebar GM, Vissink A, et al. Accuracy of fibula reconstruction using patient-specific CAD/CAM reconstruction plates and dental implants: a new modality for functional reconstruction of mandibular defects. *J Craniomaxillofac Surg.* 2015 Jun;43(5):649–657.

Schepers RH, Raghoebar GM, Vissink A, et al. Fully 3-dimensional digitally planned reconstruction of a mandible with a free vascularized fibula and immediate placement of an implant-supported prosthetic construction. *Head Neck.* 2013 Apr;35(4):E109–E114.

Semper-Hogg W, Fuessinger MA, Schwarz S, et al. Virtual reconstruction of midface defects using statistical shape models. *J Craniomaxillofac Surg.* 2017 Apr;45(4):461–466. Epub 2016 Dec 24.

Seneviratne S, Duong C, Taylor GI. The angular branch of the thoracodorsal artery and its blood supply to the inferior angle of the scapula: an anatomical study. *Plast Reconstr Surg.* 1999;104(1):85–88.

Seruya M, Fisher M, Rodriguez ED. Computer-assisted versus conventional free fibula flap technique for craniofacial reconstruction: an outcomes comparison. *Plast Reconstr Surg.* 2013 Nov;132(5):1219–1228.

Sharaf B, Levine JP, Hirsch DL, et al. Importance of computer-aided design and manufacturing technology in the multidisciplinary approach to head and neck reconstruction. *J Craniofac Surg.* 2010 Jul;21(4):1277–1280.

Shaw RJ, Brown JS. Osteomyocutaneous deep circumflex iliac artery perforator flap in the reconstruction of midface defect with facial skin loss: a case report. *Microsurgery.* 2009 Mar;29(4):299–302.

Shen Y, Sun J, Li J, et al. Special considerations in virtual surgical planning for secondary accurate maxillary reconstruction with vascularised fibula osteomyocutaneous flap. *J Plast Reconstr Aesthet Surg.* 2012 Jul;65(7):893–902.

Shipchandler TZ, Waters HH, Knott PD, et al. Orbitomaxillary reconstruction using the layered fibula osteocutaneous flap. *Arch Facial Plast Surg.* 2012 Mar-Apr;14(2):110–115.

Sinno S, Rodriguez ED. Definitive management of persistent frontal sinus infections and mucocele with a vascularized free fibula flap. *Plast Reconstr Surg.* 2017;139(1):170–175.

Smolka W, Muller-Lisse U, Sotlar K, et al. Computer-aided resection and reconstruction in a case of aneurysmal bone cyst of the mandibular condylar head. *Oral Surg.* 2015 Dec;19(4):437–442.

Sosin M, Ceradini DJ, Hazen A, et al. Total face, eyelids, ears, scalp, and skeletal subunit transplant cadaver simulation: the culmination of aesthetic, craniofacial, and microsurgery principles. *Plast Reconstr Surg.* 2016 May;137(5):845e–854e.

Steinbacher DM. Three-dimensional analysis and surgical planning in craniomaxillofacial surgery. *J Oral Maxillofac Surg.* 2015 Dec;73(12 Suppl):S40–56.

Stelter K, Andratschke M, Leunig A, et al. Computer-assisted surgery of the paranasal sinuses: technical and clinical experience with 368 patients, using the Vector Vision Compact system. *J Laryngol Otol.* 2006 Dec;120(12):1026–1032.

Stirling Craig E, Yuhasz M, Shah A, et al. Simulated surgery and cutting guides enhance spatial positioning in free fibular mandibular reconstruction. *Microsurgery.* 2015 Jan;35(1):29–33.

Swartz WM, Banis JC, Newton ED, et al. The osteocutaneous scapular flap for mandibular and maxillary reconstruction. *Plast Reconstr Surg.* 1986 Apr;77(4):530–545.

Tarsitano A, Battaglia S, Ciocca L, et al. Surgical reconstruction of maxillary defects using a computer-assisted design/computer-assisted manufacturing-produced titanium mesh supporting a free flap. *J Craniomaxillofac Surg.* 2016 Sep;44(9):1320–1326.

Taylor GI, Corlett RJ, Ashton MW. The evolution of free vascularized bone transfer: a 40-year experience. *Plast Reconstr Surg.* 2016 Apr;137(4):1292–1305.

Tepper OM, Sorice S, Hershman GN, et al. Use of virtual 3-dimensional surgery in post-traumatic craniomaxillofacial reconstruction. *J Oral Maxillofac Surg.* 2011 Mar;69(3):733–741.

Thein T, Kreidler J, Stocker E, et al. Morphology and blood supply of the iliac crest applied to jaw reconstruction. *Surg Radiol Anat.* 1997;19(4):217–225.

Thomas CV, McMillan KG, Jeynes P, et al. Use of a titanium cutting guide to assist raising the composite radial forearm free flap. *Int J Oral Maxillofac Surg.* 2013 Nov;42(11):1414–1417.

Thomas CV, McMillan KG, Jeynes P, et al. Use of a titanium cutting guide to assist with raising and inset of a DCIA free flap. *Br J Oral Maxillofac Surg.* 2013 Dec;51(8):958–961.

Ting JW, Rozen WM, Chubb D, et al. Improving the utility and reliability of the deep circumflex iliac artery perforator flap: the use of preoperative planning with CT angiography. *Microsurgery.* 2011 Nov;31(8):603–609.

Urken ML, Weinberg H, Vickery C, et al. Oromandibular reconstruction using microvascular composite free flaps. Report of 71 cases and a new classification scheme for bony, soft-tissue, and neurologic defects. *Arch Otolaryngol Head Neck Surg.* 1991 Jul;117(7):733–744.

Urken ML, Vickery C, Weinberg H, et al. The internal oblique-iliac crest osseomyocutaneous microvascular free flap in head and neck reconstruction. *J Reconstr Microsurg.* 1989 Jul;5(3):203–214; discussion 15–16.

Wang WH, Zhu J, Deng JY, et al. Three-dimensional virtual technology in reconstruction of mandibular defect including condyle using double-barrel vascularized fibula flap. *J Craniomaxillofac Surg.* 2013 Jul;41(5):417–422.

Wang YY, Zhang HQ, Fan S, et al. Mandibular reconstruction with the vascularized fibula flap: comparison of virtual planning surgery and conventional surgery. *Int J Oral Maxillofac Surg.* 2016 Nov;45(11):1400–1405.

Wang YY, Fan S, Zhang HQ, et al. Virtual surgical planning in precise maxillary reconstruction with vascularized fibular graft after tumor ablation. *J Oral Maxillofac Surg.* 2016 Jun;74(6):1255–1264.

Weitz J, Bauer FJ, Hapfelmeier A, et al. Accuracy of mandibular reconstruction by three-dimensional guided vascularised fibular free flap after segmental mandibulectomy. *Br J Oral Maxillofac Surg.* 2016 Jun;54(5):506–510.

Westermark A, Heden P, Aagaard E, et al. The use of TMJ concepts prostheses to reconstruct patients with major temporomandibular joint and mandibular defects. *Int J Oral Maxillofac Surg.* 2011 May;40(5):487–496.

Wilde F, Hanken H, Probst F, et al. Multicenter study on the use of patient-specific CAD/CAM reconstruction plates for mandibular reconstruction. *Int J Comput Assist Radiol Surg.* 2015 Dec;10(12):2035–2051.

Wilde F, Cornelius CP, Schramm A. Computer-assisted mandibular reconstruction using a patient-specific reconstruction plate fabricated with computer-aided design and manufacturing techniques. *Craniomaxillofac Trauma Reconstr.* 2014 Jun;7(2):158–166.

Wolff KD, Mücke T, von Bomhard A, et al. Free flap transplantation using an extracorporeal perfusion device: first three cases. *J Craniomaxillofac Surg.* 2016 Feb;44(2):148–154.

Xu LQ, Zhang CP, Poh EH, et al. A novel fibula osteotomy guide for mandibular reconstruction. *Plast Reconstr Surg.* 2012;129(5):861e–863e.

Yagi S, Kamei Y, Torii S. Donor side selection in mandibular reconstruction using a free fibular osteocutaneous flap. *Ann Plast Surg.* 2006 Jun;56(6):622–627.

Yu Y, Zhang WB, Liu XJ, et al. Three-dimensional accuracy of virtual planning and surgical navigation for mandibular reconstruction with free fibula flap. *J Oral Maxillofac Surg.* 2016 Jul;74(7):1503.e1–1505.e10.

Yu Y, Zhang WB, Wang Y, et al. A revised approach for mandibular reconstruction with the vascularized iliac crest flap using virtual surgical planning and surgical navigation. *J Oral Maxillofac Surg.* 2016 Jun;74(6):1285.e1–1285.e11.

Zhang WB, Yu Y, Wang Y, et al. Improving the accuracy of mandibular reconstruction with vascularized iliac crest flap: role of computer-assisted techniques. *J Craniomaxillofac Surg.* 2016 Nov;44(11):1819–1827.

Zheng GS, Wang L, Su YX, et al. Maxillary reconstruction assisted by preoperative planning and accurate surgical templates. *Oral Surg Oral Med Oral Pathol Oral Radiol.* 2016 Mar;121(3):233–238.

Zheng GS, Su YX, Liao GQ, et al. Mandible reconstruction assisted by preoperative simulation and transferring templates: cadaveric study of accuracy. *J Oral Maxillofac Surg.* 2012 Jun;70(6):1480–1485.

Zheng HP, Zhuang YH, Zhang ZM, et al. Modified deep iliac circumflex osteocutaneous flap for extremity reconstruction: anatomical study and clinical application. *J Plast Reconstr Aesthet Surg.* 2013 Sep;66(9):1256–1262.

5.3.13 Orthognathic surgery and automated splint manufacturing

Marc C Metzger, E Bradley Strong, Gido Bittermann, Rainer Schmelzeisen

1 Introduction

Good clinical results in orthognathic surgery require an accurate preoperative diagnosis and precise presurgical planning. Historically, this has been accomplished using cephalometric x-rays and plaster models. However, these techniques have limitations. Cephalometric radiographs do not provide a 3-D perspective of the patient anatomy. Orthognathic model surgery is time-consuming, labor intensive, and suffers (at least in theory) from several sources of error and inaccuracy. Additionally, many asymmetries in the craniofacial skeleton cannot be addressed with plaster models. More recently developed computer-aided technology allow surgeons to diagnose, analyze, and perform 3-D presurgical planning in a virtual environment. These applications include conventional computed tomography (CT), cone beam computed tomography (CBCT), intraoral optical scanners for virtual teeth modeling, 3-D photogrammetry, and 3-D printers. While single jaw surgery can be based on the occlusal plane of the opposite jaw, two jaw surgeries are much more complex. Computer-assisted presurgical planning has proven to be a valid alternative to plaster models [Whetten et al, 2006; Stevens et al, 2006; Miller et al, 2004; Gil et al, 2007; Mischkowski et al, 2006]. This chapter reviews the current modalities available for computer-aided presurgical planning in orthognathic surgery.

2 Data acquisition

2.1 Standard and cone beam computed tomography

Cone beam CT provides adequate bone resolution for presurgical planning, while offering a lower x-ray exposure than traditional CT (**Fig 5.3.13-1**).

Unfortunately, the reduced x-ray dosage also limits the soft-tissue resolution. If an accurate diagnosis and presurgical plan will include the assessment of the soft tissue, a traditional CT should be used. Slice thickness should be between 0.5 mm and 1.5 mm.

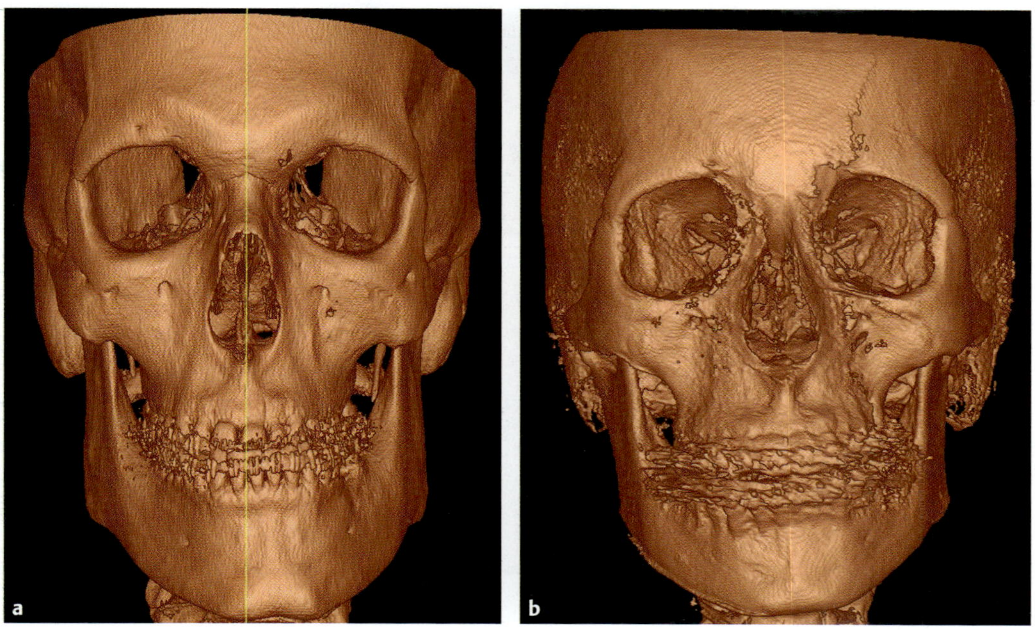

Fig 5.3.13-1a–b
a Computed tomographic (CT) view.
b Cone beam CT scan of a patient with mandibulomaxillary asymmetry.

Metallic fillings or brackets will cause artifacts that will distort the surface anatomy of the teeth. Therefore, occlusal analysis should be performed clinically and later using a surface scan of the teeth.

Transfer of digital data among surgeons, departments or institutions can be challenging. Most radiological devices generate digital imaging and communications in medicine data (DICOM). Stated simply, DICOM is the "language" used by medical imaging devices to transfer data. Patient data sets can be copied and transferred electronically or stored on hard copy modalities, such as a compact disk.

2.2 Dental scanning

It is essential to obtain a high-resolution surface scan of the teeth that can then be used to generate accurate virtual models and for fabrication of occlusal splints. Surface scans can be obtained directly with an intraoral laser scanner (**Fig 5.3.13-2**) or indirectly by obtaining plaster models and scanning them with a CT or laser scanner. The workflow varies depending on the resources available. Virtual models are generated of the upper and lower arches separately as well as both arches in occlusion (**Fig 5.3.13-3**).

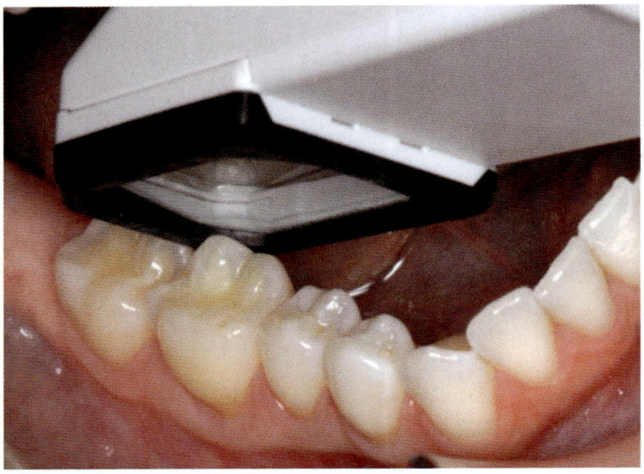

Fig 5.3.13-2 Intraoral scanning procedure (iTero scanner).

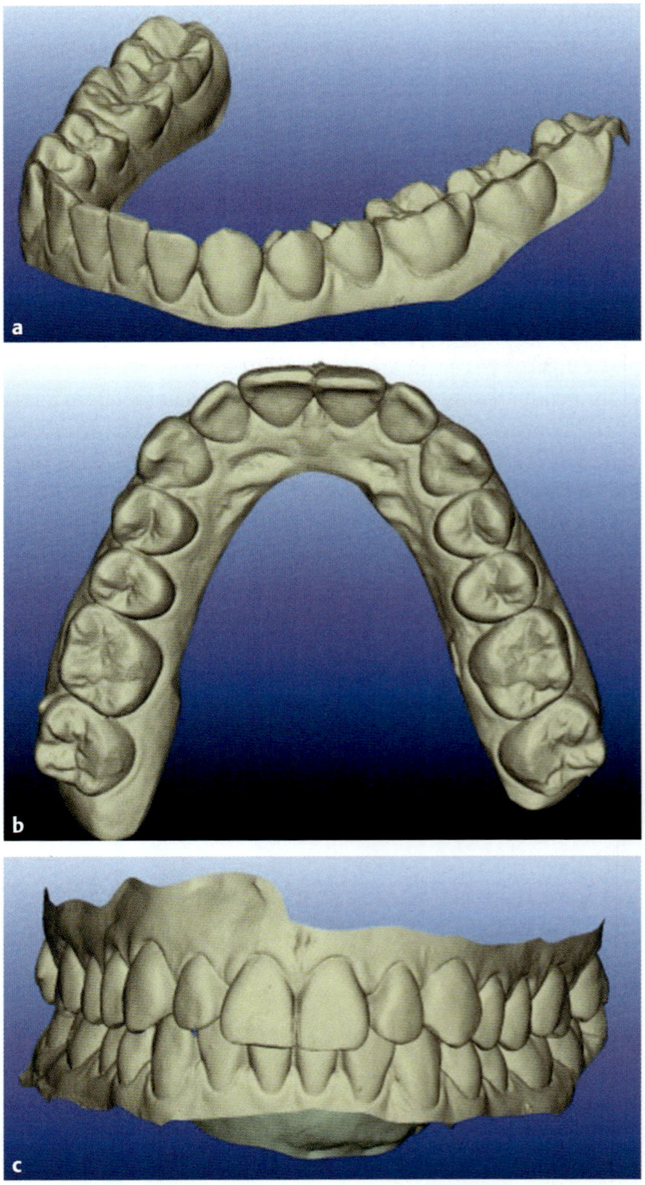

Fig 5.3.13-3a–c File of surface scan of the lower (**a**), upper (**b**) dental arch, and both scans in ideal occlusion (**c**).

2.3 Photogrammetry

While not integral to most orthognathic procedures, virtual 3-D images of the face can be useful for presurgical planning, documentation, and for patient information. Soft-tissue manipulations can be performed in the virtual environment by using additional software, such as ProPlan. However, the current software is rudimentary. It can be used to make basic modifications to the facial contour but cannot precisely predict surgical outcomes for complex orthognathic procedures.

3 Data processing

3.1 Cephalometric analysis

Accurate cephalometric analysis generally requires manual identification and placement of common cephalometric landmarks (**Fig 5.3.13-4**). Once these landmarks have been defined, software can be used for analysis of symmetry and osteotomy planning. Some common software options include Dolphine (North America, USA), Voxim (IVS-Solutions, Chemnitz, Germany), and Materialise (Leuven, Belgium).

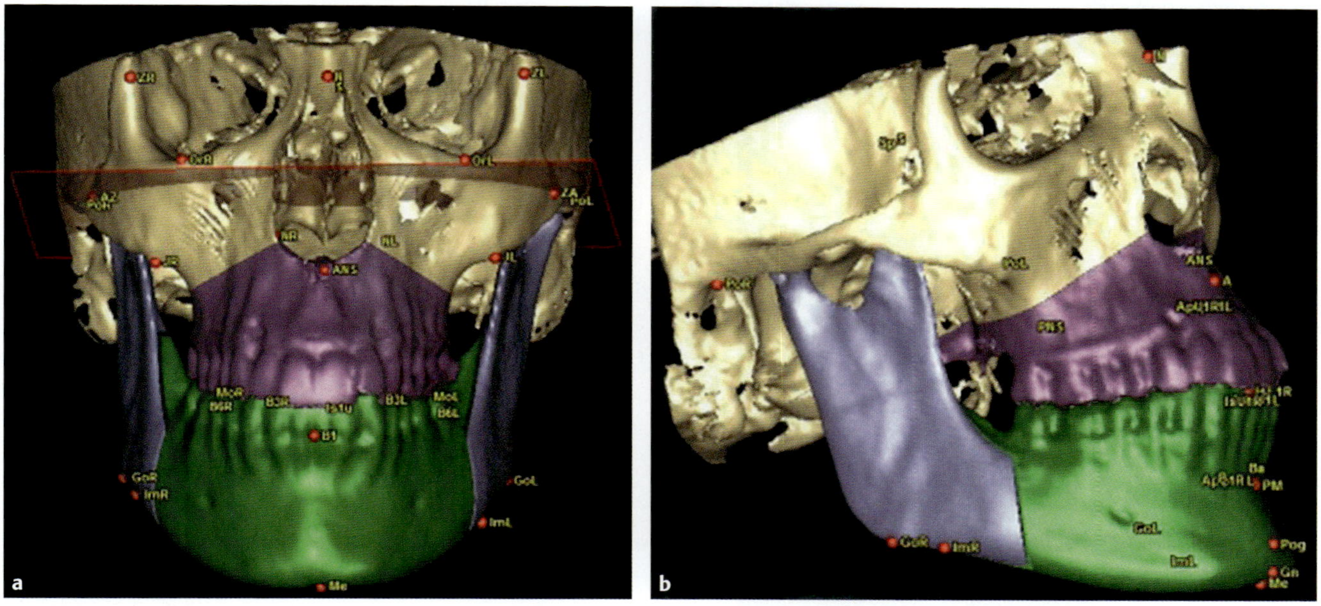

Fig 5.3.13-4a–b Manually defined cephalometric landmarks.

3.2 Data alignment

The CT data are used to generate a 3-D virtual model of the patient's skull. It is important to align the skull in true orthogonal planes (ie, axial, coronal, and sagittal) before segmentation of the virtual skull. Alignment algorithms vary depending on the software being used but most applications use the previously discussed cephalometric landmarks to align the skull.

3.3 Segmentation

The term segmentation describes the technique used to split the skull into different regions of interest. Segmentation for orthognathic surgery is performed using specific osteotomy lines. Some examples include Le Fort I osteotomy, sagittal split osteotomy, and the chin osteotomy with removal of excess bone (**Fig 5.3.13-5**). Once the bone segments have been "cut" and labeled, virtual manipulations can be performed, ie, maxillary advancement, setback, rotation, etc.

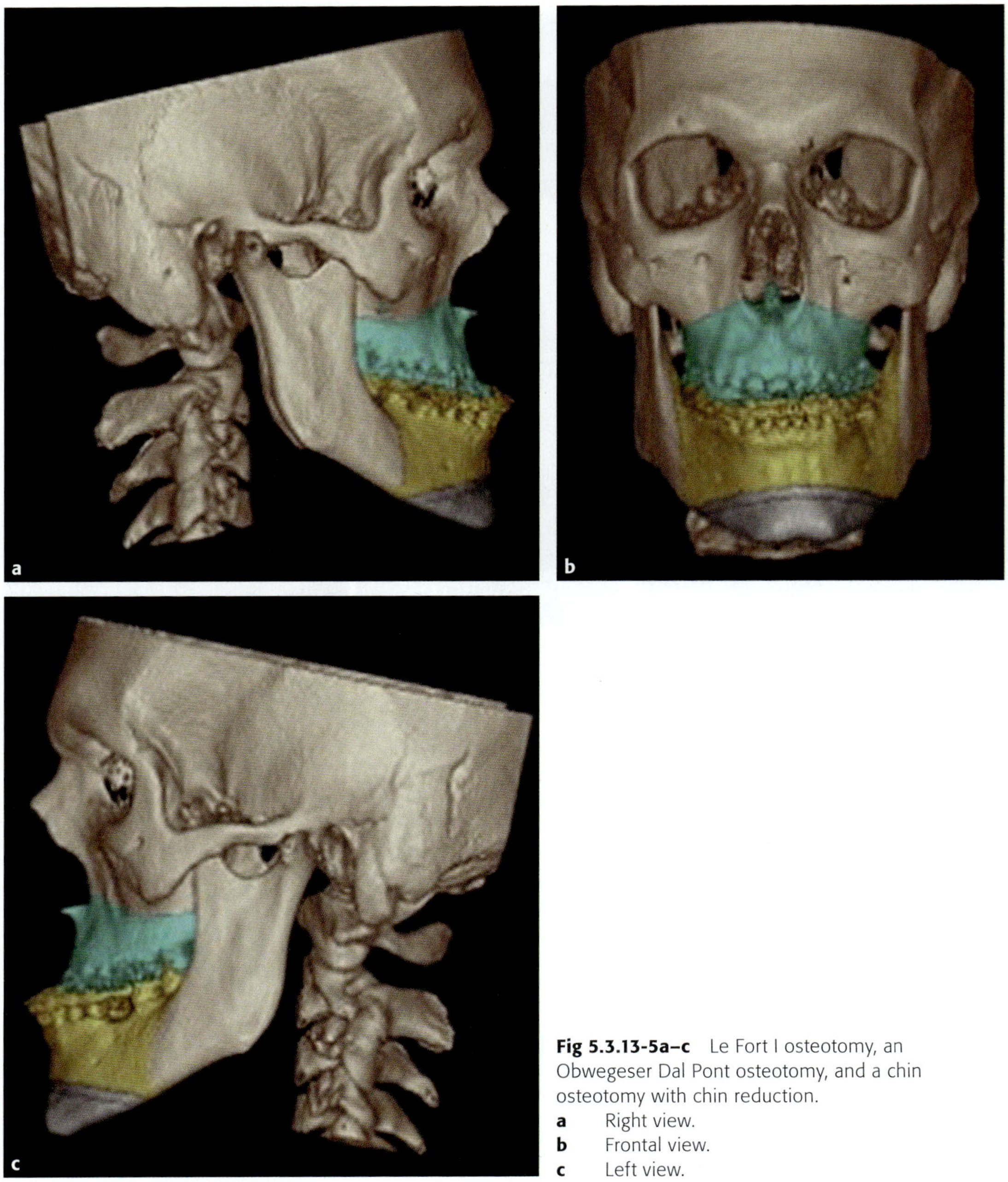

Fig 5.3.13-5a–c Le Fort I osteotomy, an Obwegeser Dal Pont osteotomy, and a chin osteotomy with chin reduction.
a Right view.
b Frontal view.
c Left view.

3.4 Data fusion

The term data fusion describes the technique of combining virtual data sets or segments to form a single data set or object. Data fusion is commonly used to overcome the problem of dental artifacts generated from dental metallic restoration materials or braces. In this scenario, a surface scan of the teeth is imported and overlayed onto the existing teeth. This fusion is then locked into place relative to the rest of the skull. It must be performed before fabrication of the splints to reduce the artifacts and to guarantee the exact fitting of the splint. The teeth surface scan with the dental arch in occlusion is only imported into the data set after the intermediate occlusion splint is prepared (**Fig 5.3.13-6**).

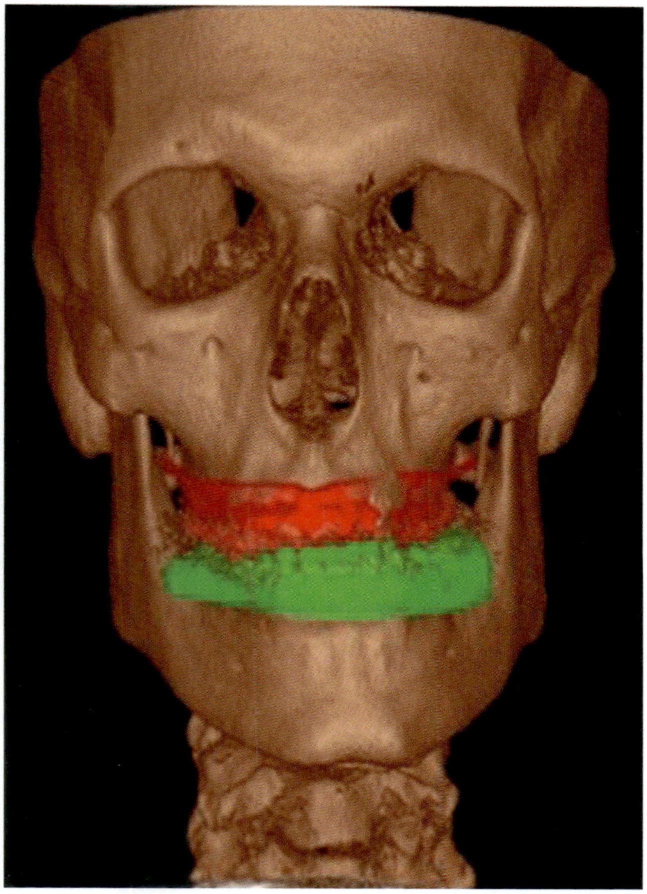

Fig 5.3.13-6 Fusion and alignment of virtual upper (red) and lower (green) dental arch with computed tomography data set.

4 Virtual corrections

4.1 Preparation of the intermediate occlusal splint

Pretreatment scanning is usually performed with the patient in full occlusion and no interocclusal space for placement of a virtual splint. The mandible can be opened virtually by defining a rotation center at each condylar head. The mandibular symphysis can then be rotated inferiorly while maintaining the occlusal relationship. If not done previously, the surface scans of the upper and lower teeth should be overlayed and fused with the maxilla and mandible. Eventually, a virtual splint can be generated (**Fig 5.3.13-7**). The virtual splint is placed on the teeth and an impression of the upper and lower dental arches is "subtracted" from the blank dental splint. The planned position of the maxilla and mandible is then transformed to the splint. Finally, the splint is fabricated on a 3-D printer.

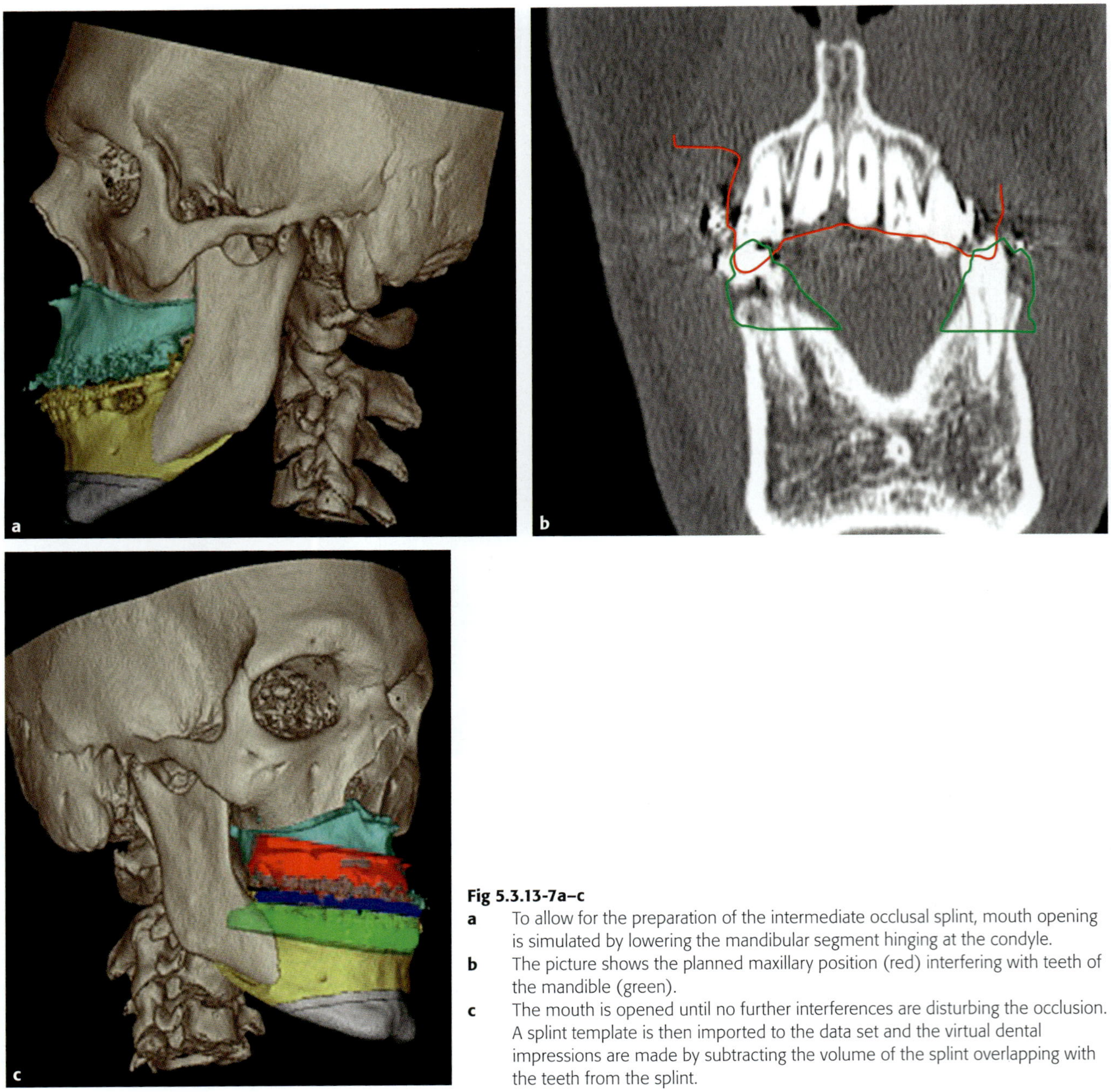

Fig 5.3.13-7a–c

a To allow for the preparation of the intermediate occlusal splint, mouth opening is simulated by lowering the mandibular segment hinging at the condyle.

b The picture shows the planned maxillary position (red) interfering with teeth of the mandible (green).

c The mouth is opened until no further interferences are disturbing the occlusion. A splint template is then imported to the data set and the virtual dental impressions are made by subtracting the volume of the splint overlapping with the teeth from the splint.

4.2 Virtual maxillary correction

After clinical examination of the patient and completion of the analysis/segmentation, the virtual skeletal corrections can be performed. Precise orientation of the maxilla should be the initial step in planning. This will affect the orientation of the mandible in 2-jaw procedures. The horizontal occlusal plane can be defined using the contact point between teeth 11 and 21, and the fissures of teeth 16 and 26. The correction of the occlusal plane, often a rotation is necessary to create facial balance, may give the impression of a horizontal maxillary deviation. Further optimization of the maxillary orientation should then be performed in the axial and sagittal views. Some maxillary rotation may be necessary to close an open bite deformity. This is most easily performed working in the sagittal view. Finally, the maxillary positions are optimized into the midsagittal orientation to find the symmetry alignment. This is most easily performed working in the axial view (**Fig 5.3.13-8**).

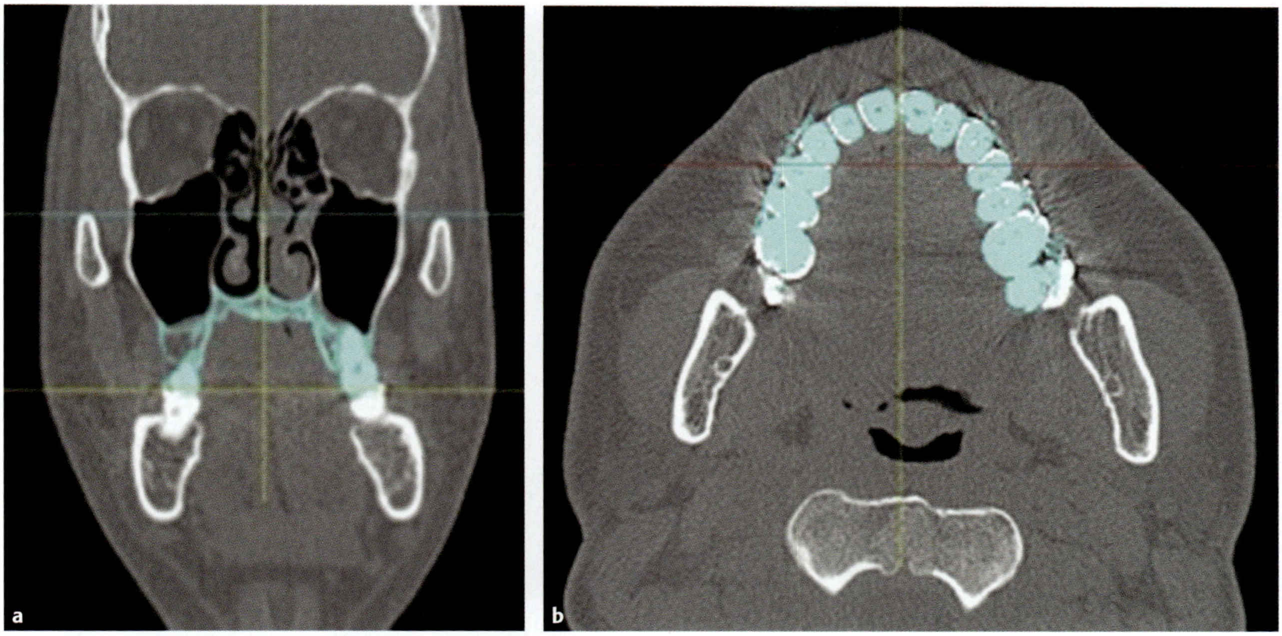

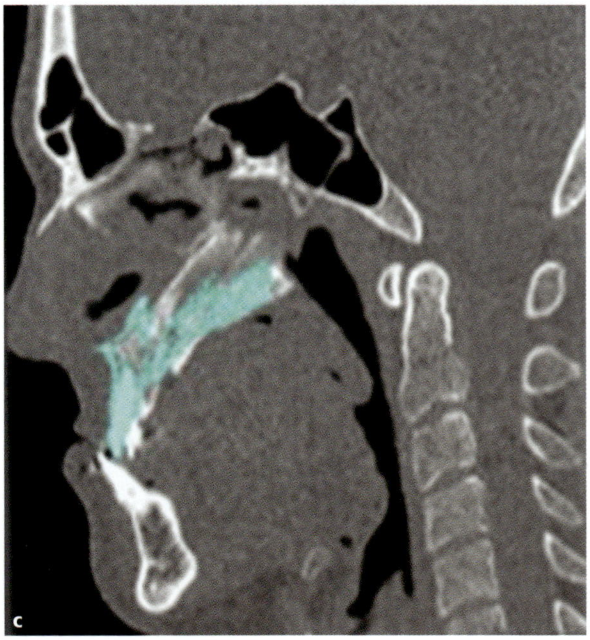

Fig 5.3.13-8a–c
- **a** Coronal view presenting the horizontal relation of the occlusal plane being in the correct position; no "roll" rotation is necessary.
- **b** In the axial view, the midline symmetry is evaluated. A clockwise rotation around the midpoint of the maxillary segment is necessary—a "yaw" rotation was performed.
- **c** The necessary anterior posterior movement is evaluated in the sagittal view. In this case an anterior movement of 5 mm is performed as determined by the cephalometric analysis and clinical investigations—an anterior "pitch" rotation was done.

4.3 Virtual mandibular correction

To evaluate the effect of the corrected position of the maxilla to the mandible, data from the teeth surface scan with teeth in the determined ideal occlusion is now imported into the data set and aligned to the planned new maxillary position (**Fig 5.3.13-9**). In a further step, it is necessary to establish a correct superposition of the mandibular teeth of the high-resolution tooth scan with the mandibular teeth of the low-resolution CT scan. This is achieved by moving the imported tooth scan until a perfect overlay with the CT has been obtained (**Fig 5.3.13-10**).

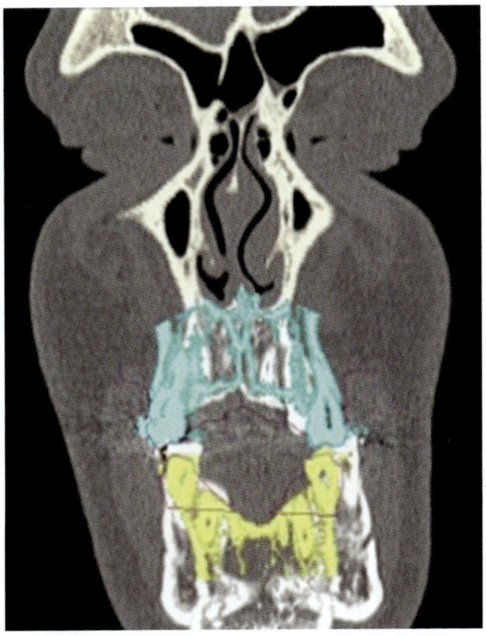

Fig 5.3.13-9 Coronal view of data set including the surface scan of upper (blue overlay) and lower (yellow overlay) dental arches in determined occlusion. Alignment to the new positioned upper dental arch was already done.

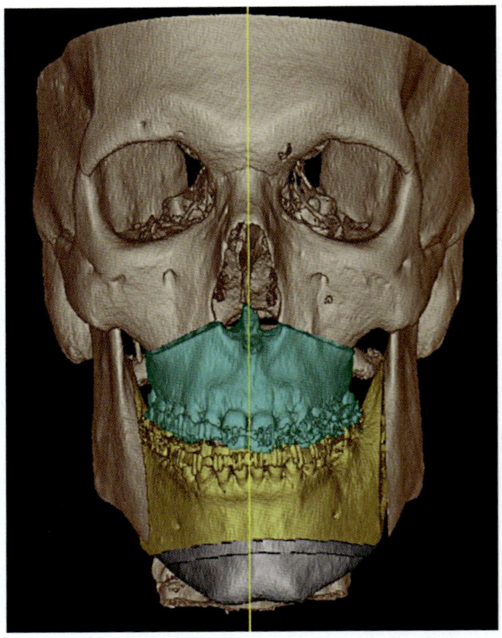

Fig 5.3.13-10 A 3-D view of the data set presenting the aligned position of the mandible using the information of the surface scan of the upper and lower dental arch in determined ideal occlusion.

The virtual planning shows a conflict between the newly positioned mandibular segment and the stationary condylar segment. Due to the "yaw" rotation, the virtual planning shows an overlap of the mandible segment and the condylar segment at the area of the sagittal split on the left side. Additional bone removal may be planned if necessary (**Fig 5.3.13-11**). If necessary, a final splint can then be produced.

4.3.1 Chin correction

Chin corrections may be indicated as part of complex mandibulomaxillary osteotomies or as stand-alone procedures. In a 3-D data set the chin position can be evaluated for projection and symmetry. Chin augmentations, correction of asymmetries, as well as chin reductions can be planned and simulated (**Fig 5.3.13-12**).

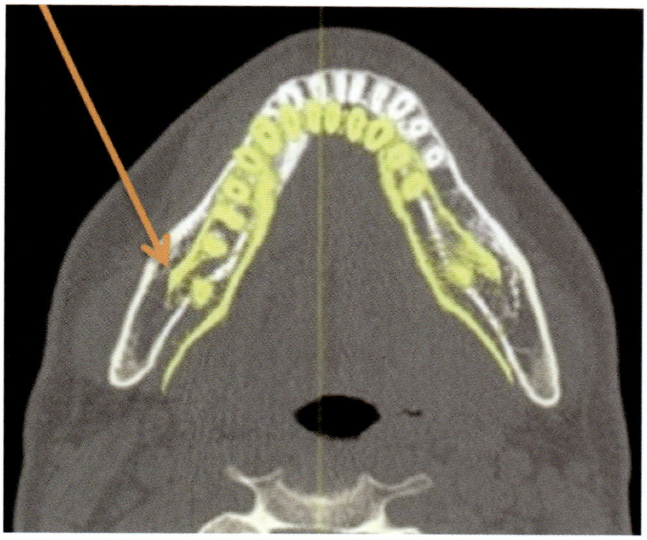

Fig 5.3.13-11 Axial view of the data set showing the new position (yellow) of the mandible in comparison with the original position (white area). The "yaw" rotation of the mandible (yellow) results in an overlap of the bone contact area with the condylar segment on the left side of the sagittal split (arrow).

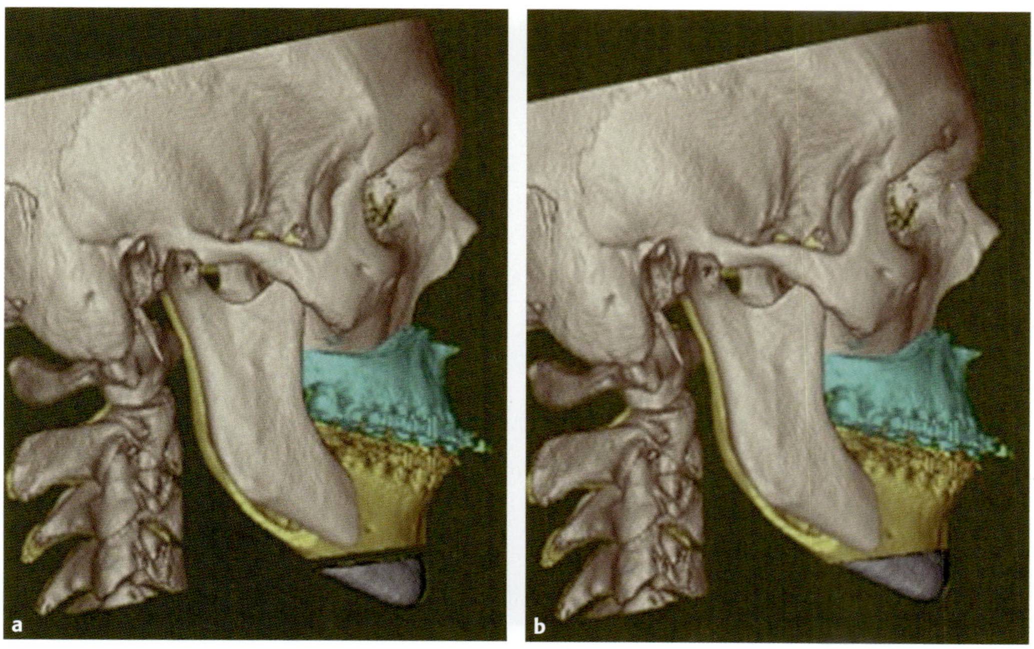

Fig 5.3.13-12a–b Planning of a chin reduction in a complex case. Side view of the 3-D data set showing the removal of a part of the chin (**a**) and the new position of the reduced chin (**b**).

5 Clinical case

The patient was a 20-year-old woman with facial asymmetry secondary to hemimandibular elongation on the right side (**Fig 5.3.13-13**).

The CT data were imported into the planning software and a 3-D virtual model was generated.

After defining the true orthogonal planes and midsagittal symmetry, the maxilla was segmented out (blue area). The occlusal plane was then defined (**Fig 5.3.13-14**). This clearly demonstrates the right-sided mandibular and maxillary hyperplasia.

In this case a clockwise rotation of the maxilla was necessary. Note the disturbing tooth contact on the left side (**Fig 5.3.13-15**), which is caused by a correction of the upper jaw and a concomitant superposition in the left side tooth area.

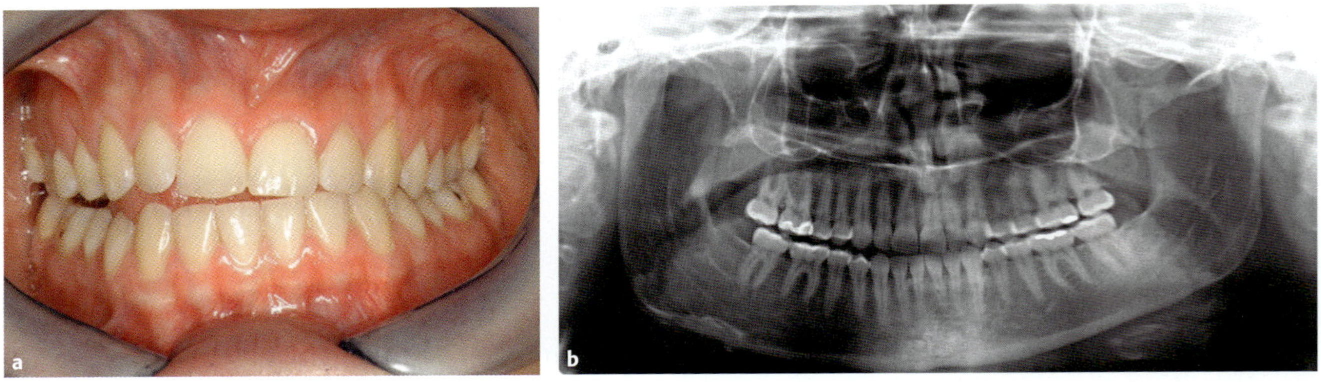

Fig 5.3.13-13a–b Patient presenting a hemimandibular elongation on the right side.
a Intraoral situation.
b Panoramic x-ray.

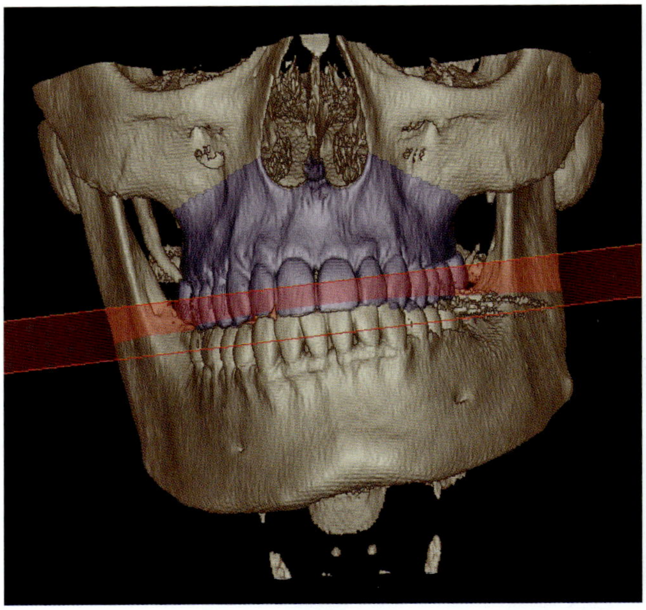

Fig 5.3.13-14 A 3-D view of the patient case. The maxilla is segmented in the Le Fort I plane for planning. The red plane visualizes the occlusion plane being not horizontal.

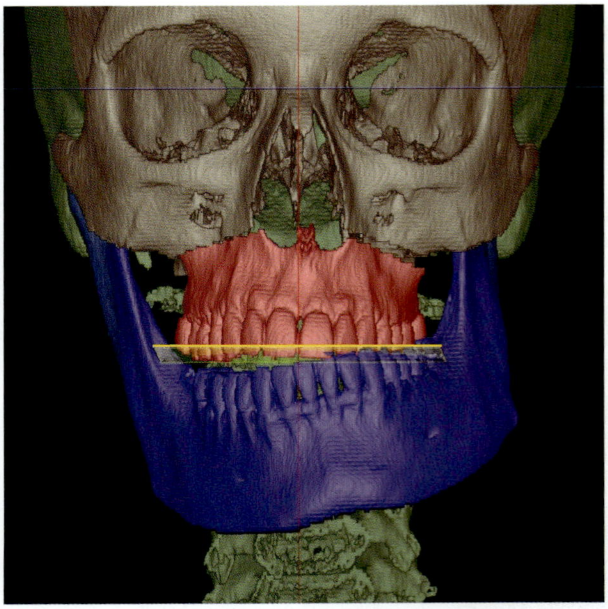

Fig 5.3.13-15 A 3-D view of the corrected position of the maxilla (red). A clockwise "roll" rotation was performed to achieve a horizontal occlusion plane (yellow).

The teeth surface scans (red and green) are then imported into the data set to overlay the existing teeth. The position of the teeth surface scans relative to the teeth of the CT scan is then locked.

To allow for the preparation of the intermediate occlusal splint, mouth opening is mimicked by lowering the mandibular segment hinging at the condyle. The mouth is opened until no further interferences are disturbing the occlusion (**Fig 5.3.13-16**).

A splint template is then imported to the data set and the virtual dental impressions are made from subtracting the volume of the splint overlapping with the teeth.

For planning of the virtual mandibular correction by condylectomy on the right side, the unaffected left mandible side was mirrored to the right side. By using the surface scan of the upper and lower dental arches in ideal occlusion, the precise position of the mandible can be determined (**Fig 5.3.13-17**).

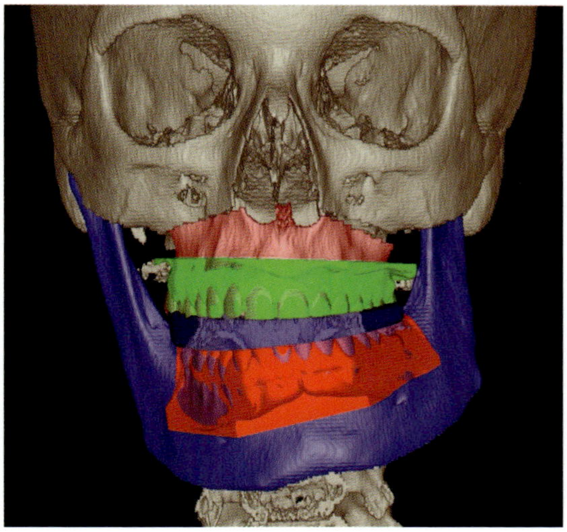

Fig 5.3.13-16 Virtual situation for producing the intermediate splint. A 3-D view of the planning after importing the scanned plaster cast models of the upper (green) and lower (red) tooth arches. A precise alignment of the tooth arches presented by the computed tomographic scan and by the surface scan was done automatically by the software.

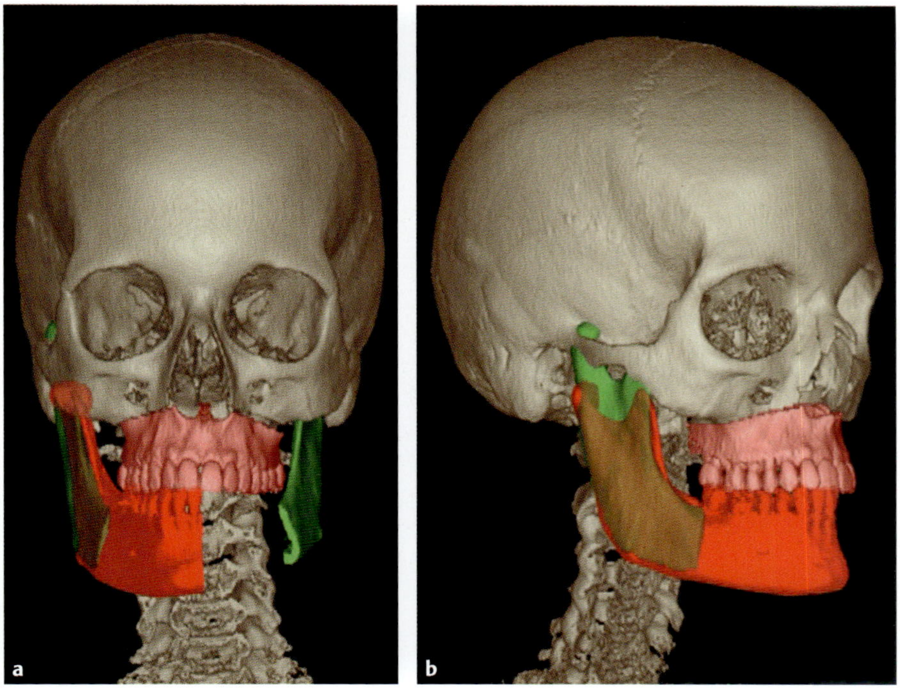

Fig 5.3.13-17a–b
a Situation after mirroring the unaffected (green ramus) left ascending ramus to the right side (red structure).
b A discrepancy of approximately 15 mm condylar length was evaluated between the original position (green right structure) and the new mandible (planned: red right structure).

The mandibular segment is then moved into occlusion with the newly positioned maxilla. A final occlusal splint was not necessary in this case. This picture shows the difference between the affected condyle and the mirrored unaffected condyle (**Fig 5.3.13-17**). In this case a 15 mm difference could be recorded.

While taking care to preserve the intraarticular disc, the condylar head was trimmed and shaved to mimic the size of the unaffected side (**Fig 5.3.13-18**). The orthognathic corrections were performed through a standard Le Fort I and a sagittal split osteotomy at the left side.

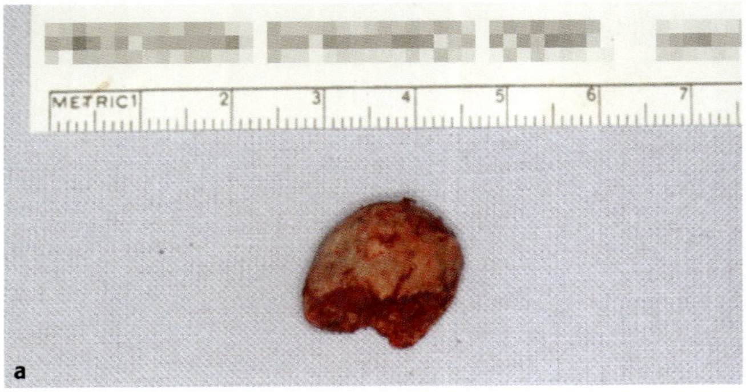

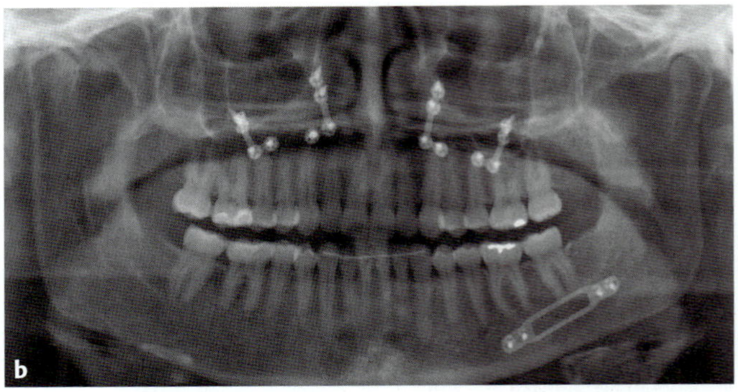

Fig 5.3.13-18a–b
a Resected condyle of the right side.
b Panoramic x-ray control after surgery.

6 Complications

Good clinical results in orthognathic surgery require an accurate preoperative diagnosis and precise presurgical planning. Virtual surgical planning enables precise analysis of a 3-D model that accurately represents the clinical situation and facilitates diagnosis and treatment planning. While single jaw surgery can be based on the occlusal plane of the opposite jaw, two jaw surgeries are much more complex. The position of the jaws is defined by orthognathic model surgery or 3-D presurgical planning in a virtual environment and coded by occlusal splints [Metzger et al, 2008]. However, these techniques have some limitations. The manufacturing of splints can be done manually by a laboratory or by virtual planning and fabrication using 3-D printers. Beside the fact that the virtual planning can be transferred precisely into an occlusal splint, several errors can occur during the planning process.

First, the midsagittal symmetry plane can be defined incorrectly. This can lead to misalignment of the occlusal plane and consequently to an incorrect maxillary and mandibular correction. To avoid this error, the patient should always be aligned in the neutral head position. A patient's profile picture during which the patient is looking in a vertical mirror is helpful to determine the neutral head position.

Second, there may be an error in the correct setting of the virtual planning levels. This could lead to an asymmetrical Le Fort I osteotomy in the upper jaw and consequently to an asymmetrical osteotomy and facial deformity. In addition, an incorrectly placed Le Fort I osteotomy line may lead to intraoperative complications, such as injury of tooth roots.

Third, metallic artifacts in the CT scan caused by dental restorations can contribute to an insufficient or inadequate overlay of 3-D data sets and result in inaccurate planning. This problem can be addressed by taking a dental laser scan from the teeth and alveolus. This information can be incorporated into the CT data. Ultimately, an intermediate splint made on this basis may lead to an unsatisfactory orthognathic correction. In addition, this can contribute to intraoperative orthognathic complications, such as irregular split patterns, nerve injury, bleedings and mechanical problems [Steenen et al, 2016; Steenen et al, 2016].

7 Summary

Computerized planning in corrective bone surgery opens up a new area for digital planning in surgery, including the manufacturing of splints, cutting guides and patient-specific implants. Up to now, it is not completely clear which subgroup of patients is likely to benefit from more sophisticated and advanced planning technology. However, many surgeons believe that the more complex cases, such as patients with facial asymmetry and complex deformities, are likely to benefit.

8 References and suggested reading

Gil JN, Claus JD, Manfro R, et al. Predictability of maxillary repositioning during bimaxillary surgery: accuracy of a new technique. *Int J Oral Maxillofac Surg.* 2007 Apr;36(4):296–300.

Metzger MC, Hohlweg-Majert B, Schwarz U, et al. Manufacturing splints for orthognathic surgery using a three-dimensional printer. *Oral Surg Oral Med Oral Pathol Oral Radiol Endod.* 2008 Feb;105(2):e1–7.

Miller RJ, Derakhshan M. Three-dimensional technology improves the range of orthodontic treatment with esthetic and removable aligners. *World J Orthodontics.* 2004 Fall;5(3):242–249.

Mischkowski RA, Zinser MJ, Kübler AC, et al. Application of an augmented reality tool for maxillary positioning in orthognathic surgery—a feasibility study. *J Craniomaxillofac Surg.* 2006 Dec;34(8):478–483.

Steenen SA, Becking AG. Bad splits in bilateral sagittal split osteotomy: systematic review of fracture patterns. *Int J Oral Maxillofacial Surg.* 2016 Jul;45(7):887–897.

Steenen SA, van Wijk AJ, Becking AG. Bad splits in bilateral sagittal split osteotomy: systematic review and meta-analysis of reported risk factors. *Int J Oral Maxillofac Surg.* 2016 Mar;45(8):971–979.

Stevens DR, Flores-Mir C, Nebbe B, et al. Validity, reliability, and reproducibility of plaster vs digital study models: comparison of peer assessment rating and Bolton analysis and their constituent measurements. *Am J Orthod Dentofacial Orthop.* 2006 Jun;129(6):794–803.

Whetten JL, Williamson PC, Heo G, et al. Variations in orthodontic treatment planning decisions of Class II patients between virtual 3-dimensional models and traditional plaster study models. *Am J Orthod Dentofacial Orthop.* 2006 Oct;130(4):485–491.

5.3.14 Interspeciality interface in head and neck oncology—current clinical use of computer-assisted surgery and future perspectives

Majeed Rana, Nils-Claudius Gellrich

1 Introduction

Head and neck oncology benefits more and more from interdisciplinary exchange of information. Personalized treatment pathways are typically defined by an interdisciplinary tumor board. Advances in image analysis methods and computer-assisted surgery have increasingly facilitated the clinical application of 3-D imaging for head and neck tumor treatment over the last decade. For adequate treatment planning for craniomaxillofacial tumors a computer-assisted analysis of 3-D image data, such as magnetic resonance imaging (MRI) and computed tomograpy (CT), is essential for tumor staging. Treatment planning is based on this information as well as on clinical data. Computer-assisted navigation technology might be a useful tool in tumor resection. The 3-D information on the origin of tumor margins or biopsies can be matched with histopathological findings, with other words geometrical and histopathological information, which can be stored digitally to improve the interdisciplinary interaction for the benefit of the patient.

2 Computer-assisted preoperative planning

Basic requirements for tumor treatment planning are CT and MRI images of the area of interest. The MRI data set is used to differentiate between tumor and healthy soft tissue, and the CT data set to visualize the hard tissue and patient bony anatomy. During the acquisition of the CT data, either four surgically inserted navigation landmarks (bony landmarks, 2.0 cross-drive titanium mini screws or an individual dental splint with additional titanium screws) are used for registration of the individual patient. These screws are used as registration points during planning and surgery. If the CT data are already provided without navigation landmarks, an additional subvolume cone beam CT with navigational landmarks is needed.

The resulting DICOM data of the patient's anatomy are imported into the planning application (iPlan, Brainlab, Feldkirchen, Germany).

After that alignment, both image data sets (CT and MRI) are coregistered by a so-called image fusion, a surface- and voxel-based matching method to have the whole multimodal information available within the previously adjusted alignment. Registration points are then planned virtually on the screw heads within the dental splint or the screws inserted in the patient's skull.

The anatomical structures and the target tumor tissue are then segmented out of the image sets. The tumor shape is outlined manually using different software tools, such as brushing, as a tumor is not automatically recognized and segmented within a patient's anatomy. The Smartbrush algorithm makes it possible to segment the structures or tumor automatically by an elastic deformation. Because of that procedure all necessary anatomical structures in the area around the tumor are identified as 3-D segmented objects. With this planning step, clearly defined anatomical representations of the patient's anatomy are available together with a target region at the tumor position for resection. All preplanned virtual patient data, objects, and trajectories are transferred to an image-guided surgery system (navigation system).

3 Intraoperative infrared-based navigation

Before surgery the patient is fixed in a Mayfield clamp or a mini tripod. A "skull reference base" with three trackable spheres is fixed with a single mini titanium screw on the patient's skull to identify the exact position and orientation of the patient. Intraoperative accuracy is checked using at least four precise navigation landmarks. An infrared-based navigation system (eg, Kick-Brainlab) is used intraoperatively.

By using a stereoscopic infrared camera, a "real-world patient's" position with its planned virtual data can be referenced and instrument positions in real time can be tracked and displayed. The patient position and anatomy is registered to the preplanned data by inserting navigational landmarks, like the above-mentioned dental splint, making sure that the markers in the splint, usually osteosynthesis screws, are oriented according to their preplanned positions. During surgery, the position of instrument tips is monitored in real time to ensure that the tumor is resected exactly at the desired position according to the preoperative virtual planning. Additionally, intraoperative landmarks are recorded (acquired) and a screenshot is done at every safety margin. The summation of these points form a point cloud, sometimes called a "tumor cloud", which is transferred to the virtual plan after surgery and helps to identify and to define the exact positions of the tumor resection at any time thereafter.

4 Postprocessing of the data set

The acquired intraoperative landmarks are postoperatively incorporated into the treatment plan. After final release of the histological findings, the individual points are color-coded according to their classification (benign/malignant). Visualization now allows for an optimized 3-D information about potential residual tumor.

4.1 Export of the data set

With iPlan the acquired point cloud can be written into the patient's DICOM data set. Only the points with tumor-positive histology are selected. These points (voxels) are allocated with a Houndsfield unit of 3,500 H. This value is far out of the traditional highest range of around 3100 H and gives a clearly defined border for easier manipulation of the original DICOM data set. It also makes fast segmentation of the point cloud possible by using threshold values.

4.2 Import into the radiation therapy simulation platform

The enhanced DICOM data set (enDICOM) can be imported into any radiation therapy planning platform. The described enDICOM is imported and superimposed with the postoperative CT scan. The well-defined high Houndsfield unit of the selected points facilitates segmentation and visualization of the additional intraoperative information and can be used to plan radiation therapy aspects.

5 Case presentation

An 81-year-old man with a residual T4a adenoid cystic carcinoma (ACC) of the maxillary sinus and nasal cavity on the left side was planned for ablative tumor surgery (**Fig 5.3.14-1**).

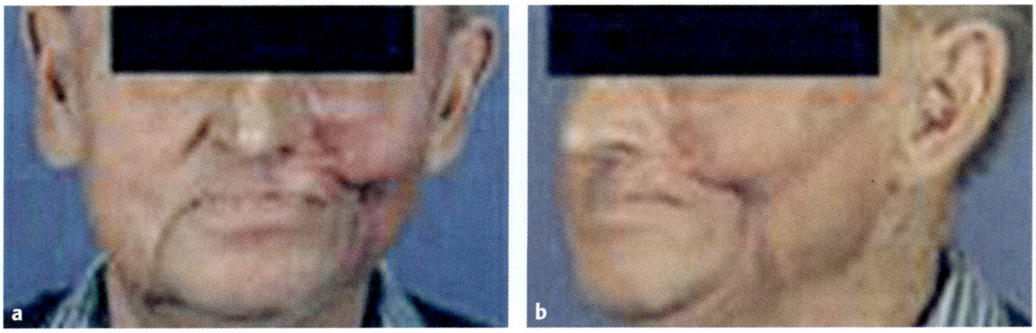

Fig 5.3.14-1a–b

a Frontal view of an 81-year-old man with a residual T4a adenoid cystic carcinoma of the cheek after tumor resection and radiochemotherapy alio loco.

b Lateral view.

After tumor resection, the position of the forceps was monitored to take specimens from the tumor margin. Additional intraoperative landmarks were acquired and a screenshot was done at every biopsy. These points (tumor cloud) were transferred to the virtual plan after surgery and helped to identify and define the exact positions of the biopsies. The specimen showed a margin between tumor and resection of less than 2 mm. In addition, positive nodes were identified in the histopathological examination after neck dissection. The intraoperatively collected data (tumor cloud) together with the histopathological findings were then forwarded to the radiation oncologist to plan adjuvant radiotherapy (**Fig 5.3.14-2**).

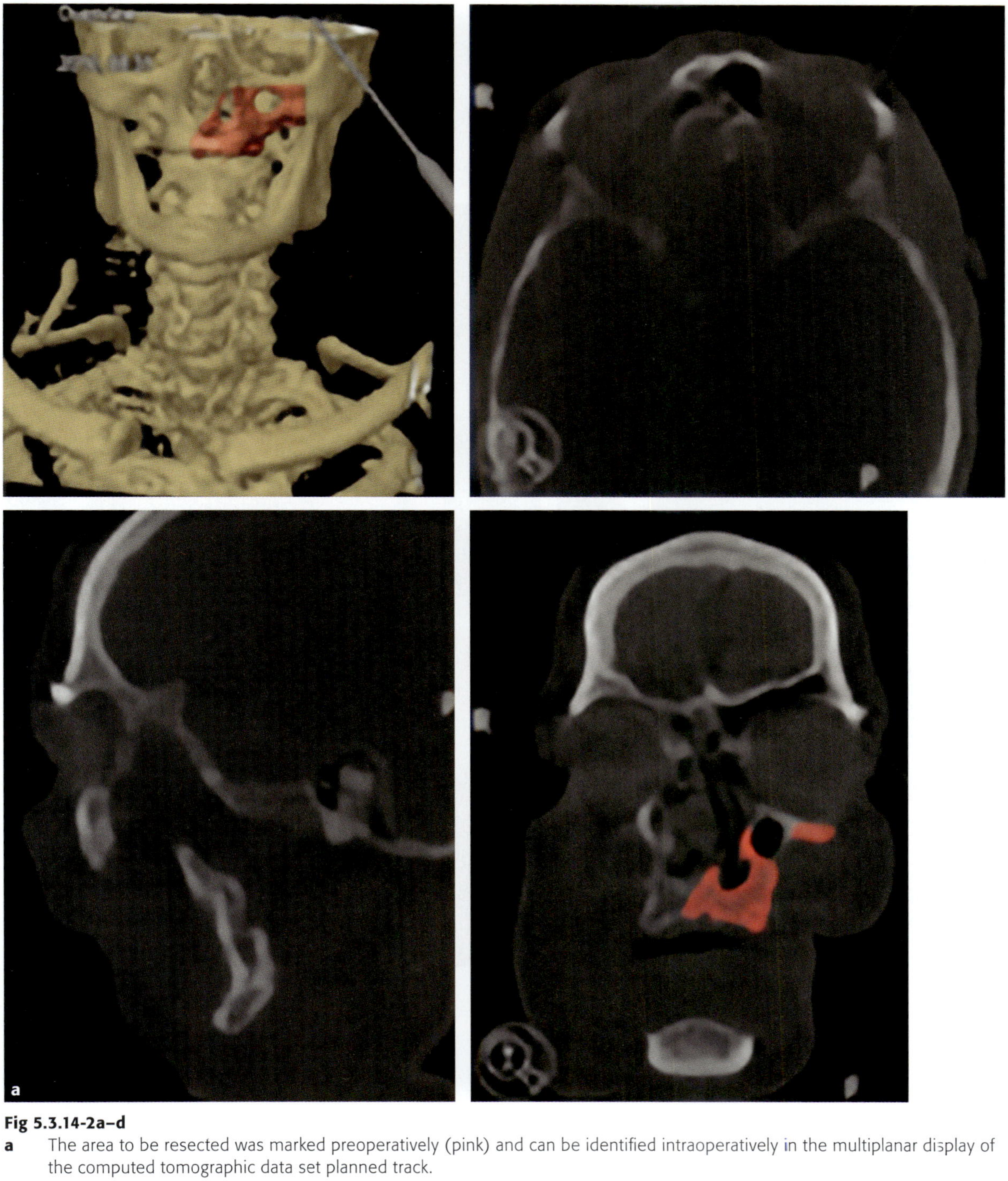

Fig 5.3.14-2a–d

a The area to be resected was marked preoperatively (pink) and can be identified intraoperatively in the multiplanar display of the computed tomographic data set planned track.

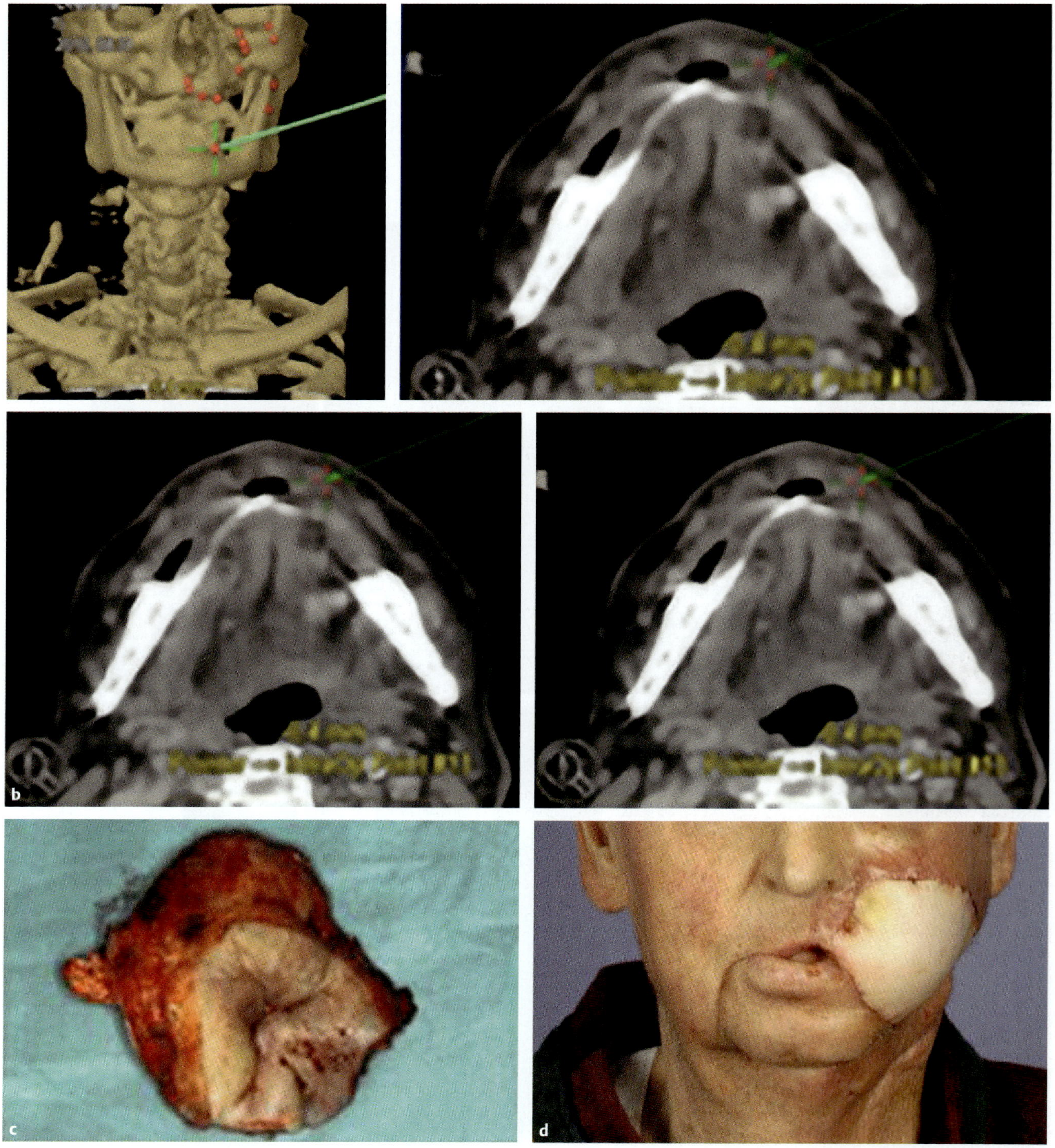

Fig 5.3.14-2a–d (cont)

b Navigation-assisted control of tumor margin. The tip (green) is pointing to the tumor, which is displayed in the multiplanar mode (axial, sagittal, and coronal), intraoperative landmarks acquired at every biopsy.

c Resected tumor of the left cheek.

d Frontal view after reconstruction with a latissimus dorsi flap 4 weeks postoperatively.

In this manner, the radiotherapy field can be matched to the postoperative tumor topography. The novel method of intraoperative mapping of the origin of specimen (biopsies, margins), either frozen sections or definite histopathological examination, allows the storage and further use of intraoperative information if needed (**Fig 5.3.14-3**).

In the field of craniomaxillofacial surgery, indications for this technique are currently limited to tumor locations within or close to hard tissue. Common head and neck malignancies affecting the floor of the mouth and tongue do not allow for the described method. An adequate soft-tissue navigation tool is a necessary precondition to use this technique. Currently, assessing resection margins intraoperatively is possible by means of frozen sections. If positive, they can be a guide to additional resection but when negative they add no information about the distance from the tumor margin.

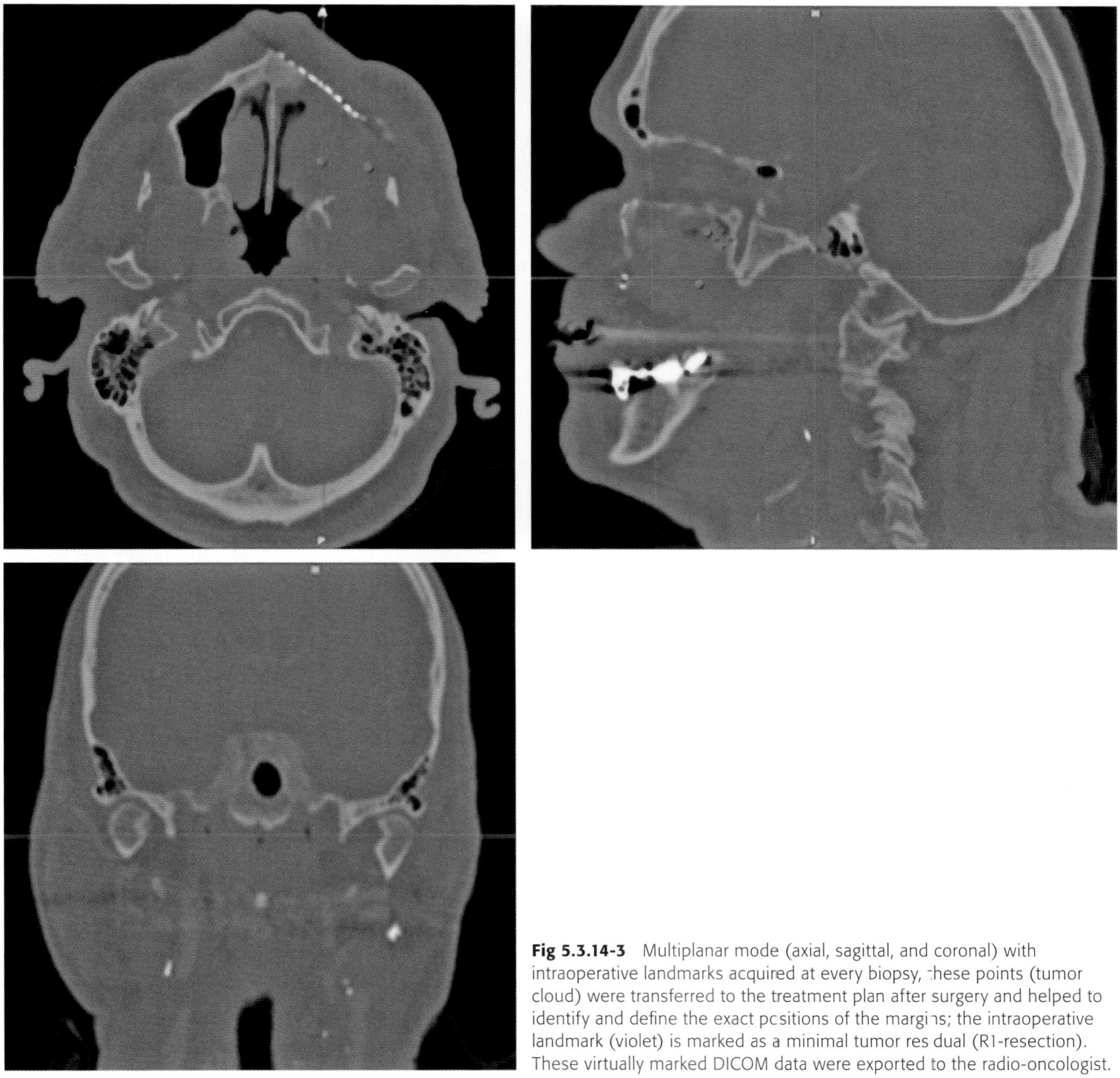

Fig 5.3.14-3 Multiplanar mode (axial, sagittal, and coronal) with intraoperative landmarks acquired at every biopsy, these points (tumor cloud) were transferred to the treatment plan after surgery and helped to identify and define the exact positions of the margins; the intraoperative landmark (violet) is marked as a minimal tumor residual (R1-resection). These virtually marked DICOM data were exported to the radio-oncologist.

6 References and suggested reading

Eckardt A, Swennen GR. Virtual planning of composite mandibular reconstruction with free fibula bone graft. *J Craniofac Surg.* 2005 Nov;16(6):1137–1140.

Essig H, Rana M, Kokemueller H, et al. Referencing of markerless CT data sets with cone beam subvolume including registration markers to ease computer-assisted surgery—a clinical and technical research. *Int J Med Robot.* 2013 Sep;9(3):e39–45.

Essig H, Rana M, Meyer A, et al. Virtual 3D tumor marking—exact intraoperative coordinate mapping improves post-operative radiotherapy. *Radiat Oncol.* 2011 Nov 16;6:159.

Gellrich NC, Schramm A, Hammer B, et al. Computer-assisted secondary reconstruction of unilateral posttraumatic orbital deformity. *Plast Reconstr Surg.* 2002 Nov;110(6):1417–1429.

Rana M, Essig H, Eckardt AM, et al. Advances and innovations in computer-assisted head and neck oncologic surgery. *J Craniofac Surg.* 2012 Jan;23(1):272–278.

Rana M, Modrow D, Keuchel J, et al. Development and evaluation of an automatic tumor segmentation tool: a comparison between automatic, semi-automatic and manual segmentation of mandibular odontogenic cysts and tumors. *J Craniomaxillofac Surg.* 2015 Apr;43(3):355–359.

Schramm A, Wilde F. [Computer-assisted reconstruction of the facial skeleton]. *HNO.* 2011 Aug;59(8):800–806. German.

5.3.15 Computer-assisted techniques in orbital surgery for thyroid eye disease

Nicholas R Mahoney, Michael P Grant

1 Introduction

Thyroid eye disease (Graves orbitopathy, thyroid-associated orbitopathy) is an inflammatory disorder seemingly resulting from acquired thyroid-stimulating hormone-receptor (TSH-R) autoimmunity. Stimulation of TSH-R positive orbital fibroblasts results in hyaluronan deposition, cellular differentiation into myofibroblasts, and activation of T-cell and mononuclear immune cells. In turn, extraocular muscle and orbital fat enlargement, tissue contraction and orbital inflammation develop. The clinical effect is a combination of periorbital swelling, proptosis, restrictive strabismus, and eyelid retraction with occasional resultant threatening of sight from compressive optic neuropathy or corneal exposure.

The disease occurs in 16 females and 3 males per 100,000 people with a predilection for fat enlargement or muscle enlargement in patients younger than 40 or older than 60 years, respectively [Burch et al, 2015; Bartley et al, 1996]. Clinical severity tends to rise and fall over 18–36 months with two-thirds of patients improving to some extent without intervention [Bartley et al, 1996]. Autoimmunity itself can be tracked measuring thyroid-stimulating immunoglobulin percentage, a bioassay measuring stimulation of TSH-induced cAMP synthesis compared with normal serum on TSH-R-transfected Chinese hamster ovary cells.

2 Surgical management

Most commonly, surgical management occurs for ocular rehabilitation in patients once inactivity is established with serial examinations and TSI monitoring. The sequence of surgical interventions in such patients is orbital decompression, strabismus surgery, eyelid retraction correction, and then blepharoplasty as indicated. Nearly all diplopia in patients existing before an extensive bony decompression will persist afterward. New diplopia can also occur in a minority of patients without preexisting strabismus. Orbital decompression, however, alters globe position and rotational angle and therefore precedes strabismus surgery. Proptosis reduction and strabismus surgery, particularly inferior rectus recession, can alter both lower and upper eyelid retraction and hence is corrected last.

Significant extraocular muscle expansion causing compression of the optic nerve posteriorly or severe proptosis resulting in exposure keratitis may require more urgent orbital decompression [Jorge et al, 2003; Kowal et al, 1994]. Generally, such patients are treated with pulse intravenous steroids but at least 25–30% will have inadequate response requiring urgent decompression. Both the radiographic findings and surgical needs of the patient with an optic neuropathy differ from those patients undergoing decompression for proptosis only and deserve special mention. Patients with compressive optic neuropathy tend to have less measured proptosis and more pronounced posterior muscle belly enlargement. The posterior inferolateral orbital configuration tends to be narrower with a larger greater wing of the sphenoid bone and optic canal tends to be bound medially by the sphenoid sinus. As the decompression needs to occur at the orbital apex and in the optic canal, including release of the annulus, an endoscopic approach to the posterior medial orbital wall and optic canal is often utilized. Alternatively, the deep medial wall can be reached once the lateral wall has been removed to allow globe lateralization. Where the medial optic canal is suboptimal, such as in the case of a fungal sphenoid sinusitis, the lateral aspect of the optic canal can also be decompressed with a frontotemporal craniotomy such as a modified orbitozygomatic approach.

2.1 Approaches to orbital decompression

At least 15 approaches are in use for orbital decompression. Complication rates (such as rates of cerebrospinal fluid leak) and proptosis reduction are the most consistently reported comparable outcome measures, and comparison of the literature suggests transconjunctival and transnasal endoscopic approaches are associated with better proptosis reduction with lower adverse-effect rates than transpalpebral and transantral approaches [Leong et al, 2009]. The best approach ultimately is determined by surgeon experience, comfort with potential complications, the amount of decompression needed, and the targets for decompression. A 3-wall decompression with removal of the floor, medial wall, and lateral wall with or without the lateral rim, is commonly needed (**Fig 5.3.15-1** and **Fig 5.3.15-2**).

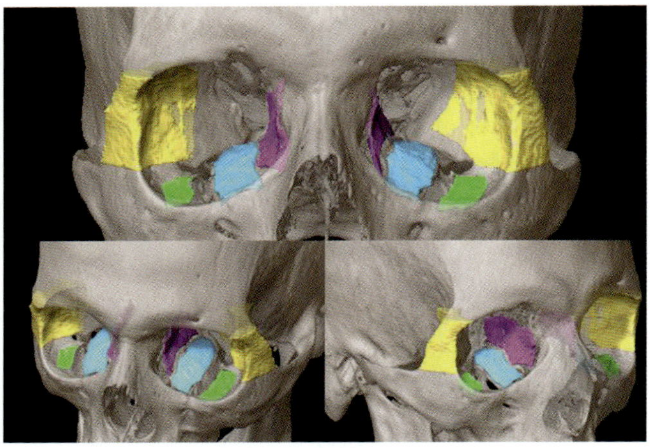

Fig 5.3.15-1 Volume-rendering demonstrating 3-wall bony decompression.

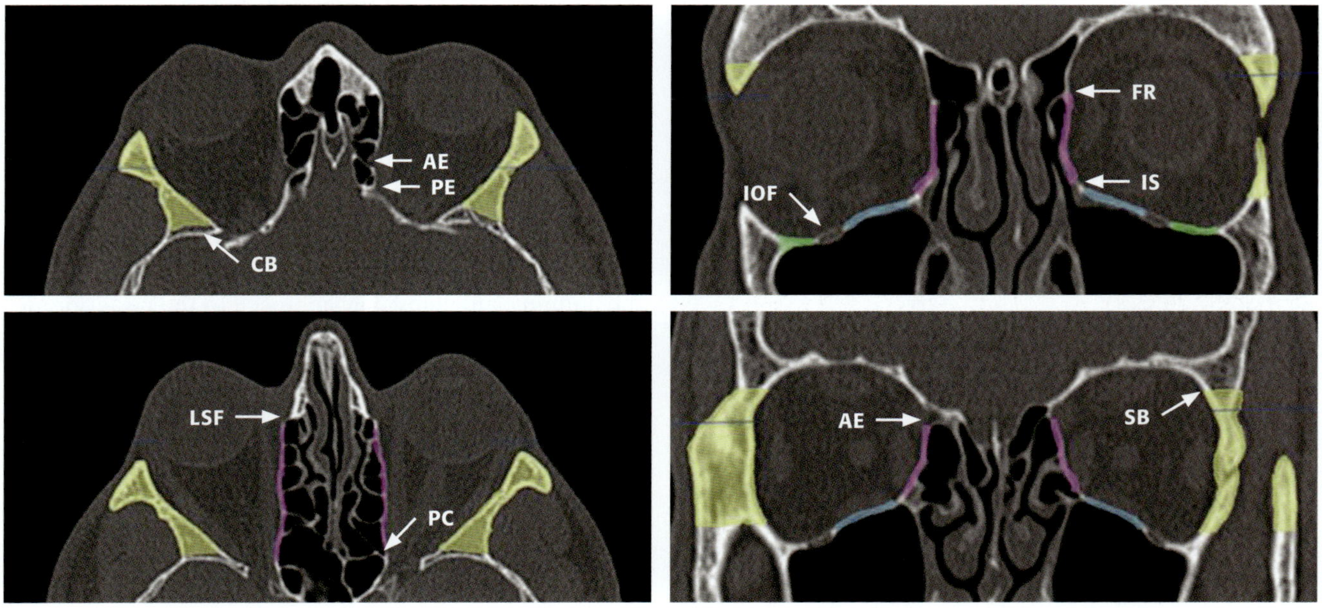

Fig 5.3.15-2 Axial and coronal images demonstrating targets for 3-wall bony decompression. CB indicates spared cortical bone at posterior lateral wall; AE, anterior ethmoid foramen; PE, posterior ethmoid foramen; IOF, infraorbital foramen; FR, limit of frontal sinus recess; IS, inframedial orbital strut; LSF, lacrimal sac fossa; PC, posterior wall of posterior ethmoid cell; and SB, superior border of lateral wall resection.

The orbital floor is often approached with a transconjunctival incision. A postseptal (fornix) incision is reliable and direct. With this approach, extraconal orbital fat is encountered and often elected to be debulked, although its removal does not affect globe position. The incision through the lower eyelid retractors, however, has little effect on lower eyelid retraction. This approach, with a sharp incision in the periosteum at the anterior edge of the orbital floor posterior to the arcus marginalis, also helps define the portion of the periorbita that will ultimately require a longitudinal relaxing incision.

An extension into a lateral canthotomy allows improved access to the inferolateral orbit. A cruciate incision through the periosteum on the lateral orbital rim centered at the lateral canthal tendon allows disinsertion of the superior and inferior crux of the lateral canthal tendon. The lateral wall can then be easily accessed.

An extension of the transconjunctival incision medially, just lateral to the caruncle, allows good access to the medial wall, particularly anteriorly. Posterior medial wall access from an anterior approach can be improved if the lateral wall rim is removed. Endoscopic access to the posterior orbital wall may be preferable in cases of optic neuropathy (**Fig 5.3.15-3**).

2.2 Computer-assisted techniques for routine decompression

2.2.1 Preoperative inspection and planning

The amount of desired proptosis reduction primarily determines the extent of bone removal. Intraconal orbital fat expansion, when present, may also be debulked. It can be estimated that every 1 cm^3 of fat removed corresponds to 1 mm of posterior globe position change. A volumetric assessment of the intraconal orbital fat can estimate the volume with a typical amount of 3–4 cm^3 targeted for removal.

On the orbital floor, the infraorbital canal can be left intact. In patients with a smaller orbit, the canal is often located laterally close to the body of the zygoma where bone removal would not contribute much toward increased orbital cavity volume. When located more centrally, often in patients with larger floor area, the floor defect size can approach the diameter of the globe and preservation of the canal prevents globe decent into the maxillary sinus.

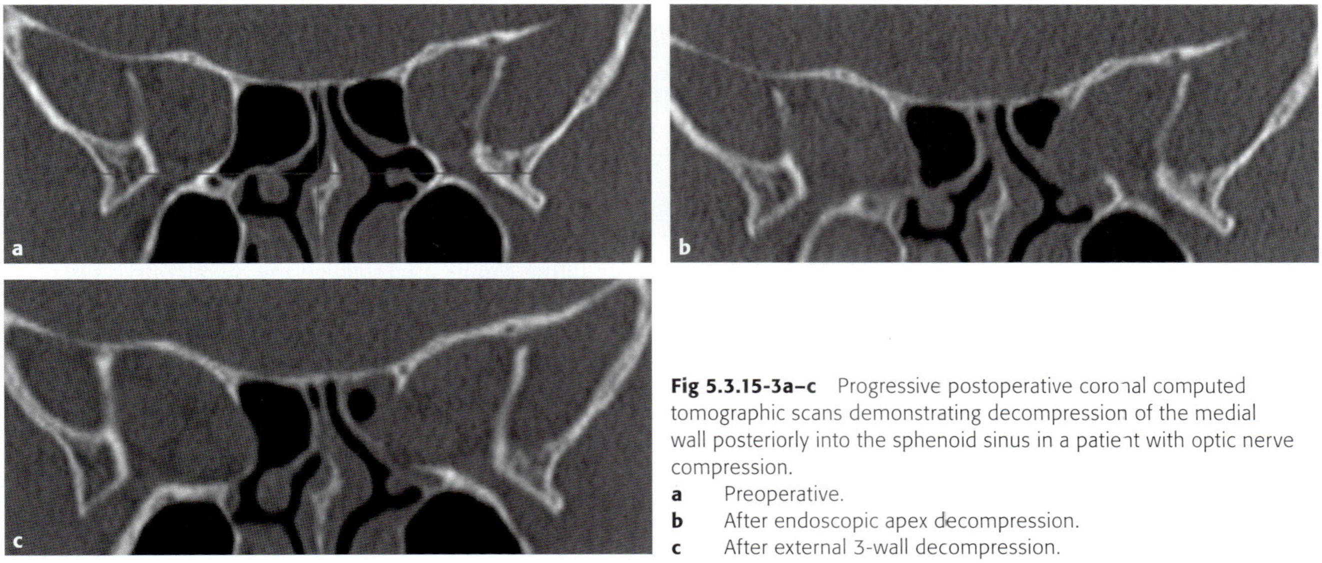

Fig 5.3.15-3a–c Progressive postoperative coronal computed tomographic scans demonstrating decompression of the medial wall posteriorly into the sphenoid sinus in a patient with optic nerve compression.

- **a** Preoperative.
- **b** After endoscopic apex decompression.
- **c** After external 3-wall decompression.

Regarding the medial wall removal, the inferomedial orbital strut should be preserved to maintain integrity of the frontomaxillary buttress. The superior extent of the medial wall resection should not extend farther superior than the frontoethmoidal suture line defined by the anterior and posterior ethmoid arteries. The artery foramen themselves can be identified in the medial wall on axial imaging at the junction of the middle cranial fossa and ethmoid sinus roof. Anterior and superior to the anterior ethmoid artery, the superior medial wall is often opposite the frontal sinus recess rather than the intracranial space. This area should also be avoided so as not to disrupt outflow of the frontal sinus. The posterior extent of the medial wall removal should account for the high variability in the ethmoid and sphenoid sinus configuration in relation to the optic canal. Decompression of the apex most often requires removal of the anterior optic canal adjacent to the sphenoid sinus. In cases without optic neuropathy, we prefer to mark our posterior limit adjacent to the most posterior ethmoid cell wall. The anterior extent should end at the posterior lacrimal crest.

Lateral wall removal is performed to a varying degree. Inspection preoperatively involves assessing the configuration and size of the greater wing of the sphenoid bone. A concave posterior lateral wall contour, associated with a narrow posterior orbit, warrants inferior lateral wall removal. Marking the posterior extent can allow preservation of a thin shell of bone over the dura to limit cerebrospinal fluid leak risk. Generally, the greater wing of the sphenoid is more cancellous bone but this thin shell of more avascular cortical bone is easy to identify. The central thin portion of the lateral wall on either side of the zygomatic-sphenoid suture should be removed. It is often thickened in patients with a proinflammatory state. Removal of the lateral wall rim from the frontozygomatic suture to the body of the zygoma, defined radiographically by an extension of the superior edge of the zygomatic arch, is effective for patients with a convex lateral wall contour, often with a wider posterior orbit. The rim can be removed entirely or advanced. When the central portion of the lateral wall or rim is removed, care must be taken to prevent the temporalis muscle from collapsing into the orbit with either pressure patching applied on the globe or a titanium expansion cage to push the muscle laterally.

With moderate disease and no strabismus, a "balanced" approach with submaximal medial and lateral bone removal is preferred. As vertical and oblique strabismus is more debilitating and difficult to correct, complete removal of the orbital floor should be done with caution. In patients requiring maximal posterior globe positioning, such as a patient with vision-threatening exposure keratopathy, the inferomedial orbital strut can be marked for removal with a plan to leave a strip of periorbita intact in this location to prevent globe subluxation.

With asymmetric disease, the lateral wall's contribution to orbital volume should be assessed. We prefer to address intraconal orbital fat first, followed by either the medial wall or lateral wall, and finally the floor if needed.

2.2.2 Intraoperative navigation

Using these principles, the targets for bone removal can be outlined as objects for intraoperative navigation. This is particularly useful to create a consistent and predictable decompression. There is added benefit from a safety perspective, specifically in avoiding optic nerve injury along the posterior medial wall and dural injury at the posterior lateral wall.

3 Postoperative comparison

Postoperative assessment of the results of an orbital decompression should not be performed until at least 3 months after surgery. Beyond posterior globe position shift, lateral rotation of the globe and thickening of the diameter of the medial rectus muscle belly can be observed and may potentiate with time (**Fig 5.3.15-4** and **Fig 5.3.15-5**). Image fusion techniques can be used to align the preoperative and postoperative scans and verification of accuracy of the preoperative target objects for bone removal can also be compared with the postoperative result.

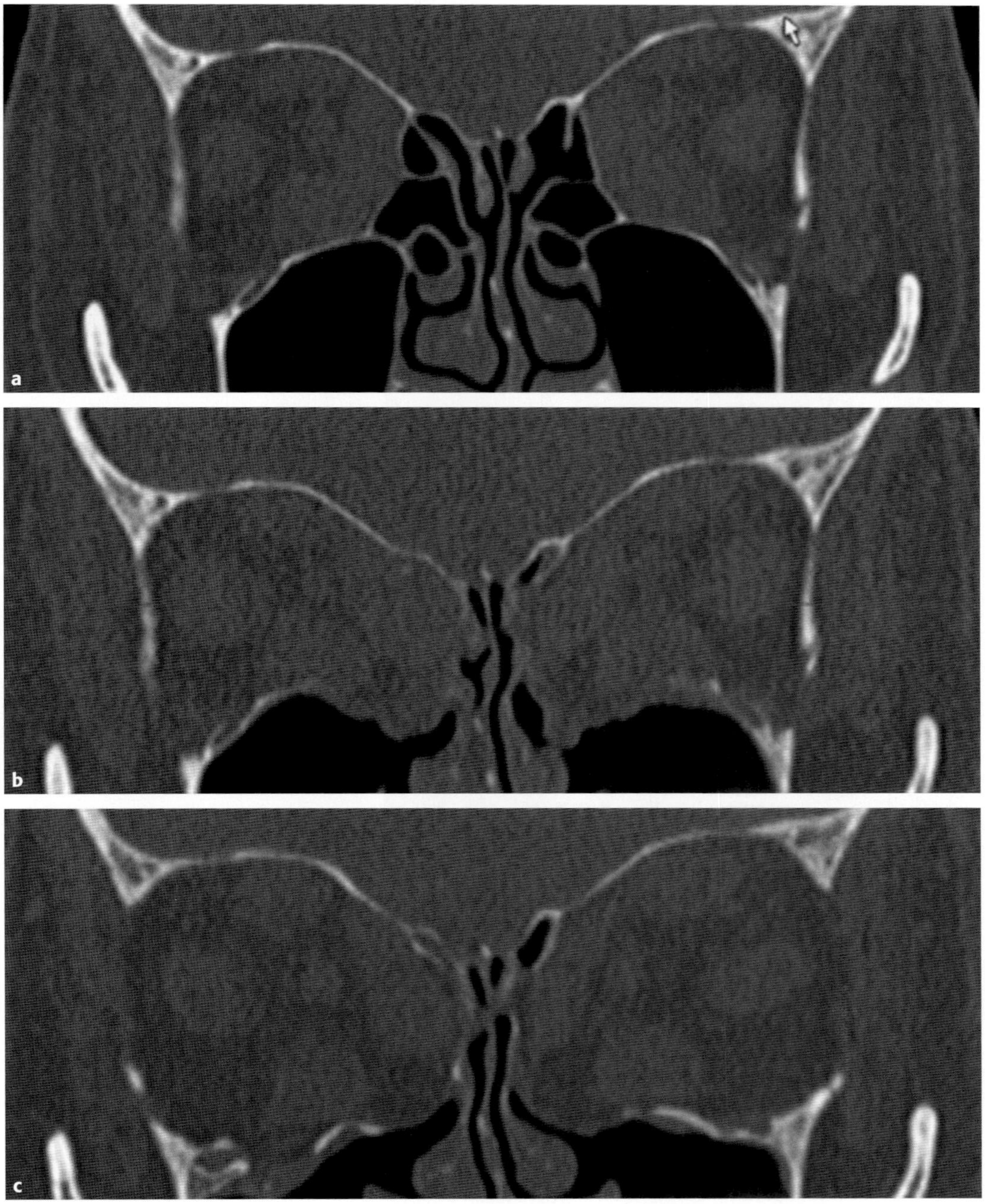

Fig 5.3.15-4a–c Progressive postoperative coronal computed tomographic scans demonstrating decompression of the medial wall, floor, and lateral wall.

a Preoperative.
b After endoscopic apex decompression.
c After external 3-wall decompression.

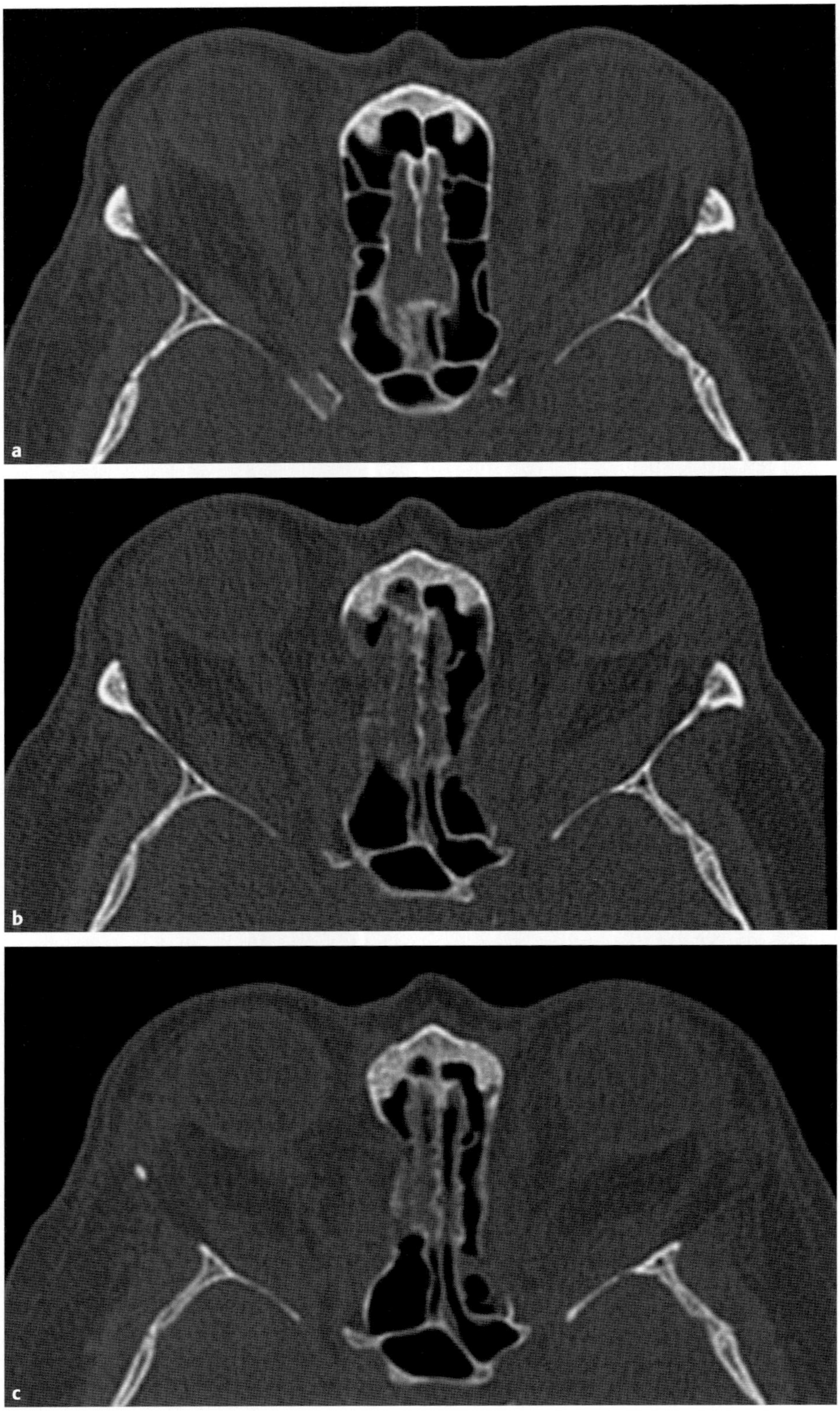

Fig 5.3.15-5a–c Progressive postoperative axial computed tomographic scans demonstrating decompression of the medial wall, floor, and lateral wall.

a Preoperative.
b After endoscopic apex decompression.
c After external 3-wall decompression.

4 Computer-assisted surgery in secondary decompressions

When inadequate decompression has been achieved or disease reactivation has resulted in worsening of proptosis, computer-assisted surgical planning can be particularly useful. Using the same preoperative planning guidelines as before, further access of the posterior lateral wall, residual floor or medial wall can be marked. As the anatomy has been disrupted by previous surgery, intraoperative navigation can provide orientation.

5 References and suggested reading

Bartley G B, Fatourechi V, Kadrmas EF, et al. Chronology of Graves' ophthalmopathy in an incidence cohort. *Am J Ophthalmol.* 1996 Apr;121(4):426–434.

Burch HB, Cooper DS. Management of Grave's disease: a review. *JAMA.* 2015 Dec 15;314(23):2544–2554.

Jorge R, Scott IU, Akaishi PM, et al. Resolution of choroidal folds and improvement in visual acuity after orbital decompression for graves orbitopathy. *Retina.* 2003;23:563–565.

Kowal L, Georgievski Z. Choroidal folds in Graves' ophthalmopathy. *Aust N Z J Ophthalmol.* 1994 Aug;22(3):216.

Leong SC, Karkos PD, Macewen CJ, et al. A systematic review of outcomes following surgical decompression for dysthyroid orbitopathy. *Laryngoscope.* 2009 Jun;119(6):1106–1115.

6 Principles and techniques for facial allotransplantation

Bernard Devauchelle, Sylvie Testelin, Stéphanie Dakpé

1 Introduction

Conventional head and neck reconstructive procedures achieve variable results in reconstruction for extensive facial defects. Often, numerous staged surgical procedures result in less optimal or unsatisfactory outcomes. In a face with extensive disfigurement, vascularized composite allotransplantation (VCA) has the potential to restore both esthetics and function. Since the first such face transplantation procedure in 2005 [Devauchelle et al, 2006], at least 37 face transplants have been performed worldwide until 2014 [Khalifian et al, 2014]. The small number is due to the complexity of the procedure, the necessary immunological suppression for organ transplantation, and the consequences of the lifelong treatment. In terms of results, this procedure is a real solution for large disfigurements from severe trauma, large malformations, or extensive benign tumors. However, it is currently achieved at a significant cost of immune suppression.

A facial VCA is a multidisciplinary operation with the need for a complex team [Dahlborg et al, 2014]. The authors specify the conditions for VCA in terms of the surgical procedure (both for recipient and donor), planning and management of the VCA, organization, immunological treatment and monitoring, some psychological and ethical features, follow-up, complications, and some thoughts on the indications for face transplantation.

2 The decision for vascularized composite allotransplantation and necessary preparations

The main prerequisite for a face transplant is when the best result can only be achieved by composite tissue beyond what can be practicably provided by local, regional or distant autogenous tissue. These characteristics include tissue type, topography and extension of defect.

There are three different steps in planning: (1) analysis and preparation of the recipient, (2) the selection of the donor and then (3) management and organization of the operative day. The patient selection is obviously essential. In France, since 2006 two teams have had the authorization to perform five facial VCA, each with the objectives of functional and morphological restitution of the face. The patient should be carefully interviewed many times. Particularly important is the evaluation of the psychological background. Reliability and compliance should be evaluated by a psychiatrist. An immunologist must define and predict the immunosuppressive protocol and the monitoring, risks and potential complications. The patient must have the capacity to follow a lifelong treatment which may have fatal consequences.

The patient is fully and carefully informed several times about all aspects of VCA and his/her consent should be obtained long before the operative day.

The preoperative imaging is determined by the type of defect but at a minimum a computed tomographic (CT) angiogram is performed and often magnetic resonance imaging. An ultrasonography of the available cervical vessels is required, and an electromyogram may be useful to evaluate the function remaining in the facial muscles and nerves. A 3-D model of the defect and modeling of the recipient bone and soft tissue should be performed to facilitate and visualize the skeletal and soft-tissue complexity of the defect (**Fig 6-1**).

A surgical navigation or computer-assisted protocol is sometimes used.

For each recipient patient, the defect is carefully analyzed and documented (eg, photography, videos, radiography, CT, 3-D printing). The transplant is then precisely defined and dissections are planned. Surgeons, residents, nurses and specialists for prosthesis fabrication are involved. Those dissections define and allow understanding of the exact size, depth (eg, muscle, nerves, bone), and extension of the transplant, with respect to the esthetic and functional units. All details, descriptions, technical points and decisions are carefully reported in a protocol which constitutes the basis of the requested document submitted to the French national agency (Agence de la Biomédicine), which controls all types of procurement. Similarly, the team manager will define the donor criteria: age, gender, blood group, skin color matching, and the necessity of "no contraindication," such as previous facial surgery, scars, or other pathologies.

The protocol for donor facial mask preparation is essential, and is performed after the facial procurement. This mask is an essential point for the family, so that they will be able to see their relative without major visible changes after transplant harvest.

As soon as the authorization of the French Agency of Biomedicine is obtained, all team members are listed for an on-call process (ie, anesthesiologist, nurses, surgeons including residents, prosthetist). The distribution of the different assignments should be decided by the responsible team leader who coordinates all steps and people. Additionally, a list of specific materials, devices, and files is prepared.

2.1 Waiting time

This period is critical because each member must be motivated to be able to be mobilized at any time. The team leader should organize and control the preparation for the operative day; the patient should be frequently contacted and regularly interviewed. Follow-up is carefully organized and the psychological, medical, and physiological goals are defined. The final decision is always with the patient, so that contact, trust and regular discussions are crucial to prepare for a smooth operative day.

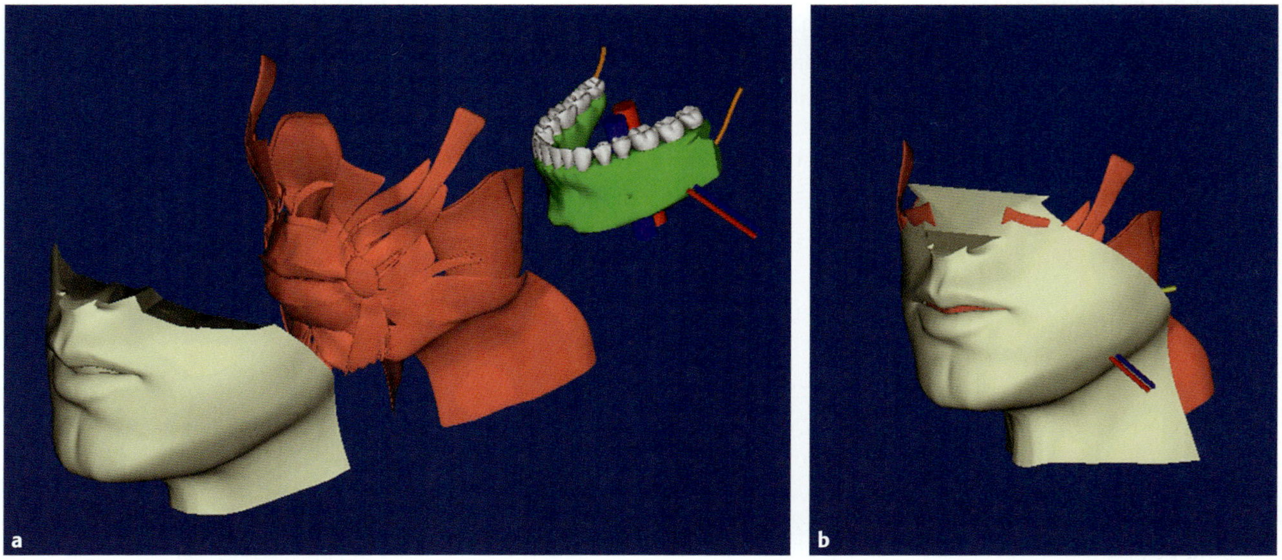

Fig 6-1a–b Digitalized model showing the three layers of the transplant: skin covering (yellow), muscle structure (red), and mandibular bone (green).

2.2 Operative day

When the leader is alerted that a corresponding potential brain-dead donor is somewhere in France, the first decision must involve analysis of a picture of the potential donor and then to accept or refuse the donor. The coordination team will ask the family, who had already accepted the organ procurement permission, if they would also accept to give a part or the whole face of their relative. In the case of a positive decision, the surgery is scheduled, and all members of the transplant team are notified to prepare and proceed according to the protocol. At the same time, the recipient patient is also contacted to come to the hospital to sign a new consent form and be prepared for surgery.

As soon as the positive answer from the donor's family is known, the patient will then receive the first immunosuppressive treatment. The decision on the timing of the operation is taken, and the distribution into two teams (one near the recipient to prepare the defect and one who will travel to the donor to harvest the face transplant) is carefully organized depending on the city and distance to the donor. The specific members and material to manufacture the donor face mask will accompany the latter part of the team near the donor. For now, there is no agreement in France to transport the brain-dead donor near to the recipient, which would make the procedure easier.

2.3 Team near the donor

For us and other transplant surgeons [Petruzzo et al, 2012] the face transplant procurement is always done first before other organs are harvested because the facial dissection should be done carefully on a body with the heart beating in the way that the face transplant will exactly match the defect as decided during the dissection procedures.

- First step—low level tracheotomy, if not previously made.
- Second step—print of the donor face to reconstitute the silicone mask for the end of the procedure.
- Third—surgical steps, depending on the size and topography; all steps will follow the preoperative dissection.
  - Precise drawing of the skin margins.
  - Skin incision and progressive dissection from upper margin to the cervical area toward the vessel dissection of the chosen vascular pedicle (ie, facial arteries, carotid arteries, external and internal jugular veins).
  - All nerves and their branches (sensory and motor) should be respected and marked to facilitate coaptation.
  - All facial muscles and ducts involved will be identified and marked.
  - In case of bone inclusion, the preoperative dissection will define the types and the orientation of the osteotomies. Problems arise if only one jaw is included in the VCA, and the recipient and donor jaw do not match. The possibility to remove and replace the opposite jaw should always be favored because of problems in the dental occlusion, which will never be better than after a bimaxillary incorporation (if a replacement of both jaws is not accepted, it will be necessary to build a temporary occlusal dental splint). The inferior alveolar nerve should be resected with a lengthening process by infratemporal dissection. For the infraorbital nerve, the removal of the infraorbital bone margin permits dissection to the pterygoid space. Teeth are often transplanted without any preparation because they belong completely to the vascularized transplant.
- The tongue and the soft palate can also be harvested. However, a careful dissection of all the suprahyoid muscles attached to the hyoid bone which can be inserted in the transplant and the muscles of the pharyngeal wall to restore the oropharyngeal motility are necessary.
- At the time of the final venous and arterial dissection (usually external carotid or its branches), the time should be noted because it constitutes the beginning of the ischemic time, which is imperative regarding the functional recovery and the vitality of the transplant.

In our group at the same time a forearm flap is also dissected as "sentinel flap" because serial skin biopsies of allogenic skin are needed for life. Thus, it was decided to perform a skin sentinel flap for biopsies to avoid any additional facial scarring.

After that the transplant is prepared with a washout by a serum solution and then conservative preparation is done, which functions as a transporting liquid and for organ preservation. A part of the team may leave the donor operating room to join the recipient operating room. In the operating room with the donor, the other teams then harvest the other organs. During that time, the prosthetist and one or two assistants prepare and build the silicone mask according to the first imprint. This includes coloration to match and respect the cadaver. After the donor surgery is completed, the restitution of the face of the donor is achieved due to an exact adaptation of the mask and a color duplicate junction prepared with specific make-up and hair arrangement to provide camouflage.

2.4 Team near the recipient

After the preoperative care is completed (premedication and immunosuppressive treatment induction), timing for the surgical launch is carefully anticipated regarding the estimated period needed for scar dissection, tumor removal, or site preparation to be on time to receive the transplant. Obviously, the distance from the place of the donor is vital to consider.

1. The first step is essential: immunosuppression with a centralized vascular approach in sterile conditions.
2. The second step is a tracheostomy, if not previously performed.
3. The third step is focused on the recipient vessel dissection according to preoperative decisions.
4. Fourth, the longer step is then removal of the scar tissue or tumor in a way to find every anatomical element around the defect (remaining muscles and nerves [sensory and motor]). Obviously, details of this step depend on the type and topography of the defect (primary resection of a benign tumor or malformation or sequalae of a traumatic case) but the quality of this dissection determines the quality of the functional recovery. In case of resection of bone structures, mandibulomaxillary fixation may be helpful to facilitate the scar tissue resection. In case of bone reconstitution, the exposure of the bone component and/or the resection of the remaining jaw are also an important part of this step particularly with respect to the further spatial harmonization of the skeletal structures. Each anatomical element should be carefully noted and labeled with colored pieces of material.
5. Fifth, for the sentinel flap insertion, the thoraco-dorsal vessels are usually chosen as recipient vessels to suture the flap in the submammary fold.

3 Transplantation

3.1 Technical aspects

When the transplant is available for the recipient, after a short preparation (dissection of the different elements after the travel), the following steps are:

1. Stabilize the bone or muscle fixation.
2. Perform the vascular anastomosis to shorten the ischemic time as much as possible.
3. Nervous and muscular coaptations are then performed from the deep to the superficial level. This is sometimes easier from the contralateral side for deep nerves like the infraalveolor nerve in its posterior position.
4. The contralateral vessels are anastomosed as soon as possible.
5. The muscles should be precisely approximated and sutured.
6. The different ducts, such as lacrimal or salivary, are carefully repaired.
7. Sutures of the mucosal planes are important for the quality of tissue repair.
8. The nasal fossae are stented by silicone tubes. There is usually no real need for drainage except in the neck area.
9. The subdermal and cutaneous layers are carefully repaired.

All surgical steps should be completed and documented by frequent pictures, and videos with a precise time notification.

3.2 Follow-up

The immediate follow-up is centered on the vascularization of the transplant. From the immunological point of view, the immunosuppressive treatment is continuously controlled according to protocol, which is followed up weekly rather than monthly and adapted to the blood controls. Psychological support is clearly defined and accomplished as an imperative criterion for a good acceptance over time. Physiotherapy is initiated and managed initially for lymphatic drainage, then sensory and motor recovery.

Long-term follow-up is based on the clinical analysis of scars and functional rehabilitation (eg, mastication, deglutition, phonation, sensation). Psychological long-term follow-up is focused on the acceptance of the transplant, the immunosuppressive treatment, and daily intake of nutrition. The immunological status is vital. The tolerance of the transplant should be checked both by a general immunological status and also to detect the rejection biopsies of sentinel flap or mucosa should be performed. Physiotherapy is at least weekly (or more often), organized near the patient's residence with a speech therapist and physiotherapist to master the synkinesis and improve the phonation, motor, and all facial functions (**Fig 6-2**).

Several other analyses or examinations are performed according to the symptoms, relevant questions, or research purposes as well as functional magnetic resonance imaging for cortical activity controls [Dubernard et al, 2013].

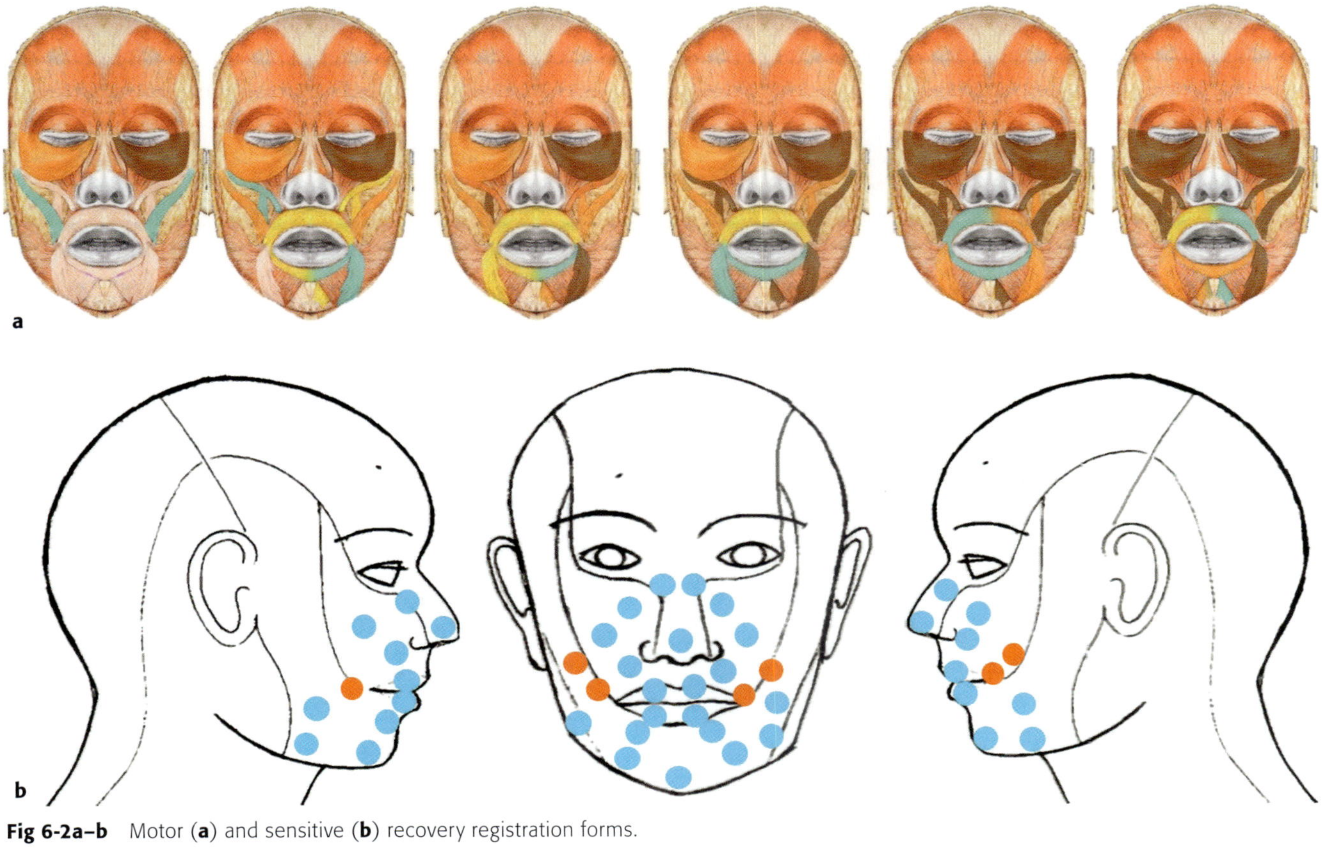

Fig 6-2a–b Motor (**a**) and sensitive (**b**) recovery registration forms.

3.3 Immunological conditions and monitoring

The initial medical status of the patient is crucial to consider and should be analyzed as soon as the decision for a VCA operation is made. The preoperative screening should include the blood group, human leukocyte antigen (HLA) criteria, and HLA-specific antibodies with a complement-dependent microlymphocytoxicity technique (Lambda cell tray, One Lambda Inc) for panel reactive antibody positivity. Many viral tests are required particularly regarding cytomegalovirus, Epstein-Barr virus, and hepatitis. The principles of the immunosuppressive treatment are based on an adaptation of the existing organ transplant protocols. The induction is generally based on polyclonal antithymocyte globulins (thymoglobulin: 1 mg/kg per day for 10 days) or anti-interleukin-2 monoclonal antibody preparation. Just after transplantation a combination of calcineurin inhibitors, like Tacrolimus (oral tablets to reach the blood concentration of 10–13 ng/mL) or Sirolimus, an antiproliferative agent like mycophenolate mofetil (Cellcept 2 g/day to be within 40–60 ng/mL) and steroids (500 mg the first day decreasing to finally reach 10 mg/day) are used in determined doses [Dubernard, 2007].

In case of acute rejection that usually occurs one or two times [Khalifian et al, 2014] in the first weeks, the treatment is slightly modified with increasing dose of steroids and sometimes tacrolimus in tapering or increasing doses. The blood rate should be carefully controlled during the first months to prevent rejection and try to avoid adverse effects.

Antimicrobial prophylaxis is induced during the surgery and then continued for several months as prophylaxis. Concerning the VCA vitality, the control is essentially based on clinical features, as there is no laboratory test except for the rejection times which should be documented by skin and mucosal biopsies. To improve tolerance, some teams propose the use of extracorporal photophoresis to decrease the dose of immunosuppression. The use of hematopoietic stem cell infusion could induce tolerance as for kidney transplantation [Hequet et al, 2008].

Those serological assessments constitute a strong regimen to control comorbidities, such as avoiding serious infections (eg, cytomegalovirus) or tumor induction (eg, Epstein-Barr virus) [Chelmonski, 2011].

4 Discussion

There are no specific considerations regarding topography except that the vascular supply of the transplant should be carefully selected. Anatomical studies have demonstrated the dependability of the cervical and facial vascular network. To our knowledge, there are no published studies of ischemic face transplant necrosis.

The most interesting and debated area of facial VCA indications is the etiology of the disfigurement.

The size and location of the defect are an important point in the discussion of this decision. The risks and comorbidities involved with immunosuppressive treatment and VCA cannot be justified in case of partial facial defects with no major functional deficits, which could be restored by classic procedures (nose reconstruction, ear reconstruction, forehead, or cheeks reconstruction). The main topography to consider is the functional triangle (lips, chin, and nose) and the orbicularis oculi depending on the amount of reconstruction of the eyelids needed.

There are three types of disfigurements:
The traumatic ones (after shotgun trauma, burns) demand a complete rehabilitation in terms of morphology and function. In the malformation cases, for which the patient has usually no reference of a "normal" face, the goal is to replace a malformed face by a face with "normal appearance." In patients with disfigurement because of tumors (exclusively benign), the priority is to remove the tumor before the restoration of the morphology and the function. The patient hopes primarily to be free of tumor.

The uncontestable indication is the traumatic case where there is no possibility of classic surgical procedures for meaningful reconstruction. The decision for face VCA should be first proposed for severe shotgun trauma. In those cases, there is often no place for classic reconstructive surgery before facial allotransplantation. In our view, classic reconstructive possibilities should remain in case of failure or rejection issues. If the selected patient has already undergone reconstruction and still presents with severe disfigurement, facial VCA can be proposed. The patient should agree to have all previous reconstructions removed. This allows the surgeons to find the uninjured anatomical structures to serve as the basis for restoring both morphology and function. It is advised to avoid removal of normal tissue or units in case of failure or rejection as the patient's condition will be worse than the original state. Animal or dog bite sequelae, explosion, large traumatic defects, or burns are certainly the best indications. Concerning extensive burn patients, the main difficulties are determining the amount of scar tissue, its depth, and the functional units involved because of cicatrized skin grafts previously done. Also, there is a risk of severe infection because of bacteria colonizing the acute care after the burn [Carty et al, 2013] (**Fig 6-3**).

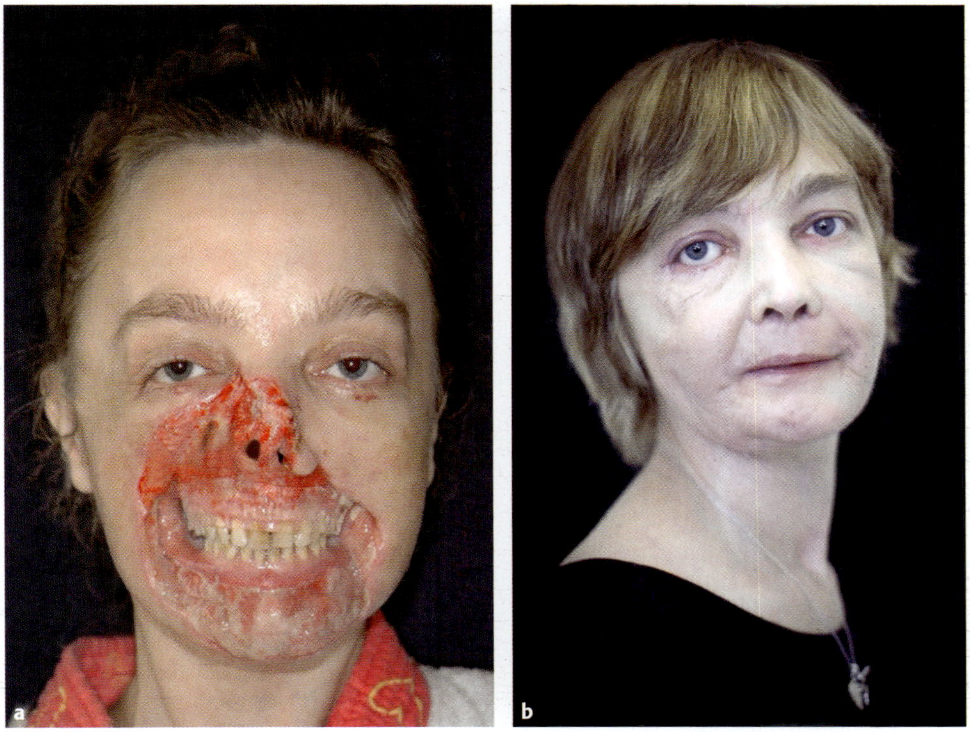

Fig 6-3a–b

a Preoperatively: first transplant patient in 2005. Facial damage after a dog bite.

b Postoperatively: 4 years result.

Malformations or benign tumors with massive deformation of the facial tissue are good indications even if the potential of the involvement of the adjacent tissue is not clearly defined. The third face transplant patient is a demonstrative case who suffers significantly from Von Recklinghausen disease. In 2007, the patient received a face transplant that changed not only his facial appearance with rehabilitation of all functions but also his way of life with good social integration. Attention should be paid at the time of surgery to the difficulty of removal of the tumor at the same time as the transplant because of the risks of blood loss, and on the challenge of the nerve anastomoses because of intrinsic malformations of the nerves themselves [Lantieri et al, 2008].

Other potentially disfiguring malformations are vascular tumors, particularly the high blood flow arteriovenous malformations with extensive and progressive disease severely involving the facial tissues. These entities are difficult to treat, embolization, surgical removal or use of certain medications (eg, steroids) have been proposed or used but reconstructive surgery outcome is often disappointing.

Due to the unpredictable course of vascular tumors, the problem is always to make the decision for surgical removal with special emphasis on the amount of resection. For the cases with lower and midface involvement, facial VCA could be a solution for reconstruction in a single procedure. The vascular malformation should be removed completely after preoperative embolization. The first case was performed in Amiens, France, in 2012, for a 52-year-old woman presenting with a huge disfiguring arteriovenous malformation involving two-thirds of the face embolized and operated on many times. The transplant included the maxilla and the mandible with the whole tongue and the muscular component of the floor of the mouth to the hyoid bone. The amount of skin included extended from the suborbital area to the tracheostomy level except for the nose. A 3-year follow-up demonstrated no recurrence of the disease and an encouraging functional rehabilitation of the mastication, swallowing, and speech. The esthetical aspect is also amazing. Note that for this patient the choice of the immunosuppressive treatment was focused preferably on anti-VEGF drugs [Devauchelle et al, 2015] (**Fig 6-4**).

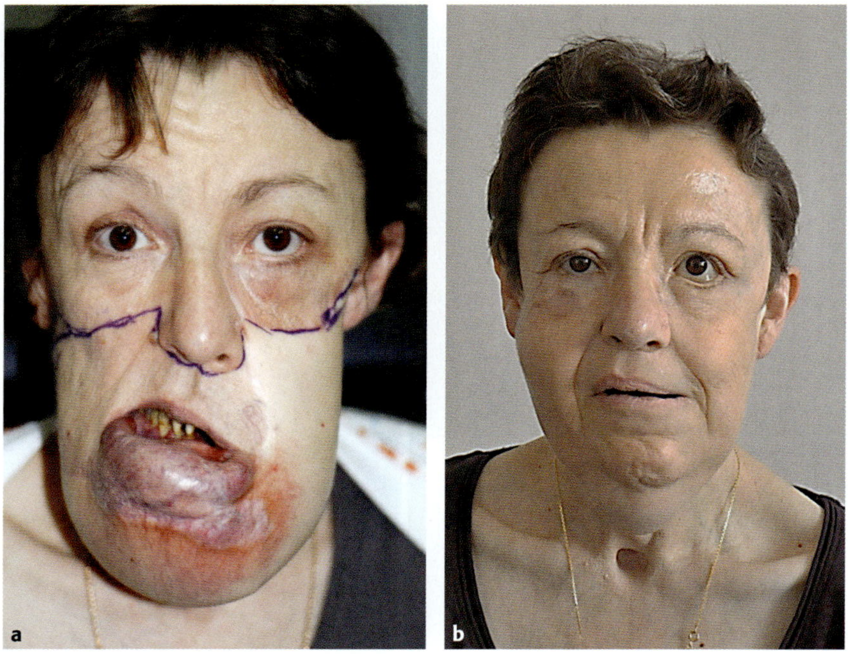

Fig 6-4a–b

a High blood flow arteriovenous malformation recurrence. Preoperatively—two-third face transplant in 2012 in Amiens, France.

b One year after facial vascularized composite allotransplantation (maxilla, mandible, tongue, soft tissues).

There is obviously no place for reconstruction after malignant tumors with facial transplantation because of the required immunosuppressive treatment and the high risk of tumor recurrence or progression. The two published cases, where unfortunate early death occurred from cancer progression, confirm the danger of recurrence with potential fatal outcome [Jiang et al, 2005]. The question of a delay until a tumor-free disease state is reached is under discussion. These patients often have sequelae of both surgery and radiotherapy with vast deficits in function and morphology. They are disabled (eg, speech, eating) and may lose all social interaction.

In the meantime, development of malignant tumors in immunosuppressed patients with facial transplants and subsequent fatal outcome has been observed. This needs to be included into the informed consent before transplantation. The indication for facial transplantation must be critically evaluated considering this possibility.

The last question regarding indications is the problem of age and especially the consideration of the indications in children. Obviously VCA is indicated for the same problems in terms of pathology. The concerns in pediatric cases are issues of growth and obviously the impact of a lifelong immunosuppressive regimen. These questions are still open and need to be addressed [Devauchelle, 2015].

5 Conclusion

In our opinion, facial VCA should be considered as an advance in terms of reconstructive surgery of the face. It presents an option to restore the face in appearance and function in a single surgery. It can only be done according to a careful plan with a team planning, organizing and performing surgery, immunological treatment, psychological preparation and follow-up of the patient. The main point is the careful selection of the patient and his/her thorough understanding, motivation, and compliance in the process. Specific attention should be paid to some technical points regarding skeletal positioning, dental occlusion, and precise nerve coaptation to avoid secondary revisions as much as possible. Another goal of future developments is a potential decrease of the immunosuppressive regimen and consequently reduction of adverse effects associated with such medications. Nevertheless, the patient should strictly adhere to the treatment and accept the close follow-up so that early treatment of acute and mild rejections may allow for a successful outcome. Presently there are no reports of continuing rejection. The sharing of data and the registration of all cases and information in the international registry of (hand and face) composite tissue transplantation are the data pool on which recommendations can be given for a well-conceived and carefully discussed decision to propose facial VCA to a patient.

6 References and suggested reading

Carty MJ, Hivelin M, Dumontier C, et al. Lessons learned from simultaneous face and bilateral hand allotransplantation. *Plast Reconstr Surg.* 2013 Aug;132(2):423–432.

Chelmoński A, Jabłecki J, Szajerka T. Insidious course of cytomegalovirus infection in hand transplant recipient: case report, diagnostics, and treatment. *Transplant Proc.* 2011 Sep;43(7):2827–2830.

Devauchelle B, Badet L, Lengelé B, et al. First human face allograft: early report. *Lancet.* 2006 Jul 15;368(9531):203–209.

Devauchelle B. Facial transplantation for pediatric disfigurements. *Monography Pediatr Surg.* 2015.

Dahlborg EJ, Diaz-Siso JR, Bueno EM, et al. The value of innovation: face and hand transplantation programs at Brigham and Women's Hospital. *Plast Reconstr Surg.* 2014 Jul;134(1).

Dubernard JM, Sirigu A, Seulin C, et al. Fifteen years later: main lessons from composite tissue allografts. *Clin Transpl.* 2013:113–119.

Dubernard JM, Lengelé B, Morelon E, et al. Outcomes 18 months after the first human partial face transplantation. *N Engl J Med.* 2007 Dec 13;357(24):2451–2460.

Hequet O, Morelon E, Bourgeot JP, et al. Allogeneic donor bone marrow cells recovery and infusion after allogeneic face transplantation from the same donor. *Bone Marrow Transplant.* 2008 Jun;41(12):1059–1061.

Jiang HQ, Wang Y, Hu XB, et al. Composite tissue allograft transplantation of cephalocervical skin flap and two ears. *Plast Reconstr Surg.* 2005 Mar;115(3):31e–35e; discussion 36e–37e.

Khalifian S, Brazio PS, Mohan R, et al. Facial transplantation: the first 9 years. *Lancet.* 2014 Dec 13;384(9960):2153–2163.

Lantieri L, Meningaud JP, Grimbert P, et al. Repair of the lower and middle parts of the face by composite tissue allotransplantation in a patient with massive plexiform neurofibroma: a 1-year follow-up study. *Lancet.* 2008 Aug 23;372(9639):639–645.

Meningaud JP, Hivelin M, Benjoar MD, et al. The procurement of allotransplants for ballistic trauma: a preclinical study and a report of two clinical cases. *Plast Reconstr Surg.* 2011 May;127(5):1892–1900.

Petruzzo P, Testelin S, Kanitakis J, et al. First human face transplantation: 5 years outcomes. *Transplantation.* 2012;93:236–240.

Index

Index

Page references with an "f" refer to the page and following pages.
Page references with a "t" refer to tables.

C

D

E

F

G

H

I

J

K

L

M

P

T